SECOND EDITION

SPINAL CORD MEDICINE

SECOND EDITION

SPINAL CORD MEDICINE

Editors

Steven Kirshblum, MD
Professor
Department of Physical Medicine and Rehabilitation
University of Medicine and Dentistry–New Jersey Medical School
Newark, New Jersey
Medical Director
Director of Spinal Cord Injury Services
Kessler Institute for Rehabilitation
West Orange, New Jersey

Denise I. Campagnolo, MD
Clinical Professor of Neurology
University of Arizona College of Medicine–Phoenix
Phoenix, Arizona
Clinical Faculty/Adjunct
Center for Adaptive Neural Systems
Arizona State University
Tempe, Arizona

Prior to January 2010
Director of Multiple Sclerosis Program
Barrow Neurology Clinics
St. Joseph's Hospital and Medical Center
Phoenix, Arizona

After January 2010
Associate Medical Director
US Medical Affairs
Biogen Idec
Weston, Massachusetts

Section Editors

Peter Gorman, MD
Associate Professor and Division Head
Division of Rehabilitation Medicine
Department of Neurology, University of Maryland School of Medicine
Chief, Division of Rehabilitation MedicineDirector, Spinal Cord Injury Service, Kernan Orthopaedics and Rehabilitation Hospital
Attending Physician, PM&R Service
VA Maryland Heathcare System
Baltimore, Maryland

Robert F. Heary, MD
Professor
Neurological Surgery
University of Medicine and Dentistry–New Jersey Medical School
Newark, New Jersey

Mark S. Nash, PhD, FACSM
Professor
Department of Neurological Surgery and Rehabilitation Medicine
Principal Investigator
The Miami Project to Cure Paralysis Director of Research
Department of Rehabilitation Medicine
University of Miami Miller School of Medicine
Lois Pope Life Center
Miami, Florida

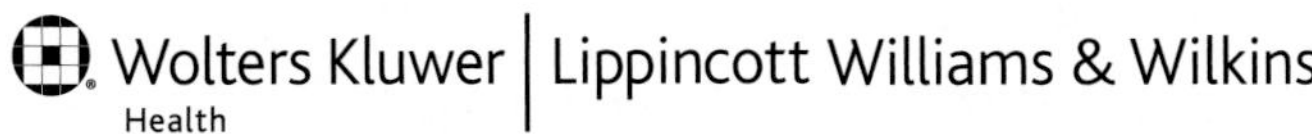

Wolters Kluwer Health | Lippincott Williams & Wilkins

Philadelphia • Baltimore • New York • London
Buenos Aires • Hong Kong • Sydney • Tokyo

Acquisitions Editor: Robert Hurley
Product Manager: Elise M. Paxson
Production Manager: Bridget Dougherty
Senior Manufacturing Manager: Benjamin Rivera
Marketing Manager: Lisa Lawrence
Design Coordinator: Doug Smock
Production Service: SPi Global

Two Commerce Square
2001 Market Street
Philadelphia, PA 19103 USA
LWW.com

Printed in China

Library of Congress Cataloging-in-Publication Data
Spinal cord medicine / editors, Steven Kirshblum, Denise I. Campagnolo. — 2nd ed.
p. ; cm.
Includes bibliographical references and index.
ISBN 978-1-60547-213-3 (hardback)
1. Spinal cord—Wounds and injuries. I. Kirshblum, Steven. II. Campagnolo, Denise I.
[DNLM: 1. Spinal Cord Injuries. 2. Spinal Cord Diseases. WL 400]
RD594.3.S6695 2011
617.4'82044—dc22

2011012877

Care has been taken to confirm the accuracy of the information presented and to describe generally accepted practices. However, the authors, editors, and publisher are not responsible for errors or omissions or for any consequences from application of the information in this book and make no warranty, expressed or implied, with respect to the currency, completeness, or accuracy of the contents of the publication. Application of the information in a particular situation remains the professional responsibility of the practitioner.

The authors, editors, and publisher have exerted every effort to ensure that drug selection and dosage set forth in this text are in accordance with current recommendations and practice at the time of publication. However, in view of ongoing research, changes in government regulations, and the constant flow of information relating to drug therapy and drug reactions, the reader is urged to check the package insert for each drug for any change in indications and dosage and for added warnings and precautions. This is particularly important when the recommended agent is a new or infrequently employed drug.

Some drugs and medical devices presented in the publication have Food and Drug Administration (FDA) clearance for limited use in restricted research settings. It is the responsibility of the health care provider to ascertain the FDA status of each drug or device planned for use in their clinical practice.

To purchase additional copies of this book, call our customer service department at (800) 638-3030 or fax orders to (301) 223-2320. International customers should call (301) 223-2300.

Visit Lippincott Williams & Wilkins on the Internet: at LWW.com. Lippincott Williams & Wilkins customer service representatives are available from 8:30 am to 6 pm, EST.

10 9 8 7 6 5 4 3 2 1

CCS1111

DEDICATIONS

Lisa S. Krivickas, MD, a former resident of ours and coauthor of the Motor Neuron Disease chapter, died on September 22, 2009, of amyotrophic lateral sclerosis (ALS). The editors dedicate this book to Lisa, in memory of her dedication to the care of patients with neuromuscular diseases, including ALS. We celebrate her career as a brilliant clinical researcher. Her courage during her personal fight against ALS will always be remembered.

Steven Kirshblum and Denise I. Campagnolo

To my mother Beverly and in memory of my father Judah who taught me the importance of caring and responsibility. To my mentors both within and outside the medical community, who have shared their wisdom, courage, and leadership, and my colleagues at Kessler Institute for Rehabilitation and UMDNJ/New Jersey Medical School, who have been a source of support for many years. To the many residents and SCI fellows I have been blessed with over the years, who challenge me to continue to grow. To my past, current, and future patients who give meaning to my work, and most importantly to my wife Anna and my children Aryeh, Rena, and Max, who give meaning to my life.

Steven Kirshblum

To my loving husband Tom, who is my strength; to my children Thomas and Emily who are the lights of my life; and to my parents Rosalie and Carmine, who have always believed in me.

Denise I. Campagnolo

To my wife Lisa for her patience with me, and children Allison and Jonathan who have grown up too fast; to the residents I teach, who allow me to continue to learn everyday; and to the patients we serve, who make all the work worthwhile.

Peter Gorman

I would like to thank Cara, Declan, and Maren whose love and support make all projects possible.

Robert F. Heary

To my wife, Lin, and my children, Carter, Bryson, and Darby. Collectively you bring light to my life, and selflessly apportion time needed to balance my roles as husband, father, and scientist. To my parents Mildred and Herbert Nash, who didn't always discern the path I would travel but trusted me enough to find my way.
I am indebted to Fredrick F. Andres, PhD, for my professional training, and for steadfast support from Drs. Ake Seiger, Richard P. Bunge, and W. Dalton Dietrich, all Scientific Directors of the Miami Project to Cure Paralysis with whom I have served. My gratitude is extended to Barth A. Green, MD, who opened the door to my scientific career.

Mark S. Nash

CONTRIBUTORS

Nduka Amankulor, MD
Department of Neurosurgery
Yale University School of Medicine
New Haven, Connecticut

Kimberly D. Anderson, PhD
Director of Education
The Miami Project to Cure Paralysis
The University of Miami
Miller School of Medicine
Miami, Florida

Alan S. Anschel, MD
Clinical Instructor of Physical Medicine and Rehabilitation
Northwestern University
Feinberg School of Medicine
Attending Physician
Spinal Cord Injury Program
Rehabilitation Institute of Chicago
Chicago, Illinois

Jacqueline Bello, MD
Professor
Department of Radiology
Montefiore Medical Center
Director, Division of Neuroradiology
Department of Radiology
Albert Einstein College of Medicine
Bronx, New York

Michael H. Berrly, MD
Past Chair
Department of Physical Medicine and Rehabilitation
Santa Clara Valley Medical Center
San Jose, California

Randal R. Betz, MD
Professor of Orthopaedic Surgery
Temple University
Chief of Staff
Shriners Hospital for Children
Philadelphia, Pennsylvania

Jessica Bloomgarden, MD
Instructor
Rehabilitation Medicine
Mount Sinai Medical Center
New York, New York

William L. Bockenek, MD
Chairman
Department of Physical Medicine and Rehabilitation
Carolinas Medical Center
Medical Director
Department of Physical Medicine and Rehabilitation
Carolinas Rehabilitation
Charlotte, North Carolina

Amy Bohn, OTR/L
The Hand & Upper Extremity Center of Georgia
Shepherd Center
Sovereign Therapy
Atlanta, Georgia
Department of Orthopaedic Surgery
Cleveland MetroHealth Medical Center
Cleveland, Ohio

Michael Bonninger, MD
Professor and Chair
Department of Physical Medicine and Rehabilitation
Associate Dean of Medical Student Research
University of Pittsburgh
Pittsburgh, Pennsylvania

Nancy L. Brackett, PhD, HCLD
Associate Professor of Neurological Surgery and Urology
The Miami Project to Cure Paralysis
University of Miami
Miller School of Medicine
Miami, Florida

Monifa Brooks, MD
Spinal Cord Injury
Kessler Institute for Rehabilitation
Clinical Instructor
University of Medicine and Dentistry
New Jersey–New Jersey Medical School
Newark, New Jersey

Anne M. Bryden, OTR/L
The Hand & Upper Extremity Center of Georgia
Shepherd Center
Sovereign Therapy
Atlanta, Georgia
Department of Orthopaedic Surgery
Cleveland MetroHealth Medical Center
Cleveland, Ohio

Anthony S. Burns, MD, MSc
Associate Professor
Division of Physiatry
Department of Medicine
University of Toronto
Medical Director
Spinal Cord Rehabilitation Program
Toronto Rehabilitation Institute
Toronto, Ontario, Canada

Denise I. Campagnolo, MD
Clinical Professor of Neurology
University of Arizona College of Medicine–Phoenix
Phoenix, Arizona
Clinical Faculty/Adjunct
Center for Adaptive Neural Systems
Arizona State University
Tempe, Arizona

Prior to January 2010
Director of Multiple Sclerosis Program
Barrow Neurology Clinics
St. Joseph's Hospital and Medical Center
Phoenix, Arizona

After January 2010
Associate Medical Director
US Medical Affairs
Biogen Idec
Weston, Massachusetts

Gregory T. Carter, MD, MS
Medical Director
Muscular Dystrophy Association
Regional Neuromuscular Center
Providence St. Peter Medical Center
Olympia, Washington

Susan Charlifue, PhD
Principal Investigator
Department of Research
Craig Hospital
Englewood, Colorado

David Chen, MD
Medical Director
Spinal Cord Injury Acute Care and Rehabilitation
Northwestern Memorial Hospital/Rehabilitation Institute of Chicago
Associate Professor of Physical Medicine and Rehabilitation
Northwestern University
Feinberg School of Medicine
Chicago, Illinois

Yuying Chen, MD, PhD
Associate Professor
Department of Physical Medicine and Rehabilitation
University of Alabama at Birmingham
Birmingham, Alabama

Rachel E. Cowan, PhD
Department of Neurological Surgery and the Miami Project to Cure Paralysis
Miller School of Medicine
University of Miami
Miami, Florida

Graham Creasey, MD
Professor
Department of Neurosurgery
Stanford University
VA Palo Alto Health Care System
Palo Alto, California

Armin Curt, MD, FRCPC
Spinal Cord Injury Center
University of Zurich
Professor and Chairman
University Hospital Balgrist
Zurich, Switzerland

Michael J. DeVivo, PhD
Professor
Department of Physical Medicine and Rehabilitation
University of Alabama at Birmingham
Birmingham, Alabama

Joel A. DeLisa, MD, MS
Professor and Chairman
Department of Physical Medicine and Rehabilitation
University of Medicine and Dentistry–New Jersey Medical School
Newark, New Jersey

Brad E. Dicianno
Assistant Professor
Department of Physical Medicine and Rehabilitation
University of Pittsburgh
Medical Director
Center for Assistive Technology
University of Pittsburgh Medical Center
Pittsburgh, Pennsylvania

Anthony F. DiMarco, PhD
Professor
Department of Physical Medicine and Rehabilitation, Physiology and Biophysics
Case Western Reserve University
MetroHealth Medical Center
Bioscientific Department
Cleveland, Ohio
Chief, Department of Medicine
University Hospitals Geauga Medical Center
Chardon, Ohio

William Donovan, MD
Professor, Chair Emeritus
Department of Physical Medicine and Rehabilitation
University of Texas Medical School
Past President, International Spinal Cord Society and American Spinal Injury Association
Co-Director, Texas SCI Model System Model System
Houston, Texas

Trevor A. Dyson-Hudson, MD
Interim Director
Spinal Cord Injury Research and Outcomes & Assessment
Research Kessler Foundation Research Center
Assistant Professor
Department of Physical Medicine and Rehabilitation
University of Medicine and Dentistry–New Jersey Medical School
Newark, New Jersey

Joaquim Farinhas, MD
Assistant Professor
Department of Radiology
Montefiore Medical Center
Department of Neuroradiology
Albert Einstein College of Medicine
Bronx, New York

Debra J. Farrell, PhD, OTR, CAAC, CRC
Department of Physical Medicine and Rehabilitation
University of Michigan Health System
Ann Arbor, Michigan

Joyce Fichtenbaum, PhD
Clinical Assistant Professor
Department of Physical Medicine and Rehabilitation
University of Medicine and Dentistry–New Jersey Medical School
Newark, New Jersey
Staff Psychologist
Department of Psychology and Neuropsychology
Kessler Institute for Rehabilitation
West Orange, New Jersey

Rebecca E. Fisher, MD
Department of Basic Medical Sciences
University of Arizona College of Medicine–Phoenix, in Partnership with Arizona State University
Phoenix, Arizona

Adam E. Flanders, MD
Department of Radiology
Thomas Jefferson University
Philadelphia, Pennsylvania

Heather M. Flett, MSc, BScPT
Lecturer
Department of Physical Therapy
University of Toronto
Advanced Practice Leader
Spinal Cord Rehabilitation Program
Toronto Rehabilitation Institute
Toronto, Ontario, Canada

Gail Forrest, PhD
Assistant Professor
Department of Physical Medicine and Rehabilitation
University of Medicine and Dentistry of New Jersey–New Jersey Medical School
Newark, New Jersey
Interim Director
Human Performance and Movement Analysis Laboratory
Kessler Foundation Research Center
West Orange, New Jersey

Nikki Fox, DO
Department of Physical Medicine and Rehabilitation
Wayne State University School of Medicine
Detroit, Michigan

Frederick Frost, MD
Associate Professor of Medicine
Department of Physical Medicine and Rehabilitation
Cleveland Clinic Lerner College of Medicine
Cleveland, Ohio

Susan V. Garstang, MD, BS
Clinical Assistant Professor
Residency Program Director
Department of Physical Medicine & Rehabilitation
University of Medicine and Dentistry–New Jersey Medical School
Newark, New Jersey
Staff Physiatrist
VA New Jersey Healthcare System
East Orange, New Jersey

David R. Gater Jr, MD, PhD
Chief, Spinal Cord Injury and Disorders
Department of VA
Hunter Holmes McGuire Medical Center
Spinal Cord Injury and Disorders Service
Richmond, Virginia

Zoher Ghogawala, MD, FACS
Clinical Assistant Professor
Department of Neurosurgery
Yale University School of Medicine
Director
Wallace Clinical Trials Center
New Haven, Connecticut

Barry Goldstein, MD
Professor
Department of Rehabilitation Medicine
University of Washington
Attending Physician
Department of Rehabilitation Medicine
Harborview Medical Center
Associate Chief Consultant
Spinal Cord Injury/Disorders Services
VACO Office of Patient Care Services
Department of VA
Seattle, Washington

Eduardo Gonzalez-Hernandez, MD
Miami Hand Center
Miami, Florida

Peter Gorman, MD
Associate Professor and Division Head
Division of Rehabilitation Medicine
Department of Neurology, University of Maryland School of Medicine
Chief, Division of Rehabilitation MedicineDirector, Spinal Cord Injury Service, Kernan Orthopaedics and Rehabilitation Hospital
Attending Physician, PM&R Service
VA Maryland Heathcare System
Baltimore, Maryland

Edwin Gulko, MD
Clinical Instructor, Radiology
Montefiore Medical Center
Department of Radiology
Albert Einstein College of Medicine
Bronx, New York

Margaret C. Hammond, MD
Physician
Department of Rehabilitation
VA Puget Sound Health Care System
Seattle, Washington

Amanda L. Harrington, MD
Department of Physical Medicine and Rehabilitation
Case Western Reserve University
MetroHealth Rehabilitation Institute of Ohio
Cleveland, Ohio

Robert F. Heary, MD
Professor
Neurological Surgery
University of Medicine and Dentistry–New Jersey Medical School
Newark, New Jersey

John A. Horton, MD
Department of Physical Medicine and Rehabilitation
University of Pittsburgh
Pittsburgh, Pennsylvania

Amitabh Jha, MD, MPH
Associate Professor
Department of Physical Medicine and Rehabilitation
University of Colorado at Denver
Research Physiatrist
Craig Hospital
Englewood, Colorado

Nanette C. Joyce, DO
Staff Physician
Department of Physical Medicine and Rehabilitation
University of California, Davis
Sacramento, California

Stephen S. Kamin, MD
Associate Professor and Acting Chair
Department of Neurology and Neurosciences
University of Medicine and Dentistry–New Jersey Medical School
Chief of Service
Department of Neurology
University Hospital
Newark, New Jersey
Attending Neurologist
Multiple Sclerosis Center at Holy Name
Holy Name Hospital
Teaneck, New Jersey

Michael W. Keith, MD
The Hand & Upper Extremity Center of Georgia
Shepherd Center
Sovereign Therapy
Atlanta, Georgia
Department of Orthopaedic Surgery
Cleveland MetroHealth Medical Center
Cleveland, Ohio

Kevin Kilgore, PhD
Adjunct Assistant Professor of Biomedical Engineering
Case Western Reserve University
MetroHealth Medical Center
Cleveland, Ohio

Steven Kirshblum, MD
Professor
Department of Physical Medicine and Rehabilitation
University of Medicine and Dentistry–New Jersey Medical School
Newark, New Jersey
Medical Director
Director of Spinal Cord Injury Services
Kessler Institute for Rehabilitation
West Orange, New Jersey

Rudi Kobetic, MS
Biomedical Engineer
Department of Research
Louis Stokes VA Medical Center
Cleveland, Ohio

John Kramer MSc, PhD (candidate)
International Collaboration on Repair Discoveries (ICORD) University of British Columbia
Vancouver, British Columbia, Canada

Andrei Krassioukov, MD, PhD, FRCPC
Professor
Division of Physical Medicine and Rehabilitation
Scientist, ICORD
Director of Autonomic Research Unit
Staff physician
Spinal Cord Program
GF Strong Rehabilitation Centre
Department of Medicine
University of British Columbia
Adjunct Professor
Department of Physical Medicine and Rehabilitation
University of Western Ontario
London, Ontario, Canada

James S. Krause, PhD
Associate Dean of Research
Department of Health Sciences and Research
Medical University of South Carolina
Charleston, South Carolina

Ilya Kupershtein, MD
Resident
Department of Orthopaedics
University of Medicine and Dentistry of New Jersey
New Jersey Medical School
Newark, New Jersey

Todd A. Linsenmeyer, MD
Associate Professor
Department of Physical Medicine and Rehabilitation
University of Medicine and Dentistry of New Jersey
New Jersey Medical School
Newark, New Jersey
Director of Urology
Kessler Institute for Rehabilitation
West Orange, New Jersey

Betty Y. Liu, MD
Assistant Professor
Center for Assistive Technology
Department of Physical Medicine and Rehabilitation
University of Pittsburgh Medical Center
Department of Rehabilitation Science and Technology
University of Pittsburgh
The Human Engineering Research Laboratories

Charles M. Lynne, MD
Department of Urology
University of Miami Miller School of Medicine
Miami, Florida

Laurie A. Malone, PhD
Lakeshore Foundation
Birmingham, Alabama

Ralph J. Marino, MD, MS
Professor
Department of Rehabilitation Medicine
Jefferson Medical College of Thomas Jefferson University
Director
Regional Spinal Cord Injury Center of the Delaware Valley
Thomas Jefferson University Hospital
Philadelphia, Pennsylvania

Isa McClure, MAPT
Clinical Specialist
Spinal Cord Injury
Kessler Institute for Rehabilitation
West Orange, New Jersey

Steven Mckenna, MD
Department of Physical Medicine and Rehabilitation
Santa Clara Valley Medical Center
Clinical Instructor (Affiliated)
Department of Medicine
Stanford University School of Medicine
Stanford, California

Michelle A. Meade, PhD
Assistant Professor
Department of Physical Medicine and Rehabilitation
University of Michigan
Chief Psychologist, Spinal Cord Injury Service
Department of Physical Medicine and Rehabilitation
University of Michigan Health System
Ann Arbor, Michigan

Jay Meythaler, MD, JD
Chairman and Professor
Department of Physical Medicine and Rehabilitation
Wayne State University
Dearborn, Michigan

Jane Mitchell, BSN, RN, CRRN CCM
Nurse Case Manager
Kessler Institute for Rehabilitation
West Orange, New Jersey

Mary Jane Mulcahey, MS, OTR/L
Director
Clinical and Outcomes Research
Shriners Hospitals for Children Philadelphia, Pennsylvania Research
Associate Professor
College of Health Professions
Department of Occupational Therapy
Thomas Jefferson University
Philadelphia, Pennsylvania

C. Raffi Najarian, MD, MPH
Department of Physical Medicine and Rehabilitation
MetroHealth Physical Rehabilitation Institute of Ohio
Cleveland, Ohio

Mark S. Nash, PhD, FACSM
Professor
Department of Neurological Surgery and Rehabilitation Medicine
Principal Investigator
The Miami Project to Cure Paralysis Director of Research
Department of Rehabilitation Medicine
University of Miami Miller School of Medicine
Lois Pope Life Center
Miami, Florida

Cindy Nead, COTA
Spinal Cord Injury Program
Kessler Institute for Rehabilitation
West Orange, New Jersey

Greg Nemunaitis, MD
Professor
Department of Physical Medicine and Rehabilitation
Case Western Reserve University School of Medicine
MetroHealth Rehabilitation Institute of Ohio
Department of Physical Medicine and Rehabilitation
Cleveland, Ohio

Kevin O'Connor, MD
Assistant Professor, Residency Training Director
Department of PM&R
Harvard Medical School Medical Director
Spinal Cord Injury Associate Medical Director
Inpatient Operations Spaulding Rehabilitation Hospital
Boston, Massachusetts

Dana A. Ohl, MD
Professor of Urology
Head, Division of Andrology and Microsurgery
Department of Urology
University of Michigan
Ann Arbor, Michigan

Ajit Pai, MD
Assistant Professor
Department of Physical Medicine and Rehabilitation
Virginia Commonwealth University
Medical Director
Polytrauma Rehabilitation Center
Physical Medicine and Rehabilitation Service
Hunter Holmes McGuire VA Medical Center
Richmond, Virginia

Allan E. Peljovich, MD, MPH
Instructor
Atlanta Medical Center
Active Staff
The Shepherd Center
Atlanta, Georgia

Conchita Q. Rader, RN, MA, CFCN, CWCN
Wound Care Coordinator
Department of Nursing
Kessler Institute for Rehabilitation
West Orange, New Jersey

Robert L. Ruff, MD, PhD
Professor
Department of Neurology and Neuroscience
Case Western Reserve University
Chief
Neurology Service
Cleveland VA Medical Center
Cleveland, Ohio

Hreday N. Sapru, PhD
Professor
Department of Neurological Surgery
University of Medicine and Dentistry–New Jersey Medical School
Newark, New Jersey

William M. Scelza, MD
Director, Spinal Cord Injury Program
Carolinas Rehabilitation
Charlotte, North Carolina

Mark Schmeler, PhD, OTR/L, ATP
Assistant Professor
Department of Rehabilitation Science and Technology
University of Pittsburgh School of Health and Rehabilitation Sciences
Pittsburgh, Pennsylvania

Stephen M. Selkirk, MD, PhD
Spinal Cord Medicine Service
Neurology Service
Louis Stokes Cleveland Department of VA Medical Center
Department of Neurology and Neurological Institute
University Hospitals of Cleveland and Case Western Reserve University
Cleveland, Ohio

Akshat Shah, MD
Chief, Spinal Cord and Orthopedic Rehabilitation
Department of Physical Medicine and Rehabilitation
Santa Clara Valley Medical Center
Assistant Clinical Professor (Affiliated)
Department of Orthopaedics
Stanford University School of Medicine
Stanford, California

Kazuko Shem, MD
Associate Chief
Department of Physical Medicine and Rehabilitation
Santa Clara Valley Medical Center
Assistant Clinical Professor (Affiliated)
Department of Orthopaedics
Stanford University School of Medicine
Stanford, California

Heather F. Smith, MD
Department of Basic Medical Sciences
University of Arizona College of Medicine–Phoenix, in Partnership with Arizona State University
Phoenix, Arizona

Jens Sønksen, MD, DMSci, PhD
Professor
University of Copenhagen
Copenhagen, Denmark
Chief Physician
Department of Urology
Herlev Hospital
Herlev, Denmark

Abhishek Srinivas, MD
Clinical Instructor
Radiology
Montefiore Medical Center
Department of Radiology
Albert Einstein College of Medicine
Bronx, New York

Ronald J. Triolo, MD
Associate Professor
Department of Orthopaedics and Biomedical Engineering
Case Western Reserve University
Senior Career Research Scientist
Department of Rehabilitation Research and Development Service
Louis Stokes Cleveland VA Medical Center
Cleveland, Ohio

Michael Vives, MD
Associate Professor
Department of Orthopaedics
University of Medicine and Dentistry–New Jersey Medical School
Newark, New Jersey

Lawrence C. Vogel, MD
Professor
Department of Pediatrics
Rush Medical College
Assistant Chief of Staff, Medicine
Shriners Hospitals for Children
Chicago, Illinois

Timothy L. Vollmer, MD
Professor of Neurology
Medical Director-Rocky Mountain MS Center
Co-Director
Rocky Mountain MS Clinic Anschutz Medical Center
University of Colorado Denver
Aurora, Colorado

Heather Walker, MD
Assistant Professor
Department of Physical Medicine and Rehabilitation
The University of North Carolina at Chapel Hill
Chapel Hill, North Carolina

Eva Widerström-Noga, DDS, PhD
Research Associate Professor
Neurological Surgery
Rehabilitation Medicine and Neuroscience Program
The Miami Project to Cure Paralysis Director of Research
Department of Rehabilitation Medicine
University of Miami Miller School of Medicine
Lois Pope Life Center
Miami, Florida

Alexandros D. Zouzias, MD
Department of Neurological Surgery
University of Medicine and Dentistry–New Jersey Medical School
Newark, New Jersey

PREFACE

The field of spinal cord injury (SCI) medicine has grown at an unprecedented rate over the last decade since the publication of the first edition of this text. We, the editors and contributors of the first edition, are delighted at the acceptance and broad use of the first edition. With recent advances in imaging, surgical techniques, and new additions in disease-modifying medications for chronic diseases, such as multiple sclerosis, the need for a second edition became clear.

This second edition of *Spinal Cord Medicine* is, as the first edition was, intended to be a comprehensive resource of spinal cord medicine for trainees, clinicians, and clinical investigators. Both traumatic and nontraumatic disorders affecting the spinal cord are detailed in corresponding chapters. The topics covered in this text again follow the blueprint of the subspecialty examination for board certification in SCI medicine.

As in the first edition, this text begins with an overview of the subspecialty of SCI medicine, followed by the important aspects of neuroanatomy and neurophysiology of the spinal cord (Chapter 2). An important evolutionary change from the first edition is the division of a single chapter (Anatomy, Mechanics, and Imaging of Spinal Injury) into two chapters. The first covers anatomy and mechanics of the spine (Chapter 3) with detailed drawings and postmortem specimens clearly illustrating the critical anatomical components of spinal integrity and the ways in which spinal stability can be compromised by trauma or disease. The second chapter is a comprehensive imaging chapter (Chapter 4) with more than 30 figures (CTs, MRIs, plain films), making it an excellent resource to understand the complex issues of imaging the spine and spinal cord.

Epidemiology of traumatic SCI is addressed in Chapter 5, and Chapter 6 supplies the reader with the most recent International Standards for examination and American Spinal Injury Association (ASIA) Impairment classification, making reference to recent revisions and clarifications made to the International Standards published in June 2011. Acute medical and surgical concerns are detailed in Chapter 7, followed by prognostication after injury (Chapter 8). The next eight chapters address the medical complications seen after SCI, organized by organ system and encompassing acute and chronic issues (Chapters 9 to 16).

Chapter 17 is a comprehensive chapter on rehabilitation, including a section devoted to the assessment of a patient's ability to drive. Wheelchair considerations are of paramount importance and are relayed in Chapter 18, followed by spinal orthotics (Chapter 19). The very challenging aspects of dual diagnosis (brain injury in combination with SCI) are addressed in Chapter 20. Then, key chapters discuss the many approaches that can help patients return to the fullest possible participation in life. These include psychological adaptations (Chapter 21) and vocational rehabilitation (Chapter 22). The next chapter solidifies the readers' understanding of sexuality after SCI (Chapter 23) and is followed by recreational and therapeutic exercise (Chapter 24).

This edition covers neuromuscular electrical stimulation (Chapter 25) and pain management issues (Chapter 26). Aging with SCI (Chapter 27) is followed by surgery for the upper extremity after injury (Chapter 28) and the concerns of the pediatric patient with SCI (Chapter 29).

The last seven chapters deal with diseases that cause nontraumatic injury to the spinal cord, including mechanical stenosis, tumors, infections, vascular and nutritional diseases, multiple sclerosis, and motor neuron disorders (Chapters 30 to 35). Acute and chronic demyelinating polyneuropathies are also covered in the last chapter, as they are a part of the subspecialty examination (Chapter 36).

The editorial board behind this book includes SCI-certified physiatrists, as well as a neurosurgeon, neurologist, and SCI scientist. They have delivered the second edition of *Spinal Cord Medicine*, which provides detail about all aspects of SCI and disease and will no doubt make an impact on the field just as the first edition did 9 years ago. We are thankful to the section editors as well as to every author of this text. Most of all, we are indebted to our readers and the patients with spinal cord disorders who are served by them.

Steven Kirshblum, MD
Denise I. Campagnolo, MD, MS

CONTENTS

CHAPTER 1 ■ THE HISTORY OF THE SUBSPECIALTY OF SPINAL CORD INJURY MEDICINE

JOEL A. DELISA AND MARGARET C. HAMMOND

The approval in 1995 of spinal cord injury (SCI) medicine as a subspecialty of the American Board of Medical Specialties (ABMS) represented the culmination of concerned efforts by many dedicated individuals over the course of decades. Formal recognition of SCI medicine has promoted more focused research efforts and improved training for physicians who care for patients with injuries and diseases of the spinal cord. As a result of this milestone, there is better cooperation and communication among the various specialties that contribute to the complex care of the SCI population. With the growing number of board-certified specialists in SCI medicine, we are likely to see more rapid application of research findings to clinical practice. Our challenge for the future is to sustain this new subspecialty by expanding the opportunities for fellowship training and recruiting clinicians dedicated to improving the care of individuals with SCI.

The steps that led to the creation of this new subspecialty were detailed by Dr. Joel DeLisa in his 16th annual Donald Munro Lecture, "Sub-specialty Certification in Spinal Cord Injury Medicine: Past, Present, and Future," presented at the 45th annual conference of the American Paraplegia Society (APS) in September 1999 (1). The groundwork for this specialty was laid by the Veterans Administration (VA) during the period following World War II. Beginning in 1943, the VA developed multidisciplinary centers devoted solely to the care of veterans with SCI. The VA currently operates 23 of these specialized facilities throughout the nation (2). Based on this model, similar centers were established in Europe, the United Kingdom, and Australia.

A comparable initiative in the private sector, the Model Spinal Cord Injury Systems (MSCIS), was implemented in the United States in 1970 to coordinate research efforts and improve the management of individuals with SCI. The MSCIS is federally funded by the Department of Education, through the National Institute on Disability and Rehabilitation Research (NIDRR). The current system includes 14 centers that are funded for the 2006 to 2011 project period (3). The APS played a pivotal role in the development of the subspecialty of SCI medicine. Formed in 1954 by physicians involved primarily in the care of patients with SCI, most of the original members were working in the VA health care system. The APS was the outcome of a movement among professionals to improve the treatment of patients with SCI and to recognize the dedication and expertise of physicians who cared for "myelopathy cases" (4).

In its early days, the APS focused exclusively on scientific, charitable, and educational endeavors. The established goals of the APS were as follows (4):

- To advance, foster, encourage, promote, and improve the care and rehabilitation of individuals with SCI
- To develop and promote research and education initiatives related to SCI
- To recognize physicians who devote their careers to SCI
- To promote the exchange of ideas among SCI professionals

The dawn of the 21st century found the APS making great strides toward its targeted goals. In 2009, the APS merged with the American Association of Spinal Cord Injury Psychologists and Social Workers (AASCIPSW) and the American Association of Spinal Cord Injury Nurses (ASSCIN), and with the formation of the Therapy Leadership Council have become the Academy of Spinal Cord Injury Professionals (ASCIP).

By the late 1970s, significant advances had been made toward understanding the physiologic changes in major organ systems that commonly occur after SCI. Moreover, promising strategies had been developed for managing post-SCI pain and for addressing the myriad psychosocial issues associated with long-term care. With this foundation in place, the APS decided to pursue the establishment of a specialty board for certification in SCI medicine, to be called the American Board of Spinal Cord Injury (ABSCI). Organized medicine, however, remained unconvinced of the need for a new, separate certification board (1). In the early 1990s, renewed efforts by the community of SCI professionals met with greater success. In 1991, a new initiative was developed to support SCI medicine as a subspecialty certificate of the American Board of Physical Medicine and Rehabilitation (ABPMR). At a conference sponsored by the Eastern Paralyzed Veterans Association (EPVA), draft proposals detailing the professional and educational requirements for this new subspecialty were prepared for both the ABMS and the Accreditation Council for Graduate Medical Education (ACGME). After extensive review and critique, these proposals were submitted to the ABMS and the ACGME. This time, the efforts were fruitful—the proposal to issue a certificate in the subspecialty of SCI medicine was approved by the ABMS in March 1995. The approval stipulated that applicants for subspecialty certification in SCI medicine must be current diplomates of a member board of ABMS and specified additional training and/or practice experience requirements (5). In recognition of the new subspecialty, the ACGME subsequently approved the program requirements for SCI medicine training programs in February 1996.

In June 1995, the EPVA awarded a 2-year grant to the ABPMR for the development of the SCI Medicine Certification Examination, support that was crucial to the success of this new venture. Over a period of 2 years, contributing writers were trained through a series of item-writing workshops held at professional meetings of the APS, the American Spinal Injury Association, the American Academy of Physical Medicine and Rehabilitation, and the American Academy of Neurology. More than 80 physicians participated in the workshop series and submitted test items for consideration by the ABPMR.

In addition to the considerable efforts devoted to generating the item bank, essential supporting documents were developed. The first edition of the *Subspecialty Certification in Spinal Cord Injury Medicine, Booklet of Information* for prospective candidates was developed in April 1997 (5). Another key document, the examination question topic outline (blueprint), was completed in January 1998 (Table 1.1).

TABLE 1.1

SPINAL CORD INJURY MEDICINE EXAMINATION OUTLINE: APPROXIMATE TARGET WEIGHTS EACH ITEM IS CLASSIFIED WITH A CODE FROM EACH OF THE THREE CLASSES: TYPES OF MYELOPATHY, PHYSIOLOGIC, COMPLICATIONS DUE TO SCI; AND CLINICAL DECISION-MAKING

I. Types of Myelopathy
  A. Traumatic (65%) (e.g., fractures, dislocations, contusions)
    1. Cervical (C1–8)
    2. Thoracic (T1–12)
    3. Lumbar (L1–5)
    4. Sacral
    5. Multiple
    6. Nonspecified
  B. Nontraumatic (25%)
    1. Motor neuron diseases
      a) Amyotrophic lateral sclerosis
      ƶ) Other motor neuron diseases
    2. Spondylotic myelopathies
      a) Spondylolysis; spondylolisthesis
      b) Spinal stenosis
      c) Disk herniation; ruptures
      d) Atlantoaxial instability
      ƶ) Other spondylotic myelopathies
    3. Infectious and inflammatory diseases
      a) Multiple sclerosis
      b) Epidural abscesses
      c) Transverse myelitis
      d) Poliomyelitis; postpoliomyelitis
      e) Osteomelitis
      f) Arachnoiditis
      g) Human immunodeficiency virus
      ƶ) Other infectious and inflammatory diseases
    4. Neoplastic diseases
      a) Malignant/metastatic tumors
      b) Nonmalignant tumors
      ƶ) Other neoplastic diseases
    5. Vascular disorders
      a) Ischemic myelopathy
      b) Arteriovenous malformations
      c) Radiation myelitis
      ƶ) Other vascular disorders
    6. Toxic/metabolic conditions
    7. Congenital/developmental disorders
      a) Myelodysplasia
      ƶ) Other congenital/developmental disorders
  C. Nonspecified/Other SCI Myelopathies (10%)
II. Physiologic Complications Due to SCI
  A. Cardiovascular (7%)
    1. Arrhythmias
    2. Ischemic hear disease
    3. Autonomic dysfunction
    4. Peripheral arterial disease
    5. [open]
    6. Deep vein thrombosis
    7. [open]
    8. Hypertension
    9. Orthostatic hypotension
    19. Applied sciences
    20. Other cardiovascular complications
  B. Pulmonary (9%)
    1. Restrictive pulmonary syndrome
    2. Pneumonia
    3. Hypoventilation/respiratory failure
    4. Pulmonary embolism
    5. Sleep disorders
    19. Applied sciences
    20. Other pulmonary complications
  C. Genitourinary (18%)
    1. Neurogenic bladder
    2. Renal impairment
    3. Urinary tract infection
    4. Sexuality and reproductive issues
    5. Lithiasis
    19. Applied sciences
    20. Other GU complications
  D. Gastrointestinal (7%)
    1. Neurogenic bowel
    2. Upper GI problems
    3. Liver dysfunction
    19. Applied sciences
    20. Other GI complications (e.g., pancreatitis)
  E. Musculoskeletal (12%)
    1. Joint complications (e.g., neuropathic, Charcot)
    2. Soft tissue complications (e.g., bursitis, contracture)
    3. Arthritis; arthritides
    4. Heterotopic ossification
    5. Demineralization (e.g., osteoporosis)
    6. Fractures (nonvertebal)
    7. Scoliosis
    8. [open]
    9. Overuse/repetitive use (e.g., rotator cuff)
    10. Spine fractures (vertebral)/dislocations
    19. Applied sciences
    20. Other musculoskeletal complications
  F. Neurological/Neuromuscular (12%)
    1. Spasticity
    2. [open]
    3. Peripheral nerve dysfunction
    4. Dysphagia
    5. Hydrocephalus
    6. Syringomyelia
    7. Autonomic dysreflexia
    19. Applied sciences
    20. Other neurological complications (e.g., coma, stroke)
  G. Integumentary (8%)
    1. Sacral ulcers
    2. Trochanteric ulcers
    3. Ischial ulcers
    20. Other/combined ulcers

TABLE 1.1

SPINAL CORD INJURY MEDICINE EXAMINATION OUTLINE: APPROXIMATE TARGET WEIGHTS (*Continued*)

- H. Systemic (8%)
    - 1. Infectious disease
    - 2. Immunosuppression
    - 3. Metabolic disorders
    - 4. Endocrine disorders
    - 5. Diabetes
    - 6. Nutrition deficiency
    - 7. Hypercalcemia
    - 8. Thermoregulation
    - 9. Lipid metabolism
    - 19. Applied sciences
    - 20. Other systemic complications (e.g., fatigue)
- I. Cognitive and Psychological (6%)
    - 1. Conversion disorders
    - 2. Communication disorders
    - 3. Depression/affective disorders
    - 4. Maladaptive behavior
    - 5. Substance abuse
    - 19. Applied sciences
    - 20. Other cognitive or psychological complications (including traumatic brain injury)
- J. Pain (8%)
    - 1. Peripheral nerve pain
    - 2. Central spinal cord pain
    - 3. Visceral pain
    - 4. Muscle and mechanical pain
    - 20. Other pain
- K. Nonspecified/Multiple Complications (5%) (including comorbidities)

III. Clinical Decision Making

- A. Patient Evaluation and Diagnosis
    - 1. Diagnostic/clinical sciences
        - a) Epidemiology
        - b) Risk factors
        - c) Etiology
        - z) Classification, other
    - 2. Physical exam, signs, symptoms
    - 3. Specific diagnostic procedures
        - a) Cardiopulmonary assessment
        - b) Urodynamics
        - c) Gait analysis
        - d) Lab studies (e.g., blood gases)
        - e) Medical imaging (e.g., x-ray, computed tomography, MRI)
        - f) Psychosocial evaluation
        - z) Other diagnostic procedures
    - 4. Functional evaluation
        - a) By level
        - b) Energy expenditure analysis
    - 5. SCI classification (ASIA)
    - 6. Prognosis
        - a) Probable complications
        - b) Life expectancy
        - c) Outcomes
- B. Electrodiagnosis (3%)
    - 1. Nerve conduction
    - 2. Electromyography
    - 3. Somatosensory evoked potential
- C. Patient Management (43%)
    - 1. Emergency care (e.g., initial care, patient transport)
    - 2. Physical agents
        - a) Heat/cryotherapy
        - b) Ultrasound
        - c) Multiple/other physical agents
    - 3. Therapeutic exercise and manipulation
        - a) Re-education; motor control
        - b) Mobility and range of motion
        - c) Strength and endurance
        - d) Multiple/other therapeutic exercises and manipulation
    - 4. Pharmacologic interventions
        - a) Analgesics
        - b) Antispasticity medications
        - c) Anti-inflammatory agents
        - d) Antibiotics
        - e) Antidepressants
        - f) Antihypertensives
        - g) Anticoagulants
        - h) Immunomodulatory agents
        - i) Bowel and bladder medications (e.g., anticholinergics, receptor blockers, colonic stimulants)
        - z) Multiple/other pharmacologic interventions
    - 5. Procedural/interventional
        - a) Surgery (including tendon transfers)
        - b) Nerve blocks (e.g., phenol, botulinum toxin)
        - c) Anesthetic injections
        - d) Serial casting
        - e) Traction/immobilization (e.g., spinal orthotics)
        - z) Multiple/other procedural/interventional
    - 6. Functional training
        - a) Mobility and ambulation
        - b) Activities of daily living
        - c) Bladder function
        - d) Bowel function
        - e) Sexual function
        - z) Multiple/other functional training
    - 7. Rehabilitation technology
        - a) Orthotics
        - b) Functional electrical stimulation
        - c) Transcutaneous electrical nerve stimulation
        - d) Ventilation
        - e) Wheelchair/seating
        - f) Communication devices
        - g) Environmental and motor vehicle adaptations
        - z) Multiple/other assistive devices
    - 8. Psychosocial issues
        - a) Relaxation therapy
        - b) Behavior modification
        - c) Psychotherapy/counseling
        - d) Patient/family education
        - e) Vocational rehabilitation
        - z) Multiple/other psychosocial issues
    - 9. Nutrition therapy
    - 10. Health care systems
        - a) Cost/unit management
        - b) Patient safety
    - 11. Ethics
    - 12. Prevention and health care maintenance
- D. Basic and Clinical Sciences (17%)
    - 1. Anatomy
    - 2. Physiology
    - 3. Pathology; pathophysiology
    - 4. Genetics
    - 5. Kinesiology; biomechanics
    - 6. Neuroregeneration
    - 7. Research and statistics
    - 20. Other basic and clinical sciences

It is evident that our colleagues endorse the purpose set forth for this certification (5). The subspecialty certification in SCI medicine offered through the ABPMR enhances the quality of care available to individuals with spinal cord dysfunction. As a result of formal specialty training in SCI medicine, we have a growing community of expert clinicians, teachers, and investigators who are equipped to achieve the following:

- Demonstrate special expertise in clinical knowledge and skill in SCI medicine
- Improve the rehabilitation and care of individuals with SCI
- Provide expert primary diagnostic and management services for complex and severe clinical problems related to SCI that require interspecialty management in SCI centers
- Support principal care providers of patients with SCI who practice in non-SCI centers, by rendering follow-up care to prevent and manage complications related to SCI

From the standpoint of future development of the profession, this relatively new subspecialty credentials accomplish the following:

- Improve the quality of teaching of SCI medicine in residency programs of related primary specialties by increasing the number of subspecialists with additional knowledge and skills in SCI medicine
- Stimulate research that addresses the problems of individuals with spinal cord dysfunction while developing potential faculty members with special interests in SCI medicine
- Improve interspecialty and interdisciplinary communication and cooperation among specialists caring for patients with SCI
- Provide access to certification in SCI medicine to diplomates of all ABMS member boards, particularly those in specialties directly related to the care of patients with SCI

The first examination in spinal cord Injury medicine was administered to 92 candidates in October 1998. Of the 80 physicians who achieved a passing score, 70 were diplomates of the ABPMR, and 10 were diplomates in other disciplines, including internal medicine, orthopaedic surgery, pediatrics, psychiatry and neurology, and urology. Today, there are 20 approved training sites for SCI fellowship programs (6). Fellows in these programs must devote a minimum of two thirds of their time to patient care, including the inpatient and outpatient settings.

TABLE 1.2

AMERICAN BOARD OF PHYSICAL MEDICINE AND REHABILITATION: 2009 SPINAL CORD INJURY MEDICINE EXAMINATION RESULTS

Exam Data Summary			
Number admissible	75		
Number taking exam	70	Initial: 17	MOC: 53
Number passing	63 (90%) (59 ABPMR, 2 ABIM, 1 ABFM, 1 ABPN)	16 (94%)	47 (89%)
Number failing	7 (10%) (7 ABPMR)	1 (6%)	6 (11%)

Summary Percentages	2009	2008	2007	2006	2005	2004	2003	2002	2001	2000	1999	1998
First-time examinees	16/16	4/4	31/41	20/23	13/15	33/36	84/85	54/56	45/48	59/63	81/92	80/92
Percent passing exam	100%	100%	76%	87%	90%	92%	98.8%	96%	94%	94%	88%	87%
Repeat examinees	0/1	3/6	1/4	2/2	0/1	0/0	2/2	3/3	1/5	9/11	6/9	
Percent passing exam	0%	50%	25%	100%	0%		100%	100%	20%	82%	66%	
Total passing	16/17 94%	7/10 70%	32/45 71%	35/39 90%	28/31 90%	33/36 92%	86/87 98.8%	57/59 96%	46/53 86%	68/74 92%	87/101 86%	80/92 87%
Accredited fellowship	16/17	4/4	10/12	5/6	3/5	14/15	9/9	9/9	8/8	8/8	4/4	
Percent passing	94%	100%	83%	83%	60%	93%	100%	100%	100%	100%	100%	
Nonaccredited fellowship	0	0	2/2	1/1	0/1	1/1	4/4	2/2	0/1	0/1	9/12	0/3
Percent passing			100%	100%	0%	100%	100%	100%	0%	0%	75%	0%
Practice track	0	3/6	20/31	29/32	25/25	18/20	73/74	46/48	38/44	60/65	74/85	80/89
Percent passing		50%	65%	91%	100%	90%	98%	96%	86%	92%	87%	90%
Number new diplomates	16	7	32	22	13	33	86	57	46	68	87	80
Total diplomates	560	544	537	505	483	470	437	351	294	248	180	93[a]
MOC examinees:	47/51	44/50	21/24	13/14	15/15							
First-time												
Percent passing exam	92%	88%	88%	93%	100%							
MOC examinees: Repeat	0/2	1/3	0/1	0	0							
Percent passing exam	0%	33%	0%									
Residents in SCIM training programs	12	14	13	9	14	18	13	13	10	8	9	3

[a]Includes 13 grandfathered physicians.

As of June 2010, the total number of diplomates certified in SCI medicine is 560 with the majority being physiatrists. Through 2009, there were 75 physicians whose primary certificate is not in PM&R. Of these, 39 are in internal medicine; 22 in psychiatry and neurology; five in pediatrics; four in family practice; two in orthopedics; and one in general surgery on or, urology, and one in colon and rectal surgery. The first opportunity to take the SCI Medicine Maintenance of Certification (MOC) examination was in 2005. The number of individuals taking the initial SCI Medicine Certification Examination is noted in Table 1.2.

References

1. DeLisa JA. Subspecialty certification in spinal cord injury medicine: past, present and future. *J Spinal Cord Med* 1999; 22(3):218–225.
2. Veterans Affairs Spinal Cord Injury and Disorders (SCI&D) Centers. Available from Veterans Health Administration SCI&D Services, 1660 S. Columbian Way (128 NAT), Seattle, WA 98108.
3. National Center for the Dissemination of Disability Research (NCDDR) Web site. Available at: http://www.ncdrr.org/rpp/hflwebres_spinal.html. Accessed October 16, 2000.
4. *Historical information re: American Board of Spinal Cord Injury.* (n.d.) Unpublished work. (Available from American Paraplegia Society, 75–20 Astoria Blvd, Jackson Heights, NY 11370.)
5. *Subspecialty certification in spinal cord injury medicine, booklet of information.* American Board of Physical Medicine and Rehabilitation. (Available from ABPMR 3015 Allegro Park Lane S Rochester, MN 55902–4139 or available on the ABPMR website www.abpmr.org actual lonk for SCI is http://www.abpmr.org/canditated/sci.html
6. https://www.abpmr.org/candidates/sci_fellowships.html

CHAPTER 2 ■ SPINAL CORD: ANATOMY, PHYSIOLOGY, AND PATHOPHYSIOLOGY

HREDAY N. SAPRU

The spinal cord receives sensory information from somatic and visceral receptors through dorsal roots, transmits this information to higher brain structures through ascending tracts, receives signals from higher centers through descending tracts, and finally transmits these signals to somatic and visceral target sites via the ventral roots. The spinal cord, therefore, is a critical component for the transmission of sensory information to the brain and for the subsequent regulation of motor and autonomic functions. In this chapter, a brief review is presented of the important anatomical features of the spinal cord, including its ascending and descending tracts (1–4). A description of several animal models of spinal cord injury (SCI) and pathophysiological correlates derived from them is also included (5,6).

COVERINGS OF THE SPINAL CORD

The coverings (meninges) of the spinal cord include the dura, arachnoid, and pia mater. Although the spinal coverings are generally similar to those of the brain, there are some differences that are listed below. The spinal dura is single layered and lacks the periosteal layer of the cranial dura. The spinal epidural space is an actual space in which venous plexuses are located and is used clinically for the administration of epidural anesthesia to produce a paravertebral nerve block. On the other hand, the cranial epidural space is a potential space that becomes filled with a fluid only in pathological conditions; normally, there is no space between the dura and the cranium. The spinal epidural space is located between the meningeal layer of the dura (there is no periosteal layer) and the periosteum of the vertebra, while the cranial epidural space (when present) is located between the periosteal layer of the dura and the cranium (Fig. 2.1).

Dura Mater

As stated earlier, the spinal dura consists of only meningeal layer and lacks the periosteal layer of the cranial dura. Rostrally, the spinal dura joins the meningeal layer of the cranial dura at the margins of the foramen magnum. The spinal epidural space separates the spinal dura from the periosteum of the vertebra and is filled with fatty connective tissue and plexuses of veins. Caudally, the spinal dura ends at the level of the second sacral vertebra (Fig. 2.2). At this level, the spinal dura becomes a thin extension (the coccygeal ligament or the filum terminale externum) and serves to anchor the spinal dura to the base of the vertebral canal.

Arachnoid

This membrane loosely invests the spinal cord and is connected to the dura via connective tissue trabeculae. Rostrally, it passes through the foramen magnum to join the cranial arachnoid, and caudally it surrounds the cauda equina (a bundle of nerve roots of all the spinal nerves caudal to the second lumbar vertebra) (Fig. 2.2). The subarachnoid space contains cerebrospinal fluid (CSF).

Pia Mater

The spinal pia is thicker as compared to the cranial pia. It is a vascular membrane and projects into the ventral fissure of the spinal cord. At intervals, toothed ligaments of pial tissue, called *dentate ligaments*, extend from the lateral surfaces of the spinal cord; these ligaments serve to anchor the spinal cord to the arachnoid and through it to the dura. As mentioned earlier, at caudal levels, spinal pia continues along the filum terminale that then anchors the spinal cord to the dura at the level of the second sacral vertebra. Rostrally, the spinal pia joins the cranial pia.

GROSS ANATOMY

The spinal cord is a long, cylindrical structure that is continuous with the medulla rostrally and ends at the rostral border of the second lumbar vertebra. At the caudal end, the spinal cord is conical in shape and is known as the *conus medullaris* (Fig. 2.2). A filament extending from the conus medullaris is called the *filum terminale*. This filament is enclosed in pia and consists of glial cells, ependymal cells, and astrocytes. As stated earlier, the caudal thin extension of spinal dura is called the *coccygeal ligament*. This ligament surrounds the filum terminale internum of the spinal cord and attaches to the coccyx in order to anchor the spinal cord.

Up through the third month of fetal life, the spinal cord occupies the whole length of the vertebral canal. After the third month, the rate of lengthening of the spinal cord is slower than the lengthening of the vertebral column. In an adult, therefore, the spinal cord occupies only the upper two thirds of the vertebral column with its caudal end located at the level of the second lumbar vertebra. For this reason, it is necessary for the lumbar and sacral nerve roots to descend some distance within the vertebral canal in order to exit from their respective intervertebral foramina. The filum terminale is surrounded by lumbosacral nerve roots to form a cluster that resembles the tail of a horse and is called the *cauda equina* (Fig. 2.2).

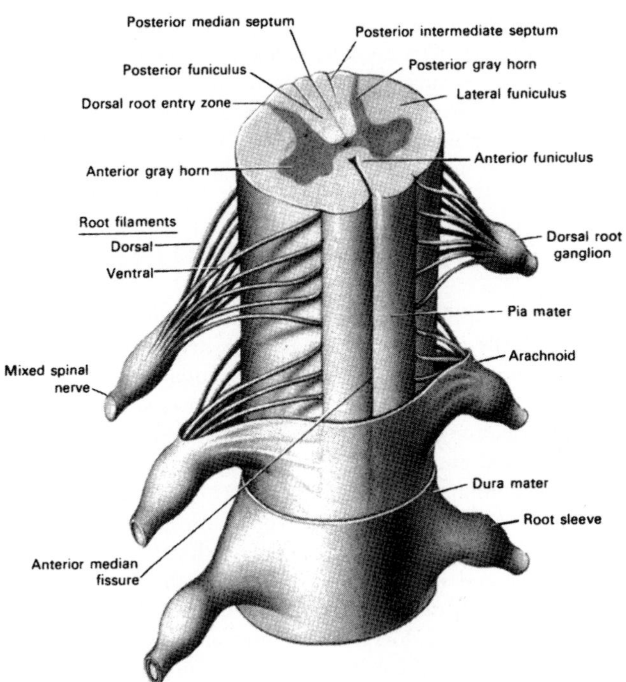

FIGURE 2.1. Coverings of the spinal cord. (From Parent A, ed. *Carpenter's human neuroanatomy*, 9th ed. Baltimore: Lippincott Williams & Wilkins, 1996:327, with permission.)

Lumbar Cistern and Lumbar Puncture

This cistern extends from the caudal end of the spinal cord located at the second lumbar vertebra to the second sacral vertebra. The subarachnoid space is widest at this site and contains the filum terminale internum and nerve roots of the cauda equina. Because of the large size of the subarachnoid space and relative absence of neural structures, this space is most suitable for the withdrawal of CSF by lumbar puncture. This procedure is used to gain specific information about the cellular and the chemical composition of the CSF in disorders such as meningitis. As noted above, the caudal end of the spinal cord in the normal adult is located at the second lumbar vertebra. A puncture is usually made between the third and the fourth lumbar vertebra, and 5 to 15 mL of the CSF is removed in order to perform the cell count, protein analysis, and microbiological studies. The patient is placed in a lateral recumbent position and the CSF pressure is measured by a manometer. Normally, the CSF pressure should be less than 200 mm of H_2O. If the intracranial pressure is high, withdrawal of CSF is contraindicated because brain tissue may get herniated through the foramen magnum.

Lesions of the Conus Medullaris and the Cauda Equina

Usually, tumors are responsible for the lesions of the conus medullaris. The symptoms of such lesions include early sphincter dysfunction, urinary incontinence, difficulty or loss of voluntary bladder emptying, enhancement of residual urine volume, lack of urge to urinate, constipation, impaired penile erection and ejaculation in males, and lack of sacral sensation (saddle anesthesia). The symptoms of lesions in the cauda equina

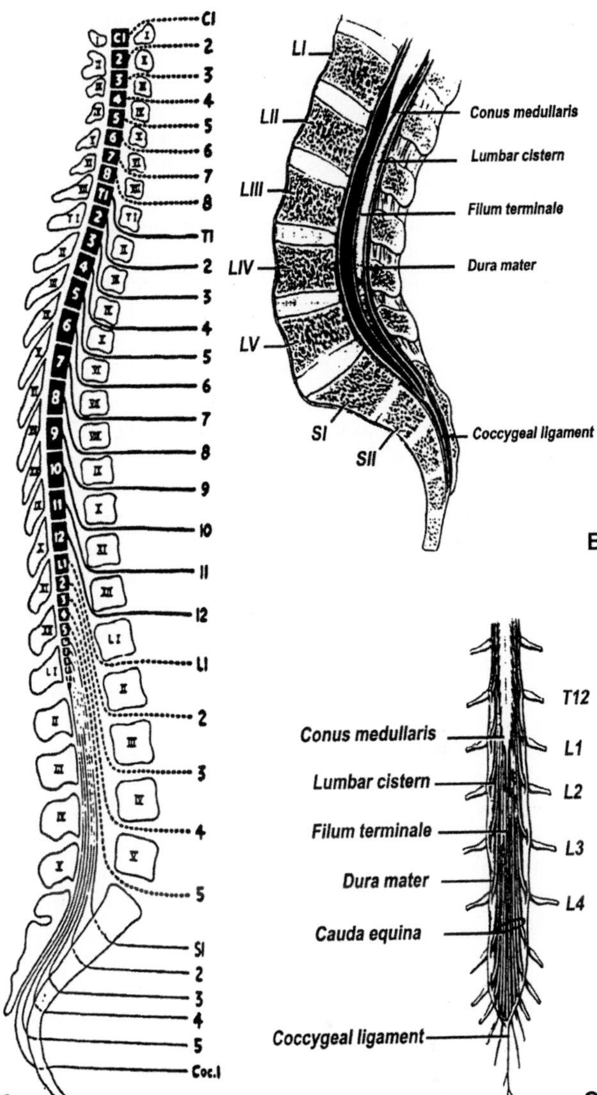

FIGURE 2.2. Bodies and spinous processes of the vertebrae and their position with reference to the spinal cord segments (**A**). Caudal part of the vertebral column showing the conus medullaris, filum terminale, cauda equina, and coccygeal ligament (**B**,**C**). (From Carpenter MB, Sutin J. *Human neuroanatomy*, 8th ed. Baltimore: Lippincott Williams and Wilkins, 1983;8 & 235, with permission.)

are related to the nerve roots involved. For example, lesions involving right L2–4 nerves will cause ipsilateral wasting and weakness of quadriceps and adductor thigh muscles, absence of knee jerk, and sensory loss in L2–4 dermatomes (4).

SPINAL NERVES

Thirty-one pairs of spinal nerves emerge from the spinal cord. At each level of the spinal cord, spinal nerves exit through the intervertebral foramina. In the thoracic, lumbar, and sacral regions of the cord, spinal nerves exit through the intervertebral foramina just caudal to the vertebra of the same name. In the cervical region, however, these nerves exit through the intervertebral foramina just rostral to the vertebra of the same name. Because there are eight cervical nerve roots and only seven cervical vertebrae, the eighth cervical spinal nerve exits through the intervertebral foramen just rostral to the first thoracic vertebra (Fig. 2.2).

Each spinal nerve consists of a dorsal root containing afferent fibers and a ventral root containing efferent fibers. The dorsal root is absent in the first cervical and coccygeal nerves. The dorsal and ventral roots travel within the dural sac surrounding the spinal cord, penetrate the dura, and then enter the intervertebral foramen. Because of the length difference between the spinal cord and the vertebral column, cervical and upper thoracic rootlets run at right angles to the spinal cord, whereas lower thoracic, lumbar, and sacral rootlets are increasingly oblique. The neurons that give rise to afferent fibers entering the spinal cord are located in the spinal ganglion (dorsal root ganglion) that resides within the intervertebral foramen.

The dorsal and ventral roots join together at a site distal to the spinal ganglion to form the common spinal nerve trunk. Usually, the following four branches (rami) arise from the common spinal nerve trunk: (a) the dorsal ramus, which innervates the muscles and the skin of the back; (b) the ventral ramus, which innervates the ventrolateral part of the body wall and all extremities; (c) the meningeal branch, formed by several small branches arising from the common nerve trunk and the ramus communicantes, which reenters the intervertebral foramen and innervates the meninges, blood vessels, and vertebral column; and (d) the ramus communicans, which consists of the white and gray portions. The white ramus communicans carries myelinated preganglionic fibers from the spinal cord to the sympathetic ganglion, while the gray ramus communicans contains the unmyelinated postganglionic fibers.

The spinal cord has two enlargements, one in the cervical and another in the lumbar region. The cervical enlargement is relatively larger than the one in the lumbar region. The cervical enlargement includes four lower cervical and the first thoracic segments. The nerve roots emerging from this enlargement form the brachial plexus that innervates the upper extremities. The lumbar plexus (comprising the nerve roots from L1 to L4) and the lumbosacral plexus (consisting of nerve roots from L4 to S2) emerge from the lumbar enlargement. The lumbar plexus innervates the lower extremities. The sacral spinal nerves emerge from the conus medullaris and contain parasympathetic and somatic motor fibers innervating the muscles of the bladder wall and the external sphincter, respectively.

INTERNAL STRUCTURE

A transverse section of the spinal cord reveals the presence of a butterfly-shaped central gray matter, which contains cell columns oriented along the rostrocaudal axis of the spinal cord (Fig. 2.3). The central gray area is surrounded by white matter consisting of ascending and descending bundles of myelinated and unmyelinated axons (tracts or fasciculi). A bundle containing one or more tracts or fasciculi is called a *funiculus*. In each half of the spinal cord, there are three funiculi: the posterior (dorsal) funiculus (located between the dorsal horn and a midline structure called the *dorsal or posterior median septum*), the lateral funiculus (located between the sites where the dorsal roots enter and the ventral roots exit from the spinal cord), and the anterior (ventral) funiculus (located between a ventral midline structure called the *anterior median fissure* and the site where the ventral roots exit). The two sides of the gray matter are connected by the gray commissure. The white commissure is located ventral to the gray commissure and contains decussating axons of nerve cells. The central canal is located in the gray commissure and is well defined in the spinal cord of the fetus and the new born. In the adult spinal cord, the lumen of the central canal may be filled with debris consisting of macrophages and neuroglial processes.

The gray matter of the spinal cord contains primarily neurons, dendrites, and myelinated and unmyelinated axons, which are either exiting from the gray matter to the white matter, or projecting from the white matter to innervate neurons located in the gray matter. The ascending and descending tracts of myelinated and unmyelinated fibers constitute the white matter.

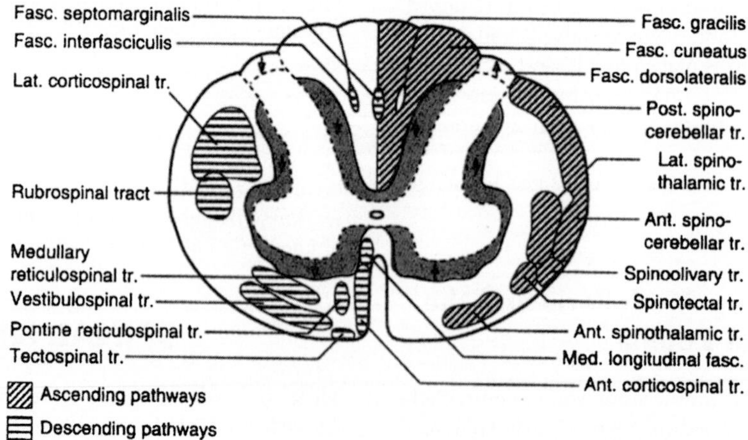

FIGURE 2.3. Ascending and descending pathways of the spinal cord. Two different types of *hatched areas* are used to differentiate ascending from descending pathway. The fasciculus proprius system (*shaded areas*) and the dorsolateral fasciculus contain both ascending and descending nerve fibers. (From Parent A, ed. *Carpenter's human neuroanatomy*, 9th ed. Baltimore: Lippincott Williams and Wilkins, 1996:401, with permission.)

SPINAL SEGMENTS

The spinal cord has been divided into 31 segments (8 cervical, 12 thoracic, 5 lumbar, 5 sacral, and 1 coccygeal) based on the existence of 31 pairs of spinal nerves. Each segment receives dorsal and ventral root filaments on each side.

Cervical Segments

As stated earlier, these are the largest segments because the amount of nerve fibers in the ascending and descending spinal tracts is greatest at this level. The anteroposterior diameter is smaller than the transverse diameter giving these segments their characteristic oval shape. Cervical segments below C5 (i.e., C5-T1) are related to brachial plexus and provide motor innervation of the upper extremities. These segments have well-developed posterior and anterior horns; the latter extend into the lateral funiculi.

Thoracic Segments

These segments are smaller than the cervical segments. All thoracic segments contain a lateral horn that includes the intermediolateral cell column where the preganglionic sympathetic neurons are located. In all thoracic segments, a prominent structure called the *dorsal nucleus of Clarke* is located medially at the base of the dorsal horn and contains large cells. At rostral levels of the thoracic cord (T1–6), both the fasciculi gracilis and the cuneatus are present, while at caudal levels, only the fasciculus gracilis is present. The spinal nerves providing motor innervation to the back and intercostal muscles (axial muscles) emerge from the rostral levels of the thoracic cord (except T1). The spinal nerves providing innervation to the abdominal muscles in addition to the axial muscles emerge from the caudal thoracic levels.

Lumbar Segments

Nerve roots emerging from the segments at L1–4 form the lumbar plexus while those emerging from L4 to S2 form the sacral plexus. The segments at L1 and L2 contain the dorsal nucleus of Clarke as well as the intermediolateral cell column and resemble lower thoracic spinal segments. The motor innervation to the large muscles in the lower extremities is provided by the lumbar segments.

Sacral Segments

These segments are relatively small and contain small amounts of white matter and abundant quantities of gray matter. The dorsal gray column is thicker due to the presence of a well-developed substantia gelatinosa. Preganglionic parasympathetic neurons innervating pelvic viscera are located along the lateral surface of the base of anterior gray horn in S2–4 sacral segments.

Coccygeal Segments

The coccygeal segment resembles the sacral segments in that the gray matter of this segment is much more developed than the white matter. It is smaller than the sacral segments.

CYTOARCHITECTURAL ORGANIZATION

The cytoarchitectural lamination of the cat spinal cord was described in detail by Rexed (7,8). A similar lamination is believed to be present in the spinal cord of all mammals (Fig. 2.4). A brief description of Rexed laminae is presented below (see also Table 2.1).

The *zone of Lissauer* (fasciculus dorsolateralis) consists of fine myelinated and unmyelinated dorsal root fibers that enter the medial portion of this zone. A large number of propriospinal fibers, which interconnect different levels of the substantia gelatinosa, are also present in this zone.

Laminae I through IV are located in the dorsal horn of the spinal cord. The cells situated in these laminae receive primarily exteroceptive (i.e., pain, temperature and tactile) inputs from the periphery. Lamina I contains terminals of dorsal root fibers mediating pain and temperature sensations that synapse, in part, on cells called the *posteromarginal nucleus*. The axons of the cells in the posteromarginal nucleus cross to the opposite side and ascend as the lateral spinothalamic tract. Immediately below lamina I lies lamina II that contains the substantia gelatinosa. The neurons in the substantia gelatinosa modulate the activity of pain and temperature afferent fibers. Activation of peripheral pain receptors results in the release of substance P and glutamate in the substantia gelatinosa. Laminae III and IV, both of which contain the proper sensory nucleus, are located in the lower aspect of the dorsal horn. The proper sensory nucleus receives inputs from the substantia gelatinosa and contributes to the spinothalamic tracts mediating pain, temperature, as well as crude touch. Lamina V neurons, which are located at the neck of the dorsal horn, receive descending fibers from the corticospinal and rubrospinal tracts and give rise to axons that contribute to the spinothalamic tracts. Lamina VI is present only in cervical and lumbar segments. It contains a medial segment that receives muscle spindle and joint afferents, and also a lateral segment that receives fibers from descending corticospinal and rubrospinal pathways. Neurons in this region are involved in the integration of somatic motor processes. Lamina VII, located in an intermediate region of the spinal gray matter, contains the nucleus dorsalis of Clarke, which extends from C8 through L3. This nucleus receives muscle and tendon afferents. Axons of this nucleus form the dorsal spinocerebellar tract, which relays this information to the ipsilateral cerebellum. Other important neurons located in lamina VII include the sympathetic preganglionic neurons, which constitute the intermediolateral cell column in the thoracolumbar cord (T1-L3), parasympathetic neurons located in the lateral aspect of sacral cord (S2–4), and numerous interneurons.

The output of alpha motor neurons is regulated by *Renshaw cells* through a mechanism called *recurrent inhibition*. Renshaw cells are interneurons that make inhibitory (glycinergic) synapses on the alpha motor neurons and receive excitatory (cholinergic) collaterals from the same neurons. When an alpha motor neuron

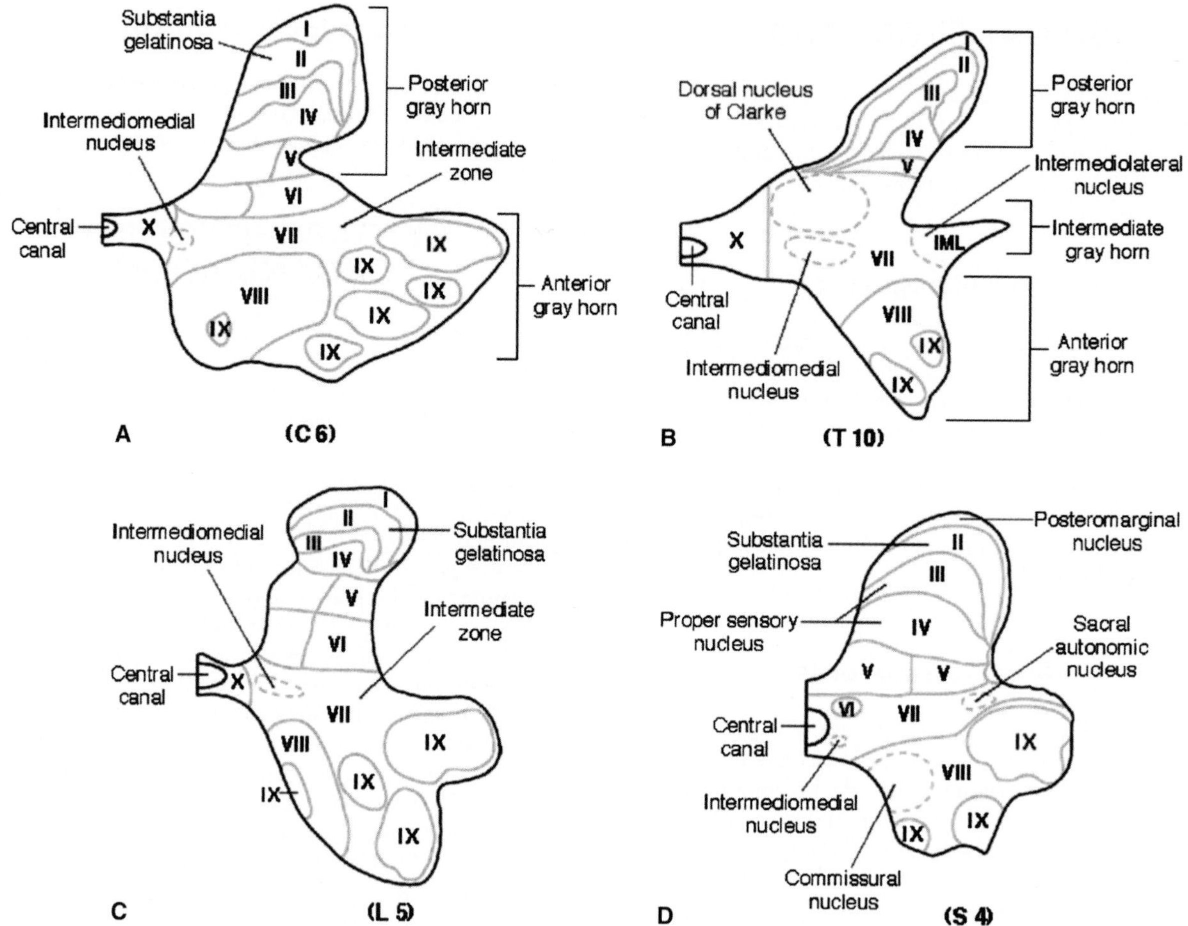

FIGURE 2.4. Structural lamination of human spinal cord segments at C6 (A), T10 (B), L5 (C), and S4 (D). (From Parent A, ed. *Carpenter's human neuroanatomy*, 9th ed. Baltimore: Lippincott Williams & Wilkins, 1996:334, with permission.)

is excited, it activates Renshaw cells via the excitatory (cholinergic) collaterals. Renshaw cells, in turn, inhibit via glycinergic synapses, the activity of the same alpha motor neuron.

Laminae VIII and IX are located in the ventral horn of the gray matter of the spinal cord. Neurons in this region, which receive inputs from the descending motor tracts from the cerebral cortex and brainstem, give rise to both alpha and gamma motor neurons that innervate skeletal muscles. Neurons in these laminae are somatotopically arranged; neurons situated in the medial aspect of the ventral horn receive afferents from the vestibulospinal and reticulospinal systems, and, in turn, innervate the axial musculature. This anatomical arrangement allows descending pathways to regulate the axial musculature (i.e., posture and balance). In contrast, neurons situated in the lateral aspect of the ventral horn receive afferents from the corticospinal and rubrospinal pathways. Axons of these neurons mainly innervate the distal musculature. This arrangement provides a basis by which these descending pathways can have a preferential influence upon the activity of the distal musculature. In the ventral horn, motor neurons are located according to the muscle that they innervate. Neurons providing innervation to the extensor muscles are located ventral to those innervating the flexors. Neurons providing innervation to the axial and limb girdle musculature are medial to those innervating muscles in the distal parts of the extremity (Fig. 2.5). In the cervical part of the spinal cord (segments C3, C4, and C5), lamina IX contains phrenic motor neurons that provide innervation to the diaphragm. Thoracic respiratory motor neurons, which innervate intercostal and other rib cage and back muscles, are located in lamina IX of the thoracic segments. The gray matter surrounding the central canal constitutes lamina X.

SPINAL CORD TRACTS

In the white matter of the spinal cord, different tracts are grouped together and are referred to as *dorsal, ventral, and lateral funiculi.* A description of these different tracts is presented below:

Long Ascending Tracts

Dorsal (Posterior) Column

The fasciculi gracilis and the cuneatus are also referred to as the *posterior (dorsal) columns.* Damage to these tracts results in symptoms that appear ipsilateral to the affected dorsal columns in the dermatomes at and below the level of the spinal cord lesion. A *dermatome* is defined as the area of skin innervated by a single dorsal root. The sensation transmitted in these tracts includes tactile (vibration, deep touch, and two-point discrimination) and

TABLE 2.1

IMPORTANT STRUCTURES IN SPINAL REXED LAMINAE

Laminae	Important structures
I	Dorsal root fibers mediating pain, temperature, touch sensations; posteromarginal nucleus
II	Substantia gelatinosa neurons mediating pain transmission
III and IV	Proper sensory nucleus that receives inputs from substantia gelatinosa and contributes to spinothalamic tracts mediating pain, temperature, and touch sensations
V	Neurons receiving descending fibers from corticospinal and rubrospinal tracts; neurons that contribute to ascending spinothalamic tracts
VI	Present only in cervical and lumbar segments; lateral segment receives descending corticospinal and rubrospinal fibers; medial segment receives afferents from muscle spindles and joint afferents
VII	Nucleus dorsalis of Clarke extending from C8 to L1 receives muscle and tendon afferents; axons from this nucleus form spinocerebellar tract; intermediolateral cell column containing sympathetic preganglionic neurons from T1 to L3; parasympathetic neurons located in S2–4 segments; Renshaw cells
VIII and IX	Located in the ventral horn; alpha and gamma motor neurons innervating skeletal muscles; neurons in medial aspect receive inputs from vestibulospinal and reticulospinal tracts and innervate axial musculature for posture and balance; neurons in lateral aspect receive inputs from corticospinal and rubrospinal tracts and innervate distal musculature; phrenic motoneurons (C3–5); thoracic respiratory neurons (thoracic levels)
X	Gray matter surrounding central canal

kinesthetic (position and movement) senses. The patient with a lesion affecting the cervical cord cannot identify an object placed in his/her hand ipsilateral to the lesion. If the lesion is located at the level of the lumbar cord, then the loss of these forms of sensation will be restricted to the ipsilateral lower limbs. The patient can perceive passive movements such as touch or pressure, and his/her movements will be poorly coordinated and clumsy because of the loss of conscious proprioception.

Fasciculus Gracilis

This tract contains long ascending fibers from the lower limbs (i.e., sacral, lumbar, and the caudal six thoracic segments) and exists at all levels of the spinal cord. Myelinated afferents from the ipsilateral dorsal root ganglion enter the dorsal funiculus, medial to the dorsal horn, and the ascending fibers occupy a medial position in the posterior (dorsal) funiculus (Fig. 2.6). Fibers from the lumbosacral regions mediating sensations from the lower limbs ascend medially, and those from higher regions ascend progressively more lateral so that fibers from the upper limbs that enter at upper thoracic and lower cervical levels can ascend in the lateral position. The neurons located in the dorsal root ganglion represent the first-order neuron. The peripheral processes of the first-order neuron innervate the pacinian (sensing tactile and vibratory stimuli) and Meissner corpuscles (sensing touch) in the skin, and proprioceptors in the joints that are involved in kinesthesia (sense of position and movement). The central processes of the first-order neuron ascend ipsilaterally in the spinal cord (i.e., the ascending fibers of first-order neuron are uncrossed) and terminate somatotopically on second-order neuron in the ipsilateral nucleus gracilis in the medulla. Axons of the second-order neuron travel ventromedially as the internal arcuate fibers and cross in the midline to form the medial lemniscus. This crossed tract ascends through the medulla, pons, and midbrain, and then terminates on the third-order neuron located in the contralateral ventral posterolateral nucleus of thalamus. Axons of the third-order neuron travel in the internal capsule and terminate in the sensorimotor cortex. The fasciculus gracilis is involved in mediating conscious proprioception that includes kinesthesia and discriminative touch.

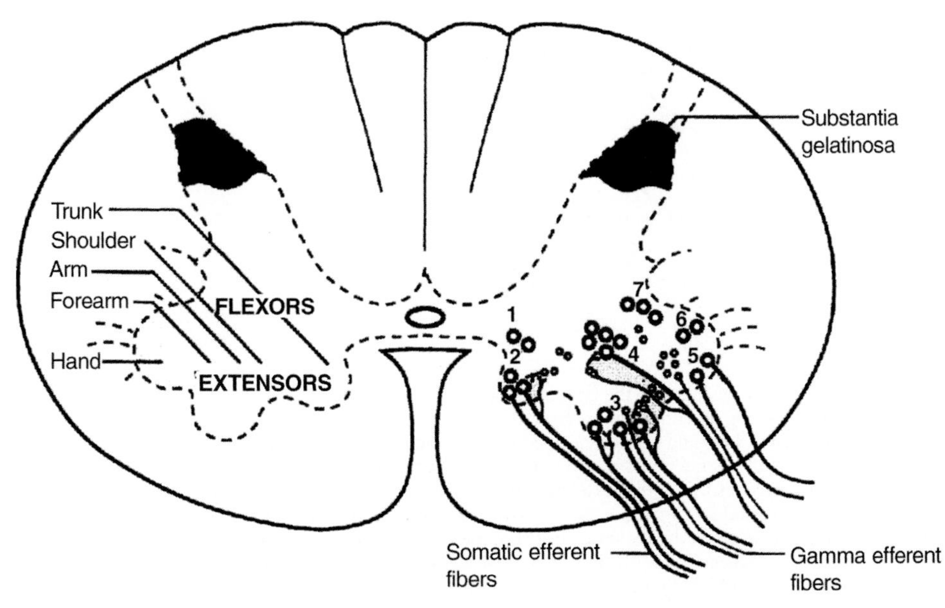

FIGURE 2.5. A diagrammatic representation of motor nuclei in anterior gray horn of a lower cervical spinal segment. Left: location of anterior horn cells that send motor axons to different muscle groups in the upper extremity. Right: different motor nuclei: (*1*) posteromedial, (*2*) anteromedial, (*3*) anterior, (*4*) central, (*5*) anterolateral, (*6*) posterolateral, (*7*) retroposterolateral. Neurons in the dotted area represent internuncial neurons. Smaller anterior horn neurons send gamma efferents to small muscle fibers of neuromuscular spindle. Somatic efferent fibers emerging from neurons located in regions *2*, *3*, and *4* send collaterals, which synapse on Renshaw cells located in the gray matter. (From Parent A, ed. *Carpenter's human neuroanatomy*, 9th ed. Baltimore: Lippincott Williams & Wilkins, 1996:344, with permission.)

Fasciculus Cuneatus

The fasciculus cuneatus exists in cervical segments and in thoracic segments above T6. It contains long ascending fibers from the upper limbs. Myelinated afferents from the dorsal root ganglion enter the dorsal funiculus medial to the dorsal horn, and the fibers ascend to occupy a lateral position in the posterior (dorsal) funiculus (Fig. 2.6). The peripheral processes of the first-order neuron innervate pacinian and Meissner corpuscles in the skin and the proprioceptors in joints. Its central processes ascend ipsilaterally to terminate on second-

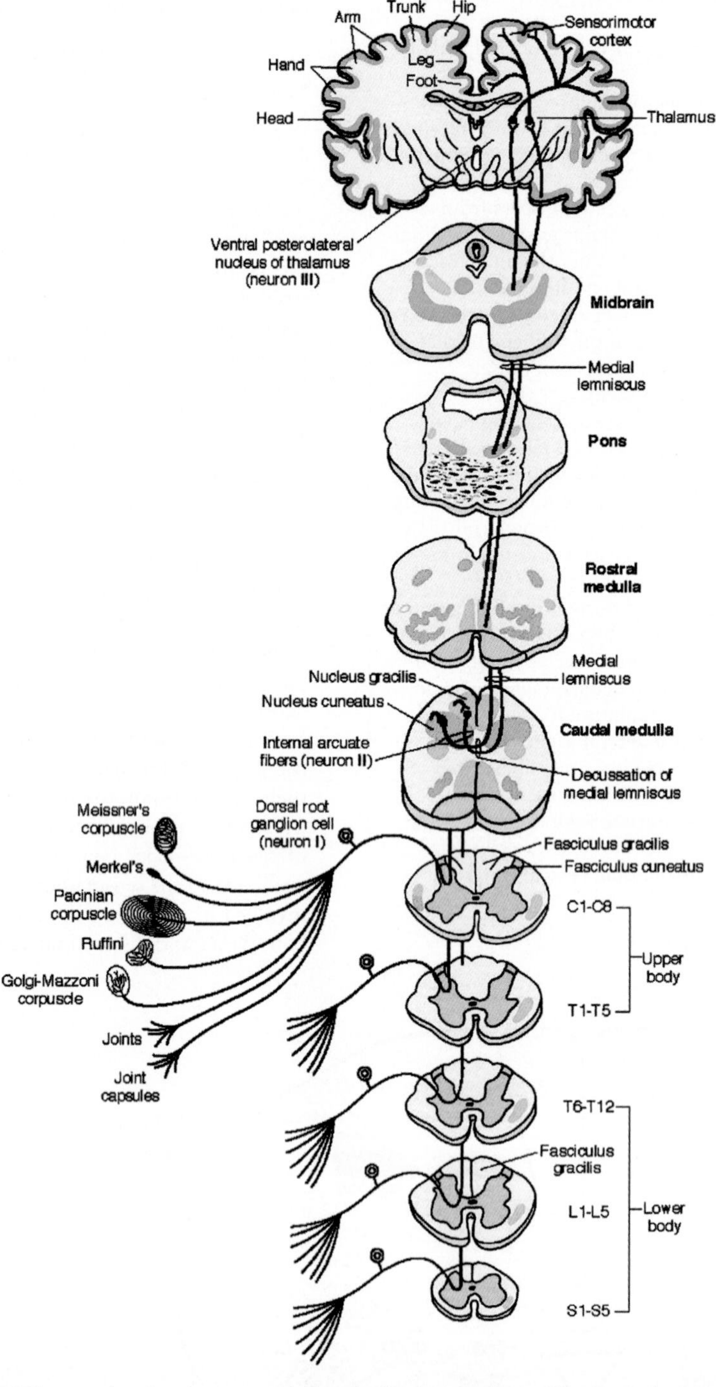

FIGURE 2.6. Diagram showing the course of fibers in the dorsal column. The fasciculus gracilis exists at all levels of the spinal cord and contains long ascending fibers from the lower limbs. The fasciculus cuneatus exists in thoracic segments above T6 (T1–6) and cervical segments (C1–8) and contains long ascending fibers from the upper limbs. The axons of second-order neurons in the nucleus gracilis and the cuneatus travel as internal arcuate fibers and cross in the midline to form the medial lemniscus, which ascends through the medulla, pons, and midbrain and terminates in the contralateral ventral posterolateral nucleus of the thalamus. Axons of third-order neurons in the thalamus travel in the internal capsule and terminate in the sensorimotor cerebral cortex. (From Siegel A, Sapru HN. *Essential neuroscience*, 2nd ed. Baltimore, MD: Lippincott Williams & Wilkins, 2011;147, with permission.)

order neurons located in the ipsilateral nucleus cuneatus of the medulla. Axons of these second-order neurons travel as internal arcuate fibers, cross the midline to form the medial lemniscus, and terminate on third-order neurons located in the contralateral ventral posterolateral nucleus of thalamus. The axons of these third-order neurons then terminate in the sensorimotor cortex. The fasciculus cuneatus is involved in mediating conscious proprioception.

Spinocerebellar Tracts

Dorsal (Posterior) Spinocerebellar Tract

The dorsal spinocerebellar tract, located in the dorsal half of the lateral aspect of the lateral funiculus of spinal cord, arises from neurons located in the nucleus dorsalis of Clarke that extends from L3 to C8. Afferent fibers arising from muscle spindles, and, to a lesser extent, Golgi tendon organs reach the nucleus dorsalis of Clarke via dorsal roots. Axons of neurons located in the nucleus dorsalis of Clarke ascend ipsilaterally (i.e., the tract is uncrossed) and reach the cerebellum by way of the inferior cerebellar peduncle where they terminate primarily in the cerebellar vermis of the anterior lobe. The tract first appears at L3 and increases in size until it reaches C8. Afferent fibers in segments caudal to L2 ascend in the fasciculus gracilis and synapse with the nucleus dorsalis of Clarke at the level of L2. The nucleus dorsalis of Clarke transmits information about muscle spindle and tendon afferents from the ipsilateral caudal aspect of the body and hind limb. The dorsal (posterior) spinocerebellar tract provides the cerebellum with information about the status of individual as well as groups of muscles, therefore enabling this region to coordinate and integrate neural signals controlling movement of individual lower limb muscles and posture.

Ventral (Anterior) Spinocerebellar Tract

The ventral spinocerebellar tract is located immediately below the dorsal spinocerebellar tract in the lateral aspect of the lateral funiculus. Neurons giving rise to this tract (second-order neurons) are located in the lateral part of the base and neck of the dorsal horn (laminae V, VI, and VII). Afferent fibers from the Golgi tendon organ reach the second-order neurons via the dorsal roots. The first-order neurons are located in the dorsal root ganglion. The axons of the second-order neurons cross in the spinal cord and ascend through the medulla to the pons. The fibers then join the superior cerebellar peduncle at the pontine level. Many of these fibers then recross and enter the cerebellum, where they terminate in the vermal region of the anterior lobe. This tract conveys information about whole limb movements and postural adjustments to the cerebellum.

Cuneocerebellar Tract

The nucleus dorsalis of Clarke does not extend to spinal segments rostral to C8. Therefore, afferent fibers entering the spinal cord rostral to this level ascend ipsilaterally in the fasciculus cuneatus and project to neurons located in the accessory cuneate nucleus located in the dorsolateral part of the medulla. Neurons located in this nucleus then give rise to the cuneocerebellar tract that is functionally related to the upper limbs. The fibers in this tract terminate in the cerebellar cortex. Thus, cuneocerebellar tract is the upper limb equivalent of the dorsal (posterior) spinocerebellar tract.

Anterolateral System of Ascending Tracts

Conventionally, the lateral spinothalamic tract is believed to transmit pain and temperature sensations, while the anterior spinothalamic tract transmits the sensation of nondiscriminative touch to the primary sensory cortex. Currently, it is believed that all components of the anterolateral ascending spinal system carry all sensory modalities (i.e., pain, temperature, and simple tactile sensations), but the pathways carrying them are different. The direct pathway, consisting of the neospinothalamic tract, mediates pain, temperature, and simple tactile sensations, while several indirect pathways mediate the affective and arousal components of these sensations. These revised concepts and new terminology for various tracts transmitting these sensations are presented below.

Direct Pathway

Neospinothalamic Tract. The neurons that give rise to this tract arise mainly from the nucleus proprius (the dorsal proper sensory nucleus) that is located in laminae III and IV. The axons of these neurons cross obliquely via the anterior white commissure to enter the contralateral white matter where they ascend in the lateral funiculus. This tract has a somatotopic organization throughout its course. Fibers arising from the lowest part of the body associated with the sacral and lumbar levels of spinal cord ascend dorsolaterally, while those arising from the upper extremities and neck in association with the cervical cord ascend ventromedially. The ascending axons synapse on third-order neurons located primarily in the ventral posterolateral nucleus of the thalamus that, in turn, project to the primary sensory cortex in the postcentral gyrus (Fig. 2.7).

Deficits following damage to direct neospinothalamic pathway on one side result in complete loss of pain (anesthesia), thermal (thermoanesthesia), and simple tactile sensations on the contralateral side of the body at and below the level of the lesion.

Loss of pain, temperature, and tactile sensations can also occur at a specific segment following damage to the area around the central spinal canal. This occurs in a condition called *syringomyelia*, in which a lesion (e.g., cavitation) occurs in or around the central canal and affects the crossing fibers from the neospinothalamic tracts on either side but only in or around the segment in which the lesion is present. Accordingly, such a disorder results in bilateral loss of pain, temperature, and simple tactile sensations at the affected segment.

The neospinothalamic tract is somatotopically organized; sacral and lumbar fibers lie dorsolateral to those of the thoracic and cervical fibers. Accordingly, a lesion within the spinal cord is likely to affect the thoracic and cervical fibers early, while the sacral and lumbar fibers would be affected late or not at all. This clinical phenomenon in which damage to the spinothalamic tracts leaves intact the pain, temperature, and simple tactile sensations in sacral dermatomes is referred to as *sacral sparing*.

When the dorsal columns as well as the anterolateral spinothalamic tracts on one side are damaged, the following phenomenon is observed. On the ipsilateral side below the level of the lesion, there is a loss of conscious proprioception, but the sensations of pain, temperature, and simple touch are preserved. On the contralateral side below the level of the lesion, the reverse is true. There is a loss of pain, temperature, and

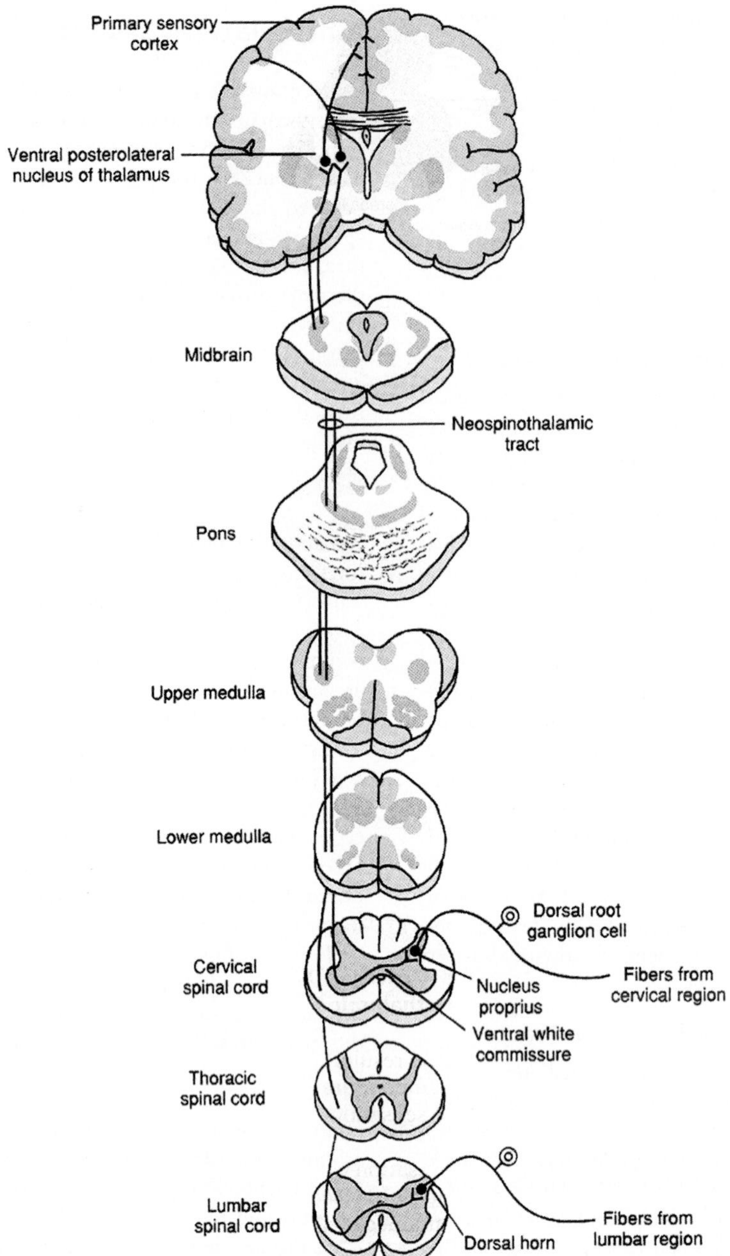

FIGURE 2.7. Direct spinothalamic pathway: the neospinothalamic tract. The peripheral processes of these dorsal root ganglion cells end as receptors sensing pain, temperature, and simple tactile sensations. The central processes of these dorsal root ganglion cells synapse with the neurons of the nucleus proprius. The axons of these second-order neurons cross via the anterior white commissure, enter the contralateral white matter, ascend in the lateral funiculus, and synapse on third-order neurons located in the ventral posterolateral nucleus of the thalamus. The axons of third-order neurons project to the primary sensory cortex. (From Siegel A, Sapru HN. *Essential neuroscience*, 2nd ed. Baltimore, MD: Lippincott Williams & Wilkins, 2011;150, with permission.)

simple tactile sensations while conscious proprioception is preserved. This is observed in Brown-Sequard syndrome.

Indirect Pathways

The indirect pathways mediate the autonomic, endocrine, motor, and arousal components of pain, temperature, and simple tactile sensations. In addition, these indirect pathways are involved in the activation of pain-inhibiting mechanisms. The axons of these neurons ascend in the spinal cord bilaterally, show poor somatotopic organization, and make multiple synapses in the reticular formation, hypothalamus, and limbic system. The following pathways are included in this system.

Paleospinothalamic Tract. The neurons of this pathway are located deep in the dorsal horn and the intermediate gray matter. Their axons ascend contralaterally as well as ipsilaterally in the ventrolateral quadrant of the spinal cord, make several synapses in the reticular formation, project to the midline and intralaminar thalamic nuclei, which, in turn, project in

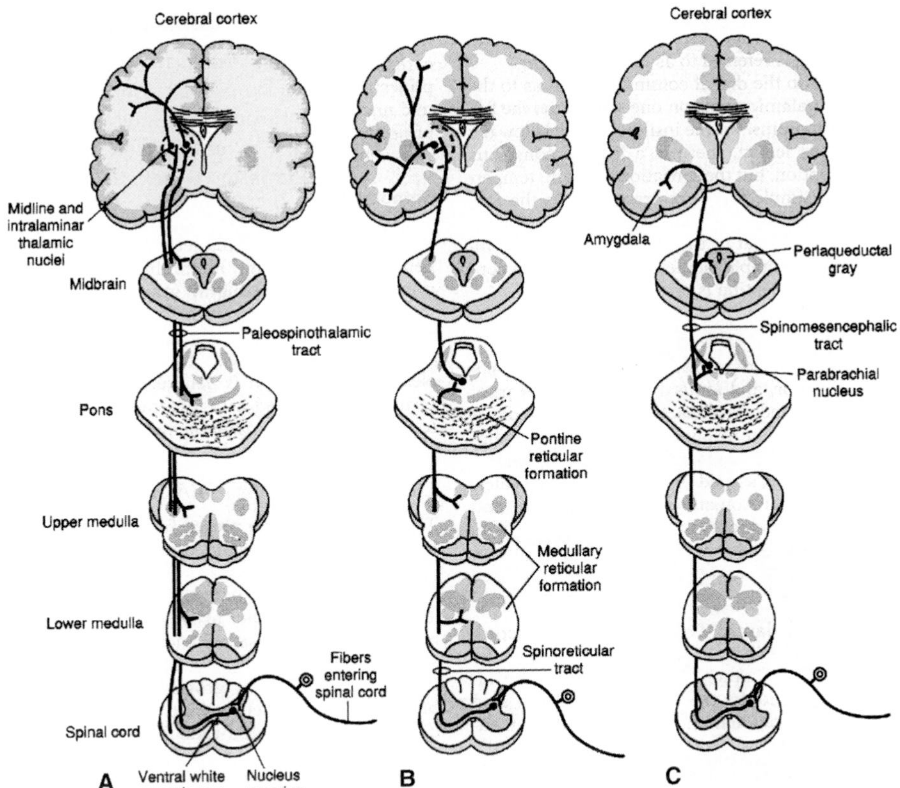

FIGURE 2.8. Indirect spinothalamic pathways. These pathways mediate the affective and arousal components of pain, temperature, and simple tactile sensations. (**A**) The ascending axons in the paleothalamic tract synapse in the brainstem reticular formation and neurons in midline and intralaminar thalamic nuclei, which then project diffusely to the cerebral cortex including the cingulate gyrus. (**B**) In the spinoreticular tract, one group of ascending axons projects to the medullary reticular formation, and the other group projects to the pontine reticular formation. The neurons in the reticular formation then project to neurons located in the midline and intralaminar thalamic nuclei. These thalamic neurons then project to the cerebral cortex. (**C**) In the spinomesencephalic tract, ascending axons terminate on the PAG neurons that, in turn, project to neurons in the amygdala via the parabrachial nuclei. (From Siegel A, Sapru HN. *Essential neuroscience*, 2nd ed. Baltimore, MD: Lippincott Williams & Wilkins, 2011;152, with permission.)

a diffuse manner to the cerebral cortex, especially the limbic regions such as cingulate gyrus (Fig. 2.8A).

Spinoreticular Tract. The neurons of this pathway are also located deep in the dorsal horn and the intermediate gray matter. The axons of these neurons project to different regions of the lower brainstem. One group of fibers terminates in the medullary reticular formation, and another ascends to the pontine reticular formation. Details concerning the origins and distributions of these pathways are not known. However, it is believed that the projections from the spinal cord to the brainstem are both crossed and uncrossed (Fig. 2.8B). A key feature about these pathways is that ascending spinoreticular fibers are believed to transmit sensory information to the reticular formation, which, in turn, activates the cerebral cortex through secondary and tertiary projections via the midline and intralaminar thalamic nuclei. The thalamocortical projections are highly diffuse and influence wide areas of the cerebral cortex. The spinoreticular fibers constitute a part of a polysynaptic system that is involved in the maintenance of the state of consciousness and awareness. Accordingly, a lesion of these fibers is likely to affect these functions.

Spinomesencephalic Tract. The neurons of this pathway are also located deep in the dorsal horn and intermediate gray matter. The axons of these neurons ascend to the midbrain where they terminate in periaqueductal gray (PAG), a region surrounding the cerebral aqueduct (Fig. 2.8C). Similar to spinoreticular fibers, details regarding the distribution of these fibers have not been clearly established. It is believed that sensory information associated with this tract is transmitted to the cerebral cortex through secondary and tertiary projections via midline and intralaminar thalamic nuclei.

Long Descending Tracts

These tracts mediate motor functions such as voluntary and involuntary movement, regulation of muscle tone, modulation of spinal segmental reflexes, as well as regulation of visceral functions. The corticospinal tract arises from the cerebral cortex and the tectospinal and rubrospinal tracts arise from the midbrain. The remaining tracts arise from different nuclear groups within the lower brainstem. These include lateral and medial vestibulospinal tracts and one reticulospinal tract that arise from the pons and the medulla. In addition, other descending pathways arising from medullary nuclei modulate autonomic functions. The corticospinal and rubrospinal pathways are mainly concerned with control over the flexor motor system and fine movements of the limbs, while the vestibulospinal and reticulospinal systems principally regulate antigravity muscles, posture, and balance.

Corticospinal Tract

The corticospinal tract arises from the cerebral cortex. The axons arising from the cortex converge in the corona radiata; descend through the internal capsule, crus cerebri, pons, and medullary pyramids; and terminate in the spinal cord (Fig. 2.9). Within the cortex, the sites from where the fibers in

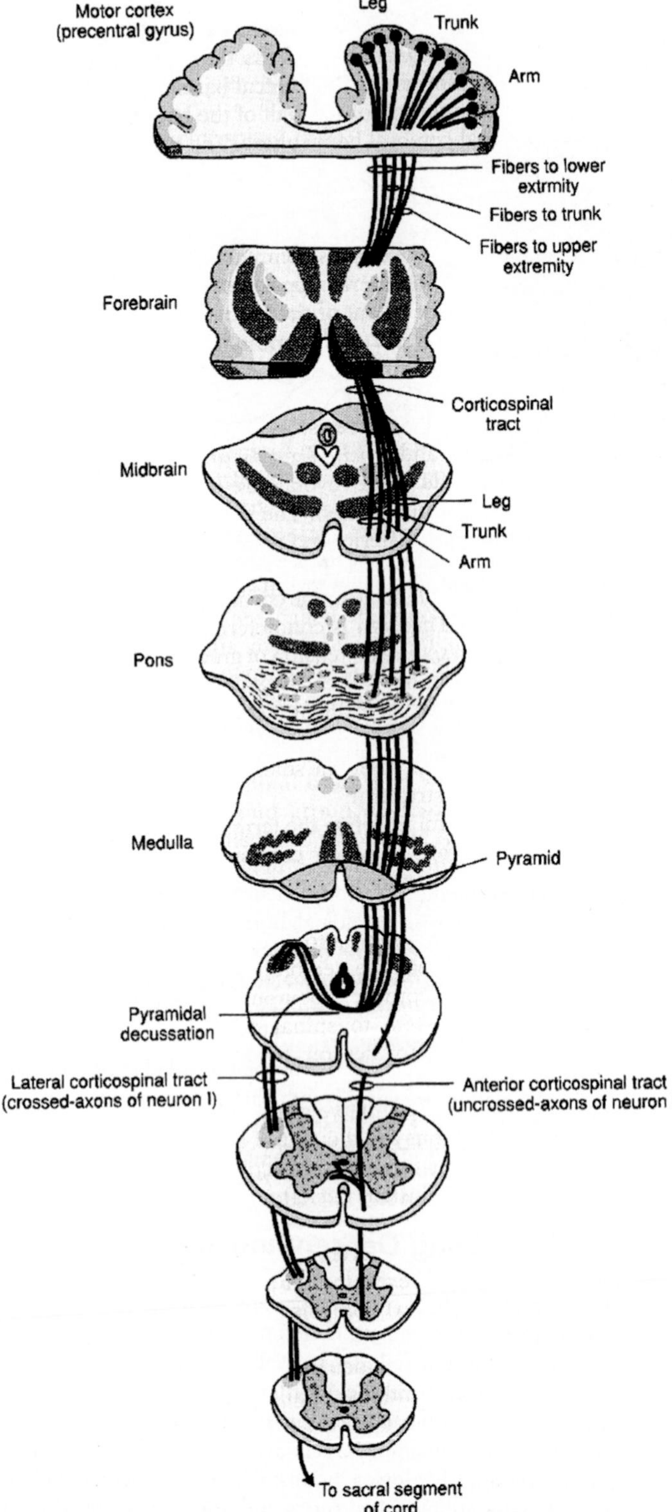

FIGURE 2.9. The corticospinal tract. This tract arises from the motor cortex (precentral gyrus), passes through the medullary pyramids, and terminates in the spinal cord. Note that a majority of corticospinal fibers cross to the contralateral side in the caudal medulla (pyramidal decussation) and descend as the lateral corticospinal tract and the remaining fibers descend ipsilaterally as anterior corticospinal tract. (From Siegel A, Sapru HN. *Essential neuroscience*, 2nd ed. Baltimore, MD: Lippincott Williams & Wilkins, 2011;153, with permission.)

this tract arise are precentral area (area 4; deeper part of lamina V), premotor and supplementary motor areas (area 6), and the postcentral gyrus (areas 3, 1, and 2). The corticospinal tract is somatotopically organized throughout its entire projection (1–4). The cells of origin functionally associated with the arm are located in the lateral convexity of the cortex, while the cells of origin functionally associated with the leg are located along the medial wall of the hemisphere. This somatotopic organization is called *cortical homunculus*. Many of these axons control fine movements of the distal parts of the extremities. At the juncture of the medulla and the spinal cord, about 90% the fibers cross to the contralateral side, forming the lateral corticospinal tract. About 8% of the fibers are uncrossed as they descend through the cord, and this pathway is called the *anterior corticospinal tract*. This tract ultimately crosses over at different segmental levels of the cord to synapse with anterior horn cells on the contralateral side. A scant 2% of the corticospinal tract remains uncrossed throughout its entire trajectory and is called the *uncrossed lateral corticospinal tract* (Fig. 2.10).

This tract controls voluntary movements of both the contralateral upper and the lower limbs. Depending upon the extent of the lesion, these functions are lost when the corticospinal tract is damaged. Following an SCI, first the affected muscles lose their tone. After several days or weeks, the muscles become spastic (i.e., they resist passive movement in one direction) and hyperreflexia occurs (i.e., the force and amplitude of the deep tendon, myotatic reflexes are increased, particularly in the legs). The superficial reflexes (abdominal, cremasteric, and normal plantar) are either lost or diminished. A Babinski sign, which usually indicates damage to the corticospinal tract, is also present. This sign is characterized by an abnormal plantar response (extension of great toe while the other toes fan out) when the sole of a foot is stroked by a blunt instrument. The normal plantar response consists of a brisk reflexion of all toes when the sole of a foot is stroked by a blunt instrument.

A lower motor neuron (LMN) is one whose cell body lies in the central nervous system (CNS) but whose axon innervates muscles or glands. An upper motor neuron (UMN) is one that descends from the cerebral cortex to the brainstem or spinal cord, or one that descends from the brainstem to the spinal cord and that synapses with an LMN. In general, an LMN is usually thought of as spinal cord motor horn cell or cranial nerve motor neuron, while UMNs are thought of as corticospinal or corticobulbar (neurons projecting from the cerebral cortex to the brainstem nuclei) neurons.

The symptoms of damage to the corticospinal tract (i.e., loss of voluntary movement, spasticity, increased deep tendon reflexes, loss of superficial reflexes, and Babinski sign) comprise an UMN paralysis. Thus, the pyramidal cells and their axons are designated as *UMNs*. The neurons located in the ventral horn of the spinal cord are designated as *LMNs*. The symptoms of LMN paralysis include loss of muscle tone, atrophy of muscles, and loss of all reflex as well as voluntary movement. Often times, after an SCI, there is an LMN injury at the level of injury, with a UMN injury to levels below the injury.

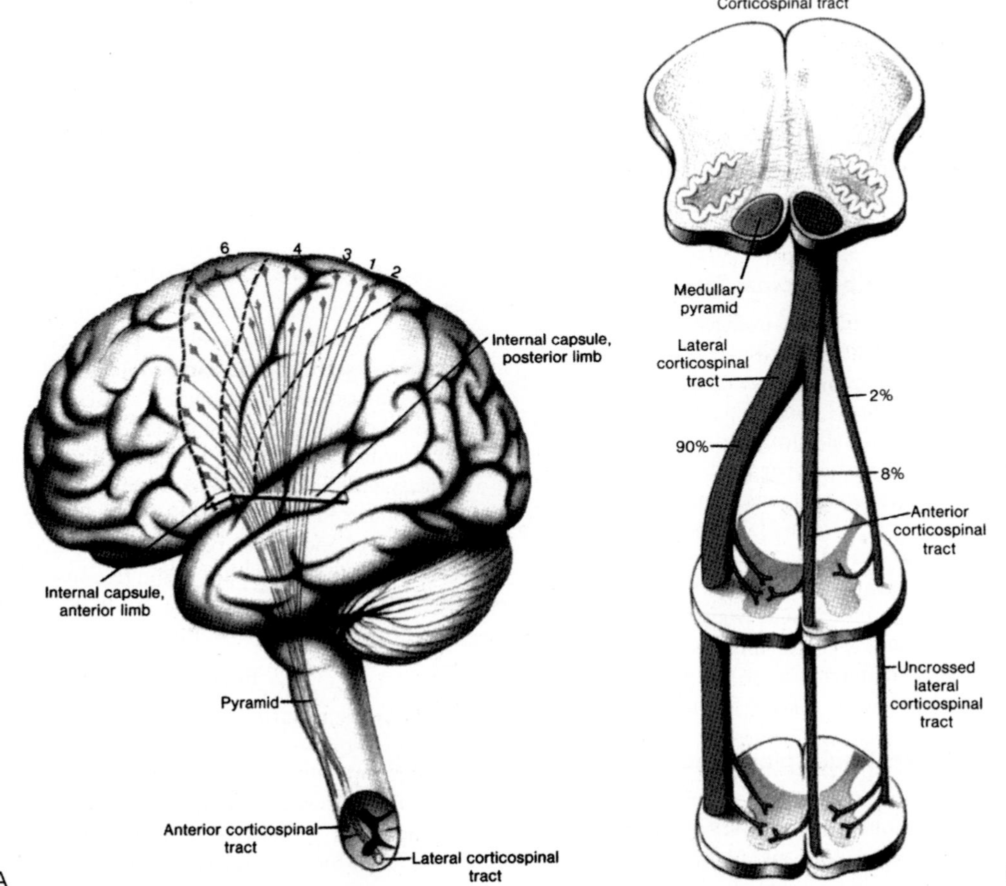

FIGURE 2.10. (A,B) Diagram showing the divisions of the corticospinal tract. (From Parent A, ed. *Human neuroanatomy*, 9th ed. Baltimore, MD: Lippincott Williams & Wilkins, 1996:384–385, with permission.)

Rubrospinal Tract

The rubrospinal tract arises from neurons called the *red nucleus* that are located in the rostral half of the midbrain tegmentum. The axons of these neurons cross the midline in the ventral midbrain (called the *ventral tegmental decussation*) and descend to the contralateral spinal cord. Fibers in the rubrospinal tract are somatotopically arranged; the cervical spinal segments receive fibers from the dorsal part of red nucleus, which in turn receive inputs from the upper limb region of sensorimotor cortex; the lumbosacral spinal segments receive fibers from the ventral half of the red nucleus, which in turn receive inputs from the leg region of sensorimotor cortex. The fibers of the rubrospinal tract enter the laminae V, VI, and VII of the spinal cord. They end on interneurons that, in turn, project to the dorsal aspect of ventral (motor) horn cells. The neurons in the red nucleus receive projections from ipsilateral cerebral cortex and contralateral deep cerebellar nuclei. Thus, the cerebral cortex and the cerebellum can influence the activity of the alpha and gamma motor neurons of the spinal cord via the rubrospinal tract that facilitates the activity of the flexor muscles and inhibits the activity of the extensor muscles. Damage to this tract is likely to compromise precise and well-controlled movements of the distal limb musculature. However, in the human nervous system, the rubrospinal tract may be of little clinical significance because it does not extend below cervical levels (9).

Tectospinal Tract

The neurons giving rise to this tract are located in the superior colliculus. The axons of these neurons descend around the PAG, cross the midline in the dorsal tegmental decussation, join the medial longitudinal fasciculus (MLF) in the medulla, and descend in the anterior funiculus of the spinal cord. They terminate in laminae VI, VII, and VIII in upper cervical segments. Since this tract is believed to aid in directing head movements in response to visual and auditory stimuli, damage to this tract is likely to affect aforementioned head movements.

Lateral Vestibulospinal Tract

The lateral vestibulospinal tract is an uncrossed tract that arises from neurons of the lateral vestibular nucleus, which is located at the border of the pons and the medulla. It descends the entire length of the spinal cord. The descending fibers enter laminae VII and VIII and terminate directly on motor neurons mainly in cervical and lumbar levels. The lateral vestibular nucleus receives inhibitory inputs from the cerebellum, and excitatory inputs from the vestibular apparatus. Impulses transmitted to the spinal cord by the lateral vestibular nucleus powerfully facilitate ipsilateral extensor motor neurons, thereby increasing extensor motor tone. Main functions of this tract are to control the muscles that maintain upright posture and balance. Therefore, maintenance of upright posture and balance will be compromised by a lesion of this tract.

Medial Vestibulospinal Tract

The medial vestibulospinal tract arises from ipsilateral and contralateral medial vestibular nuclei, descends in the ventral funiculus of the cervical spinal cord, and terminates in the ipsilateral ventral horn. Since the main function of this tract is to control the head position in association with vestibular stimulation, this function will be affected by a lesion of this tract.

Reticulospinal Tracts

The reticular formation gives rise to three functionally different fiber systems. One component of this system mediates motor functions, a second mediates autonomic functions, and a third modulates pain impulses.

Fibers arising from the medulla issue from a group of large cells located medially called the *nucleus gigantocellularis*. These cells project bilaterally to all levels of the spinal cord, and this pathway is referred to as the *lateral reticulospinal tract*. A key function of this pathway is that it powerfully suppresses extensor spinal reflex activity. In contrast, a separate reticulospinal pathway arises from two distinct nuclear groups in the medial aspect of the pons called the *nucleus reticularis pontis caudalis* and *nucleus reticularis pontis oralis*. These neurons project ipsilaterally to the entire extent of the spinal cord, but their principal function is to facilitate extensor spinal reflexes. This fiber bundle is called the *medial reticulospinal tract*.

A second group of descending reticulospinal fibers mediates autonomic functions. They arise largely from the ventrolateral medulla and project to the intermediolateral cell column of the thoracolumbar cord. This fiber system excites sympathetic preganglionic neurons in the intermediolateral cell column, which provide sympathetic innervation to visceral organs.

A third group of descending fibers modulates pain. The first limb of this pathway consists of enkephalinergic neurons that arise from the midbrain PAG and project to serotonergic neurons located in the nucleus raphe magnus of the medulla. These serotonergic neurons then project to the dorsal horn of the spinal cord, making synapse with a second group of enkephalinergic interneurons, which, in turn, synapse upon primary afferent pain fibers. Therefore, a key function of this descending fiber system is to modulate the activity of pain impulses that ascend in the spinothalamic system.

Medial Longitudinal Fasciculus

The fibers in the MLF are mainly ascending, but this bundle also contains some descending fibers. Both ascending and descending fibers arise from different vestibular nuclei (lateral, superior, medial, inferior vestibular nuclei) located in the pons. Descending fibers of the MLF are situated in the dorsal part of the ventral funiculus and project principally to upper cervical segments of the spinal cord. These fibers monosynaptically inhibit motor neurons located in the upper cervical cord. By virtue of its connections with motor neurons in the cervical cord, this pathway controls the position of the head in response to excitation by the labyrinth.

Fasciculi Proprii

The fasciculi proprii consist of ascending and descending, crossed or uncrossed, fibers that arise and end in the spinal cord. They connect different segments of the spinal cord. These fibers mediate intrinsic reflex mechanisms of the spinal cord such as the coordination of upper and lower limb movements. Signals entering the spinal cord at any segment are thus conveyed to upper or lower segments and finally transmitted to the ventral horn cells either directly or through interneurons.

SPINAL CORD AND THE AUTONOMIC NERVOUS SYSTEM

The function of the autonomic nervous system is to maintain the internal environment of the body constant (homeostasis). This system regulates involuntary functions such as blood pressure, heart rate, respiration, digestion, glandular secretion, reproduction, and body temperature. Currently, the autonomic nervous system is divided into three divisions: sympathetic, parasympathetic, and enteric (1).

Sympathetic Division

The neurons from which the outflow of the sympathetic division originates (preganglionic neurons) are located in the intermediolateral cell column of the first thoracic to second lumbar (T1-L2) spinal cord. For this reason, the sympathetic nervous system is sometimes called the *thoracolumbar division*. Generally, the axons of these preganglionic neurons exit the spinal cord through the ventral roots and enter the main trunk of the spinal nerve (Fig. 2.11). After traveling in the spinal nerve, the axons of the sympathetic preganglionic neurons exit through the white ramus and reach one of the sympathetic ganglia. The axon of the preganglionic neuron follows one or more of the following pathways:

1. The sympathetic preganglionic axon synapses upon one of the neurons (called a *postganglionic neuron*) in the paravertebral sympathetic ganglion. The axons of this postganglionic neuron (postganglionic fibers) exit through the gray ramus communicans and return to the spinal nerve. The sympathetic postganglionic fibers then innervate the target organs (e.g., a blood vessel or sweat gland).
2. The sympathetic preganglionic axons do not synapse upon any neuron in the paravertebral ganglion; they pass through the ganglion, exit through a nerve (e.g., the greater splanchnic nerve), and synapse upon a neuron in one of the prevertebral ganglia. The sympathetic postganglionic fibers exiting from the neuron in the prevertebral ganglion then innervate the target organs (e.g., segments of the gastrointestinal tract).
3. The sympathetic preganglionic axons branch; one of these branches synapses upon a neuron in a particular paravertebral ganglion, while others ascend or descend in the paravertebral sympathetic chain and synapse on neurons located in several ganglia. In this manner, one preganglionic neuron located in the intermediolateral cell column of the thoracolumbar cord innervates as many as 30 postganglionic neurons located in several paravertebral ganglia.

Sympathetic Ganglia

There are two types of sympathetic ganglia: paravertebral and prevertebral ganglia. The paravertebral ganglia (22 pairs) are located on each side of the vertebral column and are connected together by sympathetic nerve trunk, thus forming a sympathetic chain on each side (Fig. 2.12). The prevertebral ganglia (e.g., celiac and mesenteric ganglia) are located in different places in the thorax, abdomen, and pelvis. In addition, a few terminal ganglia, with short postganglionic fibers, are located in the urinary bladder and the rectum.

The sympathetic division of the autonomic nervous system is activated in stressful situations. Thus, activation of sympathetic nervous system results in pupillary dilatation and an increase in heart rate, blood pressure, blood flow in the skeletal muscles, and blood sugar. These effects are widespread because one preganglionic sympathetic axon innervates several postganglionic neurons. All of these responses prepare the individual for fight or flight. For example, increase in blood

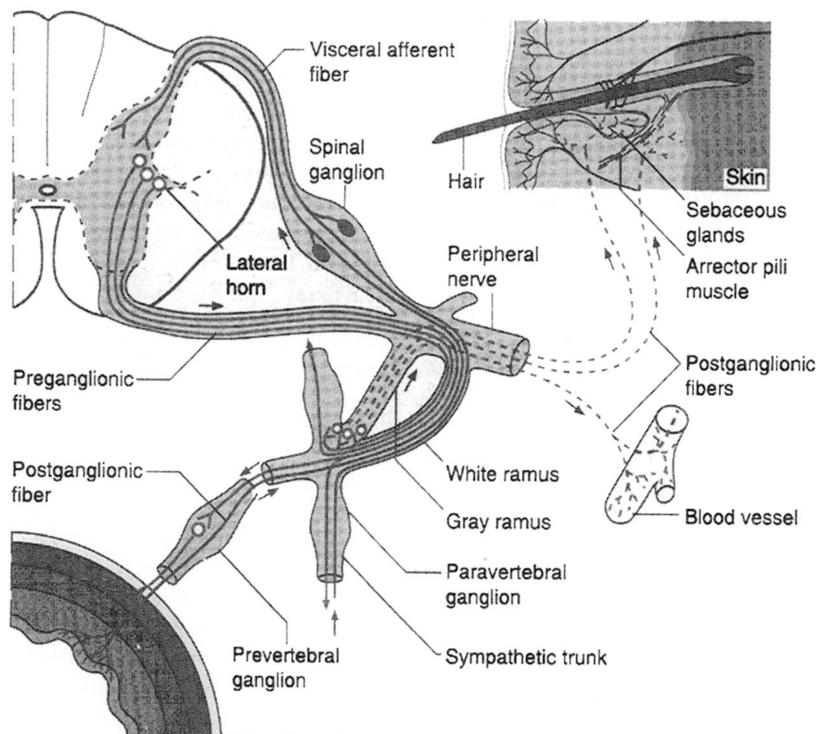

FIGURE 2.11. Diagram showing the reflex arcs of the sympathetic nervous system. (From Parent A, ed. *Human neuroanatomy*, 9th ed. Baltimore, MD: Lippincott Williams & Wilkins, 1996:295, with permission.)

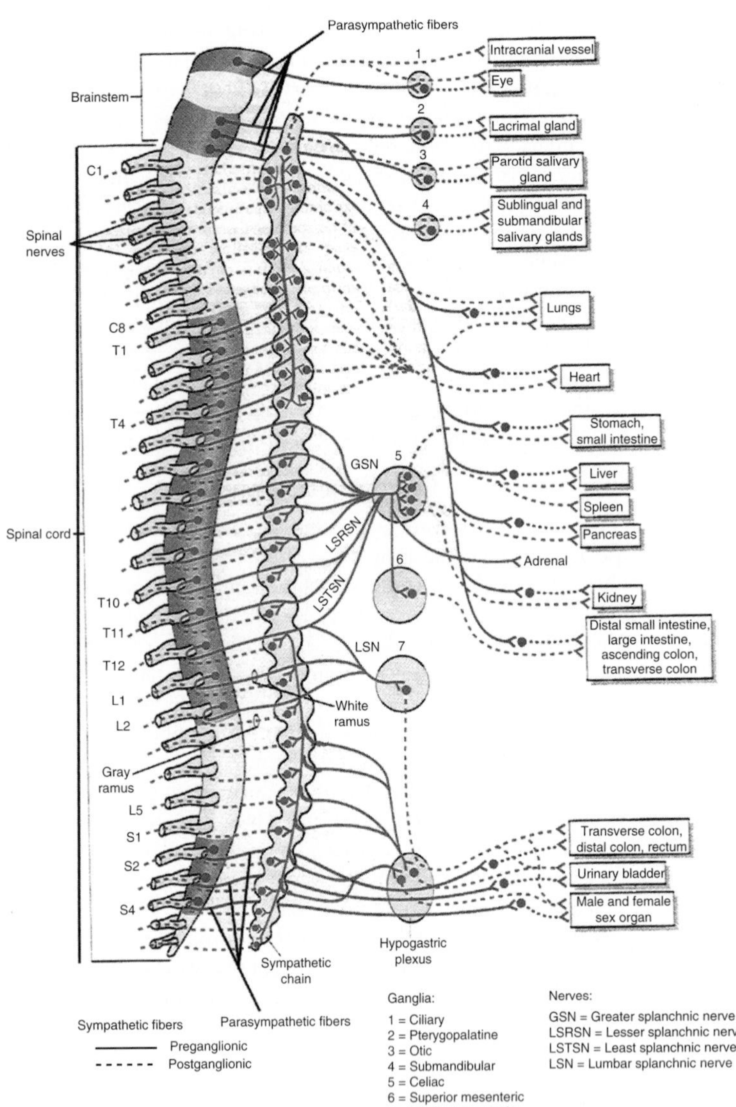

FIGURE 2.12. An overview of the sympathetic and parasympathetic components of the autonomic nervous system. C, cervical; T, thoracic; L, lumbar; S, sacral spinal segments. Ganglia: *1*, Ciliary; *2*, pterygopalatine; *3*, otic; *4*, submandibular; *5*, celiac; *6*, superior mesenteric; *7*, inferior mesenteric. Nerves: *GSN*, greater splanchnic nerve; *LSRSN*, lesser splanchnic nerve; *LSTSN*, least splanchnic nerve; *LSN*, lumbar splanchnic nerve. (From Siegel A, Sapru HN. *Essential neuroscience*, 2nd ed., Baltimore: Lippincott Williams & Wilkins, 2011;383, with permission.)

flow in the skeletal muscles will help in running away from the site of danger (flight); increase in heart rate and blood pressure will help in better perfusion of different organs; increase in blood sugar will provide energy and pupillary dilatation will provide for better vision under these circumstances. The effects of simultaneous activation of the parasympathetic division of the autonomic nervous system will complement these actions.

Parasympathetic Division

The preganglionic neurons from which the parasympathetic outflow arises are located in the brainstem (midbrain, pons and medulla oblongata) and the sacral region of the spinal cord. For this reason, this division is sometimes referred to as *craniosacral division* (Fig. 2.12).

The parasympathetic preganglionic neurons are located in the brainstem and the spinal cord. In the spinal cord, the preganglionic parasympathetic neurons are located in the intermediolateral column of the sacral spinal cord at S2–4 level. Their axons exit through the ventral roots, travel through pelvic nerves, and synapse on postganglionic neurons that are located close to or within the organs being innervated. The postganglionic parasympathetic nerve fibers are, therefore, very short compared to the sympathetic postganglionic nerve fibers.

Activation of the parasympathetic division of autonomic nervous system results in conservation and restoration of body energy. For example, decrease in heart rate brought about by the activation of parasympathetic nervous system will also decrease the demand for energy, while the increased activity of the gastrointestinal system will promote restoration of body energy. The effects of parasympathetic activation are localized and last for a short time.

Enteric Nervous System

The enteric division consists of neurons in the wall of the gut (intrinsic innervation) that regulates gastrointestinal motility and secretion. The gastrointestinal system is also controlled by sympathetic and parasympathetic innervation (extrinsic innervation). The extrinsic system can override the intrinsic system under certain situations.

Autonomic Innervation of Organs

Many organs are innervated by sympathetic as well as parasympathetic divisions (Fig. 2.12). As a rule, in most of the organs with dual innervation, activation of the parasympathetic and sympathetic divisions has antagonistic actions. Exceptions to this rule are the salivary glands where activation of either system results in an increase in the secretion of saliva; sympathetic stimulation produces viscous saliva, while parasympathetic stimulation produces watery saliva. The autonomic innervation of some selected organs, often affected by SCI, is described in the gastrointestinal, bladder, and sexuality chapters.

Neurotransmitters in the Autonomic Nervous System

Preganglionic Terminals

Within the autonomic ganglia, acetylcholine is the transmitter released at the terminals of the sympathetic as well as parasympathetic preganglionic fibers. The terminal branches of the preganglionic fibers contain vesicles (membrane-bound saclike structures) enclosing the neurotransmitter. The terminals make synaptic contacts with the postganglionic neurons located in the ganglia.

Postganglionic Terminals

The terminals of the sympathetic and parasympathetic postganglionic neurons innervate the effector cells in the target organs. At the terminals of most sympathetic postganglionic neurons, norepinephrine is the transmitter liberated with the exception of those innervating sweat glands and blood vessels of the skeletal muscles where acetylcholine is the neurotransmitter. At the terminals of all the parasympathetic postganglionic neurons, acetylcholine is the neurotransmitter liberated.

BLOOD SUPPLY OF THE SPINAL CORD

Arteries

The following major arteries supply the spinal cord (Fig. 2.13):

Posterior Spinal Arteries

The posterior spinal arteries, one on each side, are given off by the vertebral arteries as they ascend on the anterolateral surface of the medulla. They descend on the posterolateral surface of the spinal cord slightly medial to the dorsal roots.

Anterior Spinal Arteries

The anterior spinal arteries also arise from the vertebral arteries as they ascend on the anterolateral surface of the medulla. They unite to form one single artery that courses along the midline of the spinal cord.

Radicular Arteries

The radicular arteries arise from segmental levels such as ascending cervical, deep cervical, intercostal, lumbar, and sacral arteries, which, in turn, arise from the thoracic and

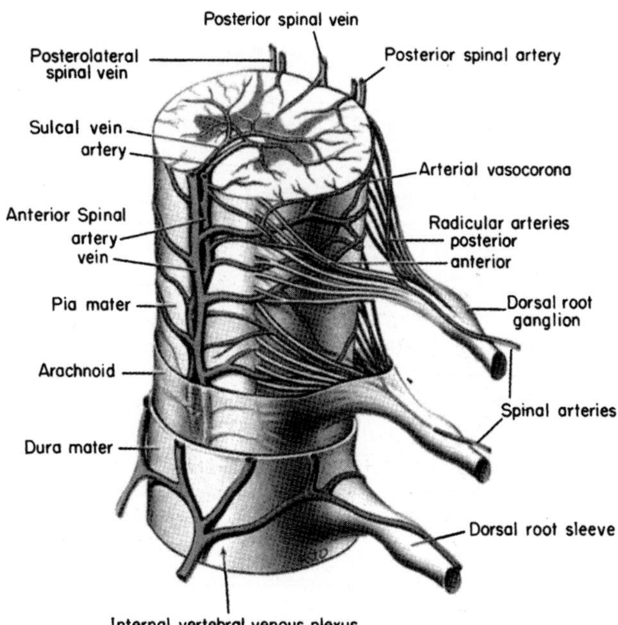

FIGURE 2.13. Diagram showing the blood supply of the spinal cord. (From Parent A, ed. *Human neuroanatomy*, 9th ed. Baltimore: Lippincott Williams & Wilkins, 1996:95, with permission.)

abdominal aorta. The radicular arteries pass through the intervertebral foramina and then bifurcate into anterior and posterior radicular arteries. These arteries provide blood supply to the thoracic, lumbar, sacral, and coccygeal regions of the spinal cord. Radicular arteries travel along the ventral roots and enter the subarachnoid space. The radicular artery present at T12-L2 supplies blood to caudal two thirds of the spinal cord. In the lumbar region of the spinal cord, one anterior radicular artery (*artery of Adamkiewicz*) is larger than others.

The cervical segments of the spinal cord are supplied by branches of the vertebral and ascending cervical arteries. Because of the dual source of blood supply, these segments are usually less vulnerable to ischemia. On the other hand, upper thoracic segments depend on radicular branches of the intercostal arteries. If one or more branches of the intercostal arteries are injured, the spinal segments T1–4 will not be adequately perfused and are vulnerable to spinal cord infarction. Similarly, spinal L1 segment is another region vulnerable to spinal infarction.

Veins

Six longitudinal veins drain the spinal cord; three are located on the ventral and three on the dorsal side (Fig. 2.13). On the ventral side, one of the three veins is located in the midline (anteromedian vein) and two others (anterolateral veins) are located along the line of attachment of the ventral roots. Branches of the sulcal veins drain both sides of the spinal cord, join, and enter the anteromedian vein. The anteromedian and anterolateral veins empty into anterior radicular veins that, in turn, empty into the anterior epidural venous plexus. On the dorsal side, one of the veins (posteromedian vein) is located in the midline and the two posterolateral veins are located along the line of attachment of the dorsal roots. The posteromedian and posterolateral veins are drained by posterior radicular veins that, in turn, empty into the posterior epidural venous plexus.

SPINAL CORD INJURY

Animal Models

Human spinal cord injuries are multifactorial and therefore it is difficult to design experimental models in which such injuries can be replicated precisely. Nevertheless, some useful data regarding the pathophysiology of SCI have been derived from animal models (5). For example, in the "weight-drop model," SCI has been experimentally induced by dropping a weight on the surface of the spinal cord (10). Recently, a more sophisticated electromechanical impactor has been developed based on the same principle (11). In the experimental "weight-drop model," some of the features of SCI resemble those observed in human SCI. For example, weight-drop injury in both experimental animals and humans causes hemorrhage and tissue necrosis, which later develops into a cyst (5). The main disadvantages of the "weight-drop model" are that the results obtained are variable (5) and the sites of injury do not simulate those observed in human SCI. For example, injury in the "weight-drop model" involves posterior cord compression, while in humans, anterior compression of the cord due to burst fractures or circumferential cord compression due to fracture dislocation is more common (5). In another model, balloon inflation in the spinal epidural space is used to induce SCI (12). In a novel approach, spinal cord vascular endothelium has been injured photochemically by injecting an organic photosensitive dye into the bloodstream (13). The spinal cord is then irradiated with a light beam of appropriate wavelength. The vascular endothelium is damaged, and the subsequent thrombosis results in ischemic lesions and vasogenic edema (13). Since the vertebral dorsal surface is adequately translucent, a laminectomy is not necessary in the model utilizing photosensitive dyes. Microsurgical procedures have also been used to produce lesions in specific spinal pathways (14).

Pathophysiology

In the spinal cord, white matter is located on the outside, while the gray matter is located on the inside. Since gray matter at any segment provides peripheral output only at that level, segmental gray matter damage compromises function restricted to that segment. On the other hand, damage to white matter at any segment causes interruption of long ascending and descending tracts and compromises function at all levels below the site if injury. Usually, injury to the spinal cord starts a series of events that result in damage to the spinal cord from the inside to outside. The gray matter is destroyed completely at the level of injury and a few segments rostral and caudal to it, while a peripheral donut-like rim of white matter remains at the level of injury (6). Mechanical trauma, including traction and compression, causes disruption of axons and neuronal membranes. Damage to the blood vessels causes hemorrhage. Spinal cord swells and occupies entire spinal canal causing compression and subsequent ischemia. Toxic chemicals are released from the disrupted neurons and axons that damage neighboring neurons (6). A summary of the pathophysiological changes that occur in a time-dependent manner secondary to SCI is presented below (5).

Ischemia

Hypoperfusion of the gray matter is a consistent feature of SCI (15). Diverse metabolites, such as serotonin, thromboxanes, platelet-activating factor, peptidoleukotrienes, and opioid peptides, have been reported to be released following SCI (5). These agents are believed to induce vasoconstriction of the vessels supplying the spinal cord and cause ischemia of the gray matter (16). The decrease in blood flow results in a decrease in oxygen tension at the site of injury (17). The contributions of ischemia to the neurological deficits following SCI remain unclear at present (18).

Edema

In experimental models of SCI, it has been observed that edema first occurs in the central part of the spinal cord and it spreads centrifugally to the white matter. The maximum formation of edema occurs during the initial stages of SCI (19).

Changes in Ionic Composition

The calcium ion concentration at the site of injury has been reported to increase within minutes after the SCI, peak at about 8 hours, and then remain elevated for at least 1 week after the injury (20–23). The increase in intra-axonal calcium has been attributed to the calcium ion entry through voltage-gated calcium channels, voltage-dependent NMDA (N-methyl-D-aspartate) receptor channels, release of calcium from intracellular storage sites such as smooth endoplasmic reticulum, and the failure of the extrusion of calcium ions via the Ca^{2+}-ATPase exchange pump. Increased calcium concentration results in the activation of phospholipase C and A2. Arachidonic acid is one of the products generated in these reactions (23). Metabolites of arachidonic acid, such as free radicals, thromboxanes, and peptidoleukotrienes, are known to cause tissue injury (24).

Calcium homeostasis is maintained in the neurons by activation of extrusion, sequestration, and buffering mechanisms. Calcium extrusion from neurons is accomplished by plasma membrane calcium ATPase (PMCAs) and the Na^+/Ca^{2+} exchanger. Sarco(endo)plasmic reticulum calcium ATPases (SERCAs) mediate sequestration of calcium into the endoplasmic reticulum. Mitochondria are also involved in maintaining calcium homeostasis in the neurons. Increase in intracellular calcium concentrations in response to malfunction of one or more of these mechanisms can induce injury mechanisms resulting in neuronal damage. PMCAs are P-type ATPases. PMCA2 and three isoforms are present in neurons. A decrease in PMCA2 transcript levels after spinal cord contusion injury (25). Based on these and other observations, it has been reported that in SCI abnormal function of PMCAs may result in impaired calcium extrusion that, in turn, may contribute to neuronal injury (26).

Another ion that is known to play a role in SCI is the potassium ion (K^+) (27). Immediately after SCI, there is an increase in extracellular K^+, which results in the depolarization of cells, leading to a conduction block. Eventually, there is a loss of K^+ in the injured spinal cord tissue due to damaged cell membranes (27).

Hydrolysis of Phospholipids and Generation of Free Radicals

Activation of phospholipases by increased calcium concentrations results in hydrolysis of phospholipids and generation of free fatty acids that, in turn, cause irreversible tissue damage (28). Activation of phospholipase A2 results in an increase in the levels of platelet-activating factor that is known to reduce blood flow and compromise the blood-CNS barrier. Phospholipid hydrolysis also results in the release of free radicals that are very reactive. Free radical reactions damage the phospholipid and cholesterol components of cell membranes (29). Since spinal cord injuries are accompanied by hemorrhage, the iron contained in hemoglobin catalyzes the oxygen radical and lipid peroxidase reactions that mediate further cell injury (5).

Role of Excitatory Amino Acids

Excitatory amino acids serve as transmitters in several different spinal pathways (30–34). The levels of excitatory amino acids such as glutamate and aspartate have been reported to be increased in response to SCI (35). Activation of glutamate receptors results in an increase in intracellular levels of Ca^{2+} that, as previously noted, has been implicated in cell death (36). This phenomenon is known as *excitotoxicity*. NMDA as well as AMPA (DL-α-amino-3-hydroxy-5-methylisoxazole-propionic acid) receptors have been implicated in this type of cell injury (37). Specific blockers for these receptors have been tested with variable success for their neuroprotective effects (38).

Inflammatory Processes

As noted earlier, the first cells to infiltrate the site of injury after spinal cord trauma are polymorphonuclear granulocytes (neutrophils) (5). The primary function of these neutrophils at the site of injury is to combat bacterial infection. However, other properties of these cells may contribute to further cellular injury. For example, neutrophils produce lysosomal enzymes and oxygen radicals that degrade the connective tissue matrix and cause tissue destruction. The reperfusion of blood into ischemic tissue has been observed to cause further tissue damage. This "reperfusion injury" is believed to be due to the mechanical obstruction caused by the reentry of neutrophils into the blood vessels in the ischemic tissue, the subsequent cytotoxic effects of neutrophils, and the infiltration of neutrophils into the parenchyma. The adhesion of leukocytes is mediated by a glycoprotein complex (integrin beta-2 subunit, CD18) on their membranes. Treatment of experimentally induced SCI with an antibody to this glycoprotein reduced tissue damage, most likely by preventing the aggregation of leukocytes in the blood vessels (39).

The appearance of neutrophils at the site of SCI is followed by appearance of phagocytic macrophages. Macrophages play a dual role at the site of injury, one involves tissue destruction and the other involves tissue repair. Their primary role is to remove cellular debris. Axonal injury results in Wallerian degeneration (i.e., degeneration of the distal nerve stump). Macrophages at the site of injury are believed to mediate the degradation of myelin by secreting neutral proteases. However, macrophages are also implicated in initiating the mitosis of Schwann cells and the proliferation of fibroblasts, which results in enhancement of the production of nerve growth factor (NGF) by nonneural tissue. Macrophages also alter the glial cell surfaces by producing a substance that permits elongation of neurites. These observations suggest that macrophages are also involved in tissue repair after spinal injury.

DIFFERENT PHASES OF TRAUMA

Acute Phase

Changes in the microvasculature of the central gray matter appear at the site of injury within minutes of the trauma and increase progressively within first few hours (5). These changes are characterized by the appearance of multifocal hemorrhages, distension of postcapillary venules with erythrocytes, and the appearance of red blood cells in perivascular spaces through damaged vascular endothelium. The endothelial cells of capillaries and postcapillary venules appear vacuolated and swollen. This damage is believed to be induced by free radicals, because pretreatment with antioxidants in experimental SCI prevented these endothelial cell abnormalities. Aneurysms and ruptured arteries appear in the lateral columns within 4 to 8 hours, and microthrombi appear in capillary size vessels within 24 hours. Some of the necrotic alterations are characterized by the presence of shrunken neurons with indistinct nuclei, loss of Nissl bodies, and swelling of rough endoplasmic reticulum. Necrotic changes occur in both glia and neurons. The neurons and the glia in the anterior horn are affected earlier than those in the posterior horn. These changes occur in the gray matter within first hours of injury. In the white matter, vacuoles appear in the myelin sheaths, and axons dilate or split giving it a spongy appearance under a light microscope (40,47).

Subacute Phase

The phase of hemorrhagic necrosis is followed by the subacute phase that is characterized by the presence of several different cell populations at the site of injury (5). Activated microglia at the site of injury exhibit an increased number of processes, an upregulation of cell surface molecules such as the histocompatibility complex class I and II antigens, the complement C3 receptor, and the macrophage activation marker ED1. This activation process, regulated by special signals such as cytokines, leads to the transformation of microglia into large phagocytic brain macrophages. At the site of injury, the astrocytes hypertrophy and proliferate, and contain an increased number of filaments consisting of glial fibrillary acidic protein. These astrocytes also exhibit increased activity of different oxidative and lysosomal enzymes. Another feature of this phase is the appearance of inflammatory cells at the site of the lesion. Within a few hours of SCI, polymorphonuclear granulocytes (neutrophils) infiltrate the lesion and the adjacent sites. Their main function is to destroy any bacteria causing infection at the injury site. These neutrophil cells have also been reported to exert cytotoxic effects on neurons; however, this view is not universally accepted. Neutrophils are attracted to the site of injury by the degradation products of hemoglobin, thrombin, and bradykinin. Other peripheral cells that appear at the site of injury include monocytes/macrophages, which are involved in phagocytosis of cell debris (41). Additional cell types found at the site of SCI include Schwann cells and fibroblasts. Schwann cells have the ability to modify their myelin sheaths and generate neurotrophic factors. Therefore, they may be involved in axonal regeneration, thus providing a basis for the physiological recovery of neurons after some types of experimental SCI (42). Fibroblasts produce basic fibroblast growth factor, a powerful angiogenic factor (43), which has been implicated in neovascularization in such injuries (44).

Late Phase

This phase, which extends over a period of weeks to months after spinal injury, follows the acute and subacute phases (5). Within a few days after the injury, phagocytic macrophages in the injured region disappear, and fluid-filled cysts (cavities surrounded by extensive scar tissue) appear. These cysts are connected to the central canal and are filled with CSF. In humans, elongated cavities are formed rostral to the injury after several months. This leads to syringomyelia (45). About a week after the spinal injury, a scar consisting of a dense network of processes is formed between the intact and the damaged tissue. This scar formation has been attributed to the accumulation of astrocytes at the margins of the lesion. Meningeal cells may also contribute to scar formation (46). The cavities formed at the site of injury are partly surrounded by white matter tissue consisting of demyelinated fibers that are incapable of conducting sensory or motor information. Demyelination is an important feature of SCI (47,48). This abnormality is responsible for impaired conduction in ascending and descending axons. Demyelination begins within 24 hours of the injury and increases progressively. Within 3 weeks, many fibers undergo Wallerian degeneration. However, there is evidence of some remyelination after experimental SCI during the late phase, although the internodes of these remyelinated axons are abnormally short and the myelination is thin. In smaller lesions, oligodendrocytes and Schwann cells may be involved in the process of remyelination, although evidence of this is scanty (49). This feature may explain the limited spontaneous recovery of function in some cases of SCI.

RECOVERY PROCESSES

Observations in Animal Studies

The pattern generators for rhythmic movements, such as walking and swimming, are located in the spinal cord (5,50). These central pattern generators (CPGs) are independent of sensory input and retain their independence even after complete deafferentation. In rats with experimentally induced injuries to the lower thoracic spinal cord, relatively few intact descending fibers (1% to 10%) are necessary to initiate functions such as postural control and locomotion. Similarly, in adult cats with spinal cord injuries at C5 level, capabilities for reaching and retrieving food were initially completely lost, but then these behaviors reappeared later. These studies suggest that mammals (e.g., cats, rats, and mice) can regain locomotion after complete or incomplete SCI via the neural circuitry called *CPGs* (50).

Observations in Human Studies

Success in the recovery of some spinal cord function in experimental animals has prompted new approaches to provide rehabilitation therapy to patients with SCI (51). It has been reported that in incomplete or complete paraplegic patients, the spinal pattern generator for locomotion can be initiated and trained (52). Impairment of motility depends on the extent of SCI. For example, it has been observed that lesions in ventral and ventrolateral funiculi do not impair motility in humans (53). On the other hand, lesions of the dorsolateral funiculi (which contain corticospinal and rubrospinal tracts) on one side combined with 90% transection on the contralateral side result in complete lower limb paralysis. However, functional recovery, such as walking, was even observed in these patients within 2 months (53). In other studies, when patients with partial spinal cord injuries with residual small sensory or motor innervation, and patients with neurologically complete spinal cord lesions (54,55) were trained on treadmills, substantial improvement in functional recovery was observed. Some of these recovered patients showed electromyograms with typical rhythmic alternating patterns in flexor and extensor muscles. In other patients, the need for weight support on the treadmill decreased gradually, and spinal walking with the aid of crutches was achieved. The following explanation has been provided for the functional improvement observed in these patients in response to the treadmill training. The functional integrity of neuronal circuits is dependent on their activity. The loss of activity is likely to result in the loss of uninjured neural connections in the spinal cord. Therefore, training on a treadmill may have prevented the loss of the uninjured spinal connections in these patients. In addition, spared descending fibers after the SCI may have, to some extent, sprouted and made functionally useful connections. Treadmill training may have also reinforced this process.

TREATMENT STRATEGIES

Spinal cord injuries create an environment that is hostile for healing and regeneration. Glial scar may be responsible for mechanical factors that prevent repair. Moreover, chemicals released from damaged myelin and glia may promote growth cone collapse and prevent axonal growth (56,57). Major inhibitors of axonal growth released from damaged myelin include neurite outgrowth inhibitor A (Nogo A) (58), myelin-associated glycoprotein (MAG) (59), and oligodendrocyte-myelin glycoprotein (OMgp) (60). Inhibitors of axonal growth released from the astrocytic scar are chondroitin sulfate proteoglycans (61). Nogo-66 receptor (NgR), also known as *Reticulon 4 receptor* (RTN4R), is a protein that is coded by the RTN4R gene. This gene also encodes the receptor for OMgp and MAG. NgR, a common receptor for the three known myelin-associated inhibitors (i.e., Nogo A, MAG, and OMgp), mediates axonal growth inhibition and may play a role in regulating axonal regeneration and plasticity in the adult central nervous system.

Irrespective of the nature of the injury, whether it is a closed contusion, open contusion, or partial transection, cell death occurs within hours, while the secondary pathological changes take place within days and weeks of injury. Therefore, early intervention is of crucial importance for a better clinical outcome. In acute SCI, the first aim should be to arrest the cascade of secondary injury processes, in order to limit the tissue damage and interrupt or reverse sensory-motor dysfunction. The second aim is focused on the rehabilitation and stabilization of the consequences of injury, and to activate residual neuronal circuits by training. This will improve the condition of living for the patient. The third aim is still in an experimental stage, and involves the enhancement of axonal regeneration by different interventions.

Current status of the treatments of spinal cord injuries has been reviewed recently (62,63). The salient features of selected strategies for treating spinal cord injuries are summarized in the following paragraphs.

Steroids

Steroids have also been used extensively in the treatment of SCI in animals and humans (64). In the National Acute Spinal Cord Injury Study (NASCIS I) (65), two groups were randomized with both groups receiving 1,000 mg bolus within 48 hours after injury. The "high-dose" and the "low-dose" groups received a maintenance dose of 1,000 mg and 100 mg of methylprednisolone, respectively, administered for 10 days. No statistical difference was found between the two regimens at 6 months or at 1 year; however, there was a trend for the patients with the higher doses of methylprednisolone to have better scores than the lower dose group (65).

Criticisms of NASCIS I included that the dose of methylprednisolone (even the high dose) used was below the theoretical therapeutic threshold believed to be about 30 mg/kg of body weight from animal models; there was no placebo arm; all types of injury were grouped together; and the doses of methylprednisolone were not based on body weight. It was also felt that treatment with methylprednisolone was started too late (started within 48 hours) after injury.

NASCIS II, initiated in 1985, was a multicenter, double-blinded, placebo-controlled study in which 487 patients were randomized (66). Inclusion criteria were an SCI diagnosis within 12 hours of injury. Exclusion criteria included nerve root or cauda equina injury only, gunshot wounds, life-threatening morbidity, pregnancy, addiction to narcotics, on maintenance steroid for any reason, age under 13 years, those who had received more than 100 mg of methylprednisolone or its equivalent or 1 mg of naloxone before admission to the study center, and those who would be difficult to follow up.

Sensation and motor status was measured at admission, 6 weeks, and 6 months. Sensation was studied using 29 dermatomal segments from C2 to S5, and tabulating the sum of 14 myotomes using the standard six-point (0 to 5) Medical Research Council scale assessed motor score. Subjects received one of the following three regimens: methylprednisolone and placebo naloxone, active naloxone, and placebo methylprednisolone, or placebo methylprednisolone and placebo naloxone.

Results of the study revealed that patients, both neurologically complete and incomplete, who received methylprednisolone within 8 hours after injury at a dosage of 30 mg/kg and maintained at 5.4 mg/kg/h for a total of 24 hours, had significantly improved neurologic (motor and sensory) recovery at 6 weeks, 6 months, and 1 year after injury. Patients treated with methylprednisolone initiated more than 8 hours after injury had no beneficial effect, and in fact did marginally worse than the placebo group. Naloxone did not have a significant effect on recovery at the dose used. The wound infection rate was 7.1% in those receiving methylprednisolone as compared to 3.3% in the placebo group, and gastrointestinal bleeding rate was 4.5% in methylprednisolone group as compared to 2.0% in the placebo group. Both of these potentially life-threatening complications although higher in the methylprednisolone group did not reach statistical significance. One of the keys to NASCIS II was the evidence that medication can improve neural recovery, thus indicating that secondary injury (injury occurring after the initial trauma to the cord) occurs.

The third study (NASCIS III), initiated in 1991, was a double-blind, randomized study with three treatment regimens (67). This includes methylprednisolone 24 hours (30 mg/kg bolus within 8 hours followed by methylprednisolone 5.4 mg/kg/h for 24 hours); methylprednisolone 48 hours (30 mg/kg bolus followed by methylprednisolone 5.4 mg/kg/h for 48 hours); and Tirilazad mesylate (TM) (30 mg/kg bolus methylprednisolone followed by TM 2.5 mg/kg every 6 hours for 48 hours). Tirilazad mesylate (Upjohn U-74006F) is a 21-aminosteroid and potent antioxidant with no glucocorticoid receptor activity that has been shown to be neuroprotective in animal SCI models. ASIA motor scores and Functional Independence measure (FIM) scores were measured at 6 weeks and 6 months. There was no true placebo group included.

Results from 499 patients recruited from 16 centers found that there was a significant improvement in motor scores in those who received 48 hours of methylprednisolone when started in the 3 to 8 hour window at 6-week and 6-month follow-up. There were no differences in sensory scores at any time between the groups. In NASCIS III, there was a twofold higher incidence of pneumonia and a fourfold higher incidence of sepsis, and sixfold high incidence of death due to respiratory complications in the 48-hour group as compared to the 24-hour group, although these differences did not reach statistical significance. Although corticosteroids are known to possess anti-inflammatory properties, their beneficial effects have been ascribed to their free radical scavenger properties (68,69) and their ability to inhibit lipid peroxidation (64).

While the above-mentioned reports provide some support for the use of steroids in acute SCI (62), it should be noted that their effectiveness and use in the treatment of SCI have been questioned in recent years (70–73). Based on critical evaluation of published studies on the use of steroids in the treatment of SCI, Hurlbert (74) concluded that methylprednisolone cannot be recommended for treating nonpenetrating (blunt) SCI. Moreover, administration of high doses of steroids for 48 hours may be harmful to the patient. Thus, the treatment of SCI with steroids should be considered investigational at the present time (74).

Lazaroids

Lazaroids (21-aminosteroids) are known to inhibit lipid peroxidation and are devoid of glucocorticoid activity (64,75). It was concluded from NASCIS III that Tirilazad was as effective as methylprednisolone in treating acute SCI when administered for 24-hour duration (76). In addition, the incidence of sepsis, pneumonia, and cardiovascular side effects was lower when Tirilazad was used. Because Tirilazad did not show efficacy superior to that of methylprednisolone in NASCIS III, it has not been adopted for neuroprotection in clinical SCI (63).

Future Strategies

A brief discussion of new and experimental drugs and procedures for the treatment of SCI, including their beneficial effects and shortcomings, is presented in the following paragraphs.

Gangliosides

Gangliosides, glycolipids present in cell membranes, are also undergoing clinical trials for treatment of acute SCI (77). Administration of a ganglioside (GM-1; 100 mg, i.v., within 72 hours of injury) in patients with acute SCI has resulted in a significant improvement in neurological function. Gangliosides have been reported to promote neurite outgrowth, regeneration, and neuronal sprouting (78–80). It is not clear yet if these properties of gangliosides are responsible for their beneficial effect in treating SCI. The results of a multicenter clinical trial of monosialo-tetrahexosylganglioside GM1 (Sygen) suggest that although this agent exerts beneficial effects in some patients with SCI, the improvement may not be statistically significant in patients with severe SCI (81,82).

Opiate Receptor Antagonists

In experimental animals, opiate receptor antagonists have also been shown to exert neuroprotective effects after SCI (64). Initial clinical trials indicated that naloxone, a nonselective opiate receptor antagonist, did not elicit a significant neuroprotective effect in patients with acute SCI (66). However, a 1-year follow-up study indicated that naloxone did elicit a significant neuroprotective effect in acute SCI in humans (69,83). The neuroprotective effects of selective opiate receptor antagonists remain to be investigated in experimental SCI models.

Fampridine

Many patients with SCI have some surviving axons within the spinal cord. However, these axons lose myelin partially and cannot conduct sensory and motor impulses properly. In demyelinated axons, exposure of large number of potassium channels results in leakage of potassium ions, causing the axon to "short circuit". Fampridine (4-aminopyridine; potassium channel blocker) has been reported to restore conduction in demyelinated nerve fibers by blocking specialized potassium channels on axons. This drug does not replace damaged myelin. Multiple studies with fampridine in multiple sclerosis and some preliminary work in SCI have shown a trend toward increased motor function in incomplete injuries and decrease in pain and spasticity (84–86). The results of a phase III clinical trial showed that administration of sustained-release oral fampridine (10 mg, twice daily, for 14 weeks) improved walking ability in some patients with multiple sclerosis (87). In January 2010, the Food and Drug Administration advisory committee had approved the marketing of fampridine (Ampyra; Acorda Therapeutics Inc.) for treatment of some patients with multiple sclerosis in order to improve their walking ability. It should be noted that there are concerns regarding some side effects (e.g., seizures) and narrow therapeutic range of Ampyra.

Enzymatic Treatments

Sialidase, an enzyme of the hydrolase class, removes important sialic acids from gangliosides, GD1a, and GD1b and renders myelin-associated glycoprotein unable to prevent axonal sprouting and regeneration. GD1a and GD1b act as axonal receptors for this myelin-associated glycoprotein. Sialidase has been reported (88) to promote growth of central nervous system neurons into peripheral nerve grafts. Therefore, this enzyme shows promise in treatment of SCI.

Chondroitinase ABC digests chondroitin sulfate proteoglycans that are released from astrocytes in injured spinal cord. These proteoglycans inhibit axonal sprouting and regeneration. Therefore, chondroitinase ABC has been used to treat SCI in order to promote sprouting and recovery of somatic and autonomic function (89–91).

Combination of Bridge and Enzymatic Treatment

Axonal growth has been reported to occur through a segment of degenerated peripheral nerve when the latter bypassed or bridged the injured region of the spinal cord (92) and recovery of motor function was observed. Recently, SCI has been treated with combination of this bridge technique with enzymatic treatment with chondroitinase ABC, and considerably improved results have been reported (93).

Glutamate Receptor Antagonists

As stated earlier, the accumulation of excess glutamate at the site of injury has been demonstrated in patients with spinal cord trauma. Administration of competitive and noncompetitive NMDA receptor antagonists has been reported to influence the pathological process in SCI (94–96). However, these antagonists have many adverse side effects, and, therefore at present, none of the competitive or noncompetitive NMDA receptor antagonists are considered to be potential therapeutic agents for treating SCI in humans. However, NBQX (an AMPA-glutamate receptor antagonist) has been shown to minimize the lesions and functional disabilities in experimental animals (97). However, limited water solubility of this drug makes its clinical use unlikely. Clinical investigations on possible use of other AMPA-receptor antagonists for treatment of stroke are underway (98). It is possible that one such drug may become available in future for treatment of SCI.

Anti-Nogo Antibodies

As mentioned earlier, Nogo A is one of the major inhibitors of axonal growth released from damaged myelin (58). Intrathecal administration of antibodies against Nogo A to rats (99) and monkeys (100,101) with damaged spinal cords has been reported to trigger axonal regeneration and functional recovery. These results have prompted phase I clinical trials using anti-Nogo antibodies in humans.

Anti-MAG Antibodies

MAG is another inhibitor of axonal growth released from damaged myelin (59). A phase I clinical trial using anti-MAG antibodies for the treatment of SCI has been started in 2007 and the results are awaited (62).

Cethrin

Cethrin is a Rho pathway antagonist. Rho is a small GTPase-associated signaling protein present in neurons. The activation of Rho elicits collapse of growth cone, retraction of neurites, and rounding of cell body (102). Rho/Rho kinase activity is increased after SCI, and this is one of the mechanisms by which regrowth of axons is prevented. The exoenzyme C3 transferase from *Clostridium botulinum* (C3) is commonly used to selectively inactivate the GTPases RhoA, RhoB, and RhoC. Cethrin is an investigational recombinant fusion protein that consists of C3 and a transport sequence that increases its ability to cross cell membranes. A phase I/IIa clinical trial of Cethrin for the treatment of SCI is ongoing (63).

Minocycline

Minocyline is a derivative of tetracycline that crosses blood-brain barrier. In the CNS, it exerts anti-inflammatory effects. This second-generation tetracycline has been reported to inhibit excitotoxicity, oxidative stress, release of proinflammatory mediators from microglia and caspase-dependent and caspase-independent pathways of neuronal death. The neuroprotective effects of minocycline have been ascribed to its ability to increase the levels of anti-inflammatory cytokine IL-10 and decrease the levels of proinflammatory TNF-α. In animal models of SCI, minocycline has been reported to exhibit neuroprotective effects. Based on these reports, minocycline may be a good candidate for starting clinical trials regarding its use in the treatment of SCI (63).

Stem Cell Transplantation

Since axonal myelination is typically lost at the site of SCI, one of the strategies for repairing this injury is to promote remyelination by using stem cells (103–105). Stem cells are able to renew themselves by mitotic cell division and differentiate into different cell types. Two main types of stem cells are embryonic stem cells and adult stem cells. Embryonic stem cells are isolated from the inner cell mass of blastocysts, while adult stem cells are present in adult tissues. Recently, mouse embryonic stem cells were used to produce oligodendrocytes that were then transplanted into the dorsal column of rat spinal cord 3 days after chemical demyelination. The latter was produced by injecting ethidium bromide into white matter that had previously been exposed to 40 Gy of x-irradiation. The transplanted embryonic stem cells survived and differentiated into mature oligodendrocytes that were capable of myelinating axons (106). In other studies on rats, fetal spinal cord cells were transplanted into the spinal cords with contusion injuries. These rats showed improvement in their gait (107). Phase I human clinical trials are undergoing to assess feasibility of using human fetal spinal cord cells to treat syringomyelia and porcine spinal cord oligodendrocyte progenitors to treat chronic traumatic SCI (103). However, it remains to be demonstrated that remyelination following transplantation is responsible for functional recovery (108).

ACKNOWLEDGMENTS

This work was supported by grants from NHLBI (HL024347–26 and HL076248–06) awarded to Dr. H. N. Sapru.

References

1. Siegel A, Sapru HN. *Essential neuroscience*, 2nd ed. Baltimore: Lippincott Williams & Wilkins, 2011: 381–406.
2. Benarroch EE, Westmoreland BF, Daube JR, et al. *Medical neurosciences*, 4th ed. New York: Lippincott Williams & Wilkins, 1999:151–223.
3. Carpenter MB, Sutin J. *Human neuroanatomy*, 8th ed. Baltimore: Lippincott Williams & Wilkins, 1983: 232–262.
4. Afifi AK, Bergman RA. *Functional neuroanatomy*. New York: McGraw-Hill, 1998:102–103.
5. Schwab ME, Bartholdi D. Degeneration and regeneration of axons in the lesioned spinal cord. *Physiol Rev* 1996;76:319–370.
6. McDonald JW, Sadowsky C. Spinal cord injury. *Lancet* 2002;359:417–425.
7. Rexed B. The cytoarchitectonic organization of the spinal cord in the cat. *J Comp Neurol* 1952;96:415–494.
8. Rexed B. A cytoarchitectonic atlas of the spinal cord in the cat. *J Comp Neurol* 1954;100:297–379.
9. Burt AM. *Textbook of neuroanatomy*. Philadelphia: WB Saunders, 1993;318.
10. Noble LJ, Wrathall R. Correlative analyses of lesion development and functional status after graded spinal cord contusive injuries. *Exp Neurol* 1989;103:34–40.
11. Bresnahan JC, Beattie MS, Todd FD, et al. A behavioral and anatomical analysis of spinal cord injury produced by a feedback-controlled impaction device. *Exp Neurol* 1987;95:548–570.
12. Tarlov IM, Klinger H. Spinal cord compression studies. *Am Med Assoc Arch Neurol Psychiatry* 1954;71: 272–290.
13. Bunge MB, Holets VR, Bates ML, et al. Characterization of photochemically induced spinal cord injury in the rat by light and electron microscopy. *Exp Neurol* 1994;127:76–93.
14. Theriault E, Tator CH. Persistence of rubrospinal projections following spinal cord injury in the rat. *J Comp Neurol* 1994;342:249–258.
15. Holtz A, Nyström B, Gerdin B. Spinal cord blood flow measured by ^{14}C-iodoantipyrine autoradiography during

and after graded spinal cord compression in rats. *Surg Neurol* 1989;31:350–360.
16. Olsson Y, Sharma HS, Pettersson A, et al. Release of endogenous neurochemicals may increase vascular permeability, induce edema and influence cell changes in trauma to the spinal cord. *Prog Brain Res* 1992;91:197–203.
17. Stokes BT, Garwood M, Walters P. Oxygen fields in specific spinal loci of the canine spinal cord. *Am J Physiol* 1981;240:H761–H766.
18. Tator CH. Hemodynamic issues and vascular factors in acute experimental spinal cord injury. *J. Neurotrauma* 1992;9:139–141.
19. Nobel LJ, Wrathall JR. Distribution and time course of protein extravasation in the rat spinal cord after contusive injury. *Brain Res* 1989;482:57–66.
20. Young W, Flamm ES. Effect of high-dose corticosteroid therapy on blood flow, evoked potentials, and extracellular calcium in experimental spinal cord injury. *J Neurosurg* 1982;57:667–673.
21. Moriya T, Hassan AZ, Young W, et al. Dynamics of extracellular calcium activity following contusion of the rat spinal cord. *J Neurotrauma* 1994;11:255–263.
22. Siesjo BK. Historical overview: calcium, ischemia, and death of brain cells. *Ann N Y Acad Sci* 1988;522:638–661.
23. Rasmussen H. The calcium messenger system (first of two parts). *N Engl J Med* 1986;314:1094–1101.
24. Xu J, Hsu CY, Junker H, et al. Kininogen and kinin in experimental spinal cord injury. *J Neurochem* 1991;57:975–980.
25. Carmel JB, Galante A, Soteropoulos P, et al. Gene expression profiling of acute spinal cord injury reveals spreading inflammatory signals and neuron loss. *Physiol Genomics* 2001;7:201–213.
26. Kurnellas MP, Nicot A, Shull GE, et al. Plasma membrane calcium ATPase deficiency causes neuronal pathology in the spinal cord: a potential mechanism for neurodegeneration in multiple sclerosis and spinal cord injury. *FASEB J* 2005;19:298–300.
27. Young W, Koreh I. Potassium and calcium changes in injured spinal cords. *Brain Res* 1986;365:42–53.
28. Faden AI, Chan PH, Longar S. Alterations in lipid metabolism, (Na^+, K^+)-ATPase activity, and tissue water content of spinal cord following experimental traumatic injury. *J Neurochem* 1987;48:1809–1816.
29. Braughler JM, Hall ED. Central nervous system trauma and stroke. 1. Biochemical considerations for oxygen radical formation and lipid peroxidation. *Free Rad Biol Med* 1989;6:289–301.
30. Chitravanshi VC, Sapru HN. NMDA as well as non-NMDA receptors mediate the neurotransmission of inspiratory drive to phrenic motoneurons in the adult rat. *Brain Res* 1996;715:104–112.
31. Chitravanshi VC, Sapru HN. NMDA as well as non-NMDA receptors in the phrenic motonucleus mediate respiratory effects of carotid chemoreflex. *Am J Physiol* 1997;272:R322–R333.
32. Sundaram K, Murugaian J, Sapru HN. Cardiac responses to the microinjections of excitatory amino acids into the intermediolateral cell column of the rat spinal cord. *Brain Res* 1989;482:12–22.
33. Sundaram K, Sapru HN. NMDA receptors in the intermediolateral column of the spinal cord mediate sympathoexcitatory responses elicited from the ventrolateral medullary pressor area. *Brain Res* 1991;544: 33–41.
34. Murugaian J, Sundaram K, Krieger AJ, et al. Relative effects of different spinal autonomic nuclei on cardiac sympathoexcitatory function. *Brain Res Bull* 1990;24:537–542.
35. Liu D, Thangnipon W, McAdoo DJ. Excitatory amino acids rise to toxic levels upon impact injury to the rat spinal cord. *Brain Res* 1991;547:344–348.
36. Choi DW. Excitotoxic cell death. *Neurobiology* 1992;23:1261–1276.
37. Wrathall JR, Choiniere D, Teng YD. Dose-dependent reduction of tissue loss and functional impairment after spinal cord trauma with AMPA/kainate antagonist NBQX. *J Neurosci* 1994;14;6598–6607.
38. Sun FY, Faden AI. High- and low-affinity NMDA receptor-binding sites in rat spinal cord: effects of traumatic injury. *Brain Res* 1994;666:88–92.
39. Clark WM, Madden KP, Rothlein R, et al. Reduction of central nervous system ischemic injury in rabbits using leukocyte adhesion antibody treatment. *Stroke* 1991;22:877–883.
40. Dusart I, Schwab ME. Secondary cell death and the inflammatory reaction after dorsal hemisection of the rat spinal cord. *Eur J Neurosci* 1994;6:712–724.
41. Perry VH, Anderson PB, Gordon S. Macrophages and inflammation in the central nervous system. *Trends Neurosci* 1993;16:268–273.
42. Li Y, Raisman G. Schwann cells induce sprouting in motor and sensory axons in the adult rat spinal cord. *J Neurosci* 1994;14:4050–4063.
43. Folkman J, Klagsbrun M. Angiogenic factors. *Science* 1987;235:442–447.
44. Blight AR. Morphometric analysis of blood vessels in chronic experimental spinal cord injury: hypervascularity and recovery of function. *J Neurol Sci* 1991;106:158–174.
45. Madsen PW, Yezierski RP, Holets YR. Syringomyelia: clinical observations and experimental studies. *J Neurotrauma* 1994;11:241–254.
46. Sievers J, Pehlemann FW, Gude S, et al. Meningeal cells organize the superficial glia limitans of the cerebellum and produce components of both the interstitial matrix and the basement membrane. *J Neurocytol* 1994;23: 135–149.
47. Blight AR, Young W. Central axons in injured cat spinal cord recover electrophysiological function following remyelination by Schwann cells. *J Neurol Sci* 1989;91:15–34.
48. Waxman SG. Demyelination in spinal cord injury. *J Neurol Sci* 1989;91:1–14.
49. Tator CH. The relationship among the severity of spinal cord injury, residual neurological function, axon counts, and counts of retrogradely labeled neurons after experimental spinal cord injury. *Exp Neurol* 1995;132:220–228.
50. Rossignol S, Dubuc R. Spinal pattern regeneration. *Curr Opin Neurobiol* 1994;4:894–902.
51. Barbeau H, Rossignol S. Enhancement of locomotor recovery following spinal cord injury. Curr Opin Neurol 1994;7:517–524.

52. Wernig A, Muller S, Nanassy A, et al. Laufband therapy based on "rules of spinal locomotion" is effective in spinal cord injured persons. *Eur J Neurosci* 1995;7:823–829.
53. Nathan PW. Effects on movement of surgical incisions into the human spinal cord. *Brain* 1994;117:337–346.
54. Dietz V, Colombo G, Jensen L, et al. Locomotor capacity of spinal cord in paraplegic patients. *Ann Neurol* 1995;37:574–582.
55. Dietz V, Colombo G, Jensen L, et al. Locomotor capacity of spinal man. *Lancet* 1994;344:1260–1263.
56. Brittis PA, Flanagan JG. Nogo domains and a Nogo receptor: implications for axon regeneration. *Neuron* 2001;30:11–14.
57. Sandvig A, Berry M, Barrett LB, et al. Myelin-, reactive glia-, and scar-derived CNS axon growth inhibitors: expression, receptor signaling, and correlation with axon regeneration. *Glia* 2004;46:225–251.
58. Caroni P, Schwab ME. Two membrane protein fractions from rat central myelin with inhibitory properties for neurite growth and fibroblast spreading. *J Cell Biol* 1988;106:1281–1288.
59. McKerracher L, David S, Jackson DL, et al. Identification of myelin-associated glycoprotein as a major myelin-derived inhibitor of neurite growth. *Neuron* 1994;13:805–811.
60. Wang KC, Koprivica V, Kim JA, et al. Oligodendrocyte-myelin glycoprotein is a Nogo receptor ligand that inhibits neurite outgrowth. *Nature* 2002;417:941–944.
61. Snow DM, Lemmon V, Carrino DA, et al. Sulfated proteoglycans in astroglial barriers inhibit neurite outgrowth in vitro. *Exp Neurol* 1990;109:111–130.
62. Onose G, Anghelescu A, Muresanu DF, et al. A review of published reports on neuroprotection in spinal cord injury. *Spinal Cord* 2009;47:716–726.
63. Baptiste DC, Fehlings MC. Pharmacological approaches to repair the injured spinal cord. *J Neurotrauma* 2006;23:318–334.
64. Seidl EC. Promising pharmacological agents in the management of acute spinal cord injury. *Crit Care Nurs Q* 1999;22:44–50.
65. Bracken MB, Collins WF, Freeman DF, et al. Efficacy of methylprednisolone in acute spinal cord injury. *JAMA* 1984;251:45–52.
66. Bracken MB, Shepard MJ, Collins WF, et al. A randomized, controlled trial of methylprednisolone or naloxone in the treatment of acute spinal cord injury. *N Engl J Med* 1990;322:1405–1411.
67. Bracken MB, Shepard MJ, Holoford TR, et al. Administration of methylprednisolone for 24 or 48 hours or tirilazad mesylate for 48 hours in the treatment of acute spinal cord injury. Results of the Third National Acute Spinal Cord Injury Randomized Controlled Trial. *JAMA* 1997;277:1597–1604.
68. Faden AI, Salzman S. Pharmacological strategies in CNS trauma. *Trends Pharmacol Sci* 1992;13:29–35.
69. Bracken MB, Shepard MJ, Collins WF, et al. Methylprednisolone or naloxone treatment after acute spinal cord injury: l-year-follow-up data. *J Neurosurg* 1992;76:23–31.
70. Nesathurai S. Steroids and spinal cord injury: revisiting the NASCIS 2 and 3 trials. *J Trauma* 1998;45:1088–1093.
71. Short DJ. High dose methylprednisolone in the management of acute spinal cord injury: a systematic review from a clinical perspective. *Spinal Cord* 2000;38:278–286.
72. Hurlbert RJ. Methylprednisolone for acute spinal cord injury: an inappropriate standard of care. *J Neurosurg* 2000;93(Suppl l):1–7.
73. Heary RF, Vaccaro AR, Mesa JJ, et al. Steroids and gunshot wounds to the spine. *Neurosurgery* 1997;41:576–583.
74. Hurlbert RJ. The role of steroids in acute spinal cord injury. *Spine* 2001;6(Suppl 24):S39–S46.
75. Clark WM, Hazel S, Coull BM. Lazaroids: CNS pharmacology and current research. *Drugs* 1995;50:971–983.
76. Bracken MB, Shepard MJ, Holford TR, et al. Methylprednisolone or tirilazad mesylate administration after acute spinal cord injury: 1 year follow up. *J Neurosurg* 1998;89:699–706.
77. Geisler FH, Dorsey Fe, Coleman WP. Recovery of motor function after spinal cord injury: a randomized, placebo-controlled trial with GM-l ganglioside. *N Engl J Med* 1991;324:1829–1838.
78. Gorio AG, Fusco M, Janigro D, et al. Gangliosides and their effects on rearranging peripheral and central neural pathways. *Cent Nerv Syst Trauma* 1984;1:29–37.
79. Sabel BA, Slavin MD, Stein DG. GM-l ganglioside treatment facilitates behavioral recovery from brain damage. *Science* 1984;225:340–342.
80. Geisler FH, Dorsey FC, Coleman WP. Past and current clinical studies with GM-l ganglioside in acute spinal cord injury. *Ann Emerg Med* 1993;22:1041–1047.
81. Geisler FH, Coleman WP, Grieco G, et al., Sygen Study Group. The Sygen multicenter acute spinal cord injury. *Spine* 2001;26:587–598.
82. Hall ED, Springer JE. Neuroprotection and acute spinal cord injury: a reappraisal. *NeuroRx* 2004;1:80–100.
83. Bracken MB, Holford TR. Effects of timing of methylprednisolone or naloxone on administration on recovery of segmental and long-tract neurological function in NASCIS 2. *J Neurosurg* 1993;79:500–507.
84. Segal JL, Brunnemann SR. 4-Aminopyridine alters gait characteristics and enhances locomotion in spinal cord injured humans. *J Spinal Cord Med* 1998;21:200–204.
85. Davis FA, Stefoski D, Rush J. Orally administered 4-AP improves clinical signs in multiple sclerosis. *Ann Neurol* 1990;27:186–192.
86. Segal JL, Brunnemann SR. 4-Aminopyridine improves pulmonary function in quadriplegic humans with longstanding spinal cord injury. *Pharmacotherapy* 1997;17:415–423.
87. Goodman AD, Brown TR, Krupp LB, et al. Sustained-release oral fampridine in multiple sclerosis: a randomised, double-blind, controlled trial. *Lancet* 2009;373:732–738.
88. Yang LJ, Lorenzini I, Vajn K, et al. Sialidase enhances spinal axon outgrowth in vivo. *Proc Natl Acad Sci USA* 2006;103:11057–11062.
89. Barritt AW, Davies M, Marchand F, et al. Chondroitinase ABC promotes sprouting of intact and injured spinal systems after spinal cord injury. *J Neurosci* 2006;26:10856–10867.
90. Bradbury EJ, Moon LD, Popat RJ, King VR, et al. Chondroitinase ABC promotes functional recovery after spinal cord injury. *Nature* 2002;416:636–640.

91. Caggiano AO, Zimber MP, Ganguly A, et al. Chondroitinase ABC1 improves locomotion and bladder function following contusion injury of the rat spinal cord. *J Neurotrauma* 2005;22:226–239.
92. David S, Aguayo AJ. Axonal elongation into peripheral nervous system "bridges" after central nervous system injury in adult rats. *Science* 1981;214:91–933.
93. Houle JD, Tom VJ, Mayes D, et al. Combining an autologous peripheral nervous system "bridge" and matrix modification by chondroitinase allows robust, functional regeneration beyond a hemisection lesion of the adult rat spinal cord. *J Neurosci* 2006;26:7405–7415.
94. Faden AI, Demediuk P, Panter SS, et al. The role of excitatory amino acids and NMDA receptors in traumatic brain injury. *Science* 1989;244:798–800.
95. Hao JX, Watson BD, Xu XJ, et al. Protective effect of NMDA antagonist MK-801 on photochemically induced spinal lesions in the rat. *Exp Neurol* 1992;118:143–152.
96. Kochhar A, Zivin JA, Mazzarella V. Pharmacologic studies of the neuroprotective actions of a glutamate antagonist in ischemia. *J Neurotrauma* 1991;8:175–186.
97. Wrathall JR, Teng YD, Choiniere D. Amelioration of functional deficits from spinal cord trauma with systemically administered NBQX, an antagonist of non-N-methyl-D-aspartate receptors. *Exp Neurol* 1996;137: 119–126.
98. Umemura K, KondoK, Ikeda Y, et al. Pharmacokinetics and safety of the novel amino-3-hydroxy-5-methylisoxazole-4-propionate receptor antagonist YM90K in healthy men. *J Clin Pharmacol* 1997;37:719–927.
99. Weinmann O, Schnell L, Ghosh A, et al. Intrathecally infused antibodies against Nogo-A penetrate the CNS and down-regulate the endogenous neurite growth inhibitor Nogo-A. *Mol Cell Neurosci* 2006;32:161–173.
100. Fouad K, Klusman I, Schwab ME. Regenerating corticospinal fibers in the Marmoset (Callitrix jacchus) after spinal cord lesion and treatment with the anti-Nogo-A antibody IN-1. *Eur J Neurosci* 2004;20: 2479–2482.
101. Freund P, Wannier T, Schmidlin E, et al. Anti-Nogo-A antibody treatment enhances sprouting of corticospinal axons rostral to a unilateral cervical spinal cord lesion in adult macaque. *J Comp Neurol* 2007;502: 644–659.
102. Jalink K, Van Corven EJ, Hengeveld T, et al. Inhibition of lysophosphatidate and thrombin-induced neurite retraction and neuronal cell rounding by ADP ribosylation of the small GTP-binding protein Rho. *J Cell Biol* 1994;126:801–810.
103. Myckatyn TM, Mackinnon SE, McDonald JW. Stem cell transplantation and other novel techniques for promoting recovery from spinal cord injury. *Transpl Immunol* 2004;12:343–358.
104. McDonald JW, Liu XZ, Qu Y, et al. Transplanted embryonic stem cells survive, differentiate and promote recovery in injured rat spinal cord. *Nat Med* 1999;5:1410–1412.
105. Kim BG, Hwang DH, Lee SI, et al. Stem cell-based cell therapy for spinal cord injury. *Cell Transplant* 2007;16:355–364.
106. Liu S, Qu Y, Stewart TJ, et al. Embryonic stem cells differentiate into oligodendrocytes and myelinate in culture and after spinal cord transplantation. *Proc Natl Acad Sci USA* 2000;97:6126–6131.
107. Stokes BT, Reier PJ. Fetal grafts alter chronic behavioral outcome after contusion damage to the adult rat spinal cord. *Exp Neurol* 1992;116:1–12.
108. Privat A, Ribotta MG, Orsal D. What is a functional recovery after spinal cord injury? *Nat Med* 2000;6:358.

CHAPTER 3 ■ SPINAL ANATOMY AND BIOMECHANICS

REBECCA E. FISHER, HEATHER F. SMITH, AND BARRY GOLDSTEIN

THE VERTEBRAL COLUMN

The vertebral column is designed to meet considerable mechanical challenges and stresses. It must combine great strength and flexibility while protecting the spinal cord and nerve roots. Rugged bones, ligaments, and muscles provide stability and strength. The column is flexible as it has many joints in close apposition, including articulations between the bodies and the intervertebral (IV) discs, and between the facets of adjacent vertebral arches. The IV discs account for approximately 25% of the total length of the vertebral column superior to the sacrum. Daily changes in the volume of the discs may result in loss of almost 1 inch in height by the end of a day. Dessication of the discs also accounts for some loss in height in old age. Aging and degenerative changes also affect the dense connective tissues of the vertebral column, resulting in increased ligamentous stiffness and osteoporosis of the vertebrae. Thickening of ligaments and joint capsules as well as degenerative bony changes may result in encroachment upon the central canal or neuroforamina. Loss of vertebral height further compounds the loss of height in the older years.

Curvatures of the Vertebral Column

In adults, the vertebral column is characterized by four alternating curvatures in the sagittal plane (Fig. 3.1). The thoracic and sacral curvatures or kyphoses are concave anteriorly and are classified as the primary curvatures of the vertebral column, having been established during fetal development. The secondary curvatures or lordoses of the vertebral column are concave posteriorly and develop during infancy. They include the cervical curvature, which develops in response to an infant learning to hold its head upright, and the lumbar curvature, which develops in response to an infant learning to sit upright and walk.

Anatomy of the Vertebrae

The vertebral column is composed of 33 vertebrae separated by IV discs. The column typically includes seven cervical, 12 thoracic, 5 lumbar, 5 sacral, and 4 coccygeal vertebrae (Fig. 3.1). By age 30, the sacral and coccygeal vertebrae fuse to form the sacrum and coccyx, respectively (1,2). The remaining 24 unfused vertebrae share a number of features.

A typical vertebra consists of a ventral body and a dorsal vertebral arch (Fig. 3.2); together they enclose the spinal cord,

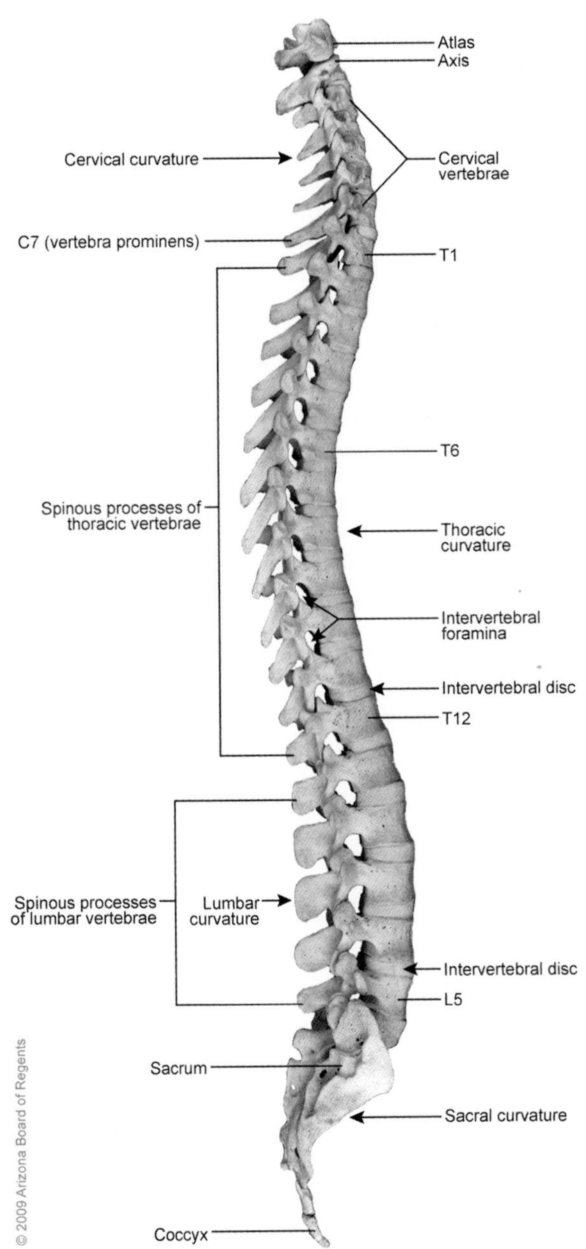

FIGURE 3.1 Vertebral column (right lateral view). Normal A-P curvatures of the adult spine. Note the anteriorly concave kyphoses of the thoracic and sacral regions, and the posteriorly concave lordoses of the cervical and lumbar regions. (Adapted from Rohen JW, Yokochi C, Lutjen-Drecoll E. *Color atlas of anatomy: a photographic study of the human body*. Baltimore, MD: Lippincott Williams & Wilkins, 2006, with permission.)

meninges, and nerve roots. Seven processes attach to each neural arch. Three processes diverge for the attachment of ligaments and muscle, the midline spinous process, and bilateral transverse processes (Fig. 3.2). Four processes, the bilateral superior and inferior articular processes, project from the junction of lamina and pedicle to join each vertebra to the two adjacent vertebrae, above and below (Fig. 3.2).

The vertebral body is located anteriorly and is attached to the adjacent IV discs superiorly and inferiorly (Figs. 3.1 and 3.2). As this part of the vertebra is largely responsible for transmitting the weight of the body, the vertebral bodies increase in size progressively from the cervical through to the lumbar regions (Fig. 3.1). The weight is transferred from the lumbar vertebrae to the pelvic girdle via the sacrum; as a result, the vertebral bodies decrease in size from the sacrum to the coccyx.

Each typical vertebra has a dense bony cortex surrounding trabecular bone and red marrow. The trabeculae are arranged in three layers disposed along the lines of force. The orientation of these layers includes the vertical layer, linking the superior and inferior surfaces, the horizontal layer, linking the lateral surfaces, and the oblique layer running from each plateau into the vertebral arch. The least amount of trabecular overlap occurs in the anterior part of the body, thus resulting in a zone of weakness, where compression fractures first occur (3). Discs of hyaline cartilage called the "vertebral end plates" cover the superior and inferior surfaces of the vertebral body (see Fig. 3.6B).

The vertebral or neural arch is located posterior to the vertebral body and is composed of two pedicles, attached to the vertebral body, and two laminae, which are fused in the dorsal midline (Fig. 3.2). The vertebral arch combines with the posterior surface of the vertebral body to form a vertebral foramen (Fig. 3.2). Collectively, the vertebral foramina of adjacent vertebrae form the vertebral canal, which houses the spinal cord, dorsal and ventral roots, the spinal meninges, and associated vasculature. The spinal nerves exit the vertebral canal via the IV foramina, passageways bounded by the superior and inferior vertebral notches of the adjacent pedicles (Figs. 3.1 and 3.2).

The vertebrae are also characterized by a number of named processes. These processes offer sites for ligament and muscle attachment and help to form joints between adjacent vertebrae and between the vertebrae and the ribs. The spinous process is located posteriorly, at the junction of the laminae, and provides a site of attachment for the extensor muscles and strong ligaments of the spine (Fig. 3.2). The transverse processes are lateral projections located at the pedicle-lamina junction (Fig. 3.2). These processes also serve as attachment sites for spinal extensor muscles; in addition, they articulate with the tubercles of the ribs in the thoracic region. Lastly, pairs of articular processes extend superiorly and inferiorly from the pedicle-lamina junction (Fig. 3.2). The superior and inferior articular facets on these processes form the facet or zygapophysial joints of the vertebral column, discussed below.

Cervical Vertebrae

The five typical cervical vertebrae (C3-7) are characterized by small vertebral bodies, transverse foramina for the passage of the vertebral arteries and veins, and superiorly and inferiorly facing articular facets (Fig. 3.3A). In a typical cervical vertebra, the ovoid body measures about twice as much from side to side as it does in its anteroposterior dimension. The bodies of the lower cervical vertebrae feature elevated superolateral margins called uncinate processes (Figs. 3.3A, see 3.9). The superior and inferior surfaces of the bodies are saddle-shaped due to these processes, which help form the uncovertebral joints (also known as the joints of Luschka or neurocentral joints), discussed below. The pedicles are short as are the relatively robust articular processes (Fig. 3.3A). Unlike the lumbar spine, the pedicles of the cervical spine project posterolaterally, thus affecting the size and shape of the central canal. The transverse processes of the cervical vertebrae feature an anterior and posterior tubercle for the attachment of levator scapulae and scalene muscles (Fig. 3.3A). Compared to other regions, the spinous processes of the cervical vertebrae are relatively short; however, the C7 vertebra is known as the vertebra prominens due to its well-developed spinous process (Fig. 3.1). The C3-6 vertebrae are characterized by bifid spinous processes in some populations (2,4). Duray et al. (4) found that males have a higher frequency of bifidity than females (e.g., 44% versus 28% for C3); however, the presence of bifid spinous processes varies even more significantly according to race, with Caucasians having a significantly higher frequency of bifidity compared to African Americans (e.g., 58% versus 14% for C3).

The C1 vertebra, or atlas, lacks a body and spinous process. Instead, the atlas consists of lateral masses united by an anterior and a posterior vertebral arch (Fig. 3.3B). The lateral masses feature concave superior articular facets that articulate

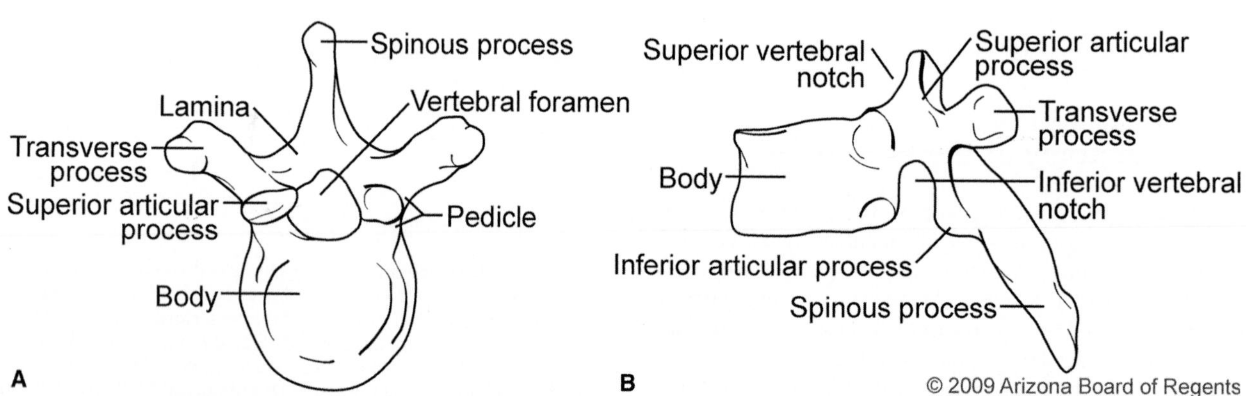

FIGURE 3.2 Features of a 'typical' vertebra. A. Superior view; B. Lateral view. (Drawing by Brent Adrian.)

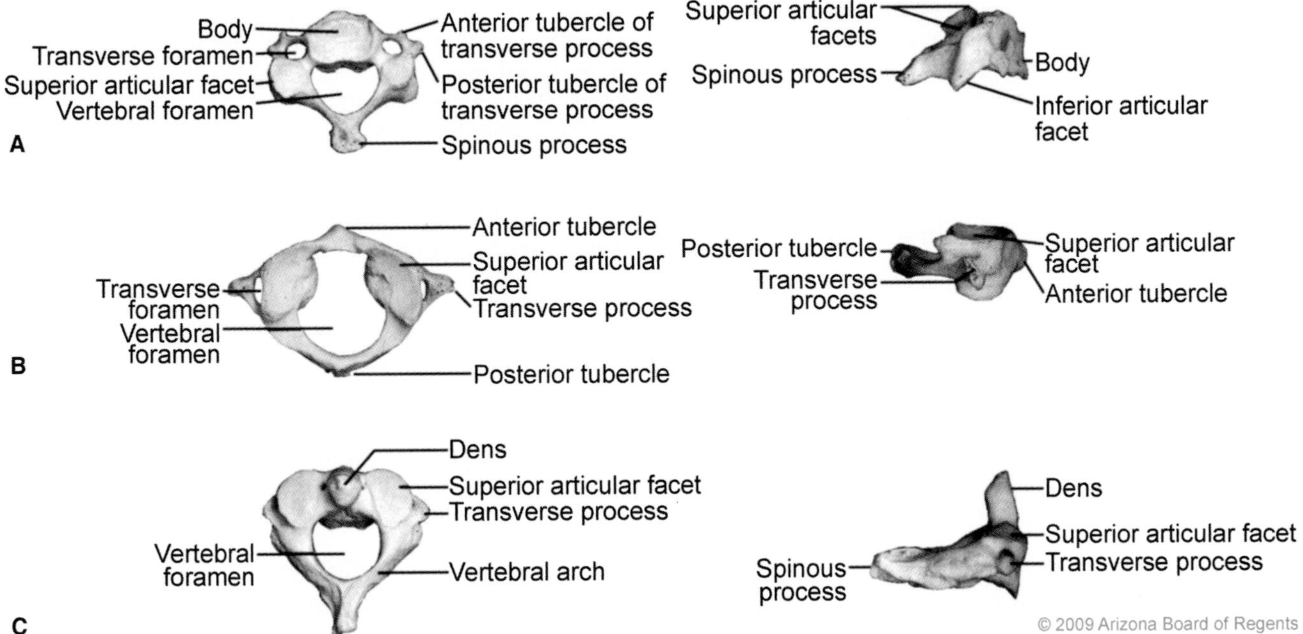

FIGURE 3.3 Cervical vertebrae (superior and lateral views). From top to bottom: **A.** Typical cervical vertebra; **B.** Atlas (C1); **C.** Axis (C2). (Adapted from Rohen JW, Yokochi C, Lutjen-Drecoll E. *Color atlas of anatomy: a photographic study of the human body*. Baltimore, MD: Lippincott Williams & Wilkins, 2006, with permission.)

with the occipital condyles of the skull. The C2 vertebra, or axis, is also distinctive. Its dens, or odontoid process, extends superiorly from the body to articulate with the anterior arch of the atlas (Fig. 3.3C). The dens represents the body of the C1 vertebra that has fused with the body of C2 during ontogeny. The axis is also characterized by well-developed, flattened superior articular facets that articulate with the inferior articular facets of the atlas (Fig. 3.3C).

Thoracic Vertebrae

The 12 thoracic vertebrae articulate laterally with the 12 pairs of ribs (Fig. 3.4). As a result, these vertebrae feature costal facets on their bodies and transverse processes (Fig. 3.4). The head of each rib articulates with the bodies of adjacent vertebrae, while the tubercle of a rib articulates with the transverse process of the vertebra (Fig. 3.4). In addition

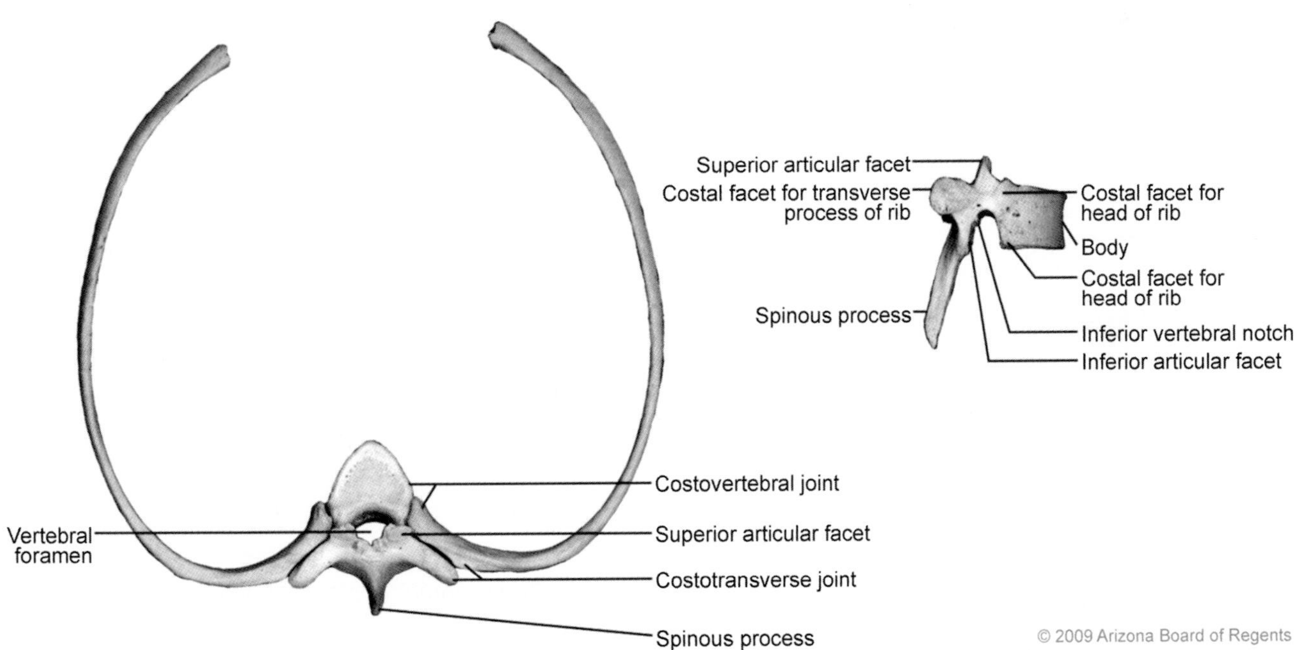

FIGURE 3.4 Thoracic vertebra and ribs (superior and lateral views). (Adapted from Rohen JW, Yokochi C, Lutjen-Drecoll E. *Color atlas of anatomy: a photographic study of the human body.* Baltimore, MD: Lippincott Williams & Wilkins, 2006, with permission.)

to the costal facets, thoracic vertebrae are characterized by inferiorly directed, slender spinous processes and anteriorly and posteriorly facing articular facets (Fig. 3.4). However, T1 is atypical in having a horizontally oriented spinous process, while T12 is also transitional in form, lacking costal facets on the inferior aspect of its body and featuring laterally oriented inferior articular facets.

Lumbar Vertebrae

The five lumbar vertebrae are distinguished by their robust kidney-shaped vertebral bodies and stout, posteriorly directed spinous processes (Fig. 3.5A). In addition, these vertebrae feature medially and laterally facing articular facets (Fig. 3.5A). The transverse processes include small accessory processes, while the superior articular processes feature mammillary processes; these processes provide attachment sites for muscles such as the multifidus and other extensor muscles of the spine.

Sacrum

The sacrum is typically formed by the fusion of five sacral vertebrae and their costal elements (Figs. 3.1 and 3.5B). The sacral promontory, an obstetrical landmark, is formed by the projecting anterior border of the S1 vertebral body (Fig. 3.5B). The vertebral canal of the lumbar spine continues inferiorly within the sacrum as the sacral canal, tapering caudally. The sacral canal ends at the sacral hiatus, bounded by the sacral cornua (Fig. 3.5B). The sacral hiatus is an important landmark for the administration of caudal epidural anesthesia. Four pairs of anterior and posterior sacral foramina transmit the ventral and dorsal primary rami of the sacral spinal nerves. The posterior foramina are easily accessible for segmental injections.

The sacrum forms the posterior wall of the pelvic cavity and its ventral, or pelvic, surface is concave and smooth. In contrast, the dorsal surface features a median sacral crest formed by the fused spinous processes, intermediate crests formed by the fused articular processes, and lateral crests formed by the fused transverse processes (Fig. 3.5B). The lateral surfaces of the sacrum, or auricular surfaces, articulate with the iliac bones, forming the sacroiliac joints (Fig. 3.5B).

The fusion of the first and second sacral vertebrae may be incomplete, which results in lumbarization of the first sacral vertebra. The sacrum may also have an additional vertebral element that may be partially or completely fused to it, this is referred to as sacralization of the fifth lumbar vertebra (1,2).

Coccyx

The coccyx is typically formed by the fusion of four coccygeal vertebrae (Fig. 3.1); however, three or five elements may be present (1,2). In addition, the first coccygeal vertebra may remain separate from the rest of the coccyx into adulthood. Compared to other primates, the coccyx is rudimentary in humans due to the lack of a tail; however, it still serves as a focal point for muscle and ligament attachment. For example, the gluteus maximus and coccygeus muscles attach here, as well as the sacrotuberous ligament.

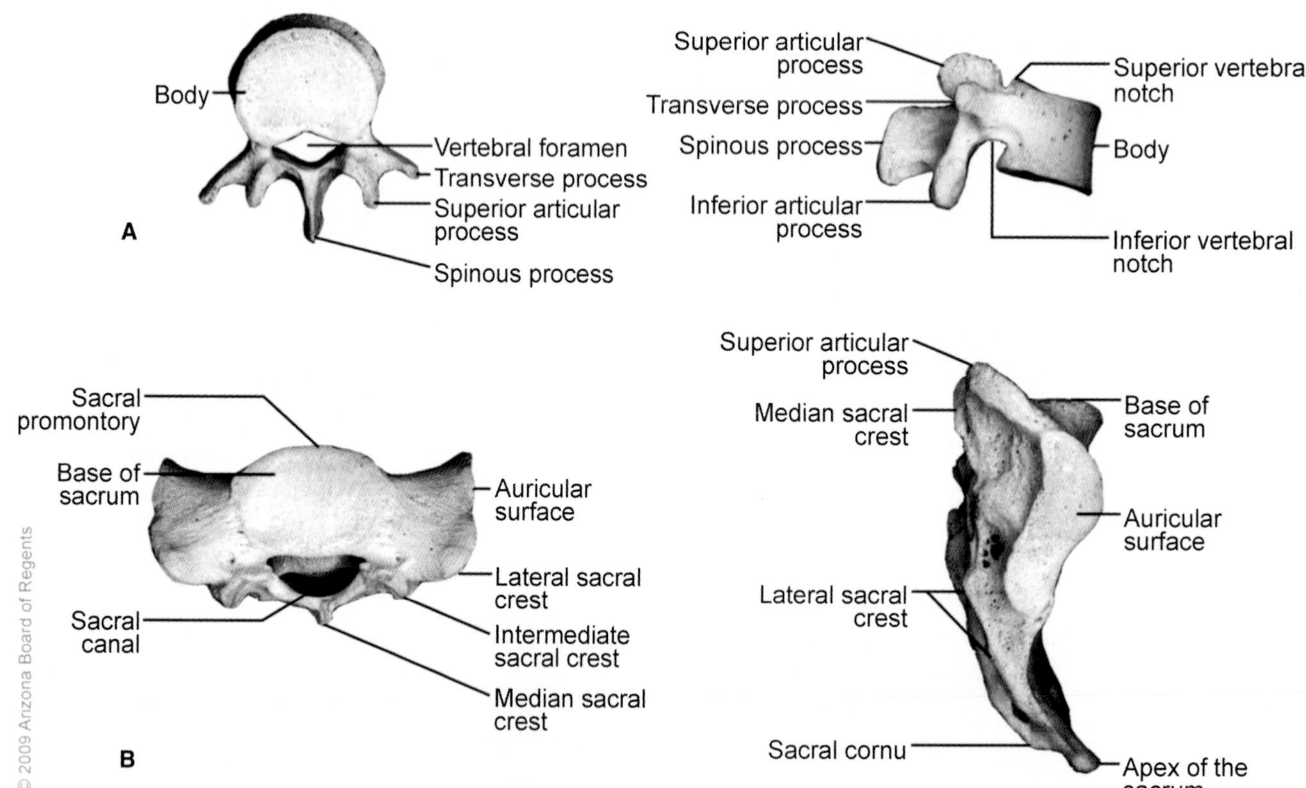

FIGURE 3.5 Lumbar vertebra and sacrum (superior and lateral views). From top to bottom: **A.** Lumbar vertebra; **B.** Sacrum. (Adapted from Rohen JW, Yokochi C, Lutjen-Drecoll E. *Color atlas of anatomy: a photographic study of the human body.* Baltimore, MD: Lippincott Williams & Wilkins, 2006, with permission.)

Joints of the Vertebral Column

The bodies of the vertebral column articulate with one another through the IV discs, whereas the vertebral arches articulate through paired facet joints.

Intervertebral Discs

Each vertebral body articulates with the adjacent vertebrae through the IV discs, forming secondary cartilaginous joints (also known as amphiarthrodial joints or symphyses) (Figs. 3.1 and 3.6). Representing 20% to 25% of the length of the vertebral column, the IV discs function as shock absorbers and provide flexibility to the spine, particularly in the cervical and lumbar regions (2). Each IV disc is composed of an outer, fibrous ring, the annulus fibrosis, and a central gelatinous core, the nucleus pulposus (Fig. 3.6). There is no IV disc between the atlas and the axis, and the sacral and coccygeal IV discs ossify progressively in adulthood. The thoracic IV discs are thin and uniform in shape, while the cervical and lumbar IV discs are thicker anteriorly, contributing to the cervical and lumbar lordotic curvatures of the vertebral column (Fig. 3.1).

Annulus Fibrosis. The annulus fibrosis is composed primarily of collagen fibers and gradually becomes differentiated from the periphery of the nucleus pulposus (Fig. 3.6). In other words, there is no delimiting membrane between the nucleus and the annulus. The fibers are attached to the peripheral margin of the adjacent vertebral bodies. The structure of the annulus has been likened to that of an onion. It consists of a series of approximately 20 concentric layers or lamellae. The collagen fibers in each layer are in a parallel arrangement oriented obliquely at about a 50-degree angle relative to the surface of the vertebrae. In each consecutive layer, the fibers are oriented in an opposite obliquity to those in the previous layer. This arrangement, where each subsequent layer runs in opposite directions, lends great stability and resistance to the outward forces from the nucleus pulposus during weight bearing (5).

Nucleus Pulposus. The nucleus pulposus is the central gelatinous portion of the IV disc (Fig. 3.6). It consists primarily of proteoglycans, water, and scant, fine, collagen fibers, similar in composition to loose connective tissue. Water is the most predominant substance in the disc, accounting for approximately 70% to 90% of the total volume, and is largely determined by the hydrophilic nature of the proteoglycans.

Functions of the IV Discs. Along with the facet joints, IV discs are primarily responsible for resisting compressive loads (Fig. 3.6B,C) (6). These loads include static loads (e.g., when standing) as well as much higher dynamic loads such as running and jumping activities. In addition to compressive

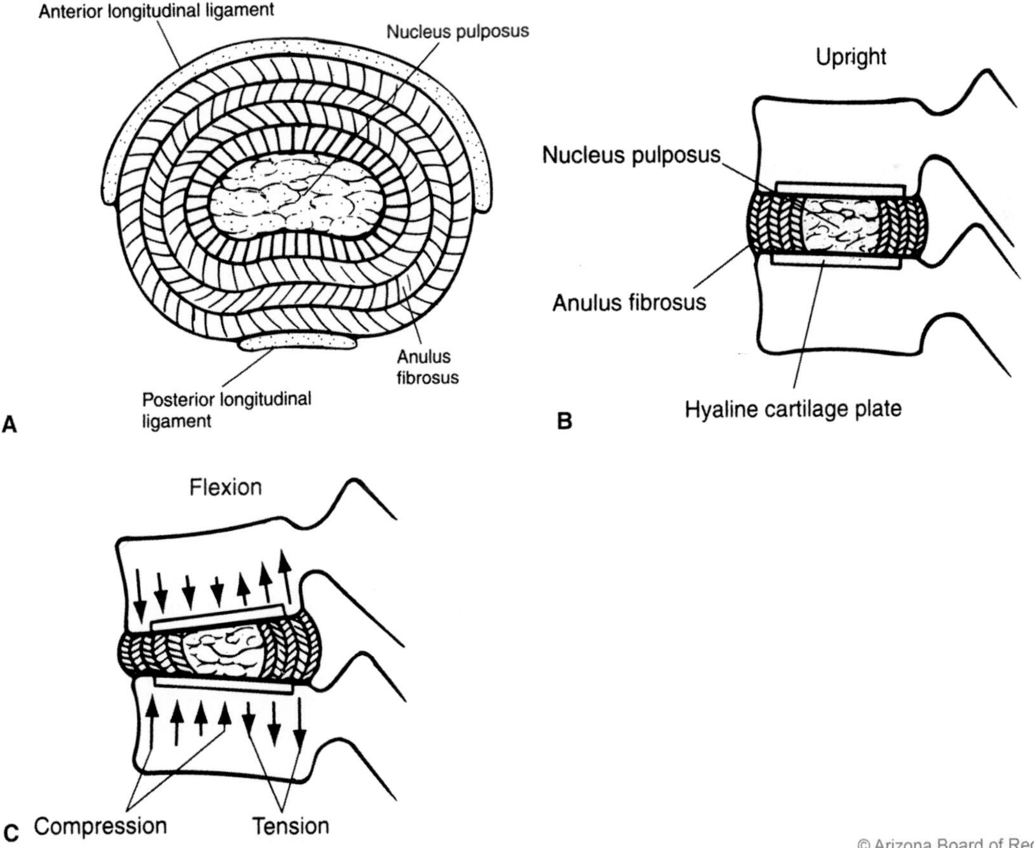

FIGURE 3.6 Intervertebral disc. A. Transverse section of intervertebral disc and its reinforcing longitudinal ligaments; **B,C.** Sagittal sections of intervertebral disc in upright and flexed positions, respectively. (Taken with permission from Kirshblum S, Campagnolo DI, DeLisa JA. *Spinal cord medicine.* Philadelphia, PA: Lippincott Williams & Wilkins, 2002.)

loads, the discs are responsible for resisting tensile and shear stresses during flexion, extension, lateral bending, and rotational movements (Fig. 3.6C).

Another function of the IV disc is to allow multiplanar motion between the rigid structural elements of the vertebral bodies. The disc functions as a swivel joint, allowing tilting, rotation, and gliding. Therefore, this joint permits flexion, and extension, lateral flexion, gliding (in the sagittal and frontal planes), and rotation (to left and right). From one region to the next, other structures constrain these movements such as the facet joints and ligaments. The nucleus pulposus behaves as a viscous fluid and in conjunction with the surrounding annulus, the disc functions as a shock absorber. Vertical loads cause the nucleus to distort uniformly in a circumferential direction, which subsequently results in distortion of the annular envelope and increases tension in the collagen fibers of the annulus (Fig. 3.6B). The healthy lumbar disc is extremely resilient to vertical loading; in fact, the bony vertebrae will often undergo fracture before there is evidence of disc injury (7,8).

Facet Joints

The facet or zygapophyseal joints of the spine are paired articular structures. Each anatomical motion segment (e.g., two contiguous vertebrae) is associated with one pair. These joints are diarthrodial planar joints in which the joint surfaces are covered with articular cartilage and the joint is enclosed by a capsule. The facet joints form an articulation between the inferior articular process of the vertebrae above and the superior articular process of the vertebrae below. The orientation of these joints determines the range of motion possible at each spinal segment.

The cervical spine is the most mobile part of the vertebral column. The facets in this region permit flexion and extension, lateral flexion, and some rotation. The articular facets of the superior articular processes face superiorly and posteriorly, while those of the inferior face inferiorly and anteriorly (Fig. 3.3A). These joints project superiorly at a 45-degree angle with the horizontal plane. In contrast, the thoracic articular facets, oriented anteriorly and posteriorly, permit rotation and some lateral flexion, but restrict flexion and extension (Fig. 3.4). The thoracic facet joints are oriented 60 degrees in the sagittal plane, although there is a gradual change from an orientation similar to the cervical spine in the upper thoracic region to one that is similar to the lumbar spine in the lower thoracic region. As a result, flexion-extension is minimal at T1-2 and maximal at T11-12, the latter facet joints being similar to the lumbar orientation. Ranges of motion are also limited in this region due to the long, inferiorly directed spinous processes of the thoracic vertebrae, as well as their articulations laterally with the ribs (Fig. 3.4).

In the lumbar spine, the shape of the superior articular facet is concave while the inferior articular facet is correspondingly convex (Fig. 3.5A). In the upper lumbar segments, the joints are vertical with a predominantly sagittal plane orientation, while in the lower lumbar segments, they are somewhat less vertical and are approximately half way between a sagittal and a coronal plane orientation. In the upper lumbar spine, the superior articular facets face medially, while the inferior articular facets face laterally (Fig. 3.5A). In the lower lumbar spine, as the orientation of the joint gradually becomes closer to the coronal plane, the superior articular facet faces both posteriorly and medially, while the superior articular facet faces anteriorly and laterally. The medially and laterally facing facets of the lumbar spine permit flexion and extension and lateral flexion, but restrict rotation.

Facet Joint Capsule. The joint capsules that enclose the facet joints are relatively tight anteriorly and more lax posteriorly (Fig. 3.7). The superior aspect of the capsule has been shown to be stretched and may be injured with axial loads, especially with the spine in extension (9). Attached to the interior surface of the joint capsule at the level of the superior and inferior joint recesses are meniscus-like structures.

Facet Joint Innervation. The facet joints and capsules are richly innervated by branches from the dorsal primary ramus as it exits the IV foramen. The dorsal primary ramus at a given segmental level sends fibers to the facet joint at that level but also to the facet joints superior and inferior to the nerve. The innervation of the facet joints and capsule is through mechanoreceptors as well as nociceptors (10,11).

Other Joints

Additional joints are found in specific regions of the spine. These include the atlanto-occipital joints, the atlanto-axial joints, the uncovertebral joints of Luschka in the cervical spine, and costovertebral joints in the thoracic spine.

Atlanto-occipital and Atlanto-axial Joints

The atlanto-occipital joints are synovial joints located between the superior articular processes of the atlas and the occipital condyles of the skull (Fig. 3.7). The primary range of motion at these joints is flexion and extension, as in nodding the head to indicate "yes." The atlanto-axial joints include three articulations between the atlas and the axis (Figs. 3.7 and 3.8). These include two lateral atlanto-axial joints, the facet joints between C1 and C2, and a median atlanto-axial joint, located between the dens, the anterior arch of the atlas, and the transverse ligament of the atlas (Fig. 3.8A). The primary range of motion at these joints is rotation, as in rotating the head to indicate "no."

Uncovertebral Joints of Luschka

The uncovertebral joints of Luschka are positioned between the inferolateral aspects of the five typical cervical vertebral bodies and the uncinate processes of the vertebra below (Fig. 3.9). The smooth articular surfaces are covered with hyaline cartilage and some authors classify them as synovial joints; however, due to the fact that these spaces appear in adolescence, it is possible that they represent degenerative fissures within the lateral aspects of the IV discs (2,12). The nerve roots pass posterior to the uncovertebral joints and anterior to the facet joints. Thus, the uncovertebral joints are in a position that prevents a disc rupture from directly compressing on the nerve root. However, osteophytes at the uncovertebral joints may compress the nerve root or the spinal cord.

Costovertebral Joints

The costovertebral joints are synovial joints located between the heads and tubercles of the ribs and the bodies and transverse processes of the thoracic vertebrae (Fig. 3.4). The head of a rib typically articulates with the costal facets of two adjacent

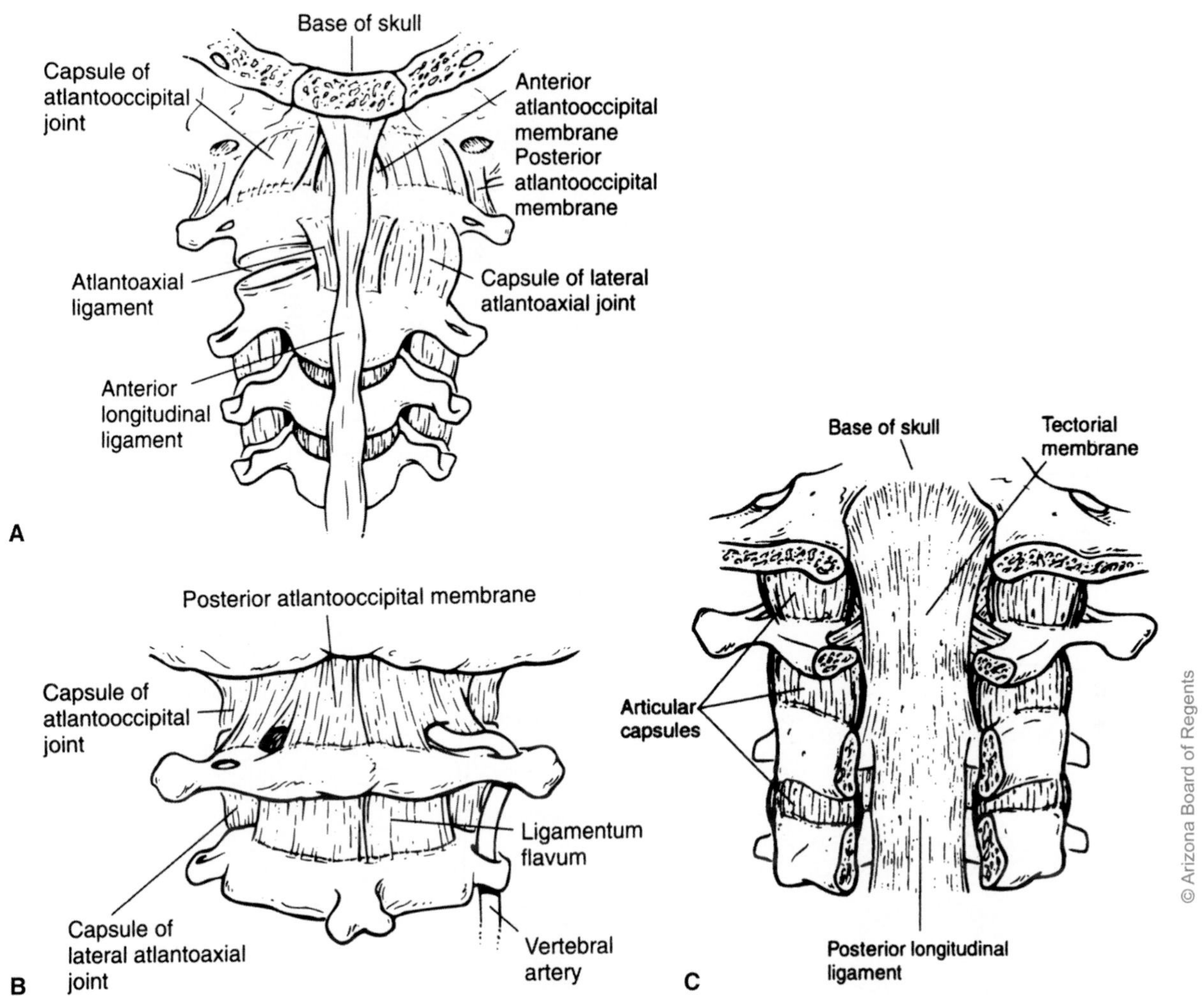

FIGURE 3.7 **Ligaments of the atlanto-occipital joints and lateral atlanto-axial joints. A.** Anterior view; **B.** Posterior view; **C.** Posterior view with vertebral arches and spinal cord removed. (Taken with permission from Kirshblum S, Campagnolo DI, DeLisa JA. *Spinal cord medicine.* Philadelphia, PA: Lippincott Williams & Wilkins, 2002.)

vertebrae as well as the intervening IV disc; however, the first and last three ribs may articulate with a single vertebral body. The tubercle of a rib typically articulates with the transverse process of its corresponding vertebra, but the last two ribs are exceptional in lacking this costotransverse articulation. The gliding movements at these joints contribute to the elevation and depression of the ribs, increasing the anterior-posterior and medial-lateral dimensions of the thoracic cavity during respiration.

Ligaments of the Vertebral Column

The spine can be viewed as a series of stacked bony elements. The column of stacked vertebrae must be held together in a manner that allows sufficient stabilization for movement in a controlled manner, while protecting neural elements. The stability of the spine is the result of tough dense connective tissues that act as check reins at the limits of range of motion; these tissues include the IV discs, the capsules of the facet joints, and the ligaments.

Spinal ligaments have different functions and constraints. First, they act to check and restrict motion at the end range. This is particularly important as the spinal cord and the spinal nerves must be protected from compressive and tensile forces. Second, spinal ligaments must allow adequate vertebral column motion without impingement of neural structures if the ligament buckles when it is slack. Third, ligaments of the spine allow fixed postural attitudes between vertebrae, minimizing the need for sustained muscular contraction. Finally, the ligaments protect and stabilize surrounding structures in the event of high-energy, high-velocity trauma. The ligaments of the vertebral column can be organized anatomically (longitudinal ligaments that span the length of the spine and segmental ligaments that span between two vertebrae) or functionally (ligaments that stabilize the IV discs and those that stabilize the vertebral arch).

Longitudinal Ligaments

The anterior longitudinal ligament (ALL) is a broad band that runs along the anterior aspect of the vertebral bodies and IV discs, and extends from the occipital bone, anterior to the foramen magnum, to the sacrum (Figs. 3.7A and 3.10A). It consists of several laminae of fibers, the deepest spanning one IV segment, while the most superficial extends over several segments. The ALL is thickest centrally, and it becomes progressively broader as it passes inferiorly. It is firmly united to the periosteum of the vertebral bodies but is free over the IV discs. This ligament limits extension of the vertebral column and anterior herniation of the nucleus pulposus (Fig. 3.10A).

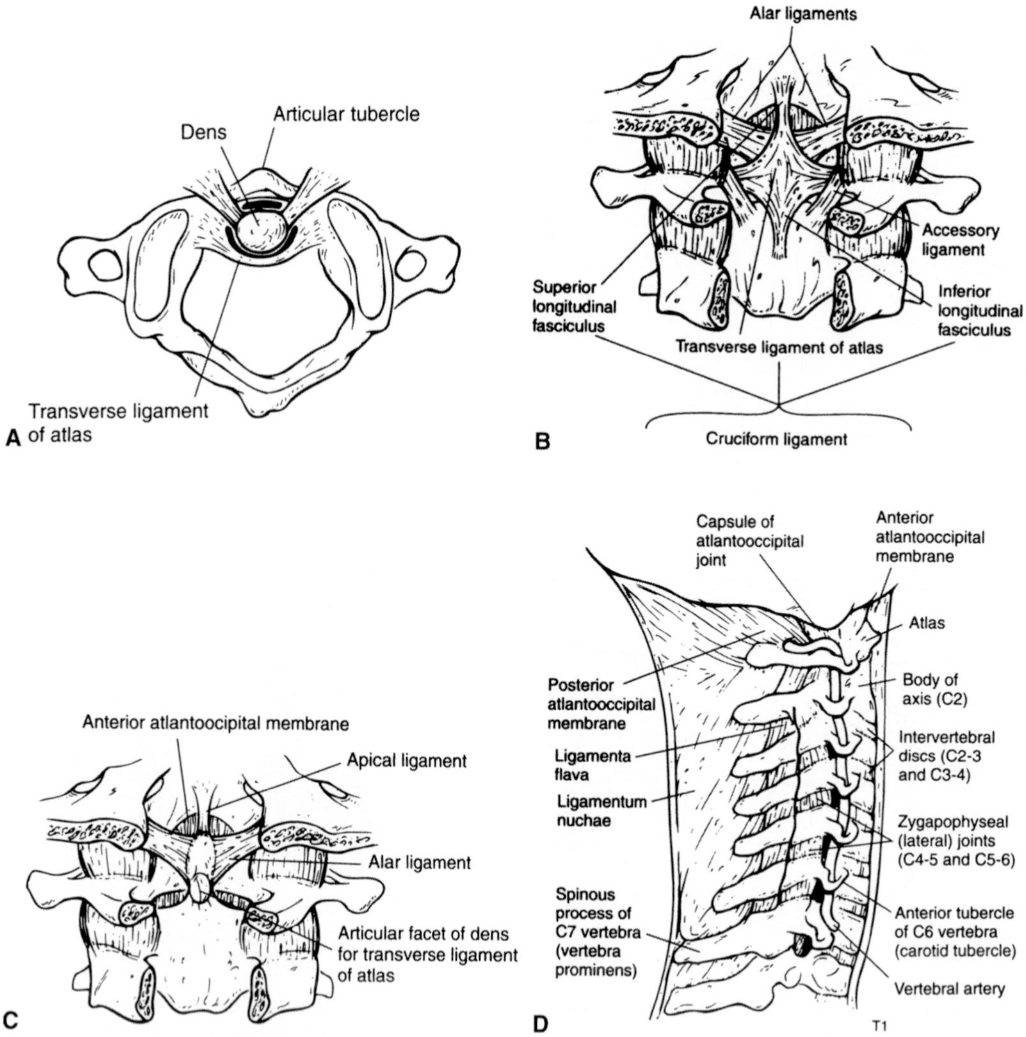

FIGURE 3.8 **Ligaments of medial atlanto-axial joints. A.** Superior view of dens with associated ligaments; **B.** Posterior view of cruciform ligament with vertebral arches and spinal cord removed; **C.** Posterior view of alar and apical ligaments with vertebral arches, spinal cord, and cruciform ligament removed; **D.** Lateral view of cervical spine ligaments. (Taken with permission from Kirshblum S, Campagnolo DI, DeLisa JA. *Spinal cord medicine.* Philadelphia, PA: Lippincott Williams & Wilkins, 2002.)

The posterior longitudinal ligament (PLL) lies on the posterior surface of the vertebral bodies and IV discs, and is therefore located within the vertebral canal (Figs. 3.7C and 3.10A,B). It is slender compared to the ALL, extending from C2 to the sacrum, narrowing gradually as it passes inferiorly. It has serrated margins, broadest over the IV discs to which it is firmly attached (Fig. 3.10B). Thus, a direct posterior herniation of the disc is uncommon, particularly in the thoracic and lumbar regions where the nucleus pulposus typically herniates in a posterolateral direction, beyond the attachment of the PLL. The PLL is also attached firmly to the superior and inferior margins of the vertebrae, but over the midportion of the vertebral bodies, it is separated by the basivertebral veins (also known as "Batson's veins" or "Batson's plexus"). This ligament limits flexion of the vertebral column. Since the PLL lies within the spinal central canal, hypertrophy and calcification of the ligament may contribute to spinal stenosis.

Segmental Ligaments

The vertebral arches are united by the ligamenta flava, intertransverse ligaments, interspinous ligaments, and supraspinous ligaments. The ligamenta flava span the distance between the laminae of adjacent vertebrae and fuse with their counterparts in the dorsal midline (Figs. 3.8D and 3.10A,C). These ligaments help form the posterior wall of the vertebral canal (Fig. 3.10C). The ligamenta flava are distinctly yellow in color from the high content of elastic fibers. Their elastic properties prevent redundancy and buckling into the central canal when the ligament is slack. The ligamenta flava help limit flexion, support the normal curvatures of the vertebral column, and due to their elasticity, assist in extending the vertebral column from a flexed position. Hypertrophy of the ligamenta flava can contribute to compression of a nerve root at the IV foramen.

Three segmental ligaments further unite and stabilize the vertebral arch: intertransverse, interspinous, and supraspinous ligaments. Along the length of the vertebral column, relatively weak intertransverse ligaments connect adjacent transverse processes. These ligaments limit lateral flexion. Interspinous ligaments unite adjacent spinous processes and are also relatively weak (Fig. 3.10A). The supraspinous ligament consists of thick, strong collagenous bands of fibrous tissue joining the tips of adjacent spinous processes (Fig. 3.10A). Cranially, the

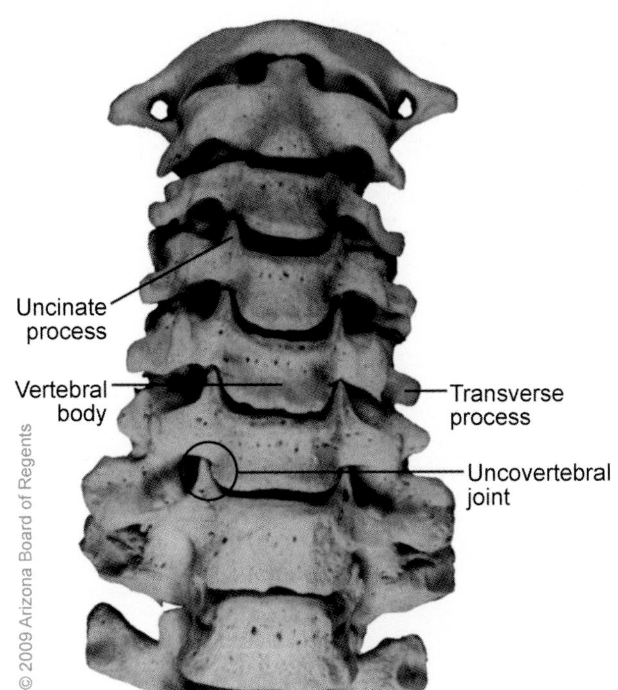

FIGURE 3.9 Cervical spine. Anterior view of the cervical spine illustrating the uncovertebral joints. (Taken with permission from Kirshblum S, Campagnolo DI, DeLisa JA. *Spinal cord medicine.* Philadelphia, PA: Lippincott Williams & Wilkins, 2002.)

supraspinous ligament merges with the ligamentum nuchae, a fibroelastic structure that extends from the external occipital protuberance to the cervical spinous processes (Fig. 3.8D). The ligamentum nuchae forms a midline raphe for the attachment of neck muscles. Both interspinous and supraspinous ligaments limit flexion of the spine.

The atlanto-occipital and atlanto-axial joints are protected by a number of specialized ligaments and membranes. The anterior and posterior atlanto-occipital membranes connect the anterior and posterior arches of the atlas with the corresponding margins of the foramen magnum (Figs. 3.7A,B and 3.8C,D). These membranes limit extension and flexion of the atlanto-occipital joints, respectively. Similarly, the anterior and posterior atlanto-axial membranes connect the anterior and posterior arches of the atlas with the lateral masses and laminae of the axis, respectively. The atlanto-axial membranes help prevent hyperextension and hyperflexion of the superior cervical spine.

The tectorial membrane is a thickened continuation of the PLL that runs from the body of the axis to the anterior margin of the foramen magnum (Fig. 3.7C). This membrane limits flexion of the superior cervical spine, and lies superficial to the cruciate, alar, and apical ligaments. The cruciate (or cruciform) ligament includes the transverse ligament of the atlas and the superior and inferior longitudinal bands (Figs. 3.8A,B). The robust transverse ligament spans the distance between the lateral masses of the axis and holds the dens in place against the anterior arch of the atlas (Fig. 3.8A,B), while the thin longitudinal bands connect the transverse ligament to the occipital bone and C2 (Fig. 3.8B). The alar ligaments extend from the lateral margins of the foramen magnum to the dens process, while the apical ligament extends from the apex of the dens to the anterior margin of the foramen magnum (Fig. 3.8C). These three ligaments help restrict the degree of rotation of the dens against the anterior arch of the atlas.

Innervation of Ligaments. The ligaments of the spine are richly innervated and may generate pain when injured, similar to ligaments found elsewhere in the body. The sinuvertebral nerve, a branch of the dorsal primary ramus, innervates all of the posterior ligaments and capsules of the facet joints. A branch of the ventral primary ramus innervates the ALL.

Spinal Muscles

The functions of spinal muscles include stabilization and movement. The spine without sufficient muscular support is extremely unstable, as seen in many neuromuscular diseases, such as spinal cord injury and muscular dystrophy (13).

Many muscle groups can move the vertebral column. Immediately anterior to the spine are primary flexor muscles, represented by longus capitis and longus colli in the neck, and psoas major in the lumbar region. Other anteriorly located muscles, such as rectus abdominus, flex the spine. Lateral flexion is performed by muscles positioned alongside the vertebral column, such as the scalenes in the neck and the abdominal obliques and transversus abdominis in the lumbar region. These muscles are all innervated segmentally by ventral primary rami.

The muscles that extend the vertebral column and skull lie posterior to the vertebrae and are innervated by dorsal primary rami (Fig. 3.11). Running the length of the spine, these muscles are known collectively as the intrinsic or extensor muscles of the back. They are also commonly referred to in clinical practice as the erector spinae muscle group. In this regard, a discrepancy exists between the muscle groups defined by anatomists and those recognized by clinicians. While clinicians often apply this term to the intrinsic back muscles as a whole, according to the *Terminologia Anatomica*, the erector spinae includes only the iliocostalis, longissimus, and spinalis muscles (14).

In the neck, the intrinsic back muscles are specialized into separate muscles for support and movement of the head. The splenius muscles (capitus and cervicis) are only found in the neck and are superficial to all of the longitudinal muscles (Fig. 3.11A). Splenius capitis and cervicis lie deep to the extrinsic muscles of the back, such as trapezius and the rhomboids. The splenius muscles arise from the ligamentum nuchae and cervical and thoracic spinous processes, and insert on the mastoid process and occipital bone (capitis) or the cervical transverse processes (cervicis). Bilateral contraction of the splenius muscles extends the cervical spine, while unilateral contraction laterally flexes and rotates the cervical spine to the ipsilateral side. The underlying longitudinal muscles are bound in position by the splenius.

The layer deep to the splenius group consists of the largest, longest, and most powerful back muscles. This layer is defined by anatomists as the erector spinae, which causes some confusion in terminology, as noted above. The erector spinae consists of three longitudinal columns of muscle (Fig. 3.11A). These columns arise from a common tendon with attachments to the iliac crest, sacrum, and lumbar spinous processes. Iliocostalis is located laterally and attaches to the ribs and cervical transverse processes. Longissimus occupies an intermediate position and attaches to the ribs, thoracic and cervical transverse processes, and mastoid process. Spinalis is located medially and connects adjacent spinous processes. Bilateral contraction of the erector spinae extends the spine, while unilateral contraction laterally flexes and rotates the spine to the ipsilateral side.

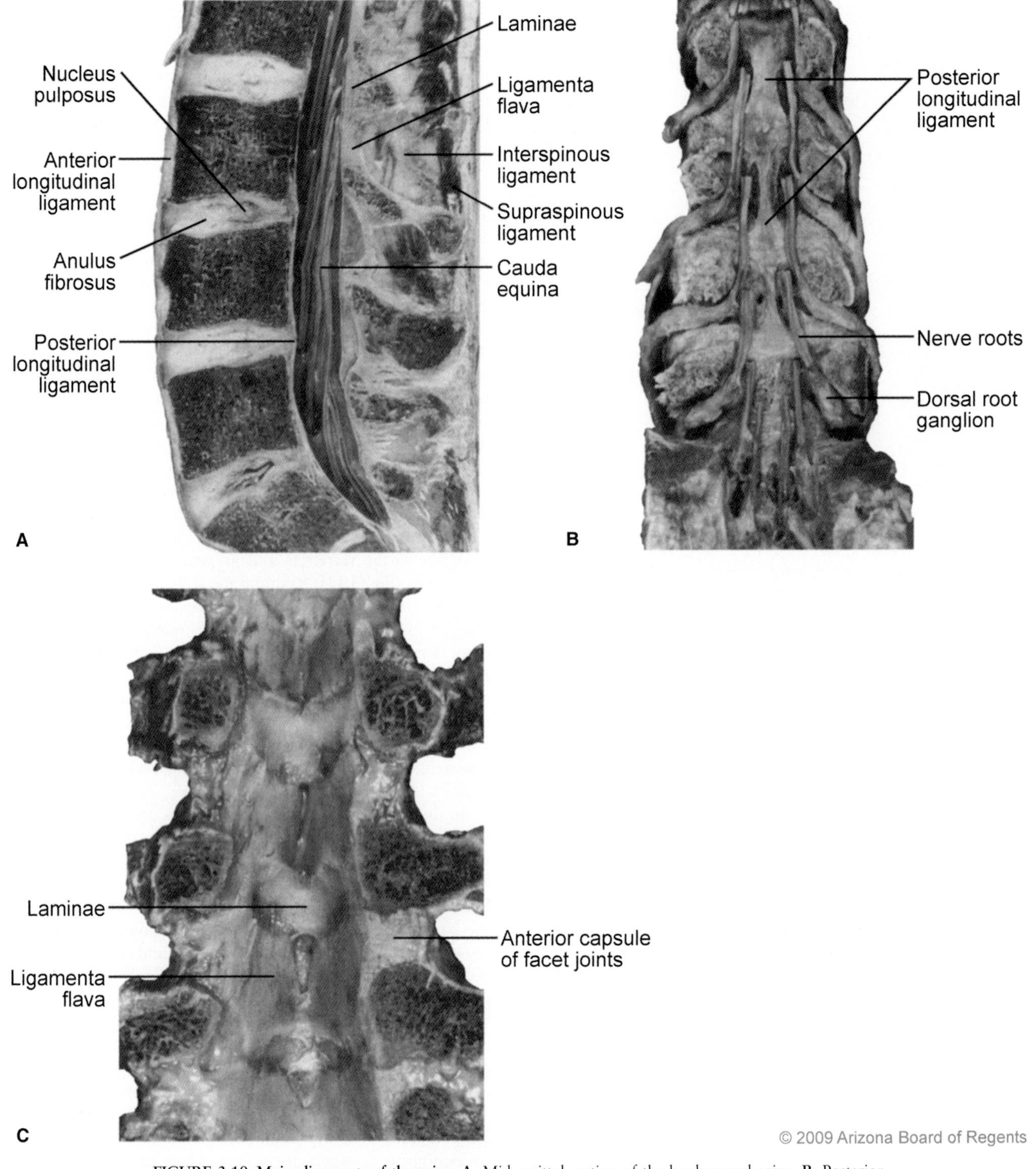

FIGURE 3.10 Major ligaments of the spine. A. Mid-sagittal section of the lumbosacral spine; **B.** Posterior view of the vertebral bodies with vertebral arches and spinal cord removed; **C.** Anterior view of the laminae and ligamenta flava with vertebral bodies and spinal cord removed. (Taken with permission from Kirshblum S, Campagnolo DI, DeLisa JA. *Spinal cord medicine*. Philadelphia, PA: Lippincott Williams & Wilkins, 2002.)

The muscle group lying deep to the erector spinae is defined as the transversospinalis group by anatomists. Named muscles include the semispinalis, multifidus, and rotatores (Fig. 3.11B). Semispinalis is present in the thoracic and cervical regions, multifidus extends along the entire column but is most developed in the lumbar region, while the rotatores are prominent in the thoracic region. Bilateral contraction of the multifidus, seminspinalis, and rotatores extends the spine, while unilateral contraction laterally flexes the spine and rotates it to the contralateral side.

The deepest layer of intrinsic back muscles consists of the levatores costarum, spanning between the ribs and transverse processes, and short muscles that run between two adjacent vertebrae (Figs. 3.9 and 3.11B). The intertransversarii join adjacent

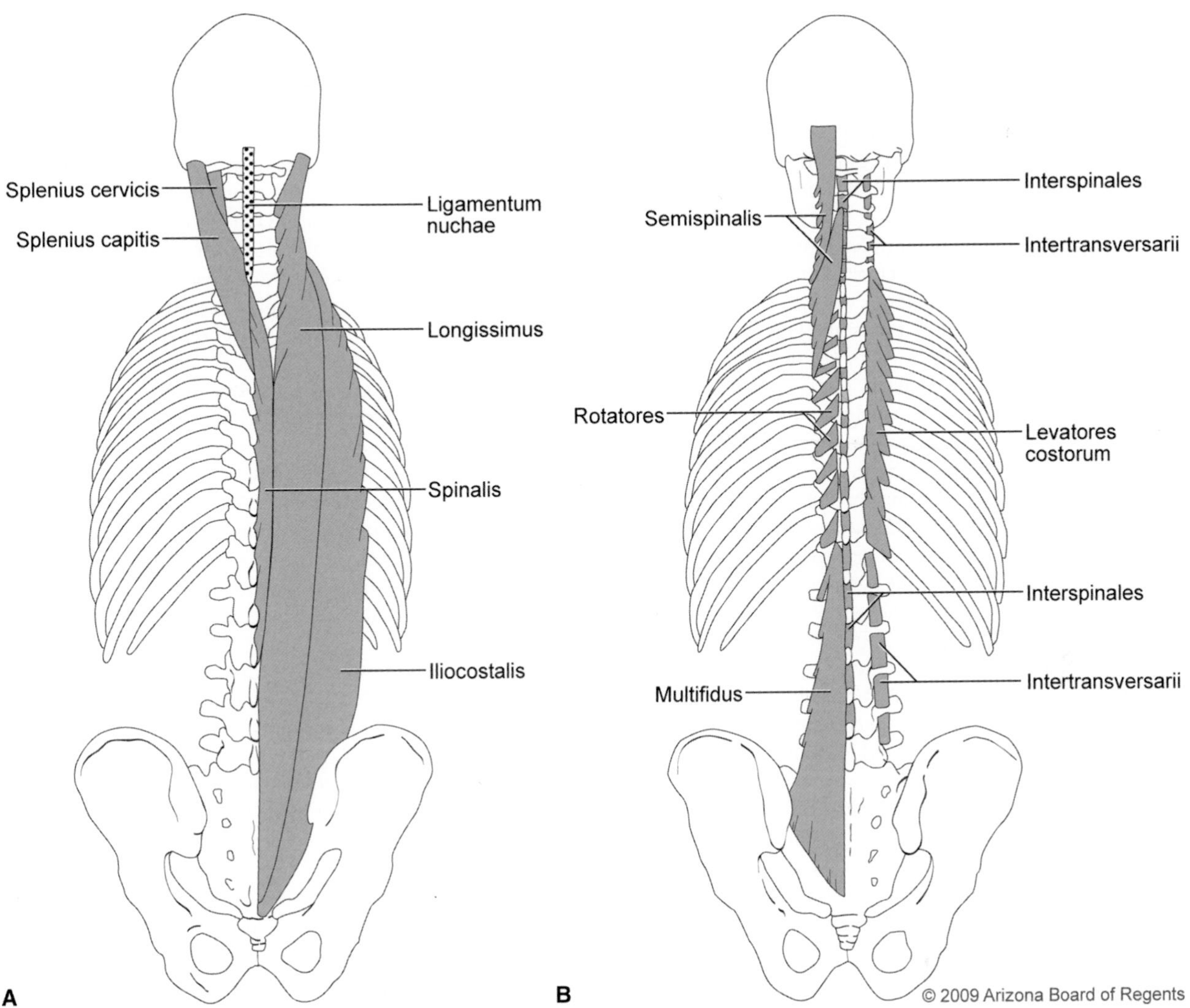

FIGURE 3.11. Muscles of the back. A. On the left, the superficial splenius muscles; on the right, the erector spinae muscles, including iliocostalis, longissimus, and spinalis; **B.** On the left, the transversospinalis muscles, including semispinalis, mulitifudus, and rotatores; on the right, the levatores costarum, intertransversarii, and interspinales muscles. (Drawing by Brent Adrian.)

transverse processes, while the interspinales extend between adjacent spinous processes (Fig. 3.11B). In the suboccipital triangle, these muscles are specialized into the rectus capitis muscles and the superior and inferior obliques. All of the deep muscles of the back are thought to be stabilizers of the vertebral column. These muscles may have a proprioceptive function as well (15).

Functions of the Spinal Muscles

Spinal muscles have several important functions. First, the muscles stabilize the spine. Although there are strong ligaments and other structures that stabilize spinal segments at end range, the muscles stabilize the spine in midrange. Therefore, in any position, muscles can contract isometrically and increase the stiffness of the vertebral column to hold in it in a particular position. Muscles are the only structures that can provide this dynamic stability in all postures. Second, the muscles produce spinal and trunk movements. These include flexion, extension, lateral bending, and rotation. Third, spinal muscles generate force to move loads. The loads on the spine and trunk vary depending on intrinsic factors such as posture, and extrinsic factors such as an external load or forces incurred during a traumatic event.

Anatomic Relationships of the Roots and Spinal Nerves

The ventral and dorsal nerve roots pass through the subarachnoid space and converge to form the spinal nerve at approximately the level of the IV foramen (Fig. 3.10B). The course of the nerve roots becomes progressively longer and more obliquely directed caudally, at more distal segmental levels. Within the dural sac, the upper cervical nerve roots tend to pass superiorly toward their spinal nerves, while the lower cervical nerve roots pass transversely or slightly inferiorly. The cervical spinal nerves occupy the IV foramen resting on top of the pedicle. In this location, they lie inferior to the level of the IV disc. Posterolateral disc prolapse is rare in the cervical region, as the discs cannot escape posterolaterally because of the uncinate processes of the vertebral bodies. If disc prolapse occurs, it is more central than in the lumbar region and consequently tends to cause cord compression.

Cord and nerve root compression in the cervical region is more commonly caused by osteoarthrosis of the uncovertebral joints. During the development of osteoarthrosis, osteophytes appear on the anterior border of the vertebral plateaus and at the level of the uncovertebral joints projecting into the confines of the IV foramen. Osteophytes also develop posteriorly from the facet joints and may compress the nerve roots. Therefore, the nerve roots may be compressed by osteophytes arising anteriorly from the uncovertebral joints and posteriorly from the facet joints (16).

In the lumbosacral regions, the nerve roots and spinal nerves travel an almost vertical course before exiting the spinal canal by passing inferior to the pedicles of the corresponding vertebrae, and exiting through the IV foramina (Figs. 3.10A,B). The IV foramina are bounded anteriorly by the posterior border of the IV disc and the adjoining parts of the vertebral bodies, superiorly and inferiorly by the pedicles of the two adjoining vertebrae, and posteriorly by the articular processes and the facet joint, which are linked by the capsular ligament and the lateral edge of the ligamentum flavum. The foramina are elliptical in shape and are approximately five times the diameter of the nerve root in the lumbar region. They are therefore large enough to easily transmit the spinal nerve, blood vessels, and nerve branches that supply the vertebral column and surrounding soft tissues. Due to the ample vertical dimension of the foramina (12 to 19 mm in the lumbar region), degenerative changes and loss of disc height tend to result in a smaller foramen yet produce little evidence of nerve compression (17,18).

In contrast, the transverse extent of foramina is much smaller (approximately 7 mm); therefore, any space-occupying lesion that narrows the transverse dimensions of the foramen (bony spur, hypertrophy of the ligamentum flavum, tumor, protruding disc) may more readily result in nerve root impingement. While these conditions are not uncommon in the cervical and lumbar regions, thoracic nerve single-level radiculopathy is extremely rare.

Anatomic Relationships of the Spinal Cord and Vertebral Canal

The spinal cord and its surrounding meninges lie in the vertebral canal. The tapered lower end of the spinal cord is the conus medullaris. The termination of the conus medullaris is at a variable level between T12 and the body of L3, most commonly ending at the L1-2 disc. From its tapered point, the conus medullaris is continued as the filum terminale. The filum terminale consists largely of glia and connective tissue elements. It is attached to the dorsum of the coccyx.

The anterior wall of the vertebral canal is formed by the vertebral bodies and the intervening discs of the vertebral column; the lateral walls by the pedicles, between which appear the IV foramina for the exit of the spinal nerves; and the posterior wall by the overlapping articular processes laterally, and medially by the laminae.

The shape of the vertebral canal is determined by the shape of the posterior aspect of the vertebral body and the orientation of the pedicles. Because the posterior border of the vertebral body is concave and the pedicles project posteriorly in the upper lumbar vertebrae, the shape of the canal is oval. In the cervical and lower lumbar regions, the posterior aspect of the vertebral bodies is slightly convex and the pedicles are more lateral in orientation, producing a triangle-shaped canal (Figs. 3.3 and 3.5). The vertebral canal in the thoracic region tends to be more circular in shape, due to the relatively more medially positioned pedicles of the thoracic vertebrae (Fig. 3.4).

The anteroposterior and the transverse diameters of the spinal cord and its meninges are considerably smaller than the diameters of the vertebral canal. This phenomenon allows for movement of the vertebral column without compressing the spinal cord or meninges. The space between the walls of the vertebral canal and the dura mater is the epidural space, which is loosely filled with fat and connective tissue that serve as padding about the cord. The epidural space also contains parts of the internal vertebral venous plexuses and the branches of the spinal arteries that supply the vertebral column, the dura, and the tissues of the epidural space. The internal vertebral venous plexus receives most of its tributaries from the large basivertebral veins draining the vertebral bodies.

Spinal stenosis is either congenital or acquired. It may occur at one or multiple levels of the spine. In the cervical spine, stenosis typically occurs in the mid or lower segments and may present with symptoms of radiculopathy or myelopathy. In the lumbar spine, spinal stenosis is most commonly observed at the L4-5 level, although it occurs at other levels as well (19). In severe lumbar stenosis, there may be symptoms of cauda equina syndrome.

Acquired spinal stenosis is caused by one or more of the following changes: disc space narrowing, spur formation from the vertebral body, hypertrophy of the facet joint, facet joint capsule, uncovertebral joint, PLL, and ligamentum flavum. Central stenosis and lateral stenosis have also been described. Central stenosis is caused by a structure that narrows the vertebral canal (e.g., posterior herniated disc, posterior vertebral body spondylophytes, or ligamentum flavum hypertrophy). Lateral stenosis typically occurs when there is loss of disc height, a posterolateral herniated disc, uncovertebral arthrosis in the cervical spine, and/or degenerative changes of the facet joints. Facet degeneration results in superior and anterior subluxation of the superior facet on the inferior facet, impinging on the pedicle above and narrowing the IV foramen. The spinal nerve that exits at this level may be entrapped.

Spinal Vasculature

The spine is associated with vasculature serving as the arterial supply and venous drainage of the muscles, ligaments, nerves, and osseous elements of the vertebral column. Due to their close anatomic relationship with the spine, these structures are at risk of damage during spinal injuries and degenerative diseases.

Spinal Branches

Spinal arterial branches supply the vertebral body and arch. The spinal branches are branches of the major cervical arteries, such as the ascending cervical artery and vertebral artery, and the segmental arteries at the corresponding level, such as the posterior intercostal and subcostal arteries, lumbar arteries, and medial and lateral sacral arteries. These branches enter the vertebral canal through the IV foramina. They subsequently divide into anterior and posterior vertebral canal branches, which supply the vertebral body and arch, respectively. The spinal branches give off radicular arteries, which travel to the dorsal and ventral nerve roots.

The venous drainage of the vertebrae and associated structures is more complicated than the arterial supply. Spinal veins contribute to two major venous plexuses along the vertebral canal, which receive blood from many smaller veins of the canal and vertebrae. The anterior and posterior internal vertebral (epidural) plexuses run superoinferiorly within the vertebral canal, while the anterior and posterior external vertebral plexuses course on the exterior of the vertebral column. Large basivertebral veins receive blood from smaller tributaries along the vertebral bodies, and drain into the vertebral venous plexuses. The IV veins drain the spinal cord and receive blood from the internal vertebral venous plexuses, and course through the IV foramina to drain into the segmental veins (in the thoracic and lumbar regions) or vertebral veins (in the cervical region).

Vertebral Arteries and Veins

Vertebral arteries, branches of the subclavian arteries, traverse the cervical region of the spine. These arteries travel superiorly through the foramina in the transverse processes of the C6 vertebra, then proceed superiorly through the transverse foramina of the remaining cervical vertebrae, including C1. (Figs. 3.3 and 3.8D). They give off spinal branches to supply the cervical vertebra, as mentioned above. Finally, they enter the skull through the foramen magnum where the left and right vertebral arteries converge to form the basilar artery, which contributes to the blood supply to the brain via the posterior aspect of the Circle of Willis.

Vertebral veins course inferiorly from the suboccipital triangle, and parallel the path of the vertebral arteries through the transverse foramina of C1-6, forming a plexus around accompanying arteries. The vertebral veins receive blood from the cervical IV veins throughout their course, and ultimately drain into the brachiocephalic veins.

References

1. Standring S. *Gray's anatomy: the anatomical basis of clinical practice.* New York: Churchill Livingstone, 2008.
2. Moore KL, Dalley AF. *Clinically oriented anatomy.* Baltimore: Lippincott Williams & Wilkins, 2005.
3. Kapandkji IA. *The physiology of joints: volume three—the trunk and the vertebral column.* Edinburgh: Churchill Livingstone, 1974.
4. Duray SM, Morter HB, Smith FJ. Morphological variation in cervical spinous processes: potential applications in the forensic identification of race from the skeleton. *J Forensic Sci*, 1999;44:937–944.
5. Cailliet R. *Low back pain syndrome*, 4th ed. Philadelphia: FA Davis Company, 1988.
6. Soderberg GL. *Kinesiology: application to pathological motion.* Baltimore: Williams & Wilkins.
7. Perey O. Fracture of the vertebral end-plate in the lumbar spine—an experimental biomechanical investigation. *Acta Orthop Scan* 1957;25(Suppl):1–101.
8. Van Dieen JH, Weinans H, Toussaint HM. Fractures of the lumbar vertebral endplate in the etiology of low back pain: a hypothesis on the causative role of spinal compression in aspecific low back pain. *Med Hypotheses* 1999;53(3):246–252.
9. El-Bohy A, Yank KH, King AI. Experimental verification of facet load transmission by direct measurement of facet/lamina contact pressure. *J Biomechanics* 1989;22: 931–941.
10. Cavanaugh JM, Ozaktay AC, Yamashita HT. Mechanisms of low back pain; a neurophysiologic and neuroanatomic study. *Clin Orthop Rel Res* 1987;335:166–180.
11. White AA, Panjabi MM. *Clinical biomechanics of the spine*, 2nd ed. Philadelphia: JB Lippincott Co, Philadelphia.
12. Bland JH, Boushey DR. Anatomy and physiology of the cervical spine. *Sem Arthritis Rheum* 1990;20:1–20.
13. Hastings JD, Ranucchi ER, Burns SP. Wheelchair configuration and postural alignment in persons with spinal cord injury. *Arch Phys Med Rehabil* 2003;84(4):528–534.
14. Whitmore I, ed. *Terminologia anatomica: international anatomical terminology.* New York: Thieme Medical Publishers, 1998.
15. Buxton DF, Peck D. Neuromuscular spindles relative to joint movement complexities. *Clin Anat* 1989;2: 211–224.
16. Macnab I, McCulloch J. *Neck ache and shoulder pain.* Maryland: Williams & Wilkins, 1994.
17. Nathan H, Feuerstein M. Angulated course of spinal nerve roots. *J Neurosurg* 1970;32:349–353.
18. Bradley WG. Disease of the spinal roots. In: Dyck PJ, Thomas PK, Lambert EH, et al., eds. *Peripheral neuropathy*, 2nd ed. Philadelphia: WB Saunders Co.
19. Kirkaldy-Willis WH, Heithoff KB, Bowen CVA, et al. Pathological anatomy of lumbar spondylosis and stenosis correlated with CT scan. In: Post MJD, ed.. *Radiologic Evaluation of the Spine.* New York: Masson Publishing, 1980.
20. Rohen JW, Yokochi C, Lutjen-Drecoll E. *Color atlas of anatomy: a photographic study of the human body.* Baltimore: Lippincott Williams & Wilkins, 2006.
21. Kirshblum S, Campagnolo DI, DeLisa JA. *Spinal cord medicine.* Philadelphia: Lippincott Williams & Wilkins, 2002.

CHAPTER 4 ■ IMAGING OF THE SPINE AND SPINAL CORD

JOAQUIM FARINHAS, ABHISHEK SRINIVAS, EDWIN GULKO, AND JACQUELINE BELLO

EPIDEMIOLOGY

An estimated 12,000 new cases of paraplegia and quadriplegia occur in the United States each year as a result of spinal cord injury (SCI) (1,2). Preexisting spinal conditions may exacerbate or predispose the patient to injury (1). Cervical spondylosis is the most common preexisting abnormality of the spinal column in SCI patients, with prevalence as high as 10% in some series (3). Spinal cord trauma may be superimposed on and exacerbated by the presence of congenital abnormalities, such as atlantoaxial instability, congenital fusions, or tethered cord and may also occur in the presence of acquired disorders such as metastatic disease, spinal arthropathies such as ankylosing spondylitis, or rheumatoid arthritis. Typically, injuries are worsened or occur with a greater frequency in the face of these associated conditions and, in some cases, may not have occurred had the associated anomaly not been present.

GENERAL IMAGING CONSIDERATIONS

In the setting of spine trauma, the role of imaging is to describe the normal anatomy of the spine. It is crucial to define the anatomic extent of trauma, by compartment, in order to best tailor treatment. The evaluation of potential associated trauma (e.g., vascular) is critical to management.

This chapter defines normal anatomy by extradural, intradural extramedullary, and intramedullary compartments. It further reviews various imaging modalities appropriate for each compartment. An understanding of spine anatomy and available imaging modalities helps the clinician appropriately triage trauma patients. Advanced imaging techniques such as high-resolution MRI, diffusion-weighted imaging (DWI), diffusion-tensor imaging (DTI), functional MRI (fMRI), and MR spectroscopy are introduced, and potential for future applications are discussed.

There are advantages and disadvantages to each imaging modality. X-ray and computed tomography (CT) are widely available and provide excellent bony detail. Rapid acquisition and reconstruction algorithms have promoted CT application to the emergency setting. Both CT and x-ray utilize ionizing radiation, an important consideration given the current awareness of cumulative radiation dose in the patient population. Potentially unstable trauma patients undergoing CT and x-ray exams are easily monitored. Although CT offers greater spatial resolution than MRI, contrast resolution is superior in MRI. The various spinal soft tissue structures are characterized by unique signal intensity. Based on this, subtle bone marrow pathology is best imaged by MRI. With respect to allergy, MR contrast agents (gadolinium-based) are better tolerated than iodinated contrast used in radiographic studies (4). In patients with renal insufficiency, gadolinium-based agents have very rarely been shown to result in nephrogenic systemic fibrosis (NSF). The FDA recommends caution to patients with moderate to end-stage renal disease (stage 4 or 5) as well as consideration of hemodialysis treatment immediately after administration of these agents in patients with chronic renal disease (5). Due to magnetic fields used in generating MR images, MR safety is of paramount importance, and precautions must be taken. Numerous resources are available delineating relative and absolute contraindications to MRI, including a more exhaustive discussion regarding NSF (5).

The clinical utility of MR contrast agents in acute trauma has not been shown (6), and case reports show that the use of gadolinium is not fully justified in the setting of acute SCI (7). Using gadolinium in MR angiography is rarely necessary in acute injury if the goal is to examine vessels for dissection or other trauma. In these cases, noncontrast MRI sequences such as 2D time-of-flight and phase-contrast sequences can provide sufficient information regarding vascular anatomy without the use of gadolinium (6).

Extradural Compartment

Anatomy

The extradural compartment of the spine includes bony vertebrae, the intervening intervertebral discs, and the ligamentous support system. Structures that often are overlooked but sometimes clinically relevant include the epidural venous plexus, segmental arteries, and epidural fat.

The vertebrae are composed of load-bearing vertebral bodies and the vertebral arch. The outer shell of the vertebral bodies is composed of hard, compact cortical bone. The inner core contains cancellous bone, marrow, and fat. The vertebral, or neural, arch is mostly composed of compact bone and protects the contents of the spinal canal. Each arch has paired pedicles, laminae, superior and inferior facets, transverse processes, and spinous processes. The characteristics of the vertebrae vary depending on their cervical, thoracic, or lumbar location (8).

The cervical spine is composed of seven vertebrae, of which two are particularly unique—the atlas (C1) and the axis (C2). The first cervical vertebra, the atlas, has no vertebral body but instead has an anterior arch connecting to the two lateral masses and a posterior arch. The central vertebral foramen of C1 is composed of a smaller anterior portion, which receives the dens of C2, and a larger posterior portion, which transmits the spinal cord and the meninges (Fig. 4.1).

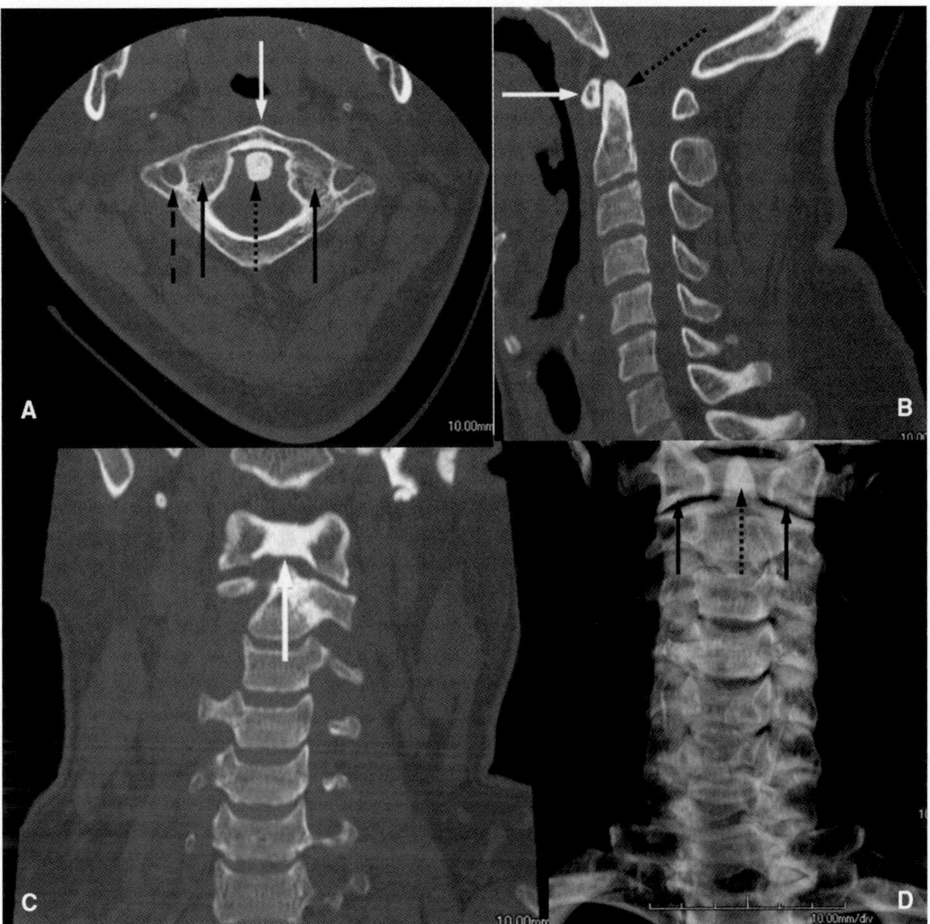

FIGURE 4.1. Axial (**A**), sagittal (**B**), coronal (**C**), and 3D (**D**) CT images of the normal bony landmarks of C1 and C2 including the lateral masses of C1 (*solid black arrows* in **A** and **D**), tip of the dens (*dotted black arrow* in **A**, **B**, and **D**), right vertebral foramen (*dashed black arrow* in **A**), and the anterior arch of C1 (*solid white arrow* in **B** and **C**).

The second cervical vertebra, the axis, is also unique with its bony projection, the dens (odontoid), arising from the vertebral body. The relationship between the axis and the atlas allows for rotational movements of the head. Also unique to the cervical spine is the presence of foramena in their transverse processes (transverse foramen or foramen transversarium), which contain the vertebral artery and vein (both entering at approximately C6) and the sympathetic plexus (Fig. 4.2).

The thoracic and lumbar vertebrae differ in their size and in their lack of transverse foramen. The thoracic vertebrae also articulate with the ribs (8) (Fig. 4.3).

The extradural compartment also includes the intervertebral discs, composed of a cartilaginous endplate, a nucleus pulposus, and an annulus fibrosis. The annulus fibrosus surrounds the nucleus pulposus and merges with the anterior and posterior longitudinal ligaments along the anterior and posterior aspects of the vertebrae. Protrusions, bulges, and herniations of the intervertebral discs may cause epidural mass effect as sequelae of trauma.

Imaging Considerations

A variety of imaging modalities are used to image the extradural compartment. The choice of modality is directed by the target tissue being evaluated for injury.

Plain Film Radiography. Due to its portability, rapidity, and accessibility, plain film radiography plays an important role in the evaluation of spine trauma. The limitations of plain film are related to technique, including issues with patient positioning and poor visualization of the craniocervical and cervicothoracic junctions. Plain film radiography is often the initial exam for the evaluation of cervical spine trauma. While the advent of multislice, rapid CT scanning may change this landscape, radiation dose remains an important consideration.

In cervical spine trauma, plain film radiography still plays a role in the evaluation of bony injury, alignment, stability during flexion and extension. Traumatic subluxations and rotational injuries are evaluated by assessing the alignment of the spinous processes (8). Appropriateness criteria for plain film radiography of the posttraumatic cervical spine have been set forth by the American College of Radiology (9):

a. Asymptomatic and alert, no cervical tenderness, no neurologic findings, no distracting injury, with or without cervical collar
   Exam: No imaging necessary
b. Alert, cervical tenderness, no neurologic findings, no distracting injury
   Exam: AP, lateral, and open-mouth radiographs

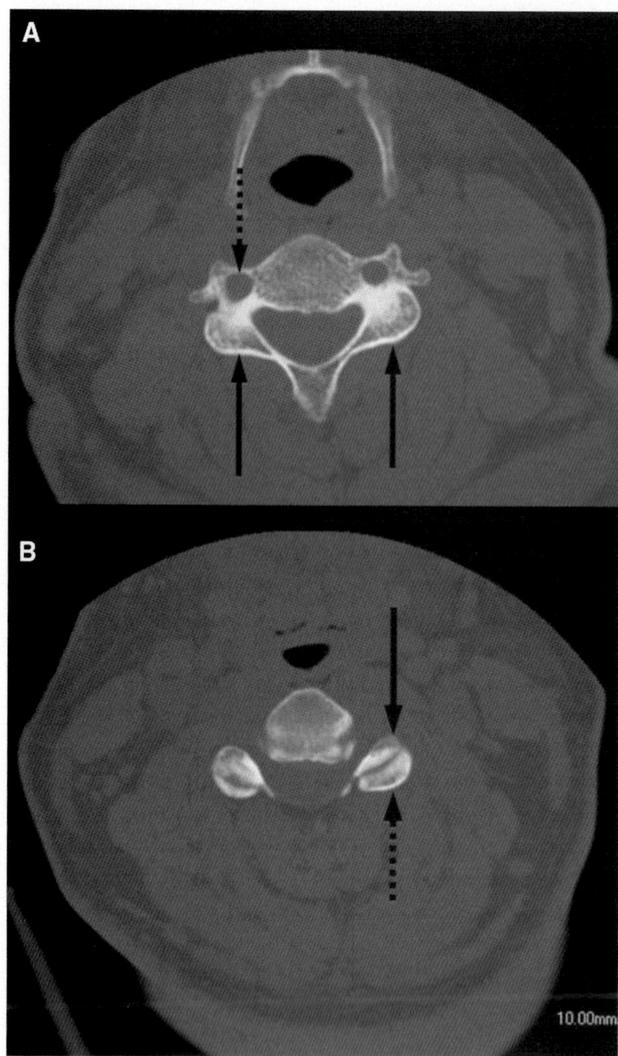

FIGURE 4.2. Axial (A) CT image of a normal midcervical vertebral body demonstrates the articular pillars (*solid black arrows*) and the right vertebral foramen (*dashed black arrow*). Axial CT (B) image of a normal midcervical vertebral body demonstrates the left superior (*solid black arrow*) and inferior (*dashed black arrow*) articular processes.

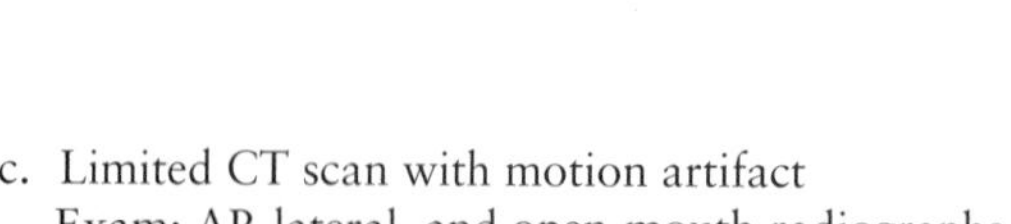

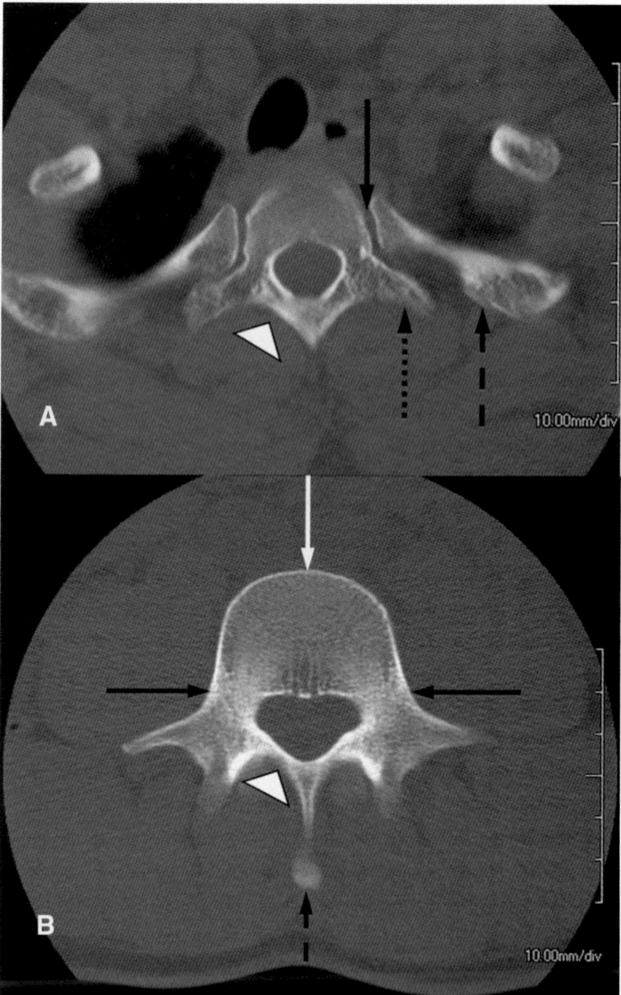

FIGURE 4.3. (A) Axial CT image of a normal upper thoracic vertebral body demonstrates the left transverse process (*dotted black arrow*), articular facet for the head of rib (*solid black arrow*), lamina (*arrowhead*) and a left rib tubercle (*dashed black arrow*). (B) Axial CT image of a normal lumbar vertebral body (*solid white arrow*) demonstrates the pedicles (*solid black arrows*), lamina (*arrowhead*) and spinous process (*dashed black arrow*).

c. Limited CT scan with motion artifact
   Exam: AP, lateral, and open-mouth radiographs

For thoracolumbar injuries, plain film radiography has similar value: additional oblique views provide a means to assess spondylolysis.

Computed Tomography. Although more costly and less accessible than plain film worldwide, CT evaluation of the spine plays an important role in certain patient populations due to its multislice capability allowing 2D and 3D reconstructions. The use of portable CT scanners is evolving in the intensive care setting. A retrospective review of plain films and CT scans in the detection of fractures was performed by Woodring and Lee. In their study, 216 patients with cervical spine fractures, they determined prospectively that plain film radiography did not detect fractures in 23% of patients and that the cervical spine injuries were unstable in 50% of cases (11).

A meta-analysis by Holmes et al. (12) further suggested that CT is superior to radiographs in the evaluation of patients at high risk for cervical injury. According to Hoffman et al. (13), such patients can be identified by a thorough physical exam. In an effort to show the utility of the physical exam in accurately stratifying which patients required imaging of the cervical spine, Hoffman et al. (13) conducted a prospective, multicenter study involving 34,069 patients. Patients were classified as having low probability of cervical injury by meeting fives rule of inclusion criteria: no midline cervical tenderness, no focal neurologic deficit, normal alertness, no intoxication, and no painful distracting injury. Their results showed that physical examination was 99% sensitive and 12.9% specific in identifying patients with cervical injury by radiography. Regardless, the two main considerations in evaluating patients with suspected cervical injury are identification of fracture(s) and assessment of spinal stability.

Appropriateness criteria for CT of the posttraumatic cervical spine have been set forth by the American College of Radiology (9):

a. Alert, cervical tenderness, paresthesias in hands/feet
   Exam: Screening CT of complete C-spine with sagittal and coronal reformatted images; MRI following CT, if indicated
b. Unconscious
   Exam: Screening CT C-spine with sagittal and coronal reformatted images
c. Impaired sensorium (including alcohol and/or drugs)
   Exam: Screening CT as above
d. Impaired sensorium and neurologic findings
   Exam: Screening CT as above; MRI following CT if indicated

Magnetic Resonance Imaging. While the bony aspects of spinal injury are best characterized by CT, MRI is complementary to CT in the evaluation of spinal ligaments and soft tissues (14). To evaluate the ligaments and the intervertebral discs within the extradural compartment, MRI is considered the best modality (6,8). Ligamentous injury can be assessed by plain film flexion and extension views; this protocol is generally safest performed 7 to 10 days after muscle spasm has subsided (6). The American College of Radiology published appropriateness criteria in 2007 stating that MRI should be the primary modality for evaluating possible spinal cord injury or compression as well as ligamentous injuries in acute cervical spine trauma (15). In patients who are medically unstable or have MRI-incompatible devices (pacemaker, ferromagnetic intracranial vascular clips, etc.), obtaining an MRI may not be feasible (10).

Adequate evaluation of the cervical, thoracic, and lumbar spine by MRI should include both fluid-sensitive and T1-weighted pulse sequences in axial and sagittal planes. A combination of gradient-recalled echo (GRE), fast spin-echo (FSE), short-Tau inversion recovery (STIR), or turbo spin-echo (TSE) sequences are used to cut down on imaging time without sacrificing image quality. Although additional sequences may result in more information, they require more time in the scanner for an acutely injured patient.

A sagittal T1-weighted sequence is obtained to identify anatomy (Fig. 4.4). On such a sequence, the cerebrospinal fluid (CSF) appears relatively hypointense (darker) to the spinal cord. The vertebral body marrow signal appears hyperintense (brighter) relative to the intervening normal discs due to normal bone marrow fat signal. The cortical margins of the vertebrae appear low in signal due to dense cortical bone and are difficult to distinguish from the hypointense longitudinal ligaments along the anterior and posterior margins. Epidural fat is bright in signal.

A sagittal T2-weighted sequence with fat suppression is obtained to evaluate spinal cord injury, ligamentous injury, and disk herniations (Fig. 4.5). In such a sequence, CSF appears bright in signal relative to the spinal cord. The vertebral bodies and the marrow-containing structures will look hypointense compared to an image without fat saturation. This sequence excels in demonstrating inflammation and reactive fluid accumulation within soft tissue structures and between ligaments. In fluid-sensitive sequences, the contrast between the CSF within the dural sac, apposed to the ligaments, makes identification of the longitudinal ligaments possible. Axial T2-weighted sequences further help to characterize the spinal cord parenchyma. Axial images are also important in evaluating the relationship of the disc to the neural elements. Signal void, due to flow, characterizes vascular structures.

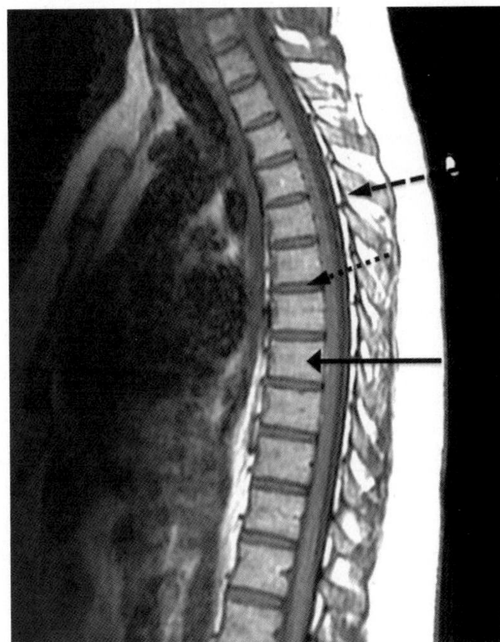

FIGURE 4.4. Sagittal T1-weighted MRI of the normal thoracic spine demonstrates the vertebral bodies (*solid arrow*) to be hyperintense relative to the intervertebral discs (*dotted arrow*) due to the marrow fat content and disc water content. Hypointense ligamentum flavum is illustrated (*dashed arrow*).

Gradient-echo sequences best demonstrate the susceptibility effect due to hemorrhage, resulting in the characteristic "blooming" artifact. This "blooming" artifact is defined as dark signal within areas of hemorrhage, secondary to magnetic susceptibility caused by the presence of hemosiderin, a product of blood breakdown. Bony fractures may sometimes appear more evident on GRE images if blood products are

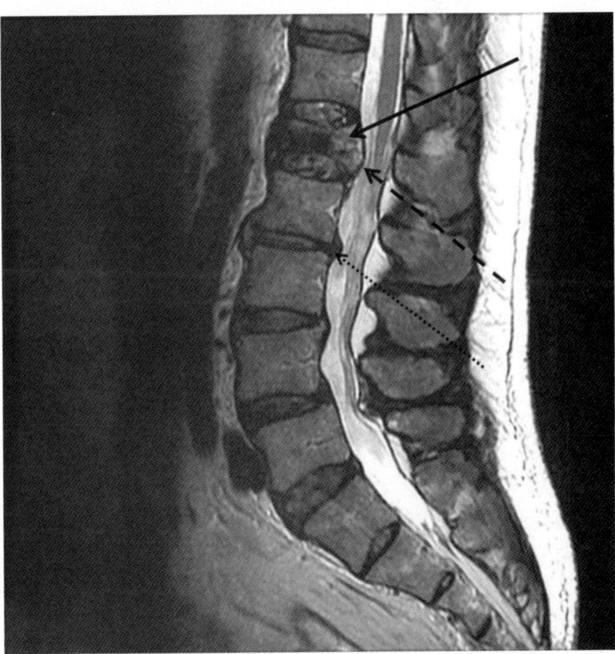

FIGURE 4.5. Sagittal T2-weighted MRI of the lumbar spine shows a compression fracture of L1 (*solid arrow*). Retropulsion of bony elements into the spinal canal displaces PLL (*dashed arrow*). Incidental L2–3 degenerative disk bulge is seen (*dotted arrow*).

present. GRE sequences can also demonstrate flow-related signal in arteries and veins. Edema in the setting of acute fracture is best demonstrated on the fluid-sensitive sequences.

In cases of cervical spine trauma, evaluation of the vertebral vessels is warranted to exclude dissection or occlusion. In such cases, noncontrast techniques such as time-of-flight or phase-contrast MR angiography provides this information noninvasively.

Extradural Injury

Atlanto-occipital Dislocation. Atlanto-occipital dislocation (AOD), caused by flexion, extension, or distraction injuries, may result in instant death, due to compression of the cardiovascular and respiratory centers of the medulla. The number of cases presenting to hospitals has increased in the last two decades due to improved emergency management (16). In the pediatric population, an increased prevalence of atlanto-occipital dislocations is attributable, in part, to injury sustained during airbag deployment (17). In AODs, the occipital condyles are distracted anteriorly, away from the superior articular surface of the atlas. The opisthion of the formen magnum is forced forward from its normal location (a line drawn vertically from the spinolaminar junction of the atlas). In addition, the basion is distracted anterior to the dens.

Multiple diagnostic techniques can be applied to the lateral cervical x-ray in the evaluation of AOD. However, a study by Harris et al. (18) found the basion-axial interval-basion-dental interval (BAI-BDI) measurement to be 100% sensitive. To measure the BAI, a line is drawn along the posterior border of the C2 anterior arch extending superiorly. A second line, which should not exceed 12 mm, is drawn perpendicular to the first toward the basion. The BDI is measured from the basion to the tip of the odontoid process and should also not exceed 12 mm (18,19) (Fig. 4.6). Currently, the BAI-BDI is the preferred method in evaluating for AOD (20). While ominous signs of AOD may not be present on plain radiographs (21), the index of suspicion is raised by the identification of prevertebral soft tissue swelling (22), or by subarachnoid hemorrhage at the craniocervical junction on CT (23) (see Chapter 7 for more on AOD).

Several studies highlight the utility of using CT and MR imaging in patients with clinically suspected AOD in the setting of normal lateral cervical x-ray. In a retrospective study of 33 patients with AOD, Horn et al. (24) developed a grading scale and treatment algorithm based on various CT and MR findings. Grade I patients, requiring external orthosis stabilization, have normal CT scans and moderate MRI findings consisting of high signal in posterior vertebral ligaments. Grade II patients, requiring spinal fixation, had one or more abnormal CT findings, or grossly abnormal MRI findings involving the occipitoatlantal joints, tectorial membrane, alar ligaments, or cruciate ligaments.

Jefferson Fracture. A Jefferson fracture, due to axial loading, compresses the C1 lateral masses between the occipital condyles and the articular facets of C2. This drives the lateral masses of C1 apart, causing fractures of its anterior and posterior arches. Fractures may be unilateral or bilateral, consisting of two to four fracture fragments. Common mechanisms of injury include diving into a shallow pool or a direct blow to the top of the head. Since fragments are expelled outward and away from the spinal cord, Jefferson fracture does not typically cause neurologic deficit if the transverse ligament remains intact (25). However, cases of neurologic impairment have been noted (26). Open-mouth radiographs can be used to diagnose Jefferson fracture; however, overestimation of lateral displacement may occur from magnification artifact Heller et al. (27). CT-reformatted coronal images at the level of the C1 lateral masses are recommended (20) (see Fig. 4.1D). To assess for Jefferson fracture, vertical lines are drawn at the lateral aspects of the C1 and C2 articular processes. The transverse distance between the two lines is measured bilaterally. The sum of the distances is noted as the total lateral mass displacement (20) (Fig. 4.7).

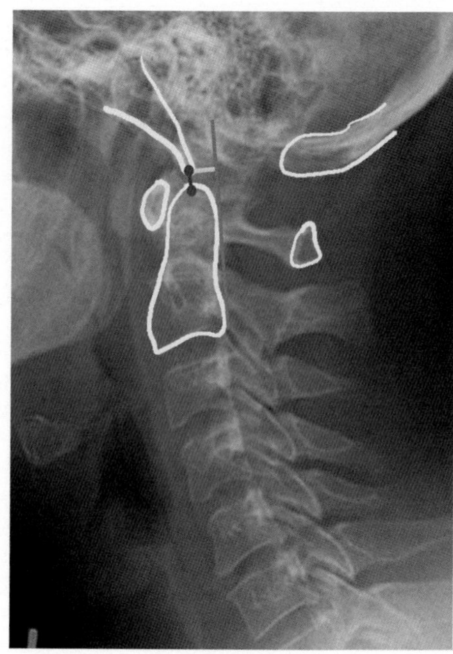

FIGURE 4.6. For measurement of BAI, a line is drawn along the posterior border of the C2 anterior arch extending superiorly (*red line*). A second line, which should not exceed 12 mm, is drawn perpendicular to the first towards the basion (*green line*). The BDI is measured from the basion to the tip of the odontoid process, and should also not exceed 12 mm (*blue line*).

Stable Jefferson fractures are almost always treated conservatively with external immobilization, and subsequent radiological follow-up imaging with dynamic flexion and extension to confirm proper fusion (29). More aggressive measures of treating a Jefferson fracture hinge on the degree of lateral displacement or instability. Levine et al. advocated for halo traction if there is 5-mm lateral displacement (30), while Spence et al. suggested surgical stabilization if displacement reached 6.9 mm (31). Disruption of the transverse atlantal ligament suggests instability of the atlas that is best seen on MRI as loss of ligamentous continuity and high signal intensity (31).

Odontoid Fractures. Odontoid fractures, accounting for roughly 55% of axis fractures (32), may result from flexion, extension, or rotational forces. Odontoid fractures are classified based on the Anderson and D'Alonzo scheme (33). Type I fractures, exceedingly rare, involve the tip of the odontoid process and are stable. Type II fractures, the most common, extend through the base of the odontoid process, are unstable, and are complicated by nonunion in roughly one third of cases (34). Type III fractures, also stable, involve the body

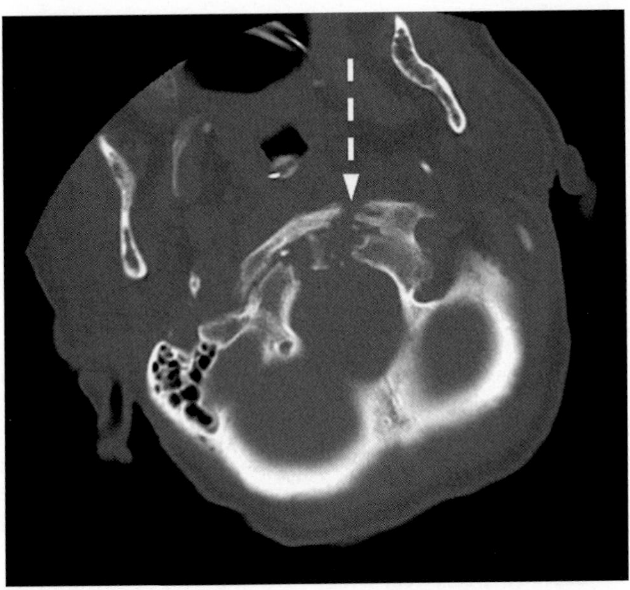

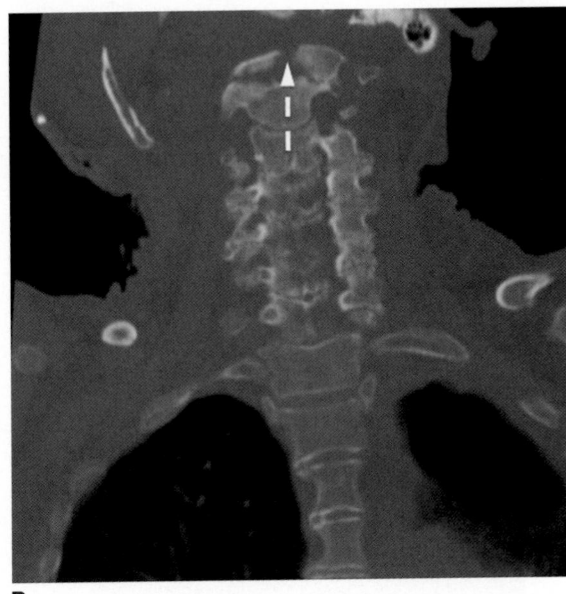

FIGURE 4.7. Axial (**A**) and coronal (**B**) CT images demonstrate a Jefferson burst fracture secondary to an axial loading injury. The fracture involves the left lateral ring of C1 (*dashed white arrow*).

of C2. Type I and Type III fractures heal spontaneously. Type II fractures at greater risk for nonunion more frequently requires surgical intervention. (See Chapter 7 for more on Type II fractures.)

In the sagittal plane, two measurements are used to evaluate odontoid fractures: fracture displacement and fracture angulation. Fracture displacement is the distance between parallel lines along the anterior border of the odontoid fragment and that of the C2 body. Fracture angulation is the angle formed by two intersecting lines: one extending inferiorly from the posterior border of the odontoid fragment and one line extending superiorly from the posterior border of the C2 body. Risk factors for Type II nonunion are initial displacement >4 mm and fracture angulation greater than 10 degrees (34).

In patients with odontoid fractures, male sex and high-velocity injury are factors associated with a higher incidence of SCI. Displacement of the odontoid fragment does not impact the likelihood of neurologic impairment (35). Patients with rheumatoid arthritis are predisposed to odontoid fractures and warrant careful evaluation in the setting of trauma (36).

Hangman's Fracture. Traumatic spondylolisthesis of the axis, known as "hangman's fracture," involves bilateral fractures through the pars interarticularis of C2. Forces tear the C2 neural arch away from its vertebral body, while the odontoid process remains intact. Common mechanisms include deceleration injuries with head impact, resulting in hyperextension and axial compression. This differs from injury incurred by hanging, which results in bilateral pedicle fractures of the C2 and complete disruption of the disc and the ligaments between C2 and C3.

These fractures have been classified by Effendi et al. (37) based on radiological findings. In Type I fractures, which are stable, the body of C2 is minimally displaced (less than 2 to 3 mm), nonangulated, and the C2/3 intervertebral disc is normal. Type II fractures involve anterior displacement of the C2 vertebral body and C2/3 disc disruption. Type III fractures result in anterior displacement of the C2 body concurrent with unilateral or bilateral C2/3 facet dislocation. Type II and III fractures are unstable, complicated by rebound hyperflexion following the initial hyperextension event. Levine et al. (38) modified the Effendi classification to subdivide Type II fractures into Type II and Type IIa. Type II fractures typically result from hyperextension and axial loading, whereas Type IIa fractures are caused by flexion and distraction. Traction used for Type II injuries could cause further distraction for a Type IIa injury (38). Currently, both Effendi Type I and Levine-Edwards Type II fractures are treated with traction and external immobilization. Levine-Edwards Type IIa and Type III fractures require rigid immobilization (39).

Evaluation of hangman's fracture is best performed by lateral cervical radiography or sagittal CT reconstruction (20). Anterior displacement of the axis is measured as the distance between two parallel lines drawn vertically from the posterior bodies of the C2 and C3 vertebrae. Angulation is calculated as the angle created by two lines extending from the inferior aspects of the C2 and C3 vertebral bodies (27).

Atlantoaxial Instability. Atlantoaxial instability results from a variety of entities causing subluxation of the atlas on the axis, rotary atlantoaxial dislocation, disruption of atlantoaxial ligaments, fracture of the odontoid process, or Jefferson fracture. The C1/2 instability may cause the dens to move posteriorly, narrowing the spinal canal with potential for cord compression. It may be secondary to hyperflexion trauma, Paget disease (40), Down syndrome (41), or inflammatory conditions affecting the synovium such as rheumatoid arthritis (42).

In the setting of trauma, the atlanto-dens interval (ADI) and posterior atlanto-dens interval (PADI) are commonly used to evaluate cervical stability. However, the reliability of ADI-PADI measurements was questioned by the Spine Trauma Study Group (20). ADI is measured as the distance between the posterior border of the anterior arch of C1 and the anterior margin of the odontoid process. It should not exceed 3 mm in normal adults (43) or 5 mm in children (44). PADI is measured as the distance between the posterior margin of the

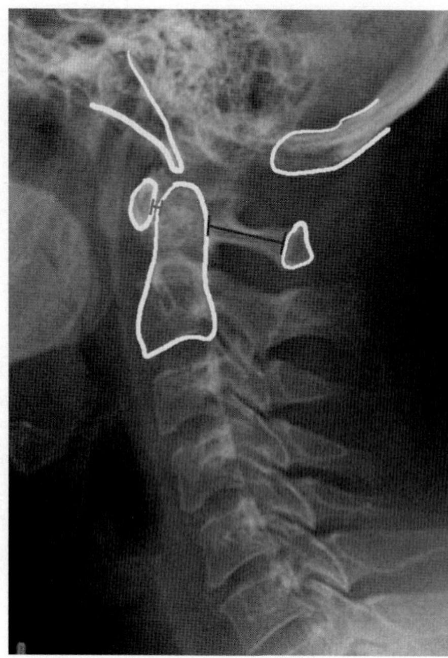

FIGURE 4.8. ADI is measured as the distance between the posterior border of the anterior arch of C1 and the anterior margin of the odontoid process (*red line*). It should not exceed 3 mm in normal adults (43) or 5 mm in children (44). PADI is measured as the distance between the posterior margin of the odontoid process to the anterior border of the posterior arch of C1 (*blue line*).

odontoid process to the anterior border of the posterior arch of C1 (Fig. 4.8).

Trauma to the Middle and Lower Cervical Spine. The subaxial cervical spine extends from C3 to C7. Due to its distinct anatomy, it is subject to different mechanisms of injury. The majority of cervical fractures and dislocations occur in the subaxial spine. Numerous classifications of subaxial cervical injury exist; no single classification is exclusively used clinically (45,46). The Subaxial Cervical Spine Injury Classification system (47) classifies subaxial cervical injuries according to neurologic status, disc-ligament-capsule complex, and morphology: compression, distraction, or translation/rotation.

Wedge Compression Fractures. These fractures due to axial loading or hyperflexion injury to the anterior vertebral body result in decreased height and destruction of the superior endplate with preservation of the inferior endplate. Most cervical compression fractures are stable; however, if axial loading is distributed evenly throughout the vertebral body, burst, lamina, and facet fractures may occur, increasing the risk of spinal instability and cord compression. The degree of compression and cervical kyphosis can be assessed using a Cobb angle measurement (48).

Flexion Teardrop Fractures. The most severe and unstable injury of the subaxial spine, the flexion teardrop fracture is a hyperflexion, axial loading injury that results in complete tearing of the anterior and posterior longitudinal ligaments. Injuries often result from diving, motor vehicle accidents, and falls. The injury produces a triangular fragment from the anterior-inferior aspect of the vertebral body, and displaces the posterior fragment toward the spinal cord causing an anterior cord syndrome with severe neurologic deficit. It is adequately seen on a lateral radiograph (49). The most common level involved is C5.

Bilateral Facet Dislocation (Perched Facets). In a flexion injury with forceful anterior subluxation, the inferior facet(s) may dislocate forward relative to the superior facets of the subjacent vertebra. Bilateral facet dislocation implies disruption of the anterior longitudinal ligament, posterior longitudinal ligament, and facet capsules (50) (Fig. 4.9). In addition, disk herniations are common (52). Among the posterior elements, the facet joints are the most critical in providing cervical stability (51). Bilateral facet dislocation frequently causes spinal instability and neurologic injury (47). The "hamburger bun" and "reverse hamburger bun" signs have been described in diagnosing facet dislocations by axial CT (53). Normally, articular facets join together to resemble two halves of a "hamburger bun," readily seen on axial CT. With facet dislocation, the halves are reversed, with convex surfaces apposed, hence the "reverse hamburger bun" sign.

Clay-Shoveler's Fracture. Named for occupational workers who shoveled heavy loads for long periods of time, this injury is an avulsion fracture of the spinous process of C6, C7, or T1. The fracture does not breach the spinolaminar junction and is stable (54). Rarely, if the fracture extends beyond the spinolaminar line, neurologic insult may result. Clay shoveler's fractures are easily visualized on a lateral radiograph, with a characteristic oblique fracture line through the spinous process (55) (Fig. 4.10). Evidence also suggests that CT imaging is superior to MRI in evaluating fractures of the cervical spine posterior elements (56).

Hyperflexion Sprain Injuries. Hyperflexion sprain injuries (anterior subluxation) result from exaggerated cervical flexion with disruption of the ligamentum flavum, supraspinous ligament, interspinous ligament, and joint capsules. Usually, the anterior longitudinal ligament is not torn. Radiologic findings include abnormal cervical kyphosis, widening of the involved interspinous space, and horizontal displacement of the subluxed vertebral body (46).

Thoracolumbar Trauma and Imaging. Most classification systems that describe fractures of the thoracolumbar spine are based on mechanism of injury, fracture pattern, or stability. However, The Three-Column Spine Concept, developed by Denis et al. (57), has gained acceptance for its simplicity and ability to predict fracture stability. The spine is divided into anterior, middle, and posterior columns. The anterior column consists of the anterior longitudinal ligament, the anterior half of the vertebral body, and the anterior disc annulus. The middle column includes the posterior half of the vertebral body, the posterior longitudinal ligament, and the posterior annulus fibrosus. The posterior column incorporates the pedicles, facets, ligamentum flavum, lamina, spinous processes, interspinous and supraspinous ligaments.

Thoracolumbar injuries involving only one column are mechanically stable. More severe injuries involving two or three columns, or with clinical neurologic signs are unstable (55,58). In a study involving 16 fresh cadavers, Panjabi et al. (59) validated the three-column theory using a high-speed

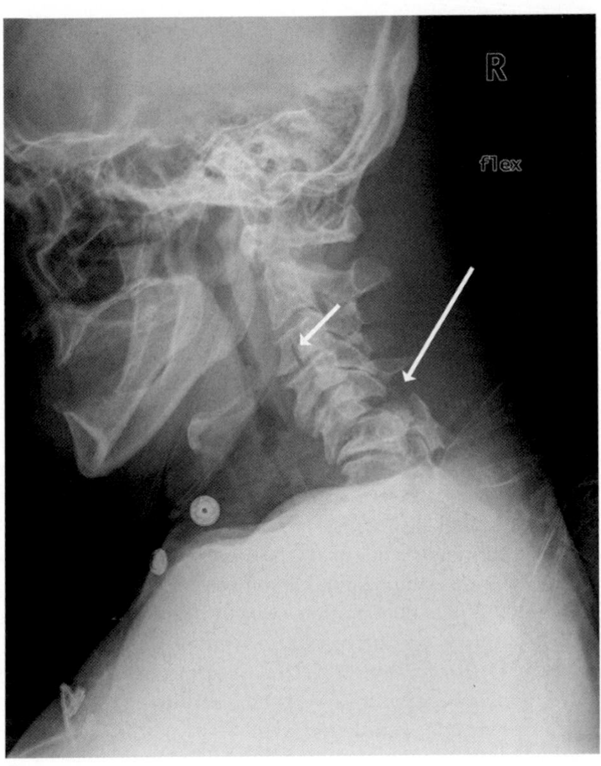

A

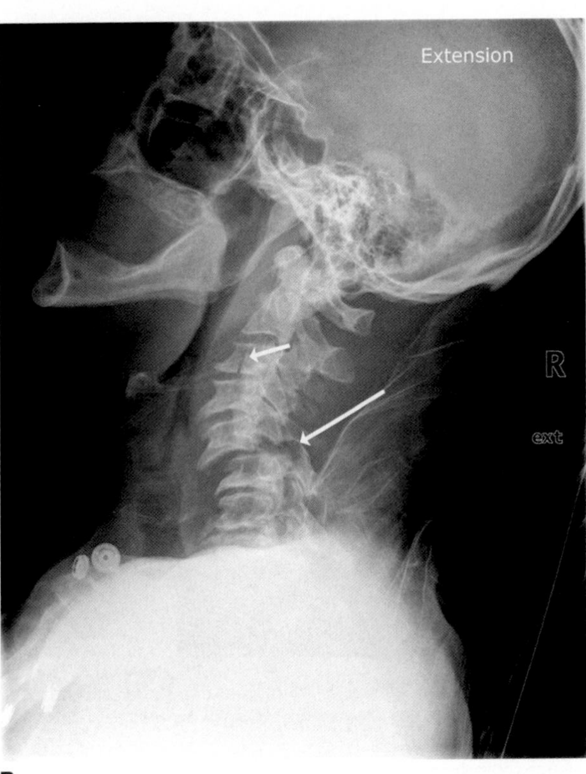

B

FIGURE 4.9. Lateral plain films of the cervical spine in flexion (A) and extension (B) demonstrate post-traumatic dislocation of the C5 facets causing anterior subluxation of the vertebral body (*long white arrow*). A vertical fracture through the anterior C3 vertebra is also seen (*short white arrow*).

trauma model. Their results supported the three-column theory and suggested that the middle column is most critical to thoracolumbar spine stability.

Hyperflexion/Compression Injury. Hyperflexion injuries account for the majority of thoracolumbar spine fractures. They result from falls in young healthy adults or in elderly patients with osteoporosis. The vertical force vector is transmitted through the nucleus pulposus during impact in a lumbar-flexed position. Consequently, the anterior vertebral body buckles, producing the common compression fracture. One or more vertebrae may be involved. There is typically less than 50% loss of vertebral body height, and the middle and posterior columns remain intact. This is a stable injury.

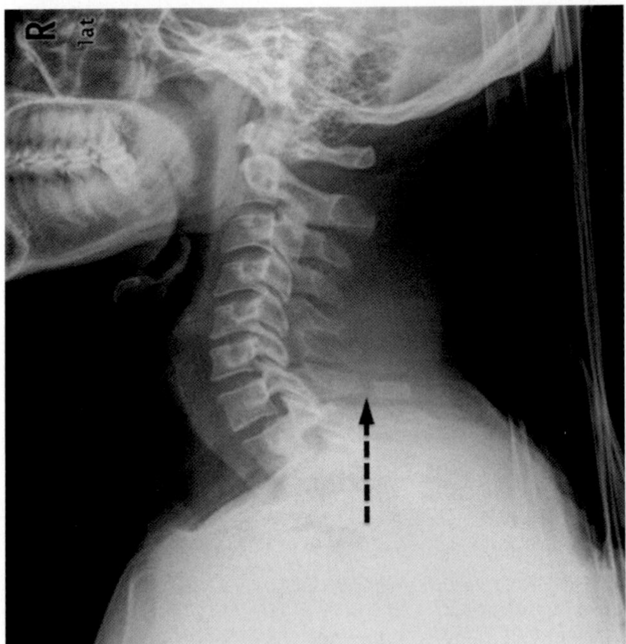

FIGURE 4.10. Lateral plain film of the cervical spine demonstrates an avulsion fracture of the C7 spinous process due to a "clay-shoveler's" fracture (*dashed black arrow*).

Flexion injuries with distraction are common among individuals involved in decelerating motor vehicle accidents while wearing a lap seatbelt, as opposed to three-point seatbelts with shoulder harness. The lap belt serves as the axis of rotation as the lower spine remains fixed, and the upper spine moves anteriorly. The result is a horizontal fracture extending from the spinous process to the vertebral body, known as the "Chance fracture" (Fig. 4.11) (60).

Traumatic kyphosis from hyperflexion injury can be estimated with the Cobb angle. The magnitude of compression can be evaluated measuring the ratio of the anterior vertebral height to the posterior vertebral height (61).

Assessment of the middle and posterior column integrity, which determine fracture stability, will influence clinical management. CT is superior to radiographs for this purpose (62). MRI best demonstrates posterior ligamentous injury, a sign of injury to the posterior column (63,64). Fat-suppressed T2-weighted images are sensitive and specific in evaluating injuries to posterior spinal ligaments (65) as well as in determining the acuity of a compression fracture.

Axial Load Injury. Axial load injuries due to vertical compression evenly distributed through the vertebral body result in a burst fracture with radial expulsion of fragments (Fig. 4.12).

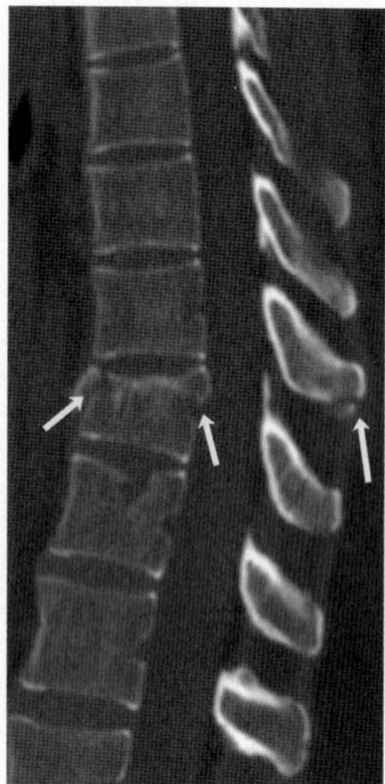

FIGURE 4.11. Chance fracture is a horizontal fracture extending from the spinous process to the vertebral body (*solid white arrows*).

Distinct from hyperflexion/compression injuries, axial load injuries commonly occur at the thoracolumbar junction, T12 and L1. Retropulsion of posterior vertebral body fragments into the spinal canal is common. Loss of vertebral body height is usually greater that 50%, both anteriorly and posteriorly. The posterior column is rarely affected. (See Chapter 7 for more imaging.)

Radiographic features of instability include widened interspinous and interlaminar distances, kyphosis greater than 20 degrees, dislocation, vertebral body height loss greater than 50%, and articular process fractures (55). The posterior border of the vertebral body is normally concave on axial CT. Subtle fracture may be diagnosed if the posterior wall appears flattened or protrudes into the spinal canal. Recently, the "reverse cortical sign" has been used to describe thoracolumbar burst fractures (66). This sign refers to the posterior fragment from a burst fracture, flipped 180 degrees, with its cancellous surface facing the spinal canal and its smooth, cortical surface facing anteriorly. The literature is conflicted as to whether the degree of spinal stenosis from a burst fracture correlates with degree of neurologic injury (67–69).

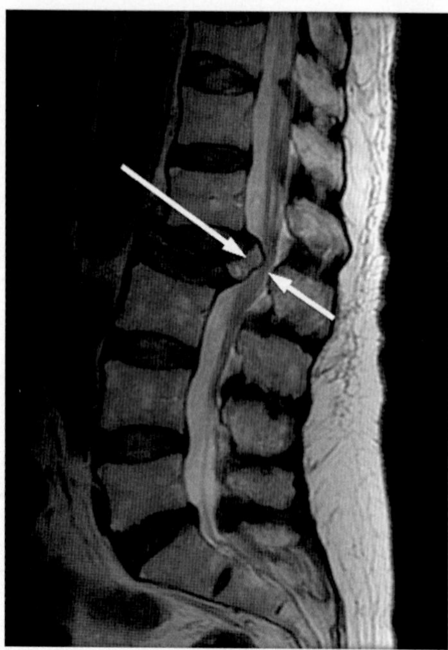

FIGURE 4.12. Sagittal T2-weighted MRI demonstrates compression fracture of L2 due to axial loading with retropulsion of bony fragment (*long white arrow*) causing severe spinal canal stenosis and cauda equina compression (*short white arrow*) in a patient status post fall, with bilateral leg weakness and perineal paresthesias.

Hyperextension Injury. Hyperextension injury results from traumatic forces to the spine causing exaggerated hyperextension. In an inverse pattern to hyperflexion injury, there is compression of the posterior elements with possible disruption of anterior spinal ligaments. The posterior column will appear grossly injured; the status of the anterior column and its ligaments will determine spinal stability. Rupture of the anterior longitudinal ligament confers spinal instability. In this setting, MRI is vital to properly visualize and assess the anterior longitudinal ligament and prevertebral soft tissue swelling. While rare, hyperextension injury poses a serious threat to patients with ankylosing spondylitis (Fig. 4.13) or diffuse idiopathic skeletal hyperostosis (70).

Shear Injury. Shear injury is caused by multidirectional force vectors with enormous kinetic energies with potential for

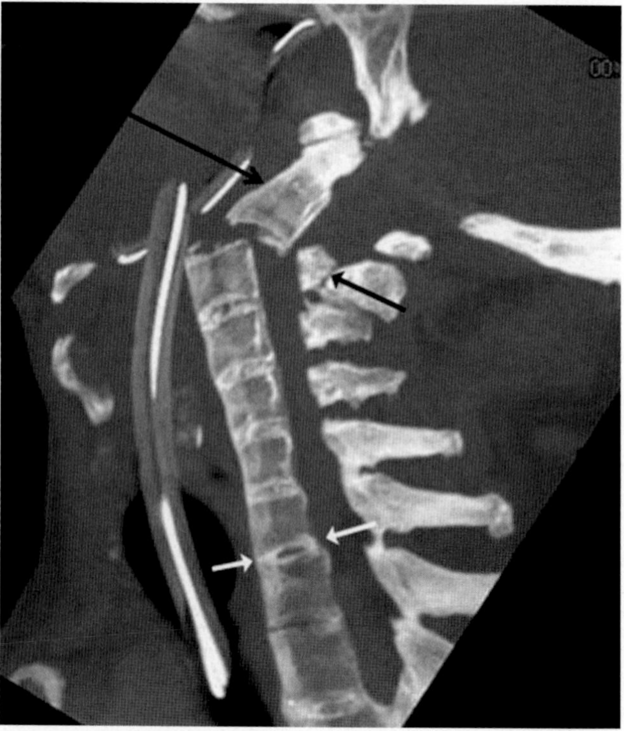

FIGURE 4.13. Sagittal reconstructed image, from a cervical spine CT in a patient with ankylosing spondylitis demonstrates fracture at the level of C2–3 with posterior displacement of C2 (*long black arrow*). A bone fragment (*short black arrow*) is seen within the spinal canal. Features of ankylosing spondylitis are present including syndesmophytes (*short white arrows*), fusing adjacent endplates creating a "bamboo spine" appearance.

disruption of all three spinal columns. Neurologic, thoracic, and abdominal injury is common. Thoracic ribs, articular facets, and transverse processes can be fractured.

Rotational Injuries. In combination with other injury that involve flexion and shearing, additional rotational force can cause asymmetric fractures of the vertebral body, articular facets, thoracic ribs, and transverse processes. The thoracolumbar spine is at risk for this injury due to greater mobility and laxity at the T12-L1 junction; patients with kyphoscoliosis or scoliosis carry additional risk (71). These fractures are unstable and cause neurologic deficit.

Sacral Fractures. Sacral fractures pose a significant challenge since they can easily be missed (72,73) and are associated with severe morbidity and neurologic sequelae. They result from high-velocity blunt trauma in healthy adults; insufficiency fractures occur in osteopenic elderly patients, metastatic disease, or in patients exposed to irradiation for pelvic malignancies (74). Sacral stress fractures may occur in runners (75–77).

Insufficiency fractures may result from low-impact trauma and present subacutely with low back pain, exacerbated by weight bearing and radiculopathy. Plain radiographs are usually inadequate to evaluate insufficiency fractures. In correlation with CT imaging, radionuclide bone scans are helpful in making the diagnosis. A characteristic "H-"shaped pattern is seen, representing symmetric bilateral radiotracer uptake in the upper sacrum (78,79). It is important to accurately and quickly diagnose sacral insufficiency fractures as they may benefit from minimally invasive treatment options (80).

The most widely accepted classification system for sacral fractures was developed by Denis et al. (81), after conducting a retrospective study of 39 cadavers and 236 patients with sacral fractures. Zone I fractures are lateral to the neural foramen near the region of the ala and occasionally damage the L5 nerve root. Zone II fractures involve the neural foramen but do not extend into the spinal canal; sciatica is often a presenting symptom. Zone III fractures extend into the central canal and are associated with saddle anesthesia, loss of sphincter tone, injury to the cauda equina, and neurogenic bladder. Zone III fractures are further subdivided into vertical or transverse fractures. Most sacral fractures are vertical, forming the basis for the Denis classification. Transverse fractures are rare but pose a serious threat of neurologic damage (82). They typically result from falls and have been called the "suicide jumper's fracture" (83).

Neurologic injury in patients with sacral fracture has been reported in 24% of zone I, 29% of zone II, 60% of vertical zone III, and 57% of transverse zone III fractures (84). Zone I and zone II fractures were found to cause unilateral lumbar or sacral radiculopathies. Zone III fractures caused more severe bilateral deficits with bowel and bladder incontinence.

It is recommended that all patients with suspected sacral trauma have standard AP radiographs of the pelvis as outlined by the Advanced Trauma Life Support Protocols. However, these imaging studies are difficult to interpret due to overlying bowel gas patterns, the anterior pelvis, and other negating factors (85). In addition, pelvic inlet and outlet radiographs are also recommended to better evaluate sacral anatomy and pelvic ring integrity.

The Spine Trauma Study Group recommends the use of coronal and sagittal reconstructed thin-sliced (1.0 to 1.5 mm) CT scans (85). Several metrics are considered when properly assessing the sacrum for trauma: anterior-posterior displacement, vertical translation, anterior-posterior translation, sagittal angulation, horizontal displacement, and spinal canal compromise. Axial CT scans with sagittal and coronal reconstructions are recommended.

Vascular Injury. The vertebral arteries, branches of the subclavian arteries, course superiorly to supply the intracranial posterior circulation as well as the spinal arteries. They enter the bony transverse foramina at the C6 level and proceed superiorly through each cervical vertebra to C1 (Fig. 4.14). This anatomy predisposes the vertebral arteries to direct injury from fractures including dissection, thrombosis, and rupture (86). A fracture through the transverse foramen may result in vertebral artery compression; the artery is also subject to stretching and tensile forces from traumatic cervical dislocations (87).

In a study of 26 patients with concomitant vertebral artery and bony cervical injury, 35% had thrombosis while 11% had dissection (88). Vertebral artery thrombosis (VAT) is highly associated with specific bony injuries such as facet dislocations and foramen fractures. One study reported that the majority of patients with vertebral artery injury on MRI/MRA were found to have unilateral facet dislocation (89). Angiography demonstrates vertebral artery injury in up to 40% of cervical subluxations (90). Early vascular intervention may prevent neurologic compromise making early diagnosis of the injury important. Cerebral angiography in patients with facet dislocations and transverse foramen fractures demonstrate the incidence of VAT to be as high as 75% and 88%, respectively (91). MRA demonstrated a lower incidence of association with 33% of foramen fractures (92).

Up to 85% of vertebral artery injuries are symptomatic. Symptoms include posterior neck pain, occipital headache, and neurologic deficit such as Wallenberg syndrome, Horner syndrome, or cerebellar signs (86). Spinal cord ischemia may also occur. Onset of symptoms may be delayed up to 1 week (93) making the initial trauma clinically occult (55).

The incidence of isolated vertebral artery injury in cervical spine trauma is unknown because patients are

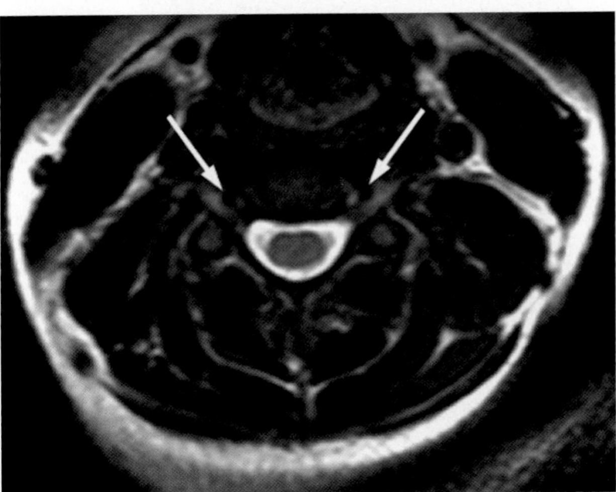

FIGURE 4.14. Axial T2-weighted MRI demonstrates signal void due to flow within vertebral arteries in the transverse foramina (*white arrows*).

usually asymptomatic (89). In a large retrospective review of 632 patients with nonpenetrating spine trauma, MRI and MRA demonstrated cervical spinal cord injury in nearly 60% of the patients with VAT (94). While VAT was more common in motor-complete (ASIA A,B) versus neurologically normal (ASIA E) patients, there was no difference in the incidence of VAT in motor-incomplete (ASIA C,D) patients compared to normal (ASIA E) patients. In a prospective series of patients admitted for blunt trauma, evaluated for vertebral artery injury with cerebral angiography (95), there was no relationship found between the grade of vertebral artery injury, neurologic deficit, and neurologic outcome. MRA of the vertebral arteries to exclude VAT after cord injury may be pertinent regardless of the neurologic examination.

In patients with suspected vascular injury, MRA/MRI is a reasonable first-line imaging modality (55,86). Catheter angiography has higher resolution, allowing for the detection of subtle arterial intimal injuries more readily than MRA, but is not always feasible (55).

In vertebral occlusion, axial MRI gradient-echo images may show hypointense clot compared to the normal flow-related signal enhancement. Alternatively, hyperintense subacute clot may be identified on T1-weighted, fat-suppressed images, compared to signal-void due to flow in the normal artery. MRA may show luminal narrowing, absence of the vessel, or absent flow distal to a dissection (Fig. 4.15). Black-blood imaging techniques (94,96) may be helpful in detection of subintimal dissection without occlusion. This technique

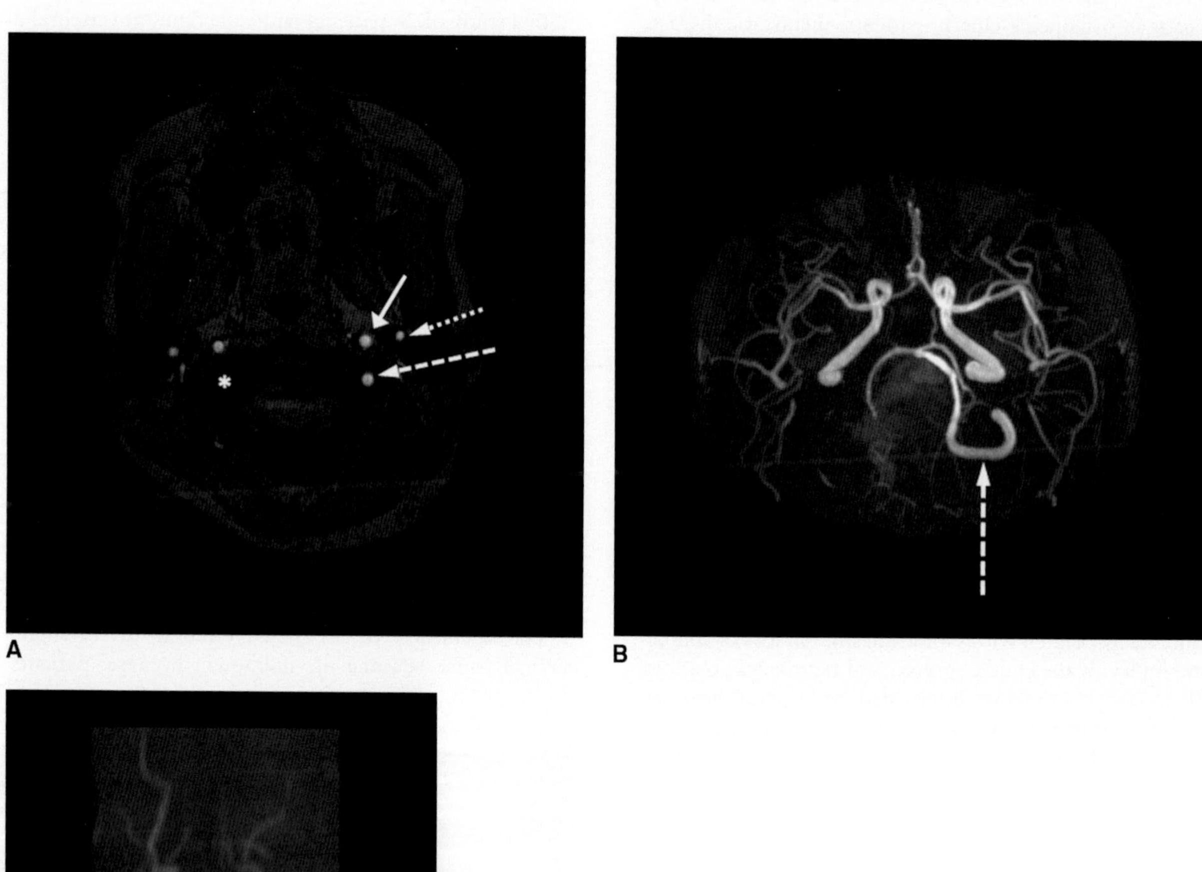

FIGURE 4.15. Axial MRA source image (**A**) demonstrates signal in the left internal carotid artery (*solid white arrow*), left external carotid artery (*dotted white arrow*), and left vertebral artery (*dashed white arrow*). There is absent signal in the expected location of the right vertebral artery (*white asterisk*). Reconstructed MRA images (**B,C**) of the vertebral arteries and Circle of Willis demonstrate normal left vertebral artery (*dashed white arrow*) and absence of the right vertebral artery. The patient is status-post trauma with severe dizziness, facial pain and left-sided numbness. Findings are compatible with a posttraumatic right vertebral artery dissection.

suppresses signal from flowing blood and surrounding tissues, causing it to appear low in signal, thus allowing distinction from high signal, subintimal clot. Follow-up imaging confirms healing (97).

Traumatic Disk Herniation. Traumatic intervertebral disc injury ranges from clinically insignificant disc bulge to disk herniation with potential for cord compression.

Prior to MRI, x-ray myelography and CT myelography were used to evaluate the relationship between an extruded disc and the thecal sac (Fig. 4.16). In patients with contraindication to MRI, CT myelography is still used in the trauma setting (55). With thin (0.625 mm) slices available on multidetector CT units, bony canal trauma and disk herniation can be demonstrated; however, disk herniation can be challenging on CT due to beam hardening artifact from adjacent bone and relatively poor tissue contrast between bone and disc tissue. MR imaging plays an important role in detecting these injuries due to its superior signal contrast between disc material and bone (10). Overall, traumatic cervical disk herniation is better evaluated by MRI than by CT or CT myelography (11,98–101).

Disk herniations are typically degenerative in the lumbar spine, while in the cervical and thoracic spine, they are more often traumatic. In thoracic injuries, up to 50% are associated with disk herniation (11). Flexion-compression and flexion-distraction injuries often result in cervical disk herniation (102). Cervical disk herniation can occur in 60% of hyperextension injuries, 47% of central cord injuries, and the majority of anterior cord injuries (99). The MRI appearance of posttraumatic and degenerative disk herniation is similar. In each case, T2 imaging demonstrates the higher signal nucleus pulposus pushed into the lower signal peripheral annulus fibrosus, which has fibers that merge with the PLL. When the nucleus pulposus extends beyond the annulus fibrosus, it compresses or distorts the ventral thecal sac. The actual tear in the annulus fibrosus allows extrusion of the nucleus pulposus resulting in cord or nerve root compression (Fig. 4.16).

In distinguishing acute disk herniation from degenerative or superimposed degenerative changes, evaluation of the disc signal may be useful. High T2-weighted signal relative to other discs often indicates hemorrhage or edema. In addition, it is useful to assess the height of the intervertebral disc space, vertebral subluxation, and associated injuries at the same level.

Cord compression from posttraumatic disk herniation is associated with more significant neurologic effect than herniation without cord compression (103,104). The presence of thecal sac compression may determine whether discectomy is performed during stabilization surgery (99,102).

Intradural, Extramedullary Compartment

Anatomy

The intradural extramedullary compartment is protected by the bony spinal canal and ligamentous surroundings. In the intervertebral portion of the canal, these contents are protected by the ligamentum flavum dorsally and the posterior longitudinal ligament ventrally (105). This compartment, bounded by the thecal sac, contains arteries, veins, the spinal cord ligaments, nerve roots, cauda equina, and the filum terminale. The cord itself is considered a separate compartment.

Like the brain, the spinal cord is covered by meninges. Tightly apposed to the cord is the pia mater. The subpial space is a potential space. Between the pia and the arachnoid is the CSF-filled subarachnoid space, continuous with the intracranial subarachnoid space. Within the subarachnoid space lies the primary vascular supply to the spinal cord, consisting of one anterior and two posterior spinal arteries (arising from the vertebral arteries), reinforced by radicular arteries (branches of segmental arteries). The subarachnoid space also contains

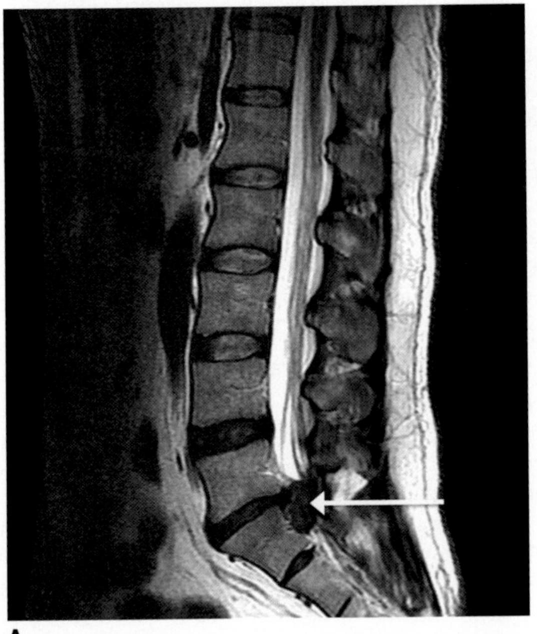

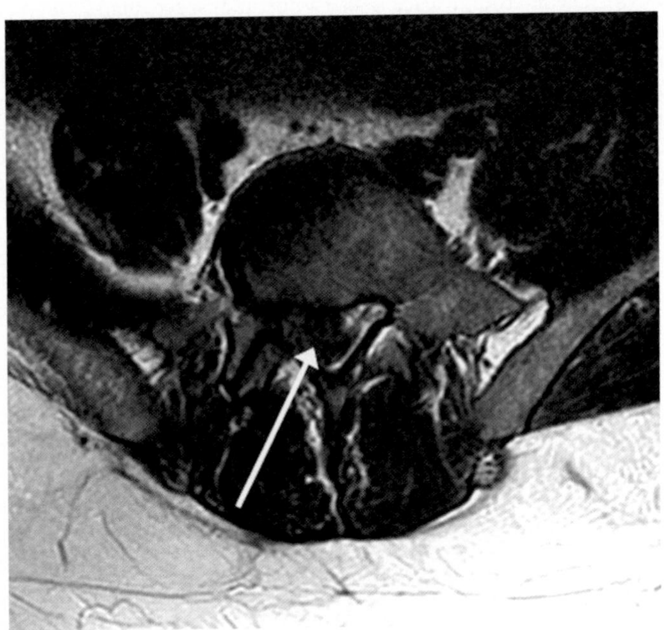

FIGURE 4.16. Sagittal T2 weighted MRI (**A**) demonstrates posttraumatic disk herniation (*white arrow*). The extruded disc completely obliterates the thecal sac. Axial T2-weighted MRI (**B**) demonstrates the extruded disc effacing CSF and impinging the right nerve root (*white arrow*).

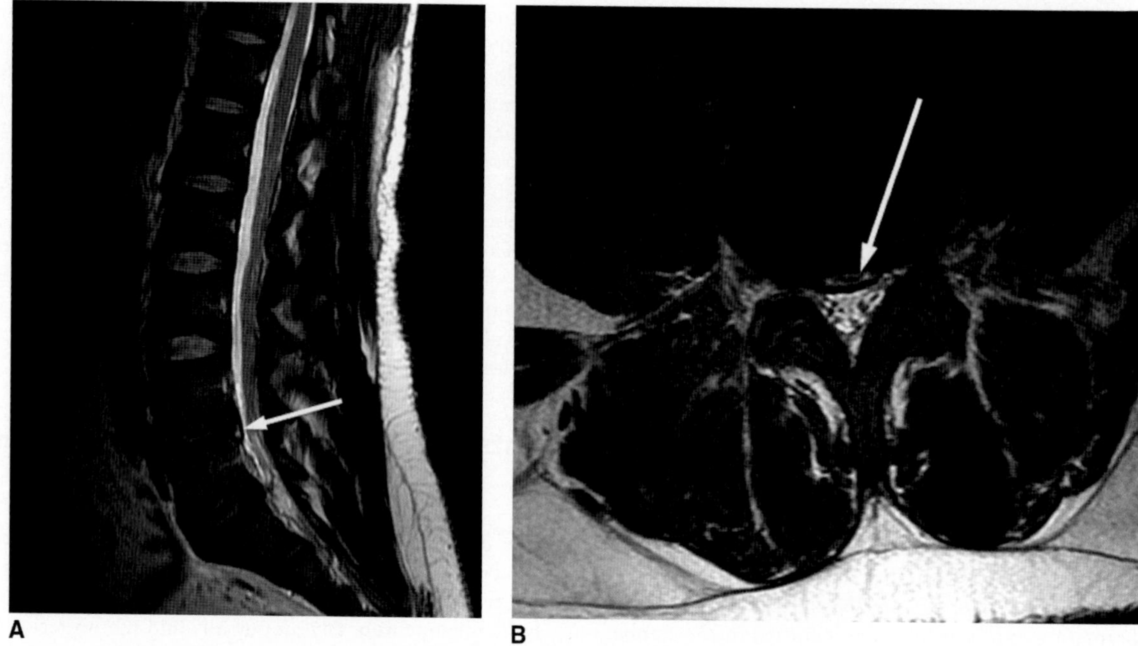

FIGURE 4.17. Sagittal (A) and Axial (B) T2-weighted MRI demonstrates an annular fissure (*white arrow*) as focal signal hyperintensity. High signal at the margin of the disc which normally has low intrinsic signal.

the spinal cord ligaments (dentate ligaments), nerves, and the filum terminale.

Immediately superficial to the subarachnoid space is the weblike, granular arachnoid. The outermost layer is the dura mater. Between the arachnoid and the dura mater is the subdural space, a potential space seen only when expanded, for example, by blood in the setting trauma. The epidural space lies superficial to the dura mater and contains a network of large thin-walled vessels, the anterior and posterior vertebral venous plexus (8). The interdural space is also a potential space, inadvertently opacified during contrast injection for CT myelography. This occurs when the bevel of the needle is positioned between the layers of the dura mater. Mentioned here only for completeness, this space rarely pertains to the trauma setting.

A complex venous drainage system exists within the intradural compartment. A central and peripheral group of radial veins drain into anastomoses on the surface of the spinal cord. The central group returns blood from the anterior horn of the spinal cord and surrounding white matter, into central veins in the anterior median fissure to form the anterior median vein. Venous drainage from the peripheral dorsal and lateral spinal cord occurs via the radial venous plexus, which empties into the coronal venous plexus on the cord surface. The coronal and median veins drain into medullary veins leaving the intradural space via the nerve root sleeve to join the epidural plexus. At the dural margin, the medullary veins have a valvelike mechanism preventing reflux into the intradural space (106).

Imaging Considerations

A 2006 evidence-based committee review by the National Institute on Disability and Rehabilitation Research Spinal Cord Injury concluded that MRI is the imaging modality of choice in evaluating spinal cord injury (107). Similarly, the American College of Radiology appropriateness criteria (2007) state that MRI should be the primary modality for evaluating spinal cord injury or compression as well as ligamentous injury in acute cervical spine trauma (108). While plain film radiography and CT are first-line modalities in evaluating bony anatomy, MRI is more sensitive in identifying the location of spinal cord injury and the degree of compression. For all spinal compartments, MRI also provides important information regarding hemorrhage, contusion, and edema in acute and subacute cord injury. MRI findings have been shown to correlate with neurologic status (109) and help establish prognosis (110,111).

Prior to the advent of MRI, evaluating injury to the spinal canal and its contents was limited to techniques unable to directly visualize the pathology (112). Techniques such as CT myelography, once used to assess the degree of cord compression, have been supplanted by MRI and MR myelography. MRI allows evaluation of the paraspinal soft tissues, integrity of intervertebral discs, ligaments, neural elements, and the spinal cord. CT myelography still has utility in patients with contraindications to MRI, as well as in the evaluation of nerve root avulsions (Fig. 4.18) and CSF leaks.

Intradural, Extramedullary Injury

Arachnoid Cyst. Arachnoid cysts are typically intradural, extramedullary, CSF-filled cysts occurring anywhere within the cerebrospinal axis. While the majority of these cysts are congenital, a small number are acquired through associations with neoplasm or resulting from adhesions occurring in the setting of hemorrhage, surgery, or infection. Typically, spinal arachnoid cysts are located dorsal to the cord in the thoracic spine. These cysts are usually secondary to a congenital or an acquired defect and may include an extradural component. Intradural spinal arachnoid cysts may also be congenital and are seen in adhesion-associated, posttraumatic and/or postinfectious settings. Pathologic samples have shown their

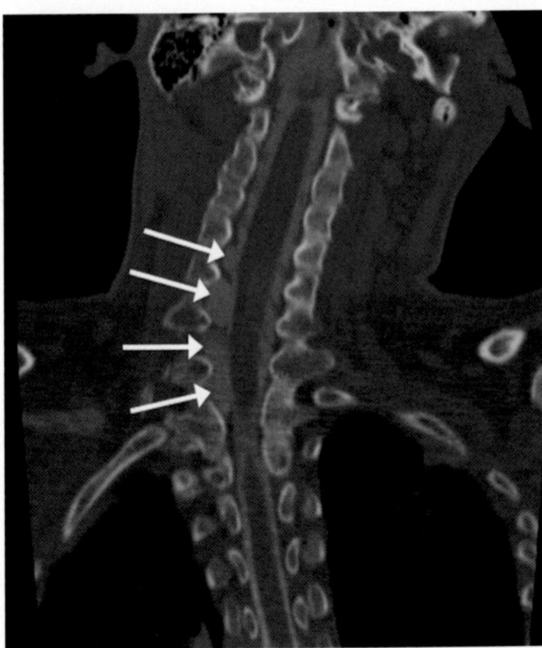

FIGURE 4.18. Coronal CT reformatted image from CT myelogram with intrathecal contrast demonstrates multiple posttraumatic meningoceles (*white arrows*) due to nerve root avulsion injuries.

walls to be formed from a splitting of the arachnoid membrane, with the inner and outer layers surrounding the cyst cavity. (113)

Arachnoid cysts are generally asymptomatic but may present with pain, paraparesis, paresthesia, hyperreflexia, and bladder/bowel incontinence. Pain symptoms may worsen with Valsalva maneuver, thought to be due to increased intracystic pressure. An association between an enlarging cyst and a worsening neurologic deficit has been demonstrated. (114)

MRI is useful in evaluating arachnoid cysts. Reliable imaging features include a nonenhancing, extramedullary loculated CSF-signal intensity collection that displaces the spinal cord or nerve roots. The cyst demonstrates CSF-signal intensity on both T1- and T2-weighted imaging. The lack of CSF flow within the cyst may give the cyst a slightly more hyperintense appearance on T1-weighted imaging. A 2D-cine phase-contrast CSF-flow study may show a sharp change in CSF flow at the cyst margin (115,116).

Intradural Hemorrhage (Subarachnoid/Subdural). Spinal subarachnoid hemorrhage (SAH) and subdural hemorrhage (SDH) are rare occurrences. Primary spinal subarachnoid hemorrhage represents approximately 1% of all SAHs. Spinal epidural hematomas are nearly four times more common than spinal SDH (Fig. 4.19) (117).

Trauma is the most common cause of spinal SAH. Spinal SAH may be isolated or secondary to spinal extension from the intracranial compartment. Spinal SAH is associated with a number of other conditions including infection, vascular malformations, hemorrhagic neoplasms, traumatic lumbar puncture, and coagulopathy. Blood within the subarachnoid space is best evaluated with MR imaging, and its appearance depends on the stage of the hemoglobin. CT may demonstrate high attenuation of blood in the subarachnoid space (118,119).

Spinal SDH occurs when blood accumulates in the potential space between the dura and the arachnoid layers. Trauma is the most common cause of spinal SDH. MR imaging demonstrates changing signal over time due to various stages of hemoglobin breakdown products. CT may demonstrate a hyperdense intradural collection of blood outlined by the epidural fat and distinct from the spinal cord (118,119).

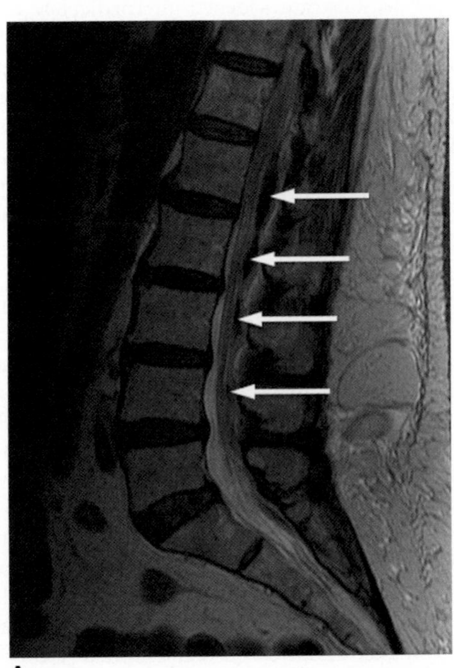

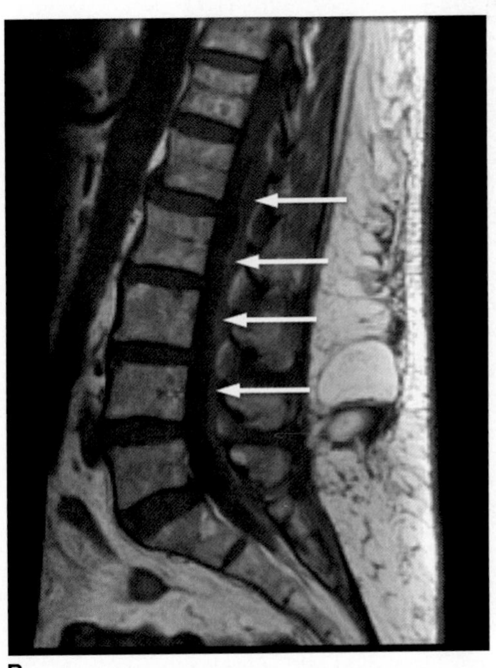

FIGURE 4.19. Sagittal T2 (**A**) and T1 (**B**) MRI demonstrate a posttraumatic epidural hematoma (*white arrows*). The acute hemorrhage is isointense on T1 and hypointense on T2 images, representing intracellular deoxyhemoglobin.

Traumatic Dural AV Fistula. Penetrating injury to the spinal canal including gunshot, stab wound, or bony trauma from fracture can rarely result in the formation of a dural arteriovenous (AV) fistula. The incidence of the traumatic AV fistula is much lower than that of spontaneous AV fistulae (120). Spinal AV fistulae are characterized by enlarged arterial feeder(s) and enlarged draining veins.

Digital subtraction angiography is considered the gold standard in the diagnosis dural AVFs, and best demonstrates the nidus and draining veins. Catheter angiography provides the access for treatment through embolization. Surgical ligation is an alternative, and definitive treatment of these lesions is the standard of care given their rapidly progressing natural history.

MR imaging may be used as an adjunct or may be the imaging modality whereby the lesion is first identified. The enlarged draining veins may appear as large signal void structures on T1-and T2-weighted imaging (Fig. 4.20). In contrast to spontaneous dural AVFs, traumatic AVFs less commonly demonstrate cord enlargement or hyperintense signal seen on T2-weighted images. Contrast-enhanced MR images may demonstrate the draining vein; however, they rarely demonstrate the nidus (119).

CSF Leak. Blunt or penetrating trauma that lacerates the dura and the arachnoid may result in traumatic spinal CSF leak. Other causes of spinal CSF leak include postoperative, post-lumbar puncture, and inadvertent meningeal puncture during epidural anesthesia (122). Identification of a CSF leak is important due to potential complications including spontaneous intracranial hypotension, headache, and meningitis, the latter occurring in 25% to 50% of untreated cases (122,123).

Imaging modalities used to evaluate CSF leak look for secondary findings suggestive of leak or directly demonstrate the leak itself. Diagnostic findings include dural thickening, engorged epidural veins, and a CSF fluid collection. Meningoceles and epidural or subdural hygromas may be seen. CT evaluation may demonstrate dilated epidural veins, appearing as anterolateral epidural "masses" on noncontrast imaging and avidly enhance with contrast. MR imaging demonstrates intraspinal or extraspinal fluid collections, isointense to CSF on T1- and T2-weighted imaging. Contrast-enhanced MR imaging may demonstrate enhancing thickened dura and intensely enhancing, enlarged venous plexus (124). The use of CT or MR myelography may be helpful in identifying the site of the leak or demonstrating arachnoid diverticula. Myelography alone is not very sensitive but, when combined with CT, has been shown to demonstrate cranial CSF fistulae with an accuracy of 22% to 100% (125). The sensitivity of CT myelography can be increased when techniques to increase the intracranial pressure, such as Valsalva maneuver, are added to the imaging protocol. MR myelography provides a less invasive method of directly evaluating a CSF leak, without requiring intrathecal injection of contrast. Using a heavily T2-weighted, fast spin-echo, fat-suppressed MR sequence, this technique exploits the inherent T2 contrast between CSF and the surrounding anatomy (124,126,127).

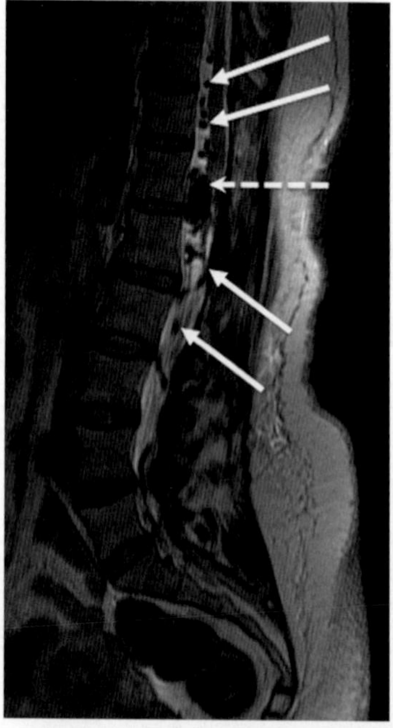

FIGURE 4.20. Sagittal T2-weighted MRI of the lower thoracic and upper lumbar spine demonstrates multiple structures devoid of signal due to flow, representing enlarged draining veins of a dural arteriovenous fistula (*solid white arrows*). A large aneurysmal vein (*dashed white arrow*) is noted.

Traumatic Dural Laceration and CSF Leak. Thoracic and lumbar compression fractures such as the "burst" fracture or laminar fracture may be associated with intradural pathology including traumatic dural laceration and CSF leak. Dural laceration may result in nerve root entrapment. If a neurologic deficit is present with a lumbar fracture, a dural laceration may be present in 25% of cases (128). Burst and laminar fractures of L3 demonstrate CSF leak or nerve root compromise in 65% of cases (129).

CT and MR imaging demonstrate bony pathology associated with dural tears, such as vertebral compression fracture involving endplates and lamina. Coronal views or AP x-ray may demonstrate widened interpediculate distance and vertical fracture through the lamina. The dural tear may be directly visualized on MR T2-weighted imaging as increased signal in the retrospinal soft tissues, with low specificity and sensitivity. Associated nerve root entrapment may be visualized on axial MR imaging. In CT myelography, intrathecal contrast is necessary to define the dural laceration and document the site of leakage. Myelography may demonstrate a CSF leak in 60% of thoracolumbar dural lacerations (130,131).

Nerve Root Avulsion Injury/Traumatic Meningocele. Traction injury to the limbs can result in permanent traumatic avulsions of the nerve roots at their attachment to the spinal cord. Nerve root avulsion predominantly occurs at the level of the cervical spine, typically a brachial plexus avulsion injury after high-speed motor vehicle accident (132). The most common sequelae of such injury include traumatic meningoceles manifesting as bulges of the arachnoid membrane through a dural tear. Conventional myelography (with or without CT) is still considered the radiologic gold standard for evaluation of meningoceles (see Fig. 4.18) (133). MR myelography, including heavily T2-weighted sequences, is also useful in evaluating meningoceles due to the high contrast resolution between CSF and surrounding soft tissue structures (Fig. 4.21A–G).

Cord Tethering. Post-traumatic spinal cord tethering results in an asymmetric appearance to the subarachnoid space. The

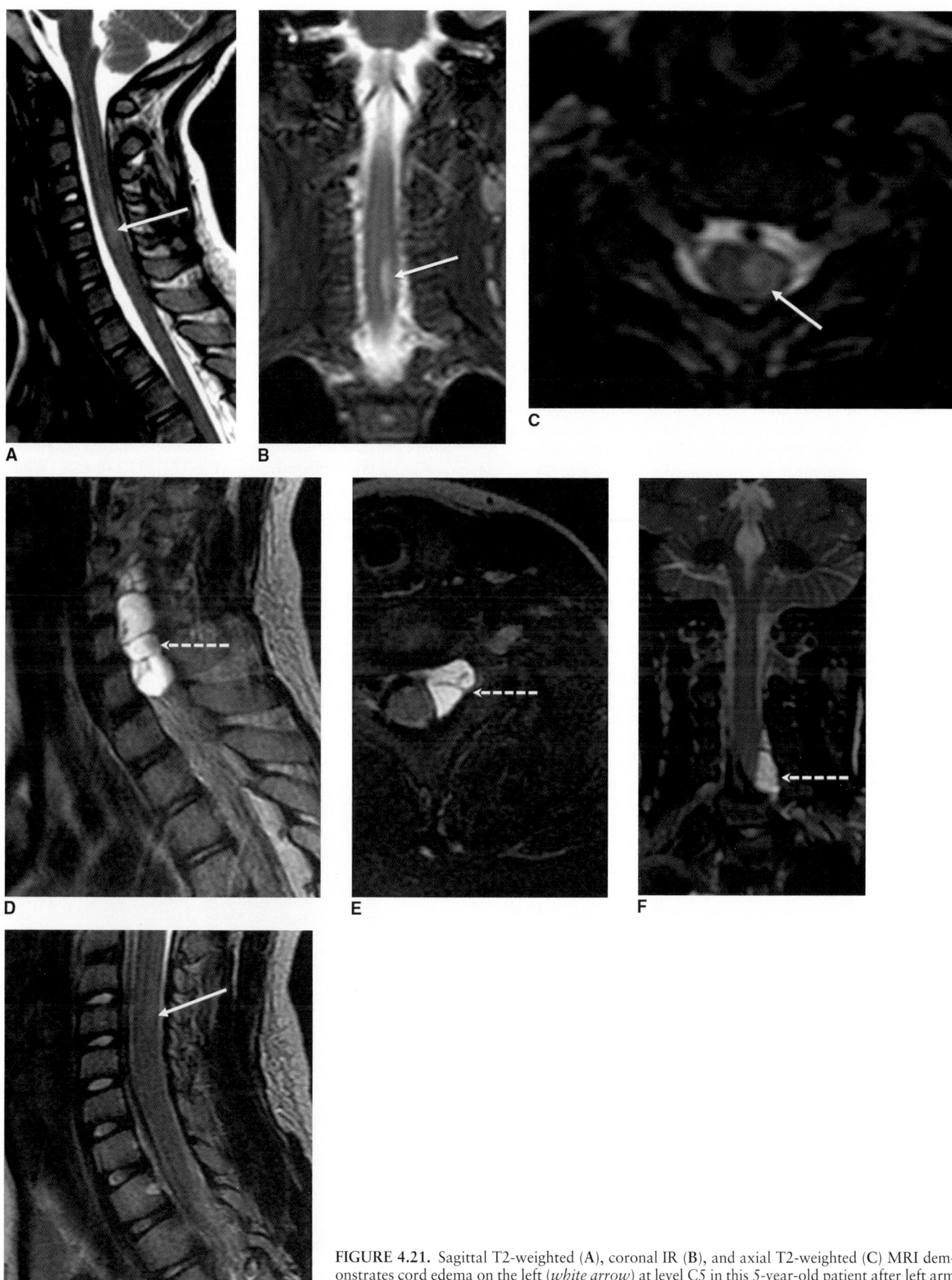

FIGURE 4.21. Sagittal T2-weighted (A), coronal IR (B), and axial T2-weighted (C) MRI demonstrates cord edema on the left (*white arrow*) at level C5 in this 5-year-old patient after left arm distraction injury. Sagittal (D), axial (E), and coronal (F) T2-weighted MRI images demonstrate the same patient 8 months after injury. Meningoceles (*dashed arrow*) are known sequelae of chronic nerve root avulsion. Sagittal T2-weighted MRI (G) demonstrates faint residual signal at the C5 level (*white arrow*) indicating near-complete resolution of the previously noted cord edema.

subarachnoid space is often obliterated dorsally, due to the patient's recumbent position; however, ventral tethering can also be seen. Myelomalacia typically coexists with tethering. The cord may appear expanded in the region of tethering due to fibrous adhesions pulling the cord apart. Direct visualization of adhesions is possible on MRI. CSF-flow studies provide information regarding the extent of adhesions and can be used postoperatively to assess normal CSF flowing the untethering procedure (134).

Intradural, Intramedullary Compartment

Anatomy

The spinal cord extends from the cervical to the lumbar region with paired spinal nerves arising at each level. The terminal portion of the cord, the conus medullaris, is located at the T12 level in the adult. Inferior to the conus, the nerve roots continue as the cauda equina with connective tissue support from an extension of pia mater termed the filum terminale. The caliber of spinal cord is prominent in two distinct regions due to the large number of exiting nerves, from C4 to T1 for the brachial plexus and T12-L4 for the lumbosacral plexus.

Mechanical trauma or traction forces may result in spinal cord injury due to compression from bone fragments, disc material, or ligaments. Trauma to the vascular supply of the cord can result in ischemic spinal cord injury. Posttraumatic spinal cord edema can rapidly progress, exacerbating the ischemia.

Imaging Considerations

Spinal cord imaging has advanced since the implementation of MRI. In the setting of trauma, MRI allows detailed visualization of cord pathology with imaging correlates predicting degree of neurologic deficit and implications for prognosis and recovery (98,100,103,110,135,136–145). These imaging correlates were first elucidated through animal models. An early rat model of spinal cord injury demonstrated that high signal on T2-weighted images correlated with edema and that low signal correlated with acute hemorrhage (55,107,146–148). In animal models, histologic analysis of the spinal cord in various stages of injury shows initial changes attributable to mechanical and vascular injury mechanisms with secondary damage due to a cascade of cytokines that expand the lesion (149). In these animal models, maximum MRI signal intensity occurs at 3 days post injury (55).

MRI findings in trauma correlate with functional outcomes. Decreased motor function has been described in lesions with greater longitudinal and cross-sectional cord involvement and evidence of central hemorrhage (7,150,151).

Injury

Trauma to the spinal cord results in primary injury to the cord or secondary cord injury due to compression or vascular compromise. Swelling, edema, and hemorrhage are components of primary cord injury and may be present individually or in any combination.

Spinal Cord Hemorrhage. Traumatic hemorrhage within the spinal cord substance is known as hemorrhagic contusion, typically centered at the point of injury, involving the central gray matter (55).

The T2-weighted MRI appearance of cord hemorrhage is lens-shaped signal hypointensity surrounded by a rim of hyperintense edema. The signal intensity of hemorrhage depends on the stage of the hemoglobin breakdown. In acute hemorrhage, deoxyhemoglobin predominates, resulting in low signal on T2-weighted and gradient-echo images (152,153). The time course of the transformation of blood products in the cord does not parallel that in the brain. The transition from deoxy- to methemoglobin takes up to 8 days or more (109,136,153) due to poor perfusion in the region of cord hemorrhage. Hours after injury, the extent of hemorrhage may expand. The temporal and spatial evolution of cord hemorrhage has been shown to increase in volume from an initial rate of 0.15% per minute up to 45% per minute within 5 hours (154) (Fig. 4.22).

In predicting clinical outcome, length of hemorrhage greater than 10 mm on sagittal MR imaging predicts complete neurologic injury (155). The location of hemorrhage and the level of injury are also closely related to outcome (98,109,136,141,155–157).

Spinal Cord Edema. Compared to cord hemorrhage, cord edema has a more favorable prognosis (136,141,144,156,158). While cord edema always accompanies cord hemorrhage, hemorrhage is not always present with edema. There is a proportional relationship between the degree of initial neurologic deficit and the length of spinal cord affected by edema (Fig. 4.23).

Edema appears hyperintense on T2-weighted MR imaging, representing fluid accumulation. The extent of edema is well defined and variable in length, existing above and below the site of injury, best seen in the sagittal MRI plane. Posttraumatic cord edema is often referred to as spinal cord "contusion" (146,157,159). Differentiating hemorrhage from edema on T1-weighted MRI sequences is difficult since both are hypointense (86).

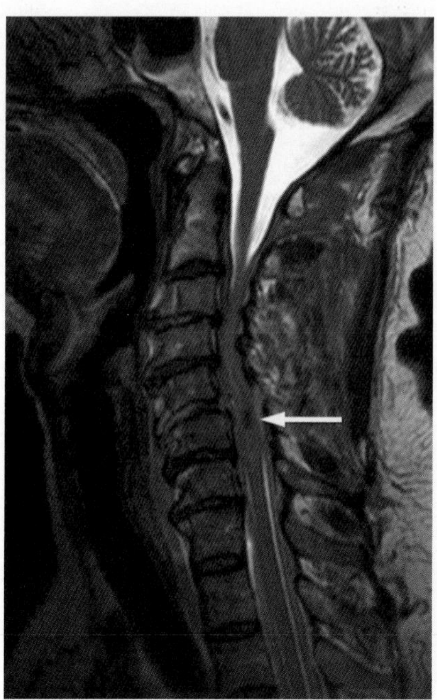

FIGURE 4.22. Sagittal T2-weighted MRI in a patient status post MVA demonstrates mild cord expansion and focal low signal within the cord (*white arrow*). This is compatible with acute hemorrhagic contusion.

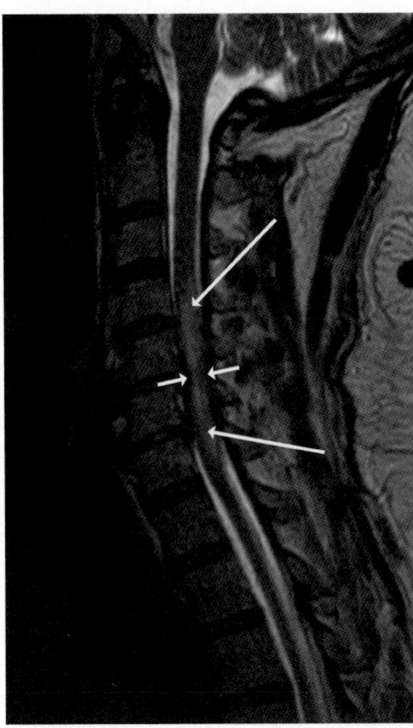

FIGURE 4.23. Sagittal T2-weighted MRI demonstrates posttraumatic spinal cord edema (*long white arrows*). Focal expansion of the spinal cord obliterates the CSF space (*small white arrows*).

Spinal Cord Swelling. In the posttraumatic spinal cord, the term "swelling" is nonspecific, referring to a focal increase in cord caliber at the level of injury. Except in the lower cervical and lumbar regions, the cord is uniform in caliber. Spinal cord swelling may demonstrate slightly lower signal than normal cord parenchyma on T1-weighted imaging, but may not demonstrate any signal abnormality (98,100,136,159). Swelling may taper rostrally or caudally from the center of injury. It may be difficult to identify in patients with inherent spinal canal stenosis. While swelling of the cord may indicate dysfunction, it does not predict the extent of injury (98,103).

Secondary Cord Damage. Compression from disk or bone elements may result in secondary cord injury as well as vascular injury. Nearly 63% of thoracic spine fractures are associated with SCI due to the relatively narrow caliber of the canal throughout that segment. T12 cord injuries are most commonly associated with paraplegia. Complete mechanical transection of the cord is uncommon, generally due to high-speed motor vehicle accidents. Cord injuries defined by the ASIA are divided into complete or incomplete lesions. Complete lesions involve loss of both motor and sensory function below the level of injury. Incomplete lesions are described by their clinical syndromes (160):

- *Central cord syndrome*
  - Following hyperextension injury to the mid and lower cervical spine, this syndrome is characterized by upper greater than lower extremity weakness, sparing sacral sensation. Spondyloarthopathy, degenerative disease, and canal stenosis are predisposing factors. The pathophysiology is due to cord compression between the vertebral body ventrally and the buckled ligamentum flavum dorsally (161). On MRI, edema is seen within the cord; the buckled ligamentum flavum is sometimes identified.
- *Anterior cord syndrome*
  - Vascular compromise of the anterior spinal artery supplying the anterior two third of the cord results in isolated motor loss due to ischemia/infarction of the anterior horn cells. In addition to motor loss below the level of injury, loss of pain and temperature sensation may occur, with sparing of the posterior column.
- *Brown-Sequard syndrome*
  - Penetrating trauma resulting in hemisection of the cord causes ipsilateral weakness, loss of proprioception and vibratory sensation secondary to disruption of the corticospinal tract and dorsal column. Temperature and pain sensation are lost on the contralateral side due to spinothalamic tract injury. MRI demonstrates hemorrhage and/or edema in the cord at the level of penetrating trauma.
- *Conus medullaris syndrome*
  - Isolated injury to the sacral spinal nerves results in this syndrome of fecal incontinence, saddle anesthesia, and areflexic bladder (55). MRI may demonstrate posttraumatic edema.
- *Cauda equina syndrome*
  - Traumatic compression of the cauda equina by bone or disc causes lower extremity weakness and perineal sensory disturbance. Relative to the spinal cord, the cauda equina is more resistant to trauma, with improved prognosis for recovery (55).

SCIWORA. Spinal cord injury without radiographic abnormality (SCIWORA) refers to spinal cord injury in the absence of radiographic abnormality on x-ray and CT. SCIWORA is limited to children; high-speed motor vehicle accidents are the most common cause (86). Cervical and thoracic levels are more frequently involved than lumbar (86). The lack of radiographic abnormality is due to ligamentous flexibility and skeletal mobility of the immature spine (162). MRI may demonstrate abnormalities not identified on CT or x-ray including ligamentous rupture, disk herniation, prevertebral hemorrhage, cord edema, cord hemorrhage, and cord transection.

Chronic Posttraumatic Evaluation. A number of patients develop neurologic symptoms weeks to years (162–166) following initial trauma, a syndrome known as posttraumatic or progressive myelopathy (155). The underlying pathology of this clinical syndrome is described by cystic lesions and/or syrinx with or without myelomalacia (167–173). MRI is the preferred modality in identifying this pathology and is important to clinical management, as early intervention may have a large impact (164,165).

Cysts and Syrinx. Posttraumatic cystic lesions within the spinal cord substance include hydromyelia and syringomyelia. Hydromyelia refers to an ependyma-lined cavity in communication with the central canal, while syringomyelia is defined as a glial-lined cavity that does not communicate with the central canal. Syringohydromyelia may include characteristics of both or may refer to an indeterminate cyst (55). Most frequently, the pathology of posttraumatic spinal cord cysts contains elements of both hydromyelia and syringomyelia. Imaging rarely distinguishes between them, and the term "syrinx" is applied (86) (Fig. 4.24).

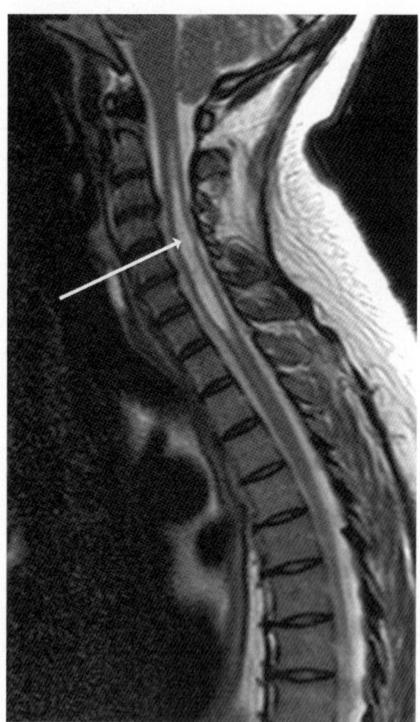

FIGURE 4.24. Sagittal T2-weighted MRI demonstrates well-circumscribed signal abnormality within the spinal cord, compatible with syrinx (*white arrow*).

Posttraumatic cyst formation occurs in 0.3% to 4% of spinal cord injuries, with a higher incidence in thoracolumbar injury (86,174–177). Symptoms from such cystic lesions include sensory and/or motor dysfunction. Pain, the most common symptom, may be exacerbated by straining, coughing, or sneezing (86,178).

Controversy and uncertainty exist over the etiology of posttraumatic cystic lesions. Two favored concepts include cavity formation and cyst extension (55). Cavity formation may be attributed to liquefaction of hematoma, cord tethering with subsequent ischemia, vascular obstruction, mechanical injury, and release of enzymes and amino acids (55). Cyst extension may occur as a result of turbulent CSF flow with a ball-valve mechanism favoring the net flow of CSF into the cyst (179).

Proper management of cystic lesions is controversial. Options include surgical decompression, shunt placement in the subarachnoid or pleural space, and untethering, creating a subarachnoid space with dural allograft (11,86,99,100,180,181). Surgery is not indicated in asymptomatic patients (55). The role of shunting in preventing cyst progression to syrinx has been debated (86). The wide spectrum of pathology and lack of long-term follow-up in patients with posttraumatic cysts limits consensus as to appropriate surgical management (55,152,182). Indications for surgical intervention and decompression are more clear in symptomatic patients with posttraumatic cystic myelopathy (152). Preoperatively, imaging plays an important role in defining cyst location and size, presence of septation(s), location of tethering, and cord compression (55).

MRI best demonstrates these well-demarcated lesions with CSF signal intensity on all MRI pulse sequences. In the setting of elevated protein, cysts may demonstrate higher signal than CSF on T1-weighted imaging. Cysts may also vary in MR signal intensity due to pulsation artifact or signal void within the cavity, which may predict enlargement (183). Cysts displaying such characteristics may actually represent a "high-pressure" syrinx, or acute expanding syrinx, more likely to improve with treatment than a "low-pressure" syrinx (184). The presence of septations is important in planning effective treatment.

Posttraumatic Myelomalacia. Posttraumatic myelomalacia has been reported in 0.3% to 2.2% of patients with chronic cord injury and may occur from 2 months to 30 years after injury (185,186). Symptoms of progressive posttraumatic myelopathy exist in patients without cystic lesions in the cord. Histologically, the cord demonstrates microcysts, reactive astrocytosis, and thickening of the pia and the arachnoid (134). Myelomalacia may be a precursor of syrinx formation (55).

MRI is the modality of choice in evaluating myelomalacia (Fig. 4.25). Ill-defined T1-weighted signal hypointensity and T2-weighted signal hyperintensity is seen within the affected cord at the level of prior injury (55,134). The caliber of the myelomalacic cord is variable, from atrophic to expanded (Fig. 4.26).

Wallerian Degeneration. Wallerian degeneration results from the separation of an axon and its myelin sheath from its nucleus after severing the nerve fiber. This degeneration begins within 24 hours and occurs distal to the site of injury. Also known as antegrade degeneration, it is usually seen above the level of injury in the dorsal column and below the level of injury in the corticospinal tracts. High T2-weighted signal may be observed in the dorsal columns rostral to the injury, as early as 7 weeks after trauma (56).

Advanced Imaging

MRI and Advanced Modalities. In the brain, DWI, DTI and tractography, MR perfusion, MR spectroscopy, and fMRI are part of the routine workup for the evaluation of strokes, tumors, inflammatory lesions, and trauma. Although equally promising for lesions of the spine, these techniques are seldom used in spine imaging due to the technical challenges limiting image quality including the magnetic inhomogeneity of structures surrounding the spinal canal, the small size of spinal structures, the craniocaudal extent of the spine, CSF and blood pulsation, respiration, swallowing, and bulk motion. In addition, the population of patients with spinal hardware requiring spinal imaging poses a challenge due to metal artifacts adjacent to the relevant anatomy (187).

Advanced imaging background. For the basic background principles of DWI, DTI, fMRI and MRI spectroscopy (MRS), the reader is referred to Lipton et al. (188).

DWI.

Application of DWI: From Brain to Cord. Anatomic MR imaging has prognostic limitations in spinal cord injury. DWI offers a potential advantage in the evaluation of spinal axonal integrity (189). Dramatic advances have been made in the study of spinal cord repair, axonal regeneration, and neuroprotection (190,191). DWI has been used to measure anisotropy, or directionality of diffusion along axons in rodent models, and may hold promise as a noninvasive method to evaluate spinal cord injury and follow response to therapy.

DWI applied to spinal cord imaging has lagged behind its application in the brain. This is, in part, due to the small size of the spinal cord requiring higher magnetic field strengths

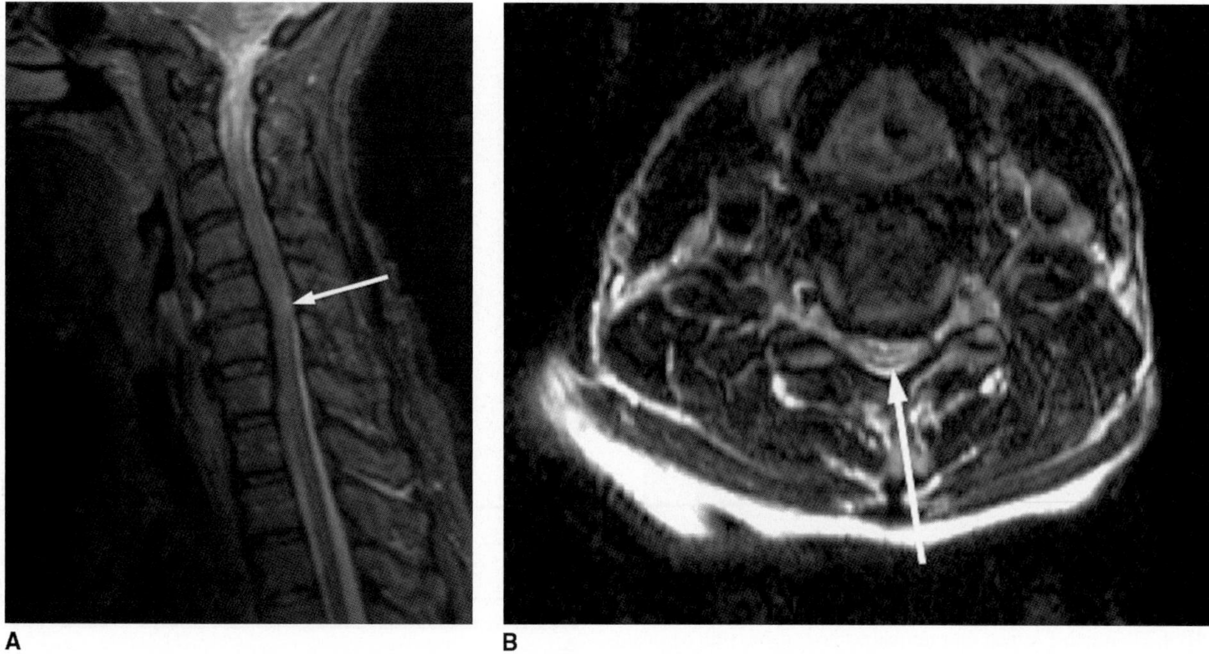

FIGURE 4.25. Sagittal MR images from STIR sequences (**A**) and axial T2-weighted image (**B**) demonstrate abnormal cord signal (*white arrows*) representing myelomalacia at the C5–6 level.

and longer imaging times to achieve diagnostic images. In vivo imaging of the spinal cord is further hindered by technical factors, including motion artifact from respiratory and cardiac activity and CSF pulsation resulting in spinal cord movement. Imaging ex vivo spinal cord specimens in experimental animal studies circumvents these issues (189).

Patients with cervical spondylosis and/or myelopathy have been evaluated using in vivo diffusion-weighted MR imaging (DWI) with apparent diffusion-coefficient (ADC) maps and apparent diffusion-tensor (ADT) maps, as an adjunct to conventional MRI and electrophysiology testing (192). DWI increases the sensitivity as well as the negative predictive value for the detection of myelopathy in patients with proven myelopathy by electrophysiology. In myelopathic patients, DWI increased the sensitivity for detection of spinal cord abnormality. Compared to spin-echo T2-weighted MR sequences, the ADC parameter is more sensitive in detecting spinal cord abnormality in cases of chronic cord compression due to cervical spondylosis.

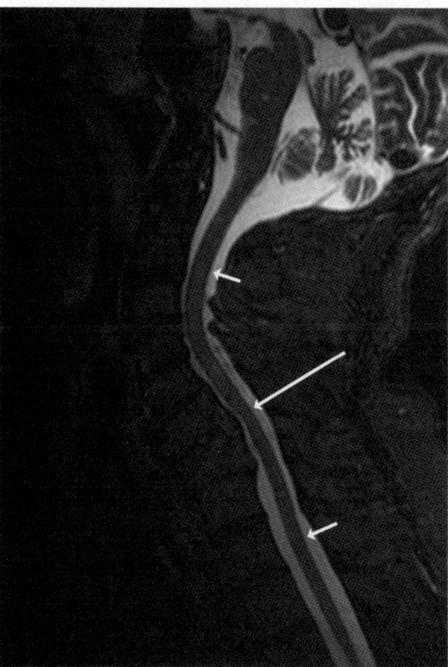

FIGURE 4.26. Sagittal MR image from STIR sequence in a patient with remote history of trauma demonstrate subtle thinning of the cord due to atrophy (*long arrow*) compared to more normal proximal and distal cord segments (*short arrows*).

Diffusion-tensor Imaging. The cylindrical anatomy and the symmetry of white matter tracts in the craniocaudal direction within spinal cord make it possible to obtain reasonably accurate longitudinal and transverse measurements of water diffusion (193).

In a rodent model of SCI, traumatized cords were scanned ex vivo with respect to DTI parameters including mean diffusivity, fractional anisotropy (FA), longitudinal and transverse apparent diffusion coefficients (lADC and tADC), and DTI tractography of both gray and white matter (Figs. 4.27–4.30). Throughout recovery, diffusion abnormalities were in regions of interest remote from the cord lesion (194). Therefore, the diffusion characteristics of the lesion alone may be inadequate in assessing the status of the spinal cord during recovery. The entire spinal cord undergoes continual change during long-term recovery from SCI over 25 weeks. This may carry implications for protocol length in future rodent SCI studies.

Additional studies have demonstrated reorganization of intracranial axons of the internal capsule and cerebral peduncle in rodents 6 weeks after SCI using fMRI activation of cortical regions where these tracts terminate (195). Contributing factors may include increased myelination, altered axonal morphology, and increased fiber density due to new sprouting.

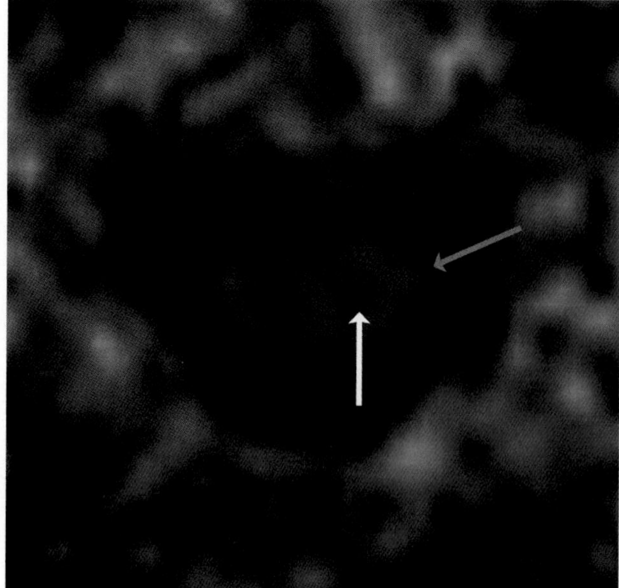

FIGURE 4.27. Axial, FA map of a normal subject, depicts direction of white matter tracts running through the cervical spinal cord. Blue color (*blue arrow*) denotes the peripheral white matter tracts running in the cephalocaudad direction (in/out of the image) with the central gray matter (*lower arrow*) void of color.

Cervical spinal cord DTI metrics in symptomatic patients after trauma (196) show ADC values to be more sensitive markers of cord injury compared to FA, relative anisotropy, and volume ratio. Changes in DTI parameters are most marked at the level of injury and reflect the severity of cord injury, especially where there may be hemorrhage. Interestingly, variation in ADC values can be demonstrated in three distinct segments of the normal cervical spinal cord. Whether this is technical, artifactual, or due to physiologic etiologies, it is an important point to consider when interpreting results.

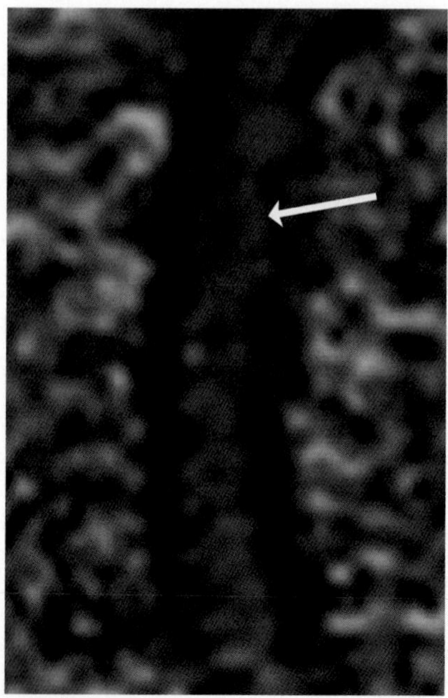

FIGURE 4.28. Sagittal, FA map of a normal subject depicts the cephalocaudad direction of white matter tracts (*arrow*) in the cervical spine.

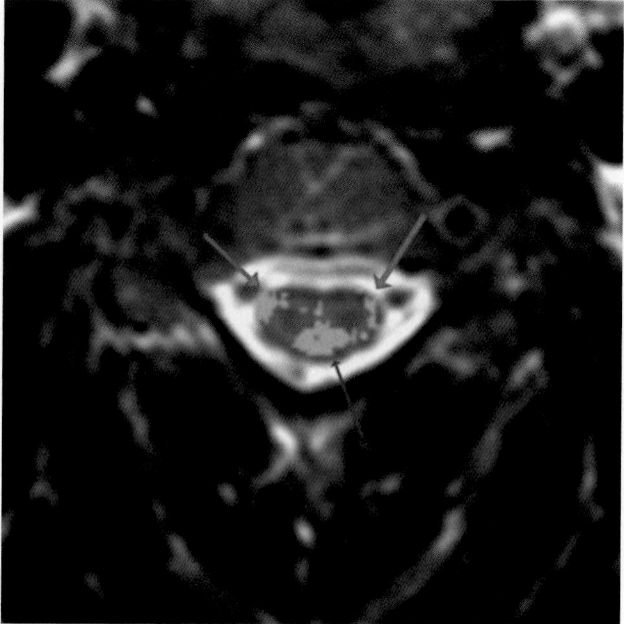

A

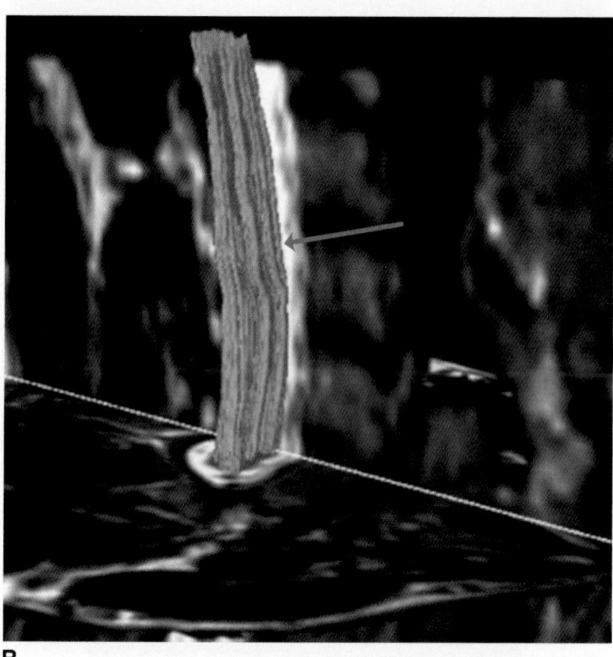

B

FIGURE 4.29. (A) Axial and (B) sagittal image demonstrating that the resulting tracts (arrow) may be mapped projections from normal 3D tractography depicts the integrity and the continuity of white matter tracts including lateral spinothalamic tracts (*upper arrows*) and posterior columns (*lower arrow*). This image is created by placing a region of interest in an area of abundant white matter, such as the cortical spinal tract in the brain. The resulting tracts may be mapped into the spinal cord.

Clinical applications of spinal DTI have demonstrated its utility in the evaluation of axonal course and integrity relative to tumor, with good results (196).

Functional MRI. Using fMRI, brain sensorimotor cortex activity has been demonstrated years following trauma in patients with

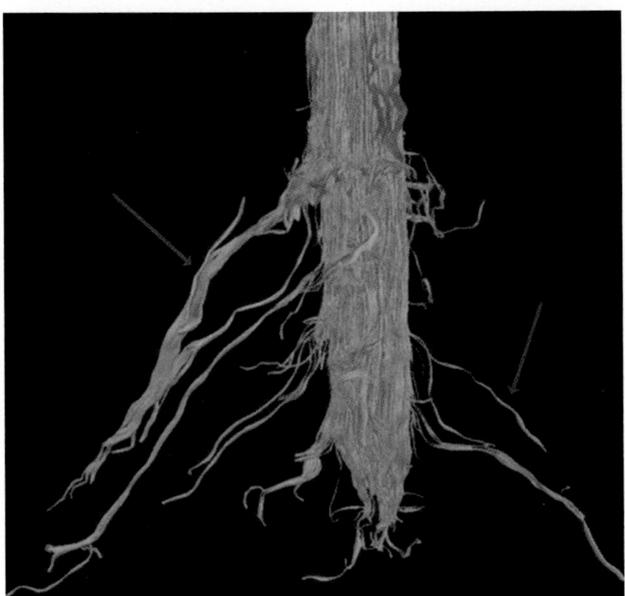

FIGURE 4.30. Normal peripheral neurography. Utilizing 3D tractography, peripheral nerve roots (*arrows*) are traced.

complete SCI between levels T6 and L1. In all patients, during attempts to move or mental imagery of the task, activation was found in cortical areas involved in motor control. Several years after injury, with some local cortical reorganization, activation of lower limb cortical networks can be generated either by the attempt to move, mental imagery of the action, or visual observation of passive sensory stimulation (197).

A rodent model has also shown reorganization in the higher centers of the brain at 4 and 8 weeks after SCI, using an fMRI paradigm involving electrical stimulation of rat paws. In normal animals, activation was seen in the contralateral somatosensory cortex. In injured animals, some degree of activation was seen in the ipsilateral cortex, thalamus, hippocampus, as well as the caudate and putamen. Significant increase in activation was observed only in the ipsilateral caudate, putamen, and thalamus. This suggests brain reorganization after spinal cord injury in the rodent (198).

fMRI is gaining ground in the evaluation of SCI treatment (199). Treatment of SCI is currently evaluated anatomically and functionally, in an attempt to correlate change in anatomy with change in function, such as ambulation. Several gaps exist in the ability to investigate the effects of various interventions on SCI recovery. Histopathological analysis of injured spinal cord tissue is not feasible in living patients. Moreover, even in animal models, it is not possible to perform serial anatomic studies of CNS injury in the same animal over time. Different cohorts of animals are typically examined at various time points after injury and intervention. This introduces intersubject variation that may confound results. In the future, fMRI in conjunction with other noninvasive imaging technology may provide visual biomarkers for spinal cord structure and function after injury (200).

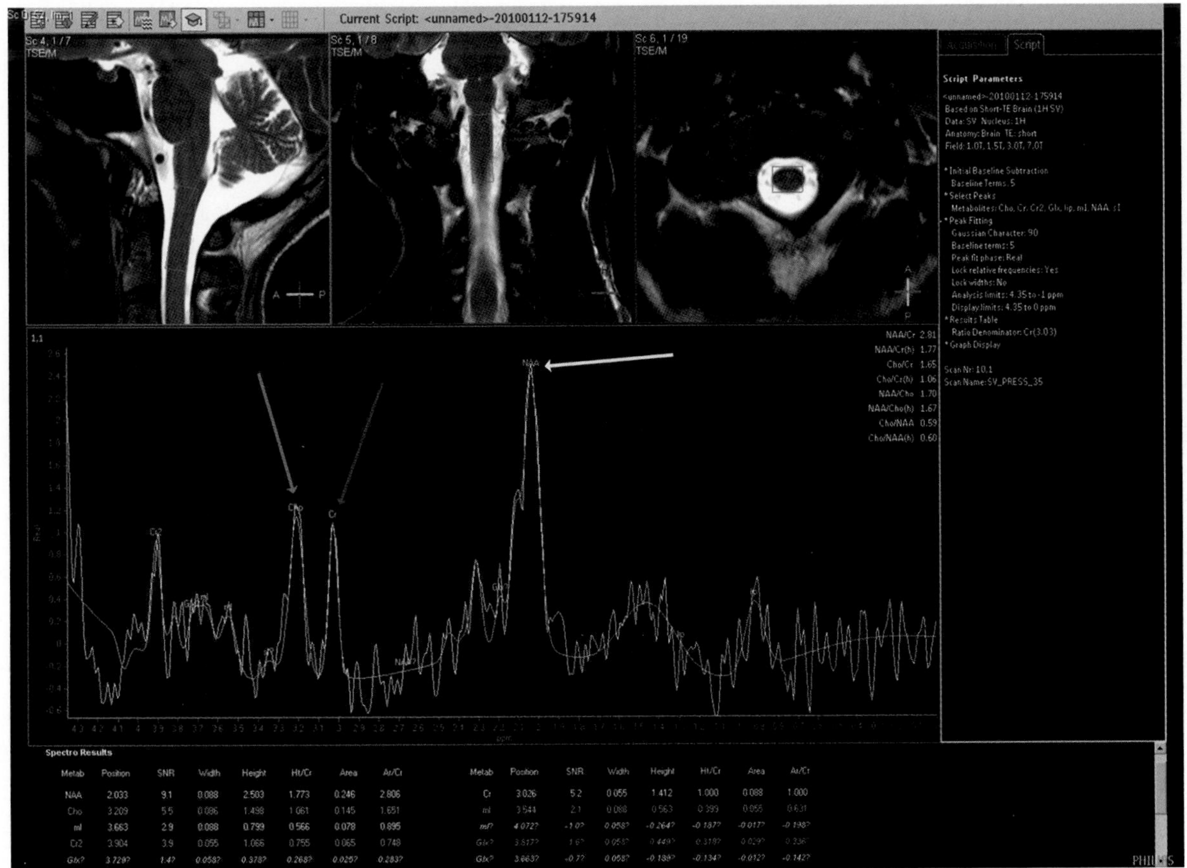

FIGURE 4.31. MR spectroscopy with PRESS excitation, cardiac gating and TE = 37 ms in a normal subject. A voxel (box, seen in three planes) has been positioned over the high cervical cord. The resultant spectrum demonstrates the normal ratio of choline (*first arrow*), creatine (*second arrow*), and *N*-acetylaspartate (*third arrow*) as commonly seen in the brain.

Spectroscopy. Following in vivo experimental traumatic SCI in rodents, phosphorus-31 (^{31}P) MRS was used to examine the ex vivo rodent cord for metabolic changes in thalamic nuclei (201). Metabolic changes in the thalamus after SCI including increases in inositol levels suggest changes in glial activity and may reflect abnormalities in both membrane metabolism and intracellular signaling mechanisms. Changes in NAA levels may indicate the response of thalamic neuronal cells to injury, including possible neuroprotective functions (201). This study also showed that both SCI and sham surgery raise NAA levels, but at different time points implying a response to different pain intensities. MRS is useful in observing metabolic changes in the thalamus that may reflect the SCI, severity of the lesion, pain response to treatment, and the extent of recovery from SCI (Fig. 4.31).

A swine model studied ^{31}P MRS in SCI with respect to myelin changes and intracellular pH to evaluate pathophysiologic events leading to secondary, nonreversible necrosis (202). In elucidating basic biochemical pathways, ^{31}P MRS allows the monitoring of intracellular pH (pHi), free magnesium, cellular bioenergetics (adenosine triphosphate, inorganic phosphate, and phosphocreatine), and myelin phospholipids. In studying the spinal cord in vivo, a nonlinkage between pH and myelin changes has been established by this technique (201,203). This supports the theory that low pH, observed in ischemia, is not the primary factor in nonreversible, secondary injury to spinal cord tissue. Trends in metabolites found by spectroscopy may help define the complex milieu in SCI that leads to secondary irreversible damage.

References

1. Sekhon LH, Fehlings MG. Epidemiology, demographics, and pathophysiology of acute spinal cord injury. *Spine* 2001;26:S2–S12.
2. National Spinal Cord Injury Statistical Center. Facts and figures at a glance. *University of Alabama at Birmingham*: Birmingham AL, 2008.
3. Tator CH, Duncan EG, Edmonds VE, et al. Changes in epidemiology of acute spinal cord injury from 1947 to 1981. *Surg Neurol* 1993;40:207–215.
4. Cochran ST, Bomyea K, Sayre JW. Trends in adverse events after IV administration of contrast media. *Am J Roentgenol* 2001;176:1385–1388.
5. Kanal E, Barkovich AJ, Bell C, et al. ACR guidance document for safe MR practices: 2007. *Am J Roentgenol* 2007;188:1447–1474.
6. Flanders A, Schwartz ED. *Spinal trauma: imaging, diagnosis, management*, 1st ed. Philadelphia: Lippincott William & Wilkins, 2007.
7. Perovitch M, Perl S, Wang H. Current advances in magnetic resonance imaging (MRI) in spinal cord trauma: review article. *Paraplegia* 1992;30:305–316.
8. Grossman RI, Yousem DM, Neuroradiology: the requisites. 2nd ed. Philadelphia: Mosby, 2003.
9. Expert Panel on Musculoskeletal Imaging ACR Appropriateness Criteria for Suspected Cervical Spine Trauma. Reston, VA: ACR, 2003.
10. Provenzale J. MR imaging of spinal trauma. *Emerg Radiol* 2007;13:289–297.
11. Woodring JH, Lee C. Limitations of cervical radiography in the evaluation of acute cervical trauma. *J Trauma* 1993;34(1):32–39.
12. Holmes JF, Akkinepalli R. Computed tomography versus plain radiography to screen for cervical spine injury: a meta-analysis. *J Trauma* 2005;58:902–905.
13. Hoffman JR, Mower WR, Wolfson AB, et al. Validity of a set of clinical criteria to rule out injury to the cervical spine in patients with blunt trauma. National Emergency X-Radiography Utilization Study Group. *N Engl J Med* 2000;343:94–99.
14. Holmes JF, Mirvis SE, Panacek EA, et al. Variability in computed tomography and magnetic resonance imaging in patients with cervical spine injuries. *J Trauma* 2002;53:524–529; discussion 530.
15. Hackney D, Daffner R. ACR appropriateness criteria on suspected spine trauma. *J Am Coll Radiol* 2007;4: 762–775.
16. Section on Disorders of the Spine and Peripheral Nerves of the American Association of Neurological Surgery. Chapter 14: Diagnosis and management of traumatic atlanto-occipital dislocation injuries. *Neurosurgery* 2002;50(Suppl):S105–S113.
17. Saveika JA, Thorogood C. Airbag-mediated pediatric atlanto-occipital dislocation. *Am J Phys Med Rehabil* 2006;85:1007–1010.
18. Harris JH Jr, Carson GC, Wagner LK, et al. Radiologic diagnosis of traumatic occipitovertebral dissociation. 2. Comparison of three methods of detecting occipitovertebral relationships on lateral radiographs of supine subjects. *Am J Roentgenol* 1994;162:887–892.
19. Harris JH Jr, Carson GC, Wagner LK. Radiologic diagnosis of traumatic occipitovertebral dissociation: 1. Normal occipitovertebral relationships on lateral radiographs of supine subjects. *Am J Roentgenol* 1994;162:881–886.
20. Bono CM, Vaccaro AR, Fehlings M, et al. Measurement techniques for upper cervical spine injuries: consensus statement of the Spine Trauma Study Group. *Spine* 2007;32:593–600.
21. Henry MB, Angelastro DB, Gillen JP. Unrecognized traumatic atlanto-occipital dislocation. *Am J Emerg Med* 1998;16:406–408.
22. Bulas DI, Fitz CR, Johnson DL. Traumatic atlanto-occipital dislocation in children. *Radiology* 1993;188:155–158.
23. Przybylski GJ, Clyde BL, Fitz CR. Craniocervical junction subarachnoid hemorrhage associated with atlanto-occipital dislocation. *Spine* 1996;21:1761–1768.
24. Horn EM, Feiz-Erfan I, Lekovic GP, et al. Survivors of occipitoatlantal dislocation injuries: imaging and clinical correlates. *J Neurosurg Spine* 2007;6:113–120.
25. Pratt H, Davies E, King L. Traumatic injuries of the C1/C2 complex: computed tomographic imaging appearances. *Curr Probl Diagn Radiol* 2008;37:26–38.
26. Bruni P, Greco R, Hernandez R, et al. Cruciate paralysis from a Jefferson's fracture. Report a case and review of the literature. *J Neurosurg Sci* 1994;38:67–72.
27. Heller JG, Viroslav S, Hudson T. Jefferson fractures: the role of magnification artifact in assessing transverse ligament integrity. *J Spinal Disord* 1993;6:392–396.
28. Hadley MN, Dickman CA, Browner CM, et al. Acute traumatic atlas fractures: management and long term outcome. *Neurosurgery* 1988;23:31–35.
29. Levine AM, Edwards CC. Treatment of injuries in the C1-C2 complex. *Orthop Clin North Am* 1986;17: 31–44.

30. Spence KF Jr, Decker S, Sell KW. Bursting atlantal fracture associated with rupture of the transverse ligament. *J Bone Joint Surg Am* 1970;52:543–549.
31. Dickman C, Greene K, Sonntag V. Injuries involving the transverse atlantal ligament: classification and treatment guidelines based upon experience with 39 injuries. *Neurosurgery* 1996;38:44–50.
32. Hadley MN, Browner C, Sonntag VK. Axis fractures: a comprehensive review of management and treatment in 107 cases. *Neurosurgery* 1985;17:281–290.
33. Anderson LD, D'Alonzo RT. Fractures of the odontoid process of the axis. *J Bone Joint Surg Am* 1974;56:1663–1674.
34. Ochoa G. Surgical management of odontoid fractures. *Injury* 2005;36(Suppl 2):B54–B64.
35. Harrop JS, Sharan AD, Przybylski GJ. Epidemiology of spinal cord injury after acute odontoid fractures. *Neurosurg Focus* 2000;8:e4.
36. Lewandrowski KU, Park PP, Baron JM, et al. Atraumatic odontoid fractures in patients with rheumatoid arthritis. *Spine J* 2006;6:529–533.
37. Effendi B, Roy D, Cornish B, et al. Fractures of the ring of the axis. A classification based on the analysis of 131 cases. *J Bone Joint Surg Br* 1981;63-B:319–327.
38. Levine AM, Edwards CC. The management of traumatic spondylolisthesis of the axis. *J Bone Joint Surg Am* 1985;67:217–226.
39. Li XF, Dai LY, Lu H, et al. A systematic review of the management of hangman's fractures. *Eur Spine J* 2006;15:257–269.
40. Tessitore E, Luzi M, Lobrinus J, et al. Cervical Paget disease of bone with spinal cord compression due to atlanto-axial instability: a case report and review of the literature. *Spine* 2008;33:E85–E89.
41. O'Connor JF, Cranley WR, McCarten KM, et al. Commentary: atlantoaxial instability in Down syndrome: reassessment by the Committee on Sports Medicine and Fitness of the American Academy of Pediatrics. *Pediatr Radiol* 1996;26:748–749.
42. Nguyen HV, Ludwig SC, Silber J, et al. Rheumatoid arthritis of the cervical spine. *Spine J* 2004;4:329–334.
43. Dickman C, Mamourian A, Sonntag V, et al. Magnetic resonance imaging of the transverse atlantal ligament for the evaluation of atlantoaxial instability. *J Neurosurg* 1991;75:221–227.
44. Fesmire F, Luten R. The pediatric cervical spine: developmental anatomy and clinical aspects. *J Emerg Med* 1989;7:133–142.
45. Harris J, Mirvis S. *The radiology of acute cervical spine trauma*, 3rd ed. Baltimore: Williams and Wilkins, 1996.
46. Moore TA, Vaccaro AR, Anderson PA. Classification of lower cervical spine injuries. *Spine* 2006;31:S37–S43; discussion S61.
47. Vaccaro AR, Hulbert RJ, Patel AA, et al. The subaxial cervical spine injury classification system: a novel approach to recognize the importance of morphology, neurology, and integrity of the disco-ligamentous complex. *Spine* 2007;32:2365–2374.
48. Bono CM, Vaccaro AR, Fehlings M, et al. Measurement techniques for lower cervical spine injuries: consensus statement of the Spine Trauma Study Group. *Spine* 2006;31:603–609.
49. Kim KS, Chen HH, Russell EJ, et al. Flexion teardrop fracture of the cervical spine: radiographic characteristics. *Am J Roentgenol* 1989;152:319–326.
50. Vaccaro AR, Madigan L, Schweitzer ME, et al. Magnetic resonance imaging analysis of soft tissue disruption after flexion-distraction injuries of the subaxial cervical spine. *Spine* 2001;26:1866–1872.
51. Pitzen T, Lane C, Goertzen D, et al. Anterior cervical plate fixation: biomechanical effectiveness as a function of posterior element injury. *J Neurosurg* 2003;99: 84–90.
52. Doran SE, Papadopoulos SM, Ducker TB, et al. Magnetic resonance imaging documentation of coexistent traumatic locked facets of the cervical spine and disc herniation. *J Neurosurg* 1993;79:341–345.
53. Daffner S, Daffner R. Computed tomography diagnosis of facet dislocations: the "hamburger bun" and "reverse hamburger bun" signs. *J Emerg Med* 2002;23:387–394.
54. Matar L, Helms C, Richardson W. "Spinolaminar breach": an important sign in cervical spinous process fractures. *Skeletal Radiol* 2000;29:75–80.
55. Schwartz ED, Flanders AE. *Spinal trauma: imaging, diagnosis, and management*. Philadelphia: Lippincott Williams & Wilkins, 2007.
56. Klein GR, Vaccaro AR, Albert TJ, et al. Efficacy of magnetic resonance imaging in the evaluation of posterior cervical spine fractures. *Spine* 1999;24:771–774.
57. Denis F. The three column spine and its significance in the classification of acute thoracolumbar spinal injuries. *Spine* 1983;8:817–831.
58. Denis F. Spinal instability as defined by the three-column spine concept in acute spinal trauma. *Clin Orthop Relat Res* 1984;189:65–76.
59. Panjabi MM, Oxland TR, Kifune M, et al. Validity of the three-column theory of thoracolumbar fractures. A biomechanic investigation. *Spine* 1995;20:1122–1127.
60. Louman-Gardiner K, Mulpuri K, Perdios A, et al. Pediatric lumbar Chance fractures in British Columbia: chart review and analysis of the use of shoulder restraints in MVAs. *Accid Anal Prev* 2008;40:1424–1429.
61. Keynan O, Fisher CG, Vaccaro A, et al. Radiographic measurement parameters in thoracolumbar fractures: a systematic review and consensus statement of the spine trauma study group. *Spine* 2006;31:E156–E165.
62. France JC, Bono CM. Initial radiographic evaluation of the spine after trauma: when, what, where, and how to image the acutely traumatized spine. *J Orthop Trauma* 2005;19:640–649.
63. Brightman RP, Miller CA, Rea GL, et al. Magnetic resonance imaging of trauma to the thoracic and lumbar spine. The importance of the posterior longitudinal ligament. *Spine* 1992;17:541–550.
64. Terk MR, Hume-Neal M, Fraipont M, et al. Injury of the posterior ligament complex in patients with acute spinal trauma: evaluation by MR imaging. *Am J Roentgenol* 1997;168:1481–1486.
65. Lee HM, Kim HS, Kim DJ, et al. Reliability of magnetic resonance imaging in detecting posterior ligament complex injury in thoracolumbar spinal fractures. *Spine* 2000;25:2079–2084.
66. Arlet V, Orndorff DG, Jagannathan J, et al. Reverse and pseudoreverse cortical sign in thoracolumbar burst

fracture: radiologic description and distinction—a propos of three cases. *Eur Spine J* 2008;18:282–287.
67. Eberl R, Kaminski A, Müller E, et al. Importance of the cross-sectional area of the spinal canal in thoracolumbar and lumbar fractures. Is there any correlation between the degree of stenosis and neurological deficit. *Orthopade* 2003;32:859–864.
68. Meves R, Avanzi O. Correlation between neurological deficit and spinal canal compromise in 198 patients with thoracolumbar and lumbar fractures. *Spine* 2005;30:787–791.
69. Mohanty SP, Bhat NS, Abraham R, et al. Neurological deficit and canal compromise in thoracolumbar and lumbar burst fractures. *J Orthop Surg* (Hong Kong) 2008;16:20–23.
70. Elgafy H, Bellabarba C. Three-column ligamentous extension injury of the thoracic spine: a case report and review of the literature. *Spine* 2007;32:E785–E788.
71. Debnath UK, Maripuri SN, Mobini B, et al. Rotational dislocation of the thoracolumbar spine. Case report and review of the literature. *J Neurosurg Spine* 2007;6:161–164.
72. Dussa CU, Soni BM. A hidden injury. *Emerg Med J* 2004;21:390–391.
73. Laasonen EM. Missed sacral fractures. *Ann Clin Res* 1977;9:84–87.
74. Rafii M, Firooznia H, Golimbu C, et al. Radiation induced fractures of sacrum: CT diagnosis. *J Comput Assist Tomogr* 1988;12:231–235.
75. Alsobrook J, Simons SM. Sacral stress fracture in a marathon runner. *Curr Sports Med Rep* 2007;6:39–42.
76. Haun DW, Kettner NW, Yochum TR, et al. Sacral fatigue fracture in a female runner: a case report. *J Manipulative Physiol Ther* 2007;30:228–233.
77. Klossner D. Sacral stress fracture in a female collegiate distance runner: a case report. *J Athl Train* 2000;35:453–457.
78. Cooper KL, Beabout JW, Swee RG. Insufficiency fractures of the sacrum. *Radiology* 1985;156:15–20.
79. Diel J, Ortiz O, Losada RA, et al. The sacrum: pathologic spectrum, multimodality imaging, and subspecialty approach. *Radiographics* 2001;21:83–104.
80. Brook AL, Mirsky DM, Bello JA. Computerized tomography guided sacroplasty: a practical treatment for sacral insufficiency fracture: case report. *Spine* 2005;30:E450–E454.
81. Denis F, Davis S, Comfort T. Sacral fractures: an important problem. Retrospective analysis of 236 cases. *Clin Orthop Relat Res* 1988;227:67–81.
82. Kim MY, Reidy DP, Nolan PC, et al. Transverse sacral fractures: case series and literature review. *Can J Surg* 2001;44:359–363.
83. Roy-Camille R, Saillant G, Gagna G, et al. Transverse fracture of the upper sacrum. Suicidal jumper's fracture. *Spine* 1985;10:838–845.
84. Gibbons KJ, Soloniuk DS, Razack N. Neurological injury and patterns of sacral fractures. *J Neurosurg* 1990;72:889–893.
85. Kuklo TR, Potter BK, Ludwig SC, et al. Radiographic measurement techniques for sacral fractures consensus statement of the Spine Trauma Study Group. *Spine* 2006;31:1047–1055.
86. Mhuircheartaigh N, Kerr J, Murray J. MR imaging of traumatic spinal injuries. *Semin Musculoskelet Radiol* 2006;10:293–307.
87. Friedman DP, Flanders AE. Unusual dissection of the proximal vertebral artery: description of three cases. *AJNR* 1992;13:283–286.
88. Willis BK, Greiner F, Orrison WW, et al. The incidence of vertebral artery injury after midcervical spine fracture or subluxation. *Neurosurgery* 1994;34:435–442.
89. Parbhoo AH, Govender S, Corr P. Vertebral artery injury in cervical spine trauma. *Injury Int J Care Injured* 2001;32:565–568.
90. Greiner FG, Orrison WW, King JN, et al. Vertebral artery injury association with cervical spine fractures. In: *Proceedings of the 29th Annual Meeting of the American Society of Neuroradiology*. Washington, DC;1991:171.
91. Wittenberg RH, Boetel U, Beyer HK. Magnetic resonance imaging and computed tomography of acute spinal cord trauma. *Clin Orthop* 1990;260:176–185.
92. Weirich SD, Cotler HB, Narayana PA, et al. Histopathologic correlation of magnetic resonance imaging signal patterns in a spinal cord injury model. *Spine* 1990;15:630–638.
93. Grossman MD, Reilly PM, Gillett T, et al. National survey of the incidence of cervical spine injury and approach to cervical spine clearance in U.S. trauma centers. *J Trauma* 1999;47:684–690.
94. Torina PJ, Flanders AE, Carrino JA, et al. Incidence of vertebral artery thrombosis in cervical spine trauma: correlation with severity of spinal cord injury. *AJNR* 2005;26:2645–2651.
95. Biffl WL, Moore EE, Elliott JP, et al. The devastating potential of blunt vertebral arterial injuries. *Ann Surg* 2000;23:672–681.
96. Friedman DP, Flanders AE, Thomas C, et al. Vertebral artery injury after acute cervical spine trauma: rate of occurrence as detected by MR angiography and assessment of clinical consequences. *Am J Roentgenol* 1995;164:443–447.
97. Sherman JL, Barkovich AJ, Citrin CM. The MR appearance of syringomyelia: new observations. *Am J Roentgenol* 1987;148:381–391.
98. Flanders AE, Schaefer DM, Doan HT, et al. Acute cervical spine trauma: correlation of MRI imaging findings with degree of neurologic deficit. *Radiology* 1990;177(1):25–33.
99. Dai L, Jia L. Central cord injury complicating acute cervical disc herniation in trauma. *Spine* 2000;25:331–335.
100. Schaefer DM, Flanders A, Northrup BE, et al. Magnetic resonance imaging of acute cervical spine trauma: correlation with severity of neurologic injury. *Spine* 1989;14:1090–1095.
101. Rizzolo SJ, Piazza MRI, Cotler JM, et al. Intervertebral disc injury complicating cervical spine trauma. *Spine* 1991;16(6):187–189.
102. Harrington JF, Likavec MJ, Smith AS. Disc herniation in cervical fracture subluxation. *Neurosurgery* 1991;29:374–379.
103. Silberstein M, Tress BM, Hennessy O. Prediction of neurologic outcome in acute spinal cord injury: the role of CT and MRI. *AJNR* 1992;13:1597–1608.
104. Rao SC, Fehlings MG. The optimal radiologic method for assessing spinal canal compromise and cord com-

pression in patients with cervical spinal cord injury. Part I: an evidence-based analysis of the published literature. *Spine* 1999;15:598–604.
105. Moore K, Dalley A, Agur A. *Clinically oriented anatomy*, 6th ed. Lippincott Williams & Wilkins, 2009.
106. Stat Dx. http://my.statdx.com; Copyright 2005–2010 Amirsys, Inc.
107. Lammertse D, et al. Neuroimaging in traumatic spinal cord injury: an evidence-based review for clinical practice and research. *J Spinal Cord Med* 2007;30:205–214.
108. Hackney D, Daffner R. ACR appropriateness criteria on suspected spine trauma. *J Am Coll Radiol* 2007;4: 762–775.
109. Bondurant FJ, Cotler HB, Kulkarni MV, et al. Acute spinal cord injury: a study using physical examination and magnetic resonance imaging. *Spine* 1990;15:161–68.
110. Schaefer DM, Flanders AE, Osterholm JL, et al. Prognostic significance of MRI in acute phase of spinal injury. *J Neurosurg* 1992;76:218–223.
111. Miyanji F, Furtan JC, Bizhan A, et al. Acute cervical traumatic spinal cord injury: MR imaging findings correlated with neurologic outcome—prospective study with 100 consecutive patients. *Radiology* June 2007;243:820–827; Published online April 12, 2007,doi:10.1148/radiol. 2433060583
112. Allen BL, Ferguson RL, Lehmann TR, et al. A mechanistic classification of closed, indirect fractures and dislocations of the lower cervical spine. *Spine* 1982;7(1):1–27.
113. Van Tassel P, Cure JK. Nonneoplastic intracranial cysts and cystic lesions. *Semin Ultrasound CT MR* 1995;16:186–211.
114. Wang MY, Levi AD, Green BA. Intradural spinal arachnoid cysts in adults. *Surg Neurol* 2003;60:49–56.
115. Sklar E, Quencer RM, Green BA, et al. Acquired spinal subarachnoid cysts: evaluation with MR, CT myelography, and intraoperative sonography. *AJNR* 1989;10:1097–1104.
116. Silbergleit R, Brunberg JA, Patel SC, et al. Imaging of spinal intradural arachnoid cysts: MRI, myelography and CT. *Neuroradiology* 1998;40:664–668.
117. Geldmacher DS, Bowen BC. Spinal cord vascular disease. In: Bradley WG, Daroff RB, Fenichel GM, et al., eds. *Neurology in clinical practice principles of diagnosis and management*, 4th ed. Philadelphia: Butterworth-Heimann, 2004:1313–22.
118. Berlis A, Scheufler KM, Schmahl C, et al. Solitary spinal artery aneurysms as a rare source of spinal subarachnoid hemorrhage: potential etiology and treatment strategy *AJNR* 2005;26:405–410.
119. Holtas S, Heiling M, Lonntoft M, et al. Spontaneous spinal epidural hematoma: findings at MR imaging and clinical correlation. *Radiology* 1996;199:409–413.
120. Cognard C, Semaan H, Bakchine S, et al. Paraspinal arteriovenous fistula with perimedullary venous drainage. *AJNR* 1995;16:2044–2048.
121. Saraf-Lavi E, Bower BC, Quencer RM, et al. Detection of spinal dural arteriovenous fistulae with MR imaging and contrast-enhanced MR angiography: sensitivity, specificity, and prediction of vertebral level. *AJNR* 2002;23:858–867.
122. Buchanan RJ, Brant A, Marshall LF. Traumatic cerebrospinal fluid fistulas. Winn HR, ed. *Youmans neurological surgery*, 5th ed. Philadelphia: WB Saunders Co., 2004:5265–5272.
123. Pearson BW. Cerebrospinal fluid rhinorrhea. In: *Otolaryngology*, 3rd ed. Philadelphia: W. B. Saunders Co, 1991:1899–1909.
124. Shetty PG, Shroff MM, Sahani DV, et al. Evaluation of high-resolution CT and MR cisternography in the diagnosis of cerebrospinal fluid fistula. *AJNR* 1998;19:633–639.
125. El Gammal T, Sobol W, Wadlington VR, et al. Cerebrospinal fluid fistula: detection with MR cisternography. *AJNR* 1998;19:627–630.
126. Jinkins JR, Rudwan M, Krumina G, et al. Intrathecal gadolinium-enhanced MR cisternography in the evaluation of clinically suspected cerebrospinal fluid rhinorrhea in humans: early experience. *Radiology* 2002;222: 555–559.
127. Matsumura A, Anno I, Kimura H, et al. Diagnosis of spontaneous intracranial hypotension by using magnetic resonance myelography. *J Neurosurg* 2000;92:873–876.
128. Carl AL, Matsumoto M, Whalen JT, et al. Anterior dural laceration caused by thoracolumbar and lumbar burst fractures. *J Spinal Disord* 2000;13:399–403.
129. Aydinli U, Karaeminogullari O, Tiskaya K, et al. Dural tears in lumbar burst fractures with greenstick lamina fractures. *Spine* 2001;26:E410–E415.
130. Pau A, Silvestro C, Carta F. Can lacerations of the thoraco-lumbar dura be predicted on the basis of radiological patterns of the spinal fractures? *Acta Neurochir* (Wien) 1994;129:186–187.
131. Silvestro C, Francaviglia N, Bragazzi R et al. On the predictive value of radiological signs for the presence of dural lacerations related to fractures of the lower thoracic or lumbar spine. *J Spinal Disord* 1991;4:49–53.
132. Shin AY, Spinner RJ, Steinmann SF, et al. Adult traumatic brachial plexus injuries. *J Am Acad Orthop Surg* 2005;13:382–396.
133. Carvalho GA, Nikkhah G, Matthies C, et al. Diagnosis of root avulsions in traumatic brachial plexus injuries: value of computerized tomography myelography and magnetic resonance imaging. *J Neurosurg* 1997;86:69–76.
134. Lee TT, Arias JM, Andrus HL, et al. Progressive posttraumatic myelomalacic myelopathy: treatment with untethering and expansive duraplasty. *J Neurosurg* 1997;86: 624–628.
135. Wittenberg RH, Boetel U, Beyer HK. Magnetic resonance imaging and computed tomography of acute spinal cord trauma. *Clin Orthop* 1990;260:176–185.
136. Kulkarni MV, McArdle CB, Kopanicky D, et al. Acute spinal cord injury: MRI imaging at 1.5T. *Radiology* 1987;164(3):837–843.
137. Schouman-Claeys E, Frija G, Cuenod CA, et al. MRI imaging of acute spinal cord injury: results of an experimental study in dogs. *AJNR* 1990;11:959–965.
138. Shimada K, Takahashi C, Satoru A, et al. Sequential MRI studies in patients with cervical cord injury but without bony injury. *Paraplegia* 1995;33:573–578.

139. Shimada K, Tokioka T. Sequential MR studies of cervical cord injury: correlation with neurological damage and clinical outcome. *Spinal Cord* 1999;37:410–415.
140. Ohta K, Fujimura Y, Nakamura M, et al. Experimental study on MRI evaluation of the course of cervical spinal cord injury. *Spinal Cord* 1999;37:580–584.
141. Marciello M, Flanders AE, Herbison GJ, et al. Magnetic resonance imaging related to neurologic outcome in cervical spinal cord injury. *Arch Phys Med Rehabil* 1993;74:940–946.
142. Flanders AE, Spettell CM, Tartaglino LM, et al. Forecasting motor recovery after cervical spinal cord injury: value of MR imaging. *Radiology* 1996;201:649–655.
143. Silberstein M, Tress BM, Hennessy O. Delayed neurologic deterioration in the patient with spinal trauma: role of MRI imaging. *AJNR* 1992;13:1373–1381.
144. Ramon S, Dominquez R, Ramirez L, et al. Clinical and magnetic resonance imaging correlation in acute spinal cord injury. *Spinal Cord* 1997;35:664–673.
145. Pollard ME, Apple DF. Factors associated with improved neurologic outcomes in patients with incomplete tetraplegia. *Spine* 2003;28:33–39.
146. Hayashi K, Yone K, Ito H, et al. MRI findings in patients with a cervical spinal cord injury who do not show radiographic evidence of a fracture or dislocation. *Paraplegia* 1995;33:212–215.
147. Hackney DB, Ford JC, Markowitz RS, et al. Experimental spinal cord injury: imaging the acute lesion. *AJNR Am. J. Neuroradiol.*, May1994;15:960–961.
148. LeMay DR, Fechner KP, Zelenock GB et al. High resolution magnetic resonance imaging of the rat spinal cord. *Neurol Res* 1996;18(5):471–474.
149. Metz GA, Curt A, van de Meent H, et al. Validation of the weight-drop contusion model in rats: a comparative study of human spinal cord injury. *J Neurotrauma* 2000;17:1–17.
150. Hackney DB, Finkelstein SD, Hand CM, et al. Postmortem magnetic resonance imaging of experimental spinal cord injury: magnetic resonance findings versus in vivo functional deficit. *Neurosurgery* 1994;35:1104–1011.
151. Hackney DB, Ford JC, Markowitz RS, et al. Experimental spinal cord injury: MR correlation to intensity of injury. *J Comput Assist Tomogr* 1994;18(3):357–362.
152. Chakeres DW, Flickinger F, Bresnahan JC, et al. MRI imaging of acute spinal cord trauma. *AJNR* 1987;8:5–10.
153. Hackney DB, Asato LR, Joseph P, et al. Hemorrhage and edema in acute spinal cord compression: demonstration by MRI imaging. *Radiology* 1986;161:387–390.
154. Bilgen M, Abbe R, Liu S. et al. Spatial and temporal evolution of hemorrhage in the hyperacute phase of experimental spinal cord injury: In vivo magnetic resonance imaging. *Magn Reson Med* 2000;43:594–600.
155. Larsson EM, Holtas S, Cronqvist S. Emergency magnetic resonance examination of patients with spinal cord symptoms. *Acta Radiol* 1988;29(1):69–75.
156. Cotler HB, Kulkarni MV, Bondurant FJ. Magnetic resonance imaging of acute spinal cord trauma: preliminary report. *J Orthop Trauma* 1988;2:1–4.
157. Blackwood W. Vascular disease of the central nervous system. In: Blackwood W, McMenemey WH, Meyer A, et al., eds. *Greenfield's neuropathology*. Baltimore: Williams & Wilkins, 1963:71–115.
158. Kulkarni MV, Bondurant FJ, Rose SL, et al. 1.5 tesla magnetic resonance imaging of acute spinal trauma. *Radiographics* 1988;8:1059–1082.
159. Kalfas I, Wilberger J, Goldberg A, et al. Magnetic resonance imaging in acute spinal cord trauma. *Neurosurgery* 1988;23:295–299.
160. Aito S, El Masry WS, Gerner HJ, et al. Ascending myelopathy in the early stage of spinal cord injury. *Spinal Cord* 1999;37:617–623.
161. Quencer RM, Bunge RP. The injured spinal cord: imaging, histopathologic clinical correlates, and basic science approaches to enhancing neural function after spinal cord injury. *Spine* 1996;21:2064–2066.
162. Kothari P, Freeman B, Grevitt M, et al. Injury to the spinal cord without radiological abnormality (SCIWORA) in adults. *J Bone Joint Surg Br* 2000;82:1034–1037.
163. Silberstein M, Tress BM, Hennessy O. Delayed neurologic deterioration in the patient with spinal trauma: role of MR imaging. *AJNR* 1992;13:1373–1381.
164. Curati WL, Kingsley DPE, Kendall BE, et al. MRI in chronic spinal cord trauma. *Neuroradiology* 1992;35:30–35.
165. Potter K, Saifuddin A. MRI of chronic spinal cord injury. *Br J Radiol* 2003;76:347–352.
166. Mani RL. Potential hazard of metal-filled sandbags in MRI imaging. *Radiology* 1992;182:286–287.
167. Hayashi K, Yone K, Ito H, et al. MRI findings in patients with a cervical spinal cord injury who do not show radiographic evidence of a fracture or dislocation. *Paraplegia* 1995;33:212–215.
168. Riviello JJ, Marks HG, Faerber EN, et al. Delayed cervical central cord syndrome after trivial trauma. *Pediatr Emerg Care* 1990;6:113–117.
169. Pang D, Wilberger JE. Spinal cord injury without radiographic abnormalities in children. *J Neurosurg* 1982;57:114–129.
170. Mendelsohn DB, Zollars L, Weatherall PT, et al. MRI of cord transection. *J Comput Assist Tomogr* 1990;14: 909–911.
171. Goldberg AL, Rothfus WE, Deeb ZL, et al. Hyperextension injuries of the cervical spine. Magnetic resonance findings. *Skeletal Radiol* 1989;18:283–288.
172. Gupta SK, Rajeev K, Khosla VK, et al. Spinal cord injury without radiographic abnormality in adults. *Spinal Cord* 1999;37:726–729.
173. Pope AM, Tarlov AR. *Disability in America: toward a national agenda for prevention*. Washington, DC: National Academy Press, 1991.
174. Smugar SS, Schweitzer ME, Hume E. MRI in patients with intraspinal bullets. *J Magn Reson Imaging* 1999;9:151–153.
175. Tartaglino LM, Flanders AE, Vinitski S, et al. Metallic artifacts on MRI images of the postoperative spine: reduction with fast spin-echo techniques. *Radiology* 1994;190:565–569.
176. Flanders AE, Tartaglino LM, Friedman DP, et al. Application of fast spin-echo MRI imaging in acute cervical spine injury. *Radiology* 1992;185:220.

177. Rockwell DT, Melhem ER, Bhatia RG. GRASE (gradient- and spin-echo) MR of the brain. *AJNR* 1999;20:1381–1383.
178. Brunberg JA, Papadopoulos SM. Technical note. Device to facilitate MRI imaging of patients in skeletal traction. *AJNR* 1991;12:746–747.
179. Van Uijen CM, den Boef JH. Driven-equilibrium radiofrequency pulses in NMR imaging. *Mag Reson Med* 1984;1:502–507.
180. Edeiken-Monroe B, Wagner LK, Harris JH. Hyperextension dislocation of the cervical spine. *Am J Radiol* 1986;146:803–808.
181. White AA III, Panjabi MM. *Clinical biomechanics of the spine*. Philadelphia: JB Lippincott, 1978.
182. Gardner E, Gray DJ. The back. In: Gardner E, Gray DJ, O'Rahilly Ronan, eds. *Anatomy*, 4th ed. Philadelphia: WB Saunders, 1975:508–540.
183. Sett P, Crockard HA. The value of magnetic resonance imaging (MRI) in the follow-up management of spinal injury. *Paraplegia* 1991;29(6):396–410.
184. Sherman JL, Barkovich AJ, Citrin CM. The MR appearance of syringomyelia: new observations. *Am J Roentgenol* 1987;148:381–391.
185. Falcone S, Quencer RM, Green BA, et al. Progressive posttraumatic myelomalacic myelopathy: imaging and clinical features. *AJNR* 1994;15:747–754.
186. Lee TT, Arias JM, Andrus HL, et al. Progressive posttraumatic myelomalacic myelopathy: treatment with untethering and expansive duraplasty. *J Neurosurg* 1997;86:624–628.
187. Vertinsky AT, Krasnokutsky MV, Augustin M, et al. Cutting-edge imaging of the spine. *Neuroimaging Clin N Am* 2007;17:117–136.
188. Lipton, Michael L: Totally Accessible MRI. A User's Guide to Principles, Technology, and Applications. Springer-Verlag New York. 2008.
189. Schwartz ED, Hackney DB. Diffusion-weighted MRI and the evaluation of spinal cord axonal integrity following injury and treatment. *Exp Neurol* 2003;184:570–589.
190. Lu J, Waite P. Spine update-advances in spinal cord regeneration. *Spine* 1999;24:926–930.
191. Schwab ME, Bartholdi D. Degeneration and regeneration of axons in the lesioned spinal cord. *Physiol Rev* 1996;76:319.
192. Demir A, Ries M, Moonen CT, et al. Diffusion-weighted MR imaging with apparent diffusion coefficient and apparent diffusion tensor maps in cervical spondylotic myelopathy. *Radiology* 2003;229:37–43.
193. Shanmuganathan K, Gullapalli RP, Zhuo J, et al. Diffusion tensor MR imaging in cervical spine trauma. *AJNR* 2008;29:655–659.
194. Ellingson BM, Kurpad SN, Schmit BD. Ex vivo diffusion tensor imaging and quantitative tractography of the rat spinal cord during long-term recovery from moderate spinal contusion. *J Magn Reson Imaging.* 2008;28:1068–1079.
195. Ramu J, Herrera J, Grill R, et al. Brain fiber tract plasticity in experimental spinal cord injury: diffusion tensor imaging. *Exp Neurol* 2008;212:100–107.
196. Vargas MI, Delavelle J, Jlassi H, et al. Clinical applications of diffusion tensor tractography of the spinal cord. *Neuroradiology* 2008;50:25–29.
197. Sabbah P, de SS, Leveque C, et al. Sensorimotor cortical activity in patients with complete spinal cord injury: a functional magnetic resonance imaging study. *J Neurotrauma* 2002;19:53–60.
198. Ramu J, Bockhorst KH, Mogatadakala KV, et al. Functional magnetic resonance imaging in rodents: methodology and application to spinal cord injury. *J Neurosci Res* 2006;84:1235–1244.
199. Ogawa S, Lee TM, Kay AR, et al. Brain magnetic resonance imaging with contrast dependent on blood oxygenation. *Proceedings of the National Academy of Sciences* 1990;87:986–988.
200. Harel NY, Strittmatter SM. Functional MRI and other non-invasive imaging technologies: providing visual biomarkers for spinal cord structure and function after injury. *Exp Neurol* 2008;211:324–328.
201. Vink R, Knoblach SM, Faden Al. ^{31}P magnetic resonance spectroscopy of traumatic spinal cord injury. *Magn Reson Med* 1987;5:390–394.
202. Akino M, O'Donnell JM, Robitaille PM, et al. Phosphorus-31 magnetic resonance spectroscopy studies of pig spinal cord injury. Myelin changes, intracellular pH, and bioenergetics. *Invest Radiol* 1997;32:383–388.
203. Faden AI, Yum SW, Lemke M, et al. Effects of TRH-analog treatment on tissue cations, phospholipids and energy metabolism after spinal cord injury. *J Pharmacol Exp Ther* 1990;255:608–614.

CHAPTER 5 ■ EPIDEMIOLOGY OF TRAUMATIC SPINAL CORD INJURY

MICHAEL J. DEVIVO AND YUYING CHEN

INTRODUCTION

Many studies of the epidemiology of traumatic spinal cord injury (SCI) in the United States have been undertaken in the past 40 years. Initially, these studies were mostly descriptive in nature, examining the demographic profile and other characteristics of persons treated at particular hospitals and rehabilitation centers (1,2). Local population–based studies of actual incidence of SCI were first conducted by Kraus et al. (3) for the northern California region and later by Griffin et al. (4) for one Minnesota county. National population–based epidemiological investigations were first conducted by Kalsbeek et al. and Bracken et al. (5,6). However, other than immediate case fatality and hospital expenses, none of these investigations included patient follow-up or any measures of treatment outcome.

In the early 1970s, the model SCI care system program was initiated with funding from what is now the National Institute on Disability and Rehabilitation Research in the United States Department of Education. As a part of this program, all funded model systems were required to contribute data on patients they treated to a national database. This database is now known as the National Spinal Cord Injury Statistical Center (NSCISC) Database and is located at the University of Alabama at Birmingham (7,8). In 1987, a similar database was established for newly injured persons treated at a Shriners Hospital SCI unit. These databases have been used extensively to develop an epidemiologic profile of new SCIs that occur each year as well as changes in that profile that have occurred over time (9–14). It has been estimated that these databases contain information on 10% to 15% of all new SCIs that occur in the United States each year (9). However, they are not population-based, and, as a result, they cannot be used to calculate incidence rates or directly assess risk factors for the occurrence of SCI. In general, when compared to population-based studies, it has been shown that persons in the NSCISC Database are representative of all SCIs except that more severe injuries, nonwhites, and injuries due to acts of violence are slightly overrepresented (9). The strength of the NSCISC and Shriners Hospital SCI databases and their unique contribution to the field of SCI epidemiology is that they were designed with a long-term follow-up component to track thousands of patients longitudinally over time for the purpose of assessing treatment outcomes.

Beginning in the 1980s, the Centers for Disease Control and Prevention began funding population-based SCI surveillance systems in many states (15–20). When combined with the more detailed information contained in the NSCISC and Shriners Hospital SCI Databases, a relatively complete description of the epidemiology of SCI in the United States can be obtained.

OVERALL INCIDENCE

Published reports of the incidence of SCI vary from 25 new cases per million population per year in West Virginia to 59 new cases per million population per year in Mississippi (18,20). Differences in SCI incidence rates among states are due to a combination of factors, including differences in population characteristics such as age, gender, and race; differences in the definition of SCI; and differences in data collection methodology. Overall, when combining information from all the state SCI registries, the incidence rate appears to be approximately 40 new cases per million population, or just over 12,000 cases per year. This figure does not include persons who die at the scene of the accident. Interestingly, although there have been shifts in the underlying causes of these SCIs over the past four decades, the overall incidence appears to have remained relatively constant (21).

Incidence of fatal SCI prior to hospitalization was reported to be 21.2 cases per million population for northern California in 1970 to 1971 and 20.8 cases per million population in Olmsted County, Minnesota, from 1935 to 1981 (3,4). However, a more recent report from the SCI population–based registry in Utah suggests that the incidence rate of fatal SCI prior to hospitalization for 1989 to 1991 was only approximately 4 cases per million population, or about 1,200 cases per year if that figure were applied nationally (17). This decrease might be due to improved emergency medical services at the scene of the accident, but incomplete reporting of cases also cannot be ruled out.

Incidence of SCI in the rest of the world is consistently lower than that in the United States, and often does not exceed 20 new cases per million population per year (22–30). Some, but not all, of this difference is due to the relatively high incidence of violence-related SCIs in the United States. Violence is a somewhat less frequent cause of SCI in many other countries.

PREVALENCE

Prevalence can be estimated in one of two ways. Given that SCI is a relatively rare condition, initial attempts to assess prevalence were by using the epidemiological formula linking prevalence to more established data on incidence and life expectancy. In 1980, using the best available data at the time, DeVivo et al. estimated SCI prevalence in the United States to be 906 persons per million population, or just under 200,000 existing cases (31). However, for this approach to be valid, both incidence and life expectancy would need to be relatively constant over time. Since life expectancy had been increasing and a current estimate was used, this approach resulted in a slight overestimate of prevalence.

The alternative approach of simply counting people with SCI was eventually undertaken only when substantial funding was provided by the Paralyzed Veterans of America. Using a sophisticated probability sampling plan of small geographic areas and institutions, Berkowitz et al. (32) conservatively estimated the prevalence of SCI in the United States to be 721 persons per million population, or approximately 176,965 persons in 1988.

More recently, Lasfargues et al. (33) combined the 1988 estimate of Berkowitz et al. with current estimates of age-sex–specific incidence and mortality to project the growth in prevalence of SCI in the United States over time. Estimated prevalence of SCI from this mathematical model was 207,129 persons in 1994; 246,882 persons in 2004; and 276,281 persons in 2014. This growth was projected to result exclusively from improved life expectancies rather than any increase in incidence. However, life expectancy has not been increasing as originally anticipated (34). Therefore, these prevalence figures may be slightly overestimated.

AGE

Several state registries have produced relatively comparable estimates of age-specific incidence rates. Typical is the state of Oklahoma, where the overall annual incidence rate of 40 cases per million population matches the national average. In Oklahoma, incidence rates are lowest for the pediatric age group (age less than 15, 6 cases per million population); highest for persons aged 15 to 19 (94 per million population); and decline steadily after age 19 to 85 per million for age 20 to 24, 71 per million for age 25 to 29, 47 per million for age 30 to 44, 32 per million for age 45 to 59, and 26 per million persons at least 60 years of age (16). Looking at actual numbers of cases rather than rates, 3% of new cases in Oklahoma occurred among persons under age 15, 47% occurred between the ages of 15 and 29, 27% occurred between the ages of 30 and 44, 12% occurred between the ages of 45 and 59, and 11% occurred at age 60 or greater.

As seen in Fig. 5.1, the distribution of age at time of injury for persons enrolled in a combined NSCISC/Shriners Hospital SCI Database is strikingly similar to the population-based data from Oklahoma. The mean age at injury for all persons in the combined database is 33.4 years (±16.7 years), the median age at injury is 29 years, and the most common age at injury is 18 years (Table 5.1). Overall, 54.4% of all persons enrolled in the combined database were aged 30 or less at the time of injury. Interestingly, the percentage of new persons enrolled in the combined database who are older than age 60 at time of injury has increased steadily from 4.7% during 1973 to 1979 to 12.9% from 2005 to 2009. This trend most likely reflects the advancing age of the general United States population, although shifts in referral patterns to model systems or changes in underlying age-specific incidence rates cannot be ruled out.

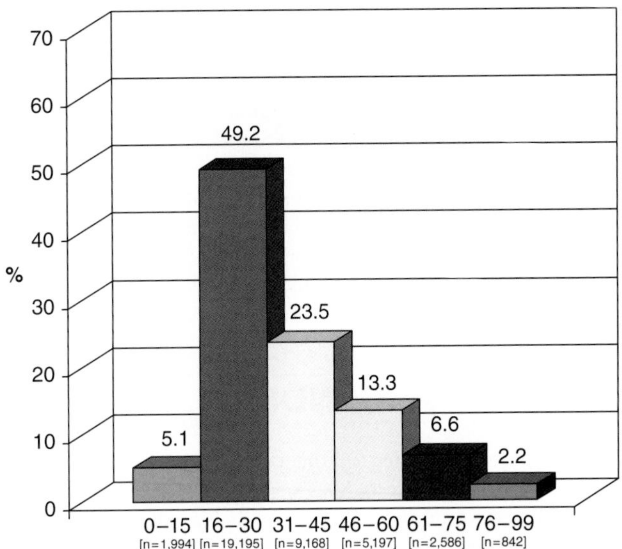

FIGURE 5.1. Age of persons enrolled in the combined NSCISC/Shriners Hospital SCI Database at time of injury (n = 38,982).

The distribution of ages at the time of injury (incident cases) is very different from the current ages of all persons who presently have an SCI (prevalent cases) because the latter is a function of both age at injury and long-term survival rates. Only the study by Berkowitz et al. (32) has attempted to estimate the

TABLE 5.1

CHARACTERISTICS OF PERSONS ENROLLED IN THE COMBINED NSCISC/SHRINERS HOSPITAL SCI DATABASE, 1973–2009

Characteristic	
Age at injury (y)	
Mean	33.4
Median	29.0
Mode	18.0
Male gender (%)	80.2
Race/ethnicity (%)	
White	65.9
African American	20.5
Native American	0.9
Asian	1.7
Hispanic	10.5
Other	0.5
Educational status at injury (%)	
Less than high school graduate	36.7
High school graduate	51.0
Associate degree	2.3
Bachelor degree	6.8
Master's degree	1.5
Doctorate	1.0
Other degree	0.7
Marital status at injury (%)	
Single—never married	52.3
Married	31.8
Divorced	9.1
Separated	3.6
Widowed	2.5
Other/unknown	0.7

current ages of people living with SCI in the United States. The median current age of all persons with SCI was estimated to be 41 years (15 years older than the median age of new cases at that time), with only 5.4% below age 25, 54.2% between ages 25 and 44, 27.8% between ages 45 and 64, and 12.7% aged 65 or greater (32). However, these estimates are now 20 years old, so the median age of all persons with SCI alive today would likely be slightly higher than it was in 1988. In fact, the average current age of all persons in the combined NSCISC/Shriners Hospital Database who were still alive in 2008 was 45 years, and 13.7% were at least 60 years of age.

GENDER

The proportion of men in the combined NSCISC/Shriners Hospital SCI Database is 80.2% (Table 5.1). This is consistent with population-based registries such as Oklahoma where 80% of SCIs occurred among men (16). Underlying annual incidence rates in Oklahoma also reflect this four to one gender ratio, with men having an incidence rate of 65 and women having an incidence rate of 16 cases per million population per year (16). This four to one gender ratio has remained remarkably consistent over time despite significant trends in age at injury, ethnicity, and etiology of injury (12,13).

Because of differential survival rates between men and women, the percentage of persons with SCI who are alive today who are men is slightly lower than the percentage of new cases that occur among men. In 1988, Berkowitz et al. (32) estimated that only 71% of prevalent cases of SCI in the United States were men, while 78.3% of persons in the combined NSCISC/Shriners Hospital SCI Database who were injured since 1973 and who are still alive in 2008 are men.

ETHNICITY

State registries consistently reveal higher incidence rates for African Americans than whites. Again, using Oklahoma as an example, the annual SCI incidence rate was 57 per million population for African Americans, 40 per million population for whites, and 29 per million for Native Americans (16). This difference between African Americans and whites is due entirely to injuries that result from acts of violence. Among African Americans, the cause-specific annual SCI incidence rate for acts of violence is 21 per million population, while the comparable figure for whites and Native Americans is only 3 per million population (16). Unfortunately, state registries have not yet published incidence rates for other racial and ethnic groups such as Asians and Hispanics.

Since 1973, 65.9% of persons enrolled in the combined NSCISC/Shriners Hospital SCI Database have been white, 20.5% African American, 10.5% Hispanic, 1.7% Asian, 0.9% Native American, and 0.5% other race (Table 5.1). However, a substantial trend has been observed in the racial distribution of persons enrolled in the combined database over time. During 1973 to 1979, 76.8% of new persons enrolled in the combined database were white, 14.3% were African American, 5.9% were Hispanic, 1.9% were Native American, and 0.9% were Asian. By comparison, between 2005 and 2009, only 66.9% of new persons enrolled in the combined database were white, while 21.2% were African American, 8.8% were Hispanic, 1.9% were Asian, and 0.5% were Native American. This trend is due in very small part to changes in the general US population. Rather, it is related to a combination of factors, including periodic changes in the identities and locations of participating model systems, changes in eligibility criteria for inclusion in the NSCISC Database, and changes in referral patterns to model systems. Given the substantial nature of this trend, some change in underlying race-specific incidence rates is also likely. However, the exact nature of any such change in race-specific incidence rates cannot be determined from these databases.

ETIOLOGY OF INJURY

Ten specific causes of traumatic SCI account for 91.4% of all new cases enrolled in the combined NSCISC/Shriners Hospital SCI Database each year. Automobile crashes rank first (35.2%), followed by falls (20.0%), gunshot wounds (14.9%), diving mishaps (6.2%), motorcycle crashes (5.6%), being hit by a falling object (2.9%), medical or surgical complications (2.6%), pedestrians being struck by motor vehicles (1.7%), bicycle mishaps (1.3%), and violent personal contact (1.0%). All other causes of SCI account for less than 1% each. Automobile crashes cause a lower percentage of cases among men than women (30.4% versus 50.2%). Conversely, men have a higher percentage of SCI than women that are due to gunshot wounds (17.3% versus 10.2%), diving mishaps (7.3% versus 2.7%), and motorcycle crashes (6.9% versus 2.0%).

Diving mishaps account for the majority of SCIs due to recreational sports reported to the combined NSCISC/Shriners Hospital SCI Database (57.7%). Snow skiing ranked second at only 5.8%, followed by football at 5.1%, surfing at 4.3%, winter sports at 4.3%, and horseback riding at 4.2%. Interestingly, SCIs due to diving, football, and trampoline mishaps have declined markedly since the initiation of the NSCISC Database in the mid-1970s, while those due to snow skiing and surfing have increased in both raw numbers and percentages (35). Football rules changes in 1976 banning deliberate "spearing" and the use of the top of the helmet as the initial point of contact in making tackles undoubtedly contributed to the decline in football-related SCIs. Similarly, removal of trampolines from schools in some states has undoubtedly contributed to the decline in trampoline-related SCIs.

It is important to keep in mind that those recreational sports activities that involve the most SCIs are not necessarily the most risky activities. To assess risk, one must know the underlying rate of exposure to that activity. For example, male gymnastics, which causes few SCIs but also has few participants, has an incidence rate of 14.3 per 100,000 athletes, while high school and college football, which cause more SCIs but also have more participants, have an incidence rate of only 1 per 100,000 athletes (36).

Neither the NSCISC nor Shriners Hospital SCI Database contains more specific information on the circumstances surrounding each SCI. However, a number of studies have been undertaken to examine the leading causes of SCI in more detail for the purpose of identifying possible preventive interventions that might be cost effective. Specific causes of SCI that have been looked at include motor vehicle crashes, gunshot wounds, diving mishaps, and falls (37–42).

Individual causes of SCI are often grouped into five categories to facilitate analysis: vehicular crashes (any type of motor

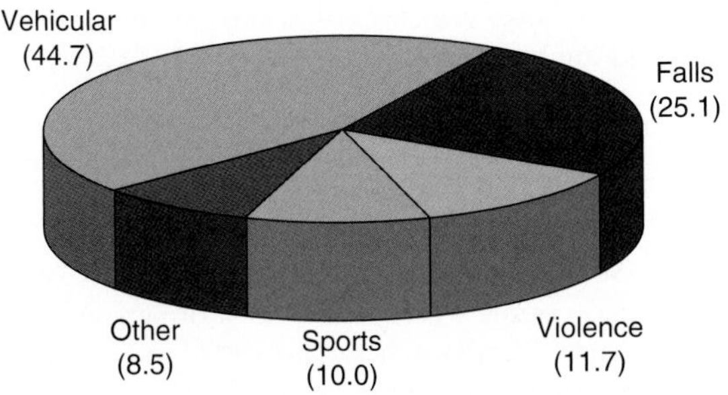

FIGURE 5.2. Grouped etiology for persons enrolled in the combined NSCISC/Shriners Hospital SCI Database between 2005 and 2009.

vehicle or bicycle), violence (gunshot wounds, stab wounds, personal contact, or explosion), recreational sports, falls, and all other causes. Fig. 5.2 reflects the distribution of grouped causes of SCI among all new persons enrolled in the combined NSCISC/Shriners Hospital SCI Database from 2005 to 2009. Overall, 44.7% of these injuries were due to vehicular crashes, 25.1% were due to falls, 11.7% were due to violence, 10.0% were due to sports, and 8.5% were due to all other causes.

A similar picture of grouped etiologies of SCI emerges from the population-based registries. In Oklahoma, 48% of SCIs are due to motor vehicle crashes, 20% are due to falls, 13% are due to recreational sports activities, 11% are due to violence, and 8% are due to other causes (16). Data from Utah are very similar to those from Oklahoma, with 49% of SCIs due to motor vehicle crashes, 21% due to falls, 16% due to recreational sports, 5% due to violence, and 9% due to other and unknown causes (17).

The most common causes of SCI in other countries are generally comparable to those observed in the United States. Typical is the case of Denmark, where 47% of SCIs are due to motor vehicle crashes, 26% are due to falls, 12% are due to recreational sports, 10% are due to acts of violence, and 5% are due to other causes (23). However, among the SCIs caused by acts of violence in Denmark, 80% result from failed suicide attempts, whereas in the United States, these injuries are usually either unintentionally inflicted (either by the individual or another person) or malicious. The pattern of causes of SCI in Taipei, Istanbul, and Spain is similar to that of Denmark (22,24,25). However, in Jordan, 29% of SCIs are due to acts of violence (almost all gunshot wounds) (27).

Grouped causes of SCI by age at time of injury for all persons enrolled in the combined NSCISC/Shriners Hospital SCI Database appear in Table 5.2. Motor vehicle crashes are the leading cause of SCI until age 60; however, beginning with the 61 to 75 year old age group, falls represent the leading cause of SCI. The percentage of SCIs due to falls increases steadily from only 7.6% among the pediatric age group to 63.7% in the oldest age group. Conversely, the percentages of SCIs due to recreational sports and acts of violence decrease with advancing age at time of injury. In the pediatric age group, recreational sports account for 20.8% and acts of violence account for 16.7% of SCIs, while in the oldest age group, the comparable figures are 0.6% and 1.0%, respectively.

There are also significant differences in causes of SCI by racial and ethnic group. Among persons enrolled in the combined NSCISC/Shriners Hospital SCI Database, 85.8% of SCIs due to recreational sports, 74.4% due to motor vehicle crashes, 69.4% due to falls, and only 23.8% due to acts of violence occur among whites.

Closer inspection of the interaction of age, gender, race, year of injury, and cause of injury reveals the rather striking pattern depicted in Fig. 5.3. Among African American and Hispanic males aged 16 to 21 at injury enrolled in the combined NSCISC/Shriners Hospital SCI Database, the percentage of persons whose SCI was due to an act of violence increased dramatically from 34.5% between 1973 and 1979 to 73.9% between 1990 and 1994 before declining to 52.0% since 2005. The comparable figures for white males aged 16 to 21 years were 4.7%, 9.0%, and 3.6%, respectively. Moreover, among adult (age 22 or older) African American and Hispanic males enrolled in the combined database, the percentage of new injuries due to acts of violence only ranged from 33.4% between 1973 and 1979 to a peak of 44.6% between 1990 and 1994 before declining again to 23.6% since 2005. Therefore, the epidemic of increased violence-induced SCIs that occurred during the late 1980s and early 1990s was limited almost entirely to African American and Hispanic males aged 16 to 21 years.

Although a portion of these trends in SCI etiology may be due to periodic changes in the identities and locations of participating model systems, changes in eligibility criteria for inclusion in the NSCISC Database, and changes in referral patterns to model systems, the magnitude of these proportional trends

TABLE 5.2

GROUPED ETIOLOGY FOR PERSONS ENROLLED IN THE COMBINED NSCISC/SHRINERS HOSPITAL SCI DATABASE BY AGE AT INJURY

	Grouped etiology (%)					
Age	Vehicular	Violence	Sports	Falls	Other	Total (%)
0–15	44.1	16.7	20.8	7.6	10.8	100.0
16–30	47.0	22.5	14.8	10.6	5.1	100.0
31–45	46.3	15.6	7.3	21.8	9.0	100.0
46–60	40.1	6.6	4.2	35.9	13.2	100.0
61–75	32.3	2.6	2.6	46.9	15.6	100.0
76–99	24.9	1.0	0.6	63.7	9.8	100.0

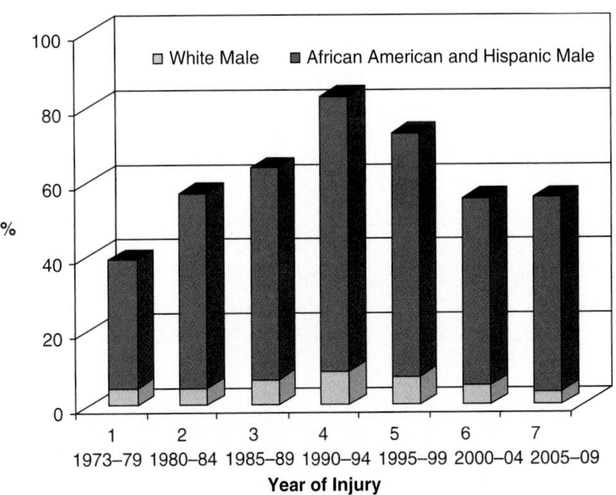

FIGURE 5.3. Percentage of 16- to 21-year-old men treated at a model system or Shriners Hospital whose SCI was due to an act of violence by racial/ethnic group and year of injury.

suggests that underlying age-sex-race-cause–specific incidence rates have changed. The overall decline in violence-induced SCI is consistent with a reduction in the violent crime rate in the United States. However, the proportion of SCI due to violence would decline if the incidence of SCI due to violence were increasing, as long as it was increasing at a slower rate than it was for other causes. Population-based studies are needed to develop a further understanding of these trends in the causes of SCI. Unfortunately, most of the population-based state registries are no longer operational due to lack of funds.

ASSOCIATED INJURIES

SCIs are often accompanied by other significant injuries. Among persons enrolled in the NSCISC Database between 1986 and 1992, 29.3% had other broken bones, 28.2% experienced loss of consciousness at least briefly after the injury, 17.8% had a traumatic pneumothorax, and 11.5% had a head injury sufficient to affect cognitive and/or emotional functioning (10).

The nature and frequency of these other injuries is significantly associated with the etiology of SCI. Among persons injured in motor vehicle crashes, 42.5% experienced loss of consciousness, 39.7% had broken bones, 18.4% had a head injury, and 16.6% had traumatic pneumothorax (10). Conversely, among persons injured in recreational sports mishaps, 22.4% had loss of consciousness, but no other associated injury occurred in more than 5% of cases (10). Not surprisingly, traumatic pneumothorax is most common among persons injured by acts of violence (35.9% of cases), but other associated injuries are relatively rare among these persons (10).

There have been two detailed investigations of the incidence and risk factors of extraspinal fractures associated with acute SCI (43,44). Overall, extraspinal fractures occurred in 28% of all new SCIs, with rib/sternum fractures most common, followed by upper extremity, lower extremity, and skull fractures (43,44). These extraspinal fractures were most common among SCIs caused by motor vehicle crashes and among persons with thoracic and lumbosacral injuries (44).

TIME OF INJURY

Traumatic SCI occurs with greater frequency on weekends than other days of the week, with 19.3% of persons enrolled in the NSCISC Database between 1994 and 1998 being injured on Saturday and another 17.2% being injured on Sunday (12). The least common injury days are Tuesday (11.3%) and Wednesday (11.4%). This pattern is typical of other types of injuries as well.

Substantial seasonal variation also exists in the incidence of SCI, with peak incidence occurring in July (10.9% of persons enrolled in the combined NSCISC/Shriners Hospital SCI Database), followed closely by August and June. The lowest incidence of SCI occurs in February (6.1%). This seasonal pattern in SCI incidence is much more pronounced in the northern part of the United States where seasonal variation in climate is greater. The increased incidence of SCI in the summer months is due mostly to higher frequencies of diving and other sports and recreational mishaps, and increased motor vehicle–related injuries secondary to greater summertime vehicular use. Interestingly, with the proportional decrease in SCIs due to sports and recreational activities described earlier, seasonal variation in overall SCI incidence has also declined in recent years (12).

NEUROLOGIC LEVEL AND EXTENT OF LESION

Neurologic level of injury is defined as the lowest level of the spinal cord with both intact sensory and motor function bilaterally. Figure 5.4 reflects the distribution of neurologic levels of lesion at time of discharge from model system or Shriners Hospital inpatient rehabilitation programs. Overall, 53.8% of persons

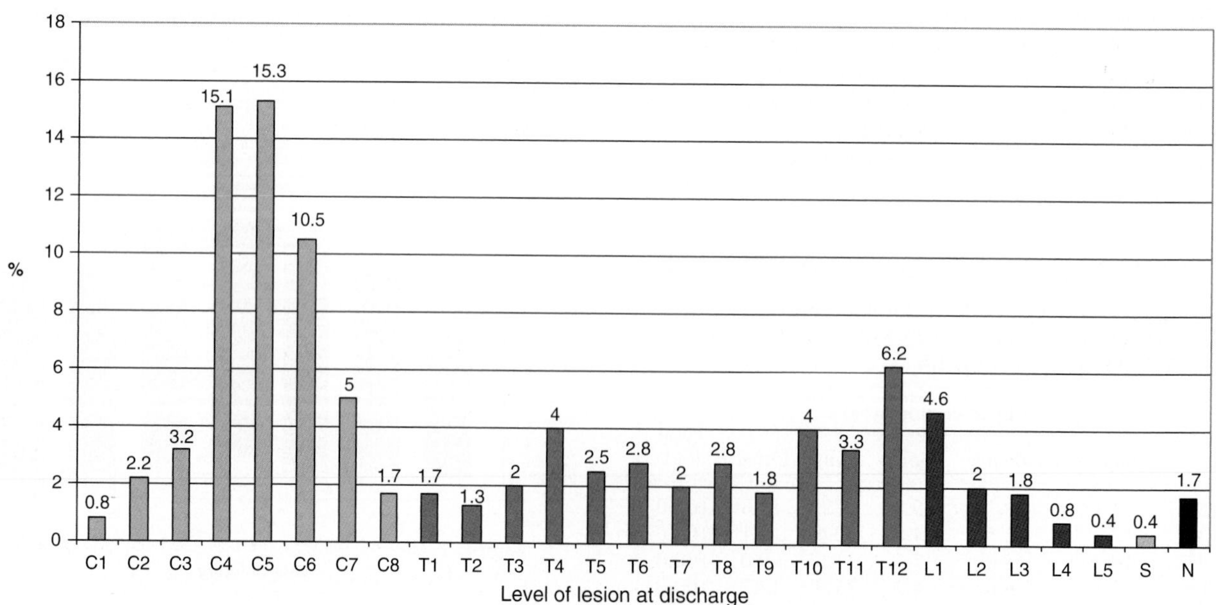

FIGURE 5.4. Percentage of persons enrolled in the combined NSCISC/Shriners Hospital SCI Database by neurologic level of lesion at discharge.

in the combined NSCISC/Shriners Hospital SCI Database have cervical lesions, 34.4% have thoracic lesions, and 10.0% have lumbosacral lesions. The fifth cervical segment is the most common lesion level at discharge (15.3%), followed by C4 (15.1%), C6 (10.5%), T12 (6.2%), C7 (5.0%), and L1 (4.6%).

Extent of injury is typically assessed using the five category American Spinal Injury Association Impairment Scale (AIS) (45). At time of discharge from inpatient rehabilitation, 52.0% of persons enrolled in the combined NSCISC/Shriners Hospital SCI Database had neurologically complete injuries (AIS Classification A), 10.3% had incomplete injuries with sensory sparing (AIS Classification B), 10.8% had incomplete injuries with nonfunctional motor capabilities below the lesion level (AIS Classification C), 25.2% had incomplete injuries with functional motor capabilities below the lesion level (AIS Classification D), and 1.7% had essentially complete neurologic recovery (AIS Classification E). Thoracic injuries are most likely to be neurologically complete (75.6% of T1-6 lesions and 65.3% of T7-12 lesions), while most lower level lesions are AIS D injuries (51.3% of lumbar lesions and 85.1% of sacral lesions). Cervical injuries are usually classified as either AIS A (42.5% for C1-4, 38.4% for C5-8) or AIS D (33.1% for C1-4 and 35.0% for C5-8).

Based on logistic regression analysis of the NSCISC Database, the odds of having a cervical injury relative to a lower injury level increase significantly with advancing age at time of injury, male gender, and when the injury is due to sports or recreational activities. There has also been a trend toward increased likelihood of cervical injury since 1994 (12). Neurologically complete (AIS A) injuries are more likely to occur as a result of acts of violence and among younger age groups. However, the proportion of incomplete injuries has not decreased significantly since the mid-1970s when the NSCISC Database was initiated (12).

Since severity of injury is a function of both neurologic level and extent of lesion, these two measures are often grouped together. Excluding AIS E, one common method of grouping neurologic level and extent of lesion is to create four categories as follows: complete tetraplegia (C1-8 AIS A), incomplete tetraplegia (C1-8 AIS BCD), complete paraplegia (T1-S5 AIS A), and incomplete paraplegia (T1-S5 AIS BCD). Using this grouping approach, the most frequent combination at discharge from inpatient rehabilitation among persons enrolled in the NSCISC Database is incomplete tetraplegia (32.1%), followed by complete paraplegia (26.8%), complete tetraplegia (21.3%), and incomplete paraplegia (19.8%).

Etiology of injury is strongly associated with neurologic group. About half of motor vehicle crashes (56.2%) result in tetraplegia (31.6% incomplete and 24.6% complete). A somewhat similar pattern emerges for falls, with 55.8% resulting in tetraplegia (38.3% incomplete and 17.5% complete). However, acts of violence usually result in paraplegia (42.3% complete and 25.4% incomplete), while recreational sports–related SCIs almost always result in tetraplegia (43.3% incomplete and 42.1% complete).

MARITAL STATUS

It is not surprising given the relatively young age at which most SCIs occur that 52.3% of persons enrolled in the NSCISC Database have never been married at the time of their injury (Table 5.1). Moreover, only 31.8% have intact marriages at the time of injury, with the remainder being either separated, divorced, or widowed. Among those who were at least 15 years of age at the time of injury, 32.1% of persons in the NSCISC Database have still never married 20 years after SCI. The annual marriage rate after SCI is 59% below that of the general population of comparable age, gender, and marital status (never married versus previously married) (46). The annual divorce rate during the first 3 years after SCI is 2.3 times normal, and for those marriages that occur after injury, the divorce rate is still 1.7 times normal (47,48).

Factors associated with increased likelihood of marriage after SCI include being a college graduate, having been previously divorced, having paraplegia rather than tetraplegia, being ambulatory, being independent in activities of daily living, and living in a private residence. There has been no trend in marriage rates among persons with SCI over the existence of the NSCISC Database (46). Factors associated with divorce among persons with SCI who were married at the time of injury are younger age, being female, being African American, having no children, having a prior marriage ending in divorce, and being nonambulatory (47). Factors associated with divorce among marriages that occur after SCI include being male, having less than a college education, having a previous marriage end in divorce, and having a thoracic injury level (48).

LEVEL OF EDUCATION

In general, the SCI population is not well educated. Among persons enrolled in the combined NSCISC/Shriners Hospital SCI Database, only 63.3% have at least completed high school (Table 5.1), whereas 83.0% are at least 19 years of age at the time of their injury. Moreover, very few have degrees beyond high school (2.3% associate degree, 6.8% bachelor degree, 1.5% master's degree, 1.0% doctorate, and 0.7% other degree). Among persons enrolled in the NSCISC Database who were in the 9th to the 11th grades at the time of their injury, 46.5% completed a high school diploma within 5 years of injury. However, among those who had a high school diploma at the time of their injury, only 13.6% completed a post–high school degree within 5 years. These low levels of educational attainment can magnify the difficulty in adjusting to one's disability and obtaining subsequent employment.

OCCUPATIONAL STATUS

The majority of persons enrolled in the NSCISC Database who are between the ages of 16 and 59 are employed in the competitive labor market at the time of injury (64.2%). Another 15.0% of new SCIs in this age range occur among students. However, 16.3% of new SCIs in this age range occur among the unemployed, a figure that is substantially above the typical unemployment rate of the United States general population during the past 25 years. Many of the model systems are located in large urban areas where unemployment is typically more common. Nonetheless, high rates of unemployment prior to injury are problematic because of the strong correlation between preinjury and postinjury employment status (49–51).

Virtually all studies of employment after SCI have focused on either obtaining employment or current employment status rather that maintaining employment over time. Fig. 5.5 depicts occupational status by time postinjury and neurologic level of

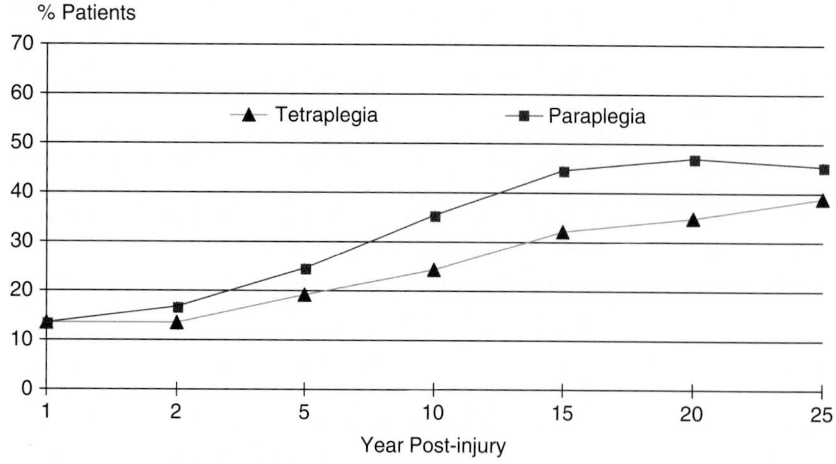

FIGURE 5.5. Percentage of persons enrolled in the NSCISC Database who are employed by neurologic level of lesion and year postinjury.

injury for persons currently aged 16 to 59 who are enrolled in the NSCISC Database. The percentage of persons with tetraplegia who are employed in the competitive labor market increases steadily with time from 13.4% at the first anniversary of injury to 38.9% at the 25th anniversary of injury. Among persons with paraplegia, the percentage employed in the competitive labor market is only slightly higher, ranging from 13.6% 1 year after injury to 47.1% 20 years after injury. Most of those who are employed have full-time rather than part-time jobs (49,50,52).

Predictors of increased likelihood of postinjury employment include younger age, being male, being white, higher level of formal education, higher reported intelligence quotient, greater functional capability, having a less severe injury, being employed at the time of injury, having greater motivation to return to work, having a nonviolent injury etiology, being able to drive, and greater elapsed time postinjury (49–56). Persons who return to work within the first year of injury usually return to the same job with the same employer, while those who return to work after more than 1 year has elapsed usually acquire a different job with a different employer, often after retraining (57). The most common types of jobs that persons with SCI obtain are professional/technical jobs and clerical/sales jobs (52,57).

Estimates of prevalence of current employment for persons enrolled in the NSCISC Database have also been produced. At the time of their most recent evaluation, 27% of persons with SCI were presently employed, but this varied substantially by neurologic level and extent of injury (49). Among persons with AIS A, B, or C injuries, 13.7% of persons with C1-4 injury levels, 22.7% of persons with C5-8 injury levels, and 28.5% of persons with thoracic, lumbar, or sacral injuries were presently employed (49). Among persons with neurologically incomplete AIS D injuries at any level, 38.7% were presently employed (49).

DISCHARGE PLACEMENT

Among all persons enrolled in the NSCISC Database, 88.7% are discharged to a private residence and an additional 1.4% are discharged to a group living situation within the community. Only 6.8% are discharged to another acute care hospital or nursing home, 0.6% are discharged to other environments, and the remaining 2.5% die during hospitalization. Overall, among those who are actually discharged alive, 92.4% have historically been discharged back into the community, either in a private residence or group living situation.

Discharge back into the community is one patient outcome measure on which model systems differ from other hospitals and rehabilitation centers. Among 4,961 persons treated in 1999 at facilities participating in the Uniform Data System for Medical Rehabilitation (UDSMR) program, only 81% were discharged back into the community, with 8% being discharged to long-term care facilities, 7% being discharged to acute or subacute care hospitals, and another 2% being discharged to other rehabilitation facilities (58).

Significant predictors of nursing home discharge include having a cervical injury without useful motor functional capability below the injury level (AIS A, B, or C), being ventilator dependent, older age, being unmarried, being unemployed, being from a region of the United States other than the southeast, having an indwelling urethral catheter or external catheter bladder drainage, having either Medicaid or health maintenance organization (HMO) insurance, being dependent in performing activities of daily living, and being nonambulatory (59). There has also been a significant trend toward an increasing percentage of persons being discharged to nursing homes with the advent of shorter inpatient rehabilitation lengths of stay and older average ages of persons with SCI at the time of their injury (59,60). Between 1973 and 1979, 5.5% of persons enrolled in the NSCISC Database were discharged to a nursing home or other hospital. However, 11.0% of persons in the NSCISC Database who were injured since 2005 have been discharged to a nursing home or other hospital. Nonetheless, this is still below the 1999 UDSMR report of 17% discharges to long-term care facilities or other hospitals (58). Of those who are initially discharged to a nursing home, about one third eventually move to a community residence (61).

Ten years after injury, approximately 98% of persons enrolled in the NSCISC Database who are still alive are still residing in private residences within the community (62). Age is the most significant predictor of long-term nursing home residence, with 12.4% of persons aged 61 to 75 and 22.2% of persons who are at least 76 years of age residing in a nursing home at the time of their most recent anniversary of injury (63). During the first few years after injury, most persons who spend time in a nursing home eventually return to the community rather than spend the entire year in that institution; however, after the third anniversary of injury, full-year stays become more common (61).

LIFE EXPECTANCY

Life expectancy of persons with SCI remains below normal. Among persons admitted to a model system within 24 hours of injury, the mortality rate during the first year after injury has been conservatively estimated at 6.3% (64). Mortality during postinjury year 2 has been estimated at only 1.7%, with a further decline to about 1.2% per year thereafter (64). Significant predictors of mortality during the first year after injury include advanced age, being male, being injured by an act of violence, having a higher injury level (particularly C4 or above), having a neurologically complete injury, being ventilator dependent, and having either Medicare or Medicaid third-party sponsorship of care (65). There has also been a substantial decline in first-year mortality rates over time such that after adjusting for other differences in patient characteristics, the odds of dying for persons injured between 2002 and 2006 were 56% lower than for persons injured between 1973 and 1981 (66).

The same factors that predict mortality during the first year after injury also predict increased likelihood of dying during subsequent years, albeit with somewhat reduced impact (65). Additional predictors of higher mortality rates in later years following SCI include lower satisfaction with life, poor health, emotional distress, being more dependent, poor self-rated adjustment to disability, family income below the poverty line, and poor community integration (67,68). Interestingly, the substantial declines observed in mortality rates during the first year after injury have not been observed in subsequent years (34,65,66,69).

Most striking is the case of ventilator-dependent persons for whom first-year mortality rates have been reduced by 92% from their very high rates in the 1970s (69). However, mortality rates in postinjury years 2 and beyond have not improved, perhaps because deaths that would previously have occurred in the first year have simply been postponed into the next few years rather than longer postinjury (69). Interestingly, the average age in 2008 of chronic ventilator-dependent persons enrolled in the NSCISC Database who were still alive was only 38 years, while age at injury for newly injured ventilator-dependent persons was 43 years. This is because age-specific mortality rates for ventilator-dependent persons are so high once patients reach their 40s that few survive to reach their 50s. Therefore, most of those who are still alive are those who were injured at very young ages or who were injured only a few years ago. By comparison, persons who were not ventilator dependent and were still alive averaged 45 years of age in 2008.

Using a variety of analytic techniques and the combined NSCISC/Shriners Hospital SCI Database, life expectancy estimates for persons with SCI have been developed and periodically updated (65,69–73). These estimates are typically based on neurologic level of injury, degree of injury completeness, age at injury, and ventilator dependency. Separate tables have been developed beginning at either the time of injury or the first anniversary of injury, with the latter reflecting slightly higher life expectancies due to removing the higher mortality rate during the first year after injury. The similarity of results using these different analytic techniques serves to enhance the validity of these life expectancy estimates.

The latest life expectancy estimates from the NSCISC Database beginning at the first anniversary of injury appear in Table 5.3. An abridged version of this table is updated annually on the NSCISC web site at www.spinalcord.uab.edu.

TABLE 5.3

LIFE EXPECTANCY FOR PERSONS WITH SCI TREATED AT MODEL SYSTEMS WHO SURVIVE AT LEAST 1 YEAR POSTINJURY BY AGE, NEUROLOGIC CATEGORY, AND VENTILATOR STATUS

	Life expectancy (y)					
		Not ventilator dependent				
				Tetraplegia		
Current age (y)	No SCI[a]	Motor functional, any injury level	Paraplegia	C5-8	C1-4	Ventilator dependent, any injury level
10	68.5	62.6	54.9	49.9	45.9	33.0
15	63.6	57.7	50.0	45.1	41.1	28.5
20	58.8	53.0	45.5	40.8	36.9	25.1
25	54.0	48.4	41.1	36.6	32.9	22.0
30	49.3	43.7	36.7	32.3	28.8	18.7
35	44.5	39.1	32.2	28.0	24.8	15.4
40	39.9	34.5	27.9	23.9	20.8	12.2
45	35.3	30.1	23.8	20.1	17.2	9.5
50	30.9	25.9	20.0	16.6	14.0	7.2
55	26.6	21.9	16.4	13.3	11.0	5.3
60	22.5	18.1	13.1	10.3	8.4	3.6
65	18.7	14.6	10.1	7.8	6.1	2.4
70	15.1	11.4	7.6	5.6	4.3	1.4
75	11.9	8.6	5.4	3.8	2.8	0.6
80	9.1	6.2	3.6	2.4	1.6	<0.1

[a]Values for persons with no SCI are taken from the 2004 US Life Tables for the general population.

These estimates are not adjusted for gender, race, presence of preexisting medical conditions, or other factors that significantly affect long-term survival. Therefore, Table 5.3 should only be used as a rough guide for estimating the life expectancy of any individual. It can also be used to track progress in prognosis following SCI by comparison to previous life expectancy estimates. More detailed life expectancy tables are being developed by the NSCISC under the auspices of a grant from the Paralyzed Veterans of America and should be available on the NSCISC web site toward the end of 2009. Nonetheless, these tables will still need to be interpreted cautiously in light of any individual's overall medical condition.

As seen in Table 5.3, life expectancy is almost normal for persons with incomplete motor-functional (AIS D) injuries but declines steadily as injury severity increases. Interestingly, in general, as age increases within each neurologic category, the percentage reduction in life expectancy also increases. For example, among persons with high-level (C1-4) tetraplegia who survive the first year after injury, life expectancy is 67.0% of normal for a 10-year-old person, 58.4% of normal for a 30-year-old person, 45.3% of normal for a 50-year-old person, and 28.5% of normal for a 70-year-old person.

Similar life expectancy tables have been produced for persons with SCI in Great Britain, Denmark, Australia, and Canada (74–77). Life expectancies following SCI appear to be quite comparable in those countries to the experience in the United States. The Canadian study is of particular interest because it also assesses health expectancy, revealing that for persons aged 25 to 34 at injury, on average, 79.3% of the remaining life expectancy should be accompanied by overall good health, with declining health presumably occurring during the last few years of life expectancy (77).

CAUSES OF DEATH

Primary (underlying) causes of death for all persons enrolled in the NSCISC Database who subsequently died of a known cause appear in Table 5.4. Diseases of the respiratory system are the leading cause of death following SCI, accounting for 22.0% of all deaths. Of deaths due to respiratory diseases, 70.1% are specifically due to pneumonia. Heart disease ranks second at 19.6%, with 7.8% being hypertensive or ischemic in nature and 11.8% being attributed to other types of heart disease. However, heart disease is somewhat overestimated as a cause of death because more than half of the "other heart diseases" reflect heart attacks that occur in young persons with no apparent underlying heart or vascular disease. Therefore, this probably reflects poor quality of cause of death data and reporting practices on many death certificates of persons with SCI rather than true underlying heart disease. The mortality rate for ischemic heart disease is approximately six times normal for persons aged 30 years or less, but only 30% increased for persons aged 31 to 60 years, and not significantly elevated in persons over 60 years of age (70). Additional study is needed to assess the impact of heart disease among long-term survivors of SCI.

TABLE 5.4

PRIMARY (UNDERLYING) CAUSE OF DEATH FOR PERSONS WITH SCI TREATED AT MODEL SYSTEMS ($N = 4{,}321$)

ICD9CM codes	Primary cause of death	%
460–519	Diseases of the respiratory system	22.0
420–429	Other heart disease	11.8
000–139	Infective and parasitic diseases	10.4
400–414	Hypertensive and ischemic heart disease	7.8
140–239	Neoplasms	7.3
E800–E949	Unintentional injuries	5.7
415–417	Diseases of pulmonary circulation	4.6
520–579	Diseases of the digestive system	4.6
780–799	Symptoms and ill-defined conditions	4.0
430–438	Cerebrovascular disease	3.8
580–629	Diseases of the genitourinary system	3.8
E950–E959	Suicides	3.7
E980–E989	Subsequent trauma of uncertain nature (unintentional/suicide/homicide)	2.7
240–279	Endocrine, nutritional, metabolic, and immunity disorders (includes AIDS)	1.7
320–389	Diseases of the nervous system and sense organs	1.7
440–448	Diseases of the arteries, arterioles, and capillaries	1.4
E960–E969	Homicides	1.2
290–319	Mental disorders	0.5
451–459	Diseases of veins, lymphatics, and other diseases of the circulatory system	0.3
710–739	Diseases of the musculoskeletal system and connective tissue	0.3
280–289	Diseases of blood and blood-forming organs	0.2
740–759	Congenital anomalies	0.1
E970–E979	Legal intervention	0.1
	Total known causes of death	100.0

Infective and parasitic diseases (10.4%) are the next leading cause of death behind respiratory and heart disease. These are virtually always cases of septicemia (94.2%) and are usually associated with either pressure ulcers, urinary tract or respiratory infections. Often, the source of septicemia is not identified on death certificates.

The next most common cause of death is cancer (7.3%). The most common location of cancer is the lung (28.1% of fatal cancer cases), followed by bladder (7.3%), colon/rectum (7.3%), prostate (5.7%), and digestive system (5.4%). Diseases of pulmonary circulation (95.9% of which are cases of pulmonary emboli) account for 4.6% of deaths. Deaths due to pulmonary emboli usually occur prior to discharge from acute care and rehabilitation, and decline sharply with the passage of time after injury.

External causes of death such as unintentional injuries, suicide, homicide, and legal intervention account for a combined 13.3% of deaths following SCI. Among these deaths, unintentional injuries are slightly more common than suicides and considerably more common than other external causes. The suicide rate is about five times that of the general population of comparable age, gender, race, and length of follow-up (78). Suicide risk is highest during the first 5 years after SCI, highest for persons with neurologically complete paraplegia, and higher for whites than African Americans (78).

Other causes of death following SCI include diseases of the digestive system (4.6%), symptoms and ill-defined conditions (4.0%), diseases of the genitourinary (GU) system (3.8%), and cerebrovascular disease (3.8%). The decline in deaths due to GU system diseases is particularly striking since this was the leading cause of death in persons with SCI 40 years ago.

In addition to considering the most common causes of death, it is also important to consider the frequency of these causes of death in relation to the general population of comparable age, gender, and race but without SCI. Overall, it has been conservatively estimated that deaths due to septicemia among persons with SCI occur at 64.2 times the normal rate, while deaths due to diseases of pulmonary circulation occur at 47.1 times the normal rate, and deaths due to pneumonia and influenza occur at 35.6 times the normal rate (70). Conversely, the mortality rates for ischemic heart disease and cancer in persons with SCI are similar to those of the general population, although some specific cancer mortality rates such as that of bladder cancer are elevated (70,79).

During the first month after injury, most deaths are due to either pneumonia (300 times the normal rate), pulmonary embolism (500 times the normal rate), symptoms and ill-defined conditions (275 times the normal rate), or septicemia (500 times the normal rate) (80). However, these extraordinarily high cause-specific mortality multiples decline rapidly after the first month postinjury. For example, after the fifth postinjury year, the mortality rate for pneumonia is reduced to 19 times normal, while the septicemia mortality rate is 46.7 times normal, and the pulmonary embolism mortality rate is 8.9 times normal (70).

Pneumonia is by far the leading cause of death for persons with tetraplegia (24.7% of deaths for C1-4 injuries and 19.7% of deaths for C5-8 injuries), while heart disease (16.1%), septicemia (13.2%), and suicide (11.5%) are more common among persons with paraplegia (70). Among persons with incomplete motor-functional (AIS D) injuries at any neurologic level, heart disease again ranks as the leading cause of death (24.1%), followed by pneumonia (11.0%) (70).

LIFETIME COSTS

Managed care and other cost containment pressures have had a dramatic effect on the way in which persons with SCI are initially treated. Median length of stay in acute care for persons enrolled in the NSCISC Database has decreased from a peak of 24 days from 1973 to 1979 to 12 days from 2005 to 2008, while median length of stay in inpatient rehabilitation has decreased from a peak of 98 to 37 days over that same time period. Conversely, in Europe, lengths of hospital stay following SCI remain high. For example, in Denmark, acute care length of stay averages about 2 months and average rehabilitation length of stay ranges from 5 months for persons with motor incomplete paraplegia to 9.5 months for persons with motor complete tetraplegia (23).

Among persons enrolled in the NSCISC Database from 2002 to 2006, average acute care charges adjusted to 2005 dollars were $204,441 and average inpatient rehabilitation charges were an additional $107,325 (66). By comparison, average charges for persons enrolled in the NSCISC Database from 1973 to 1981 (in 2005 dollars) were $72,507 for acute care and $146,957 for inpatient rehabilitation (66). Average charges per day in constant 2005 dollars for acute care rose during that same period from $2,613 to $11,444, while average charges per day for rehabilitation rose from $1,380 to $2,471, reflecting increased intensity of service (66).

Table 5.5 depicts average first-year and annual expenses in 2008 dollars for persons with SCI over their remaining lifetime by neurologic level and extent of injury. These estimates are derived from a study of model system patients performed between 1988 and 1990 and updated for inflation by using the Medical Care Component of the Consumer Price Index (81). These charges only include items that are directly related to the SCI; other medical expenses that would be encountered in the absence of SCI were not counted. Moreover, items that might have been needed or at least desirable but that were not acquired were not counted. However, an appropriate value was assigned to items that were received free of charge and those items were counted. Lost wages, fringe benefits, and other indirect costs are not included in these estimates. These indirect costs frequently exceed the direct costs seen in Table 5.5 (52,81).

Average first-year charges range from $801,161 for persons with C1-4 injury levels (excluding incomplete motor functional injuries) to $236,109 for persons with incomplete motor functional injuries at any level, while average annual charges for the remainder of life are estimated to range from $143,507 to $16,547 for those same two groups of patients. More detailed predictive models reveal that persons who are ventilator dependent will experience even higher average charges in 2008 dollars of $1,079,069 in the first year after injury and $423,388 per year for the remainder of their life (81). These estimates of first-year and annual charges are relatively consistent with results obtained from population-based studies after conversion of those results to 2008 dollars (52,82).

A detailed categorization of these charges has been reported previously (81). During the first year, most charges result from inpatient acute care and rehabilitation, although significant charges are also often incurred for attendant care after discharge, durable equipment, and environmental modifications, particularly for persons with cervical injuries. Recurrent annual

TABLE 5.5

AVERAGE ANNUAL EXPENSES AND PRESENT VALUE OF LIFETIME DIRECT COSTS OF CARE FOR PERSONS WITH SCI TREATED AT MODEL SYSTEMS BY NEUROLOGIC CATEGORY AND AGE AT TIME OF INJURY[a]

	Average annual expenses		Estimated lifetime costs	
	First year	Each subsequent year	25 y.o.	50 y.o.
C1-4	$801,161	$143,507	$3,160,137	$1,860,390
C5-8	$517,356	$58,783	$1,786,836	$1,131,560
T1-S5	$292,740	$29,789	$1,055,869	$720,169
AIS D	$236,109	$16,547	$704,344	$510,452

[a]In 2008 dollars discounted at 2%.

charges are mostly for attendant care and rehospitalizations, although other items such as durable equipment, outpatient services, medications, supplies, and in some instances, substantial nursing home charges are also incurred (81,83).

The estimated present value of average lifetime direct costs of SCI in 2008 dollars using a real discount rate of 2% for persons injured at age 25 and 50 by neurologic level and extent of injury also appears in Table 5.5. At age 25, the present value of lifetime direct costs of care is estimated to be $3,160,137 for persons with C1-4 injury levels and $704,344 for persons with incomplete motor functional injuries at any level. Estimates of present value of lifetime costs at age 50 are lower because of the lower life expectancy of these persons.

Estimates of average first year and annual charges for SCIs of different etiologies have also been reported (84). First-year and annual recurring charges are highest for SCI resulting from sports mishaps because they almost always result in cervical injuries and for motor vehicle crashes that often involve other injuries in addition to the SCI that require more intensive acute care and may delay rehabilitation. Based on a 2% real discount rate, estimated present value of total annual aggregate direct costs in the United States that could be avoided if all new SCIs could be prevented was reported to be $7.7 billion in 1995 dollars or $12.7 billion if adjusted to 2008 dollars (84). Because they are the most frequent cause of injury, motor vehicle crashes accounted for just under half of that total aggregate cost, followed by acts of violence, falls, sports, and all other causes. These estimates of SCI costs by etiology are more useful when considered from a public health or primary prevention perspective than are estimates based on injury severity.

CONCLUSION

A broad understanding of the epidemiology of SCI has emerged from a variety of sources, including the NSCISC Database, the Shriners Hospital SCI Database, the state population-based registries, and other studies conducted both within and outside the United States. Future efforts should be directed toward attempts to standardize data collection and combine these data sources in ways that take full advantage of the unique strengths of each available database. This process is now well underway with the development of International SCI Data Sets (85–90).

References

1. Wilcox NE, Stauffer ES, Nickel VL. A statistical analysis of 423 consecutive patients admitted to the spinal cord injury center, Rancho Los Amigos Hospital, 1 January 1964, through 31 December 1967. *Paraplegia* 1970;8:27–35.
2. Fine PR, Kuhlemeier KV, DeVivo MJ, et al. Spinal cord injury: an epidemiologic perspective. *Paraplegia* 1979;17:237–250.
3. Kraus JF, Franti CE, Riggins RS, et al. Incidence of traumatic spinal cord lesions. J Chron Dis 1975;28:471–492.
4. Griffin MR, Opitz JL, Kurland LT, et al. Traumatic spinal cord injury in Olmsted County, Minnesota, 1935–1981. *Am J Epidemiol* 1985;121:884–895.
5. Kalsbeek WD, McLaurin RL, Harris BSH, et al. The national head and spinal cord injury survey: major findings. *J Neurosurg* 1980;53(Suppl):19–31.
6. Bracken MB, Freeman DH, Hellenbrand K. Incidence of acute traumatic hospitalized spinal cord injury in the United States, 1970–1977. *Am J Epidemiol* 1981;113:615–622.
7. Stover SL, DeVivo MJ, Go BK. History, implementation, and current status of the national spinal cord injury database. *Arch Phys Med Rehabil* 1999;80:1365–1371.
8. DeVivo MJ, Go BK, Jackson AB. Overview of the national spinal cord injury statistical center database. *J Spinal Cord Med* 2002;25:335–338.
9. DeVivo MJ, Rutt RD, Black KJ, et al. Trends in spinal cord injury demographics and treatment outcomes between 1973 and 1986. *Arch Phys Med Rehabil* 1992;73:424–430.
10. Go BK, DeVivo MJ, Richards JS. The epidemiology of spinal cord injury. In: Stover SL, DeLisa JA, Whiteneck GG, eds.. *Spinal cord injury: clinical outcomes from the model systems*. Gaithersburg: Aspen, 1995:21–55.
11. Vogel LC, DeVivo MJ. Pediatric spinal cord injury issues: etiology, demographics and pathophysiology. *Top Spinal Cord Inj Rehabil* 1997;3(2):1–8.
12. Nobunaga AI, Go BK, Karunas RB. Recent demographic and injury trends in people served by the model spinal cord injury care systems. *Arch Phys Med Rehabil* 1999;80:1372–1382.
13. Jackson AB, Dijkers M, DeVivo MJ, et al. A demographic profile of new traumatic spinal cord injuries: change

and stability over 30 years. *Arch Phys Med Rehabil* 2004;85:1740–1748.
14. DeVivo MJ, Vogel LC. Epidemiology of spinal cord injury in children and adolescents. *J Spinal Cord Med* 2004;27(Suppl):S4–S10.
15. Acton PA, Farley T, Freni LW, et al. Traumatic spinal cord injury in Arkansas, 1980 to 1989. *Arch Phys Med Rehabil* 1993;74:1035–1040.
16. Price C, Makintubee S, Herndon W, et al. Epidemiology of traumatic spinal cord injury and acute hospitalization and rehabilitation charges for spinal cord injuries in Oklahoma, 1988–1990. *Am J Epidemiol* 1994;139:37–47.
17. Thurman DJ, Burnett CL, Jeppson L, et al. Surveillance of spinal cord injuries in Utah, USA. *Paraplegia* 1994;32:665–669.
18. Woodruff BA, Baron RC. A description of nonfatal spinal cord injury using a hospital-based registry. *Am J Prev Med* 1994;10:10–14.
19. Johnson RL, Gabella BA, Gerhart KA, et al. Evaluating sources of traumatic spinal cord injury surveillance data in Colorado. *Am J Epidemiol* 1997;146:266–272.
20. Surkin J, Colley Gilbert BJ, Harkey HL, et al. Spinal cord injury in Mississippi: findings and evaluation, 1992–1994. *Spine* 2000;25:716–721.
21. Glick T. Spinal cord injury surveillance: is there a decrease in incidence? [abstract]. *J Spinal Cord Med* 2000;23(Suppl):61.
22. Chen CF, Lien IN. Spinal cord injuries in Taipei, Taiwan, 1978–1981. *Paraplegia* 1985;23:364–370.
23. Biering-Sorensen F, Pedersen V, Clausen S. Epidemiology of spinal cord lesions in Denmark. *Paraplegia* 1990;28: 105–118.
24. Garcia-Reneses J, Herruzo-Cabrera R, Martinez-Moreno M. Epidemiological study of spinal cord injury in Spain 1984–1985. *Paraplegia* 1991;28:180–190.
25. Karamehmetoglu SS, Unal S, Karacan I, et al. Traumatic spinal cord injuries in Istanbul, Turkey: an epidemiological study. *Paraplegia* 1995;33:469–471.
26. Schonherr MC, Groothoff JW, Mulder GA, et al. Rehabilitation of patients with spinal cord lesions in The Netherlands: an epidemiological study. *Spinal Cord* 1996;34:679–683.
27. Otom AS, Doughan AM, Kawar JS, et al. Traumatic spinal cord injuries in Jordan—an epidemiological study. *Spinal Cord* 1997;35:253–255.
28. Martins F, Freitas F, Martins L, et al. Spinal cord injuries—epidemiology in Portugal's central region. *Spinal Cord* 1998;36:574–578.
29. Ahoniemi E, Alaranta H, Hokkinen EM, et al. Incidence of traumatic spinal cord injuries in Finland over a 30-year period. *Spinal Cord* 2008;46:781–784.
30. O'Connor PJ. Forecasting of spinal cord injury annual case numbers in Australia. *Arch Phys Med Rehabil* 2005;86:48–51.
31. DeVivo MJ, Fine PR, Maetz HM, et al. Prevalence of spinal cord injury: a reestimation employing life table techniques. *Arch Neurol* 1980;37:707–708.
32. Berkowitz M, Harvey C, Greene CG, et al. *The economic consequences of traumatic spinal cord injury*. New York: Demos, 1992.
33. Lasfargues JE, Custis D, Morrone F, et al. A model for estimating spinal cord injury prevalence in the United States. *Paraplegia* 1995;33:62–68.
34. Strauss DJ, DeVivo MJ, Paculdo DR, et al. Trends in life expectancy after spinal cord injury. *Arch Phys Med Rehabil* 2006;87:1079–1085.
35. DeVivo MJ. Head neck injuries in industries and sports. In: Yoganandan N, Pintar FA, Larson SJ, et al., eds. *Frontiers in head and neck trauma: clinical and biomechanical*. Amsterdam: IOS Press, 1998:92–100.
36. Clarke KS. Spinal cord injuries in organized sports. *Model Systems SCI Digest* 1980;2:9–17.
37. Kraus JF, Franti CE, Riggins RS. Neurologic outcome and vehicle and crash factors in motor vehicle related spinal cord injuries. *Neuroepidemiology* 1982;1:223–238.
38. Wigglesworth EC. Motor vehicle crashes and spinal cord injury. *Paraplegia* 1992;30:543–549.
39. Fine PR, Stafford MA, Miller JM, et al. Gunshot wounds of the spinal cord: a survey of literature and epidemiologic study of 48 lesions in Alabama. *Ala J Med Sci* 1976;13:173–180.
40. Weingarden SI, Graham PM. Falls resulting in spinal cord injury: patterns and outcomes in an older population. *Paraplegia* 1989;27:423–427.
41. DeVivo MJ. Prevention of spinal cord injuries resulting from falls. *J Spinal Cord Med* 2000;23(Suppl):15–16.
42. DeVivo MJ, Sekar P. Prevention of spinal cord injuries that occur in swimming pools. *Spinal Cord* 1997;35: 509–515.
43. Wang CM, Chen Y, DeVivo MJ, et al. Epidemiology of extraspinal fractures associated with acute spinal cord injury. *Spinal Cord* 2001;39:589–594.
44. Chen Y, DeVivo MJ. Epidemiology of extraspinal fractures in acute spinal cord injury: data from the model spinal cord injury care systems, 1973–1999. *Top Spinal Cord Inj Rehabil* 2005;11(1):18–29.
45. Marino RJ, Barros T, Biering-Sorensen F, et al. International standards for neurological classification of spinal cord injury. *J Spinal Cord Med* 2003;26(Suppl):S50–S56.
46. DeVivo MJ, Richards JS. Marriage rates among persons with spinal cord injury. *Rehabil Psychol* 1996;41:321–339.
47. DeVivo MJ, Fine PR. Spinal cord injury: its short-term impact on marital status. *Arch Phys Med Rehabil* 1985;66:501–504.
48. DeVivo MJ, Hawkins LN, Richards JS, et al. Outcomes of post-spinal cord injury marriages [published erratum appears in *Arch Phys Med Rehabil* 1995;76:397]. *Arch Phys Med Rehabil* 1995;76:130–138.
49. Krause JS, Kewman D, DeVivo MJ, et al. Employment after spinal cord injury: an analysis of cases from the model spinal cord injury systems. *Arch Phys Med Rehabil* 1999;80:1492–1500.
50. DeVivo MJ, Rutt RD, Stover SL, et al. Employment after spinal cord injury. *Arch Phys Med Rehabil* 1987;68: 494–498.
51. Pflaum C, McCollister G, Strauss DJ, et al. Worklife after traumatic spinal cord injury. *J Spinal Cord Med* 2006;29:377–386.
52. Berkowitz M, O'Leary PK, Kruse DL, et al. *Spinal cord injury: an analysis of medical and social costs*. New York: Demos, 1998.

53. James M, DeVivo MJ, Richards JS. Postinjury employment outcomes among African-American and white persons with spinal cord injury. *Rehabil Psychol* 1993;38: 151–164.
54. Krause JS, Anson CA. Employment after spinal cord injury: relation to selected participant characteristics. *Arch Phys Med Rehabil* 1996;77:737–743.
55. McShane SL, Karp J. Employment following spinal cord injury: a covariance structure analysis. *Rehabil Psychol* 1993;38:27–40.
56. Hess DW, Ripley DL, McKinley WO, et al. Predictors for return to work after spinal cord injury: a 3-year multicenter analysis. *Arch Phys Med Rehabil* 2000;81:359–363.
57. Young JS, Burns PE, Bowen AM, et al. Spinal cord injury statistics: experience of the regional spinal cord injury systems. Phoenix (AZ): Good Samaritan Medical Center, 1982.
58. Deutsch A, Fiedler RC, Granger CV, et al. The uniform data system for medical rehabilitation report of patients discharged from comprehensive medical rehabilitation programs in 1999. *Am J Phys Med Rehabil* 2002;81:133–142.
59. DeVivo MJ. Discharge disposition from model spinal cord injury care system rehabilitation programs. *Arch Phys Med Rehabil* 1999;80:785–790.
60. Fiedler IG, Laud PW, Maiman DJ, et al. Economics of managed care in spinal cord injury. *Arch Phys Med Rehabil* 1999;80:1441–1449.
61. Dijkers MP, Abela MB, Gans BM. The aftermath of spinal cord injury. In: Stover SL, DeLisa JA, Whiteneck GG, eds. *Spinal cord injury: clinical outcomes from the model systems*. Gaithersburg: Aspen, 1995:185–212.
62. DeVivo MJ, Richards JS, Stover SL, et al. Spinal cord injury: rehabilitation adds life to years. *West J Med* 1991;154:602–606.
63. DeVivo MJ, Shewchuk RM, Stover SL, et al. A cross-sectional study of the relationship between age and current health status for persons with spinal cord injuries. *Paraplegia* 1992;30:820–827.
64. DeVivo MJ, Stover SL, Black KJ. Prognostic factors for 12-year survival after spinal cord injury. *Arch Phys Med Rehabil* 1992;73:156–162.
65. DeVivo MJ, Krause JS, Lammertse DP. Recent trends in mortality and causes of death among persons with spinal cord injury. *Arch Phys Med Rehabil* 1999;80:1411–1419.
66. DeVivo MJ. Trends in spinal cord injury rehabilitation outcomes from model systems in the United States: 1973–2006. *Spinal Cord* 2007;45:713–721.
67. Krause JS, Sternberg M, Lottes S, et al. Mortality after spinal cord injury: an 11-year prospective study. *Arch Phys Med Rehabil* 1997;78:815–821.
68. Krause JS, DeVivo MJ, Jackson AB. Health status, community integration, and economic risk factors for mortality after spinal cord injury. *Arch Phys Med Rehabil* 2004;85:1764–1773.
69. Shavelle RM, DeVivo MJ, Strauss DJ, et al. Long-term survival of persons ventilator dependent after spinal cord injury. *J Spinal Cord Med* 2006;29:511–519.
70. DeVivo MJ, Stover SL. Long-term survival and causes of death. In: Stover SL, DeLisa JA, Whiteneck GG, eds. *Spinal cord injury: clinical outcomes from the model systems*. Gaithersburg: Aspen, 1995:289–316.
71. DeVivo MJ, Ivie CS. Life expectancy of ventilator-dependent persons with spinal cord injuries. *Chest* 1995;108:226–232.
72. Strauss D, DeVivo MJ, Shavelle R. Long-term mortality risk after spinal cord injury. *J Insurance Med* 2000;32: 11–16.
73. Shavelle RM, DeVivo MJ, Paculdo DR, et al. Long-term survival after childhood spinal cord injury. *J Spinal Cord Med* 2007;30(Suppl):S48–S54.
74. Frankel HL, Coll JR, Charlifue SW, et al. Long-term survival in spinal cord injury: a fifty year investigation. *Spinal Cord* 1998;36:266–274.
75. Hartkopp A, Bronnum-Hansen H, Seidenschnur AM, et al. Survival and cause of death after traumatic spinal cord injury: a long-term epidemiological survey from Denmark. *Spinal Cord* 1997;35:76–85.
76. Yeo JD, Walsh J, Rutkowski S, et al. Mortality following spinal cord injury. *Spinal Cord* 1998;36:329–336.
77. McColl MA, Walker J, Stirling P, et al. Expectations of life and health among spinal cord injured adults. *Spinal Cord* 1997;35:818–828.
78. DeVivo MJ, Black KJ, Richards JS, et al. Suicide following spinal cord injury. *Paraplegia* 1991;29:620–627.
79. Stonehill WH, Dmochowski RR, Patterson AL, et al. Risk factors for bladder tumors in spinal cord injury patients. *J Urol* 1996;155:1248–1250.
80. DeVivo MJ, Kartus PL, Stover SL, et al. Cause of death for patients with spinal cord injuries. *Arch Intern Med* 1989;149:1761–1766.
81. DeVivo MJ, Whiteneck GG, Charles ED. The economic impact of spinal cord injury. In: Stover SL, DeLisa JA, Whiteneck GG, eds. *Spinal cord injury: clinical outcomes from the model systems*. Gaithersburg: Aspen, 1995: 234–271.
82. Johnson RL, Brooks CA, Whiteneck GG. Cost of traumatic spinal cord injury in a population-based registry. *Spinal Cord* 1996;34:470–480.
83. Ivie CS, DeVivo MJ. Predicting unplanned hospitalizations in persons with spinal cord injury. *Arch Phys Med Rehabil* 1994;75:1182–1188.
84. DeVivo MJ. Causes and costs of spinal cord injury in the United States. *Spinal Cord* 1997;35:809–813.
85. Biering-Sorensen F, Charlifue S, DeVivo M, et al. International spinal cord injury data sets. *Spinal Cord* 2006;44:530–534.
86. DeVivo M, Biering Sorensen F, Charlifue S, et al. International spinal cord injury core data set. *Spinal Cord* 2006;44:535–540.
87. Biering-Sorensen F, Craggs M, Kenelley M, et al. International lower urinary tract function basic spinal cord injury data set. *Spinal Cord* 2008;46:325–330.
88. Biering-Sorensen F, Craggs M, Kenelley M, et al. International urodynamic basic spinal cord injury data set. *Spinal Cord* 2008;46:513–516.
89. Alexander MS, Biering-Sorensen F, Bodner D, et al. International standards to document remaining autonomic function after spinal cord injury. *Spinal Cord* 2009;47:36–43.
90. Widerstrom-Noga E, Biering-Sorensen F, Bryce T, et al. The international spinal cord injury pain basic data set. *Spinal Cord* 2008;46:818–823.

CHAPTER 6 ■ ASSESSMENT AND CLASSIFICATION OF TRAUMATIC SPINAL CORD INJURY

STEVEN KIRSHBLUM, KIM ANDERSON, ANDREI KRASSIOUKOV, AND WILLIAM DONOVAN

ASSESSMENT OF SPINAL CORD INJURY

The most accurate way to neurologically assess a person who has sustained a spinal cord injury (SCI) is to perform a standardized neurological examination as endorsed by the International Standards for Neurological Classification of Spinal Cord Injury (ISNSCI) Patients (1), also commonly referred to as the *International Standards*. These standards provide basic definitions of the most common terms used by clinicians in the assessment of SCI and describe the neurological examination (Table 6.1). The examination and classification of a person with SCI are two different skills and, therefore, will be described separately.

The International Standards are not intended to be a substitute for a complete neurological examination nor are they meant to be used to predict individual functional outcomes or neurologic recovery. Rather, they were developed to document selected neurologic parameters at the time the exam is conducted (2). Subsequently, they have been used by many for prognostication for large groups of persons with SCI and research.

In the Standards, the neurological examination of the person with SCI has two main components, sensory and motor, with required and optional elements th at should be recorded on a standardized flow sheet (Fig. 6.1). The required elements allow the determination of the sensory, motor, and neurologic levels; generation of sensory and motor index scores; determination of the completeness of the injury; as well as classification of the impairment. The rectal examination, which tests for voluntary anal contraction (VAC) and deep anal pressure (DAP) (previously called deep anal sensation), is part of the required components of the examination. Optional elements include aspects of the neurological examination that may better describe the patients' clinical condition but are not used for numerical scoring. To learn how to use the *International Standards*, a web-based instructional course (InStep) is available through the American Spinal Injury Association (ASIA) (www.asialearningcenter.com). The reference manual published in 2003 (3) is no longer up-to-date. The International Standards were revised in june 2011 (1), and these changes are reflected in this chapter. A recent article also highlighted some of these changes (2).

Sensory Examination

The sensory exam is performed on 28 key dermatomes (Fig. 6.1), each tested for pinprick (sharp/dull discrimination) and light touch (LT) appreciation on both sides of the body as well as DAP as part of the rectal examination. These points were adapted from Austin (4) and consensus among experienced spinal cord physicians. A three-point scale [0–2] is used, with the face as the normal control point. Testing is performed with the patient's eyes closed or vision blocked, so the patient cannot identify the site being tested. For the pinprick examination, the patient must be able to distinguish between the pin (sharp edge) and dull (rounded) edge of a disposable safety pin. Absent sensation, which includes the inability to distinguish between the sharp and the dull edges of the pin, yields a score of 0. A score of 1 (impaired) for PP testing is given when the patient can distinguish between the sharp and the dull edges of the pin, but the intensity of the sharpness is different (greater or lesser) as compared with the face. If there is a question whether the patient can definitively discriminate between the pin and the dull edges, 8 out of 10 correct answers is considered accurate (3), as this reduces the probability of correct guessing to less than 5.0%. The score of 2 (normal or intact) is given only if the intensity of sharpness is the same as on the face. For light touch, a tapered wisp of cotton (i.e. from a cotton tip applicator) is used with a score of 2 (intact) being the same touch sensation as on the face and 1 (impaired) if less than on the face. The cotton tip swab should be stroked across the skin moving over a distance not to exceed one centimeter. A score of 0 (absent) is used if there is no appreciation of sensation.

When testing the digits for dermatomes C6-8, the dorsal surface of the proximal phalanx should be tested. For the chest and abdomen, sensory testing should be performed at the mid-clavicular line. The C4 dermatome comes down low on the upper part of the chest, even as far as the T3 interspace. When sensory loss begins at, or just above, the nipple line (T4 dermatome), careful sensory testing at key points on the upper limbs is essential to properly determine a sensory level, rather than just assuming a T3 sensory level. In a patient who has absent T1 and T2 sensation with apparently preserved T3, T3 should be scored as absent if there is no sensation at T4. For persons in whom it may be difficult to identify the T3 and T4 dermatomes (i.e., patients who are obese or women with large breasts), the T3 and T4 intercostal spaces can be verified by palpation of the anterior ribs rather than relying on the nipple line; for T3, the intercostal space below the 3rd rib. An alternative method of locating T3 is palpating the manubriosternal joint, which is at the level of the second rib. At that point, moving slightly lateral to palpate the second rib and continuing to move in a caudal direction will locate the third rib and the corresponding intercostal space just below it (2). It is extremely important to test the S4-5 dermatome (less than 1 cm lateral to the mucocutaneous junction) for both PP and

TABLE 6.1

GLOSSARY OF KEY TERMS

Key muscle groups: **Ten muscle groups that are tested as part of the standardized spinal cord examination.**

Root level	Muscle group
C5	Elbow flexors
C6	Wrist extensors
C7	Elbow extensors
C8	Long finger flexors
T1	Small finger abductors
L2	Hip flexors
L3	Knee extensors
L4	Ankle dorsiflexors
L5	Long toe extensor
S1	Ankle plantarflexors

Dermatome: The area of the skin innervated by the sensory axons within each segmental nerve (root).

Myotome: The collection of muscle fibers innervated by the motor axons within each segmental nerve (root).

Motor level: The most caudal key muscle group that is graded 3/5 or greater with the segments cephalad graded normal (5/5) strength.

Motor index score: Calculated by adding the muscle scores of each key muscle group; a total score of 100 is possible. It is now recommended to separate the motor scores into two scores; one for the upper limb and one for the lower limb.

Sensory level: The most caudal dermatome to have normal sensation for both pinprick/dull and LT on both sides.

Sensory index score: Calculated by adding the scores for each dermatome; a total score of 112 is possible for each PP (sharp/dull discrimination) and LT modalities.

NLI: The most caudal level at which both motor and sensory modalities are intact.

Complete injury: The absence of sensory and motor function in the lowest sacral segments (i.e., no sacral sparing).

Incomplete injury: Preservation of motor and/or sensory function below the neurologic level that includes the lowest sacral segments. (i.e., presence of sacral sparing)

Skeletal level: The level at which, by radiological examination, the greatest vertebral damage is found.

ZPP: Used only with complete injuries, refers to the dermatomes and myotomes caudal to the motor and sensory levels that remain partially innervated. The most caudal segment with some sensory and/or motor function defines the extent of the ZPP.

Source: International Standards (1).

LT, as this represents function of the most caudal aspect of the sacral spinal cord. If accurate sensory testing in any dermatome cannot be performed, (i.e., cast or bandage in place, burn, amputation), "NT" (not testable) should be recorded on the work sheet, or an alternate location within the dermatome can be tested with notation that an alternate site was used.

To test for DAP, a rectal digital examination is performed. The patient is asked to report any sensory awareness with firm pressure of the examiner's digit on the rectal walls, innervated by the somatosensory components of the pudendal nerve (S4/5), and consistently perceived pressure is recorded as either present (yes) or absent (no) on the work sheet. A technique more recently described recommends pressure applied using the thumb to gently squeeze the anus against the inserted index finger (5). The technique avoids moving viscera that might be innervated by autonomic nerves when testing somatic sensation (2). Testing for DAP is important, especially in patients who have absent PP and LT sensation in the S4-5 dermatome, as this may be the only evidence of a clinically incomplete SCI. One of teh new revisions of 2011, is that in patients who have LT or PP at the S4-5 dermatome, examination of DAP is not required as the patient already has a designation for a sensory incomplete injury, although this is still recommended to complete the worksheet (1). The rectal exam is still required, however, to test for voluntary anal contraction.

Optional elements of the sensory examination include joint movement appreciation and position sense, and awareness of and deep pressure/deep pain. Joint movement appreciation and position sense can be tested in the upper (little finger at the proximal interphalangeal joint, thumb, and wrist) and lower extremities (great toe, ankle, and knee). Scoring is as follows: 0 (absent)—if unable to report joint movement correctly; 1 (impaired)—if consistently correct (8/10) on large movements of the joints but inconsistent on small movements of the joints (10 degrees or less); 2 (normal)—if consistently correct on small movements of joints; and NT—if the patient is unable to understand and follow directions or if unable to test the joint (i.e., cast or amputation). Deep pressure/pain appreciation of the limbs is only tested if other sensory modalities are absent and performed by applying firm pressure for 3 to 5 seconds at different locations (wrist, nail bed of the thumb, little finger, small and great toe, or ankle) after establishing a baseline with the patient by applying pressure using the index finger or thumb on the chin. Scoring is 0 (absent) if no pressure is felt peripherally and 1 (present) if felt reliably when pressure is applied.

Motor Examination

The required elements of the motor examination consist of testing 10 key muscles, 5 in the upper limb and 5 in the lower limb on each side of the body Table 6.1. Other muscles are also clinically important but are viewed as optional in that they do not contribute to the motor index scores or levels. It is recommended (although at the discretion of the examiner) (2) that the muscles be examined in a rostral to caudal sequence, starting with the elbow flexors (C5 tested muscle) and finishing with the ankle plantarflexors (Sl muscle). Testing of all key muscles during the initial as well as the follow-up examinations are performed with the patient in the supine position, to allow for a valid comparison of scores throughout the phases of care, and graded and recorded on the standard work sheet, on a six-point scale from 0 to 5 (6). For purposes of inter-rater reliability, it has been recommended that only whole numbers (rather than pluses and minuses) be used when comparing data (especially for research) from one institution to another. In order to be confident that a true change in strength has occurred, muscle grades should change more than one full grade (7).

While there is a clear distinction for each root level during sensory testing (one site per dermatome tested), the myotomes are not as clearly delineated. Although each of the key muscles has one root listed, usually two segments innervate these muscles (i.e., for biceps—C5 and C6). The key muscles have been chosen because of their consistency for being innervated primarily by the segments indicated and for their ease of testing in the supine position. If a particular muscle has a grade of 3/5, it is considered to have full innervation by at least the more cephalad nerve

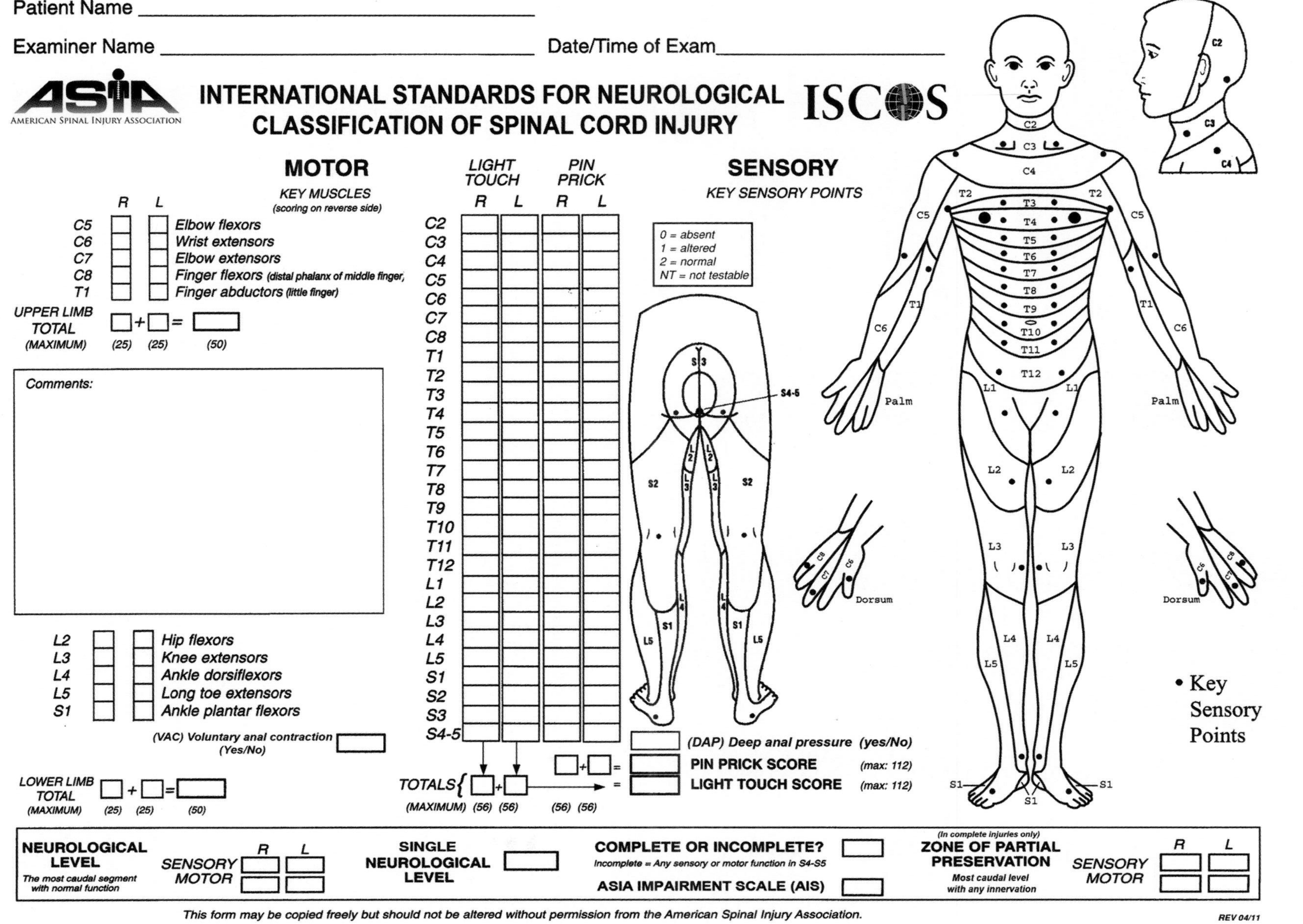

Patient Name ______________________________

Examiner Name ______________________________ Date/Time of Exam ______________________________

ASIA AMERICAN SPINAL INJURY ASSOCIATION

INTERNATIONAL STANDARDS FOR NEUROLOGICAL CLASSIFICATION OF SPINAL CORD INJURY

ISCOS

MOTOR

KEY MUSCLES (scoring on reverse side)

	R	L	
C5			Elbow flexors
C6			Wrist extensors
C7			Elbow extensors
C8			Finger flexors (distal phalanx of middle finger)
T1			Finger abductors (little finger)

UPPER LIMB TOTAL (MAXIMUM) ☐ + ☐ = ☐ (25) (25) (50)

Comments:

	R	L	
L2			Hip flexors
L3			Knee extensors
L4			Ankle dorsiflexors
L5			Long toe extensors
S1			Ankle plantar flexors

(VAC) Voluntary anal contraction (Yes/No) ☐

LOWER LIMB TOTAL (MAXIMUM) ☐ + ☐ = ☐ (25) (25) (50)

SENSORY

KEY SENSORY POINTS

	LIGHT TOUCH R	LIGHT TOUCH L	PIN PRICK R	PIN PRICK L
C2				
C3				
C4				
C5				
C6				
C7				
C8				
T1				
T2				
T3				
T4				
T5				
T6				
T7				
T8				
T9				
T10				
T11				
T12				
L1				
L2				
L3				
L4				
L5				
S1				
S2				
S3				
S4-5				

TOTALS ☐ + ☐ = ☐ ☐ + ☐ = ☐

(MAXIMUM) (56) (56) (56) (56)

0 = absent
1 = altered
2 = normal
NT = not testable

(DAP) Deep anal pressure (yes/No) ☐

PIN PRICK SCORE (max: 112) ☐

LIGHT TOUCH SCORE (max: 112) ☐

NEUROLOGICAL LEVEL		R	L
The most caudal segment with normal function	SENSORY	☐	☐
	MOTOR	☐	☐

SINGLE NEUROLOGICAL LEVEL ☐

COMPLETE OR INCOMPLETE? ☐
Incomplete = Any sensory or motor function in S4-S5

ASIA IMPAIRMENT SCALE (AIS) ☐

(In complete injuries only) ZONE OF PARTIAL PRESERVATION		R	L
Most caudal level with any innervation	SENSORY	☐	☐
	MOTOR	☐	☐

This form may be copied freely but should not be altered without permission from the American Spinal Injury Association.

REV 04/11

FIGURE 6.1. ASIA flow sheet.

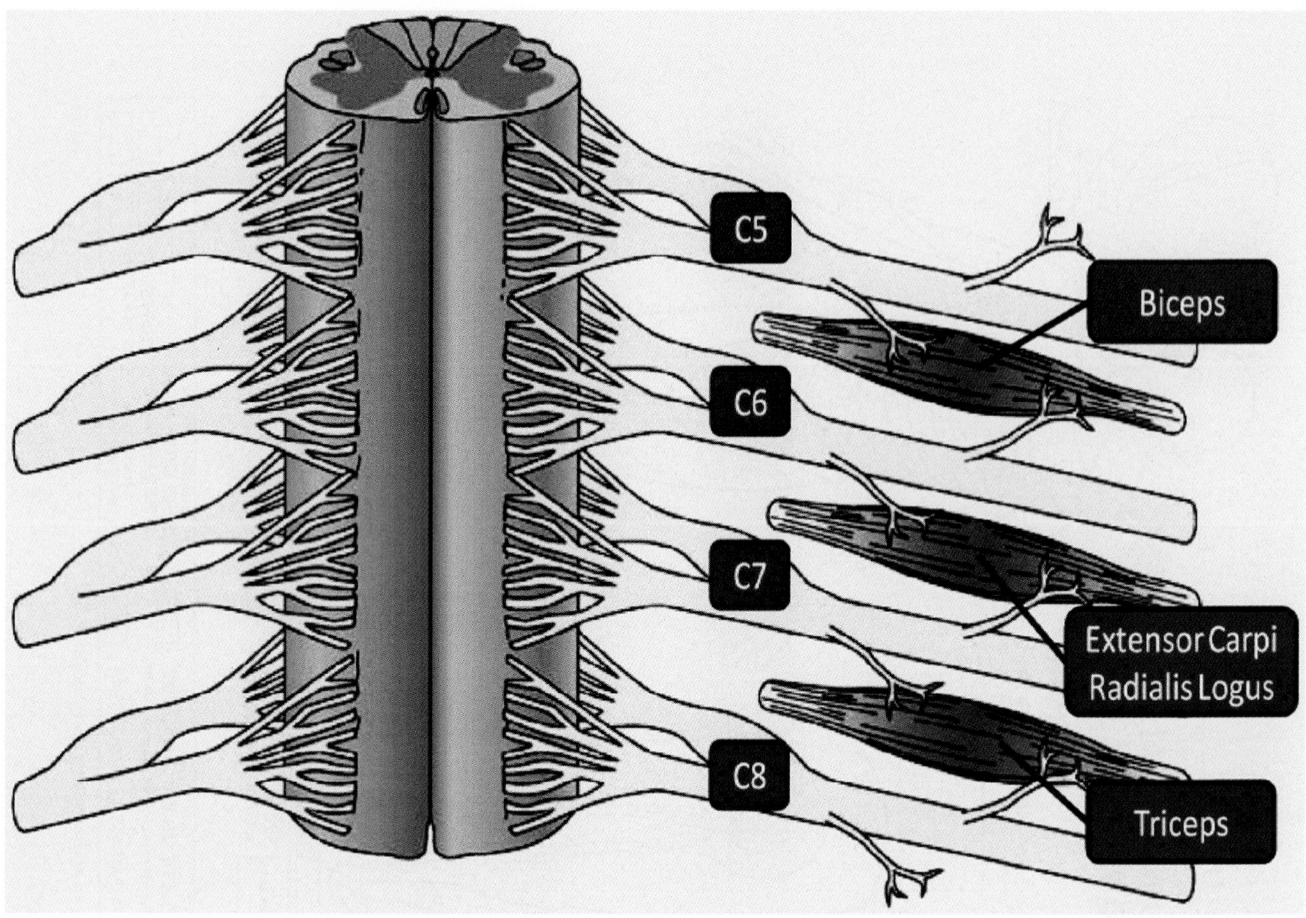

FIGURE 6.2. Muscle innervation by level of injury.

root segment and is considered useful for functional activities. A muscle initially graded as normal (5/5) would be considered to be fully innervated by both spinal root segments (Fig. 6.2).

Placing the joints in the proper position during MMT and stabilizing above and below the joint tested are important especially if the muscles do not have antigravity strength. This will also help prevent confusion from substitution movements of other muscles that may occur. Examples include wrist extension mimicked by forearm supination; elbow extension by external rotation of the shoulder with the patient flexing the elbow and then relaxing; long finger flexion by wrist extension (tenodesis); finger abduction by finger extension; hip flexion by abdominal or adductor muscle contraction; and ankle dorsiflexion by long toe extension. Proper positioning is also important when grading muscles for antigravity strength (1). The InStep training videos are recommended to visualize all of these positions.

Often, the patient's clinical condition may prevent the completion of an accurate examination. Limiting factors such as pain and deconditioning may be present such that the patient only grades a 4/5. If the examiner feels that the patient would otherwise have normal strength, the muscle should be graded as a 5* to indicate that inhibiting factors were present and documented in the comment box on the work sheet. When the patient is not fully testable for any reason, including spasticity that prevents accurate stabilization of the joint, uncontrolled clonus, severe pain, or a fracture present limiting the exam, the examiner should record "NT" instead of a numerical score. If a contracture limits less than 50% of the normal range, then the muscle is graded through its available range subject to the same criteria of the 0 to 5 scale (2). If the contracture limits greater than 50% of the normal range, then the muscle should be graded as "NT." Other examples when "NT" should be recorded include if the patient is unable to participate in the exam because of cognitive status (i.e., comatose from an associated traumatic brain injury); has an injury to the brachial or lumbosacral plexi; or a limb immobilized because of a fracture.

In a patient with a potentially unstable spine, care must be taken when performing MMT. When examining a newly injured individual with a lesion below T8, the hip should not be flexed passively or actively beyond 90 degrees, as this may place too great a kyphotic stress on the lumbar spine (1). In a patient who may have an unstable spine or be in too much pain to lift up his or her leg, MMT should be tested isometrically by placing a hand on the patients thigh just above the knee while asking the patient to lift his or her leg while the examiner offers resistance to movement. The examiner can then grade the force (without allowing for flexion) between 2 and 5. If the patient has only minimal movement, the examiner should palpate over the more superficial hip flexors (i.e., sartorius, rectus femoris) rather than the iliopsoas, as the iliopsoas is too deep to palpate (3).

VAC is tested as part of the motor examination by sensing contraction of the external anal sphincter (innervated by somatic motor components of the pudendal nerve from S2-S4) around the examiner's finger (by requesting the patient to "squeeze as if hold back a bowel movement") and graded as either present (yes) or absent (no). It is important not to confuse a reflex contraction of the anal sphincter (bulbocavernosus [BC] reflex) with voluntary contraction. During the rectal examination, one should also document the presence or absence of DAP, as previously described.

A number of optional muscles (diaphragm, deltoids, abdominal muscles, medial hamstrings, and hip adductors) may also be tested, which may be helpful in determining motor sparing of certain regions of the spinal cord and motor incompleteness, but are not used to obtain a motor index score (3). The diaphragm can be tested by measurement of the vital capacity but may also be tested under fluoroscopy. Movement of the hemidiaphragm two or more interspaces generally indicates normal function, and movement of one interspace is considered impaired. The deltoid, while important with respect to function as it provides a major contribution for reach of the upper extremity, is not used for motor scoring because it cannot properly be tested in the supine position. Beevor sign can test the abdominal muscles (innervated by T6-12). While asking the patient to flex the head and neck (a half sit-up or crunch), if the patient has a lesion between T9 and T11 the umbilicus will move rostrally since the upper abdominal muscles are innervated at and above T10. A negative Beevor sign (no movement of the umbilicus with trunk flexion) is present when the abdominal muscles have full innervation or total absence of abdominal innervation. Palpating the abdominals during the test helps distinguish between these, as no movement with no palpable contraction is a sign of absence of innervation (lesion above T7). This test should not be performed during the acute stages of thoracic/lumbar injuries. The hip adductor muscle, while not used as part of the motor score, is an important muscle to monitor as it is often the first muscle to recover in the lower extremity.

CLASSIFICATION OF SPINAL CORD INJURY

Until recent years, there was confusion regarding the definitions of the neurological and functional deficits of SCI. It was therefore difficult to measure clinically and scientifically the outcome of different treatments. Using a standard method of neurological assessment is important to help determine the course of recovery and the effect of interventions in the treatment of SCI (8).

There have been many systems developed for the classification of SCI that have been based on bony patterns of injury, mechanism of injury, neurological function, and functional outcome (9–16). A history of the classifications used in SCI is reviewed elsewhere (17). In 1969, Frankel described a five-grade system of classifying traumatic SCI, with a division into "complete" and "incomplete" injuries (18). In 1982, the ASIA published a booklet *Standards for Neurological Classification of SCI* (19) that defined basic terms and examination in SCI, as well as described a number of anatomically incomplete clinical syndromes. Other scales and examination techniques have also been described (20–23), some that utilize additional muscle groups, such as used in the NASCIS trials (22,23). El Masry et al. (24), however, found the ASIA and the NASCIS motor scoring systems comparable in representing motor deficits and recovery. Since fewer muscles were required to be tested in the ASIA Standards, this was recommended.

TABLE 6.2

ASIA IMPAIRMENT SCALE

A = Complete: No motor or sensory function is preserved in the sacral segments S4-5.
B = Incomplete: Sensory but not motor function is preserved below the neurological level and includes the sacral segments S4-5 AND no motor function is preserved more than 3 levels below the motor level on either side of the body.
C = Motor function is preserved below the neurological level**, and more than half of the key muscles below the single neurological level have a muscle grade less than 3 (Grades 0–2).
D = Incomplete: Motor function is preserved below the neurological level**, and **at least half** (half or more) of key muscles below the neurological level have a muscle grade of ≥ 3.
E = Normal: Motor and sensory function are normal.

Note: **For an individual to receive a grade of C or D, i.e. motor incomplete status, they must have either 1) voluntary anal sphincter contraction or 2) sacral sensory sparing (at S4-5 or DAP) with sparing of motor function more than 3 levels below the motor level for that side of the body. The Standards at this time allows even non-key muscle function more than 3 levels below the motor level to be used in determining motor incomplete status (AIS B vs. C) (1).

Definitions and classifications over the years have changed with multiple revisions of the Standards. This includes the muscles tested, areas of key dermatomes, terminology used, and the classification itself. In 1992, the *ASIA Impairment Scale* (AIS) (25) replaced the Frankel classification and was revised in 1996 (26), 2000 (27), and 2002, with reprints in 2006 and 2008, and the newest revisions in 2011 (1) (Table 6.2). The 1996 standards were endorsed by the International Medical Society of Paraplegia (IMSOP), now the International Spinal Cord Society (ISCoS), and thereafter became known as the *International Standards for Neurological and Functional Classification of Spinal Cord Injury* or just termed the *International Standards*. In 2000, when the FIM was removed from the standards, the term 'Functional' was removed (27).

DEFINITIONS OF TERMS IN SCI

Tetraplegia, preferred to the term *quadriplegia*, is defined as impairment or loss of motor and/or sensory function in the cervical segments of the spinal cord due to damage of neural elements within the spinal cord. It does not include brachial plexus lesions or injury to the peripheral nerves outside the neural canal (1). Tetraplegia results in impairment of function in the arms as well as possibly the trunk, legs, and pelvic organs. *Paraplegia* refers to an impairment of motor and/or sensory function in the thoracic, lumbar, or sacral segments of the spinal cord secondary to damage of neural elements within the spinal canal. With paraplegia, neurologic function in the upper extremities is spared, but depending on the level of injury, the trunk, legs, and pelvic organs may be involved. Paraplegia can also refer to cauda equina and conus medullaris injuries, but not lumbar-sacral plexus lesions or injuries to peripheral nerves outside the neural canal. The terms *quadriparesis* (tetraparesis) and *paraparesis* are discouraged because they describe incomplete lesions imprecisely.

The *sensory level* is the most caudal dermatome to have normal (score of 2) sensation for both PP and LT on both sides of the body. This is determined by a grade of 2 (normal/intact), in all dermatomes beginning with C2 and extending caudally to the first segment that has a score of less than 2 for either light touch or pinprick. The intact dermatome level located immediately above the first dermatome level with impaired or absent light touch or pin sensation is designated as the sensory level. Since the right and left sides may differ, the sensory level should be determined for each side. Testing will generate up to four sensory levels per dermatome: R-pin, R- light touch, L-pin, L-light touch. For a single sensory level, the most rostral of all is taken. If sensation is abnormal at C2, the sensory level is designated as C1 (not C0) (1). If sensation is intact through S4-5, the sensory level should be recorded as intact ("INT") rather than as S4-5. If the patient is unable to reliably appreciate sensation when tested on the face, then NT should be recorded and no sensory level is given. *Sensory index scoring* is calculated by adding the scores for each dermatome, for a total score possible of 112 (56 on each side) for pinprick and for LT. If "NT" has been documented at any level, then a sensory score cannot be calculated. The sensory score provides a means of numerically documenting changes in sensory function.

The *motor level* is defined as the lowest key muscle that has a grade of at least 3, provided the key muscles represented by segments above that level are graded as 5 (1,2). The motor level may differ by side of the body; a single motor level would be the more rostral of the two. If "NT" has been documented as part of the exam, and this muscle is required for determination of the motor level, the designation of the motor level for that side should be deferred.

For myotomes that are not clinically testable by MMT (i.e., above C4, T2-L1, and S2-5), the motor level is presumed to be and recorded the same as the sensory level if testable motor function above that level is normal as well. For example, if the sensory level is C4, and there is no C5 motor function strength (or strength graded as ≥3), the motor level is C4. In a case where the C5 motor function is graded <3 on both sides of the body, with a sensory level on the left at C4 and on the right C3 (the right C4 dermatome is impaired); the motor level on the left would be C5 and on the right C3. Since the C4 dermatome on the right is impaired, it is presumed that the C4 myotome is also impaired. Therefore, the motor level is designated as C3, since the patient does not meet the criteria of having a key muscle function (in this case, the C5 muscle) ≥3/5 with the levels above (in this case C4) scoring as normal. On the left side, the C4 dermatome is normal, so the C4 myotome is considered normal and as a result the left motor level is C5. If all upper limb key muscle functions are intact, with intact sensation to T6, the sensory level as well as the motor level is recorded as T6. Lastly, if with a T6 sensory level, the T1 muscle function is graded a 3 instead of a 5, while T6 is still the sensory level, the motor level would be T1, as all the muscles above the T6 level cannot be considered normal.

It is important to recognize and document if neurologic injury is unrelated to SCI. For example, in a patient with a thoracic level injury who also has a brachial plexus injury, a note should be made in the comment box on the worksheet to correctly classify the patient's spinal level of injury, rather than assigning a higher level due to a non-SCI related injury.

Motor index scoring is calculated by adding the muscle scores of each key muscle group. In the past, a total motor score of 100 (25 for each extremity) was calculated, but it is no longer recommended to add the upper and lower limb scores together. Rather, it is recommended to separate the motor scores into two scores: one for the upper limb and one for the lower limb (1). The motor score provides a means of numerically documenting changes in motor function. If "NT" has been documented, then a motor index score cannot be calculated. Pluses and minuses are not considered for motor index scoring.

The *Neurologic Level of Injury* (NLI) refers to the most caudal segment of the cord with intact sensation and antigravity muscle function and is determined for the right and left sides, and for motor and sensory functions. Therefore, up to four different levels are possible (i.e., motor and sensory for the right and left sides of the body), and if so, it is recommended to record each separately, to present a clearer picture of the patient's status. Motor and sensory levels are the same in less than 50% of complete injuries, and the motor level may be multiple levels below the sensory level at 1 year postinjury (28,29).

The single neurological level is the single most caudal level at which both motor and sensory modalities are intact on both sides of the body (i.e., the highest of all the levels). If the motor level is C7 and the sensory level is C8, the overall single NLI is C7. The single NLI is used when determining the AIS grade differentiating AIS C from D.

The motor level and upper extremity motor index score better reflect the degree of function as well as the severity of impairment and disability, relative to the NLI, after motor complete tetraplegia (28). This is because the sensory level may place the neurologic level more cephalad, thereby incorrectly implying poorer function.

The *zone of partial preservation* (ZPP) is defined as the dermatomes and myotomes caudal to the sensory and motor levels that remain partially innervated in an individual with a neurologically complete (AIS A) injury (see later). The ZPP should be recorded on the work sheet by documenting the most caudal segment with some sensory and/or motor function bilaterally. A single segment for each ZPP rather than the entire range of partially innervated segments should be documented. For example, if the right sensory level is C5 and some sensation extends to C8, then C8 is recorded in the right sensory ZPP block on the form. For ZPP description, motor function does not follow sensory function (i.e., in a case of a T6 level of injury, impaired sensation at T7 does not mean there is impaired motor function at T7). If there is no ZPP (no partially innervated segments below a motor or sensory level), the motor or sensory level should be entered as the ZPP (1). With an incomplete injury, the ZPP is not applicable and "NA" is placed.

A neurological *complete* injury is defined as the absence of sensory and motor function in the lowest sacral segments (no sacral sparing), and an *incomplete* injury as partial preservation of sensory and/or motor function as determined by examination of the most caudal segment (S4-5) (*sacral sparing*). Sacral sparing is tested by LT and PP at the anal mucocutaneous junction (S4/5 dermatome) on both sides, as well as testing VAC of the external anal sphincter (the motor aspect) and DAP as part of the rectal examination. If any of these are present (representing sacral sparing), intact or impaired, even on one side, the individual has an incomplete injury. According to this definition, a patient with cervical SCI can have sensory and motor function in the trunk or even in the legs, but unless sacral sparing is present, the injury is classified as 'complete' with a large ZPP. When sacral sparing is used to define

TABLE 6.3

STEPS TO AIS CLASSIFICATION

1. Determine sensory levels for right and left sides.
   Sensory level = "Most caudal segment of the spinal cord where both PP and LT are normal and all rostral segments are normal." Start from top of the worksheet, and go down until you see a "1" or "0" for either LT or sharp/dull, and go up one level. That is the sensory level.
2. Determine motor levels for right and left sides.
   Motor level = "The lowest key muscle that has a grade of at least 3, providing that the key muscles ... above that level ... are normal."
   Note: In regions where there is no myotome to test, the motor level is presumed to be the same as the sensory level, if testable motor function above that level is also normal.
3. Determine the single neurological level.
   Note: This is the lowest segment where motor and sensory function is normal on both sides, and is the most cephalad of the 4 levels (2 sensory; 2 motor) determined in steps 1 and 2.
   Single neurological level = The most rostral of sensory and motor levels.
   For example, if
   Sensory level: Right C4; Left C5
   Motor level: Right C5; Left C6
   Then, single neurological level = C4.
4. Determine whether the injury is complete or incomplete (sacral sparing).
   Sacral sparing = sensory or motor function in the sacral segments, S4-5.
   - Sensory function = S4-5 dermatome or DAP.
   - Motor function = voluntary anal sphincter.
5. Determine AIS grade:
   a. Is injury *incomplete*? NO, AIS = A. Record ZPP.
      If the injury is complete, the worksheet will read "N-0-0-0-0-N."
   b. If YES, is injury *motor incomplete*? NO, AIS = B.
      (*Yes = voluntary anal sphincter contraction or motor function more than three levels below the motor level on a given side with sensory sacral sparing.*)
   c. If YES, are at least half (half or more) of the key muscles below the (single) neurological level graded 3 or better? NO, AIS = C.
   d. If yes, AIS = D.
   e. If sensation and motor function is normal in all segments, AIS = E.

Note: AIS E is used in follow-up testing when an individual with a documented SCI has recovered normal function. If at initial testing no deficits are found, the individual is neurologically intact; the AIS does not apply.

incompleteness, motor recovery is significantly more likely to occur than when it is not (30). The *sacral sparing* definition of the completeness of the injury was adopted by the neurological standards committee in 1992 (25). Prior to this, an injury was considered "incomplete" if motor or sensory function extended more than three levels below the injury (19). The sacral sparing definition is considered a more stable definition, because fewer patients convert from incomplete to complete status over time postinjury. In addition, this offers an improved prognostication for improving from sensory incomplete to motor incomplete status as only 13% of patients with the older definition improved from admission to discharge from a motor complete sensory incomplete status to a motor incomplete status, in contrast to 54% utilizing the sacral sparing definition (3,30).

The *AIS* has five grades, which are listed in Table 6.2. The determination of the AIS is described in Table 6.3.

AIS A: Motor and sensory complete—no sacral sparing including PP or LT sensation at any of the S4-5 dermatomes; no VAC and no DAP. In this case, a ZPP is documented on the flow sheet. If the injury is complete, the worksheet will read "N-O-O-O-O-N" across the bottom—"no" for VAC, the four 0s for no S4-5 sensation for LT or PP modalities on either side of the body, and "no" for anal sensation (2).

AIS B: Sensory incomplete. Sacral sparing of sensory function (either LT or PP at S4-5, or DAP present), and there is no VAC or motor function more than three levels below the *motor* level on either side of the body.

AIS C: Motor incomplete, which can be determined by the presence of

1. Sacral sparing of motor function (i.e., VAC)
2. Sacral sparing of sensation (as described above) with motor function present in *more* than three levels below the *motor* level on either side. Motor function in this case includes all voluntary muscles below the motor level, not only the key muscles (1,3). The use of non-key muscles is somewhat controversial, and research in this area is warranted. A computerized classification program has been developed utilizing this schema (31).

If a patient has a sensory incomplete lesion and absence of all the key muscle groups below the level, however, voluntary sphincter contraction, the individual is classified as an AIS C. In a case like this, however, one should be careful that he or she is feeling the anal sphincter rather than contracting gluteal muscles or a reflex sphincter contraction. When in doubt, the patient should be scored as not having voluntary power of the anal sphincter (3).

AIS D: Motor incomplete status as above, with half or more of the key muscles below the *single NLI* are graded on MMT 3.

It is important to note that to distinguish AIS C versus D, the motor scores below the *single NLI* are used, whereas to distinguish between an AIS B versus a C, the *motor level* on each side of the body is utilized. The reason for using the motor level

TABLE 6.4

CLASSIFICATION EXAMPLES

1. C5-5, C6-5, and all distal muscles 0. (Motor level?)
2. C5-5, C6-5, C7-3, C8-3, T1-0. (Motor level?)
3. C5-5, C6-5, C7-5, C8-4, T1-4. (Motor level?)
4. All UE key muscles are 5/5. LE muscle groups are 0. Sensory level is T6. (Motor level?)
5. C5-8 muscles are 5; T1 is 3. Sensory level is T6; nothing below. (Motor and NLI?)
6. Intact sensation to T12 and absent below. UE key muscles are 5. L2-3, L3-1, all others-0. (Motor level?)
7. Intact sensation through L2, with impaired sensation below (including S4-5). UE strength is normal. Right L2-4, L3-3, L4-1, L5-0, and S1-0. On the left L2-5, L3-4, L4-2, L5, and S1-0. No VAC is present (AIS grade?)
8. Normal sensation to C7, absent below, with present DAP. Key muscles C5-C7 -5, C8-3, T1-1, L2-2, L3-4, L4-1, L5 on the left is 1 and 4 on the right, S1-4 bilaterally with present VAC. (Sensory, motor, single NLI and AIS grade?)

Answers:

1. Motor level is C6.
2. Motor level is C7, since it is the lowest muscle to test at least 3/5 with the next rostral muscle testing normal (5/5).
3. Motor level is C8, because the C8 is the lowest key muscle to test at least 3/5 with the next most rostral key muscle testing normal. While the T1 muscle is 4/5, the level above it is not normal.
4. Motor level is T6. Since all of the UE muscles are intact, the motor level is determined by the sensory level.
5. Motor and NLI are T1. In this case, motor level does not defer to the sensory level since there is a definitive motor level at T1. One only defers to the sensory level if a motor level cannot be clarified on its own. If T1 muscle graded a 5, then the motor and NLI would be T6.
6. Motor level is T12. Since the L1 dermatome is not normal, despite the L2 motor level having at least grade 3 strength, the next most rostral level (L1) does not meet the criteria of being presumed normal.
7. AIS B. In order to be classified as an AIS C, motor function must extend more than three levels caudal to the motor level. This patient would need to have voluntary motor function extending to the S1 myotome or anal sphincter contraction to be considered an AIS C.
8. Sensory level—C7. Motor level is C8. The single NLI is C7. There are 14 key muscles below this neurological level. Since exactly ½ of the muscles below the single NLI have a grade ≥3, the patient has an AIS D classification.

to distinguish an AIS B versus C is to avoid the possible situation when a patient may regain sensation in one more caudal level that would falsely change the AIS from "C" to a "B." For example, if a patient initially had a motor level of C5 and a sensory level of C4 with sensory sparing at S4/5 and some motor sparing only in C6-8, using the neurologic level, this patient would qualify for AIS C (since C8 motor is more than three levels below the neurologic level [C4]). If the patient regains normal sensation over time in the C5 dermatome, the neurologic level changes to C5 and the patient would revert from an AIS C to B because C8 is no longer more than three levels below the neurologic level, indicating "worsening" despite neurologic improvement. This is avoided by using the motor level, since the designation is independent of the sensory level. Once a patient is classified as having a motor incomplete injury, it is important to determine if he or she should be classified as an AIS C or D. He or she is classified as an AIS C if more than half of the key muscles below the single NLI are graded less than 3/5.

AIS E: All components of the standardized neurological examination are normal. The grade E is used in follow-up when testing an individual with a previously documented SCI that has recovered normal function. If at initial testing no neurological deficits are found, then the AIS does not apply.

See Table 6.4 for examples of determining the motor, sensory, and NLI.

Having a well-defined classification of SCI allows clinicians and researchers to study the effect of drug and rehabilitation interventions and determine prognosis. The AIS is currently the most valid and reliable classification to assess SCI and is used by the Model System Spinal Cord Injury database.

RELIABILITY OF EXAMINATION

The motor and sensory examination and the classification of patients with SCI according to the International Standards have been found to be reliable and sensitive to change, most especially in patients with neurologically complete injuries (32–35). Cohen et al. (31) found high reliability of the LT, PP, and motor examinations; inter-rater reliability values ranged from 0.96 to 0.98 and intra-rater reliability values were 0.98 to 0.99. Marino et al. (32) also demonstrated that the motor and sensory examination is reliable, with inter-rater reliability of the motor exam of 0.97, LT – 0.96, and PP – 0.88, when conducted by trained examiners. PP scores had the lowest reliability, possibly because of the need to differentiate sharp from dull sensation.

The reliability of individual dermatome and myotome scores is less than for summed scores. Jonnson et al. (34) reported that inter-rater reliability of dermatome and myotome scores was weak in incomplete SCI patients. However, in this study, they used the unweighted kappa statistic, which requires exact agreement, rather than the weighted kappa, which is more appropriate for ordinal scales. The kappa statistic is a chance-corrected measure of agreement, and the weighted kappa gives partial credit for scores that are close to each other but not exactly the same. Savic et al. (35) used both the weighted and the unweighted kappa statistics to evaluate agreement in myotome scores for two examiners, using 45 individuals with SCI. For individual myotomes, the unweighted kappa values ranged from 0.60 to 0.94, while weighted kappa values were above 0.93 for all muscles except the biceps.

In summary, there is generally good test-retest agreement for individual and summed myotome scores, particularly for individuals with complete SCI. When present, most differences are within one muscle grade for skilled examiners. Dermatome scores are more variable. Regardless, scores for individual dermatomes are consistent enough that summed scores still show excellent reliability. It is recommended that while overall the examination results are reliable, one should not place too much weight on a change of a single dermatome or muscle when applying the Standards (36). Rather, follow-up examinations are recommended.

In the pediatric population, Mulcahey et al. found that the examination was not reliable in children younger than 4 years of age (37). Children younger than 10 were distressed by the PP exam, and motor scores in children under the age of 15 and sensory scores in children under the age of 5 showed good reliability although with wide confidence intervals (CI), somewhat limiting their usefulness (37). A larger study of 187 subjects found intra-rater agreement on LT, PP and motor scores in children over age 6 with neurologically complete injuries, with wider CI in those with incomplete injuries (38). Vogel et al. reported on the agreement of repeated anorectal examinations in the pediatric population that agreement on repeated PP and LT sensation at S4-5 was good for all age groups and types of injury (tetra/paraplegia) (5). For deep pressure and VAC, there was strong agreement in the 6- to 11-year and 16- to 21-year age groups, but weaker agreement in the 12- to 15-year age group. VAC had the lowest CI values. Subjects with tetraplegia had greater agreement relative to those with paraplegia, perhaps because young children with tetraplegia have neurological complete injuries. These findings therefore do not necessarily support the use of the anorectal exam in all children/youth for designation of injury severity or clinical research trials (5).

CLINICAL SYNDROMES OF SPINAL CORD INJURY

A number of neurological incomplete clinical syndromes of SCI are frequently referred to in the literature that include central cord, Brown-Sequard, anterior cord, posterior cord, conus medullaris, and cauda equina syndromes. The original definitions of these syndromes have remained for the most part unchanged, except central cord syndrome, which is no longer considered to be caused by hemorrhage into the spinal cord as originally described and may be predominantly due to a white matter lesion (39–42).When this syndrome is accompanied by lower motor neuron (LMN) findings in the UEs, there is also gray matter involvement (43).

Central Cord Syndrome (CCS) is the most common of the incomplete injuries, accounting for approximately 50% of incomplete injuries and 9% of all traumatic SCI. This applies almost exclusively to cervical injuries and is characterized by motor weakness in the UEs greater than the lower extremities, in association with sacral sparing (40). At the level of injury, there is LMN weakness as well as sensory loss, with upper motor neuron (UMN) paralysis below the lesion level. In addition to the motor weakness, other features include bladder dysfunction and varying sensory loss below the level of the lesion. CCS most frequently occurs in older persons with cervical spondylosis who suffer a hyperextension injury, most commonly from a fall, followed by motor vehicle crashes. However, CCS may occur in persons of any age and is associated with other etiologies, predisposing factors, and injury mechanisms. The postulated mechanism of injury involves compression of the cord both anteriorly and posteriorly by degenerative changes of the bony structures, with inward bulging of the ligamentum flavum during hyperextension in an already narrowed spinal canal (40–45). CCS can occur with or without fracture or dislocation.

The pathophysiology of the upper limbs being more affected relative to the lower limbs has been postulated to be from location of motor tracts of the upper limbs located more centrally, with the lower limbs more peripherally located (40,44). MRI evidence has revealed that this clinical pattern may not be based on locations of the arm and leg fibers within the corticospinal tract, but rather that this tract carries fibers that mainly innervate distal limb musculature, and therefore, the functional deficits are more pronounced in the hands when the tract is the primary site of damage (46).

There is no consensus regarding the diagnostic criteria for traumatic CCS (47,48). In an online worldwide survey of spine surgeons, it was found that there is a wide range of definitions used to define CCS (48). It has been proposed that a difference of at least 10 points of UEMS and LEMS be present as a clear diagnostic criteria, but additional studies are needed (47,48).

CSS usually has a favorable prognosis (45). The typical pattern of recovery occurs earliest and to the greatest extent in the lower extremities, followed by bowel and bladder function, upper extremity (proximal), and then intrinsic (distal) hand function. Penrod et al. have noted that the prognosis for functional recovery of ambulation, activities of daily living (ADL), and bowel and bladder function is dependent upon the patient's age, with a less optimistic prognosis in older patients relative to younger patients (49,50). Patients less than 50 years of age are more successful in achieving independent ambulation than older patients (87% to 97% versus 31% to 41%). Similar differences were seen between the younger and the older patients in independent bladder function (83% versus 29%), independent bowel function (63% versus 24%), and dressing (77% versus 12%). However, persons with initial neurological examinations (within 72 hours) with a classification of AIS D tetraplegia, prognosis for recovery of independent ambulation is excellent, even for those whose age is greater than 50 (52).

A syndrome with similar clinical features of upper extremity paresis or paralysis, with minimal to no lower extremity involvement is *cruciate paralysis*, first described by Bell (53). This may occur with fractures of C1 and C2, with neurological compromise at the cervicomedullary junction (54). In CCS, the injury is usually localized in the mid to lower segments of the cervical spinal cord (i.e., C4-5), while in cruciate paralysis, the damage is higher, with respiratory insufficiency occurring in roughly 25% of patients. A number of reports have appeared in the literature with cases suspected with this diagnosis (55–58). The prognosis for cruciate paralysis is good, with most patients demonstrating complete recovery. Wallenberg proposed an anatomical explanation for this clinical syndrome (59), suggesting that the decussation of the fibers to the upper limb lay in a more rostral, medial, and ventral location in the cervicomedullary junction compared to a more lateral and caudal location of the lower limb decussating fibers. Therefore, injury to the canal where the upper extremity fibers travel alone after decussation causes preferential injury to the upper limbs. Neuroanatomical evidence to support this hypothesis, however, has not been found (60).

A variation of CCS, with only a few case reports reported, is the presence of motor sparing in the absence of all sensation (49,61). This variation does not meet the criteria of CCS, as there is no sparing of sacral sensation. Prognosis is difficult to determine given the limited information, but from the case report (61), the patient did develop some sensory recovery (at ~ 3 months) and regain the ability to ambulate short distances (personal communication with the author).

Brown-Sequard Syndrome (BSS) involves a hemisection of the spinal cord, consisting of asymmetric paresis with hypoalgesia more marked on the less paretic side and accounts for 2% to 4% of all traumatic SCI (62–64). In the classic presentation of BSS, there is (a) ipsilateral loss of all sensory modalities at the level of the lesion, (b) ipsilateral flaccid paralysis *at* the level of the lesion, (c) ipsilateral loss of position sense and vibration *below* the lesion, (d) contralateral loss of pain and temperature *below* the lesion, and (e) ipsilateral motor loss (UMN) *below* the level of the lesion. Neuroanatomically, this is explained by the crossing of the spinothalamic tracts in the spinal cord, as opposed to the corticospinal and dorsal columns, which decussate in the brainstem. Only a limited number of patients have the pure form of BSS. Much more common is a presentation with some features of the Brown-Sequard and Central Cord syndrome, with a relative ipsilateral hemiplegia with a relative contralateral hemianalgesia. This is referred to as *Brown-Sequard like* or *Brown-Sequard Plus Syndrome*. Although BSS has traditionally been associated with knife injuries, a variety of etiologies, including those that result in closed spinal injuries with or without vertebral fractures, may be the cause. In addition, neoplastic causes as well as intramedullary inflammatory lesions, such as in multiple sclerosis, can result in partial or complete BSS.

Despite the variation in presentation, considerable consistency is found in the prognosis of BSS. Recovery takes place in the ipsilateral proximal extensors and then the distal flexors (68,69). Motor recovery of any extremity having a pain/temperature sensory deficit occurs before the opposite extremity, and these patients may expect functional gait recovery by 6 months. Of all the spinal cord syndromes, patients with BSS have the greatest prognosis for functional outcome and potential for ambulation. Seventy-five to ninety percent of patients ambulate independently at discharge from rehabilitation, and nearly seventy percent perform functional skills and ADL independently (45,63,65). The most important predictor of function is whether the upper or the lower limb is the predominant site of weakness: when the upper limb is weaker than the lower limb, patients are more likely to ambulate at discharge (65). Recovery of bowel and bladder function is also favorable, with continence achieved in 82% and 89%, respectively, in one study (65).

The *Anterior Cord Syndrome* (ACS) accounts for 2.7% of traumatic SCI, and involves a lesion affecting the anterior two thirds of the spinal cord while preserving the posterior columns. ACS may occur from retropulsed disc or bone fragments (70), direct injury to the anterior spinal cord, or most commonly with vascular injury or occlusion of the anterior spinal artery, which provides the blood supply to the anterior spinal cord (71). This can occur during surgery to the aorta (especially with clamping above the renal artery) or other processes that could decrease blood flow to the spinal cord (i.e., vertebral burst fracture). There is a variable loss of motor as well as PP sensation with a relative preservation of LT, proprioception, and deep-pressure sensation. Usually, patients with ACS have only 10% to 20% chance of muscle recovery, and even in those with some recovery, there is poor muscle power and coordination (72).

The *Posterior Cord Syndrome* is the least frequent of incomplete SCI syndromes and has been omitted from recent versions of the International Standards (1,26,27). It is characterized by preservation of pain, temperature, and touch appreciation with varying degrees of motor preservation, and an absence of all dorsal column function. Prognosis for ambulation is poor, secondary to the propioceptive deficits.

Conus Medullaris and Cauda Equina Injuries

The conus medullaris, which is the terminal segment of the adult spinal cord, lies at the inferior aspect of the L1 vertebrae (see Chapter 2 for details). The segment above the conus medullaris is termed the *epiconus*, consisting of spinal cord segments L4-S1. Nerve roots then travel from the conus medullaris caudally, as the cauda equina. Lesions of the epiconus, or upper part of the conus medullaris, will affect the lower lumbar roots supplying muscles of the lower part of the leg and foot, with sparing of reflex function of sacral segments. The BC reflex and micturition reflexes are preserved, representing an UMN or a suprasacral lesion. Spasticity will most likely develop in sacral innervated segments (toe flexors, ankle plantarflexors, and hamstring muscles). Recovery is similar to other UMN spinal cord injuries (Table 6.5).

Lower conus medullaris lesions affecting neural segments S2 and below will present with LMN deficits of the anal sphincter and bladder due to damage of the anterior horn cells of S2-4. Bladder and rectal reflexes are diminished or absent, depending on the exact level and extent of the lesion. There is paralysis of the bladder detrusor muscle due to destruction of the preganglionic

TABLE 6.5

COMPARISON OF DIFFERENT LEVEL OF LESIONS

Symptom	Epiconus	Conus medullaris	Cauda equina
Fracture level	**T12 and above**	**T12/L1-2**	**Below L2**
Pain	Uncommon	Uncommon	Very common and may be severe
Bowel/bladder reflexes	Present (UMN syndrome)	Absent[a] most commonly (LMN syndrome)	Absent (LMN syndrome)
Anal and BC reflex	Present	Absent[a] (LMN syndrome)	Absent (LMN syndrome)
Muscle tone	Increased (UMN syndrome)	(LMN syndrome)[b]	Decreased (LMN syndrome)
MSRs	Increased[c]	(LMN syndrome)[b]	Decreased (LMN syndrome)
Symmetry of weakness	Yes	Yes	No
Sensation	In dermatomal distribution	Absent in saddle distribution and may be dissociated	In root distribution
Recovery prognosis	Limited	Limited	Possible

[a]Unless a high conus lesion

[b]Depends if nerve roots are affected. If so, then is decreased.

[c]Ankle plantarflexors and hamstrings, not knee jerks.

MSR, muscle stretch reflexes; UMN, upper motor neuron; LMN, lower motor neuron.

parasympathetic (PS) fibers, with retention of urine and overflow incontinence. In men, there is failure of penile erections and ejaculation due to the destruction of the preganglionic PS neurons and the somatic motor ventral horn cells, respectively. Emission of semen can still occur, since the motor fibers to the ductus deferens and seminal vesicles have sympathetic innervation. Motor strength in the legs and feet may remain intact if the nerve roots (L3-S2) are not affected. The lumbar nerve roots may be spared partially or totally in the conus medullaris; referred to as *root escape*. If the roots are affected as they travel with the sacral cord in the spinal column, this will result in LMN damage, with diminished or absent reflexes. In some conus injuries, the knee reflexes may be preserved, but the ankle reflexes affected. In low conus lesions, the S1 segment is not involved, and therefore, the ankle reflexes are normal, a finding accounting for most instances of failure to make the diagnosis. Due to the small size of the conus medullaris, lesions are more likely to be bilateral as compared to those of the cauda equina. With conus medullaris lesions, recovery is limited.

Injuries below the L1 vertebral level do not cause injury to the spinal cord, but rather to the cauda equine (CE) or nerve rootlets supplying the lumbar and sacral segments of the skin and muscle groups referred to as *Cauda Equina Syndrome* (CES). This usually produces flaccid paralysis (due to LMN injury) and atrophy of the LEs (L2-S2), varying sensory loss in a radicular pattern, with bowel and bladder involvement (S2-4), and areflexia of the knee, ankle, and plantar reflexes. The patient may have spared sensation in the perineum and/or LEs but have complete paralysis. In cauda injuries, there is loss of anal and BC reflexes, as well as impotence. Cauda equina injuries are usually asymmetric, possibly because the rootlets are more mobile than the cord.

Cauda equina injuries have a better prognosis for recovery than UMN spinal cord injuries. This is most likely due to the fact that the nerve roots are more resilient to injury and because many of the biochemical processes that occur in the spinal cord and produce secondary damage occur to a much less extent in the nerve roots. CE injuries may represent a neuropraxia or an axonotomesis and demonstrate progressive recovery over a course of weeks and months. As the cauda equina rootlets are histologically peripheral nerves, regeneration can occur.

Separation of cauda equina and conus lesions in clinical practice is difficult, because the clinical features of these lesions overlap (see Table 6.5). Isolated conus lesions are rare since the roots forming the CE are wrapped around the conus. Traumatic SCI will likely produce a combination syndrome or a pure cauda equina lesion. The conus may be affected by a fracture of L1, whereas a fracture of L2 or lower impinges solely on the CE. Sacral fractures as well as fractures of the pelvic ring also damage the CE, as well as the sacral plexus. Bullet wounds can penetrate the bony structures to traumatize the cauda and conus. Intrinsic tumors of the conus medullaris can selectively damage the conus.

Some differences between these lesions are noted in Table 6.5. Pain is uncommon in conus lesions but is frequently a complaint in CES. Sensory abnormalities occur in a saddle distribution in conus lesions and, if there is sparing, there is usually dissociated loss with a greater loss of pain and temperature while sparing touch sensation. In cauda equina lesions, sensory loss occurs more in a root distribution and is not dissociated.

Cauda equina lesions can be considered as multiple radiculopathies and as such electrodiagnostic studies may be helpful in the diagnosis. Sensory nerve action potentials in lesions that are proximal to the dorsal root ganglia should remain normal, whereas in CE lesions they will be affected. The electromyographic abnormalities in cauda lesions would be widespread and bilateral (but asymmetrical). Other methods of studying root or nerve function (H-reflexes, F waves, root stimulation, somatosensory evoked potentials) may be used to aid in diagnosis. Conus medullaris lesions should cause significant electrical abnormalities only where the LMNs are affected. In that case, abnormalities may be present in muscles supplied by S2-4 levels (such as the anal sphincter).

SCI syndromes can be the result of both traumatic and nontraumatic etiologies. CCS and conus medullaris syndromes are most likely due to falls, whereas motor vehicle crash is the primary etiology for BSS. In contrast, anterior cord and posterior cord syndromes are more frequently the result of a nontraumatic injury. CES is almost equally due to traumatic and nontraumatic etiologies (45).

DISCOMPLETE INJURIES

Neurological pathways within the spinal cord may be spared even after a neurologically complete injury. The term *discomplete injury* was introduced by Dimitrijevic et al. (73,74) to describe a clinically complete SCI with neurophysiological evidence of residual function and connectivity between above and below the injury. Other studies have shown that some communication between segments above and below the injury is possible even in clinically complete SCI (74–78).

Finnerup et al. (78) performed quantitative sensory testing (including thermal stimulation, pressure, pinch and pain sensitivity) in 24 subjects with AIS A (with no sparing of voluntary motor function or preserved PP or LT sensation below the injury) and found that 50% had vague localized sensation to the stimuli. All patients had no cortical response to lower extremity (posterior tibial nerve) SSEP. There was no relationship between the presence of this sensory perception with the level of injury or etiology. There was also no correlation between the presence of sensory perception with the presence or severity of spasticity or chronic neuropathic pain (78).

Neuropathological studies found a similar percentage (50%) of anatomical discomplete injuries in persons with functional complete injuries (75,77). Prolonged painful or repetitive stimuli may pass through axons in the injured cord when a threshold is exceeded (78). It is not clear however where this spared information travels or what the preservation of these pathways represents. Knowledge of retained neural communication across a spinal injury may have consequences for treatment strategies aimed at enhancing function or collateral sprouting of surviving axons and further study is needed.

INTERNATIONAL STANDARDS TO DOCUMENT REMAINING AUTONOMIC FUNCTION AFTER SPINAL CORD INJURY

Individuals with SCI not only face paralysis, but lifelong problems with a variety of autonomic dysfunctions including abnormal blood pressure and heart rate, sweating, and temperature dysregulation (79,80). Until recently, the impact of an SCI on a person's neurological function was evaluated through the use of only motor and sensory assessment that is a part of the

International Standards that does not examine the status of a person's autonomic function. In order to address this deficiency, the ASIA and the ISCoS commissioned a group of international experts to develop a common strategy to document remaining autonomic neurologic function (81). Some of the challenges in studying autonomic dysfunctions following SCI include the complexity and organization of the autonomic nervous system (ANS) and its involvement in the control of almost every bodily system, making it difficult to select appropriate clinical tests for individuals with SCI; limited experience in the clinical assessment of autonomic dysfunctions in individuals with SCI; a lack of uniform operational definitions of autonomic dysfunction; and difficulty in evaluating the ANS regarding bladder, bowel, and sexual function during a bedside examination. There is relatively limited information on the relationship between the level and completeness of the SCI lesion and the degree of autonomic dysfunction (82). The goal of the Autonomic Standards is to describe the impact of SCI on particular organ systems function in a succinct document in conjunction with the International Standards. These standards are not meant to provide recommendations for treatment of specific organ systems. Rather, they will allow clinicians and researchers to appreciate possible autonomic dysfunctions and to be able to describe the effects of SCI on bowel, urinary bladder, sexual, cardiovascular, bronchopulmonary, sudomotor, and other autonomic functions.

COMPONENTS OF THE INTERNATIONAL AUTONOMIC STANDARDS

The autonomic standards contain four components: general autonomic, urinary bladder, bowel, and sexual functions (Fig. 6.3). A general anatomic diagnosis is utilized to document the overall impact of SCI on different autonomic functions. A classification chart allows the description of the autonomic control of cardiovascular, bronchopulmonary, and sudomotor function, including thermoregulation on a single form. The chart also allows for the examiner to describe and grade the neurologic control of lower urinary tract (LUT), bowel, and sexual responses. Finally, this form allows documenting detailing of urodynamic evaluation that should be completed on all patients (Fig. 6.3).

ASIA
AMERICAN SPINAL INJURY ASSOCIATION

ISCoS

AUTONOMIC STANDARDS ASSESSMENT FORM

Patient Name: ______________

Anatomic Diagnosis: (Supraconal □, Conal □, Cauda Equina □)

General Autonomic Function

System/Organ	*Findings*	*Abnormal conditions*	*Check mark*
Autonomic control of the heart	Normal		
	Abnormal	Bradycardia	
		Tachycardia	
		Other dysrhythmias	
	Unknown		
	Unable to assess		
Autonomic control of blood pressure	Normal		
	Abnormal	Resting systolic blood pressure below 90 mmHg	
		Orthostatic hypotension	
		Autonomic dysreflexia	
	Unknown		
	Unable to assess		
Autonomic control of sweating	Normal		
	Abnormal	Hyperhydrosis above lesion	
		Hyperhydrosis below lesion	
		Hypohydrosis below lesion	
	Unknown		
	Unable to assess		
Temperature regulation	Normal		
	Abnormal	Hyperthermia	
		Hypothermia	
	Unknown		
	Unable to assess		
Autonomic and Somatic Control of Broncho-pulmonary System	Normal		
	Abnormal	Unable to voluntarily breathe requiring full ventilatory support	
		Impaired voluntary breathing requiring partial vent support	
		Voluntary respiration impaired does not require vent support	
	Unknown		

Lower Urinary Tract, Bowel and Sexual Function

System/Organ		*Score*
Lower Urinary Tract		
Awareness of the need to empty the bladder		
Ability to prevent leakage (continence)		
Bladder emptying method __________ (specify)		
Bowel		
Sensation of need for a bowel movement		
Ability to Prevent Stool Leakage (Continence)		
Voluntary sphincter contraction		
Sexual Function		
Genital arousal (erection or lubrication)	Psychogenic	
	Reflex	
Orgasm		
Ejaculation (male only)		
Sensation of Menses (female only)		

2 = Normal function, 1=Reduced or Altered Neurological Function 0=Complete loss of control NT=Unable to assess due to preexisting or concomitant problems

Urodynamic Evaluation

System/Organ	*Findings*	*Check mark*
Sensation during filling	Normal	
	Increased	
	Reduced	
	Absent	
	Non-specific	
Detrusor Activity	Normal	
	Overactive	
	Underactive	
	Acontractile	
Sphincter	Normal urethral closure mechanism	
	Normal urethral function during voiding	
	Incompetent	
	Detrusor sphincter dyssynergia	
	Non-relaxing sphincter	

Date of Injury______________ Date of Assessment______________ Examiner______________

This form may be freely copied and reproduced but not modified (Sp Cord, 2009, 47, 36-43)
This assessment should use the terminology found in the International SCI Data Set
(ASIA and ISCoS - http://www.asia-spinalinjury.org/bulletinBoard/dataset.php)

FIGURE 6.3. International Autonomic Standards.

Autonomic nervous system: anatomy and function. The ANS commonly is subdivided into two major parts: the sympathetic and the parasympathetic components (83). Most of the visceral organs are innervated by both components of the ANS (83,84). The sympathetic and PS systems are integrated functionally with each other within the central nervous system and provide balanced regulation of innervated organs. (For greater details, see Chapter 2.) The level and the severity of injury to these pathways result in a variety of autonomic dysfunctions depending on the altered supraspinal control of the sympathetic and parasympathetic nervous systems (85). Certain cortical structures, and the hypothalamus, contribute to regulation of the autonomic circuits within the brainstem and spinal cord. These cerebral structures should be intact morphologically, but there may be functional alterations following SCI.

THE AUTONOMIC STANDARDS ASSESSMENT FORM

Anatomical classification. An anatomical classification to describe the impact of SCI on urinary bladder, bowel, and sexual function is recommended. Terms include supraconal, conal, and cauda equina. Supraconal refers to those injuries occurring above the conus medullaris. In general, supraconal injuries cause an overactive or UMN pattern of damage affecting LUT, bowel, and sexual functions. Conal injuries often cause a mixed lesion to LUT, bowel, and sexual functions with a resultant overactive or acontractile picture. Cauda equine (CE) injuries generally cause an acontractile or LMN picture affecting LUT, bowel, and sexual functions.

It should be noted that the anatomical classification for autonomic function is intended to ultimately be used in conjunction with the International Standards (ISNSCI). Thus, in addition to using the above terminology, the examiner should provide information on the completeness of injury as determined by the preservation of perianal and anal sensation and VAC, and the type of reflex activity present, as described in the Autonomic Standards.

Assessment of General Autonomic Function

A documentation of remaining general autonomic function should be provided via checks in the appropriate boxes in the table entitled General Autonomic Function (Fig. 6.3). The information is determined based on a combination of neurologic examination and clinical history.

Heart rate dysfunctions: The recognition and assessment of cardiac dysrhythmias include documentation of bradycardia or heart rate under 60 beats per minute (bpm) and tachycardia or heart rate over 100 bpm. Other dysrhythmias should also be documented.

Blood pressure dysfunctions: Abnormalities of arterial blood pressure (BP) include supine hypertension (BP > 140/90 mm Hg) and supine hypotension (systolic BP < 90 mm Hg). Orthostatic hypotension is a symptomatic or asymptomatic decrease in BP, usually exceeding 20 mm Hg systolic or 10 mm Hg diastolic on moving from the supine to an upright position (86). Symptoms include dizziness, headache or "coat hanger" neck ache, and fatigue (87,88).

Autonomic dysreflexia is a constellation of signs and/or symptoms in SCI at and above T6 in response to noxious or nonnoxious stimuli below the level of injury defined by an increase in SBP (≥20 mm Hg above baseline), which may include one of the following symptoms: headache, flushing and sweating above the level of the lesion, vasoconstriction below the level of the lesion, and dysrhythmias (79,80). This syndrome may or may not be symptomatic and may occur at any period following SCI (89–91) (see Chapter 9).

Sweating dysfunctions: Abnormalities of sudomotor function including hyperhydrosis or nonphysiological sweating in response to noxious/non-noxious stimuli, positioning, etc. and hypohydrosis, diminished sweating below the level of the injury in response to a rise in temperature should be documented (92,93).

Temperature dysfunctions: Temperature dysregulation or an elevation or decrease in body temperature without signs of infection may result from exposure to environmental temperature change and should be documented (94,95). A decrease in body temperature has been divided into subnormal temperatures (95.8°F to 97.7°F; 35.4°C to 36.5°C), and hypothermia (less than 95.8°F; 35.4°C) (96). Hyperthermia or *Quad fever* refers to presentation with temperatures often exceeding 40°C (101.5°F), although only a mild elevation in core temperature may be present. Quad fever is a diagnosis of exclusion and other sources must be ruled out as sources of fever before quad fever can be diagnosed (97).

Bronchopulmonary dysfunctions: The autonomic components related to bronchopulmonary control are not easily tested at bedside; however, it is important to document the respiratory capacity of individuals with SCI (98,99). Therefore, the need for complete or partial ventilatory assistance should be documented under bronchopulmonary control.

Assessment of Urinary Bladder, Bowel, and Sexual Function

Information related to urinary, bowel, and sexual function is recorded in the table entitled lower urinary tract, bowel, and sexual function and is based on the clinical examination and history (Fig. 6.3). Responses include normal [2] when there is no change in neurologic control with respect to a specific function, reduced or altered [1] neurologic control with regards to a specific function, absent [0] neurologic control with regards to a specific function, and unable to assess a specific function [not testable = NT].

For the LUT, it is strongly recommended that urodynamics be routinely performed following SCI, although not all persons with SCI will have this performed early after injury. Clinicians benefit from being able to communicate information regarding the patient's ability to perceive sensations related to bladder filling and voluntary control of voiding. The assessment listed is recommended until a urodynamic evaluation can be performed. Furthermore, the clinician should consult the International Data Sets in SCI for more information on recommended urologic assessments and procedures (100,101). Acknowledging the limitations of patient self-report, it is recommended that awareness of the need to empty the bladder (sensation) is documented, followed by the ability to prevent leakage (continence). The bladder emptying method should be recorded.

For bowel function, the sensation of the need for a bowel movement is recorded. Continence of stool, that is, the ability to prevent an accidental bowel movement, should be recorded followed by documentation of the presence of VAC.

For sexual function, it is recommended that the presence of psychogenic genital arousal (penile erection or vaginal lubrication) is first recorded followed by documentation of reflex genital arousal. Ability to achieve orgasm is recorded. The presence of antegrade ejaculation is documented for males. The ability to sense menses (cramping, pain, etc.) relative to before injury is documented for females.

Urodynamic Evaluation

The urodynamic assessment is based on the clinical examination and observations made during urodynamic studies. There are three sections to the assessment: sensation during filling, detrusor activity, and sphincter function.

Sensation during filling has five possible choices and is dependent on specific information that can only be obtained via urodynamics. The time points and associated data must be documented when performing urodynamics after SCI (101,102). The time points include the first sensation of bladder filling, the first desire to void, and the strong desire to void.

Normal bladder sensation can be determined by these three defined points noted during filling cystometry and evaluated in relation to the bladder volume at that moment and in relation to the individual's symptomatic complaints. Increased bladder sensation is defined, during filling cystometry, as an early first sensation of bladder filling (or an early desire to void) and/or an early strong desire to void, which occurs at low bladder volume and which persists. Reduced bladder sensation is defined, during filling cystometry, as diminished sensation throughout bladder filling. Absent bladder sensation means that, during filling cystometry, the individual has no bladder sensation. Nonspecific bladder sensations, during filling cystometry, may make the individual aware of bladder filling, for example, abdominal fullness or vegetative symptoms.

Assessment of detrusor function is the next variable that should be documented through performance of urodynamics. Four separate types of detrusor function are defined for purposes of documentation: normal detrusor function, detrusor overactivity, detrusor underactivity, and acontractile detrusor. Normal detrusor function allows bladder filling with little or no change in pressure, and no involuntary phasic contractions occur despite provocation. Normal detrusor function in the voiding phase is achieved by a voluntarily initiated continuous detrusor contraction that leads to complete bladder emptying within a normal time span and in the absence of obstructions. Detrusor overactivity is a urodynamic observation characterized by involuntary detrusor contractions during the filling phase that may be spontaneous or provoked. Detrusor overactivity in the case of SCI is generally neurogenic detrusor overactivity, and it is recommended this term be used in lieu of *detrusor hyperreflexia*. Idiopathic detrusor overactivity can also occur without defined cause. Detrusor underactivity is defined as a contraction of reduced strength and/or duration, resulting in prolonged bladder emptying and/or a failure to achieve complete bladder emptying within a normal time span. Finally, an acontractile detrusor is one that cannot be demonstrated to contract during urodynamic studies.

The final area that should be documented based on urodynamics is that of urethral sphincter function. Normal urethral closure mechanism maintains a positive urethral closure pressure during bladder filling even in the presence of increased abdominal pressure, although it may be overcome by detrusor overactivity. Normal urethral function during voiding is defined as a urethral sphincter that opens and is relaxed continuously to allow the bladder to be emptied at a normal pressure. Incompetent urethral closure mechanism is defined as one that allows leakage of urine in the absence of a detrusor contraction. Detrusor sphincter dyssynergia is defined as a detrusor contraction concurrent with an involuntary contraction of the urethral and/or periurethral striated muscle during voiding. Occasionally, flow may be prevented altogether. *Nonrelaxing internal sphincter* is defined as obstruction during voiding that usually occurs in individuals with sacral or cauda equina lesions, such as meningomyelocele, and is characterized by a nonrelaxing, obstructing urethra resulting in reduced urine flow.

Overall, the Autonomic Standards assessment is a new system to document the impact of SCI on autonomic function and should be used in conjunction with the ISNSCIS. The Autonomic Standards assessment is meant to complement information available in the respective International SCI Data Sets. Thus, the degree of detail in the Autonomic Standards is significantly less than that of the data sets, which are designed to serve as a complete patient record for persons with SCI (103,104).

THE FUNCTIONAL EVALUATION

To accurately describe the impact of the SCI on an individual and to monitor functional progress, it is necessary to use descriptive terms and a standard measure of ADL. The World Health Organization (WHO) has defined terms that are frequently used when functional deficits are discussed (International Classification of Functioning, Disability, and Health = ICF); losses or abnormalities of bodily function and structure (impairments), limitations of activities (previously referred to as *disabilities*), and restriction in participation (previously referred to as *handicaps*) (105). *Impairment* is any loss or abnormality of bodily structure or of a physiological or psychological function, such as paralysis. Restriction or lack of ability to perform an *activity* in the nature and extent of functioning within the range considered normal (resulting from an impairment) may refer to the inability to walk from the paralysis. *Restrictions in participation* (handicap) refers to a disadvantage for a given individual, resulting from an impairment and limitation of activity that prevents the fulfillment of a role that is normal (depending on age, gender, and social and cultural factors) for that individual, such as paralyzed and unable to walk and, therefore, unable to return to one's previous work and avocational pursuits.

Several outcome measures are available to measure impairment, activity, and participation, though not all of them are recommended for use in SCI. During the past few years, there have been several expert panels formed to review multiple categories of SCI outcome measures with the goal being to identify the most valid and reliable measures. Detailed reviews and recommendations have been published for physiological functional recovery (106) and participation (107). A summary review and recommendations for all of the categories of SCI outcome measures have been recently published (108).

The most commonly used measures, as well as the most recently recommended, for a comprehensive functional evaluation are summarized below in relation to physiologic function, psychologic function, and participation.

Classification of Impairments and Limitations of Activities

Physiologic Function

The *Modified Barthel Index* evaluates an individual's ability to perform 10 tasks related to self-care, continence, and mobility, with a scale range of 0 to 100 (109). The MBI was not designed specifically for SCI and, as such, has weaknesses. It does not address the easiest and hardest tasks that individuals with SCI may face, such as respiratory management and ground-wheelchair transfers, and it is not sensitive to changes in continence management. The MBI has been shown to have validity and reliability in SCI, with the exception of the bladder and bowel items, but has little clinical utility.

The *Functional Independence Measure* (FIM) was initially developed in 1983 to 1984 to measure functional ability in daily activities and was designed for the *disabled population in general*, not specifically for persons with SCI (110). The FIM is the most widely used functional assessment instrument for disability in the United States and, as such, has been demonstrated to be a valid and reliable instrument for many disabilities. There are concerns, however, regarding its usefulness in SCI (106).

The FIM consists of 18 items (13 motor and 5 cognitive) clustered into six areas: self-care; sphincter control of bladder and bowel; mobility (transfers); locomotion; communication; and social recognition (111,112). Each of these 18 functions is evaluated using a seven-point scale with respect to independence. The scale used assigns to each subscore a value of 1 to 7 that describes the "burden of care" associated with the individual engaging in each activity (1 is the highest burden, 7 the lowest). "Burden of care" refers to the amount of time and or energy that is provided by another person or the use of an assistive device when the individual with a disability engages in each target activity. An assistive device, for example a brace or an adapted telephone, is viewed as adding an additional potential burden of care; that is, if the device were not available, assistance from another person would be needed. The sum of all items represents the total FIM score, ranging from 18 (least independent) to 126 (most independent), which projects the cost of the disability in terms of safety and a person's dependence on others or technological devices, to achieve and maintain a certain quality of life.

The most significant limitation of the FIM in the SCI population is that it lacks sensitivity to change in many areas. The locomotion items are the least sensitive to change, in contrast to the transfer items of the FIM (113–117). Further, the FIM is less sensitive to small gains compared with the QIF (118) in persons with tetraplegia, less sensitive to walking recovery than the Walking Index for Spinal Cord Injury (WISCI) (119), and less sensitive to functional changes in SCI than the SCIM (113,114). It has also been shown that the cognitive domain may be inappropriate for use in SCI (120,121).

There have been significant attempts to utilize the FIM in the SCI population. The FIM was used in NASCIS 3 to attempt to measure functional change (122). In fact, the FIM was added to the Standards in 1992 but was subsequently removed in the 2000 revisions (27). Upon recent review of the entire literature of SCI functional outcome measures, an expert panel has concluded that the FIM is a valid and reliable instrument to measure burden of care only (106). However, it is not suitable for detecting small but functionally significant amounts of change in the SCI population and is not recommended as an outcome measure for clinical trials.

The *Spinal Cord Independence Measure (SCIM-III)* is a scale that was developed specifically for people with SCI in order to evaluate their performance of ADL and to make functional assessments that are sensitive to changes relevant to this population (113). The SCIM scores a task higher when it is accomplished with less assistance, fewer aids, or less medical compromise (123). The SCIM has been modified three times, and the most recent version (123,124) is comprised of 19 items in three subscales, which are (a) self-care (6 items, subscore 0 to 20), (b) respiration and sphincter management (4 items, subscore 0 to 40), and (c) mobility (9 items, subscore 0 to 40). The total score ranges from 0 to 100.

The SCIM has been tested in the traumatic and nontraumatic SCI populations as well as at acute and chronic time points (114). It has been shown to be a valid and reliable measure of overall functional ability specific to SCI (113,123,124). The SCIM has also been shown to be more sensitive to change than the FIM for persons with SCI (113,123,125–127). The majority of work regarding the SCIM has been published by the original creators of the instrument. A consensus was recently published by a panel of experts in the field of functional recovery suggesting that the SCIM was the most appropriate tool for assessing global disability and function in SCI, but it was also recommended that further assessments of the validity, reliability, sensitivity, and utility of the SCIM be performed independent of the creators of the tool (106). A recent multicenter trial in the US found that the SCIM III is a reliable and valid measure of functional change in SCI (128). Recommendations were made to improve scoring instructions and a few modifications to the scoring categories to reduce variability between raters and enhance clinical utility.

Walking Index for Spinal Cord Injury (WISCI): To more precisely measure walking capacity after incomplete SCI, the WISCI was developed for use in clinical studies and then modified to the WISCI II (129). The WISCI II is a 21-point scale that takes into consideration the use of walking aids, braces, and physical assistance during a 10-m walk. A higher score represents less impairment.

Studies have demonstrated that the WISCI has validity and reliability and is sensitive to change (118,128,130,131). It has been recommended by experts in the field that the most comprehensive assessment of ambulation would include evaluations of speed, endurance, and functional capacity and would require the use of a combination of tests, such as the WISCI II and the 10-Meter Walk Test (108).

Quadriplegia Index of Function (QIF): The QIF was developed specifically to detect small, clinically relevant changes in function in individuals with a cervical SCI (132). The QIF consists of 10 categories of function (wheelchair mobility, transfers, bed activities, grooming, bathing, feeding, dressing, bladder program, bowel program, and understanding personal care) with subdivisions within each category. Weights are assigned for each category in the QIF, for a total score, after calculation, up to 100. A shorter form of the QIF has also been developed and tested (133).

The QIF has been shown to be more sensitive to change than the Barthel Index (132) and the FIM (118,134). It has also been demonstrated that there is a stronger correlation between the QIF and the ASIA Upper Extremity Motor Score (UEMS) than between the FIM and the ASIA UEMS (118,134). The QIF has not yet been compared with the SCIM.

The QIF has been shown to be valid and reliable for what it was designed to test (118,132,134). The main limitation of the QIF is that its use is limited to the nonambulatory, tetraplegic population because it only focuses on activities requiring hand function. However, it is recommended that the QIF continue to be developed and tested as an outcome measure specific to the upper extremity.

The *Capabilities of Upper Extremity (CUE) instrument* was designed to measure UE functional limitations in individuals with tetraplegia (135). This instrument is a 32-item questionnaire that assesses the difficulty in performing certain actions with the UE (with one or both hands) including reaching and lifting, pulling and pushing, wrist, hand and finger, and bilateral actions. It was found to be able to distinguish between different levels of tetraplegia more than one level apart and was correlated with ASIA motor scores and the FIM. Few studies have published results utilizing the CUE since its inception, and further work is needed to determine its sensitivity to change in function.

The *Canadian Occupational Performance Measure (COPM)* is a client-centered outcome tool. It was designed for occupational therapists to use to assess client-identified problems in the areas of self-care, productivity, and leisure (136). It is administered as a semistructured interview that follows a five-step process to identify individual problems. Two scores are generated, one for performance and one for satisfaction with performance. The COPM can be used to identify longitudinal changes in performance on self-selected problems and to capture the degree of satisfaction associated with those changes. There have been studies demonstrating sensitivity to change (137), reliability (138), validity (139–141), and clinical utility (142). There have also been studies utilizing the COPM as an outcome measure for the SCI population (143–146). Overall, there is growing use of the COPM in clinical practice and in research across multiple disabilities. Though not specifically designed for SCI, the COPM could potentially be utilized as a powerful outcome tool in clinical trials in an effort to measure subject satisfaction with therapeutic interventions.

Graded and Redefined Assessment of Strength, Sensibility, and Prehension (GRASSP): Likely to become the most comprehensive functional assessment tool for the arm and hand, the GRASSP is being developed as a clinical research tool that is responsive to change and would track the extent of spontaneous recovery or possible outcomes of a surgical or pharmacological intervention in a clinical trial (108). The GRASSP evaluates changes within the motor and sensory systems, as well as qualitative and quantitative components of prehension to relate impairment level changes to complex hand function tasks (147). The GRASSP is currently undergoing international reliability and validity testing.

Benzel Classification: Benzel et al. (148) described a slightly more detailed classification than the AIS, in which functional motor individuals (Frankel D) were divided into three categories. Categories include the inability to independently walk, walking limited to 25 ft, and unlimited walking. There are a total of seven, rather than five categories. While utilized in the Sygen trial (149), this scale has otherwise not been widely used.

PSYCHOLOGICAL FUNCTION

Quality of Life

A recent review of health-related quality-of-life (QoL) outcome measures was conducted by a group of clinicians and rehabilitation psychologists (108). They defined QoL for SCI as a "multidimensional construct that includes physical functioning, functional ability, emotional functioning, and satisfaction with life" and recommended the scales discussed below.

Short Form–36/Short Form–12 (SF-36/SF-12): The SF-36/SF-12 measures are the most widely used and reflect both health status, including physical functioning, physical and emotional role limitations, bodily pain, general health, vitality, social functioning, and mental health. However, the SF-36/SF-12 measures were developed for the nondisabled (150) and do not account for SCI-related physical limitations. There are concerns regarding their validity that remain to be addressed as well as modifications regarding wording and weighting of items.

Sickness Impact Profile (SIP-68): The original SIP was developed as a measure of general health–related functional status (151). The shortened SIP-68 consists of 68 items in six subscales (somatic autonomy, mobility control, psychologic autonomy and communication, emotional stability, mobility range, and social behavior). Multiple studies have demonstrated the SIP-68 to be a valid and reliable questionnaire, but there are concerns regarding sensitivity to changes in health status and potential ceiling effects in the mental subscales.

The *Satisfaction with Life Scale (SWLS)* is a measure of life satisfaction as a cognitive judgmental process (152). There are five items, each scored from 1 (strongly disagree) to 7 (strongly agree). There are multiple reliability and validity studies in the SCI population with normative data from Model SCI Systems. One negative attribute of the SLWS is that it taps into only one domain within the health related QoL framework.

Several instruments are currently in development but deserve mention. The Patient Reported Outcomes Measurement Information System (PROMIS), the Neuro-QoL, and the related SCI-QoL instruments are in development, using a grounded theory approach to guide their development and large-scale field testing. Plans are to develop these measures using computerized adaptive technology as they cover issues relevant to individuals with SCI.

Classification of Restrictions on Participation

Participation

Participation is defined by the WHO as "involvement in life situations" (105). An evidence-based review of participation outcome measures relevant for use in clinical practice and research involving SCI was recently conducted (107), and the recommended tools are summarized below.

Craig Handicap Assessment and Reporting Technique (CHART): The CHART is the most widely used instrument and it assesses 32 items in six WHO domains of handicap, including physical independence, cognitive independence, mobility, occupation, social integration, and economic self-sufficiency (153). There are a significant amount of validity and reliability data available regarding the use of the CHART in SCI populations (107). There are two limitations of the CHART, however. One, it was developed prior to the establishment of the WHO ICF concept of participation. Thus, it was based on the previous WHO concept of handicap. However, it has been shown to correlate with the ICF participation codes (154). Two, the CHART is a quantitative measure of an individual's performance of normative life roles. It does not assess an individual's satisfaction or subjective assessment of life roles nor does it include an individual's personal preferences.

Assessment of Life Habits (LIFE-H): The LIFE-H is also based on societal norms of participation, like the CHART, but it is a more qualitative measure. It is based on the Disability Creation Process (DCP) definition of participation, which takes into account the interaction between personal and environmental factors (155). The LIFE-H is made up of 240 items across 12 domains (nutrition, fitness, personal care, communication, housing, mobility, responsibility, interpersonal relation, community, education, employment, recreation). It has been demonstrated to have validity and reliability in the SCI population (156); however, it is not widely used. It is thought that the reasons underlying its lack of use are that the DCP conceptual framework is not widely known and that it is somewhat burdensome to administer due to its length (107).

Impact on Participation and Autonomy (IPA): The IPA is different from the CHART and LIFE-H in that it measures participation as well as choice in decision making from the perspective of the individual (157). It is comprised of 32 items spanning five domains (autonomy indoors, autonomy outdoors, family role, social relations, paid work and education). It also takes into account how problematic the restrictions on participation are for the individual (158). The IPA is a newer outcome measure; thus, there are few validation studies available for the SCI population (159,160).

Four other promising measures of participation are recommended to be monitored for their applicability to SCI (107), and those are the Participation Measure for Post-Acute Care (PM-PAC) (161), the Participation Survey/Mobility (PARTS/M) (162), the PAR-PRO (163), and Community Participation Indicators (CPI) (164).

References

1. American Spinal Injury Association: International Standards for Neurological Classification of Spinal Cord Injury. Revised 2011. Atlanta, GA.
2. Waring WP, Biering-Sorenson F, Burns S, et al. 2009 review and revisions of the International Standards for neurological classification of spinal cord injury. *J Spinal Cord Med* 2010;33(4):346–352.
3. American Spinal Injury Association. *Reference manual for the International standards for neurological classification of spinal cord injury*. Chicago, IL: American Spinal Injury Association, 2003.
4. Austin GM. *The spinal cord: basic aspects and surgical consideration*. 2nd ed. Springfield, IL: Thomas, 1972:762.
5. Vogel LC, Vogel L, Samdani A, et al. Intra-rater agreement of the anorectal exam and classification of injury severity in children with spinal cord injury. *Spinal Cord* 2009;47(9):687–691.
6. Daniels L, Worthingham C. *Muscle testing techniques of manual examination*. 5th ed. Philadelphia, PA: WB Sanders, 1986.
7. Hinderer KA, Hinderer SR. Muscle strength development and assessment in children and adolescents. In: Ringdal K, ed. *International perspectives in physical therapy: vol on muscle strength*. Edinburgh, UK: Churchill Livingstone, 1992:20.
8. Ditunno JF, Graziani V, Tessler A. Neurological assessment in spinal cord injury. *Adv Neurol* 1997;72:325–333.
9. Michaelis LS. International inquiry on neurological terminology and prognosis in paraplegia and tetraplegia. *Paraplegia* 1969;7:1–5.
10. Cheshire DJE. A classification of the functional end-results of injury to the cervical spinal cord. *Paraplegia* 1970;8:70–73.
11. Maroon JC, Alba AA. Classification of acute spinal cord injury, neurological evaluation, and neurosurgical considerations. *Crit Care Clin* 1987;3:655–677.
12. Allen BL, Ferguson RL, Lehman TR, et al. A mechanistic classification of the lower cervical spine. *Spine* 1982;7:1–27.
13. Bracken MB, Webb SB, Wagner FC. Classification of the severity of acute spinal cord injury: implications for management. *Paraplegia* 1977–78;15:319–326.
14. Roaf R. International classification of spinal injuries. *Paraplegia* 1972;10:78–84.
15. Chehrazi B, Wagner FC, Collins WF, et al. A scale for evaluation of spinal cord injury. *J Neurosurg* 1981;54:310–315.
16. Jochheim KA. Problems of classification in traumatic paraplegia and tetraplegia. *Paraplegia* 1970;8:80–82.
17. Kirshblum SC, Donovan W. Neurological assessment and classification of traumatic spinal cord injury. In: Kirshblum SC, Campagnolo D, DeLisa JE, eds. *Spinal cord medicine*. Philadelphia, PA: Lippincott/Williams and Wilkins, 2002:82–95.
18. Frankel HL, Hancock DO, Hyslop G, et al. The value of postural reduction in initial management of closed injuries of the spine with paraplegia and tetraplegia. *Paraplegia* 1969–70;7:179–192.
19. American Spinal Injury Association. *Standard for neurological classification of spinal injured patients*. Chicago, IL: ASIA, 1982.
20. Lucas JT, Ducker TB. Motor classification of spinal cord injuries with mobility, morbidity and recovery indices. *Am J Surg* 1979;45:151–158.
21. Bracken MB, Hildreth N, Freeman DH, et al. Relationship between neurological and functional status after acute spinal cord injury: an epidemiological study. *J Chronic Dis* 1980;33:115–125.
22. Bracken MB, Collins WF, Freeman DF, et al. Efficacy of methylprednisolone in acute spinal cord injury. *JAMA* 1984;251:45–52.
23. Bracken MB, Shephard MJ, Collins WF, et al. A randomized controlled trial of methylprednisolone or naloxone in the treatment of acute spinal cord injury: results of the second national acute spinal cord injury study. *N Engl J Med* 1990;332:1405–1411.
24. El Masry WS, Tsubo M, Katoh S, et al. Validation of the American spinal injury association (ASIA) motor score and the national acute spinal cord injury study (NASCIS) motor score. *Spine* 1996;21:614–619.
25. American Spinal Injury Association/International Medical Society of Paraplegia (ASIA/IMSOP).*International standards for neurological and functional classification of spinal cord injury patients (revised)*. Chicago, IL: American Spinal Injury Association, 1992.
26. American Spinal Injury Association/International Medical Society of Paraplegia. *International standards for neurological and functional classification of spinal cord injury patients*. Chicago, IL. 1996.
27. American Spinal Injury Association/International Medical Society of Paraplegia. *International standards for neurological classification of spinal cord injury patients*. Chicago, IL. 2000
28. Marino RJ, Rider-Foster D, Maissel G, et al. Superiority of motor level over single neurological level in categorizing patients. *Paraplegia* 1995;33:510–513.

29. Waters RL, Adkins R, Yakura J, et al. Motor and sensory recovery following complete tetraplegia. *Arch Phys Med Rehabil* 1993;74:242–247.
30. Waters RL, Adkins RH, Yakura JS. Definition of complete spinal cord injury. *Paraplegia* 1991;29:573–581.
31. Chafetz RS, Prak S, Mulcahey MJ. Computerized classification of neurologic injury based on the international standards for classification of spinal cord injury. *J Spinal Cord Med* 2009;32:532–537.
32. Cohen ME, Bartko JJ. Reliability of the ISCSCI-92. In: Ditunno JF, Donovan WH, Maynard FM, eds. *Reference manual for the international standards for neurological and functional classification of spinal cord injury*. Chicago, IL: ASIA, 1994:59–66.
33. Marino RJ, Jones L, Kirshblum S, et al. Reliability and repeatability of the motor and sensory examination of the international standards for neurological classification of spinal cord injury. *J Spinal Cord Med* 2008;31: 166–170.
34. Jonnson M, Tolback A, Gonzalez H, et al. Inter-rater reliability of the 1992 international standards for neurological and functional classification of incomplete spinal cord injury. *Spinal Cord* 2000;38:675–679.
35. Savic G, Bergstom EM, Frankel HL, et al. Inter-rater reliability of motor and sensory examinations performed according to American Spinal Injury Association standards. *Spinal Cord* 2007;45:444–451.
36. Marino RJ. Neurological and functional outcomes in spinal cord injury: review and recommendations. *Top Spinal Cord Inj Rehabil* 2005;10:51–64.
37. Mulcahey MJ, Gaughan J, Betz RR, et al. The International standards for neurological classification of spinal cord injury: reliability of data when applied to children and youths. *Spinal Cord* 2007;45:452–459.
38. Chafetz RS, Gaughan JP, Vogel LC, et al. The International Standards for Neurological Classification of Spinal Cord Injury: Intra-rater agreement of total motor and sensory scores in the pediatric population. *J Spinal Cord Med* 2009;32:157–161.
39. Bing R. *Compendium of regional diagnosis in affection of the brain and spinal cord*. 2nd ed. New York, NY: Rebman CO, 1921.
40. Schneider RC, Cherry GR, Patek H. Syndrome of acute central cervical spinal cord injury with special reference to mechanisms involved in hyper-extension injuries of cervical spine. *J Neurosurg* 1954;11:546–577.
41. Quencer RM, Bunge RP, Egnor M, et al. Acute traumatic central cord syndrome: MRI pathological correlations. *Neuroradiology* 1992;34:85–94.
42. Bunge RP, Puckett WR, Becerra JL, et al. Observation on the pathology of human spinal cord injury: a review and classification of 22 new cases with details from a case of chronic cord compression with extensive focal demyelination. *Adv Neurol* 1993;59:75–89.
43. Kakulas BA, Bedbrook GM. Pathology of injuries of the vertebral column. In: Vinken PJ, Bruyn GW, eds. *Handbook of clinical neurology*. Vol 25. Amsterdam, The Netherlands: N. Holland Pub Co., 1976:27–42.
44. Taylor AR. The mechanism of injury to the spinal cord in the neck without damage to the vertebral column. *J Bone Joint Surg Br* 1951;33-B:543–547.
45. Mckinley W, Santos K, Meade M, et al. Incidence and outcomes of spinal cord injury clinical syndromes. *J Spinal Cord Med* 2007;30:215–224.
46. Levi AD, Tator CH, Bunge RP. Clinical syndromes associated with disproportionate weakness of the upper versus the lower extremities after cervical spinal cord injury. *Neurosurgery* 1996;38:170–185.
47. Pouw MH, van Middlendorp JJ, van Kempen A, et al. Diagnostic criteria of traumatic central cord syndrome. Part 1. A systematic review of clinical descriptors and scores. *Spinal Cord* 2010;48:652–656.
48. Van Middendorp JJ, Pouw MH, Hayes LCC, et al. Diagnostic criteria of traumatic central cord syndrome. Part 2. A questionnaire survey among spine specialists. *Spinal Cord* 2010;48:657–663.
49. Merriam WF, Taylor TKF, Ruff SJ, et al. A reappraisal of acute traumatic central cord syndrome. *J Bone Joint Surg Br* 1986;68:708–713.
50. Penrod LE, Hegde SK, Ditunno JF. Age effect on prognosis for functional recovery in acute, traumatic central cord syndrome. *Arch Phys Med Rehabil* 1990;71:963–968.
51. Roth EJ, Lawler MH, Yarkony GM. Traumatic central cord syndrome: clinical features and functional outcomes. *Arch Phys Med Rehabil* 1990;71:18–23.
52. Burns SP, Golding DG, Rolle WA, et al. Recovery of ambulation in motor incomplete tetraplegia. *Arch Phys Med Rehabil* 1997;78:1169–1172.
53. Bell HS. Paralysis of both arms from injury of the upper portion of the pyramidal decussation with "cruciate paralysis". *J Neurosurg* 1970;33:376–380.
54. Dickmen CA, Hadley MN, Pappas CTE, et al. Cruciate paralysis: a clinical and radiographic analysis of injuries to the cervicomedullary junction. *J Neurosurg* 1990;73:850–858.
55. Erlich V, Snow R, Heier L. Confirmation by magnetic resonance imaging of Bells' cruciate paralysis in a young child with Chiari type I malformation and minor head trauma. *Neurosurgery* 1989;25:102–105.
56. Marano SR, Calica AB, Sonntag VKH. Bilateral upper extremity paralysis (Bells Cruciate Paralysis) from a gunshot wound to the cervicomedullary junction. *Neurosurgery* 1986;18:642–644.
57. Schneider RC, Crosby EC, Russo RH, et al. Traumatic spinal cord syndromes and their management. *Clin Neurosurg* 1973;20:424–492.
58. Hatzakis M, Bryce N, Marino R. Case report: cruciate paralysis, hypothesis for injury and recovery. *Spinal Cord* 2000;38:120–125.
59. Wallenberg A. Anatomischer Befund in einem als "acute bulbaraffection (embolie der cerebellar post inf sinista?)" beschreiben falle. *Arch Phychiatr* 1901;34:923–959.
60. Pappas CTE, Gibson AR, Sonntag VKH. Decussation of hind-limb and fore-limb fibers in monkey corticospinal tract: relevance to cruciate paralysis. *J Neurosurg* 1991;75:935–940.
61. Kowalske KJ, Herbison GJ, Ditunno JF, et al. Spinal cord injury syndrome with motor sparing in the absence of all sensation. *Arch Phys Med Rehabil* 1991;72:932–934.
62. Bohlman HH. Acute fractures and dislocations of the cervical spine. An analysis of three hundred hospitalized patients and review of the literature. *J Bone Joint Surg* 1979;61A:1119–1142.

63. Bosch A, Stauffer ES, Nickel VL. Incomplete traumatic quadriplegia—a ten year review. *JAMA* 1971;216:473–478.
64. Brown-Sequard CE. Lectures on the physiology and pathology of the central nervous system and the treatment of organic nervous affections. *Lancet* 1868;2:593–595, 659–662, 755–757, 821–823.
65. Roth EJ, Park T, Pang T, et al. Traumatic cervical Brown-Sequard and Brown-Sequard plus syndromes: the spectrum of presentations and outcomes. *Paraplegia* 1991;29:582–589.
66. Tattersall R, Turner B. Brown-Sequard and his syndrome. *Lancet* 2000;356:61–63.
67. Koehler PJ, Endtz LJ. The Brown Sequard syndrome—true or false? *Arch Neurol* 1986;43:921–924.
68. Graziani V, Tessler A, Ditunno JF. Incomplete tetraplegia: sequence of lower extremity motor recovery. *J Neurotrauma* 1995;12:121.
69. Little JW, Halar E. Temporal course of motor recovery after Brown-Sequard spinal cord injuries. *Paraplegia* 1985;23:39–46.
70. Bauer RD, Errico TJ. Cervical spine injuries. In: Errico TJ, Bauer RD, Waugh T, eds. *Spinal trauma*. Philadelphia, PA: JB Lippencott, 1991:71–121.
71. Cheshire WP, Santos CC, Massey EW, et al. Spinal cord infarction: etiology and outcome. *Neurology* 1996;47:321–330.
72. Bohlman HH, Ducker TB. Spine and spinal cord injuries. In: Rothman RH, ed. *The spine*. 3rd ed. Philadelphia, PA: WB Saunders, 1992:973–1011.
73. Dimitrijevic MR. Neurophysiology in spinal cord injury. *Paraplegia* 1987;25:205–208.
74. Sherwood AM, Dimitrijevic MR, Mckay WB. Evidence of subclinical brain influence in clinically complete spinal cord injury: discomplete SCI. *J Neurol Sci* 1992;110: 90–98.
75. Bunge RP, Puckett WR, Becrerra JL, et al. Observations on the pathology of human spinal cord injury. A review and classification of 22 new cases with details from a case of chronic cord compression with extensive focal demyelination. *Adv Neurol* 1993;59:75–89.
76. Dimitrijevic MR, Dimitrijevic MM, Faganel J, et al. Suprasegmentally induced motor unit activity in paralyzed muscles of patients with established spinal cord injury. *Ann Neurol* 1984;16:216–621.
77. Kakulas BA. The applied neuropathology of human spinal cord injury. *Spinal Cord* 1999;37:79–88.
78. Sabbah P, Leveque C, Pfefer F, et al. Functional MR imaging and traumatic paraplegia: preliminary report. *J Neuroradiol* 2000;27:233–237.
79. Finnerup NB, Glydensted C, Fuglsang-Fredrickson A, et al. Sensory perception in complete spinal cord injury. *Acta Neurol Scan* 2004;109:194–199.
80. Krassioukov A, Claydon VE. The clinical problems in cardiovascular control following spinal cord injury: an overview. *Prog Brain Res* 2006;152:223–229.
81. Mathias CJ, Frankel HL. Autonomic disturbances in spinal cord lesions. In: Bannister R, Mathias CJ, eds. *Autonomic failure, a textbook of clinical disorders of the autonomic nervous system*. Oxford Medical Publications, 2002:839–881.
82. Alexander MS, Biering-Sorensen F, Bodner D, et al. International standards to document remaining autonomic function after spinal cord injury. *Spinal Cord* 2008.
83. Low PA. Testing the autonomic nervous system. *Semin Neurol* 2003;23:407–421.
84. Krassioukov AV, Weaver LC. Physical medicine and rehabilitation: state of the art reviews. In: Teasell R, Baskerville VB, eds. *Anatomy of the autonomic nervous system*. Philadelphia, PA: Hanley & Belfus, Inc., Medical Publishers, 1996:1–14.
85. Lefkowitz RJ, Hoffman BB, Taylor P. Neurohumoral transmission: the autonomic and somatic motor nervous system. In: Gilman AG, Rall TW, Nies AS, et al., eds. The pharmacological basis of therapeutics. New York, NY: Pergamon Press, 2007:84–121.
86. Furlan JC, Fehlings MG, Shannon P, et al. Descending vasomotor pathways in humans: correlation between axonal preservation and cardiovascular dysfunction after spinal cord injury. *J Neurotrauma* 2003;20:1351–1363.
87. Consensus statement on the definition of orthostatic hypotension, pure autonomic failure, and multiple system atrophy. The Consensus Committee of the American Autonomic Society and the American Academy of Neurology. *Neurol* 1996;46:1470.
88. Claydon VE, Steeves JD, Krassioukov A. Orthostatic hypotension following spinal cord injury: understanding clinical pathophysiology. *Spinal Cord* 2006;44: 341–351.
89. Cariga P, Ahmed S, Mathias CJ, et al. The prevalence and association of neck (coat-hanger) pain and orthostatic (postural) hypotension in human spinal cord injury. *Spinal Cord* 2002;40:77–82.
90. Kirshblum SC, House JG, O'connor KC. Silent autonomic dysreflexia during a routine bowel program in persons with traumatic spinal cord injury: a preliminary study. *Arch Phys Med Rehabil* 2002;83:1774–1776.
91. Linsenmeyer TA, Campagnolo DI, Chou IH. Silent autonomic dysreflexia during voiding in men with spinal cord injuries. *J Urol* 1996;155:519–522.
92. Ekland MB, Krassioukov AV, McBride KE, et al. Incidence of autonomic dysreflexia and silent autonomic dysreflexia in men with spinal cord injury undergoing sperm retrieval: implications for clinical practice. *J Spinal Cord Med* 2008;31:33–39.
93. Krassioukov AV, Karlsson AK, Wecht JM, et al. Assessment of autonomic dysfunction following spinal cord injury: rationale for additions to the International Standards for Neurological Assessment. *J Rehabil Res Dev* 2007;44:103–112.
94. Head H, Riddoch G. The automatic bladder, excessive sweating and some other reflex conditions in gross injuries of the spinal cord. *Brain* 1917;40:188–263.
95. Colachis SC, Otis SM. Occurrence of fever associated with thermoregulatory dysfunction after acute traumatic spinal-cord injury. *Am J Phys Med Rehabil* 1995;74:114–119.
96. Schmidt KD, Chan CW. Thermoregulation and fever in normal persons and in those with spinal-cord injuries. *Mayo Clin Proc* 1992;67:469–475.
97. Khan S, Plummer M, Martinez-Arizala A, et al. *J Spinal Cord Med* 2007;30:27–30.

98. Krassioukov AV, Karlsson AK, Wecht JM, et al. *J Rehabil Res Dev* 2007;44:103–112.
99. Linn WS, Spungen AM, Gong H, et al. Forced vital capacity in two large outpatient populations with chronic spinal cord injury. *Spinal Cord* 2001;39:263–268.
100. Schilero GJ, Grimm DR, Bauman WA, et al. Assessment of airway caliber and bronchodilator responsiveness in subjects with spinal cord injury. *Chest* 2005;127:149–155.
101. Biering-Sorensen F, Craggs M, Kennelly M, et al. International lower urinary tract function basic spinal cord injury data set. *Spinal Cord* 2008;46:325–330.
102. Biering-Sorensen F, Craggs M, Kennelly M, et al. International urodynamic basic spinal cord injury data set. *Spinal Cord* 2008;46(7):513–516.
103. Abrams P, Cardozo L, Fall M, et al. The standardization of terminology of lower urinary tract function: report from the International Standardisation Sub-committee Continence Society. *Neurourol Urodyn* 2002;21:167–178.
104. DeVivo M, Biering-Sorensen F, Charlifue S, et al. International spinal cord injury core data set. *Spinal Cord* 2006;44:535–540.
105. Biering-Sorensen F, Charlifue S, DeVivo M, et al. International spinal cord injury data sets. *Spinal Cord* 2006;44:530–534.
106. World Health Organization. *International classification of functioning, disability, and health*. Geneva, Switzerland: World Health Organization, 2001.
107. Anderson K, Aito S, Atkins M, et al. Functional recovery measures for spinal cord injury: comparison by a multi-national work group. *J Spinal Cord* Med 2008;31: 133–144.
108. Magasi SR, Heinemann AW, Whiteneck GG; Quality of Life/Participation Committee. Participation following traumatic spinal cord injury: an evidence-based review for research. *J Spinal Cord Med* 2008;31(2):145–156.
109. Alexander MS, Biering-Sorensen F, Bodner D, et al. International standards to document remaining autonomic function after spinal cord injury. *Spinal Cord* 2009;47(1):36–43.
110. Shah S, Vanclay F, Cooper B. Predicting discharge status at commencement of stroke rehabilitation. *Stroke* 1989(20):766–769.
111. Hamilton BB, Granger CV, Sherwin FS. A uniform national data system for medical rehabilitation. In: MJ Fuhrer, ed. *Rehabilitation outcomes: analysis and measurement*. Baltimore, MD: Brooks, 1987:137—147.
112. Functional Independence Measure. In: Ditunno JF, Donovan WH, Maynard FM, eds. *Reference manual for the International standards for neurological and functional classification of spinal cord injury*. Chicago, IL: ASIA, 1994:53–57.
113. *Guide for the uniform data set for medical rehabilitation (adult FIM) Version 5.1*. Buffalo, NY: State University of New York at Buffalo, 1997.
114. Catz A, Itzkovich M, Agranov E, et al. SCIM—spinal cord independence measure: a new disability scale for patients with spinal cord lesions. *Spinal Cord* 1997(35):850–856.
115. Catz A, Itzkovich M, Agranov E, et al. The spinal cord independence measure (SCIM): sensitivity to functional changes in subgroups of spinal cord lesion patients. *Spinal Cord* 2001(39):97–100.
116. Dodds TA, Martin DP, Stolov WC, et al. A validation of the functional independence measurement and its performance among rehabilitation inpatients. *Arch Phys Med Rehabil* 1993(74):531–536.
117. Middleton JW, Truman G, Geraghty TJ. Neurological level effect on the discharge functional status of spinal cord injured persons after rehabilitation. *Arch Phys Med Rehabil* 1998(79):1428–1432.
118. Middleton JW, Harvey LA, Batty J, et al. Five additional mobility and locomotor items to improve responsiveness of the FIM in wheelchair-dependent individuals with spinal cord injury. *Spinal Cord* 2006(44):495–504.
119. Yavuz N, Tezyurek M, Akyuz M. A comparison of two functional tests in quadriplegia: the Quadriplegia index of function and the functional independence measure. *Spinal Cord* 1998(36):832–837.
120. Morganti B, Scivoletto G, Ditunno P, et al. Walking index for spinal cord injury (WISCI): criterion validation. *Spinal Cord* 2005(43):27–33.
121. Ditunno JF, Cohen ME, Formal CS, et al. Functional outcomes in spinal cord injury. In: Stover SL, DeLisa J, Whiteneck GG, eds. *Spinal cord injury: clinical outcomes from the model system*. Gaithersburg, MD: Aspen, 1995:170–184.
122. Hall KM, Werner P. Characteristics of the functional independence measure in traumatic spinal cord injury. *Arch Phys Med Rehabil* 1999;80:1471–1476.
123. Bracken MB, Shephard MJ, Holford TR, et al. Administration of methylprednisolone for 24 or 48 hours or tirilazad mesylate for 48 hours in the treatment of acute spinal cord injury: results of the third national acute spinal cord injury randomized controlled trial. *JAMA* 1997;277:1597–1604.
124. Catz A, Itzkovich M, Tesio L, et al. A multi-center International study on the spinal cord independence measure, version III: Rasch psychometric validation. *Spinal Cord* 2007(45):275–291.
125. Itzkovich M, Gelernter I, Biering-Sorensen F, et al. The spinal cord independence measure (SCIM) version III: reliability and validity in a multi-center international study. *Disabil Rehabil* 2007;29(24):1926–1933.
126. Catz A, Greenberg E, Itzkovich M, et al. A new instrument for outcome assessment in rehabilitation medicine: spinal cord injury ability realization measurement index. *Arch Phys Med Rehabil* 2004(85):399–404.
127. Grijalva I, Guizar-Sahagun G, Castaneda-Hernandez G, et al. Efficacy and safety of 4-aminopyridine in patients with long-term spinal cord injury: a randomized, double-blind, placebo-controlled trial. *Pharmacotherapy* 2003(23):823–834.
128. Anderson KD, Acuff ME, Arp BG, et al. United States (US) multi-center study to assess the validity and reliability of the Spinal Cord Independence Measure (SCIM III). *Spinal Cord*. 2011;49(8):880–5.
129. Ditunno JF, Ditunno PL, Graziani V, et al. Walking index for spinal cord injury (WISCI): an international multicenter validity and reliability study. *Spinal Cord* 2000;38:234–243.
130. Dittuno PL, Dittuno JF Jr. Walking index for spinal cord injury (WISCI II): scale revision. *Spinal Cord* 2001;39(12):654–656.
131. Kim MO, Burns AS, Ditunno JF Jr, et al. The assessment of walking capacity using the walking index for spinal

cord injury: self-selected versus maximal levels. *Arch Phys Med Rehabil* 2007;88:762–767.

132. JF Ditunno, G Scivoletto, M Patrick, et al. Validation of the walking index for spinal cord injury in a US and European clinical population. *Spinal Cord* 2008;46:181–188.
133. Gresham GE, Labi MLC, Dittmar SS, et al. The quadriplegia index of function (QIF): sensitivity and reliability demonstrated in a study of thirty quadriplegic patients. *Paraplegia* 1986;24:38–44.
134. Marino RJ, Goin JE. Development of a short form quadriplegia index of function scale. *Spinal Cord* 1999;37:289–296.
135. Marino RJ, Huang M, Knight P, et al. Assessing self care status in quadriplegia: comparison of the quadriplegia index of function (QIF) and the functional independence measure (FIM). *Paraplegia* 1993;31:225–233.
136. Marino RJ, Shea JA, Steinman MG. The capabilities of upper extremity instrument: reliability and validity of a measure of functional limitation in tetraplegia. *Arch Phys Med Rehabil* 1998;79:1512–1521.
137. Law M, Baptiste S, McColl M, et al. The Canadian occupational performance measure: an outcome measure for occupational therapy. *Can J Occup Ther* 1990;57:82–87.
138. Law M, Polatajko H, Pollock N, et al. Pilot testing of the Canadian occupational performance measure: clinical and measurement issues. *Can J Occup Ther* 1994;6:191–197.
139. Eyssen IC, Beelen A, Dedding C, et al. The reproducibility of the Canadian occupational performance measure. *Clin Rehabil* 2005;19:888–894.
140. McColl MA, Paterson M, Davies D, et al. Validity and community utility of the Canadian occupational performance measure. *Can J Occup Ther* 2000;67:22–30.
141. Ripat J, Etcheverry E, Cooper J, . A comparison of the Canadian Occupational Performance Measure and the Health Assessment Questionnaire. *Can J Occup Ther* 2001;68:247–253.
142. Dedding C, Cardol M, Eyssen IC, et al. Validity of the Canadian occupational performance measure: a client-centred outcome measurement. *Clin Rehabil* 2004;18:660–667.
143. Toomey M, Nicholson D, Carswell A. The clinical utility of the Canadian occupational performance measure. *Can J Occup Ther* 1995;62:242–249.
144. Mulcahey MJ, Betz RR, Kozin SH, et al. Implantation of the freehand system during initial rehabilitation using minimally invasive techniques. *Spinal Cord* 2004;42:146–155.
145. Mulcahey MJ, Lutz C, Kozin SH, et al. Prospective evaluation of biceps to triceps and deltoid to triceps for elbow extension in tetraplegia. *J Hand Surg [Am]*. 2003;28:964–971.
146. Samuelsson KA, Tropp H, Gerdle B. Shoulder pain and its consequences in paraplegic spinal cord-injured, wheelchair users. *Spinal Cord* 2004;42:41–46.
147. Effing TW, van Meeteren NL, van Asbeck FW, et al. Body weight-supported treadmill training in chronic incomplete spinal cord injury: a pilot study evaluating functional health status and quality of life. *Spinal Cord* 2006;44:287–296.
148. Kalsi-Ryan S. Quantification, sensitivity and reliability for the sensory module of the graded and redefined assessment of sensibility strength and prehension (GRASSP) hand measure. ASIA Annual Meeting June 2007 (poster presentation), Tampa Bay, FL.
149. Benzel EC, Larson SJ. Functional recovery after decompressive spine operation for cervical spine fractures. *Neurosurgery* 1987;20:742–746.
150. Geisler FH, Coleman WP, Greico G, et al.; Sygen Study Group. The Sygen multicenter acute spinal cord injury study. *Spine* 2001;26(24 Suppl):S87–S98.
151. Ware JE, Sherbourne CD. The MOS 36 item short form health survey (SF-36). I. Conceptual framework and item selection. *Med Care* 1992;30:473–483.
152. Bergner M, Bobbitt RA, Carter WB, et al. The sickness impact profile: development and final revision of a health status measure. *Med Care* 1981;19:787–805.
153. Diener E, Emmons RA, Larsen RJ, et al. The satisfaction with life scale. *J Pers Assess* 1985;49:71–75.
154. Whiteneck GG, Charlifue SW, Gerhart KA, et al. Quantifying handicap: a new measure of long-term rehabilitation outcomes. *Arch Phys Med Rehabil* 1992;73:519–526.
155. Perenboom RJ, Chorus AM. Measuring participation according to the International classification of functioning, disability, and health (ICF). *Disabil Rehabil* 2003;25:577–587.
156. Fougeyrollas P, Noreau L, Bergeron H, et al. Social consequences of long-term impairments and disabilities: conceptual approach and assessment of handicap. *Int J Rehabil Res* 1998;21:127–141.
157. Dumont C, Bertrand R, Fougeyrollas P, et al. Rasch modeling and the measurement of social participation. *J Appl Meas* 2003;4:309–325.
158. Cardol M, de Haan RJ, van den Bos GAM, et al. The development of a handicap assessment questionnaire: the impact on participation and autonomy (IPA). *Clin Rehabil* 1999;13:411–419.
159. Cardol M, de Haan RJ, de Jong BA, et al. Psychometric properties of the impact on participation and autonomy questionnaire. *Arch Phys Med Rehabil* 2001;82: 210–216.
160. Larsson Lund M, Nordlund A, Nygård L, et al. Perceptions of participation and predictors of perceived problems with participation in persons with spinal cord injury. *J Rehabil Med* 2005;37:3–8.
161. Lund ML, Fisher AG, Lexell J, et al. Impact on participation and autonomy questionnaire: internal scale validity of the Swedish version for use in people with spinal cord injury. *J Rehabil Med* 2007;39:156–162.
162. Gandek B, Sinclair SJ, Jette AM, et al. Development and initial psychometric evaluation of the participation measure for post-acute ace (PM-PAC). *Am J Phys Med Rehabil* 2007;86:57–71.
163. Gray DB, Hollinsworth HH, Stark SL, et al. Participation survey/mobility: psychometric properties of a measure of participation for people with mobility impairments and limitations. *Arch Phys Med Rehabil* 2006;87:189–197.
164. Ostir GV, Granger CV, Black T, et al. Preliminary results for the PRO-PAR: a measure of home and community participation. *Arch Phys Med Rehabil* 2006;87:1043–1051.
165. Hammel J, Magasi S, Heinemann A, et al. What does participation mean? An insider perspective from people with disabilities. *Disabil Rehabil* 2008;30(19): 1445–1460.

CHAPTER 7 ■ ACUTE MEDICAL AND SURGICAL MANAGEMENT OF SPINAL CORD INJURY

ROBERT F. HEARY, ALEXANDROS D. ZOUZIAS, AND DENISE I. CAMPAGNOLO

Traumatic spinal cord injury (SCI) is a complex, multifactorial process with an estimated incidence of approximately 12,000 new cases per year in the United States alone (1). The initial management of new-onset SCI can mean the difference between functional recovery and lifelong dependence. While the inciting trauma causes unavoidable direct mechanical damage to neuronal elements, further injury is now known to occur as a result of an intricate pathophysiologic cascade. Reducing or eliminating the severity of this secondary insult has emerged as a potential goal in early treatment. Accordingly, the most critical concepts in the evolving SCI paradigm remain early recognition of injury, immediate in-field stabilization, aggressive and timely resuscitation, and avoidance of further deterioration via medical complications or improper handling. Once stabilized, a subgroup of SCI patients may benefit from early decompression of the neuronal elements, although this remains heavily debated (2,3). This chapter covers the principles of prehospital management, immediate emergency department (ED) evaluation and care, radiographic appraisal, and biomechanical stabilization. In addition, potential surgical strategies and new technical developments in spinal surgery are briefly discussed.

INITIAL FIELD ASSESSMENT/ PREHOSPITAL CARE

The most common causes of traumatic SCI, in descending order of frequency, are as follows: motor vehicle crashes (MVC), falls, violence, and sports injuries. In younger SCI patients, accidents and sports injuries (most commonly diving) account for the majority of injuries sustained. Falls remain a common cause of SCI pathology in individuals over 45 or with underlying diseases such as osteoporosis or ankylosing spondylitis. Intentionally inflicted trauma, either blunt or penetrating, remains a significant cause of SCI in urban locales. Overall, accidents account for almost half (44.5%) of new-onset cases within the United States (4).

Early recognition is a key to the ensuing management of SCI. At any accident scene, the first responders will most likely be emergency medical technicians. These individuals are trained in extrication, immobilization, and primary survey. More advanced in-field care is delivered by EMT paramedics, who are ACLS-trained, and can secure airways via intubation, place peripheral lines for access, and administer intravenous medications in the case of cardiac arrest. Both primary and secondary responders must remain aware at all times of the potential for an unstable SCI in the polytrauma patient. Since 5% to 10% of unconscious MVC victims have concomitant cervical spine injuries, responders should treat all unresponsive patients as having an SCI until proven otherwise (5). Should a focal neurological deficit (failure to move an extremity, complaints of numbness, or paresthesias) be noted at the scene, it should immediately be reported to the receiving personnel upon arrival to a trauma center.

The main goals of the initial field assessment are establishment of an adequate airway, breathing, and circulation. As with all standard trauma protocols, the airway remains the highest priority. Field responders should avoid neck hyperextension during placement of an endotracheal (ET) tube; the jaw-thrust maneuver and inline cervical immobilization must be used in the case of an unconscious patient (6). Adequate ventilation is key in the initial critical minutes to hours following injury to prevent hypoxemia and thus secondary ischemia in the spinal cord. Supplemental oxygen should be administered in all patients. Bleeding in the field is managed with manual compression and pressure dressings; foreign bodies should not be removed outside of the hospital due to the potential for rapid exsanguination. Hypotension is initially treated with intravenous fluids via two large-bore peripheral venous catheters (7).

Proper handling and stabilization in the field remain of paramount importance once the primary survey is completed and the surroundings are established to be safe. In the case of a car-crash victim, extrication can be prolonged and particularly dangerous in the case of a high-level SCI. If the patient remains sitting in the vehicle when found, a hard cervical collar of adequate size should be fitted by one responder as manual stabilization is held by an assistant. After the cervical spine is secured, extrication can be carried out. Techniques for transfer include the four-man lift, the scoop stretcher, and the Kendrick Extrication Device (KED). Unlike a short spine board, a KED uses a series of vertical bars to fully immobilize the head and the spine during removal, including along the axis of rotation (8). It should be noted that these methods are time intensive and appropriate only for patients deemed to be stable with a controlled environment; unstable patients should be removed using rapid extrication techniques and manual inline stabilization (9). Once withdrawn safely from the wreckage, the subject should be immobilized on a standard rigid spine board for definitive transport. In the case of an ejection or of a pedestrian struck and found supine, logroll techniques should be used to maneuver the patient onto a long hardboard. Ideal positioning on a backboard is to have the patient covered fully from head to feet and strapped down at the forehead, thorax, and extremities. The head and the spine should be maintained in neutral alignment. Occipital padding should be used as needed; pediatric patients less than 6 years of age may require an occipital recess given their increased head size in relation to the torso. Lateral head rotation can be prevented with standard head blocks, improvised rolled blankets, and tape for reinforcement (10).

Diving accidents in which the SCI victim is still immersed should be managed with multiple rescuers floating the patient supine and ensuring support at the occipital, cervical, and lower thoracolumbar regions. Once in shallow water, a spine board should be slipped beneath the patient and secured as previously detailed, with board and patient removed together from the water's edge for further transport. In the case of a football-related injury in which SCI is suspected, protective gear such as the helmet and shoulder pads should not be removed in the field (11). Face masks, however, should be removed as expeditiously as possible, and cut away if necessary, due to the potential for rapid airway compromise (12). Inline manual traction should be applied in these cases.

Growing levels of evidence in the recent literature support the early transfer of stabilized SCI patients to specialized centers, which may or may not be part of the regional level I trauma center (13). Additionally, patients with SCI plus multisystem injuries may benefit from immediate transfer to a level I trauma center rather than initial management at a lower tier center (14). Actual methods of transportation depend on patient stability, distance to be covered, and local traffic conditions. Short distances (less than 50 miles) can be managed via an ambulance. For greater distances (50 to 150 miles) or during periods of traffic congestion, a helicopter is preferred. Transport to remote centers (greater than 150 miles) is optimally handled by fixed-wing aircraft (15).

ED/TRAUMA MANAGEMENT

The initial ED team to evaluate the SCI patient in the trauma bay should be multidisciplinary and include the traumatologist or the general surgeon, the anesthesiologist, the neurological surgeon, the orthopaedic surgeon, the ED physician, the respiratory technician, and trained nursing personnel. Primary goals of this group are to maintain airway patency, prevent hypoxemia, normalize vital signs, and ensure the maintenance of spinal stability and normal alignment. A recent consortium guidelines published discusses many of the medical and surgical issues discussed below (16).

A rigid backboard is critical for transportation, but once at the hospital, transfer of the patient onto a firm padded surface while maintaining good spinal alignment is important to protect skin from pressure ulcer development, optimally within the first 2 hours. Baseline skin assessment should be performed and documented when the patient is removed from backboard. If the patient must remain on rigid board, the skin over bony prominences should be maintained with padding, and the skin inspected every 30 minutes if possible. Potential secondary objectives may include administration of therapeutic agents to prevent further neuronal cell death as well as early and rapid reduction to remove compressive forces from the neuraxis. Clear and effective channels of communication must exist between all members of the group. If the trauma team deems it necessary to intubate an unstable or intoxicated patient, ideally the spinal surgeon should be informed and present in order to establish a baseline neurological examination prior to induction by anesthesia. Should this prove unfeasible, chemical paralysis must be reversed as soon as possible to perform a detailed neurological assessment and to eliminate the possibility of a missed SCI.

Following the initial mechanical insult in SCI, catecholamines are released with a transient hypertensive phase. Depending on the rapidity of transport, SCI patients may present to the ED with elevated systolic blood pressures. This stage is brief, however, and is followed by what is defined as spinal shock. Spinal shock is defined as temporary loss of spinal reflex activity occurring below a total or near-total SCI and implies flaccid paralysis and loss of deep tendon reflexes below the level of the cord injury (17). Care must be taken to differentiate this condition from neurogenic shock, which manifests as concurrent hypotension, bradycardia, and hypothermia. These cardiovascular manifestations are common in patients with a neurological level of injury at or above T6. Physiologically, the mechanism of action is thought to be diminished levels of sympathetic outflow with cervical or high thoracic injuries, leaving parasympathetic influences unopposed. Loss of sympathetically mediated vascular tone ensues; when injuries are located above T1, unchecked vagal activity can induce heart rates less than 60 beats/min (18,19). Bradycardia can be present even with simultaneous blood loss and hypovolemic shock, necessitating a thorough evaluation and exclusion of all sources of potential bleeding.

Fluid resuscitation is the preferred initial management of hypotension in the SCI patient, regardless of the source. If not placed in the field, a Foley catheter should be inserted on arrival to the trauma bay for urinary drainage; the detrusor muscle will display the same flaccid paralysis as the extremities in acute SCI. Furthermore, an indwelling catheter is critical for accurate measurement of output to optimize therapy. Urine output in adequate fluid resuscitation should be greater than 30 mL/h in adults. As a general guideline, a 1.5 to 2.0 L bolus of crystalloid administered over the first hour should be adequate to achieve this endpoint. In the face of persistent hypotension following fluid challenge, care must be taken to differentiate the underlying cause. Due to an impaired ability to mediate vasoconstriction, patients in neurogenic shock may be at increased risk of capillary leak and pulmonary edema with continuous fluid administration. In this population, early use of vasopressors is preferred over further intravenous infusion. Central venous catheterization can be performed rapidly and safely in the trauma bay as part of the initial hospital workup to aid in determining volume status.

Maintenance of the mean arterial pressure (MAP) at greater than 85 mm Hg has been associated with improved neurologic outcomes for cervical and upper thoracic injuries in a widely referenced study by Vale and colleagues (20). Monitoring of the MAP via arterial lines should be carried out in all SCI patients. Initial vasopressors for hypotensive, bradycardic SCI patients can include dopamine (2.5 to 5 µg/kg/min), which has both alpha- and beta-agonist properties, with norepinephrine (Levophed, 0.01 to 0.2 µg/kg/min) as a potential secondary agent if required. Phenylephrine (Neosynephrine) is not an appropriate initial choice in the SCI patient as it is a pure alpha agonist and can worsen an already preexisting bradycardia (21). In some SCI cases, transvenous pacing may be required in the acute period (5).

Patients who arrive intubated or who require in-house intubation due to compromised respiratory function should have a nasogastric tube placed as soon as possible to prevent emesis and potential aspiration. In the setting of facial trauma with midface or anterior basal skull fractures, an orogastric tube should be used instead. If an SCI patient is not currently intubated, the level of injury should be rapidly assessed and forced vital capacity (FVC) measured. An FVC of greater than 1.5 L indicates an adequate level of inspiratory muscle strength. Less than 1 L is alarming and typically a harbinger of ventilatory failure; airway protection and mechanical ventilation should be instituted. Patients with an FVC between 1 and 1.5 L should be carefully observed and serially assessed as this is considered borderline. All SCI patients with levels of injury above T12 may have difficulty clearing pulmonary secretions. High cervical tetraplegics may have no cough or gag, and thus be at high risk for aspiration or mucous plugging. Prophylactic intubation (ideally by an anesthesiologist under fiberoptic conditions) may be indicated in this subset of SCI patients.

Once the patient has been appropriately resuscitated and stabilized, a thorough neurologic evaluation must be performed. History of any central nervous system disorders or spinal issues predisposing to SCI (cervical stenosis, ankylosing spondylitis, ossification of the posterior longitudinal ligament) should be obtained from either the patient or the family. A careful motor and sensory assessment as per the criteria set forth by the American Spinal Injury Association should be documented (see Chapter 6.) It is recommended that a physician specializing in SCI (i.e., physiatrist board certified in SCI Medicine) be part of the trauma team to recommend appropriate treatment as well as perform the exam. This initial examination provides an immediate baseline against which any subsequent changes in neurological status can be compared. Any physical anomalies noted on the primary survey such as paraspinal tenderness or abrupt step-offs should also be noted. Both the primary survey and the neurological assessment can serve to guide the focus of further spinal imaging.

Signs of traumatic brain injury (TBI), as well as abdominal, intrathoracic, pelvic trauma, and peripheral bone fractures should be sought. The acute treatment team should assess and document early and frequently for any evidence of TBI in the form of loss of consciousness by use of the Glasgow coma scale and posttraumatic amnesia (by using the Galveston Orientation and Amnesia Test (GOAT) or equivalent. Early identification will help facilitate acute management (i.e., agitation) and rehabilitation planning. For extraspinal (i.e., long bone) fractures that present along with the acute SCI, surgery should occur as warranted as they are not pathological in nature (16). If managed conservatively, great care should be taken to avoid circumferential casts to allow for monitoring of insensate skin.

A careful evaluation for thoracic, abdominal, and pelvic injury should be performed in all patients with acute SCI. These are more common in persons sustaining thoracolumbar injuries versus cervical injuries (10% versus 4%) (16). As the physical examination is not as reliable in this situation, diagnostic modalities such as ultrasound and CT scanning are required. Injuries to the aorta may occur with high-energy trauma (22) more common with upper thoracic injury (23). If present, urgent repair may be required (16).

Priapism is a common finding during the early period after SCI and is usually self-limited (few hours) without the need for treatment (16). There is no evidence that urethral catheterization should be avoided. If pripaism is prolonged, urology consultation should be considered.

RADIOGRAPHIC ASSESSMENT

The standard trauma series for spine injury has traditionally consisted of cross-table lateral and anteroposterior views of the cervical and thoracolumbar spine. This protocol has undergone significant evolution, however, with the expanded availability of rapid computed tomography (CT) scanning. Current trauma literature indicates the superiority of CT evaluation over plain radiography in patients considered at high risk for cervical SCI (24). Computed tomography not only allows more facile identification of fractures that might have been missed with plain radiographs but also provides views of the entire spinal axis that can be reconstructed to further characterize malalignments not well appreciated on axial imaging alone. As there is a range of 10% to 40% incidence of noncontiguous spinal fractures in the setting of trauma, careful inspection of the entire spinal column is necessary once a single fracture is identified (6,16,25). In a study of the National Trauma Databank, 13% of persons with a cervical spine fracture had a thoracic or lumbar fracture (26) supporting the practice of imaging the complete spine when a cervical fracture is identified (16). Additionally, approximately 47% of spine trauma and 65% of SCI patients will have concomitant injuries such as TBI or long-bone fractures, necessitating further radiographic workup (27).

Plain radiographs can provide further detail regarding specific areas of the spinal axis (assessment of the cervicothoracic junction on swimmer's view, open mouth cervical spine views to assess the lateral masses of C1 and the odontoid process) and should be inspected carefully for signs of soft tissue swelling. Increases in diameter of the prevertebral soft tissues can indicate ligamentous disruption and may be the only sign of an otherwise subtle fracture or fracture dislocation. In adult patients, retropharyngeal soft tissue diameter should be no more than 10 mm at C1 and 7 mm at C2 through C4. Below C5-6, retrotracheal soft tissue should be no more than 22 mm in diameter (28). Flexion-extension views of the cervical spine can also be used to assess for instability and possible ligamentous injury; this assumes no distracting injuries and a patient who is not intoxicated or obtunded. Dynamic studies should not be obtained in an acute fashion or in a patient with neurological deficits.

Should an SCI become evident, the decision must then be made by the assessing surgeon whether to defer immediate intervention such as closed reduction with traction or open surgical intervention in favor of further radiographic workup such as magnetic resonance imaging (MRI). Advantages of early MRI include identification of ligamentous injuries that might contraindicate traction, such as occipitoatlantal (OA) dissociation, or that might guide the surgical approach to be undertaken in the case of a cervical injury. In particular, short tau inversion recovery sequences on MRI can be highly sensitive for detection of occult ligamentous injuries in the cervical spine (29). Disadvantages include the time investiture needed to obtain the study, which may be quite involved in the case of an intubated polytrauma SCI patient. Arguments have been put forth in the literature both for and against MRI prior to skeletal traction or open decompression and stabilization

(30–32). An emerging consensus would appear to indicate that early cervical traction to relieve mechanical compression is relatively safe in the awake SCI patient without preexisting cervical stenosis; obtunded patients who cannot cooperate with serial neurological examinations should undergo early MRI prior to reduction. Postreduction, patients should undergo MRI to exclude the possibility of cord compression from disk herniation (33).

The timing of diagnostic radiographic imaging studies ultimately depends on the neurological status of the SCI patient at the time of presentation to the hospital. Neurologically intact patients should undergo the full diagnostic workup of the admitting institution, which can include plain radiographs in addition to more advanced modalities such as CT and MRI. In the case of patients unable to undergo MRI due to indwelling pacemakers or body habitus, myelography may be indicated. Patients with an incomplete SCI (ASIA Impairment Scale [AIS] classes B through D) and a stable neurological examination are treated identically to intact patients with a thorough diagnostic workup. In the relatively rare case of an incomplete SCI with progressive neurological deterioration, emergent treatment is indicated and the radiographic evaluation may be deferred. SCI patients with a complete (AIS A) injury present a challenging case for the evaluating surgeon and the role of early intervention versus further workup continues to be debated. (See later for detailed discussion.)

MEDICAL AND PRESURGICAL INTERVENTIONS

Ancient records from the *Edwin Smith Surgical Papyrus* (c. 1700 BC) reveal that Egyptian physicians characterized SCI as an "ailment not to be treated" and recommended withholding water from spinal cord–injured soldiers (34). Hippocrates further confirmed the dismal prognosis for SCI with paralysis, although he developed rudimentary forms of traction in an attempt to realign spinal deformity without evidence of cord injury (35). Modern advances in emergency in-field protocols, critical care medicine, and the development of targeted SCI centers have significantly increased survival in this patient population. Attention has now been turned toward the development of strategies to maximize potential neurological recovery.

Closed reduction with skeletal traction remains one of the fastest modalities to relieve mechanical compression in the cervical spine when applied appropriately to selected SCI patients. A thorough historical and radiographic workup is essential prior to institution of cervical traction; certain conditions such as ankylosing spondylitis and OA dislocation are absolute contraindications. As previously discussed, the decision whether or not to seek advanced imaging prior to application of traction remains contested. At the authors' institution, the paradigm has been toward early and rapid reduction prior to MRI, particularly in cases of complete SCI or incomplete SCI with progressive neurological deterioration.

Traction is accomplished with the SCI patient placed in either a Stryker frame or a Roto-Rest bed. Gardner-Wells tongs or a halo ring is applied using local anesthetic. For straight traction, optimal pin insertion is 1 cm superior to the pinna of the ear. If flexion or extension is desired, the pins can be placed posteriorly or anteriorly, respectively. Initial weight application is 5 lb, with additional 5 lb-increments until reduction is achieved. The presence of prior cervical fusion may require a slower increase in weight. A neurologic evaluation must be performed and documented after each increase in weight, and a lateral radiographic imaging study must be obtained. Cotler described applying up to 140 lb to reduce dislocation in awake and cooperative patients (36). Once reduction is confirmed radiographically, either with plain radiographs or tomography, 10 to 20 lb of weight is used to maintain reduction. The patient is brought to the operating room for open stabilization once medically stabilized and once the necessary personnel are available.

Several pharmacologic agents have been proposed and evaluated for their potential to improve neurologic recovery in SCI survivors. Methylprednisolone remains the most prominent following the publication of the National Acute Spinal Cord Injury Studies (NASCIS-I to III) (37–39). Since publication of the NASCIS-II results, methylprednisolone (initial bolus dose of 30 mg/kg followed by 5.4 mg/kg/h maintenance dose for 23 hours) has been considered standard of care. However, the scientific integrity of these studies has been reevaluated based on quality of evidence. A review by Hurlbert has expressed that both NASCIS-II and NASCIS-III were well-designed and executed trials, but the data from NASCIS-III were weak and minimally compelling (40). Further systematic meta-analysis concluded that the use of 24-hour methylprednisolone remains experimental and the use of 48-hour methylprednisolone is potentially harmful, with neither being recommended for routine treatment (41). The senior author does not use steroids in the treatment of acute SCI. Current SCI guidelines put forth by the American Association of Neurological Surgeons state that "Methylprednisolone… is recommended as an option in the treatment of patients with acute spinal cord injuries that should be undertaken with the knowledge that the evidence suggesting harmful side effects is more consistent than any suggestion of clinical benefit" (42). Steroids are not administered to persons who present neurologically intact and should be stopped if neurologic symptoms have resolved to reduce deleterious side effects (16).

Despite initial indications holding promise, neither tirilazad mesylate (a lazaroid assessed in NASCIS-III) nor GM-1 ganglioside has shown statistically significant improvement in clinical functionality following injury (39,43). Local hypothermia may display some neuroprotective qualities in regards to secondary injury, but currently remains impractical outside of specialized centers (44,45). Current proposed neuroprotective agents ongoing preclinical trials in the process of transitioning to the clinical arena include minocycline, the Rho antagonist BA-210 (Cethrin), potassium channel blockers, anti-NOGO monoclonal antibodies, and embryonic stem cells (46,47). Current significant medical interventions in regard to SCI recovery remain prehospital recognition, aggressive resuscitation with targeted MAP greater than 85 mm Hg in the acute injury period, injury stabilization, and prevention of ensuing neurological or systemic complications.

As the third leading cause of SCI in the United States, civilian GSWs deserve special attention in regards to medical management. Unlike closed high-impact injuries, GSWs and stab wounds generally do not produce spinal instability and thus rarely require surgical stabilization (48). Management includes careful inspection of entrance and exit wounds in order to determine whether cerebrospinal fluid (CSF) leakage is present. Plain radiographs and CT scans are used to assess the degree of bony injury and adjacent soft tissue damage; injury to nearby vascular structures may necessitate angiography. Penetrating objects such as knives within the spinal canal should be removed in the operating room under direct visualization; the extent of thoracic or abdominal injury must be known prior. Bullets that traverse the abdominal viscera have an increased risk of infection within the central nervous system and should be treated with broad-spectrum antibiotics for 7 days (49). Tetanus prophylaxis should be routinely administered in the ED. Surgery is rarely indicated with a penetrating SCI. Indications include to close a CSF fistula or to decompress the spinal cord in cases when a foreign body, bone fragment or expanding hematoma is causing progressive neurologic deterioration. Bullets do not have to be removed during the course of a spinal decompression; however, if the bullet is felt to be causing neuronal compression and is accessible, removal should be attempted (50). Neurologic recovery following GSWs is generally poor, and complete injury can result from bullets that do not enter the spinal canal due to the surrounding blast effect. Steroids have shown no benefit in regards to penetrating injuries, and their use has been associated with an increased incidence of spinal and extraspinal infection (50).

SURGICAL MANAGEMENT

The timing of surgical treatment for patients with acute SCI is controversial. Conflicting reports exist in the medical literature stating whether surgery should be performed acutely or whether it is more appropriate to delay and allow the neural elements to "cool off." Marshall et al. (51), in 1987, published a large and widely quoted study indicating that the rate of neurologic complications was higher in patients undergoing surgery during the first 5 days following the inciting trauma, compared to a second group that underwent delayed (greater than 6 days postinjury) spinal surgery. Subsequently, Vaccaro et al. (52) in 1997 undertook a prospective study on acute cervical SCI. These authors were unable to demonstrate a significant difference in neurologic outcome between patients who received early (defined as within 72 hours) and late (defined as 5 days or later) surgery. Both studies have been subjected to intense criticism, however, regarding methodology and design. In the study by Marshall et al., decompressive laminectomy through a dorsal approach was frequently performed alone as the procedure of choice. While acceptable and reasonable in the 1980s, present management of traumatic SCI has evolved beyond this paradigm with the development of sophisticated spinal instrumentation. Criticism of the Vaccaro study rests on the definition of "early" surgery as within a 72-hour period from the initial traumatic event. Some critics felt that this allowed an excessive lapse of time and that a more stringent definition of early surgery should be within 24 hours or less of the primary injury.

Within the spinal surgery community, proponents of early surgery continue to maintain that it offers an advantage to patients with an acute SCI. This concept has never been proven in a randomized, prospective study. Fehlings and Perrin performed an evidence-based review of the literature in 2006 to evaluate the rationale and indications for timing of decompressive surgery after acute nonpenetrating SCI. They determined that experimental animal studies have consistently shown benefit to early decompressive surgery after SCI, and that recent analysis demonstrated surgery within 24 hours may result in statistically better outcomes (53). Evidence from the ongoing Surgical Treatment for Acute Spinal Cord Injury Study also supports this belief, with 1-year results demonstrating that 24% of patients who underwent decompressive surgery within 24 hours had a two grade or greater improvement in ASIA Impairment Scale versus 4% of those patients receiving delayed treatment (54,55). Long-term follow-up is forthcoming from this multicenter trial.

The sole unanimously agreed upon principle in the management of the acute SCI patient is that early surgery is indicated in the face of progressive evolving neurologic deterioration; this situation is uncommon in clinical practice. However, if a patient with a documented neurological baseline examination proceeds to develop a subsequent deficit, immediate surgical intervention is indicated. In all other cases, the choices of emergent, urgent, and elective surgery are supportable.

Any discussion of the surgical management of acute SCI requires an understanding of spinal stability. White and Panjabi have, in the most widely accepted theory regarding spinal instability, defined clinical instability as "the loss of the ability of the spine, under physiologic loads, to maintain its pattern of displacement so that there is no initial or additional neurological deficit, no major deformity, and no incapacitating pain." This definition is applicable to all levels of the spine (56).

Radiographic criteria have been established for the diagnosis of clinical spinal instability. Denis in 1983 published the widely accepted three-column theory for thoracolumbar fractures. In this theory, the spine is divided into three columns (Fig. 7.1). The anterior column is composed of the anterior vertebral body, the anterior longitudinal ligament (ALL), and the anterior half of the annulus fibrosus. The middle column is made up of the posterior vertebral body, the posterior longitudinal ligament (PLL), and the posterior half of the annulus fibrosus. The posterior column includes all of the posterior elements (including the pedicles). According to this theory, spinal instability is deemed to be present if any two of the three columns are violated (57).

Benzel introduced the concept of the instantaneous axis of rotation (IAR). In work published from Benzel's biomechanics laboratory, the principles of force and motion affecting the thoracolumbar spine are set forward. Forces on the spine are defined as acting through vectors, and failure modes of the spine occur depending on the direction and relative location of the IAR (58). Understanding these concepts allows the spine surgeon to select the most biomechanically sound and advantageous stabilization procedure to be performed.

Injuries to the spine or spinal cord are the result of failure of the bony elements, ligamentous supporting structures, and surrounding musculature. An understanding of the basic underlying principles is key to surgical treatment. Primarily ligamentous injuries (such as facet dislocations) require internal stabilization procedures. These injuries have high failure rates when external orthoses are attempted as the sole treatments. The most common external orthoses used in the cervical spine are halo vest immobilization and hard cervical collars. In the thoracolumbar spine, common external orthoses include a thoracolumbosacral orthosis (TLSO) or a body cast. Stable

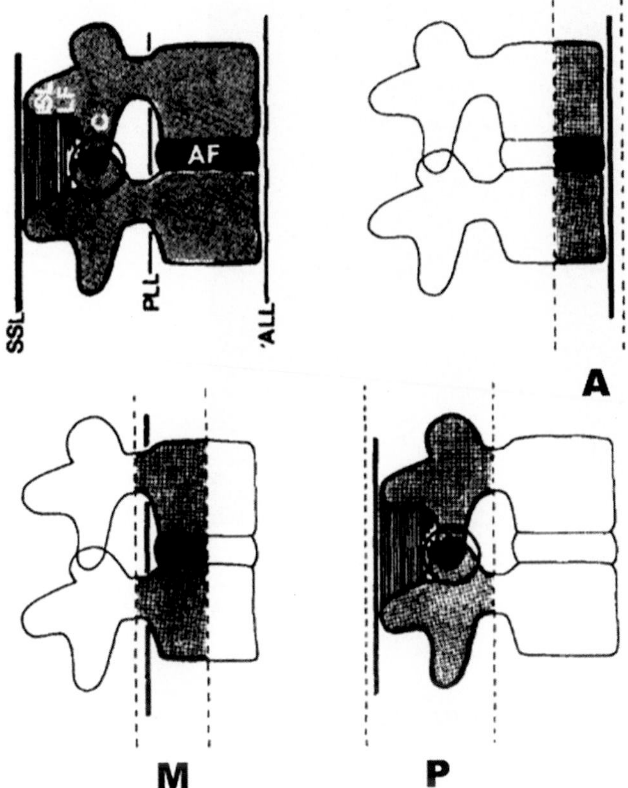

FIGURE 7.1. The three column spine. *P*, posterior column; *M*, middle column; *A*, anterior column; *SSL*, supraspinous ligament; *PLL*, posterior longitudinal ligament; *ALL*, anterior longitudinal ligament; *AF*, annulus fibrosus. (From, Denis F. The three-column spine and its significance in the classification of acute thoracolumbar spinal injuries. *Spine* 1983;8:817–831, with permission.)

fractures of the bony elements can heal with external bracing alone if the ligamentous structures are not significantly disrupted. Unstable fractures require open surgical intervention with internal stabilization; this is frequently the case in SCI.

The primary goal of surgery in acute SCI is adequate decompression of the neural elements. Either an anterior or a posterior approach may accomplish this; each individual case depends on both the comfort and expertise of the operating surgeon as well as the specific injury to be addressed. The most common etiology of SCI results from retropulsion of bone fragments or disc material from a ventral location into the spinal canal. This injury pattern favors an anterior approach to decompress the neural elements. Reconstruction of the anterior column following decompressive surgery also holds biomechanical advantages related to the IAR. However, anterior surgery for trauma is not always advisable at certain locations of the spine, including the occipitocervical complex, upper thoracic spine, and lower lumbar regions. Posterior surgery, which only secures the posterior elements, such as hook-rod constructs, is at a biomechanical disadvantage and requires longer construct lengths for adequate stability. The usage of instrumentation, which allows three-column fixation, such as pedicle screw placement, allows for more robust and shorter segmental stabilization.

Following decompression, the spine requires stabilization and fusion. Autologous bone remains the gold standard in trauma cases, which can frequently be harvested from the iliac crest. Allograft bone can also be used in anterior surgery, along with carbon fiber cages or trabecular metal for anterior column support.

Surgical instrumentation, or hardware, is used as an adjunct to fixate bones so that fusion may occur. It is essential to understand that this instrumentation is only a *temporary* device meant to facilitate the eventual bony fusion; without the development of this long-term fusion, the construct will eventually fail, leading to a pseudarthrosis. An external orthosis can be utilized in addition to the internal stabilization, depending on the preferences of the operating surgeon and the initial pattern of injury. When an external orthosis is used, it is typically maintained for 3 months or the length of time required to radiographically demonstrate bony fusion in both complete and incomplete SCI patients. The type of orthotic chosen depends on the level of spinal injury; for the occipital to C2 levels, either the halo vest or a hard cervical collar is used. For C3 to C7, a hard cervical collar is appropriate. At T1 to T4, a cervicothoracic orthosis such as the Minerva or SOMI brace is used. From T4 to L2, a TLSO is used; at L3 and below, a lumbosacral (LSO) orthotic can be worn, with the attachment of a hip-thigh spica attachment to ensure adequate immobilization of the low lumbar and sacral spine (59) (see Chapter 19).

SPINAL INJURIES

Occipital-Atlantoaxial Complex

The occipitocervical complex is responsible for approximately 50% of neck rotational movement. Fractures in this region may be singular or occur in combination, and the surgical stabilization procedure necessary depends on the overall stability of various injuries, with the least stable segment determining the mode of therapy. OA dislocation is frequently a fatal event. It can be assessed via CT scanning or on lateral cervical radiographs with numerous craniometric lines devised to define normal occipital anatomic locations with respect to the cervical spine. The *Powers ratio*, set forth by Powers et al. (60) in 1979, may be used to define OA dislocation. Cervical traction is absolutely contraindicated in this instance. Should the patient survive the initial insult, the surgical treatment of choice is a posterior occipitocervical fusion.

Atlas (C1) fractures were initially described by Sir Geoffrey Jefferson in 1920 and are commonly referred to as *Jefferson burst fractures* (61). The mechanical pattern of injury is frequently axial loading, and these are usually stable injuries without neurologic deficit that can be treated with external orthoses. Unstable Jefferson burst fractures are defined by Spence et al. (62) as having more than 7 mm of combined overhang of the C1 lateral masses on open-mouth odontoid radiographs (rule of Spence). This radiographic finding indicates probable transverse ligament disruption, which can be confirmed on MRI, and is treated with posterior surgical stabilization.

Fractures of the dens, or odontoid fractures, are classified into three types. Type I fractures are the rarest and involve only the tip of the odontoid process. Type II odontoid fractures are much more common, especially in the elderly, and involve a transverse fracture through the base of the dens at its junction with the C2 vertebral body (Fig. 7.2). Type III odontoid fractures are injuries that extend from the base of the odontoid into the vertebral body proper. Type I fractures

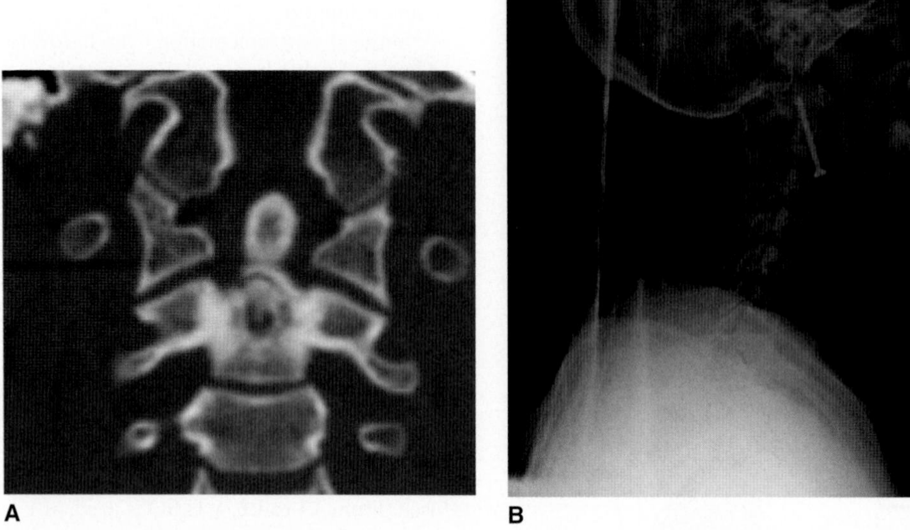

FIGURE 7.2. A: Coronal computed tomography demonstrating a type II dens fracture in a 24-year-old female following a motor vehicle collision. B: Lateral radiograph demonstrating treatment of the same fracture using an odontoid screw.

typically require no intervention. Type III odontoid fractures are usually treated with an external orthosis (either halo vest or hard cervical collar) for 3 months. Type II odontoid fractures have a high incidence of nonunion when external immobilization alone is used. With less than 6-mm displacement of the fracture, a 10% nonunion rate was observed; however, with greater than 6-mm displacement, the nonunion rate approaches 70% (63). In such cases, definitive management with surgical intervention may be recommended. External immobilization alone is reserved for patients with concomitant injuries or medical conditions that preclude surgery or make the intraoperative risks unacceptably high. Anterior surgery for type II odontoid fractures frequently involves odontoid screw fixation to preserve C1-2 motion with fusion occurring between the base of C2 and the odontoid peg. This technique is only feasible with fractures less than 6 months old and requires an intact transverse ligament (64). Alternative surgical options include C1 and C2 posterior stabilization and fusion. This may be achieved using the older wiring techniques described by Gallie and modified by Brooks (both of which require an intact C1 posterior arch) or by C1-2 transarticular screw placement described by Grob and Magerl in 1987, in which screws are placed through the lateral mass of C2 into the lateral mass of C1 for atlantoaxial segmental immobilization (65–67). The latter technique, however, cannot be used in the presence of fixed subluxation of C1 on C2 or in the case of an aberrant pathway of the vertebral artery. As an alternative method, polyaxial screws can be inserted into the lateral masses of C1 and the pars or pedicle of C2, followed by rod fixation (Harms technique) (68). Pedicle fractures of C2 are frequently bilateral and are referred to as *hangman's fractures*. These are also frequently stable injuries without associated neurological deficits, and can be treated with external orthoses such as a halo vest or hard cervical collar. Instability can be indicated by significant sagittal translation or angulation of the C2 vertebral body and can be approached surgically via either an anterior C2-3 discectomy and fusion or a posterior C1-2 fusion, as described above.

Subaxial Cervical Spine (C3 Through C7)

Fractures and subluxations in this region are frequently associated with SCI. Injuries confined to the bony anatomy without neurologic compression may heal with external orthoses alone; patients with SCI secondary to fractures frequently have associated ligamentous injuries that allow spinal cord compression. These patients require open surgical intervention to decompress the cord and fuse the unstable spinal segments.

The most common burst fracture in the subaxial cervical spine occurs at the C5 level. These injuries are typically associated with bony retropulsion compressing the spinal cord and are best treated with anterior surgery. Cervical traction is usually applied as previously discussed, and the surgery itself usually involves a corpectomy (vertebral body resection) with a minimum width of 15 mm. This allows adequate decompression of the cervical cord, which typically has a width of 13 mm at these levels. Following the bony resection, a strut graft (usually autologous iliac crest) is used for anterior column reconstruction and stabilization is achieved via a screw-plate system. Since initial description by Caspar in 1989, a multitude of individual anterior cervical instrumentation systems have become available, and the choice of construct is based on operator familiarity (69). As with upper cervical spine injuries, external orthoses may be used to augment the construct and fusion.

Subluxations of the cervical spine can involve unilateral or bilateral facet injuries. Most commonly, the C5-6 level is affected by the subluxation. In the case of a unilateral facet injury ("jumped" or "perched" facet), the patient typically does not sustain a complete SCI. More frequently, these injuries are associated with nerve root deficits at the level of the facet subluxation, although incomplete SCI may be present. The treatment involves application of cervical traction in order to realign the spinal elements, with the timing of advanced imaging controversial, as previously discussed. Bilateral facet subluxations are associated with complete (AIS A) SCI (Fig. 7.3). Following reduction in traction, open stabilization is indicated; if traction is unsuccessful in reducing the injury,

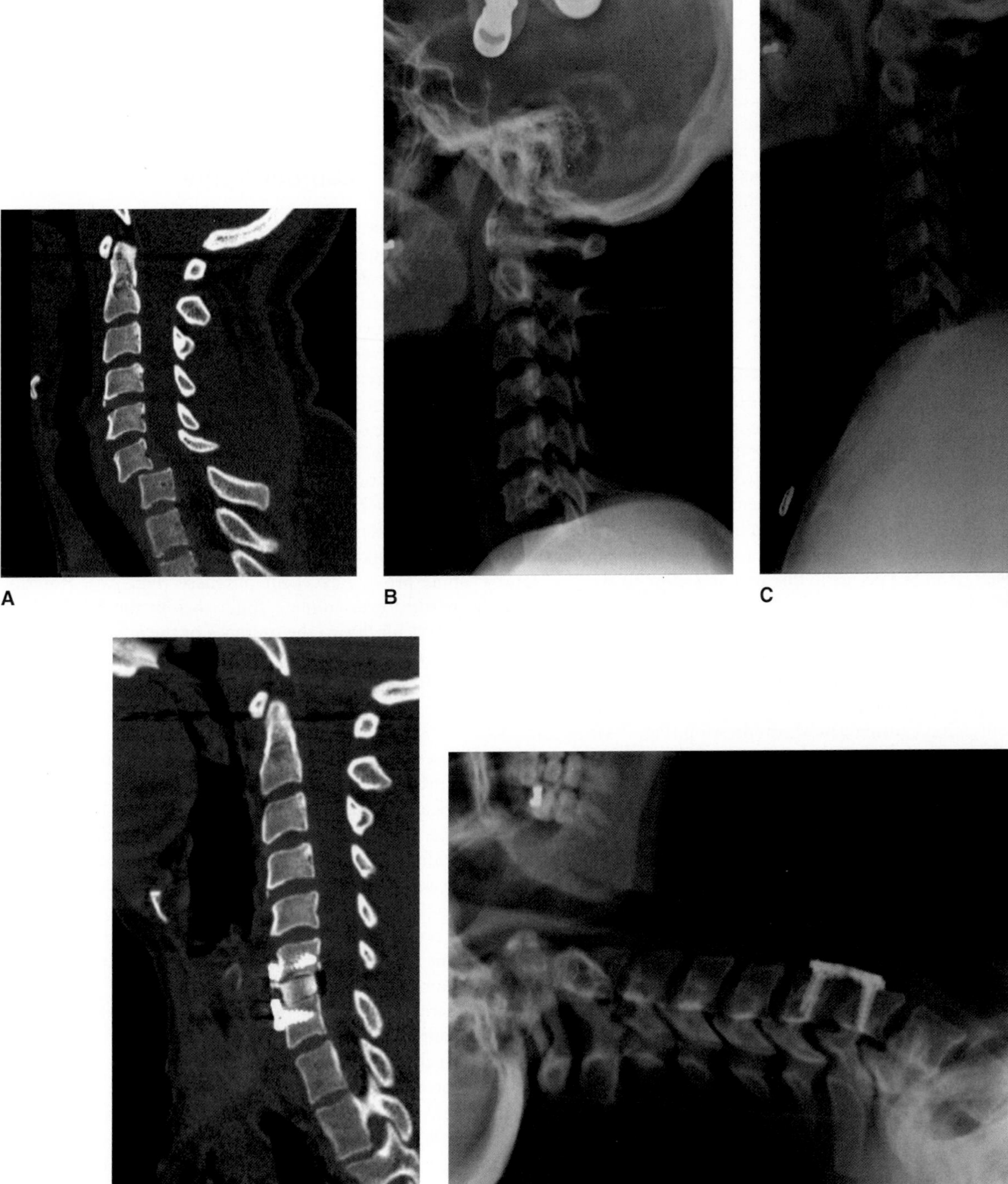

FIGURE 7.3. **A:** Computed tomography demonstrating severe C6 on C7 anterolisthesis with bilateral jumped and locked facets. The patient is a 33-year-old female who sustained a fall down stairs and complained of inability to move her lower extremities to emergency responders. Her neurological examination in the trauma bay was notable for no voluntary lower extremity movement and diminished rectal tone. Based on these findings, the decision was made to forego further advanced imaging and reduce the patient immediately with cervical skeletal traction. Lateral cervical spine radiographs before (**B**) and after (**C**) reduction with 90 lb of traction. The patient was then taken to the OR for a C6-7 anterior cervical diskectomy and fusion with a screw-plate system and iliac crest autograft. **D:** Computed tomography taken 24 hours postoperatively, showing maintenance of reduction with good cervical lordosis. **E:** Lateral cervical spine radiograph taken 3 months postoperatively showing early graft incorporation. The patient has made an excellent clinical recovery and is now ambulating independently.

open reduction must be performed in the operating room. If there is a herniated disk or bony injury causing cord compression anteriorly, an anterior decompressive procedure with fusion and screw-plate fixation is indicated. In the absence of these findings, either an anterior or a posterior approach may be used. Posterior techniques include decompression and multilevel fixation with bone graft and lateral mass screws, as well as pedicle screw fixation at the C7 level should the bony anatomy permit. Older techniques include interspinous wiring with bone grafting.

Thoracic Spine

The most common thoracic spinal injury involves fractures of the T12 vertebra; this may or may not be associated with acute SCI. Possibly due to the increased stability afforded this region by the presence of stabilizing ribs and intercostal musculature, subluxations in the lower thoracic spine are uncommon. Fractures in the upper thoracic spine can result from the use of seat belt restraints, which place a flexion moment of force in this region upon impact in a motor vehicle collision. The upper thoracic spine is a vascular watershed area with poor blood supply; as a result, if an SCI occurs in this area, it is more likely to be neurologically complete.

Following determination of the stability of a thoracic spinal injury, unstable injuries are treated with stabilization and fusion procedures. Decompression may be required when bony elements have retropulsed into the spinal canal, or in the case of subluxation causing neural compression (Fig. 7.4). In the lower thoracic spine, either an anterior or a posterior approach may be employed. Anterior surgery is performed via a thoracotomy or a thoracoabdominal approach, and usually involves corpectomy with anterior column reconstruction. Bone grafting and screw-plate or screw-rod constructs are used to allow for short-segment stabilization and reconstruction. Cages filled with auto- or allograft can also be used to facilitate fusion. Anterior surgery in the upper thoracic spine can be technically challenging and involve scapular disarticulation or a trans-sternal approach. Posterior thoracic surgery can involve laminectomy at the injured segment, followed by multilevel fixation. The use of pedicle screw fixation in the thoracic spine has allowed for biomechanically advantageous three-column stabilization; some newer percutaneous instrumentation systems have become increasingly popular for lower thoracic spine surgeries. This has resulted in the falling out of favor of previous hook and rod segmental constructs. Spinal orthotics (TLSO) are typically worn for 3 months after stabilization for both complete and incomplete SCI patients.

Flexion-distraction type fractures, also known as *Chance fractures*, occur most commonly at the lower thoracolumbar spine. Previously associated with lap belts in motor vehicle accidents, with the addition of shoulder restraints to safety belts the majority of these fractures are now due to thoracic hyperflexion from a fall or crush injury. Radiographically, these fractures will display horizontal vertebral splitting extending from the lamina through the pedicles and into the vertebral body. The anterior column may display a wedge-shaped compression deformity with distraction of the posterior elements. These are frequently three-column injuries and commonly require operative stabilization with transpedicular fixation, with potential corpectomy and grafting of the anterior vertebral body depending on the degree of kyphosis and bony retropulsion (70). There is a strong association of intra-abdominal injury with a Chance fracture, especially in the pediatric population, and visceral trauma should always be carefully excluded when one is diagnosed (71,72).

Lumbar Spine

In the lumbar region, the most common cause of SCI is L1 burst fracture. Frequently, these occur as a result of falls from a considerable height and are associated with injury to both the conus medullaris and the cauda equina. Injuries to the lower lumbar segments are considered nerve root injuries that involve the cauda equina. Bowel and bladder function may be affected. As previously stated, there is no proven benefit to treatment with steroid medications in the lower lumbar spine. Surgical treatment of upper lumbar injuries can involve corpectomy of the involved vertebral body followed by anterior column reconstruction and stabilization with a screw-plate or screw-rod construct. Posterior surgery involves decompression of the affected neural elements followed by pedicle screw fixation and rod stabilization; the large pedicles of the lower lumbar spine provide excellent purchase (Fig. 7.5). Anterior surgery in the lower lumbar spine (below the L3 level) is extremely difficult due to the presence of the great vessels and the iliopsoas muscles. At the L1 and the L2 levels, the anterior approach is frequently used.

Additional Surgical Issues

In many cases of severe polytrauma, multiple spinal segments may be injured independently (6). Under such circumstances, major surgical stabilizing procedures may need to be staggered due to concerns of critical care or systemic medical comorbidities. Additionally, some SCI disruptions in trauma patients may be so severe as to require both anterior and posterior approaches to decompress and stabilize the spine adequately. Whenever possible, all stabilizations should be ideally completed in one sitting so as to mobilize the patient more quickly following surgical stabilization.

Laminectomy alone is rarely indicated in acute spine trauma resulting in SCI. Should the predominant neural insult result from dorsal compression with relative preservation of the anterior elements, laminectomy may be the procedure of choice. However, this is more likely to occur with penetrating rather than blunt trauma.

In regards to anesthetics, it is recommended to avoid the use of succinylcholine after the first 48 hours post-SCI, due to the risk of fatal hyperkalemic response to succinylcholine from upregulation of acetylcholine receptors on denervated muscle (16). This is unlikely to occur in the first 48 hours after injury.

SCI Medical Consultants

The rehabilitation team (including the SCI Medicine board certified physician) should be involved in the care of the patient with SCI as early as possible. Assuring focus and communication regarding SCI Medicine–specific areas including medical, physical, psychological, and social issues are critical.

The specific medical issues will be covered in the subsequent chapters by organ system. A few key issues will briefly be described that are important in the first few days after SCI.

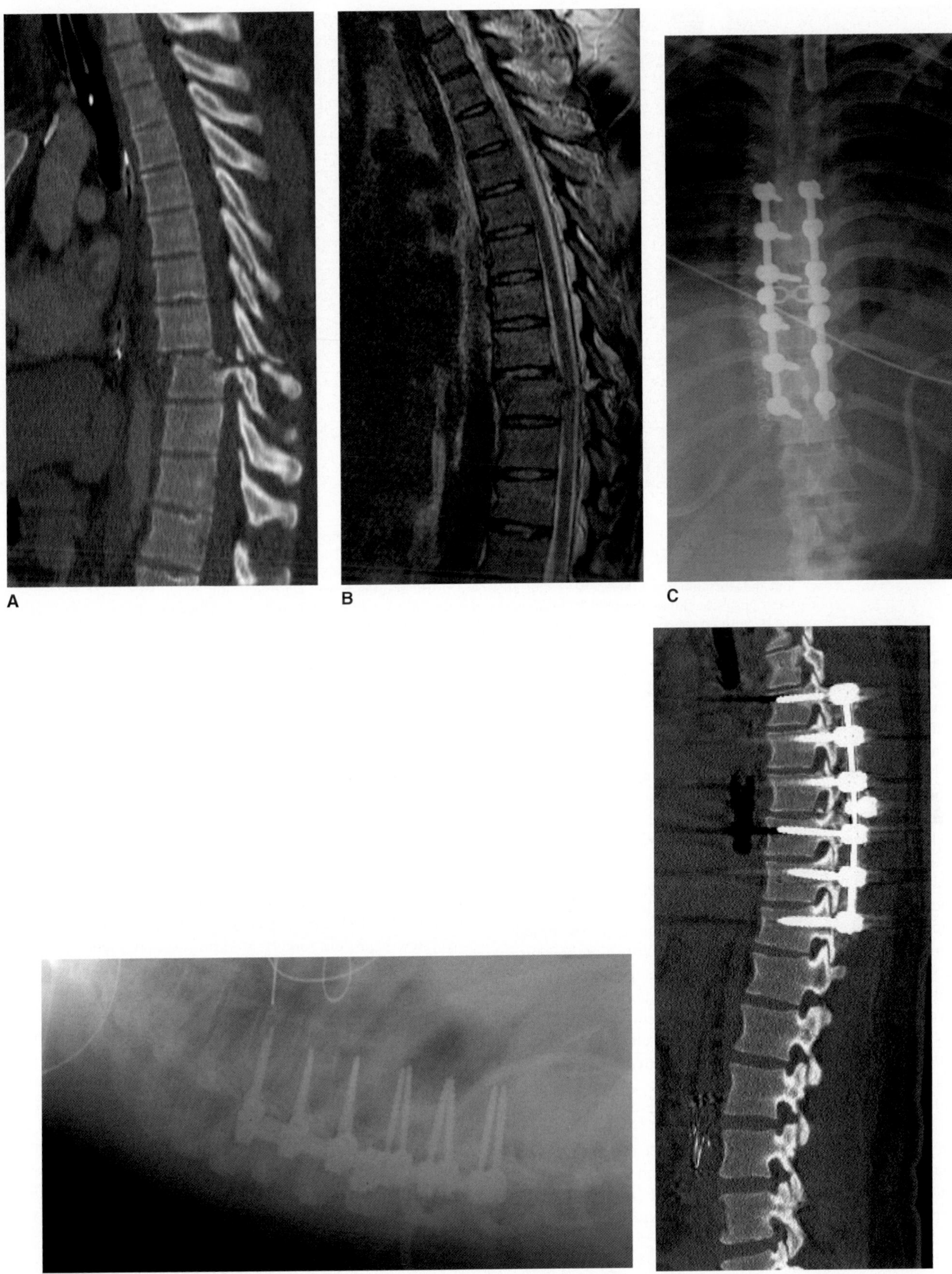

FIGURE 7.4. Computed tomography (A) and magnetic resonance imaging (B) demonstrating fracture-subluxation of T8 on T9, with an associated T9 pedicle fracture. Note the posterior T2 hyperintensity on MRI, indicative of ligamentous disruption. The patient is a 25-year-old male who presented as a pedestrian struck with multisystem injuries. He underwent decompression and posterior thoracic instrumentation using pedicle screws and rods. Anteroposterior (C) and lateral (D) radiographs, as well as computed tomography (E) demonstrate restoration of sagittal alignment.

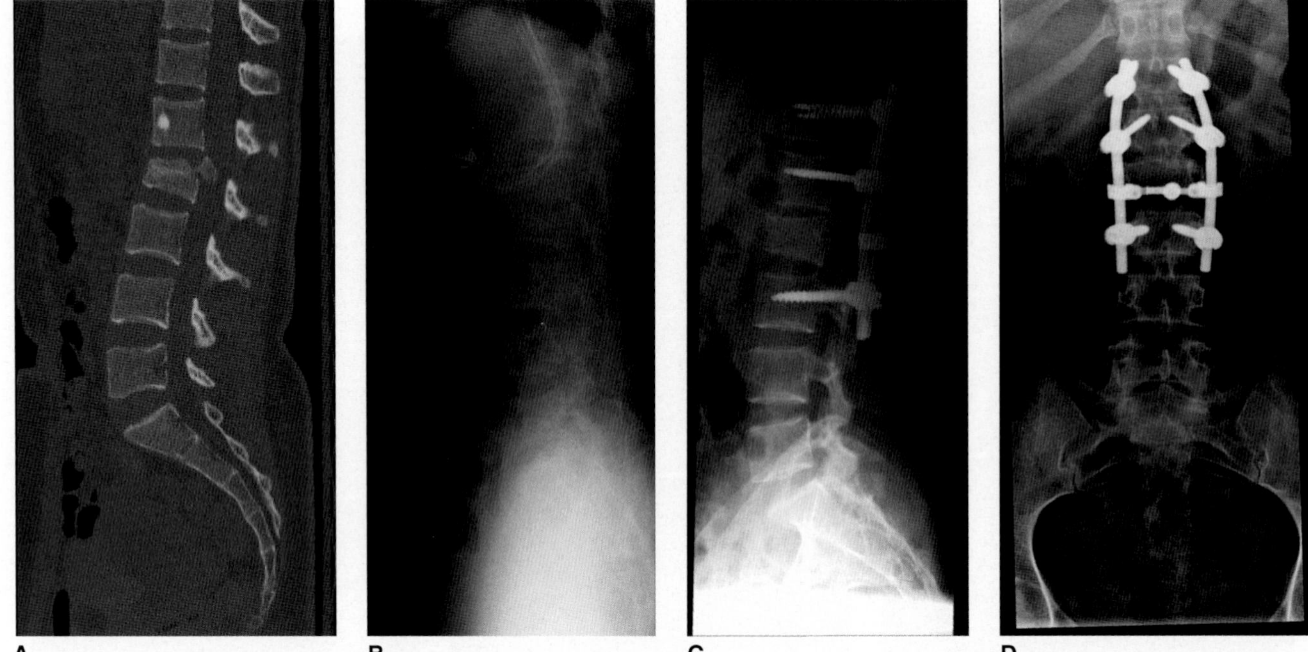

FIGURE 7.5. Computed tomography (A) and lateral radiographs (B) demonstrating an L2 burst fracture with significant bone fragment retropulsion. The patient is a 22-year-old female who jumped out of a window to escape a home fire. She landed on her feet and immediately felt a sharp pain in her lower back, but did not note any other deficits and presented to the trauma center neurologically intact. She underwent posterior thoracolumbar decompression and fusion from T12 to L3 and has done well postoperatively, with an excellent radiographic result (C,D).

Extraspinal fractures (i.e., long bone fractures) that occur concurrent with the SCI should usually undergo fixation as early as possible to facilitate early rehabilitation. Caution should be taken to protect the skin postoperatively, especially in insensate areas (16).

The nutritional needs of the acutely injured patient are important. Enteral nutrition should be initiated as tolerated within 24 to 48 hours, using the semirecumbent position when possible to prevent aspiration (16). If enteral feeds cannot be initiated, parenteral nutrition should be. Gastrointestinal prophylaxis should be initiated. The use of appropriate pressure reduction mattresses and protocols for turning the patients to reduce the incidence of pressure ulcers cannot be overstated. Deep vein thrombosis prophylaxis is also of critical importance (see Chapter 9). Current consensus is that pharmacological prophylaxis should be initiated within 72 hours unless there are contraindications such as an acute bleed. The use of low molecular weight heparin has shown to be effective, although should be held the day of surgery, and restarted 1-day post spinal surgery if there are no bleeding concerns. Vena cava filters should be used in persons who are contraindicated for pharmacological prophylaxis or very high level of injury (16,73). Vena cava filters should not be used however as a primary prophylaxis (74). Permanent filters are associated with a rate of up to 36% frequency of development of a DVT (75,76), so a temporary filter may be more appropriate. The presence of a vena cava filter is a relative contraindication to manually assisted cough techniques (quad coughing) for clearance of bronchial secretions, especially early after placement (16).

Education of patients when possible and families is important to begin early and the rehabilitation team plays important roles in this education process, as well as to begin assessing the rehabilitation services that will be needed after the acute hospitalization.

CONCLUSION

The events of the first hour following the initial injury are frequently held to determine the course of neurological outcome following acute SCI. Despite great strides in improving patient survival, improvements in functional outcome remain incremental. As previously discussed, timing of surgery remains controversial. At the current time, there is no uniform consensus as to early versus late surgery; it remains our belief, however, that early reduction with traction and early decompression and stabilization are advantageous to the acute SCI patient. Brief forays have been made into the principles of spinal stabilization and a broad overview regarding surgery at various spinal segments has been described. In summary: when surgery is planned to treat a patient with SCI, the primary goal of the operation is decompression of the neural elements. Secondarily, the intent is to stabilize and fuse the spine for long-term recovery. In the case of a complete neurologic injury, surgery is performed to allow for earlier mobilization, possibly prevent the development of chronic pain and posttraumatic syringomyelia, improve posture, and assist with more expeditious entry into the rehabilitation process. If there is an incomplete SCI or the patient is neurologically intact with an unstable injury, the purpose of surgery is to decompress and stabilize the spinal canal, prevent any neurologic deterioration or deformity, and preserve as much functionality as can be saved.

References

1. Facts and figures: National Spinal Cord Injury Statistical Center. *J Spinal Cord Med* 2008;31:119–120.
2. McKinley W, Meade MA, Kirshblum S, et al. Outcomes of early surgical management versus late or no surgical

intervention after acute spinal cord injury. *Arch Phys Med Rehabil* 2004;85:1818–1825.
3. Fehlings MG, Perrin RG. The role and timing of early decompression for cervical spinal cord injury: update with a review of recent clinical evidence. *Injury* 2005;36 (Suppl 2):B13–B26.
4. DeVivo MJ. Epidemiology of traumatic spinal cord injury. In: Kirshblum S, Campagnolo DI, DeLisa JA, eds. *Spinal cord medicine*. Baltimore, MD: Lippincott Williams & Wilkins, 2002:69–81.
5. Cohen M. Initial resuscitation of the patient with spinal cord injury. *Trauma Q* 1993;9:38–43.
6. Vaccaro AR, An HS, Betz RR, et al. The management of acute spinal trauma: pre-hospital and in-hospital emergency care. *Instr Course Lect* 1997;46:113–125.
7. Bernhard M, Gries A, Kremer P, et al. Spinal cord injury (SCI)—prehospital management. *Resuscitation* 2005; 66:127–139.
8. Howell JM, Burrow R, Dumontier C, et al. A practical radiographic comparison of short board technique and Kendrick Extrication Device. *Ann Emerg Med* 1989;18: 943–946.
9. Bernhard M, Helm M, Aul A, et al. Preclinical management of multiple trauma. *Anaesthesist* 2004;53:887–904.
10. De Lorenzo RA, Olson JE, Boska M, et al. Optimal positioning for cervical immobilization. *Ann Emerg Med* 1996;28:301–308.
11. Waninger KN. On-field management of potential cervical spine injury in helmeted football players: leave the helmet on! *Clin J Sport Med* 1998;8:124–129.
12. Kleiner DM, Almquist JL, Bailes J, et al. Prehospital care of the spine-injured athlete: a document from the Inter-Association Task Force for appropriate care of the spine-injured athlete. Dallas, TX: Inter-Association Task Force for Appropriate Care of the Spine-Injured Athlete, 2001.
13. Bagnall AM, Jones L, Richardson G, et al. Effectiveness and cost-effectiveness of acute hospital based spinal cord injuries services: systematic review. *Health Technol Assess* 2003;7(iii):1–92.
14. Demetriades D, Martin M, Salim A, et al. The effect of trauma center designation and trauma volume on outcome in specific severe injuries. *Ann Surg* 2005;242: 512–519.
15. Slucky AV, Eismont FJ. Treatment of acute injury of the cervical spine. *J Bone Joint Surg Am* 1994;76:1882–1896.
16. Early acute management in adults with spinal cord injury: clinical practice guidelines for health-care professionals. Consortium for *J Spinal Cord Med.* 2008;31(4): 408–479.
17. Atkinson PP, Atkinson JL. Spinal shock. *Mayo Clin Proc* 1996;71:384–389.
18. Garstang SV, Miller-Smith SA. Autonomic system dysfunction after spinal cord injury. *Phys Med Rehabil Clin N Am* 2007;18:275–292, vi-vii.
19. Furlan JC, Fehlings MG. Cardiovascular complications after acute spinal cord injury: pathophysiology, diagnosis and management. *Neurosurg Focus* 2008;25:E13.
20. Vale FL, Burns J, Jackson AB, et al. Combined medical and surgical treatment after acute spinal cord injury: results of a prospective pilot study to assess the merits of aggressive medical resuscitation and blood pressure management. *J Neurosurg* 1997;87:239–246.
21. Kee VR. Hemodynamic pharmacology of intravenous vasopressors. *Crit Care Nurse* 2003;23:79–82.
22. Murakami R, Tajima H, Ichikawa K, et al. Acute traumatic injury of the distal descending aorta associated with thoracic spine injury. *Eur Radiol* 1998;8(1):60–62.
23. Sturm JT, Hynes JT, Perry JF. Thoracic spinal fractures and aortic rupture: a significant and fatal association. *Ann Thorac Surg* 1990;50(6):931–933.
24. Gale SC, Gracias VH, Reilly PM, et al. The inefficiency of plain radiography to evaluate the cervical spine after blunt trauma. *J Trauma* 2005;59:1121–1125.
25. Qaiyum M, Tyrell PN, McCall IW, et al. MRU detection of unsuspected vertebral injury in acute spinal trauma: incidence and significance. *Skeletal Radiol* 2001;30: 299–304.
26. Winslow JE, Hensberry R, Bozeman WP, et al. Risk of thoracolumbar fractures doubled in victims of motor vehicle collisions with cervical spine fractures. *J Trauma* 2006;61(3):686–687.
27. Savitsky E, Votey S. Emergency department approach to acute thoracolumbar spine trauma. *J Emerg Med* 1997;15:49–60.
28. DeBenhe K, Havel C. Utility of prevertebral soft tissue measurements in identifying patients with cervical spine injury. *Ann Emerg Med* 1994;24:1119–1124.
29. Saifuddin A. MRI of acute spinal trauma. *Skeletal Radiol* 2001;30:237–246.
30. Grauer J, Vaccaro A, Lee J, et al. The timing and influence of MRI on the management of patients with cervical facet dislocations remains highly variable: a survey of members of the Spine Trauma Study Group. *J Spinal Disord Tech* 2009;22:96–99.
31. Wimberley DW, Vaccaro AR, Goyal N, et al. Acute quadriplegia following closed traction reduction of a cervical facet dislocation in the setting of ossification of the posterior longitudinal ligament: case report. *Spine* 2005;30:E433–E438.
32. Grant GA, Mirza SK, Chapman JR, et al. Risk of early closed reduction in cervical spine subluxation injuries. *J Neurosurg* 1999;90:13–18.
33. Vaccaro AR, Falatyn SP, Flanders AE, et al. Magnetic resonance evaluation of the intervertebral disc, spinal ligaments, and spinal cord before and after closed traction reduction of cervical spine dislocations. *Spine* 1999;24:1210–1217.
34. Breasted JH. *Edwin Smith surgical papyrus*. Chicago, IL: University of Chicago Press, 1930.
35. Heary RF, Madhavan K. The history of spinal deformity. *Neurosurgery* 2008;63(3 Suppl):5–15.
36. Cotler JM, Herbison GJ, Nasuti JF, et al. Closed reduction of traumatic cervical spine dislocation using traction weights up to 140 pounds. *Spine* 1993;18:386–390.
37. Bracken MB, Collins WF, Freeman DF, et al. Efficacy of methylprednisolone in acute spinal cord injury. *JAMA* 1984;251:45–52.
38. Bracken MB, Shepard MJ, Collins WF, et al. A randomized controlled trial of methylprednisolone or naloxone in the treatment of acute spinal cord injury: results of the Second National Acute Spinal Cord Injury Study. *N Engl J Med* 1990;322:1405–1411.
39. Bracken MB, Shepard MJ, Holford TR, et al. Methylprednisolone or tirilazad mesylate administration

after acute spinal cord injury: 1-year follow up. Results of the Third National Acute Spinal Cord Injury randomized controlled trial. *J Neurosurg* 1998;89:699–706.
40. Hurlbert RJ. Methylprednisolone for acute spinal cord injury: an inappropriate standard of care. *J Neurosurg* 2000;93:1–7.
41. Hurlbert RJ. The role of steroids in acute spinal cord injury: an evidence-based analysis. *Spine* 2001;26:S39–S46.
42. Hadley MN, Walters BC, Grabb PA, et al. Guidelines for the management of acute cervical spine and spinal cord injuries. *Clin Neurosurg* 2002;49:407.
43. Geisler FH, Coleman WP, Grieco G, et al. The Sygen multicenter acute spinal cord injury study. *Spine* 2001;26: S87–S98.
44. Kwon BK, Mann C, Sohn HM, et al. Hypothermia for spinal cord injury. *Spine J* 2008;8:859–874.
45. Inamasu J, Nakamura Y, Ichikizaki K. Induced hypothermia in experimental traumatic spinal cord injury: an update. *J Neurol Sci* 2003;209:55–60.
46. Chen MS, Huber AB, van der Haar ME, et al. Nogo-A is a myelin-associated neurite outgrowth inhibitor and an antigen for monoclonal antibody IN-1. *Nature* 2000;403:434–439.
47. Simonen M, Pedersen V, Weinmann O, et al. Systemic deletion of the myelin-associated outgrowth inhibitor Nogo-A improves regenerative and plastic responses after spinal cord injury. *Neuron* 2003;38:201–211.
48. Bono CM, Heary RF. Gunshot wounds to the spine. *Spine J* 2004;4:230–240.
49. Roffi RP, Waters RL, Adkins RH. Gunshot wounds to the spine associated with a perforated viscus. *Spine* 1989;14:808–811.
50. Heary RF, Vaccaro AR, Mesa JJ, et al. Steroids and gunshot wounds to the spine. *Neurosurgery* 1997;41: 576–583.
51. Marshall LF, Knowlton S, Garfin SR, et al. Deterioration following spinal cord injury: a multicenter study. *J Neurosurg* 1987;66:400–404.
52. Vaccaro AR, Daugherty RJ, Sheehan TP, et al. Neurologic outcome of early versus late surgery for spinal cord injury. *Spine* 1997;22:2609–2613.
53. Fehlings MG, Perrin RG. The timing of surgical intervention in the treatment of spinal cord injury: a systematic review of recent clinical evidence. *Spine* 2006;31:S28–S35.
54. Fehlings MG, Arvin B. The timing of surgery in patients with central spinal cord injury (editorial). *J Neurosurg Spine* 2009;10:1,2.
55. Fehlings MG, Aarabi B, Dvorak M, et al. A prospective multicenter trial to evaluate the role and timing of decompression in patients with cervical spinal cord injury: initial one-year results of the STASCIS study. 76th Annual Meeting, American Association of Neurological Surgeons; 28 April, 2008; Chicago, IL.
56. White AA, Panjabi MM. *Clinical biomechanics of the spine*. 2nd ed. Philadelphia, PA: Lippincott, 1990.
57. Denis F. The three column spine and its significance in the classification of acute thoracolumbar spinal injuries. *Spine* 1983;8:817–831.
58. Resnick DK, Weller SJ, Benzel EC. Biomechanics of the thoracolumbar spine. *Neurosurg Clin North Am* 1997;8:455–469.
59. Benzel EC, Larson SJ. Postoperative stabilization of the posttraumatic thoracic and lumbar spine: a review of concepts and orthotic techniques. *J Spinal Disord* 1989;2:47–51.
60. Powers B, Miller MD, Kramer RS, et al. Traumatic anterior atlanto-occipital dislocation. *Neurosurgery* 1979;4:12–17.
61. Jefferson G. Fracture of the atlas vertebra: report of four cases, and a review of those previously recorded. *Br J Surg* 1920;7:407–422.
62. Spence KF Jr, Decker S, Sell KW. Bursting atlantal fragment associated with rupture of the transverse ligament. *J Bone Joint Surg Am* 1978;60:279–284.
63. Hadley MN, Browner C, Sonntag VK. Axis fractures: a comprehensive review of management and treatment in 107 cases. *Neurosurgery* 1985;17:281–290.
64. Apfelbaum RI, Lonser RR, Veres R, et al. Direct anterior screw fixation for recent and remote odontoid fractures. *J Neurosurg* 2000;93:227–236.
65. Gallie WE. Fractures and dislocation of the cervical spine. *Am J Surg* 1939;46:495–499.
66. Brooks AL, Jenkins EB. Atlanto-axial arthrodesis by the wedge compression method *J Bone Joint Surg Am* 1978;60:279–284.
67. Grob D, Magerl F. Surgical stabilization of C1 and C2 fractures (German), *Orthopade* 1987;16:46–54.
68. Harms J, Melcher RP. Posterior C1-C2 fusion with polyaxial screw and rod fixation. *Spine* 2001;26:2467–2471.
69. Caspar W, Barbier DD, Klara PM. Anterior cervical fusion and Caspar plate stabilization for cervical trauma. *Neurosurgery* 1989;25:491–502.
70. Triantafyllou SJ, Gertzbein SD. Flexion distraction injuries of the thoracolumbar spine: a review. *Orthopedics* 1992;15:357–364.
71. Tyroch AH, McGuire EL, McLean SF, et al. The association between Chance fractures and intra-abdominal injuries revisited: a multicenter review. *Am Surg* 2005;71:434–438.
72. Mulpuri K, Reilly CW, Perdios A, et al. The spectrum of abdominal injuries associated with Chance fractures in pediatric patients. *Eur J Pediatr Surg* 2007;17:322–327.
73. Clinical practice guidelines: prevention of thromboembolism in spinal cord injury. *J Spinal Cord Med* 1997;20:259–283.
74. Geerts WH, Pineo GF, Heit JA, et al. Prevention of venous thromboembolisms: the seventh ACCP conference on antithrombotic and thrombolytic therapy. Chest 2004;126(Suppl 3):338s–400s.
75. Duperier T, Mosenthal A, Swan KG, et al. Acute complications associated with greenfield filter insertion in high-risk trauma patients. *J Trauma* 2003;54:545–549.
76. PREPIC Study Group. Eight year follow up of patients with permanent vena cava filters in the prevention of pulmonary embolism: The PREPIC randomized study. *Circulation* 2005;112:416–422.

CHAPTER 8 ■ PREDICTING OUTCOME FOLLOWING TRAUMATIC SPINAL CORD INJURY

ANTHONY S. BURNS, RALPH J. MARINO, ADAM E. FLANDERS, JOHN KRAMER, HEATHER FLETT, AND ARMIN CURT

INTRODUCTION

Understanding and establishing prognosis is central to the delivery of effective and efficient rehabilitation following traumatic spinal cord injury (SCI). As patients emerge mentally and emotionally from the acute phase of their injury, they begin to question how their lives will be impacted. Patients want to know whether they will be able to walk, work, perform self-care activities, achieve sexual intimacy, and have children. It is the responsibility of the SCI clinician to accurately convey information about prognosis and, in partnership with the patient, develop goals compatible with anticipated recovery.

Patients, family members, and health care providers also need accurate information to begin the process of planning for postdischarge care and identifying required resources. As resources for health care become increasingly scarce, clinicians are often asked to justify the appropriateness of medical and rehabilitation interventions to third-party payers. In order to serve as effective advocates, clinicians need to be familiar with the literature on neurological recovery following SCI.

Current and future efforts to move SCI rehabilitation forward also require a firm understanding of the nature and extent of natural recovery following SCI. In the absence of such an understanding, it will be impossible to differentiate therapeutic effects from natural recovery and confirm the efficacy of new interventions. For these reasons, it is imperative that we continue to advance our understanding of what determines natural recovery following SCI.

Therefore, with the overarching goal of providing the reader with a broad overview of prognosis and outcomes following SCI, this chapter reviews the variables that impact the performance of an accurate neurological assessment, describes the magnitude and timing of natural recovery following traumatic SCI, clarifies the outlook for specific outcomes such as ambulation, summarizes the role of imaging and clinical neurophysiology, and concludes with a brief overview of the underlying mechanisms of recovery.

ASSESSING INJURY SEVERITY FOLLOWING TRAUMATIC SCI

The determination of prognosis and expected outcomes is predicated on performing an accurate examination according to the International Standards for Neurological Classification of SCI (1) (see Chapter 6 for details). The most important determinant of long-term prognosis is whether an injury is clinically complete or incomplete. The International Standards define SCI as complete when there is a complete absence of sensory and motor function in the lowest sacral segment ("sacral sparing"). This has been shown to be the most reliable and clinically useful definition (2). In comparison, an incomplete injury is characterized by the presence of "sacral sparing" (sensory and/or motor function at S4-5). This definition is intuitive in that in order for sacral sparing to be present, some signals have traversed the entire length of the spinal cord as would be expected with an incomplete block. After it has been determined whether the injury is complete or incomplete, injury severity is graded using the American Spinal Injury Association Impairment Scale (AIS) (see Chapter 6).

Relationship Between Timing of Assessment and Prognosis

Often, the question is raised as to whether or not an accurate assessment can be performed in the early stages after injury. Stauffer (3) cautioned against making a prognosis during spinal shock. Most clinicians characterize spinal shock as the absence of reflexes; however, it is rare for individuals to be admitted with the absence of all reflexes (4). In actuality, the evolution of reflexes following injury may be more relevant to prognosis than the term *spinal shock* and the accompanying presence or absence of reflexes (4). As an example, the emergence and persistence of a delayed plantar response (DPR) is associated with a particularly poor prognosis for ambulation (4).

Admittedly, examinations performed in the emergency room can be difficult and may lead to error; however, it is still important to perform an examination as soon as possible for documentation purposes, and to establish a baseline for monitoring improvement or decline in neurological status. When performing an assessment in this context, the assessor should be aware that there are factors that can affect the accuracy of an early examination. Burns et al. (5) assessed factors that affect the reliability of the initial assessment, when performed within 1 to 2 days of injury. There was a higher rate of conversion (complete to incomplete), at both 1 week and 1 year after injury, in patients who had one or more of the following factors: (a) mechanical ventilation; (b) intoxication, chemical sedation, or paralysis; (c) closed head injury; (d) psychiatric illness; (e) language barrier; (f) severe pain; or (g) cerebral palsy. None of the clinically complete patients without these factors converted to motor incomplete by 1 year, while 13% (3/23) of patients with at least one factor did. The results suggest that the risk of misclassification is higher when there are variables present that limit reliable communication and participation by the subject.

For the purposes of long-term prognostication, it has been recommended that the neurological examination be performed at least 72 hours after injury (6), as prior studies suggest that the 72-hour examination is superior to the first day examination (7,8). This baseline has been utilized in several studies examining recovery following SCI (9–11). Another common baseline interval for predicting recovery is 1-month postinjury (12–15). Historically, the 1-month time point corresponded closely with the timing of admission to a rehabilitation facility, but recently managed care and medical reform in the United States have led to shorter lengths of stay for acute hospitalization. Regardless, when determining prognosis, the clinician should be aware of the baseline utilized in the medical literature being referenced (16,17). The reliability of the examination is detailed in Chapter 6. Given the likelihood that future pharmacological and surgical trials will require early intervention postinjury (within 12 to 24 hours), further studies are needed to validate the reliability of the early examination.

NATURAL RECOVERY FOLLOWING TRAUMATIC SCI

Complete SCI

Conversion ("Complete" to "Incomplete")

People with complete SCI are classified as AIS grade A. In this subset of patients, recovery of motor function distal to the zone of injury is uncommon, and when it does occur tends to be minimal and nonfunctional. One study using data from the U.S. Model Spinal Cord Injury System found that 13% of AIS grade A patients admitted within 1 week of injury converted to incomplete status by 1 year (18). However, only 2.3% of initially complete patients progressed to AIS grade D, where the majority of muscles below the injury level had antigravity or greater strength. Compared to the Model Systems study, two studies using a 1-month baseline examination reported complete (AIS A; Fig. 8.1) to incomplete (AIS B, C, D) conversion rates ranging from 4% to 10% (12,13). As expected, conversion rates were lower for the studies using 1-month baseline examinations, as conversions occurring 0 to 30 days postinjury would not be captured.

Recent literature has reported higher rates of conversion between initial and follow-up examinations. A comprehensive review of the existing literature by the International Campaign for Cures of Spinal Cord Injury Paralysis (ICCP) reported a conversion rate of approximately 20% at 1 year postinjury, with 10% converting to AIS B and an additional 10% regaining some volitional motor function (AIS C and D) (19). In the same report, it was noted that the conversion rate of AIS A to AIS B or D was twice as high for tetraplegics compared to paraplegics. The reasons for this are unclear; however, possibilities include compromised communication with tetraplegics (e.g., intubation) or greater mechanical force associated with trauma to the thoracic spine. A recent evaluation of the European Multicenter study about Spinal Cord Injury (EMSCI) reported that 70% of persons presenting as AIS A (within 15 days) remained AIS A at 1 year, with 17.3% improving to AIS B, 5.8% to AIS C, and 7.2% to AIS D (20). It is interesting but unclear why recent studies have reported have higher rates of conversion from complete to incomplete injury. In the only study of late conversion (after the 1-year time frame), 5.6% (32/571) of complete injuries exhibited conversion between 1 and 5 years postinjury (21), though it should be noted that only six individuals showed "functional" recovery (AIS D) and there was evidence that three were likely coded incorrectly.

As discussed above, the circumstances and reliability of the neurological assessment also impact conversion rates. One study (5) reported a complete to incomplete conversion rate of 11.3% (6/53) by 1 year postinjury. Three subjects regained sacral sparing of sensation (AIS B) and three subjects regained volitional motor function below the zone of injury, two to AIS C and one to AIS D. However, when analysis excluded sub-

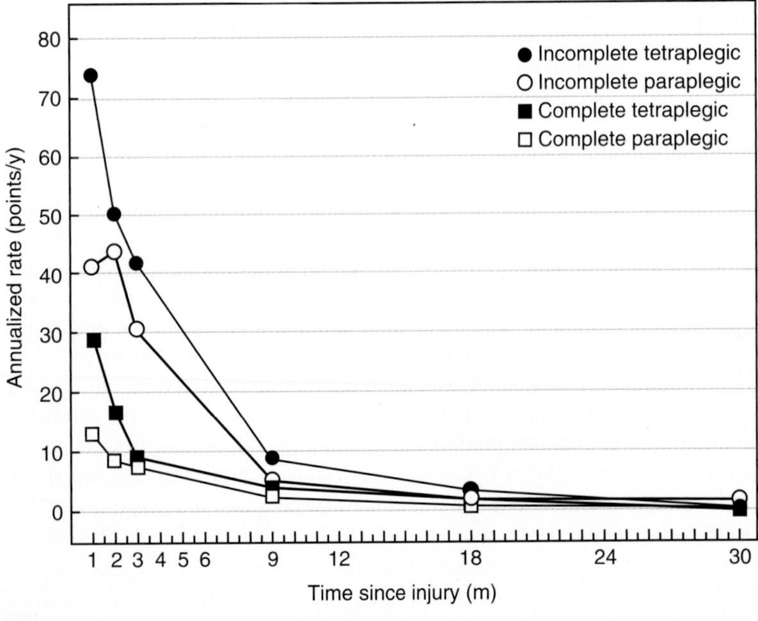

FIGURE 8.1. Recovery rates of ASIA motor scores for persons with incomplete and complete paraplegia and tetraplegia based on neurological classification at 1 month. (Copyright 1998 by Eastern Paralyzed Veterans Association; Reprinted from Water RL, Adkins R, Yakura J, et al. Donald Munro Lecture: functional and neurologic recovery following acute SCI. *J Spinal Cord Med* 1998;21:195–199. with permission.)

jects with factors that could affect exam reliability, only 2 of 30 individuals (6.7%) converted from complete to incomplete status, with both subjects improving to AIS grade B; motor function remained absent below the zone of injury in all subjects. In comparison, for the subjects with factors affecting exam reliability, 4 of 23 (17.4%) individuals converted from complete to incomplete, with three subjects developing volitional motor function (AIS grade C or D) by 1 year.

Magnitude of Neurorecovery (Tetraplegia)

In the context of complete tetraplegia, the chance of motor recovery in the lower extremities (LE) is low (less than 10%) if the patient remains motor and sensory complete for more than 1 month postinjury (13). In addition, when LE motor function develops, it is usually not functional. Despite this, recovery in the upper extremities (UE) is very important as this helps determine the level of functional independence with activities of daily living. In order for a muscle to have "useful" motor function, it is generally accepted that the muscle must have at least antigravity strength (≥grade 3 of 5).

One approach to predicting recovery is to determine the likelihood that the initial motor level will descend. In contrast to recovery below the zone of injury, most individuals with complete tetraplegia experience local recovery within two to three segments of the initial neurological level. In one study, it was observed that if motor strength was at least a grade 2 at a given motor level (C5—biceps) by 1 week postinjury, all patients eventually gained functional strength (≥3/5) at the next motor level (C6—extensor carpi radialis) (22). The majority of individuals with complete tetraplegia will gain at least one motor level, although there are differences dependent on the initial motor level. If the initial motor level is C4, 70% will gain C5 motor function; the corresponding rates for C5 to C6 and C6 to C7 are 75% and 85%, respectively (10). In a study of 24 motor complete C4 and C5 tetraplegics, Browne et al. (23) studied the relationship between the characteristics of sensory preservation at C5 and motor recovery in the adjacent C6 myotome (extensor carpi radialis). All subjects had initial ECR strength of less than 3/5. Fourteen of fifteen subjects with at least partial preservation of pinprick/light-touch discrimination at C5 recovered functional strength (≥3/5) in the extensor carpi radialis (C6), compared to two of nine subjects without C5 pinprick/light-touch discrimination.

Other studies have focused on the relationship between the initial strength in a muscle and the magnitude of long-term recovery in the same muscle. Studies in complete tetraplegia have found that greater than 90% of muscles presenting with grade 1/5 or 2/5 strength, 1 week to 1 month after injury, will eventually recover to ≥3/5 strength (13,24,25). In contrast, muscles with 0/5 strength 1 month after injury and located one neurological level below the most caudal level with motor function regained ≥3/5 strength in only 27% of cases at 1 year postinjury (13). Muscles two levels below the most caudal level with motor function (1 month postinjury) regained ≥3/5 strength in only 1% of cases. Finally, recovery is rare in muscles that are 0/5 at 1-month postinjury and more than two levels below the most caudal level with volitional motor function at 1 month, being seen in less than 1% of cases (13).

Magnitude of Neurorecovery (Paraplegia)

In comparison to tetraplegia, neurological status is relatively static following complete paraplegia. Using a 1-month baseline examination, Waters reported that in 73% (108/148) of individuals with paraplegia, the neurological level of injury (NLI) did not change at 1 year postinjury (12). Only two patients recovered greater than two levels. None of the patients with an initial neurological level above T9 regained LE motor function. In cases where active lower abdominal muscles were observed, 26% of hip flexors recovered to grade 3/5 or greater at 1 year. In a recent secondary analysis of data from the Sygen (GM1-ganglioside) multicenter trial, Harrop et al.(26) reported a median change of 1.48 points for pinprick (PP) and 1.40 for light touch (LT) at 1 year follow-up. Overall, greater than 70% of the sensory levels were unchanged from baseline assessment at 1 year postinjury.

Incomplete SCI

Magnitude of Neurorecovery

In comparison to complete injuries, recovery following incomplete injuries is often substantial. One multicenter study compared the descent of the motor level in complete and incomplete tetraplegics (10). Greater than 90% of incomplete injuries gained at least one additional motor level in the UEs compared to 70% to 85% of complete injuries. Waters prospectively studied recovery in incomplete tetraplegia and paraplegia using a 1-month baseline examination (14,15). Using the International Standards, he reported that the magnitude of LE recovery is relatively constant regardless of the initial NLI. As reviewed in Chapter 6, the International Standards identify five key muscles in each UE and five key muscles in each LE. Each muscle is graded from 1 to 5 and the maximum lower extremity motor score (LEMS) is 50 for the lower extremities. For incomplete tetraplegics and paraplegics, there was approximately a 12- to 14-point increase in LEMS from 1-month to 1-year postinjury and minimal additional improvement during year 2. The exception being sensory incomplete tetraplegics without sharp/dull discrimination, who failed to demonstrate any lower extremity motor recovery. For tetraplegics, UE motor scores improved 11 points during year 1 with little additional improvement by 2 years postinjury. A recent study from the EMSCI reported relative recovery for incomplete AIS grades (27). Relative recovery is the percentage of possible recovery observed and is based on the initial assessment. It is calculated using the equation: follow-up composite motor score–baseline composite motor score/maximum possible composite motor score–baseline composite motor score. In accordance with the International Standards, the maximum possible composite motor scores are 100 points for tetraplegia and 50 points for paraplegia. Relative recovery was as follows: AIS B (tetra = 24%, para = 30%), AIS C (tetra = 63%, para = 58%), and AIS D (tetra = 73%, para = 67%).

Waters studies also described the relationship between the strength of individual muscles at 1 month and the long-term recovery (14,15). In incomplete paraplegia, 85% of muscles that were 1/5 or 2/5 at 1 month recovered to ≥3/5 by 1 year. In comparison, for muscles that were 0/5 at 1 month, 55% (117/212) recovered some volitional control, but only 26% (55/212) recovered "motor useful" (≥3/5) function. The study on incomplete tetraplegia found a similar relationship between strength present at 1 month and magnitude of long-term recovery (14).

Specific Syndromes (See Chapter 6 for Details)

The anterior cord syndrome is characterized by the relative preservation of light-touch and proprioception in the absence of volitional motor function and the ability to differentiate pinprick and light touch. The syndrome predominantly affects the spinothalamic (pain and temperature) and the corticospinal (motor) tracts, both located in the anterior two thirds of the human spinal cord, while sparing the posterior columns (light touch and proprioception). Motor recovery is poor in these individuals in comparison to other incomplete patients (9,14,28). Central cord syndrome is characterized by disproportionately more motor impairment in the upper compared to the LE. Prior studies have reported that 57% to 86% of patients with this syndrome will ambulate independently (29,30). Penrod et al. (31) assessed the impact of age in central cord syndrome and noted that 97% (29/30) of patients younger than 50 years of age ambulated compared to 41% (7/17) of patients older than 50 years. In another study of central cord syndrome, Foo (32) reported that only 31% of patients ambulated, although the mean age of study subjects was 65 years, providing further evidence for the importance of age. Brown-Sequard syndrome is due to injury to predominantly one side of the cord. This results in ipsilateral loss of proprioception and volitional motor function and contralateral loss of pin (pain) and temperature. The prognosis is also favorable with this syndrome and almost all patients will ambulate successfully (29,31,33). It has been theorized that uncrossed axons in the contralateral cord facilitate recovery (34).

Timing of Recovery

Following incomplete and complete SCI, the majority of neurological recovery occurs during the first 6 to 9 months (Fig. 8.2) (12–15,25,35). Afterward, the rate of improvement rapidly drops off with a plateau being reached 12 to 18 months postinjury with little additional improvement. Early improvement in neurological status is also associated with greater recovery than slow improvement (36). Late recovery following complete SCI, defined as motor recovery after 1 year after injury, can occur but is generally of small magnitude and nonfunctional (21).

Patterns of Reflex Recovery following SCI

Ko et al. (4) described the pattern of reflex recovery following SCI and its implications for prognosis. In most cases, the DPR is the first reflex observed followed by the bulbocaver-

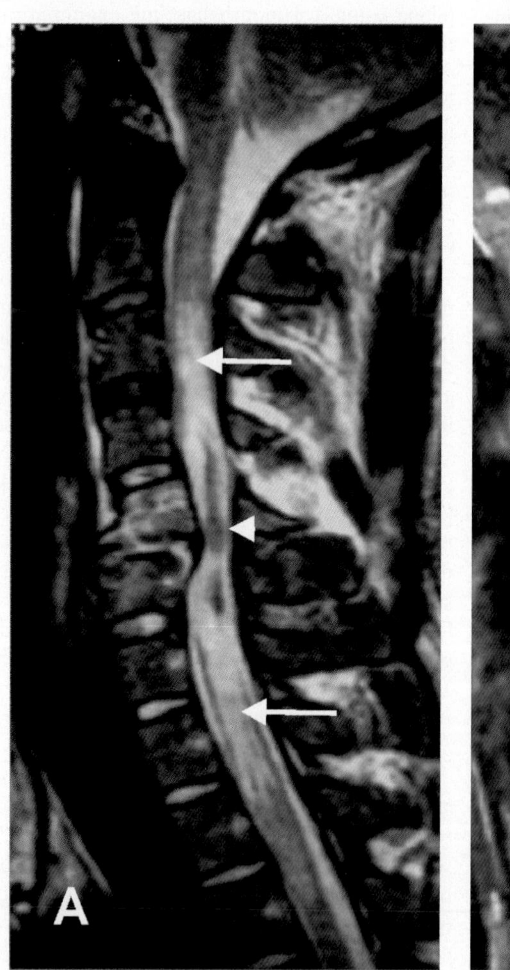

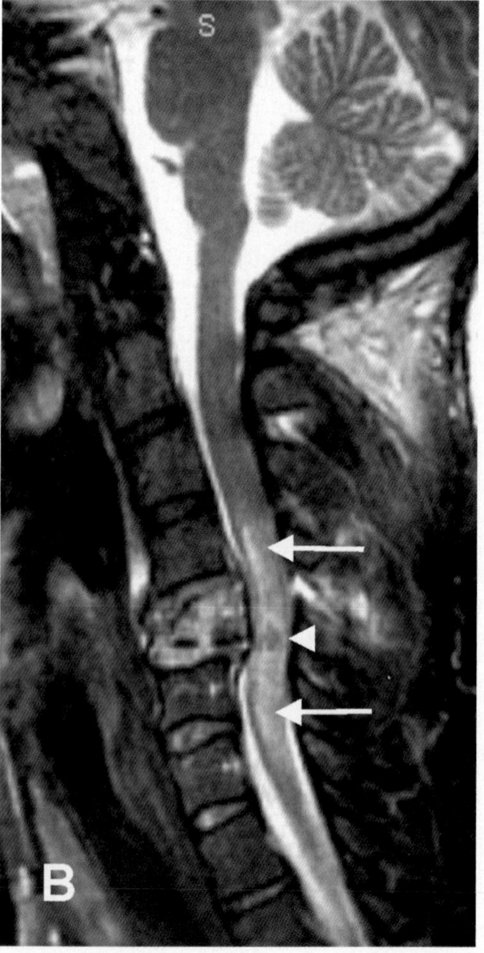

FIGURE 8.2. Representative magnetic resonance (MR) imaging for two SCI patients with clinically complete cervical spinal cord injuries (AIS A). **A:** T2-weighted sagittal MR image in a 20-year-old male. **B:** T2-weighted sagittal MR image in a 29-year-old. Both individuals had significant intramedullary hemorrhage, which is associated with clinically complete injury. *Arrowheads*, intramedullary hemorrhage, *arrows*, intramedullary edema.

nosus and cremasteric, respectively, within the first few days of injury. Deep tendon reflexes such as ankle jerks and knee jerks reemerge 1 to 2 weeks postinjury. The DPR is a transient and pathologic reflex unmasked by severe SCI, and it gradually dissipates with the emergence of the Babinski sign. The DPR is evoked by stroking with a blunt instrument upward from the heel toward the toes along the lateral sole of the foot, then continuing medially across the volar aspect of the metatarsal heads. Afterward, the toes flex and relax in a delayed fashion. It was present in 31/31 complete injuries (versus 9/22 incomplete injuries) and persisted for an average duration of 14.3 days. The DPR has particular value as a prognostic indicator. In 24/31 complete subjects, the DPR persisted greater than 7 days, whereas only one incomplete subject manifested a DPR for greater than 7 days.

Calancie et al. (37) systematically studied recovery of deep tendon reflexes in 229 subjects with acute SCI. Several novel findings were described. Without exception, the crossed adductor was never observed in individuals who remained motor complete. In contrast, only three individuals with motor incomplete and cervical SCI failed to demonstrate the crossed adductor response when follow-up exceeded 12 weeks. For two of these subjects, volitional motor function was limited to the abductor hallucis muscle (toe flexion) of one foot. The presence of the crossed adductor response therefore accurately predicted the preservation of axons spanning the injury site. For the duration of follow-up, amplitudes of deep tendon reflexes were diminished in motor-complete compared to motor-incomplete subjects. Using a combination of deep tendon reflex amplitudes and the presence or absence of crossed adductor response, the investigators were able to identify with 100% accuracy which individuals would remain motor complete.

Ambulation Following SCI (See Chapter 17 for Details)

Prognostic Indicators

Not surprisingly, injury severity is an important predictor of walking post-SCI. Individuals with complete injuries (AIS A) rarely walk (8,12,13), and when they do, it often requires the use of cumbersome orthoses, prohibitive energy expenditure, and is thus not sustained long term (38,39). Individuals who present with sensory incomplete SCI (AIS B) have a better prognosis for walking, although there is still considerable variability; 20% to 50% of individuals initially classified as AIS B recover the ability to walk by 1 year (8,9,40–42). For AIS B injuries, the nature of sensory sparing is important (9,40,42). In one study of 27 individuals with AIS B SCI, 8 of 9 individuals with partial preservation of pinprick/light-touch discrimination (within 24 hours of injury) became functional ambulators at rehabilitation discharge, compared to 2 of 18 individuals with only light-touch preservation (9). The largest study (n = 131) of AIS B injuries to date, a secondary analysis of the Sygen (GM1-ganglioside) trial, confirmed the prognostic value of pinprick preservation (42). Both sacral (S4-5) pinprick preservation at 4 weeks postinjury and baseline LE pinprick preservation were associated with an improved prognosis for walking. Forty percent of individuals with LE pinprick preservation were functional ambulators at 1 year compared to 16% of individuals without.

The initial presence of motor function below the neurological level postinjury is also a positive predictor for walking. Burns et al. (43) studied the relationship between initial AIS grade (≤72 hours postinjury) and ambulation in individuals with motor-incomplete tetraplegia. They found that 67% of AIS C and 100% of AIS D patients were able to walk by rehabilitation discharge. Recently, the relationship between AIS grade at rehabilitation admission and walking outcomes at discharge has also been examined. Similar trends were found with 15% of AIS B, 28% to 40% of AIS C, and 67% to 75% of AIS D patients able to walk at discharge (44,45).

The extent of LE motor function is also a strong predictor of walking (15,46–48). Waters et al. (15,46) found that 1-month LEMS correlated closely with walking status at 1 year. In fact, 87% of incomplete tetraplegics and 100% of incomplete paraplegics who had LEMS ≥10 by 1 month were community ambulators at 1 year. They also demonstrated that incomplete paraplegics who initially had ≥2/5 hip flexor or knee extensor strength in one leg regained sufficient motor recovery in other musculature to enable community walking by 1 year. Achieving ≥3/5 knee extensor strength within 2 months has also been shown to predict functional ambulation at 6 months (49).

A recent report from the EMSCI initiative evaluated the prognostic value of sacral sparing during the acute phase for independent ambulation during the chronic phase (50). For sacral sparing criteria, the presence of deep anal sensation (acute phase) did not contribute significantly to the prognosis of long-term walking, whereas preservation of LT and PP at S4-5 as well as voluntary anal contraction did.

The specific level of injury does not necessarily predict walking ability (45); however, distinctions have been found between paraplegic and tetraplegic individuals. To achieve comparable walking function, tetraplegics require greater LEMS compared to paraplegics (51). Ambulation rates at 1 and 2 years postinjury are also higher for incomplete paraplegics versus incomplete tetraplegics (76% versus 46%) (14,15). This has been attributed to greater trunk muscle and upper extremity impairments in tetraplegics and therefore a reduced ability to utilize ambulation aids.

Age also impacts walking prognosis. As described above, 97% of individuals with central cord syndrome who are less than age 50 walked at discharge compared to only 41% ≥ age 50 (31). In another study of incomplete tetraplegics, older AIS C individuals (≥ age 50) were again less likely to walk at rehabilitation discharge (42% versus 91%) (43). Kay (45) did not find the same age effect with AIS C individuals; however, individuals over age 50 with AIS D injuries were less likely to walk at discharge (55% versus 79%).

Determinants of Walking following an SCI

Understanding the key determinants and characteristics of walking in SCI helps predict not only the likelihood but also the extent of walking. Given that walking is a complex task, it should be considered along a continuum from several perspectives and not dichotomously. Determinants of walking are factors that allow an individual to walk and navigate safely and efficiently in such a way that when the factor becomes insufficient it prevents or limits walking (52,53). The characteristics of the patient population influence which determinants are most significant. Following SCI, the majority of walking determinants relate to injury severity, particularly the extent of LE motor function; however, other common impairments such as spasticity, balance, and proprioception also play a role in walking ability, yet their relative contributions are not known.

There is strong evidence that lower extremity motor function is not only an important predictor of walking outcome but also a major determinant of walking status at a given point in time. Both composite and individual muscle strength scores have been shown to correlate with walking status. Several authors have demonstrated significant relationships between LEMS and walking status (46,54,55). Individuals with LEMS ≤ 20 were limited household ambulators meaning they walked slower, with increased heart rate and energy expenditure and greater peak axial load on assistive devices, whereas a LEMS ≥ 30 was associated with community ambulation (46). Proximal LE muscle strength is particularly important (39). Significant correlations have been demonstrated between composite scores of proximal LE muscles and walking outcomes such as the Timed Up & Go, 6-minute walk test, and the 10-m walk tests (54). Kim et al. (55) found that proximal muscle strength, particularly of the less affected side, was an important determinant of walking ability. Specifically, strength of the less affected hip flexor accounted for 50% of the variance in walking speed and 6-minute walk distance, whereas the strength of the less affected hip extensors accounted for 64% of community ambulatory capacity. In contrast to previous studies (39,49), knee extensor strength was not related to ambulatory capacity although the generally high knee extensor strength of these subjects (≥3/5) likely accounts for this difference.

In the normal gait and stroke literature (56), truncal control has been identified as being very important for walking, yet in SCI, little data exist to support this empiric notion. This is likely due to the omission of trunk muscle function from the International Standards as well as the complexity of measuring the function of these muscles. Balance is also very important following SCI. In a recent study by Scivoletto et al. (54), the Berg Balance Scale was the only significant predictor of walking ability in individuals with chronic SCI, as measured using the Walking Index for Spinal Cord Injury and the 6-minute walk. In fact, compared to LEMS, balance had higher correlations to all walking tests. In this same study, spasticity was found to negatively affect walking speed and Timed Up & Go performance. Other authors have also found an inverse relationship between spasticity and walking (39,57). Finally, impairments in LE proprioception are common following SCI and have been found to impact walking (39,58).

Walking ability in individuals with SCI is highly heterogeneous; however, several common characteristics have been identified. Studies have found that individuals with SCI walk slower (59,60), have less capacity to increase walking speed (61), walk less efficiently (59,60,62), and require greater attentional demand (63). Consideration also needs to be given to the broad range of factors influencing community walking such as assistance required (physical and assistive devices) and the ability to generate sufficient speed (1.06 to 1.22 m/s) to cross a street (60), manage curbs and uneven terrain, and walk sufficient distances (342 m) in the community (64). In summary, walking is a common goal following SCI, which can be attained by certain individuals depending on the severity of their injury, extent of lower extremity motor function, age, and other impairments. It is important to consider the key predictors, determinants, and characteristics of walking in SCI in order to provide accurate and comprehensive information to patients, families, and others.

Relationship of Injury Level to Functional Outcomes

In 1955, Long (65) related functional capacity to level of injury. In the interim, others have also documented a relationship between injury level and eventual functional outcomes (66,67). To further assist clinicians, the Consortium for Spinal Cord Medicine published clinical practice guidelines summarizing expected outcomes following traumatic SCI (68). For the purpose of describing expected function, it has been shown that motor level is superior to the single neurological level (11). Outcomes by level of injury are detailed in Chapter 17.

THE ROLE OF IMAGING FOR PROGNOSIS AND FUNCTIONAL RECOVERY

Magnetic resonance imaging (MRI) has contributed more than any other imaging modality to our understanding of natural history following SCI, and the clarity with which MRI is able to depict the anatomy of the spinal cord is unmatched. Specifically, MRI has made it possible to assess intracanalicular and paraspinal soft tissues, including the spinal cord itself (69–79). Despite this, the clinical indications for performing an MRI evaluation of the spine in the setting of trauma are controversial, and in the absence of a neurological deficit, the routine use of MRI may be unwarranted. MRI, however, is helpful in the acute period for excluding occult ligamentous/soft tissue injury, vertebral thrombosis, and for confirmation of bone injury age. MRI has also been used to exclude a neurological injury in uncooperative, obtunded, or malingering patients. There is unequivocal agreement that an MRI examination in the acute period is warranted in any patient who has a persistent neurological deficit following spinal trauma (75,76,80).

MRI Findings of SCI

MRI allows clinicians to visualize intramedullary hemorrhage and edema. In animal studies, the combination of MRI lesion length, cord caliber, and extent of white matter preservation (in cross section) has been shown to be related to both functional status and pathologic findings at autopsy (81–83). The MRI appearance of experimentally induced SCI has also been used to explain the variability in functional deficit among animals subjected to identical injuries (81).

Spinal Cord Hemorrhage

Posttraumatic spinal cord hemorrhage (i.e., hemorrhagic contusion) is defined as the presence of a discrete focus of hemorrhage within the substance of the spinal cord (intramedullary). The most common location is within the central gray matter of the spinal cord, centered at the point of mechanical impact (70,72,74,78,84,85). Drawing from experimental and autopsy studies, the underlying lesion is most often hemorrhagic necrosis of the spinal cord. True hematomyelia is rare (85).

Immediately following injury, deoxygenated hemoglobin (deoxyhemoglobin) is the most common hemoglobin species generated (70,72,75,78,85–87). The presence of deoxyhemoglobin in the spinal cord substance is depicted on high field strength scanners as a discrete area of hypointensity on T2-weighted and gradient echo images (69–72,74,78,80,84,87,88). These findings represent hemorrhagic necrosis of the spinal cord (72,74,89,90). Free radicals and oxidative stress in the lesion site eventually cause deoxyhemoglobin to evolve to methemoglobin, a form of hemoglobin unable to carry oxygen, which is characterized by the iron in the heme group being in the Fe^{3+} state as opposed to the normal Fe^{2+} state. In the brain, methemoglobin appears approximately 3 to 5 days after an initial hemorrhage. In the spinal cord, conversion to intracellular methemoglobin may be delayed for 8 days or more following injury, due to local hypoxia/hypoperfusion and delayed degradation of deoxyhemoglobin. After conversion to methemoglobin, the hemorrhagic component of the SCI is depicted as increased signal on T1-weighted images.

Parenchymal hemorrhage likely develops rapidly in the spinal cord after injury. In animal models, hemorrhage was found in 12.5% of the cross-sectional area of the lesion epicenter initially, increasing exponentially to approximately 25% of the epicenter cross section within hours of injury (91). The rate of change in volume of hemorrhage was initially 0.15% per minute, with a maximal rate of 45% per minute within 5 hours after injury.

Spinal Cord Edema

Spinal cord edema is defined on MRI as a focus of abnormal high signal intensity on T2-weighted images (80). This signal abnormality is thought to reflect a focal accumulation of intracellular and interstitial fluid in response to injury (71,72,74–77,79,80,92,93). Extent of edema is best defined using the midsagittal long TR image. Axial T2-weighted images offer supplemental information regarding the involvement of specific structures in cross section. Edema typically involves a variable length of spinal cord above and below the level of injury, with discrete boundaries adjacent to uninvolved parenchyma. Spinal cord edema is invariably associated with some degree of spinal cord swelling. Posttraumatic spinal cord hemorrhage always coexists with spinal cord edema; however, the converse is not always true, that is, edema can occur without MRI evidence of intramedullary hemorrhage. In the setting of trauma, edema within the spinal cord has been referred to as a contusion or a hemorrhagic contusion when blood products are present (84,86,88,90,94). Cord edema alone connotes a more favorable prognosis than cord hemorrhage (74,84,94–96).

Factors affecting the length of spinal cord edema include age and the time from injury to imaging. Patient age is inversely proportional to length of spinal cord edema (97), while time to imaging is directly proportional to edema length. In patients with complete cervical SCI, length of spinal cord edema increases approximately one vertebral segment every 30 hours during the first 72 hours postinjury (98). While it is not known how long it takes for edema to first develop after traumatic SCI, following cerebral infarction, it takes approximately 6 hours to detect signal abnormalities on T2-weighted images. Recently, Aoyama et al. (99) described a patient who fell and sustained a complete SCI at the C4 level. An MRI taken 120 minutes after injury had no signal changes in the cord on T1- or T2-weighted images. A postoperative MRI 8 hours after injury detected increased signal on T2-weighted images in the same area where intraoperative ultrasound indicated a hyperechoic lesion.

Clinical Significance of Spinal Cord MRI Findings

The anatomic location of the hemorrhage corresponds closely to the neurologic level of injury (NLI), and the presence of intramedullary hemorrhage implies a poor prognosis (70,72,74,84,87,95,100) (see Figure 8.2). Boghosian et al. (101) found that the upper boundary of hemorrhage showed a stronger correlation to the NLI than either the upper boundary of edema or the lesion epicenter. Use of multiple regression analysis suggested that the combination of lesion epicenter and edema length was the best predictor of NLI (101). Patients with Brown-Sequard syndrome following blunt cervical trauma often have edema limited to the hemicord on the side of greater weakness (102). Patients with central cord syndrome typically have evidence of cord edema but not hemorrhage at the level of injury (103). Therefore, MRI measures may be used as an objective measure of the NLI and can suggest the pattern and severity of injury when determination by clinical examination is not possible.

The imaging parameters associated with neurological deficit and prognosis are spinal cord hemorrhage, spinal cord edema, and spinal cord compression. Using multiple regression analysis, Flanders et al. (104) assessed the utility of MRI for predicting motor function independent of the initial clinical evaluation. Initial motor scores, the presence of hemorrhage, and the length of edema were independent predictors of final motor score and the proportion of muscles with useful function at 1 year. The addition of MRI parameters to the initial clinical information improved the predictive power of the model by 16% for the UE and 34% for the LE.

Spinal Cord Hemorrhage

It was initially thought that detection of intramedullary hemorrhage was predictive of a complete SCI (72). However, the increased sensitivity and spatial resolution of current MRI techniques has shown that small amounts of hemorrhage are identifiable in incomplete lesions. Subsequently, it has been shown that the severity of neurological deficits is determined by the extent of cord edema and cord hemorrhage, in addition to presence or absence (88). Therefore, the basic construct has been altered such that the detection of a sizable focus of blood (greater than 10 mm in length on sagittal images) in the spinal cord is typically indicative of a complete neurological injury (94). Recently, Boldin et al. (105) found that patients with hemorrhages, which measured greater than 4 mm in cranial-caudal length, showed no clinical improvement at follow-up. Patients with hemorrhages measuring less than 4 mm had incomplete injuries and showed clinical improvement at follow-up. While the number of subjects was small and the authors were unable to control for time to clinical follow-up or time to imaging, their data suggest that there may be an absolute threshold for lesion size that predicts neurological recovery.

Schaefer et al. (106) correlated the appearance of the admission MRI to change in total motor scores. Tetraplegic patients with hemorrhagic lesions failed to show significant improvement in motor scores at follow-up. In a similar study of 24 tetraplegic subjects, Marciello et al. (95) correlated the presence or absence of intramedullary hemorrhage to changes in upper and lower extremity motor scores. For patients with spinal cord hemorrhage, only 16% of upper extremity muscles and 3% of lower extremity muscles improved to a useful grade

(≥3/5) at follow-up, and only 7% of patients improved one or more motor levels. In comparison, for patients without MRI evidence of spinal cord hemorrhage, 73% of upper extremity and 74% of lower extremity muscles improved to a useful grade and 78% of subjects improved one or more levels.

Spinal Cord Edema

Cord edema alone connotes a more favorable prognosis than cord hemorrhage (74,84,94–96). In addition, the length of spinal cord edema is directly proportional to the initial neurological deficit (72,88). Schaefer et al. (88,106) reported that cord edema that extended for more than the span of one vertebral segment was associated with greater initial deficits than smaller areas of edema. These investigators also reported that patients with only edema had a greater improvement in total motor score compared to patients with hemorrhage. In addition, patients with small areas of edema (less than one vertebral segment in length) demonstrated the largest improvement in total motor score (72% recovery), whereas larger areas of edema showed less recovery (42%). This finding was confirmed by Flanders et al. (104) in a study of 104 cervical SCI patients followed for 1 year postinjury. Individual manual muscle test scores were recorded for the UE and LT at acute hospital admission and 12 months postinjury. Motor recovery rates for the upper and lower extremities were also determined. The injured spinal cord segment was measured using a unique method, which quantified spinal cord hemorrhage and edema relative to known anatomic landmarks. Lesion length was directly proportional to neurological impairment at the time of injury ($p < 0.001$). Nonhemorrhagic MRI (edematous) lesions were associated with higher motor recovery rates in the LE and UE and had a higher proportion of muscles with useful motor function.

Spinal Cord Compression

Silberstein et al. (100) reported that findings associated with severe spine trauma such as spinal fractures, subluxation, ligamentous injury, prevertebral swelling, and epidural hematoma were associated with severe clinical deficits at presentation and a poor prognosis. In contrast, Flanders et al. (72) found that the presence of fractures, disk herniation, and ligamentous injury was not predictive of the neurological deficit; however, the presence of residual spinal cord compression by bone, disc, or fluid was predictive of a hemorrhagic spinal cord lesion. Such findings suggest that residual compression may be an important factor in determining recovery and provide some support for the controversial concept of early decompression following SCI (69,72,107).

Clearly, there is a relationship between extent of spinal cord compression and neurological injury (108). Rao and Fehlings (109) performed a critical, evidence-based analysis of the existing literature. Reviewed studies contained both quantitative and qualitative assessments of the spinal canal and spinal cord dimensions. Preexisting midsagittal canal stenosis (developmental or congenital) was associated with a more severe neurological deficit following cervical injury, most notable when midsagittal canal diameter was 10 mm or less. In another study of cervical SCI, the anteroposterior diameter of the spinal canal was again smaller in patients with complete (10.5 mm) and incomplete injuries (13.1 mm) compared to patients with no deficits (16.7 mm) (110). Hayashi et al. (111) found that 30% of patients with severe spinal cord compression (defined as a 2/3 reduction in spinal cord diameter) had a complete motor deficit at the time of injury compared to 20% of patients with mild spinal cord compression (defined as less than 1/3 reduction in spinal cord diameter). More importantly, 90% of patients with mild spinal cord compression improved by one or more AIS grades compared to 30% for patients with severe spinal cord compression.

Recently, Miyanji et al. (112) used quantitative assessment to determine whether MRI correlated with initial neurological status and clinical outcomes in 100 consecutive cervical SCI patients. Complete motor and sensory deficits were associated with spinal cord compression and spinal canal compromise and a higher incidence of intramedullary hemorrhages, lesion length, soft tissue injury, stenosis, and cord swelling. Initial cord compression, intramedullary hemorrhage, and extent of cord swelling were predictive of poor neurological outcomes at follow-up. Interestingly the subjects with incomplete SCI (ASIA grade B, C, or D) or minimal deficits (ASIA grade E) had a mean lesion length of 20 mm or less, whereas those in the patients with complete injuries had a mean length of 40 mm.

Limitations of Conventional MRI in the Evaluation of Spinal Cord Injury

MRI is currently the best imaging modality for the evaluation of spinal cord parenchyma; however, it does not differentiate edema from axonal injury. While MRI provides valuable information about location and basic injury characteristics, water content (edema) and hemorrhage do not necessarily reflect axon integrity and function. This limitation is apparent in animal models of SCI. Following a spinal cord contusion in adult rats, there was no correlation between magnitude of neurological recovery and lesion size (volume), whether evaluated by T2-weighted abnormal signal (edema) or T2 hypointensity (hemorrhage) (93). In another study using adult rat spinal contusions, water content and T2 signal did not always change significantly in injured areas (113); therefore, conventional MRI techniques may underestimate the degree of injury. Additionally, some small areas of hemorrhage may not be visible on T2 images. The utility of imaging of chronic SCI has been limited to assessing posttraumatic syringomyelia and myelomalacia (114–119).

Advanced MRI techniques such as diffusion MRI, functional MRI (fMRI), and MR spectroscopy (MRS) could provide important information about function and axonal integrity of damaged spinal cord parenchyma. To date, however, the clinical application of these techniques has been limited. The technical challenges are substantial, specifically the small size of the spinal cord, its close proximity to bony structures, and reduction in image quality due to pulsation of cerebrospinal fluid and respiratory motion. Despite this, preliminary studies show promise (120–122); however, larger definitive studies are still needed to clarify the role of diffusion MRI for predicting function and neurological recovery.

THE ROLE OF NEUROPHYSIOLOGICAL TESTING FOLLOWING SCI

Following SCI, neurophysiological testing complements standard bedside clinical assessments by objectively assessing neural substrates and identifying underlying neuropathology (i.e., demyelination and degeneration). For patients who are unable to cooperate with the clinical examination, electrophysiological testing provides important information about the condition of the spinal cord. Currently, electrophysiological testing is not used to determine the appropriateness of surgical intervention following acute SCI, where, in any case, the primary goals are to alleviate spinal cord compression (e.g., spinal canal encroachment) and stabilize the spine (e.g., unstable vertebral fracture). Postoperative electrophysiological recordings can detect adverse changes in spinal cord or nerve function, and thereby stimulate further diagnostic testing (27).

With new therapeutic interventions on the horizon, there will be an increasing need for measures that (a) provide proof of specific mechanisms of recovery in humans (i.e., inducing repair and/or increased neural plasticity) and (b) are sensitive and responsive to change. While functional outcomes, such as ambulation, will be key endpoints for human SCI trials, such an emphasis will not explain the underlying neurophysiology of how an intervention induced a beneficial effect. For these reasons, neurophysiological testing will play an important and complementary role in future clinical study. The application of neurophysiological techniques to assess various characteristics of SCI pathology is summarized in Figure 8.3 and Table 8.1.

Evoked Potentials

Dorsal Columns

Electrical stimulation of mixed peripheral nerves and the recording of accompanying cortical responses, using electroencephalography, yield somatosensory evoked potentials (SSEPs). SSEPs are complementary to sensory and motor scores, and can help clinicians determine the prognosis for functional outcomes, such as ambulation (tibial), grasping (median/ulnar), and bladder and sexual function (pudendal) (47,123–129). SSEPs recorded during the early period after trauma also provide important information about the clinical completeness of SCI. While not routinely performed as part of the diagnostic workup following SCI, SSEPs are particularly useful in cases of possible conversion disorder, malingering, coma, etc. In the setting of tetraplegia, the absence of tibial and pudendal SSEPs corresponds reliably to a clinically complete injury (no preservation of sacral sensory function) in almost all patients. The findings are associated with very limited functional recovery below the NLI, similar to prognosis based on clinical examination.

Following incomplete SCI, amplitudes are reduced and latencies increased, findings that reflect sensitivity to partial

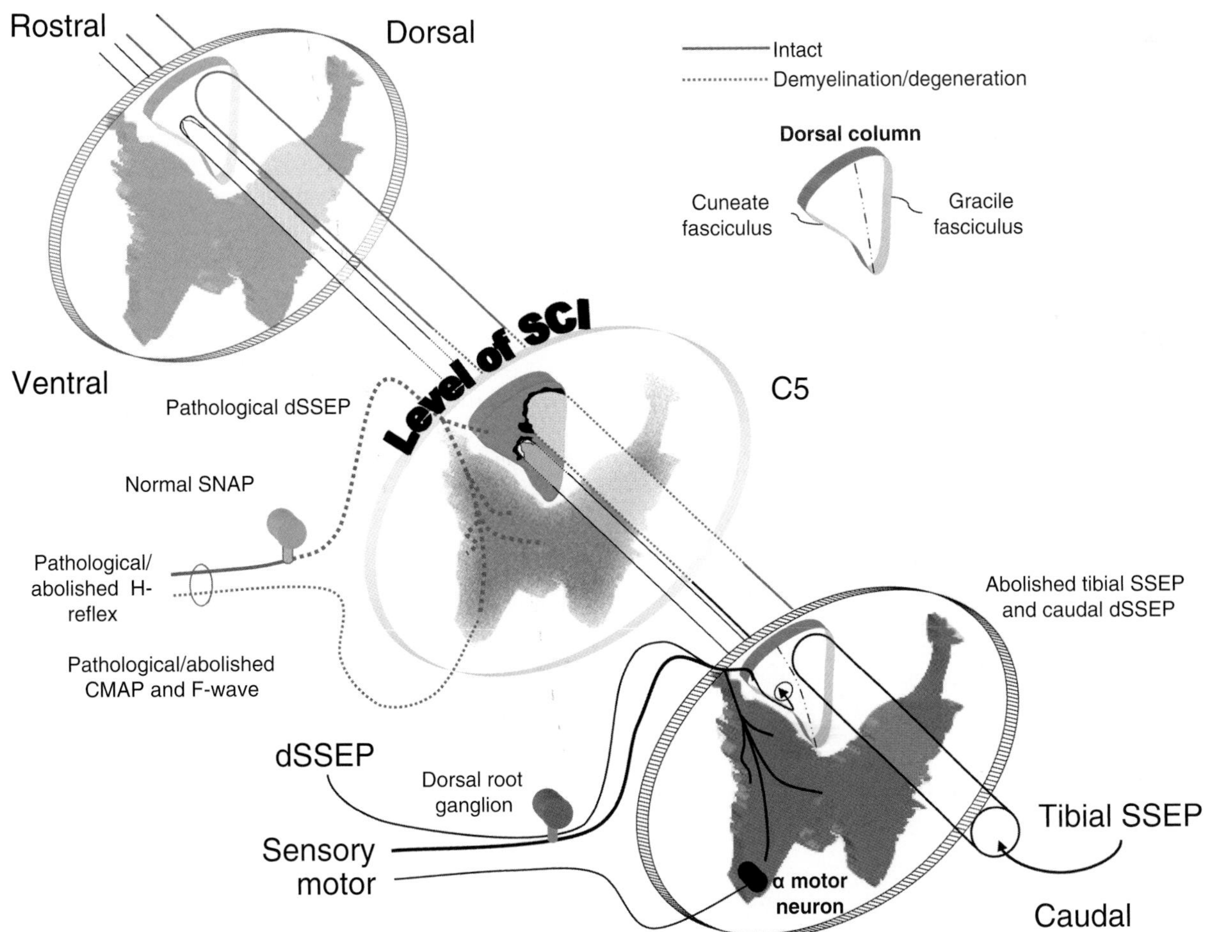

FIGURE 8.3. Segmental neurophysiological approaches, such as spinal reflexes, NCS, and dSSEPs, are important for describing pathology of nerve fibers near the level of SCI, whereas longitudinal, such as conventional evoked potential investigation (only SSEP shown here), provides information regarding the extent of disruption of ascending and descending nerves fibers through the injury. The application of both types of approaches may be necessary to address changes within spinal cord segments and across the level of injury. (*Note:* the dorsal root ganglion, unlike the alpha motor neuron, is outside of the spinal cord and therefore not prone to degeneration following spinal canal pathologies).

TABLE 8.1

FUNCTIONAL, CLINICAL, AND NEUROPHYSIOLOGICAL OUTCOMES OF LONGITUDINAL PATHWAYS AFFECTED BY SCI

	Pathological SCI outcomes		
Spinal cord tract	**Functional**	**Clinical (ISNCSCI)**	**Neurophysiological**
Dorsal column	Paresthesia	Absent/impaired light touch rating[a]	Abolished/increased SSEP onset latency
Corticospinal tract	Muscle weakness	Paralysis/reduced upper/lower limb motor score	Abolished/increased MEP central motor conduction time, reduced amplitude
Sympathetic nerve fibers	Autonomic dysreflexia and orthostatic hypotension	None	Abolished SSR
Spinothalamic tract	Thermoanesthesia, hypersensitivity/neuropathic pain	Absent/impaired pin prick rating[a]	Abolished/increased LEP/CHEPS onset latency

[a]According to patient perception.

ISNCSCI, International Standards for Neurological Classification of Spinal Cord Injury.

disruption and demyelination of axons ascending through the dorsal columns and traversing the injured segment. Normal SSEP latencies (tibial and pudendal) are associated with the functional recovery of ambulation in patients with tetraplegia and paraplegia. The presence of preserved latencies improves our ability to predict long-term ambulation and hand function (median and ulnar), in comparison to solely measuring motor scores in accordance with International Standards.

Corticospinal Tracts

Motor evoked potentials (MEPs) are induced in the motor cortex using transcranial magnetic stimulation, and the accompanying responses recorded in peripheral muscle using electromyography (EMG). Conduction times through the corticospinal tracts are markedly increased and amplitudes reduced by pathology in individuals with incomplete SCI. The relationship of MEP findings to prognosis for motor control and functional independence is similar to what has been described for SSEPs. MEP abnormalities of the abductor digiti minimi and anterior tibialis are associated with a poorer prognosis for functional recovery of hand function and ambulation, respectively, and the absence of MEPs below the NLI corresponds closely to complete SCI (49,130). MEPs are also helpful for diagnosing spinal cord syndromes, such as anterior cord syndrome, which is characterized by poor functional outcomes and complete motor paralysis. This is due to the fact that the injury is predominantly anterior, which corresponds to the anatomical location of the primary motor pathway, the corticospinal tract. As a result, MEPs may be absent or show marked abnormalities while SSEPs (dorsal columns) are comparatively preserved.

Spinothalamic Tracts

The future application of neurophysiological testing to small diameter axons in the spinothalamic tracts is promising. Such techniques could provide important insights into hypersensitivity and neuropathic pain beyond what can be obtained using alternative techniques (e.g., semiquantitative thermal sensory testing). Case reports have described subclinical pathology in individuals with SCI who have undergone testing using laser evoked potentials (LEPs) to assess small diameter C-fibers (131,132). The recent development of contact heat evoked potential stimulation (CHEPS), which utilizes rapid heating (70°C/s) and cooling (40°C/s), should further improve the clinical applicability of small diameter fiber evoked potentials by resolving safety concerns associated with LEPs (i.e., skin and eye burns). In SCI patients, CHEPS have been applied to assess the impairment of spinothalamic conduction at and below the level of lesion and to quantify changes in cortical responses to physiological heat stimuli (132).

Sympathetic Nerve Fibers

Sympathetic axons descending from supraspinal structures are also affected following SCI, compromising autonomic functions such as bowel, bladder, sexual, and cardiovascular control. The integrity of autonomic axons can be assessed via the Sympathetic Skin Response (SSR), which is induced by electrical stimulation and recorded using standard clinical EMG equipment. This noninvasive technique involves the application of an arousal stimulus (i.e., controlled electrical shock, loud noise, cold pressure, inspiratory gasp), which stimulates supraspinal autonomic control centers in the hypothalamus. Autonomic centers, in turn, evoke an electrodermal response in skin that can be recorded (133). Following SCI, an arousal stimulus (electrical) is applied above the NLI, and the presence or absence of the SSR is recorded using active electrodes placed on the palms or alternatively the feet (e.g., above and below the level of a thoracic SCI). The SSR is severely affected or abolished below the level of complete SCI among individuals who experience bouts of autonomic dysreflexia (134). The findings from these studies demonstrate the involvement of disrupted autonomic fibers in the development of autonomic dysreflexia. The sacral SSR is also a valuable neurophysiological method for predicting sexual and bladder function following SCI (135–138), and hence provides quantifiable parameters for important autonomic functions not considered by the International Standards.

Segmental Spinal Cord Innervation

The segmental neurophysiological assessment of the spinal cord is of considerable relevance because SCI is rarely constrained to one level; instead, involvement is typically diffuse and varies over multiple levels. Dermatomal somatosensory evoked potentials (dSSEPs) have been applied in individuals with SCI to study segmental innervation comprising the sensory afferents that enter the spinal cord via the posterior root, project into the dorsal horn, and ascend in the dorsal column (130,139). dSSEPs can assess the integrity of specific dermatomal levels and when applied over multiple radicular levels in a segmental rostral to caudal approach, can define the neurophysiological sensory level of SCI. This approach lends itself to quantification, through the measurement of latencies and amplitudes, and is thus more objective compared to the subjective scoring employed by the current International Standards. Cervical myotomes can be assessed in a similar fashion by recording MEPs from targeted upper limb musculature, in order to complement the manual muscle examination (140). Segmental MEPs of paravertebral and intercostal musculature are also emerging as a means to assess thoracic myotomes (141).

Nerve Conduction Studies

Sensory and Motor Nerves

Profound changes in peripheral nerve function can occur in conjunction with SCI. Electrophysiological approaches to examine peripheral nerve injury are useful following SCI to differentiate CNS and PNS pathology. Compound motor (CMAP) and sensory nerve action potentials (SNAP) are particularly relevant for the diagnosis of peripheral nerve injury during the acute stage of SCI, when the interpretation of clinical observations is complicated by spinal shock, as well as for decisions regarding rehabilitation (e.g., functional electrical stimulation which requires intact peripheral motor nerves). Peripheral injuries can occur acutely during the course of traumatic SCI (i.e., brachial plexus injury) or chronically, such as with long-term wheelchair usage. Both conditions can manifest as diminished CMAP and SNAP amplitudes and conduction velocities (142). Central pathology of the spinal cord can also lead to acute and chronic alpha motoneuron insults and accompanying CMAP abnormalities. Specifically, pathological processes affecting the ventral gray matter and its motor neurons (i.e., spinal compression, ischemic lesions, and syringomyelia) can induce Wallerian degeneration of motor axons. Deterioration of CMAP amplitudes can be seen within 10 days of injury. The dorsal root ganglion is not affected by pathology confined to the spinal canal (Fig. 8.3); therefore, sensory nerve conduction studies are often normal in the setting of severe spinal cord malacia (i.e., massive spinal cord infarction) or cauda equina lesions (142–145). In addition, CMAPs can be helpful for assessing lesions of the conus medullaris or the cauda equina (145).

Spinal Reflexes

The H-reflex is a true reflex arc and is analogous to the muscle tendon stretch reflex. It therefore requires the collective integrity of (a) sensory afferents to the spinal cord, (b) synapses with motor neurons in the ventral gray, and (c) motor efferents to peripheral muscle. Supramaximal electrical stimulation of a peripheral nerve abolishes the H-reflex and yields an M-wave coupled with a variable, low-amplitude F-wave. The F-wave is a late response due to antidromic conduction of the initial peripheral nerve stimulation, accompanying depolarization of alpha motor neurons, and the eventual propagation of action potentials back to the peripheral muscle, which in turn are detected as a "late response."

H-reflexes are variably affected caudal to longstanding SCI. There is conflicting evidence for altered H- to M-wave ratios, chronic neuronal hyperexcitability, and a potential neural mechanism mediating the clinical presentation of spasticity (146–148). Recently, the H-reflex modulation has received considerable attention as a method to study changes in underlying neurophysiology following interventional body-weight support treadmill training (149–152). The strongest clinical application of the electrophysiological measurement of spinal reflexes following SCI has been to monitor spinal shock. In the context of spinal shock, F-waves in particular demonstrate markedly reduced amplitudes and low persistence (number of responses to a given number of stimulations) caudal to SCI. These findings are associated with flaccid paralysis and the absence of deep tendon reflexes, and recovery parallels the reemergence of tendon reflexes (143,152,153).

MECHANISMS OF RECOVERY FOLLOWING SCI

Following SCI, the ability of spared neurons to regenerate and replace lost neuronal connections is limited at best (154). Therefore, an important compensatory mechanism involves maximizing the function of uninjured structures and pathways in order to compensate for lost tissue. This process is termed *neuroplasticity* and is the primary mechanism of recovery following SCI. Neuroplasticity has been defined as "...an adaptive reorganization of the neural pathways occurring after injury that acts to restore some of the lost function" (155). This "rewiring" is increasingly recognized as a major mechanism for recovery following central nervous system injury, including the spinal cord (155–161). Specific mechanisms that mediate neuroplasticity involve altered excitability of neurons, extension of axons and the formation of new connections between neurons, and modulation of the efficacy of synaptic transmission between neurons.

Neuroplasticity is particularly important for incomplete SCI where there is partial preservation of the communication between the brain and the body. Human motor activity requires three components: (a) initiation of a motor signal in the motor cortex, (b) propagation of the signal through the spinal cord, and (c) activation of motor neurons, which results in the conduction of an action potential to peripheral skeletal muscle. Because of this fact, both the brain and the spinal cord can contribute to recovery following SCI. It is known that following human and experimental SCI, physiologic and anatomic alterations occur in both the cortex and the spinal cord, including changes in cortical representation of body parts and formation of new circuits in the spinal cord (162–170). As an example, regions of the brain that control body areas, which retain some communication, enlarge and shift in location (166,167,171,172). In the spinal cord, axons can sprout above the lesion and, by making connections on neurons that have maintained viable descending axons, form new circuits that can bypass partial lesions and mediate recovery (167,170). Because of neuroplasticity, marked recovery can occur, following experimental SCI, with as little as 10% of the axons spared (173–178).

Peripheral mechanisms such as intramuscular sprouting and muscle fiber hypertrophy likely play an important role in facilitating local recovery within the zone of partial preservation (ZPP). Nakamura (179) reported that motor function fully recovers after mild incomplete cervical SCI in rats despite irreversible changes in motor neurons at the injured site. In another study, Nakamura (180) found evidence of marked motor unit reorganization in the zone of injury. Rather than being randomly dispersed, muscle fibers were grouped by fiber type. This was interpreted to represent peripheral axon sprouting from innervated muscle fibers to neighboring denervated fibers, resulting in the incorporation of denervated muscle fibers into larger, homogeneous motor unit territories. Electrophysiological studies in humans have also demonstrated motor unit reorganization following SCI. Findings include increased motor unit forces, large electromyographic (EMG) potentials, and densely innervated motor unit territories within the zone of injury (181,182). Marino et al. (183) used single-fiber EMG to study muscles in the zone of injury following human SCI and reported evidence consistent with peripheral sprouting. All of the above studies support the concept of significant motor unit reorganization within the ZPP following SCI, and compensatory sprouting by spared motor neurons likely plays a prominent role in the process.

References

1. Marino RJ, Barros T, Biering-Sorensen F, et al. International standards for neurological classification of spinal cord injury. *J Spinal Cord Med* 2003;26(Suppl 1):S50–S56.
2. Waters RL, Adkins RH, Yakura JS. Definition of complete spinal cord injury. *Paraplegia* 1991;29:573–581.
3. Stauffer ES. Diagnosis and prognosis of acute cervical spinal cord injury. *Clin Orthop Relat Res* 1975(112):9–15.
4. Ko HY, Ditunno JF Jr, Graziani V, et al. The pattern of reflex recovery during spinal shock. *Spinal Cord* 1999;37:402–409.
5. Burns AS, Lee BS, Ditunno JF Jr, et al. Patient selection for clinical trials: the reliability of the early spinal cord injury examination. *J Neurotrauma* 2003;20:477–482.
6. Whiteneck G, Adler C, Bidddle AK, et al. *Outcomes following traumatic spinal cord injury: clinical practice guidelines for Health-care professionals*. Washington, DC: Paralyzed Veterans of America, 1999.
7. Brown PJ, Marino RJ, Herbison GJ, et al. The 72-hour examination as a predictor of recovery in motor complete quadriplegia. *Arch Phys Med Rehabil* 1991;72: 546–548.
8. Maynard FM, Reynolds GG, Fountain S, et al. Neurological prognosis after traumatic quadriplegia. Three-year experience of California Regional Spinal Cord Injury Care System. *J Neurosurg* 1979;50:611–616.
9. Crozier KS, Graziani V, Ditunno JFJ, et al. Spinal cord injury: prognosis for ambulation based on sensory examination in patients who are initially motor complete. *Arch Phys Med Rehabil* 1991;72:119–121.
10. Ditunno JFJ, Cohen ME, Hauck WW, et al. Recovery of upper-extremity strength in complete and incomplete tetraplegia: a multicenter study. *Arch Phys Med Rehabil* 2000;81:389–393.
11. Marino RJ, Rider-Foster D, Maissel G, et al. Superiority of motor level over single neurological level in categorizing tetraplegia. *Paraplegia* 1995;33:510–513.
12. Waters RL, Yakura JS, Adkins RH, et al. Recovery following complete paraplegia. *Arch Phys Med Rehabil* 1992;73:784–789.
13. Waters RL, Adkins RH, Yakura JS, et al. Motor and sensory recovery following complete tetraplegia. *Arch Phys Med Rehabil* 1993;74:242–247.
14. Waters RL, Adkins RH, Yakura JS, et al. Motor and sensory recovery following incomplete tetraplegia. *Arch Phys Med Rehabil* 1994;75:306–311.
15. Waters RL, Adkins RH, Yakura JS, et al. Motor and sensory recovery following incomplete paraplegia. *Arch Phys Med Rehabil* 1994;75:67–72.
16. Kirshblum SC, O'Connor KC. Predicting neurologic recovery in traumatic cervical spinal cord injury. *Arch Phys Med Rehabil* 1998;79:1456–1466.
17. Burns AS, Ditunno JF. Establishing prognosis and maximizing functional outcomes after spinal cord injury: a review of current and future directions in rehabilitation management. *Spine* 2001;26:S137–S145.
18. Marino RJ, Ditunno JF Jr, Donovan WH, et al. Neurologic recovery after traumatic spinal cord injury: data from the Model Spinal Cord Injury Systems. *Arch Phys Med Rehabil* 1999;80:1391–1396.
19. Fawcett JW, Curt A, Steeves JD, et al. Guidelines for the conduct of clinical trials for spinal cord injury as developed by the ICCP panel: spontaneous recovery after spinal cord injury and statistical power needed for therapeutic clinical trials. *Spinal Cord* 2007;45:190–205.
20. Speiss MR, Muller RM, Rupp R, et al. Conversion in ASIA impairment scale during the first year after traumatic spinal cord injury. *J Neurotrauma* 2009;26(11): 2027–2036.
21. Kirshblum S, Millis S, McKinley W, et al. Late neurologic recovery after traumatic spinal cord injury. *Arch Phys Med Rehabil* 2004;85:1811–1817.
22. Ditunno JFJ, Sipski ML, Posuniak EA, et al. Wrist extensor recovery in traumatic quadriplegia. *Arch Phys Med Rehabil* 1987;68:287–290.
23. Browne BJ, Jacobs SR, Herbison GJ, et al. Pin sensation as a predictor of extensor carpi radialis recovery in spinal cord injury. *Arch Phys Med Rehabil* 1993;74:14–18.
24. Fischer CG, Noonan VK, Smith DE, et al. Motor recovery, functional status, and health related quality of life in patients with complete spinal cord injuries. *Spine* 2005;30:2200–2207.
25. Ditunno JFJ, Stover SL, Freed MM, et al. Motor recovery of the upper extremities in traumatic quadriplegia: a multicenter study. *Arch Phys Med Rehabil* 1992;73:431–436.
26. Harrop JS, Maltenfort MG, Geisler FH, et al. Traumatic thoracic ASIA A examinations and potential for clinical trials. *Spine* 2009;34(23):2525–2529.
27. Curt A, van Hedel HJ, Klaus D, et al.; EM-SCI Study Group. Recovery from a spinal cord injury: significance of compensation, neural plasticity, and repair. *J Neurotrauma* 2008;25:677–685.

28. Foo D, Subrahmanyan TS, Rossier AB. Post-traumatic acute anterior spinal cord syndrome. *Paraplegia* 1981;19:201–205.
29. Bosch A, Stauffer ES, Nickel VL, et al. Incomplete traumatic quadriplegia. A ten-year review. *JAMA* 1971;216:473–478.
30. Merriam WF, Taylor TK, Ruff SJ, et al. A reappraisal of acute traumatic central cord syndrome. *J Bone Joint Surg Br* 1986;68:708–713.
31. Penrod LE, Hegde SK, Ditunno JFJ. Age effect on prognosis for functional recovery in acute, traumatic central cord syndrome. *Arch Phys Med Rehabil* 1990;71(12): 963–968.
32. Foo D. Spinal cord injury in forty-four patients with cervical spondylosis. *Paraplegia* 1986;24(5):301–306.
33. Taylor RG. Incomplete spinal cord injuries with Brown-Sequard phenomena. Gleave JRW. *J Bone Joint Surg Br* 2000;39:438–450.
34. Little JW, Halar E. Temporal course of motor recovery after Brown-Sequard spinal cord injuries. *Paraplegia* 1985;23:39–46.
35. Waters RL, Adkins R, Yakura J, et al. Donald Munro Lecture: functional and neurologic recovery following acute SCI. *J Spinal Cord Med* 1998;21:195–199.
36. Ishida Y, Tominaga T. Predictors of neurologic recovery in acute central cervical cord injury with only upper extremity impairment. *Spine* 2002;27:1652–1658.
37. Calancie B, Molano MR, Broton JG. Tendon reflexes for predicting movement recovery after acute spinal cord injury in humans. *Clin Neurophysiol* 2004;115: 2350–2363.
38. Cerny D, Waters R, Hislop H, et al. Walking and wheelchair energetics in persons with paraplegia. *Phys Ther* 1980;60:1133–1139.
39. Hussey RW, Stauffer ES. Spinal cord injury: requirements for ambulation. *Arch Phys Med Rehabil* 1973;54:544–547.
40. Katoh S, el Masry WS. Motor recovery of patients presenting with motor paralysis and sensory sparing following cervical spinal cord injuries. *Paraplegia* 1995;33: 506–509.
41. Stover SL, DeLisa JA, Whiteneck GG. *Spinal cord injury: clinical outcomes from the model systems*, 1st ed. Gaitherburg, MD: Aspen Publishers, 1995.
42. Oleson CV, Burns AS, Ditunno JF, et al. Prognostic value of pinprick preservation in motor complete, sensory incomplete spinal cord injury. *Arch Phys Med Rehabil* 2005;86:988–992.
43. Burns SP, Golding DG, Rolle WA Jr, et al. Recovery of ambulation in motor-incomplete tetraplegia. *Arch Phys Med Rehabil* 1997;78:1169–1172.
44. Dobkin BH, Apple D, Barbeau H, et al. Methods for a randomized trial of weight-supported treadmill training versus conventional training for walking during inpatient rehabilitation after incomplete traumatic spinal cord injury. *Neurorehabil Neural Repair* 2003;17: 153–167.
45. Kay ED, Deutsch A, Wuermser LA. Predicting walking at discharge from inpatient rehabilitation after a traumatic spinal cord injury. *Arch Phys Med Rehabil* 2007;88: 745–750.
46. Waters RL, Adkins R, Yakura J, et al. Prediction of ambulatory performance based on motor scores derived from standards of the American Spinal Injury Association. *Arch Phys Med Rehabil* 1994;75:756–760.
47. Curt A, Dietz V. Ambulatory capacity in spinal cord injury: significance of somatosensory evoked potentials and ASIA protocol in predicting outcome. *Arch Phys Med Rehabil* 1997;78:39–43.
48. Curt A, Keck ME, Dietz V. Functional outcome following spinal cord injury: significance of motor-evoked potentials and ASIA scores. *Arch Phys Med Rehabil* 1998;79:81–86.
49. Crozier KS, Cheng LL, Graziani V, et al. Spinal cord injury: prognosis for ambulation based on quadriceps recovery. *Paraplegia* 1992;30:762–767.
50. van Middendorp JJ, Hosman AJ, Pouw MH; EM-SCI Study Group. Is determination between complete and incomplete traumatic spinal cord injury clinically relevant? Validation of the ASIA sacral sparing criteria in a prospective cohort of 432 patients. *Spinal Cord* 2009;47(11):809–816.
51. Wirz M, van Hedel HJ, Rupp R, et al. Muscle force and gait performance: relationships after spinal cord injury. *Arch Phys Med Rehabil* 2006;87:1218–22.
52. Nadeau S, Gravel D, Olney SJ. Determinants, limiting factors and compensatory strategies in gait. *Crit Rev Phys Rehabil Med* 2001;13:1–24.
53. Barbeau H. Locomotor training in neurorehabilitation: emerging rehabilitation concepts. *Neurorehabil Neural Repair* 2003;17:3–11.
54. Scivoletto G, Romanelli A, Mariotti A, et al. Clinical factors that affect walking level and performance in chronic spinal cord lesion patients. *Spine* 2008;33:259–264.
55. Kim CM, Eng JJ, Whittaker MW. Level walking and ambulatory capacity in persons with incomplete spinal cord injury: relationship with muscle strength. *Spinal Cord* 2004;42:156–162.
56. Michael KM, Allen JK, Macko RF. Reduced ambulatory activity after stroke: the role of balance, gait, and cardiovascular fitness. *Arch Med Rehabil* 2005;86: 1552–1556.
57. Krawetz P, Nance P. Gait analysis of spinal cord injured subjects: effects of injury level and spasticity. *Arch Phys Med Rehabil* 1996;77:635–638.
58. Winchester PK, Querry R, Mosby J, et al. Prediction model for change in gait speed following body weight supported treadmill training. *J Spinal Cord Med* 2006;29:256.
59. Waters RL, Lunsford BR. Energy cost of paraplegic locomotion. *J Bone Joint Surg Am* 1985;67:1245–1250.
60. Lapointe R, Lajoie Y, Serresse O, et al. Functional community ambulation requirements in incomplete spinal cord injured subjects. *Spinal Cord* 2001;39:327–335.
61. Pepin A, Ladouceur M, Barbeau H. Treadmill walking in incomplete spinal-cord-injured subjects: 2. Factors limiting the maximal speed. *Spinal Cord* 2003;41:271–279.
62. Waters RL, Yakura JS, Adkins RH. Gait performance after spinal cord injury. *Clin Orthop Rel Res* 1993:87–96.
63. Lajoie Y, Barbeau H, Hamelin M. Attentional requirements of walking in spinal cord injured patients compared to normal subjects. *Spinal Cord* 1999;37:245–250.
64. Robinett CS, Vondran MA. Functional ambulation velocity and distance requirements in rural and urban communities. A clinical report. *Phys Ther* 1988;68:1371–1373.

65. Long C. Functional significance of spinal cord lesion level. *Arch Phys Med Rehabil* 1955;36, 249–255.
66. Welch RD, Lobley SJ, O'Sullivan SB, et al. Functional independence in quadriplegia: critical levels. *Arch Phys Med Rehabil* 1986;67:235–240.
67. Zafonte RD, Demangone DA, Herbison GJ. Daily self-care in quadriplegic subjects. *Neurol Rehabil* 1991;1:17–24.
68. Consortium for Spinal Cord Medicine. Outcomes following traumatic spinal cord injury: clinical practice guidelines for health-care professionals. Washington, DC: Paralyzed Veterans of America, 1999.
69. Beers GJ, Raque GH, Wagner GG, et al. MR imaging in acute cervical spine trauma. *J Comput Assist Tomogr* 1988;12:755–761.
70. Bondurant FJ, Cotler HB, Kulkarni MV, et al. Acute spinal cord injury. A study using physical examination and magnetic resonance imaging. *Spine* 1990;15: 161–168.
71. Chakeres DW, Flickinger F, Bresnahan JC, et al. MR imaging of acute spinal cord trauma. *Am J Neuroradiol* 1987;8:5–10.
72. Flanders AE, Schaefer DM, Doan HT, et al. Acute cervical spine trauma: correlation of MR imaging findings with degree of neurologic deficit. *Radiology* 1990;177:25–33.
73. Goldberg AL, Daffner RH, Schapiro RL. Imaging of acute spinal trauma: an evolving multi-modality approach. *Clin Imaging* 1990;14:11–16.
74. Kulkarni MV, McArdle CB, Kopanicky D, et al. Acute spinal cord injury: MR imaging at 1.5 T. *Radiology* 1987;164:837–843.
75. Mirvis SE, Geisler FH, Jelinek JJ, et al. Acute cervical spine trauma: evaluation with 1.5-T MR imaging. *Radiology* 1988;166:807–816.
76. Sett P, Crockard HA. The value of magnetic resonance imaging (MRI) in the follow-up management of spinal injury. *Paraplegia* 1991;29:396–410.
77. Tracy PT, Wright RM, Hanigan WC. Magnetic resonance imaging of spinal injury. *Spine* 1989;14:292–301.
78. Weirich SD, Cotler HB, Narayana PA, et al. Histopathologic correlation of magnetic resonance imaging signal patterns in a spinal cord injury model. *Spine* 1990;15:630–638.
79. Wittenberg RH, Boetel U, Beyer HK. Magnetic resonance imaging and computer tomography of acute spinal cord trauma. *Clin Orthop Relat Res* 1990;(260):176–185.
80. Goldberg AL, Rothfus WE, Deeb ZL, et al. The impact of magnetic resonance on the diagnostic evaluation of acute cervicothoracic spinal trauma. *Skeletal Radiol* 1988;17:89–95.
81. Hackney DB, Finkelstein SD, Hand CM, et al. Postmortem magnetic resonance imaging of experimental spinal cord injury: magnetic resonance findings versus in vivo functional deficit. *Neurosurgery* 1994;35:1104–1111.
82. Hackney DB, Ford JC, Markowitz RS, et al. Experimental spinal cord injury: MR correlation to intensity of injury. *J Comput Assist Tomogr* 1994;18:357–362.
83. Metz GA, Curt A, van de MH, et al. Validation of the weight-drop contusion model in rats: a comparative study of human spinal cord injury. *J Neurotrauma* 2000;17:1–17.
84. Cotler HB, Kulkarni MV, Bondurant FJ. Magnetic resonance imaging of acute spinal cord trauma: preliminary report. *J Orthop Trauma* 1988;2:1–4.
85. Schouman-Claeys E, Frija G, Cuenod CA, et al. MR imaging of acute spinal cord injury: results of an experimental study in dogs. *Am J Neuroradiol* 1990;11:959–965.
86. Hackney DB, Asato R, Joseph PM, et al. Hemorrhage and edema in acute spinal cord compression: demonstration by MR imaging. *Radiology* 1986;161:387–390.
87. Sato T, Kokubun S, Rijal KP, et al. Prognosis of cervical spinal cord injury in correlation with magnetic resonance imaging. *Paraplegia* 1994;32:81–85.
88. Schaefer DM, Flanders A, Northrup BE, et al. Magnetic resonance imaging of acute cervical spine trauma. Correlation with severity of neurologic injury. *Spine* 1989;14:1090–1095.
89. Blackwood W. Vascular disease of the central nervous system. In: Blackwood W, Meyer A, Norman RM, eds. *Greenfield's neuropathology*. Baltimore, MD: Williams & Wilkins, 1963:71–115.
90. Kalfas I, Wilberger J, Goldberg A, et al. Magnetic resonance imaging in acute spinal cord trauma. *Neurosurgery* 1988;23:295–299.
91. Bilgen M, Abbe R, Liu SJ, et al. Spatial and temporal evolution of hemorrhage in the hyperacute phase of experimental spinal cord injury: in vivo magnetic resonance imaging. *Magn Reson Med* 2000;43:594–600.
92. Perovitch M, Perl S, Wang H. Current advances in magnetic resonance imaging (MRI) in spinal cord trauma: review article. *Paraplegia* 1992;30:305–316.
93. Falconer JC, Narayana PA, Bhattacharjee MB, et al. Quantitative MRI of spinal cord injury in a rat model. *Magn Reson Med* 1994;32:484–491.
94. Ramon S, Dominguez R, Ramirez L, et al. Clinical and magnetic resonance imaging correlation in acute spinal cord injury. *Spinal Cord* 1997;35:664–673.
95. Marciello MA, Flanders AE, Herbison GJ, et al. Magnetic resonance imaging related to neurologic outcome in cervical spinal cord injury. *Arch Phys Med Rehabil* 1993;74:940–946.
96. Kulkarni MV, Bondurant FJ, Rose SL, et al. 1.5 tesla magnetic resonance imaging of acute spinal trauma. *Radiographics* 1988;8:1059–1082.
97. Leypold BG, Flanders AE, Schwartz ED, et al. The impact of methylprednisolone on lesion severity following spinal cord injury. *Spine* 2007;32:373–378.
98. Leypold BG, Flanders AE, Burns AS. The early evolution of spinal cord lesions on MR imaging following traumatic spinal cord injury. *Am J Neuroradiol* 2008;29: 1012–1016.
99. Aoyama T, Hida K, Akino M, et al. Ultra-early MRI showing no abnormality in a fall victim presenting with tetraparesis. *Spinal Cord* 2007;45:695–699.
100. Silberstein M, Tress BM, Hennessy O. Prediction of neurologic outcome in acute spinal cord injury: the role of CT and MR. *Am J Neuroradiol* 1992;13:1597–1608.
101. Boghosian G, Leypold BG, Flanders AE, et al. Predicting the neurological level of injury with MRI following cervical spinal injury. Radiological Society of North America (RSNA) Annual Meeting; 2006; Chicago, IL.
102. Miranda P, Gomez P, Alday R, et al. Brown-Sequard syndrome after blunt cervical spine trauma: clinical

and radiological correlations. *Eur Spine J* 2007;16: 1165–1170.
103. Quencer RM, Bunge RP. The injured spinal cord: imaging, histopathologic clinical correlates, and basic science approaches to enhancing neural function after spinal cord injury. *Spine* 1996;21:2064–2066.
104. Flanders AE, Spettell CM, Tartaglino LM, et al. Forecasting motor recovery after cervical spinal cord injury: value of MR imaging. *Radiology* 1996;201:649–655.
105. Boldin C, Raith J, Fankhauser F, et al. Predicting neurologic recovery in cervical spinal cord injury with postoperative MR imaging. *Spine* 2006;31:554–559.
106. Schaefer DM, Flanders AE, Osterholm JL, et al. Prognostic significance of magnetic resonance imaging in the acute phase of cervical spine injury. *J Neurosurg* 1992;76:218–223.
107. Harrington JF, Likavec MJ, Smith AS. Disc herniation in cervical fracture subluxation. *Neurosurgery* 1991;29:374–379.
108. Fehlings MG, Rao SC, Tator CH, et al. The optimal radiologic method for assessing spinal canal compromise and cord compression in patients with cervical spinal cord injury. Part II: Results of a multicenter study. *Spine* 1999;24:605–613.
109. Rao SC, Fehlings MG. The optimal radiologic method for assessing spinal canal compromise and cord compression in patients with cervical spinal cord injury. Part I: An evidence-based analysis of the published literature. *Spine* 1999;24:598–604.
110. Kang JD, Figgie MP, Bohlman HH. Sagittal measurements of the cervical spine in subaxial fractures and dislocations. *J Bone Joint Surg Am* 1994;76:1617–1628.
111. Hayashi K, Yone K, Ito H, et al. MRI findings in patients with a cervical spinal cord injury who do not show radiographic evidence of a fracture or dislocation. *Paraplegia* 1995;33:212–215.
112. Miyanji F, Furlan JC, Aarabi B, et al. Acute cervical traumatic spinal cord injury: MR imaging findings correlated with neurologic outcome—prospective study with 100 consecutive patients. *Radiology* 2007;243:820–827.
113. Ford JC, Hackney DB, Alsop DC, et al. MRI characterization of diffusion coefficients in a rat spinal cord injury model. *Magn Reson Med* 1994;31:488–494.
114. Milhorat TH, Johnson RW, Milhorat RH, et al. Clinicopathological correlations in syringomyelia using axial magnetic resonance imaging. *Neurosurgery* 1995;37:206–213.
115. Jinkins JR, Reddy S, Leite CC, et al. MR of parenchymal spinal cord signal change as a sign of active advancement in clinically progressive posttraumatic syringomyelia. *Am J Neuroradiol* 1998;19:177–182.
116. Quencer RM, Sheldon JJ, Post MJ, et al. MRI of the chronically injured cervical spinal cord. *Am J Roentgenol* 1986;147:125–132.
117. Schurch B, Wichmann W, Rossier AB. Post-traumatic syringomyelia (cystic myelopathy): a prospective study of 449 patients with spinal cord injury. *J Neurol Neurosurg Psychiatry* 1996;60:61–67.
118. Schwartz ED, Falcone SF, Quencer RM, et al. Posttraumatic syringomyelia: pathogenesis, imaging, and treatment. *Am J Roentgenol* 1999;173:487–492.
119. Bodley R. Imaging in chronic spinal cord injury—indications and benefits. *Eur J Radiol* 2002;42:135–153.
120. Hesseltine SM, Law M, Babb J, et al. Diffusion tensor imaging in multiple sclerosis: assessment of regional differences in the axial plane within normal-appearing cervical spinal cord. *Am J Neuroradiol* 2006;27:1189–1193.
121. Demir A, Ries M, Moonen CT, et al. Diffusion-weighted MR imaging with apparent diffusion coefficient and apparent diffusion tensor maps in cervical spondylotic myelopathy. *Radiology* 2003;229:37–43.
122. Shanmuganathan K, Gullapalli RP, Zhuo J, et al. Diffusion tensor MR imaging in cervical spine trauma. *Am J Neuroradiol* 2008;29:655–659.
123. Curt A, Rodic B, Schurch B, et al. Recovery of bladder function in patients with acute spinal cord injury: significance of ASIA scores and somatosensory evoked potentials. *Spinal Cord* 1997;35:368–373.
124. Curt A, Dietz V. Electrophysiological recordings in patients with spinal cord injury: significance for predicting outcome. *Spinal Cord* 1999;37:157–165.
125. Iseli E, Cavigelli A, Dietz V, et al. Prognosis and recovery in ischaemic and traumatic spinal cord injury: clinical and electrophysiological evaluation. *J Neurol Neurosurg Psychiatry* 1999;67:567–571.
126. Rowed DW, McLean JA, Tator CH. Somatosensory evoked potentials in acute spinal cord injury: prognostic value. *Surg Neurol* 1978;9:203–210.
127. Hayes KC, Wolfe DL, Hsieh JT, et al. Clinical and electrophysiologic correlates of quantitative sensory testing in patients with incomplete spinal cord injury. *Arch Phys Med Rehabil* 2002;83:1612–1619.
128. Jacobs SR, Yeaney NK, Herbison GJ, et al. Future ambulation prognosis as predicted by somatosensory evoked potentials in motor complete and incomplete quadriplegia. *Arch Phys Med Rehabil* 1995;76:635–641.
129. Curt A, Dietz V. Traumatic cervical spinal cord injury: relation between somatosensory evoked potentials, neurological deficit, and hand function. *Arch Phys Med Rehabil* 1996;77:48–53.
130. Cheliout-Heraut F, Loubert G, Masri-Zada T, et al. Evaluation of early motor and sensory evoked potentials in cervical spinal cord injury. *Neurophysiol Clin* 1998;28:39–55.
131. Iannetti GD, Truini A, Galeotti F, et al. Usefulness of dorsal laser evoked potentials in patients with spinal cord damage: report of two cases. *J Neurol Neurosurg Psychiatry* 2001;71:792–794.
132. Wydenkeller S, Wirz R, Halder P. Spinothalamic tract conduction velocity estimated using contact heat evoked potentials: what needs to be considered. *Clin Neurophysiol* 2008;119:812–821.
133. Vetrugno R, Liguori R, Cortelli P, Montagna P. Sympathetic skin response: basic mechanisms and clinical applications. *Clin Auton Res* 2003;13:256–270.
134. Curt A, Weinhardt C, Dietz V. Significance of sympathetic skin response in the assessment of autonomic failure in patients with spinal cord injury. *J Auton Nerv Syst* 1996;61:175–180.
135. Rodic B, Curt A, Dietz V, et al. Bladder neck incompetence in patients with spinal cord injury: significance of sympathetic skin response. *J Urol* 2000;163: 1223–1227.

136. Schmid DM, Schurch B, Hauri D. Sildenafil in the treatment of sexual dysfunction in spinal cord-injured male patients. *Eur Urol* 2000;38:184–193.
137. Schmid DM, Reitz A, Curt A, et al. Urethral evoked sympathetic skin responses and viscerosensory evoked potentials as diagnostic tools to evaluate urogenital autonomic afferent innervation in spinal cord injured patients. *J Urol* 2004;171:1156–1160.
138. Schurch B, Curt A, Rossier AB. The value of sympathetic skin response recordings in the assessment of the vesicourethral autonomic nervous dysfunction in spinal cord injured patients. *J Urol* 1997;157:2230–2233.
139. Kramer JL, Moss AJ, Taylor P, et al. Assessment of posterior spinal cord function with electrical perception threshold in spinal cord injury. *J Neurotrauma* 2008;25:1019–1026.
140. Shields CB, Ping ZY, Shields LB, et al. Objective assessment of cervical spinal cord injury levels by transcranial magnetic motor-evoked potentials. *Surg Neurol* 2006;66:475–483.
141. Cariga P, Catley M, Nowicky AV, et al. Segmental recording of cortical motor evoked potentials from thoracic paravertebral myotomes in complete spinal cord injury. *Spine* 2002;27:1438–1443.
142. Nogajski JH, Engel S, Kiernan MC. Focal and generalized peripheral nerve dysfunction in spinal cord-injured patients. *J Clin Neurophysiol* 2006;23:273–279.
143. Curt A, Keck ME, Dietz V. Clinical value of F-wave recordings in traumatic cervical spinal cord injury. *Electroencephalogr Clin Neurophysiol* 1997;105: 189–193.
144. Curt A, Dietz V. Neurographic assessment of intramedullary motoneuron lesions in cervical spinal cord injury: consequences for hand function. *Spinal Cord* 1996;34:326–332.
145. Rutz S, Dietz V, Curt A. Diagnostic and prognostic value of compound motor action potential of lower limbs in acute paraplegic patients. *Spinal Cord* 2000;38: 203–210.
146. Schindler-Ivens SM, Shields RK. Soleus H-reflex recruitment is not altered in persons with chronic spinal cord injury. *Arch Phys Med Rehabil* 2004;85:840–847.
147. Little JW, Halar EM. H-reflex changes following spinal cord injury. *Arch Phys Med Rehabil* 1985;66:19–22.
148. Nakazawa K, Kawashima N, Akai M. Enhanced stretch reflex excitability of the soleus muscle in persons with incomplete rather than complete chronic spinal cord injury. *Arch Phys Med Rehabil* 2006;87:71–75.
149. Trimble MH, Behrman AL, Flynn SM, et al. Acute effects of locomotor training on overground walking speed and H-reflex modulation in individuals with incomplete spinal cord injury. *J Spinal Cord Med* 2001;24:74–80.
150. Phadke CP, Wu SS, Thompson FJ, et al. Comparison of soleus H-reflex modulation after incomplete spinal cord injury in 2 walking environments: treadmill with body weight support and overground. *Arch Phys Med Rehabil* 2007;88:1606–1613.
151. Muller R, Dietz V. Neuronal function in chronic spinal cord injury: divergence between locomotor and flexion- and H-reflex activity. *Clin Neurophysiol* 2006;117: 1499–1507.
152. Hiersemenzel LP, Curt A, Dietz V. From spinal shock to spasticity: neuronal adaptations to a spinal cord injury. *Neurology* 2000;54:1574–1582.
153. Leis AA, Kronenberg MF, Stetkarova I, et al. Spinal motoneuron excitability after acute spinal cord injury in humans. *Neurology* 1996;47:231–237.
154. Yiu G, He Z. Glial inhibition of CNS axon regeneration. *Nat Rev Neurosci* 2006;7:617–627.
155. Bradbury EJ, McMahon SB. Spinal cord repair strategies: why do they work? *Nat Rev Neurosci* 2006;7:644–653.
156. Dietz V, Harkema SJ. Locomotor activity in spinal cord-injured persons. *J Appl Physiol* 2004;96:1954–1960.
157. Edgerton VR, Tillakaratne NJ, Bigbee AJ, et al. Plasticity of the spinal neural circuitry after injury. *Annu Rev Neurosci* 2004;27:145–167.
158. Blesch A, Tuszynski MH. Spontaneous and neurotrophin-induced axonal plasticity after spinal cord injury. *Prog Brain Res* 2002;137:415–423.
159. Schwab ME. Increasing plasticity and functional recovery of the lesioned spinal cord. *Prog Brain Res* 2002;137:351–359.
160. Wolpaw JR, Tennissen AM. Activity-dependent spinal cord plasticity in health and disease. *Annu Rev Neurosci* 2001;24:807–843.
161. Raineteau O, Schwab ME. Plasticity of motor systems after incomplete spinal cord injury. *Nat Rev Neurosci* 2001;2:263–273.
162. Turner JA, Lee JS, Schandler SL, et al. An fMRI investigation of hand representation in paraplegic humans. *Neurorehabil Neural Repair* 2003;17:37–47.
163. Corbetta M, Burton H, Sinclair RJ, et al. Functional reorganization and stability of somatosensory-motor cortical topography in a tetraplegic subject with late recovery. *Proc Natl Acad Sci USA* 2002;99:17066–17071.
164. Mikulis DJ, Jurkiewicz MT, McIlroy WE, et al. Adaptation in the motor cortex following cervical spinal cord injury. *Neurology* 2002;58:794–801.
165. Turner JA, Lee JS, Martinez O, et al. Somatotopy of the motor cortex after long-term spinal cord injury or amputation. *IEEE Trans Neural Syst Rehabil Eng* 2001;9: 154–160.
166. Bruehlmeier M, Dietz V, Leenders KL, et al. How does the human brain deal with a spinal cord injury? *Eur J Neurosci* 1998;10:3918–3922.
167. Bareyre FM, Kerschensteiner M, Raineteau O, et al. The injured spinal cord spontaneously forms a new intraspinal circuit in adult rats. *Nat Neurosci* 2004;7: 269–277.
168. Raineteau O, Fouad K, Bareyre FM, et al. Reorganization of descending motor tracts in the rat spinal cord. *Eur J Neurosci* 2002;16:1761–1771.
169. Curt A, Alkadhi H, Crelier GR, et al. Changes of non-affected upper limb cortical representation in paraplegic patients as assessed by fMRI. *Brain* 2002;125(Pt 11): 2567–2578.
170. Weidner N, Ner A, Salimi N, et al. Spontaneous corticospinal axonal plasticity and functional recovery after adult central nervous system injury. *Proc Natl Acad Sci USA* 2001;98:3513–3518.
171. Fouad K, Pedersen V, Schwab ME, et al. Cervical sprouting of corticospinal fibers after thoracic spinal cord

injury accompanies shifts in evoked motor responses. *Curr Biol* 2001;11:1766–1770.

172. Dobkin BH. Spinal and supraspinal plasticity after incomplete spinal cord injury: correlations between functional magnetic resonance imaging and engaged locomotor networks. *Prog Brain Res* 2000;128:99–111.
173. Bregman BS, Kunkel-Bagden E, Schnell L, et al. Recovery from spinal cord injury mediated by antibodies to neurite growth inhibitors. *Nature* 1995;378:498–501.
174. Liu Y, Kim D, Himes BT, et al. Transplants of fibroblasts genetically modified to express BDNF promote regeneration of adult rat rubrospinal axons and recovery of forelimb function. *J Neurosci* 1999;19:4370–4387.
175. Wall PD. The sensory and motor role of impulses travelling in the dorsal columns towards cerebral cortex. *Brain* 1970;93:505–524.
176. Fehlings MG, Tator CH. The relationships among the severity of spinal cord injury, residual neurological function, axon counts, and counts of retrogradely labeled neurons after experimental spinal cord injury. *Exp Neurol* 1995;132:220–228.
177. Eidelberg E, Straehley D, Erspamer R, et al. Relationship between residual hindlimb-assisted locomotion and surviving axons after incomplete spinal cord injuries. *Exp Neurol* 1977;56:312–322.
178. Blight AR. Cellular morphology of chronic spinal cord injury in the cat: analysis of myelinated axons by line-sampling. *Neuroscience* 1983;10:521–543.
179. Nakamura M, Fujimura Y, Yato Y, et al. Changes in choline acetyltransferase distribution in the cervical spinal cord after reversible cervical spinal cord injury. *Paraplegia* 1994;32:752–758.
180. Nakamura M, Fujimura Y, Yato Y, et al. Muscle reorganization following incomplete cervical spinal cord injury in rats. *Spinal Cord* 1997;35:752–756.
181. Yang JF, Stein RB, Jhamandas J, et al. Motor unit numbers and contractile properties after spinal cord injury. *Ann Neurol* 1990;28:496–502.
182. Thomas CK, Broton JG, Calancie B. Motor unit forces and recruitment patterns after cervical spinal cord injury. *Muscle Nerve* 1997;20:212–220.
183. Marino RJ, Herbison GJ, Ditunno JF Jr. Peripheral sprouting as a mechanism for recovery in the zone of injury in acute quadriplegia: a single-fiber EMG study. *Muscle Nerve* 1994;17:1466–1468.

CHAPTER 9 ■ CARDIOVASCULAR AND AUTONOMIC DYSFUNCTIONS AFTER SPINAL CORD INJURY

SUSAN V. GARSTANG AND HEATHER WALKER

INTRODUCTION

Disruption of the intact spinal cord involves not only pathways of the somatic nervous system carrying voluntary motor and sensory signals but also autonomic pathways of both the sympathetic and the parasympathetic nervous system (PNS). Impaired regulation of the autonomic nervous system (ANS) leads to many of the clinical features seen after spinal cord injury (SCI), including altered cardiovascular and thermoregulatory functions, as well as altered function of end organs such as the bowel and bladder.

Immediately after SCI, the disruptions in ANS functions are clearly manifest. Depending on the level of injury, signs of ANS dysfunction include alterations in heart rate and blood pressure, as well as impaired temperature regulation and pulmonary dysfunction. Initially after injury, patients may have hypothermia, and marked bradycardia and hypotension; arrhythmias are not uncommon in the acute period, both bradyarrhythmia and tachyarrhythmia. After the first 2 to 6 weeks, these fluctuations in cardiovascular control lessen in severity. In addition, after acute SCI, there is an elevated risk of thromboembolism, which is multifactorial and persists for several months postinjury. Chronically, patients may still have altered cardiovascular responses, often manifested by autonomic dysreflexia in patients with injury levels above T6, as well as orthostasis, impaired temperature regulation, and response to exercise.

AUTONOMIC NERVOUS SYSTEM ANATOMY

An understanding of the ANS structure and function is essential to fully comprehend the effects of derangements in this system. The ANS has three divisions, the sympathetic nervous system (SNS), the PNS, and the enteric nervous system. Disruption to the spinal cord primarily involves the sympathetic and PS divisions. The level of SCI is one of the main determinants of which division of the ANS is effected, as well as the severity of the injury to the cord itself. It is possible to predict the alterations in ANS response by a thorough understanding of the anatomy.

The sympathetic and parasympathetic divisions of the ANS are often found to serve opposing regulatory roles. The pathways by which the signals travel consist of effector organs, efferent pathways, integration centers in the central nervous system (CNS), afferent pathways, and sensory receptors (1). With the exception of the cranial parasympathetic division, impulses are carried in the spinal cord and then exit the cord after synapsing with interneurons in the CNS. These interneurons, termed "preganglionic neurons," traverse the ventral roots and terminate in an ANS ganglion outside the CNS (2). There is another synapse in the ANS ganglion, where effector neurons originate. These neurons, termed "postganglionic neurons," then travel to the effector organs.

The PNS has cell bodies in the visceral brainstem nuclei and the 2nd to 4th sacral (S2-4) segments of the spinal cord and thus is often referred to as the "craniosacral division" of the ANS. The cranial nerve fibers are carried with cranial nerves III, VII, IX, and X and innervate structures in the head and neck, as well as thoracic and abdominal viscera. The preganglionic PS fibers that originate in the sacral segments innervate the descending colon and pelvic organs. The efferent impulses to the sacral cord are carried from the brainstem in the lateral reticulospinal tract. Most preganglionic PS fibers synapse in the inferior mesenteric ganglion, but some continue without synapsing through the hypogastric nerves to reach the vesical plexus in the bladder wall (3).

The cell bodies of the SNS are located in the intermediolateral or intermediomedial cell columns of the spinal cord. The preganglionic fibers exit the cord and join the ventral roots of T1 to L2; thus, the SNS is often referred to as the "thoracolumbar division" of the ANS. Note that variations in level of origin do occur, and preganglionic fibers from as high as C7 to as low as L4 have been demonstrated (3). All sympathetic preganglionic fibers above the diaphragm synapse in the paravertebral ganglion of the sympathetic chain. Below the diaphragm, these fibers may synapse in the sympathetic chain, or in collateral (prevertebral) ganglia located near the viscera (3). These postganglionic fibers travel with major arteries to their effector organs, or form visceral nerves such as the cardiac nerves.

The heart has both sympathetic and PS innervation. The cardiac sympathetic preganglionic and postganglionic neurons synapse in the middle cervical and stellate ganglia (4). The parasympathetic fibers to the heart originate in the dorsal motor nucleus of the vagus nerve and in the nucleus ambiguus of the medulla oblongata. These fibers travel in the recurrent laryngeal nerves and vagus nerve and join the sympathetic cardiopulmonary nerves to form the ventral and dorsal cardiopulmonary plexuses (5,6). The cardiac nerves (three large and several small) emerge from these plexuses to innervate the atria, ventricles, and the conduction system. The PS fibers synapse with postganglionic cells on the epicardial surface or within the walls of the heart near the SA or AV node.

AUTONOMIC NERVOUS SYSTEM PHYSIOLOGY

The ANS regulates many aspects of circulation including vascular resistance, heart rate, and stroke volume; these in turn determine cardiac output and arterial blood pressure. Feedback from afferent pathways is used to regulate the frequency and force of cardiac contraction, as well as control vasoconstriction or vasodilation. The control of cardiovascular function occurs via a complex system of feedback loops that modulate SNS and PNS output.

Sympathetic outflow to the vasculature is excitatory, while the parasympathetic role tends to be inhibitory. The arterial baroreceptors located in the carotid sinuses and aortic arch respond to an increase in arterial pressure by inhibition of the spinal sympathetic excitatory tract, stimulation of the spinal sympathetic inhibitory tract, and stimulation of the parasympathetic preganglionic nerves (1). In addition, there is sympathetic excitatory input to the nucleus tractus solitarius from the arterial chemoreceptors, ergoreceptors in skeletal muscle, and cardiopulmonary receptors (2).

Conversely, the arterial baroreceptors respond to a decrease in arterial pressure by increasing activity of sympathetic excitatory nerves and decreasing activity of PS nerves. In addition, parasympathetic afferents from the aortic arch and carotid baroreceptors provide opposing inhibitory input to the nucleus tractus solitarius via cranial nerves IX (glossopharyngeal) and X (vagus) (7).

The ANS also controls heart rate and rhythmicity. The sinoatrial (SA) node is under direct influence of both the sympathetic and the PS nervous systems. Sympathetic input increases the rate at which the SA node generates action potentials, and parasympathetic input decreases the rate of action potential generation (8).

The SNS exerts primary control of blood flow to the skin, kidneys, and splanchnic organs (9). Activation of the SNS can produce an 80% reduction in flow in the splanchnic circulation and cause a large shift of blood to the central circulation (9). This shift in blood volume is a key determinant of the elevation in blood pressure that is seen during episodes of autonomic dysreflexia. In addition, the sympathetic control over circulating blood volume in various vascular beds is part of the mechanism that regulates systemic vascular resistances and cardiac filling pressure. The final outcome of all these processes is regulation of stroke volume and cardiac output, which in turn have major influences on arterial blood pressure.

ALTERATIONS IN ANS FUNCTION AFTER SCI

SCI interrupts the connections between the supraspinal regulatory centers and the effector organs, which interferes with both afferent and efferent signal transmission. The level and extent of SCI determine the amount of reduction or absence of autonomic control. Many of the major cardiovascular functions are associated with segmental outflow from several levels, such as the outflow to the heart or the splanchnic outflow; thus, injuries often cause partial reduction in function. Sympathetic control of the blood vessels in the limbs and skin, as well as the regulation of the sweat glands, tends to be regionalized to more limited levels of the spinal cord (see Table 9.1).

The main sympathetic regulatory center in the CNS is in the rostroventrolateral medulla, where supraspinal control of the SNS originates (10). Descending sympathetic input from this supraspinal center travels through the cervical spinal cord, and then intraspinal interneurons synapse with the sympathetic preganglionic neurons starting at T1. Therefore, SCI above T1 interrupts the transmission of signals from the medulla to the thoracic spinal cord; more severe injuries result in poorer conduction of descending signals (11). Autopsies in patients with cervical SCI who clinically manifested severe cardiovascular abnormalities revealed marked loss of axons in the dorsal aspects of the lateral funiculus, which is thought to be the location of the descending vasomotor pathways (11,12).

TABLE 9.1

SPINAL CORD LEVELS OF SYMPATHETIC AND PARASYMPATHETIC OUTFLOW

CNS or spinal cord level	ANS division	Ganglion	Nerve	Organs innervated
Dorsal motor nucleus of cranial nerve X	PNS	n/a	Vagus nerve Cardiac nerves	Heart, lungs, abdominal viscera, ascending and transverse colon
T1-4	SNS	Middle cervical and stellate	Cardiac nerves	Heart Lungs
T3-L3 (but mainly T5-9)	SNS	Superior mesenteric (but doesn't synapse)	Lesser splanchnic nerve	Adrenal medulla
T5-11	SNS	Celiac and superior mesenteric	Greater and lesser splanchnic nerves	Abdominal viscera Ascending and transverse colon
L1-3	SNS	Inferior mesenteric	Lumbar splanchnic nerves	Descending colon and rectum, kidney, bladder, uterus, external genitalia
S2-4	PNS	n/a	Pelvic splanchnic nerves	Descending colon and rectum, bladder, uterus, external genitalia

CNS, central nervous system; ANS, autonomic nervous system; PNS, parasympathetic nervous system; SNS, sympathetic nervous system; n/a, not applicable.

The sympathetic innervation to the heart is from T1 to T4, including innervation to the myocardium and SA and AV nodes. Thus, injuries between T1 and T4 have partial innervation to the heart, and injuries below T4 have complete innervation to the heart. If the level of SCI is below T4, normal cardiac responses are maintained; however, vascular tone and control of blood pressure will still be under local regulation. Because the PS innervation to the heart is via the vagus nerve, which does not travel in the spinal cord, the only supraspinal input to the heart in injuries above T1 is PS in nature.

Sympathetic outflow to the splanchnic organs originates primarily from T5 to T9 via the greater splanchnic nerve to the celiac ganglion (although there are splanchnic efferents from T5 to L2). This outflow regulates most of the blood flow in the splanchnic circulation. Injuries below T5 have some ability to regulate splanchnic flow, and this control increases with more distal levels of injury. Damage to the spinal cord above T5 impairs the ability of the splanchnic beds to vasodilate, thus reducing the ability of the blood to pool in the splanchnic circulation. This lack of compensatory response to an elevation in blood pressure is part of the pathogenesis of autonomic dysreflexia, which occurs in persons with SCI at T6 and above.

Sympathetic responses to events are regulated by the effects of the SNS on the heart and vasculature, as well as by the actions of the SNS on the adrenal medulla. This then leads to the release of circulating hormones such as epinephrine, which has effects both locally and at distant sites in many organs. SCI impairs the sympathetic response to exercise or stress if the level of injury is above T9. The major outflow of sympathetic efferents to the adrenal medulla is from T5 to T9, although these efferents can originate as high as T3 and as low as L3.

The sympathetic regulation of the blood vessels in the limbs and skin, as well as the regulation of the sweat glands, tends to be more regionalized than the major outflows and functions listed above. Sweat glands receive dual innervation from both adrenergic and cholinergic fibers; however, cholinergic stimulation provokes the largest response (2,13). Sweat glands from spinal segments T2-4 supply sweat glands on the head and neck; T2-8 supply the glands of the upper limbs, T6-10 supply the trunk, and T11-L2 supply the lower limbs (2,13). Autonomic innervation to the dermatomes extends several levels above and below the corresponding somatic levels. Only injuries below L2 have minimal effects from SNS dysregulation.

When there is a loss of supraspinal connections to the SNS, particularly in injuries above T1, homeostasis is achieved via local and spinal reflex control. There is evidence that after SCI spinal circuits are capable of generating some sympathetic reflex activity (14). Sympathetic preganglionic neurons show spontaneous activity after SCI in the absence of input and function as "spinal sympathetic interneurons" (15). There is also peripheral alpha-adrenoceptor hyperresponsiveness, which is thought to contribute to the propensity for autonomic dysreflexia. Interestingly, sympathovagal balance appears to be maintained, secondary to a decrease in sympathetic activity that is paralleled by a decline in PS activity (16).

The lack of descending sympathetic input leads to low resting blood pressure, orthostatic hypotension, and loss of diurnal fluctuation of BP (17). In normally innervated people, there is a typical nocturnal decrease in BP, which is not seen in persons with cervical SCI (18). In addition, the 24-hour plasma norepinephrine level in individuals with SCI shows little diurnal variation.

CARDIOVASCULAR ALTERATIONS AFTER ACUTE SCI

At the moment of SCI, there is a disruption in central sympathetic control due to interruption of the descending pathways that travel in the spinal cord. In animal models, within minutes after injury, there is a systemic pressor response, which is thought to be due to both the outflow of epinephrine from the adrenal medulla and a generalized burst of sympathetic activity (19). Spinal cord transection creates an initial increase of norepinephrine, with associated increased systemic vascular resistance, hypertension, increased left ventricular (LV) ejection fraction, and bradycardia with escape arrhythmias (20–23). Guha et al. used a murine compression injury model and showed that upper thoracic SCI is characterized by a brief hypertensive peak (2 to 3 minutes in their model) (24). All animal models demonstrate that profound hypotension follows this initial hypertensive phase.

In humans and animals, this period of neurogenic shock is characterized by hypotension, bradycardia, and hypothermia (25). Neurogenic shock results from both a reduction in sympathetic activity below the level of injury and the loss of supraspinal control to the regions below the injury. This is substantiated by low plasma epinephrine, norepinephrine, and urinary metabolite measurements after SCI (26). Neurogenic shock is one component of the spinal shock syndrome, defined as the period after injury characterized by a marked reduction or abolition of sensory, motor, or reflex function of the spinal cord below the level of injury (27).

Studies in the feline model of SCI show that the loss of direct sympathetic input to the heart appears to be the primary reason for decreased cardiac output, with a marked decrease in both heart rate and contractility (28). In the rat model of SCI, hypotension and bradycardia occur, which is presumed due to unopposed vagal tone leading to nitric oxide release and vasodilation (29,37). In addition, vagal stimulation may also depress cardiac function and impair ventricular filling by slowing atrioventricular conduction and altering the synchronicity of the atrial and ventricular contractions.

The pathophysiology of acute SCI is thought to be due in part to spinal cord ischemia and its subsequent effects on the spinal cord (30). This ischemia is thought to be due to both local factors such as the direct effects of the SCI and focal vasospasm leading to loss of autoregulation of spinal cord blood flow, and systemic factors such as hypotension leading to decreased spinal cord blood flow and perfusion. Several studies have looked at maintenance of adequate systolic blood pressure as an important way to improve prognosis after acute SCI, based on the reduction of cord ischemia (31).

Hypotension

The extent and severity of the blood pressure and heart rate changes appear to correlate with the location and severity of the SCI. In a group of 71 persons with SCI, 68% of individuals with complete tetraplegia (21 of 31) had hypotension (defined as SBP < 90 mm Hg), while none of the motor-incomplete tetraplegics or paraplegics met the criteria for hypotension (32). The supine mean arterial pressure (MAP) in recently injured persons with cervical SCI averages 57 mm Hg, as compared to 82 mm Hg in supine non–cord-injured persons (33).

Recently published guidelines on blood pressure management after acute SCI (based on review of existing Class III evidence) conclude that providing blood pressure support to keep the MAP > 85 to 90 mm Hg improves neurological outcomes (31). The duration of blood pressure support was chosen arbitrarily at 5 to 7 days based on similar data in patients after traumatic brain injury. All articles describe the use of some type of invasive vascular monitoring such as central venous pressure or Swan Ganz catheter monitoring to determine fluid status, followed by initial volume resuscitation with crystalloid, and then colloid (whole blood or plasma) as indicated. If MAP remains below 85, most studies use pressors, typically a beta-agonist, followed by an alpha-agonist (34). However, it should be noted that no standard practice exists in this area.

Several studies have looked at persons after SCI with close management of hemodynamic parameters. Tator et al. studied 144 patients with SCI who were treated with attention to the management of respiratory failure and aggressive treatment of hypotension with crystalloid and whole blood or plasma transfusion (35). They compared outcomes with a cohort of 358 patients who were treated at their center prior to institution of the above treatment principles. Overall morbidity and mortality were reduced, as were costs and length of stay; these improvements were attributed to the improved respiratory management and avoidance of hypotension. This study was flawed by use of historical control, and lack of certainty of which interventions were helpful due to nonspecific outcome measures.

Levi et al. (36) treated 50 patients with acute cervical SCI with a protocol that focused on improved cardiac output and keeping MAP > 90 mm Hg, by use of invasive monitoring along with volume and pressor support. 82% of patients had volume-resistant hypotension requiring pressor within the first 7 days of treatment, which was 5.5 times more common in those with motor-complete injuries. These patients had a reduced peripheral vascular resistance index, with 58% having values below normal; half the patients also had a reduced systemic vascular resistance index. The authors note that no patient with a motor-complete injury and marked deficits in these vascular indices experienced significant neurological recovery at 6 weeks.

Vale et al. (37) managed a cohort of 77 patients with acute SCI with invasive monitoring and blood pressure support to maintain a MAP > 85 mm Hg for 7 days postinjury. The average pretreatment MAP for the neurologically complete (ASIA Impairment Scale [AIS]) A) cervical patient was 66 mm Hg. Nine of ten cervical ASIA A patients required pressor to meet the MAP goal, and 52% of the incomplete cervical injuries needed pressors. Only 9 of 29 thoracic level patients needed pressors to meet the MAP goal of greater than 85. Minimal morbidity was associated with the use of invasive monitoring or pressors. Reported outcomes were very good; 3 of 10 cervical AIS A patients regained ambulatory function, and 23 of 25 patients with incomplete cervical SCI were ambulatory at 1 year. The authors reported improved neurological outcomes based on this strategy, but with lack of specificity of intervention and without a control group, further study is needed.

Hypotension after acute SCI is caused by loss of vasomotor tone and pooling of blood in the peripheral and splanchnic vasculature. Ball et al. recommend volume resuscitation of 1 to 2 L, with caution not to infuse excess volume in a normovolemic patient (38). The interruption of the sympathetic cardioaccelerator fibers causes the heart to be unable to compensate for increased venous return with an increase in heart rate; thus, the only change that can occur is an increase in stroke volume (which may not be attainable). Thus, use of a vasopressor with both alpha and beta-adrenergic actions (such as dopamine or norepinephrine) is physiologically thought to be ideal, to give the heart the chronotropic support as well as counteracting the lack of sympathetic tone to the vessels. This strategy may help to prevent complications associated with volume overload such as pulmonary edema, which is very common after acute SCI due to aggressive volume resuscitation in an effort to treat hypotension.

Zach et al. (39) used volume expansion and monitoring of central venous pressure in order to maintain blood pressure for 7 days in a cohort of 117 patients with acute SCI. 62% of the patients with cervical injuries neurologically improved, and 38% were unchanged; no patient with a cervical injury worsened. Patients who were admitted within 12 hours of injury were more likely to improve than those admitted later (after 48 hours). The authors concluded that early management and close attention to maintaining an acceptable blood pressure improve prognosis. As in other previously mentioned studies, these results were limited by lack of a comparison group.

Wolf et al. managed patients with acute cervical bilateral facet dislocations by monitoring and maintaining a MAP above 85 mm Hg for 5 days, in combination with immediate reduction (either open or closed) of the cervical spine (40). They reported neurological improvement in 21% of patients with complete and 62% of patients with incomplete cervical injuries. The authors conclude that their management protocol improved outcomes after acute cervical SCI. The study was limited by lack of a control group.

In summary, hypotension is common after cervical SCI. Patients with complete cervical SCI require vasopressor support more frequently than either those with incomplete SCI or those with level of injury in the thoracic or lumbar neurology levels (41). There is no accepted standard for the type of vasopressor to be used. Based on nonrandomized studies, generally 5 to 7 days of support is necessary. A recent systematic review did not find high-level evidence to support neurological improvements in those with MAP of less than 85 and those with MAP less than 90 (41).

Bradycardia

Bradycardia is common in patients with cervical SCI, due to a preponderance of vagal tone and a lack of descending sympathetic input. This bradycardia typically lasts for 2 to 6 weeks postinjury; however, episodes of persistent bradycardia after that time can be seen in persons with severe injuries (42). Lehmann et al. (32) studied 71 consecutive patients after acute traumatic SCI and found that all 31 with severe cervical SCI (Frankel A and B) had persistent bradycardia (less than 60 beats per minute). The severe cervical group also had more marked bradycardia (pulse less than 45), hypotension with SBP < 90 mm Hg, supraventricular arrhythmias (predominantly atrial fibrillation), and primary cardiac arrest. 29% of patients in the severe cervical group required repeated injections of atropine or a transvenous pacer, while none in the other groups did.

In the cohort described in Lehmann's study, primary cardiac arrest occurred in 5 of 31 patients, all of whom were Frankel A

(32). All had shown some cardiovascular abnormality, including hypotension and persistent bradycardia in all five, a need for pressor therapy in four, a need for atropine in three, and both prior tachyarrhythmias and new AV block in two. Three of the cardiac arrests had a fatal outcome. The frequency of bradyarrhythmias peaked on day 4 after injury and subsided over the first 10 days. The cardiovascular abnormalities (including hypotension and bradycardia) resolved within 2 to 6 weeks. The etiology of the cardiovascular abnormalities seen after acute cervical SCI is presumed to be secondary to a lack of sympathetic innervation to the heart in patients with cervical SCI. Evidence to support this includes low baseline serum catecholamines, a subnormal rise in heart rate with atropine, the prevention of bradyarrhythmias with low-dose sympathomimetics, and the ability of unopposed vagal tone to cause bradycardia, sinus arrest, AV block, and atrial fibrillation.

Hypoxia stimulates a sympathetic response through the pulmonary inflation reflex and a vagal response through carotid body chemoreceptor activation (43). Severe bradycardia and sinus arrest have been reported to occur after vagal stimulation such as tracheal suctioning in persons with tetraplegia (43–45). While in non-SCI individuals the sympathetic response dominates and produces tachycardia in the presence of hypoxia, in persons with cervical SCI the response to hypoxia is paradoxical bradycardia. This is thought to be due to the lack of responsiveness of the SNS that normally counteracts the rise in vagal tone with suctioning or other maneuvers (including defecation or even turning). The treatment of bradyarrhythmias with atropine is only partially and transiently effective, which is consistent with the lack of sympathetic tone as the cause rather than excessive parasympathetic tone. Use of low-dose isoproterenol was suggested by Lehmann et al., which reportedly eliminated the sinus pauses (32). Intravenous aminophylline has been shown to be useful in treating severe symptomatic bradycardia and prevent pacemaker placement when given after acute SCI (46). The hypothesized mechanism is by increasing cyclic adenosine monophosphate and activating the sympathoadrenal system. Several other clinical cases also support the use of aminophylline as well as theophylline for the treatment of bradycardia in persons with acute tetraplegia (47,48).Whitman et al. (49) found that resolution of symptomatic bradycardia was associated with maintaining therapeutics levels of serum theophylline (1.9 to 3.4 mg/L).

Ruiz-Arango et al. reported on three cases of patients with cervical SCI who required permanent pacemaker implantation (50). All cases were patients with injuries at C5 or above, who had episodes of hypoxia leading to profound bradycardia and asystole, and cardiac arrhythmias requiring temporary pacing. In this case series, the most common arrhythmia was bradycardia, but patients also had AV block (first-degree and Mobitz II), atrial fibrillation, sinus arrest with sinus pauses, and asystole. Two of these patients had asystole after vagal stimulation, necessitating resuscitation. Bilello (19) reported on 83 patients with tetraplegia whom they divided into two groups, a high cervical group (C1-5) and the low cervical group (C6-7). All patients with tetraplegia had hypotension (SBP < 90) and bradycardia (HR < 50), but while 24% of the high group needed cardiovascular interventions such as pressors, chronotropes, and cardiac pacing, only 5% of the low group required these interventions. There were two patients who required permanent pacemakers, both in the high cervical group.

In summary, bradycardia is common in persons with cervical SCI. Hypoxia should be avoided and atropine should be used both reactively and prophylactically for procedures known to cause vagal stimulation. Recommendations for implantation of permanent pacemakers in individuals with cervical SCI and persistent cardiovascular abnormalities are not clear, and the literature in this area is limited to case reports.

Respiratory Impairments

In addition to the cardiovascular consequences of SCI, there is also involvement of the pulmonary system due to the loss of supraspinal sympathetic control. These pulmonary impairments are in addition to those created by the lack of innervation to respiratory musculature, which causes ventilatory difficulties or problems with secretion clearance. The pulmonary vascular bed has rich sympathetic innervation, and the lack of sympathetically mediated bronchodilation may exacerbate respiratory difficulties. In addition, neurogenic pulmonary edema occurs not uncommonly after acute SCI, due to leaky pulmonary capillaries worsened by volume overload from resuscitation.

Immediately after traumatic SCI, there is an increase in blood pressure, resulting in increased systemic and pulmonary vascular pressures. This results in a shift of blood from the high-resistance systemic circulation to the low-resistance pulmonary circulation (51). In addition, aggressive fluid resuscitation may lead to hypervolemia, which is not uncommon due to the inability to gauge fluid status in an acutely injured patient with severe hypotension (52). Marked increases in pulmonary vascular pressures and in pulmonary blood volume then produce neurogenic pulmonary edema because of the hydrostatic effect of increased pulmonary capillary pressure (53). After the transient pulmonary vascular hypertension subsides, the patient is left with abnormal pulmonary capillary permeability, which contributes to the persistence of pulmonary edema (51). Interestingly, neurogenic pulmonary edema has been reported to occur with autonomic dysreflexia, which supports the theory that a massive sympathetic discharge is the initiating event in neurogenic pulmonary edema (54).

Levi et al. (36) studied the altered response of the pulmonary vascular bed after cervical SCI in 50 patients with acute cervical SCI. These authors noticed that patients with a low pulmonary vascular resistance index (PVRI) were less likely to recover any neurologic function than patients with a higher pulmonary or systemic vascular resistance index. They also found that these patients have a reduced response to conventional volume challenge, which improves with small amounts of dopamine. They hypothesized that the poor prognosis for patients with low PVRI is a reflection of the severity of the SCI, and that the pulmonary vascular bed is more sensitive to the effects of the lack of sympathetic innervation seen in cervical SCI.

POSTACUTE CARDIOVASCULAR RESPONSES

The emergence from spinal shock is marked by the return of neuronal activity in the spinal cord interneurons (55). Spinal shock typically persists 4 to 6 weeks, but there is still a lack of clarity regarding the definition of the end of spinal shock, with different reflexes recovering at different times. For example, reflexes such as the deep plantar and the bulbocavernosus reflex return within the first 48 hours after SCI, while deep tendon reflexes take 2 weeks to return postinjury, and bladder reflexes may take even longer to develop (14). Several studies have noted the return of heart rate and blood pressure to near-normal values within 5 to 7 days of lower cervical and upper thoracic SCI (56,57). However, even after the acute phase of SCI, there continue to be alterations in cardiovascular function due to the lack of connection between CNS regulatory centers and the effector organs of the ANS.

In general, after the acute phase of injury, basal systolic and diastolic blood pressure in tetraplegics remains about 15 mm Hg lower than in normal subjects, due to the interruption of supraspinal sympathetic input (43). As would be expected, an inverse relationship between level of injury and blood pressure has been found, which is thought to be the result of the lack of sympathetic vasoconstrictor influences below the level of injury (58). In persons with chronic tetraplegia, supine blood pressure is lower than in non–cord-injured persons, with loss of the nocturnal circadian fall of blood pressure (59). In addition, there are low basal levels of plasma noradrenaline and adrenaline. Krum et al. (60) measured blood pressure and heart rate variability over a 24-hour period, in persons with cervical SCI as compared noninjured controls. They found that nighttime blood pressures (BPs) were the same in both groups, but daytime BPs were higher in non–cord-injured persons, even when postural changes were eliminated. The findings support the absence of normal diurnal variation in sympathetic activity in persons with tetraplegia.

Other cardiovascular alterations that are seen after acute SCI include changes in heart rate and cardiac output. Individuals with midthoracic cord injuries have elevated heart rates both at rest and with activity when compared to non–cord-injured persons. In addition, those with SCI have lower stroke volumes at rest and with activity than non–cord-injured persons (61). The lower stroke volume is due to decreased venous return from regions below the level of injury, which is both from lack of effective muscle pumping action and lack of sympathetic vasoconstrictor tone (8). The elevated heart rate may be to compensate for the reduced stroke volume.

In persons with chronic SCI, vascular adaptations are seen, most of which have been shown to occur within the first 6 weeks after injury. These include a 30% reduction in femoral artery diameter, with a reduction in blood flow and volume, and doubling of stress levels in the femoral artery with increased basal shear rate levels and flow-mediated dilation (62). The change in limb volume due to muscle atrophy is proportional and parallels the time course of the arterial changes, suggesting a hypothetical link between muscular and arterial adaptations.

de Groot et al. (63) determined that the dimensions of the left atrium, left ventricle, and vena cava are all reduced in persons with cervical SCI. These changes are hypothesized to occur due to a variety of factors including vascular atrophy with resultant reduced total blood volume, reduced cardiac filling, and lower stroke volume and cardiac output. In addition, cardiac preload is decreased due to pooling of blood in the lower extremities, as well as low systolic blood pressure, and lower heart rate. All these factors may contribute to lower LV wall stress and subsequent cardiac atrophy. Nash found that LV wall atrophy is common in persons with chronic tetraplegia, but that exercise causes remodeling and an increase in LV mass (64).

Changes in Circulating Catecholamines

Present SNS activity can be assessed using free plasma catecholamine measurements, due to their short half-life. Plasma noradrenaline levels reflect sympathetic nerve functioning, while plasma adrenaline levels reflect adrenomedullary function (25,65,66). Individuals with tetraplegia have low basal levels of both noradrenaline and adrenaline (67,68). Individuals with injuries between T1 and T5 have low levels of adrenaline, indicating impaired release of catecholamines from the adrenal medulla (67,69). With exercise, persons with cervical level injuries do not have augmentation of catecholamines, those with lesions from T1 to T5 have increased noradrenaline but not adrenaline, and those with lesions below T5 have an increase in both catecholamines (70). This is again consistent with the known spinal level of innervation of the sympathetic outflow to the adrenal medulla.

ORTHOSTATIC HYPOTENSION

Blood pressure control depends on tonic activation of the SNS by means of descending input from supraspinal structures (14). In non-SCI persons, assumption of upright posture is associated with pooling of blood in the lower extremities, which reduces cardiac output. This causes a decline in blood pressure, which is sensed by the aortic and carotid sinus baroreceptors. This causes a decrease in the rate of afferent inhibitory action potentials to the medullary vasomotor center via the glossopharyngeal and vagus nerves (2). In response, there is sympathetic activation through descending spinal tracts that causes vasoconstriction and also results in PS inhibition (25).

Orthostatic hypotension is defined as a decrease in systolic blood pressure of more than 20 mm Hg or a decrease in diastolic blood pressure of more than 10 mm Hg with upright posture, or head-up tilt to 60 degrees for at least 3 minutes (7). This is typically accompanied by symptoms, including fatigue, weakness, dizziness, light-headedness, blurred vision, dyspnea, and/or nausea (71,72). The frequency and severity of these symptoms are not necessarily related to absolute BP. In one study, 74% of spinal cord–injured persons had orthostasis, but only 41% of cord-injured persons with orthostatic hypotension were asymptomatic (73). Orthostasis is often more severe acutely, but persists for some patients chronically, and may in fact worsen many years postinjury (71).

Many changes after SCI contribute to the development of orthostasis. Because SCI interrupts the excitatory descending sympathetic input from the rostroventrolateral medulla, there is resulting low resting blood pressure, loss of BP autoregulation, and disturbed vascular reflex control (74). In addition, there is decreased venous return, decreased ventricular end-diastolic filling pressure and stroke volume, and decreased cardiac output and arterial blood pressure (75–77). Persons with SCI above T6 also lose the ability to vasoconstrict in the splanchnic vascular bed, which contributes to loss of the ability to autoregulate blood pressure. Even in patients with injury levels below T6, there is still loss of reflex vasoconstriction in the skeletal muscle bed, which may lead to orthostatic hypotension (although usually not as pronounced as in those with higher levels) (58). In addition, venous pooling in the lower extremities occurs due to lack of the beneficial effects of the venous pumping action of active muscle contractions. All of these changes predispose to orthostatic hypotension after SCI.

Persons with SCI tend to tolerate orthostasis well, perhaps due to changes in cerebral autoregulation that maintain cerebral blood flow and oxygenation, despite greater decrease in MAP and stroke volume than non–cord-injured (78,79). There is usually no loss of consciousness with orthostasis, except in recently injured persons with tetraplegia, or in those with chronic tetraplegia after a period of recumbancy. Studies in persons with tetraplegia reveal the ability to autoregulate cerebral perfusion at lower systemic blood pressures than non–cord-injured persons.

Persons with cervical SCI have a slight increase in heart rate during head-up tilt, due to decreased baroreceptor activity causing a reduction in vagal tone. However, the heart rate does not typically go above 100 beats per minute, due to the interrupted SNS (80). This is different from non–cord-injured individuals, who may become tachycardic with hypotensive episodes. Plasma noradrenaline levels do not rise with head-up tilt, as expected due to the impaired ability to activate the SNS reflexively in response to a fall in blood pressure. However, there are a variety of other mechanisms that help the person with tetraplegia adapt to orthostatic challenges. The release of renin occurs independently of sympathetic stimulation, probably secondary to the fall in renal perfusion pressure (80). This results in the formation of angiotensin II, which is a vasoconstrictor and also facilitates the release of aldosterone from the adrenal cortex. Aldosterone causes retention of sodium and water, which in turn increases intravascular volume (81). Vasopressin (antidiuretic hormone) also is released, which causes fluid retention and decreased urine output during prolonged head-up tilt.

The return of lower extremity (LE) spasticity can counter the LE venous pooling and may reduce the incidence of orthostasis in those with chronic SCI. Other mechanisms that decrease the degree of orthostatic hypotension experienced by persons with chronic SCI include vigorous renal vasoconstriction and some autonomy of spinal vasomotor reflexes (14).

The management of orthostasis is discussed in detail in a review by Claydon et al. (82). Physical methods, including compression wraps to the legs and an abdominal binder donned prior to sitting up help to prevent venous distension and prolonged pooling of blood in the LEs, should be tried to mitigate orthostasis. Repeated postural changes on a tilt table or a high back reclining wheelchair also lessen the drop in BP. Maintaining adequate fluid intake is important and one should not be started on fluid restriction for an IC bladder program until the symptoms have improved. Avoiding diuretics such as alcohol and caffeine, and partaking in small meals to minimize postprandial hypotension are recommended. Sleeping with the bed head raised by 10 to 20 degrees should be encouraged to increase plasma volume and orthostatic tolerance.

Pharmacologic agents are added to the treatment regimen if the above interventions do not resolve the symptoms. Sodium chloride tablets (1 g four times per day) or catecholamines such as midodrine hydrochloride (2.5 to 10 mg three times per day) are used. If ineffective, a salt-retaining mineralcorticoid such as fludrocortisone (0.05 to 0.1 mg daily) can be added (83–85). The medication should be given approximately 1 hour prior to activity known to cause hypotensive episodes. Patients should be monitored closely for hypertension when taking these medications.

Chronic low resting BP may interfere with participation in activities that may provoke symptoms and impact quality of life. Chronic hypotension may have a deleterious effect upon the patient's long-term health, as low resting systolic BP (less than 110 mm Hg) is associated with fatigue and can lead to deficits in cognitive performance (82). These patients may also be at greatest risk for other cardiovascular abnormalities.

AUTONOMIC DYSREFLEXIA

Autonomic dysreflexia (AD) is a potentially life-threatening emergency that can occur in individuals with SCI at the level of T6 and above, and has been reported in patients with SCI as low as T8-10 (54,86). This condition has previously been referred to as autonomic hyperreflexia, paroxysmal hypertension, and sympathetic hyperreflexia (87–90). AD is characterized by elevation in blood pressure accompanied by a symptom complex commonly including headache, flushing and sweating above the level of injury, and piloerection below the level of injury (91,92). This reaction is provoked by increased sympathetic outflow in response to a noxious stimulus below the level of SCI, most frequently due to bladder or bowel distention. Early recognition and management of AD is extremely important, as dramatic elevation in blood pressure can be associated with seizures, intracranial hemorrhage, and even death in the SCI population.

Historically, AD has been reported to occur 48% to 85% of patients with tetraplegia or high paraplegia (91,93); however, some studies have reported a much lower incidence of AD. This is possibly a reflection of the shorter hospital lengths of stay in patients with SCI within recent years, as AD typically presents between 6 months and 1 year after injury, with 92% of cases presenting within the first year (91). Ragnarsson et al. (94) reported a 15.4% incidence of AD during the acute phase in patients with tetraplegia. Although AD does not routinely present acutely following SCI, Krassioukov et al. (95) reported a 5.7% incidence of early-onset AD within the first month after injury in patients with cervical SCI, with the earliest presentation 4 days postinjury.

AD occurs most commonly in individuals with complete SCI, but can also occur in those with incomplete SCI. Helkowski et al. reported that the incidence of AD in patients with AIS A SCI was significantly higher than in those patients with incomplete SCI (25% versus 10%). Further analysis of AD in incomplete SCI revealed an incidence of 12% in patients with AIS B, 13% in patients with AIS C, and 6% in patients with AIS D SCI. The time from injury to onset of AD ranged from 3.5 weeks to 6 months (96).

Pathophysiology

Autonomic dysreflexia is precipitated by a noxious stimulus below the level of lesion that is transmitted to the spinal cord by intact peripheral nerves. The inciting factor most commonly is bladder distention, but AD can arise from multiple other stimuli including fecal impaction, ingrown toenails, medical procedures, and pressure ulcers. The afferent impulses from the noxious stimulus ascend through the dorsal columns and spinothalamic tracts and cause a massive sympathetic discharge below the level of injury. The majority of splanchnic outflow is mediated through the T5 through L2 segments of the spinal cord (97,98). Activation of the sympathetic system causes release of neurotransmitters including norepinephrine and dopamine, which in turn cause regional vasoconstriction of the splanchnic vessels, leading to systemic hypertension. In an intact spinal cord, the sympathetic response is mediated by descending inhibitory input from supraspinal centers (97); however, in the individual with SCI, there is loss of this inhibitory control. Additional mechanisms may also contribute to the exaggerated sympathetic response, including formation of abnormal synapses from axonal sprouting around the injury site, and development of sympathetic receptor site within the spinal cord and the periphery (99).

The sympathetically induced elevation in blood pressure is sensed by the carotid sinus and aortic body, and subsequently, compensatory mechanisms are initiated in an attempt to correct the systemic hypertension. The SA node of the heart is activated by vagus nerve input, which may potentially result in reflex bradycardia, though this sign is not present in all patients experiencing AD and has been reported in as few as 10% of patients (100). The reflex bradycardia is ineffective at lowering blood pressure; however, because according to Poiseuille law, the pressure within a tube is only affected linearly by change in flow rate (slowed heart rate), but is affected to the fourth power by changing the radius (vasoconstriction of the vessels) (101). In addition to the reflex bradycardia, there is a general increase in parasympathetic activity above the level of the spinal cord lesion, resulting in vasodilation of the vasculature above the lesion (92) (Fig. 9.1).

Signs and Symptoms

Classic signs and symptoms of AD include an increase in blood pressure 20 to 40 mm Hg above baseline, bilateral pounding headache, piloerection and pallor below the level of injury, with flushing and sweating above the level of lesion. These clinical features associated with autonomic dysreflexia can be

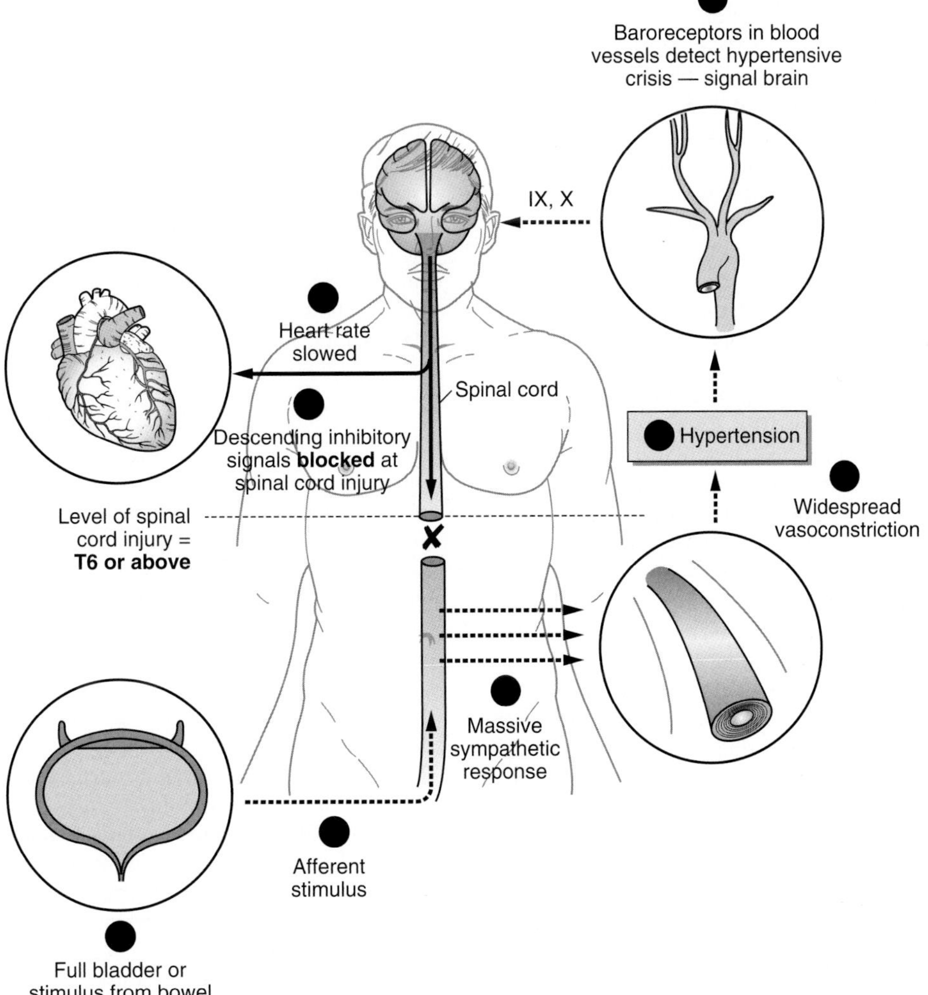

FIGURE 9.1. A diagram illustrating how autonomic dysreflexia occurs in a person with spinal cord injury. The afferent stimulus, in this case a distended bladder, triggers a peripheral sympathetic response, which results in vasoconstriction and hypertension. Descending inhibitory signals, which would normally counteract the rise in blood pressure, are blocked at the level of the spinal cord injury. The roman numerals (*IX, X*) refer to cranial nerves. (Adapted from Blackmer J. Rehabilitation medicine: 1. Autonomic dysreflexia. *CMAJ* 2003;169(9):931–935).

TABLE 9.2

SIGNS AND SYMPTOMS

Signs and symptoms of autonomic dysreflexia and autonomic etiology		
Sympathetic nervous system	**Parasympathetic nervous system**	**Nonspecific**
Systemic hypertension	Bradycardia	Anxiety
Chest pain	Cardiac arrhythmias	Nausea
Urinary retention and visceral spasm	Sweating above level of injury	Metallic taste
Pallor below level of injury	Flushing above level of injury	Respiratory distress
Piloerection below level of injury	Nasal congestion	
Blurred vision due to pupillary dilatation		

explained by the response below and above the spinal lesions to the sympathetic and PS systems, respectively. Sympathetically induced vasoconstriction below the level of spinal cord lesion decreases blood flow to this region, resulting in the pallor of the skin below the level of lesion that is commonly seen, and piloerection from sympathetic input to the hair follicles. Parasympathetically induced vasodilation of the pain-sensitive intracranial vasculature and the vasculature above the level of spinal cord lesion results in increased blood flow to these areas, causing pounding headache and flushing/above the level of injury (92). Other symptoms of AD can include generalized anxiety, nasal congestion due to vasodilation of the nasal mucosa, nausea, and blurred vision due to pupillary dilatation in individuals with injury above T1 (see Table 9.2).

Episodes of AD can result in extreme elevations of blood pressures as high as 250 to 300 mm Hg systolic and 200 to 220 mm Hg diastolic (102). These extreme elevations of blood pressure can cause end-organ damage and can potentially be fatal. Serious, potentially life-threatening complications of AD include seizures (103,104), intracerebral hemorrhage (104,105), and even death (104–106). There are case reports of other various complications including hypothermia resulting from excessive reflex sweating during AD episodes (107), reversible posterior leukoencephalopathy due to sudden elevation in blood pressure (108), and neurogenic pulmonary edema (54).

Although AD poses the risk of severe morbidity and mortality, some disabled athletes attempt to induce AD in order take advantage of the increased cardiac output due to elevation of blood pressure, which theoretically enhances the athlete's performance. Athletes who induce AD for performance enhancement, referred to as "boosting," typically do so by overdistending the bladder, wearing tight leg straps or by sitting on sharp objects. One study in wheelchair distance racers revealed that the average time in athletes inducing AD was 10% faster than those athletes who did not report boosting. Voluntary boosting is considered unethical and illegal by the International Paralympic Committee Medical and Anti-Doping Code (109).

Inciting Events

Any noxious stimulus below the level of injury can trigger AD; however, bladder distention is the most common cause and is responsible for 75% to 85% of cases (91). The bladder may become overdistended due to a kink in the Foley catheter or insufficient frequency of intermittent catheterization program resulting in high bladder volumes. The second most common cause of AD is from bowel distention due to fecal impaction, accounting for 13% to 19% of cases (91). Other potential causes include pressure ulcers (110,111), ingrown toenails (91), sperm retrieval (112,113), ejaculation (114) among others (see Table 9.4). There are reports of silent AD occurring during voiding (115) and urological procedures (115,116), as well as during bowel programs (117). Furusawa et al. (118) reported significant increases in blood pressure during insertion of rectal medication, digital stimulation, and manual evacuation of stool during performance of routine bowel program in patients with cervical SCI. They later reported that the use of topical anesthesia with instillation of lidocaine jelly into the rectal vault prior to the initiation of bowel programs in subjects with cervical SCI significantly decreased the mean maximal increase in systolic BP (119).

Treatment

Due to the serious nature of this disorder, it is of the utmost importance that AD be recognized and treated as soon as possible. The Consortium for Spinal Cord Medicine published clinical practice guidelines on the acute management of AD, which were last revised in 2001, detailing the appropriate recognition and treatment of AD (120). Individuals at risk for development of AD should be thoroughly educated on the symptoms associated with AD and appropriate treatment so that they may assist with early diagnosis and treatment should they experience this disorder. The individual's blood pressure should be checked immediately once signs and symptoms of AD are recognized. If the systolic and diastolic blood pressures are noted to be 20 to 40 mm Hg above baseline for that individual (15 to 20 mm Hg elevation in adolescents, 15 mm Hg elevation in children), one should initiate the treatment protocol for AD (see Table 9.3). If the individual is lying supine during the episode, he should immediately be repositioned to sit upright, allowing the orthostatic response to assist with lowering the blood pressure. All constricting clothing, including abdominal binders and elastic stockings, should be removed immediately to assist with blood pooling into the lower extremities. The individual's blood pressure and pulse should be monitored frequently (every 2 to 5 minutes) while the survey is initiated to determine the underlying etiology of the AD episode.

TABLE 9.3

TREATMENT PROTOCOL

Treatment protocol for autonomic dysreflexia
1. Sit the patient upright 2. Loosen tight clothing, remove abdominal binder and GES 3. Monitor blood pressure and heart rate every 2–5 min 4. If Foley catheter is in place, check for kinks or blockage. Flush with 10–15 mL of saline if necessary 5. If no Foley catheter, instill 2% lidocaine jelly into the urethra and catheterize 6. If symptoms are present and SBP > 150, administer antihypertensive agent 7. If symptoms are present and SBP < 150, manually disimpact and perform bowel program after instillation of 2% lidocaine jelly into the rectum 8. If symptoms persist despite above treatment, search for other inciting factor (see Table 9.4)

The urinary system should be evaluated first, as bladder distention is responsible for the majority of cases of AD. If the individual has an indwelling catheter, it should be checked for possible kinks or constrictions that could be interfering with drainage. If no kink is detected but the catheter appears to be blocked, it should be gently flushed with 10 to 15 mL of body temperature normal saline (5 to 10 mL in children, 10 to 15 mL in adolescents). If the catheter does not drain, it should be replaced, or if the individual does not have an indwelling urinary catheter, he should be catheterized after instillation of 2% lidocaine jelly into the urethra. If there is no evidence of bladder distention, fecal impaction should be suspected, as this is the second most common cause of AD. If the systolic blood pressure is less than 150 mm Hg, lidocaine jelly should be instilled into the rectal vault, and then the rectal vault should be checked for stool, and manually disimpacted if possible. If evaluation of the bladder and bowel does not reveal the cause of the episode of AD, less common causes should be investigated, including ingrown toenails, fractures, heterotopic ossification, and others (see Table 9.4).

For patients with a systolic BP above 150 mm Hg, the use of an antihypertensive agent with rapid onset and short duration of action should be considered. Various medications have been used including nitrates, nifedipine, hydralazine, mecamylamine, prazosin, diazoxide, captopril, clonidine, and phenoxybenzamine (121). Of these agents, immediate-release nifedipine (bite and swallow administration) and nitrates (topical paste or sublingual) are the most commonly utilized (121). Blood pressure should be monitored closely after administration of an antihypertensive agent once the episode of AD has passed, as the patient is at risk for reflex hypotension.

AD can occur in pregnant women and can be difficult to differentiate from preeclampsia. The morbidity in both disorders is related to the hypertension, and it is therefore important to control the blood pressure. Treatment recommendations for management of AD in pregnant patients were addressed in the revised version of the clinical practice guidelines (120). According to these guidelines, consideration for referral to an experienced obstetrician may be indicated to assist with choice of antihypertensive medication or management of recurrent or life-threatening episodes of AD, AD occurring in the third trimester of pregnancy, or other concerning signs such as vaginal bleeding or possible onset of labor (122) (see Chapter 23).

Following resolution of the acute episode of AD, the individual's blood pressure should be monitored over the next 2 hours to ensure that the episode has resolved, and that the decrease in blood pressure was not just due to the administration of an antihypertensive agent. Once the inciting factor

TABLE 9.4

ETIOLOGIES AND PRECIPITANTS OF AUTONOMIC DYSREFLEXIA

Urogenital system
Bladder distention
Catheterization
Urinary tract infection
Testicular torsion
Scrotal compression
Epididymitis
GU instrumentation
Sexual intercourse
Sexually transmitted diseases
Ejaculation
Electroejaculation
Vibratory stimulation–induced ejaculation
Menstruation
Labor and delivery
Gastrointestinal system
Bowel distention
Appendicitis
Erosive gastritis
Gastric reflux
Gastric and duodenal ulcers
Peritoneal irritation
Cholecystitis, cholelithiasis
Enemas
Hemorrhoids
Anal fissure
GI instrumentation
Skin
Pressure ulcer
Ingrown toenails
Sunburn
Blisters
Constrictive clothing
Contact with sharp objects
Extremities
Heterotopic ossification
Deep venous thrombosis
Fracture
Joint dislocation
Electrical stimulation
Other
Boosting
Excessive caffeine intake
Excessive alcohol intake
Substance abuse
Surgical procedures
Pulmonary emboli

is discovered, appropriate adjustments must be made to the individual's treatment plan in order to attempt to prevent future episodes of AD from that precipitating factor. Appropriate documentation of the episode is necessary, including presenting signs and symptoms, treatments, and their response. If the episode of AD does not resolve, or the inciting factor is not discovered, consideration should be made to admit the patient for further observation and workup.

THROMBOEMBOLIC DISORDERS IN SCI

The development of deep vein thrombosis (DVT) is a well-established medical complication in patients with acute SCI. Studies based solely on clinical parameters in acutely injured SCI patients have revealed the presence of DVT in approximately 14% to 16% of patients (123–125). With the use of more sensitive measures, including duplex ultrasound, venography, and ^{125}I fibrinogen scans, the incidence of DVT has been estimated to be 47% to 100% without prophylaxis (125–128). The development of DVT has been seen as early as 72 hours postinjury (129), with peak incidence within 2 weeks of injury (130,131). Venous thrombosis is a significant cause of morbidity and mortality in the acutely injured population. Chemoprophylaxis should be initiated soon after injury to decrease the risk of DVT and PE. Duplex ultrasound has been shown to be a reliable, cost-effective screening tool in traumatic SCI patients at admission to rehabilitation (132–136). Studies using duplex ultrasound surveillance at rehabilitation admission have shown the incidence of DVT in patients with acute SCI to be 11.6% to 13% at time of admission (134,135). Early detection and treatment of DVT in the SCI population is of utmost importance in order to avoid severe complications such as pulmonary embolism, which has been shown to occur in 8% to 14% of patients with acute SCI (126,130,131).

Etiology

Individuals with SCI have a high incidence of thromboembolic disorders because they meet the criteria for clot formation described by Virchow: stasis, hypercoagulability, and endothelial injury (137). The stasis component of Virchow's triad is due to the loss of muscle tone with the onset of paralysis and immobility in SCI. The loss of the active calf muscle pump in the LEs leads to venous stasis. Frieden et al. (138) demonstrated decreased venous outflow in the LEs as measured by venous occlusion plethysmography in patients with SCI without DVT when compared to able-bodied controls. Rouleau and Gertin (139) found that following experimental transection of the spinal cord in mice the diameter of the femoral and saphenous veins was increased 1.5 fold. These investigators hypothesized that the increased diameter of the deep vein size would decrease the blood flow velocity and subsequently increase the risk for thrombus formation.

In addition to venous stasis, patients with SCI are also at risk for thromboembolic disorders due to a hypercoagulable state following injury. In the noninjured individual, homeostasis is maintained by balanced activity between fibrin deposition and fibrinolysis. Studies have shown that following SCI there are alterations in levels of various regulatory proteins involved in the clotting cascade, including antithrombin III, plasma homocysteine, and inhibitors of plasminogen activator-1, as well as evidence of increased platelet aggregation and decreased fibrinolytic activity (126,136–142). The combination of these factors is responsible for the hypercoagulable state experienced by individuals with SCI.

Some of these factors are present acutely and remain in the chronic time frame. For example, Frisbie (140) noted decreased fibrinogen half-life and increased fibrinogen uptake in acute and chronic SCI patients compared to controls, indicating ongoing thrombotic activity. Ersoz et al. (141) found that collagen-induced platelet aggregation remained elevated when compared to controls in patients 12 to 48 weeks after SCI. Lastly, levels of tissue plasminogen activator (tPA), a measure of fibrinolytic activity, were measured in patients with SCI 1 to 6 months post-SCI, and there was no difference in tPA levels as a function of time. These findings indicated that fibrinolytic potential did not improve in the first 6 months following injury (142). Winther noted increased euglobulin clot lysis time in patients with cervical SCI of at least 2 years' duration compared to age-matched controls, indicating decreased fibrinolytic activity at this time point (143).

Screening

Venous thrombosis is a significant cause of morbidity and mortality in the acutely injured SCI population. Early detection and treatment of DVT in the SCI population is important in order to avoid severe complications such as PE. Historically, several modalities have been used to diagnose DVT, including ^{125}I Fibrinogen scanning, impedance plethysmography (IPG), and also venography, which is considered the gold standard for diagnosis of DVT. Duplex ultrasound is frequently utilized for the diagnosis of DVT, as it is a relatively inexpensive, noninvasive test. Duplex ultrasound has been proven effective in the detection of DVT, with sensitivity and specificity ranging from 98% to 100% and 75%to 100%, respectively (132,133).

Powell et al. (134) evaluated the appropriateness of obtaining screening duplex exams in the SCI population at admission to rehabilitation and found 11.6% were diagnosed with a DVT. Kadyan et al. (135) noted that the incidence of DVT at admission to rehabilitation was 8.7%; of those patients with initial negative dopplers, 4.8% were later noted to have DVT and 4.8% developed pulmonary emboli. Both studies reached the conclusion that obtaining screening dopplers at admission to rehabilitation is clinically indicated in the high-risk SCI population.

D-dimer levels have been shown to provide good negative predictive value for DVT in the general population (144,145), but poor specificity for diagnosing DVT. Roussi et al. (146) studied d-dimer levels for diagnosis of DVT in patients with SCI, and noted that d-dimer levels were normal in only 31% of patients but were elevated in all patients diagnosed with DVT. These investigators concluded that normal d-dimer levels have good negative predictive value and may limit the need for further workup, including duplex ultrasound, in some patients with SCI.

Furlan et al. conducted a systematic review investigating the utility of screening for DVT in the SCI population, with various screening modalities including the use of d-dimer, duplex ultrasound, ^{125}I Fibrinogen scanning, and IPG. The frequency of DVT in these studies varied from 5.3% to 38.6%. The investigators found that in order to prevent one death due to asymptomatic DVT, 71 to 260 SCI patients would need to be screened. Based on their findings, they were unable to conclude whether routine screening for DVT should be performed in the acute SCI population (147).

Kadyan et al. evaluated the cost effectiveness for obtaining screening duplex ultrasound in SCI patients. They noted a 10.3% incidence of DVT in their population of SCI patients undergoing duplex exam at time of admission. Using a statistical model previously described by Meythaler (148), these investigators determined that the use of screening duplex ultrasound at admission to rehabilitation is cost effective (136).

DVT Prophylaxis

Various chemoprophylactic agents have been investigated to prevent DVT/PE, including low-dose and adjusted-dose heparin, low molecular weight heparins (LMWH), and oral agents such as aspirin, dipyridamole, and warfarin. The effectiveness of mechanical agents in the prevention of DVT/PE, including gradient elastic stockings (GES), external compression devices, electrical stimulation (ES), and inferior vena cava (IVC) filters, has also been evaluated.

Prior to the mid-1970s, measures were not taken to prevent venous thrombosis, and patients were simply treated if DVT or PE were detected. Watson initiated a chemoprophylactic regimen that consisted of heparin 5,000 units subcutaneous (sc) given every 12 hours for the first month after SCI, followed by anticoagulation using warfarin (with a goal INR of 2 to 3) during the second and third months following SCI, with the goal of decreasing the incidence of venous thrombosis in patients with SCI. He reported that there was a significant decrease in the incidence of venous thromboembolic disorders and death when using this regimen (123).

Green et al. compared the effectiveness of external pneumatic calf compression (EPCC) when used alone or in combination with antiplatelet agents (aspirin 300 mg twice daily and dipyridamole 75 mg three times daily). These investigators found a significantly lower rate of DVT in those subjects who were randomized to receive the combination of antiplatelet agents and EPCC (149).

In a later prospective study, Green et al. compared fixed, low-dose heparin versus adjusted-dose heparin in the prevention of thromboembolism in subjects with SCI. The low-dose fixed heparin group received 5,000 units sc twice daily, while the adjusted-dose heparin group received doses that prolonged the activated partial thromboplastin time (aPTT) to a goal of 1.5 times control. The patients in the adjusted-dose heparin group were noted to have a significantly lower incidence of DVT (7% versus 31%); however, they were at a higher risk of bleeding (150).

Mechanical methods for prevention of DVT have been investigated in patients with SCI when used alone and in conjunction with chemoprophylactic agents. Winemiller et al. published a case cohort study of patients with SCI admitted to their hospital from 1976 to 1995. They reported the effectiveness of sequential compression devices and GES in reducing the risk of thromboembolism (RR: 0.5, CI: 0.28 to 0.90). These investigators also noted a trend toward decreased risk of DVT with the use of heparin therapy; however, these results did not reach statistical significance (151). Merli et al. reported on the use of GES and external pneumatic compression in combination with low-dose heparin in motor-complete or nonfunctional motor-incomplete SCI patients within 48 hours of injury. When compared to a previous control group, the investigators reported a significant reduction in incidence of venous thrombosis with the use of combined mechanical and pharmacological prophylaxis; there was a 5.2% incidence of DVT in the study group compared to 35.3% in the control group (152).

ES is another mechanical modality that has been investigated for the prevention of venous thrombosis. Merli et al. compared the use of low-dose heparin alone or in combination with ES applied to the tibialis anterior and gastrocnemius 23 hours per day to control patients who received only saline injections without mechanical or pharmacological prophylaxis. These investigators found that the incidence of DVT as determined by ^{125}I fibrinogen scanning and venography was 47% in the placebo group, 50% in the low-dose heparin group; however, the incidence of DVT in the group receiving both low-dose heparin and ES was significantly lower, at only 6.7% (126).

LMWH are noted to have better absorption and less variability in the anticoagulant response. The effectiveness of several different LMWH's in prevention of venous thrombosis has been investigated. Green et al. reported on the safety and efficacy of logiparin in patients with acute motor-complete SCI. Patients were randomized and received either standard heparin 5,000 units subcutaneous three times daily or the LMWH, logiparin, 3,500 anti-Xa units subcutaneously once daily. None of the subjects in the LMWH group developed venous thrombosis, while 7 of 21 patients (34.7%) in the standard heparin group developed DVT or PE; two of these patients died from PE (129).

Aito et al. studied the effect of nadroparine, an LMWH, used in combination with GES and external sequential pneumatic compression of the lower extremities in patients admitted to their center and initiated within 72 hours from trauma compared to patients who were admitted and started on the protocol between 8 and 28 days after SCI. These investigators found that the incidence of DVT was only 2% in those patients admitted early and started on the protocol within 72 hours of SCI. This finding was significantly lower than the incidence of DVT in the group of patients admitted and started on the protocol at 8 days or later; 26% of this group was found to have a DVT (153).

Enoxaparin is another LMWH that has also been studied in the SCI population. Deep et al. performed a retrospective review of 276 patients admitted to their center, 146 of whom were neurologically intact, the other 130 patients had sustained an SCI. All patients received GES and enoxaparin 40 mg subcutaneously once daily from time of admission until the patients "were able to be out of bed for at least 4 hours per day for physical rehabilitation" (154), although the time of initiation was variable if the patient presented to another center initially. These investigators reported that in the neurologically intact group no subjects developed DVT, and only one of the 146 patients developed pulmonary embolism; however, that subject had not received enoxaparin until 6 days after injury. In the SCI group, only 2 of 130 patients developed DVT while on enoxaparin, and 4 of 130 and 1 of 130 developed DVT and PE, respectively, after being taken off enoxaparin, as per protocol. Enoxaparin was well tolerated, with only one reported complication of possible intraspinal bleeding; no other bleeding complications were noted (154).

Standard low-dose heparins have been compared to LMWHs. Thumbikat et al. reported on a retrospective review of two groups of patients who received either heparin with transition to warfarin (INR 2 to 3) or enoxaparin (20 mg or 40 mg daily) in addition to GES and passive movements to the lower extremities. Anticoagulation was discontinued in both groups once the patients were "mobile in a wheelchair for several hours each day undergoing physical rehabilitation" (155). These researchers found that 4% of patients receiving the heparin/warfarin regimen developed venous thrombosis. In the enoxaparin group, 25% of the patients receiving the 20-mg dose and 9.4% of the patients receiving 40-mg dose developed venous thrombosis. Six of the thirteen thrombotic events in the enoxaparin group occurred after the prophylaxis had been stopped. Bleeding complications necessitating cessation of chemoprophylaxis occurred in 8% of the group receiving warfarin, which was higher than the 4.2% bleeding complication rate in the enoxaparin group (155).

The Spinal Cord Injury Thromboprophylaxis Investigators further evaluated prevention of venous thromboembolism following SCI in a two-part, multicenter study conducted during the acute hospitalization immediately following SCI, and subsequently during the inpatient rehabilitation phase. Patients were randomized to receive either heparin 5,000 units sc every 8 hours plus intermittent pneumatic compression (IPC) for at least 22 hours per day, or enoxaparin 30 mg sc every 12 hours without IPC. The study protocol was initiated within 72 hours of injury, and for patients undergoing surgical procedures only a single dose of heparin or enoxaparin was held preoperatively and the medications were restarted within 24 hours postoperatively. Bilateral venography and duplex ultrasound were performed at 2 weeks. Findings from the first phase of this two-part study suggested that the safety and efficacy of both protocols were similar (156). Upon completion of the first phase of the study, subjects without evidence of venous thromboembolism continued on to the rehabilitation phase of the study. Those subjects initially randomized to the heparin plus IPC group continued to receive heparin 5,000 units subcutaneous every 8 hours, but IPC was discontinued. The subjects in the enoxaparin group continued to receive enoxaparin at a lower dose of 40 mg subcutaneous daily. This second phase of the study revealed that the enoxaparin group had fewer episodes of new venous thromboembolism (8.5% enoxaparin group, 21.7% heparin group). Both interventions were found to be safe in this population, with only 1.2% of patients in each group discontinued from the study for bleeding complications (157).

Several studies have also compared the effectiveness of different LMWHs, as well as effectiveness of different doses of a single LMWH. Hebbeler et al. performed a retrospective chart review to evaluate the effectiveness of enoxaparin 30 mg twice daily compared to enoxaparin 40 mg sc once daily to patients admitted to an acute inpatient rehabilitation hospital and found that both regimens had equivalent efficacy; the incidence of DVT noted to be 2.0% in the patients receiving twice-daily enoxaparin compared to 1.25% in the once-daily group. Bleeding complications were also noted to be similar between groups, with a reported complication rate of 4.1% in the twice-daily group and 6.3% in the once-daily group (158). Chiou-Tan et al. compared the efficacy and safety of dalteparin 5,000 units sc once daily and enoxaparin 30 mg sc every 12 hours in a group of patients with complete or incomplete SCI, recruited within 3 months of injury in a prospective, open-labeled study. Duplex ultrasound was not routinely obtained in patients, however was performed if a patient was suspected of having a DVT. They reported similar rates of DVT and bleeding in both study groups; 6% incidence of DVT in those receiving enoxaparin versus 4% incidence of DVT in dalteparin group and 4% bleeding rate in enoxaparin group versus 2% bleeding complications in those receiving dalteparin. This study was limited by lack of standard screening duplex ultrasound in all patients and potentially delayed recruitment following acute SCI (159). Slavik et al. later reported results from a retrospective cohort study comparing the safety and efficacy of dalteparin 5,000 units sc daily versus enoxaparin 30 mg sc every 12 hours in patients with acute SCI or major orthopaedic trauma. The findings from this study suggested that enoxaparin was superior to dalteparin in prevention of venous thromboembolic event (incidence of DVT/PE 1.6% in enoxaparin group, 9.7% in dalteparin group). No differences in major or minor bleeding or mortality were noted between enoxaparin and dalteparin (major bleeding 6.4% versus 6.9%; minor bleeding 64% versus 69%; mortality 4.8% versus 6.9%) (160).

Given the strong evidence supporting the superior efficacy of the LMWHs compared to unfractionated heparin and other agents, many SCI centers use LMWH for DVT prophylaxis in patients with SCI. The Consortium for Spinal Cord Medicine Clinical Practice Guidelines (161) recommends that chemoprophylaxis should be initiated within 72 hours after SCI and continued for 8 weeks in patients with uncomplicated motor-complete SCI (AIS A and B). The FDA recently asked manufacturers of LMWH (enoxaparin, dalteparin, and ardeparin) and the heparinoid danaparoid to include in their product labeling a black-box warning of an increased risk of epidural or spinal hematoma in patients undergoing neuraxial anesthesia or spinal procedures, or in those with a history of spinal surgery (162). Therefore, initiation of LMWH may be delayed at the discretion of the treating physician based on risks and benefits of use of LMWH. Those patients with motor-complete SCI who have other risk factors placing them at higher risk for thromboembolism (lower limb fracture, previous thrombosis, cancer, heart failure, obesity, age over 70, or presence of an IVC filter) should receive chemoprophylaxis for 12 weeks. Patients with AIS C SCI should receive chemoprophylaxis up to 8 weeks, and those with AIS D injuries should receive chemoprophylaxis while remaining in the hospital (161).

Inferior Vena Cava Filters

The routine use of IVC filters for the prevention of PE is becoming more commonplace in trauma patients, including those with SCI. Several types of filters are available, including permanent and retrievable IVC filters. Several studies have been published evaluating the safety and efficacy of IVC filter placement in patients at high risk for thromboembolic events. Khansarinia et al. studied the use of prophylactic placement of Greenfield filters in trauma patients. These investigators found a significantly lower rate of PE in the group receiving prophylactic placement of the Greenfield filter (0% had a PE) compared to the control group that did not undergo filter placement (13 of 216 patients were diagnosed with PE, 9 of which were fatal) (163). Wojcik et al. reported their findings from a long-term follow-up study after the placement of IVC filters in trauma patients. High-risk patients with contraindication to chemoprophylaxis for DVT prevention had IVC filters placed for prophylactic purposes. Of these patients, none developed PE; however, 44% were noted to develop DVT after placement of IVC filter (164).

Although IVC filters have been shown to be effective in the prevention of PE in trauma patients at high risk for thromboembolism, placement of IVC filters carries the risk of potential complications. Early complications can include post-procedural bleeding, vessel penetration, malposition of the filter, and failure of filter opening. Complications can also arise weeks to months after IVC filter placement and can include IVC thrombosis, PE, venous stasis, and migration of IVC filter (165). Tetraplegic patients receiving assisted cough may be at increased risk for IVC filter migration (166).

Although several studies have evaluated the effectiveness of prophylactic placement of IVC filters in trauma patients, the literature on this topic regarding patients with SCI is relatively sparse. Maxwell et al. reported that the use of routine prophylactic IVC filter placement is not appropriate in all SCI patients. They analyzed data from SCI patients identified from the trauma registry of their regional center and noted a relatively low incidence of DVT and PE (9.0% and 1.8%, respectively) among their subjects. Maxwell noted that many of these patients were receiving chemoprophylaxis in accordance with the standards set forth by the Consortium for Spinal Cord Medicine Clinical Practice Guidelines (161) and proposed that prophylactic IVC filter placement is not appropriate for all SCI patients given the relatively low incidence of DVT/PE in SCI patients treated with chemoprophylactic agents. These investigators indicated that IVC filter placement may be appropriate in those SCI patients with contraindication to chemoprophylaxis, or those with long bone fractures, which significantly increases the risk of DVT (167). In a review article investigating the use of IVC filters in SCI patients, Johns et al. support the consideration of prophylactic IVC filter placement in those SCI patients with contraindication to early chemoprophylaxis with LMWH (168). The Consortium for Spinal Cord Medicine Clinical Practice Guidelines published in 1997 recommends that IVC filter placement should be performed in patients with contraindication to use of anticoagulation or those who have failed chemoprophylaxis. In addition, it is recommended that those patients with SCI who have poor cardiopulmonary reserve and those with complete high cervical lesions (C2, C3) receive prophylactic IVC filter placement (161). Gorman et al. recently reported increased relative risk of DVT in individuals with acute SCI who underwent prophylactic IVC filter placement. In their retrospective review of 112 patients they noted that 54 of the patients received a prophylactic IVC filter and 58 did not have an IVC filter placed. Of the patients who received prophylactic IVC filters, 11 (20.4%) were noted to develop a DVT during rehabilitation, while only 3 (5.2%) of the patients without IVC filters developed DVT ($p = 0.021$). Only one patient was diagnosed with a PE during rehabilitation, and this individual was in the group that received a prophylactic IVC filter following acute SCI (169). Further studies are necessary to determine the appropriateness of routine prophylactic placement of IVC filters in the SCI population.

Treatment of DVT or PE in persons with SCI is similar to those without SCI, except that the duration of anticoagulation may be longer. Clinical practice guidelines for the treatment of DVT in the non–spinal cord-injured population typically recommend LMWH for the initial inpatient treatment of DVT, with either unfractionated heparin or LMWH for the treatment of PE (170). LMWH was shown in a recent systematic review to be modestly superior to unfractionated heparin at preventing recurrent DVT. Patients with transient risk factors may not benefit from more than 3 months of treatment for DVT, while persons with SCI usually are given 6 months of treatment (171).

Chronically, DVT is seen less frequently than after acute SCI; with an incidence of 2.1% at 1-year follow-up, 1% at 2-year follow-up, and 0.5% at 5-year follow-up (172). These rates are still higher than the general population, in which the risk of DVT is 0.1% (173). The risk of thromboembolism increases in persons with chronic SCI who become medically ill or undergo surgery; thus, prophylaxis is recommended (174).

TEMPERATURE REGULATION

Spinal cord injuries affect the body's ability to regulate temperature in varying environments. While central temperature mechanisms are unaffected by SCI, there is impairment in the ability to regulate body temperature due to loss of connection between the hypothalamus and the tissues that aid in temperature regulation (i.e., muscles, sweat glands) below the level of injury. In addition, there is interruption of the afferent pathways from the peripheral temperature receptors below the level of SCI that feedback information to the hypothalamus on the condition of the body. In persons with SCI above T6, there is a complete loss of shivering, thermoregulatory sweating, and no peripheral circulatory adjustment (vasoconstriction/dilation) below the lesion. Individuals with SCI have lower core temperatures in the cold than non-SCI individuals, resulting in the term "partial poikiliotherms" (175). When they are exposed to warm environments, their body temperatures will rise giving a false impression of being febrile. Patients should be educated in avoidance of extreme temperatures (including sun protection and frostbite protection) as their body temperatures will tend toward the temperature of their environment, with potentially dangerous outcomes such as heat stroke or hypothermia. However, patients with cervical injuries may have very high fevers (up to 109°F) in response to infection due to lack of thermoregulatory abilities in response to a febrile state, but these are not "central fevers" and must be differentiated from high fevers after brain injury with hypothalamic damage. There is some evidence of spinal reflex–mediated sweating, but this remains a matter of debate (176). In paraplegics, deep or central temperature receptors sensitive to cold are able to initiate shivering above the level of the SCI. These receptors can act independently of the temperature of the skin above the SCI (177).

CONCLUSION

The ANS plays a key role in the regulation of many physiologic processes, with mediation by supraspinal control from centers in the CNS. SCI is associated with alterations in autonomic regulation, with level of injury playing a key role in many of the subsequent derangements that occur. Above T1,

SCI causes a complete disruption of the sympathetic pathways, and results in a variety of problems typically seen in the acute phase of injury including bradycardia, neurogenic pulmonary edema, arrhythmias, and hypotension. SCI above T6 causes an altered splanchnic outflow, which causes hypotension and altered vascular regulation. Patients with injuries at T6 and above are also prone to autonomic dysreflexia and its associated complications, also due to the loss of descending sympathetic inhibition and the inability to use the splanchnic vascular beds for volume regulation. Even persons with injuries below T6 have changes in cardiovascular response as consequences of the altered ANS regulation, although the effects of this dysregulation are less severe in lower levels of injury. Spinal cord injuries also are associated with a markedly increased risk of thromboembolic events, due to venous stasis and alterations in platelet aggregation and fibrinolysis that lead to a hypercoagulable state. While some of the issues mentioned above resolve or diminish in severity in time after SCI, many persons with SCI may have persistent orthostasis and intermittent episodes of autonomic dysreflexia on an ongoing basis, as well as impaired temperature regulation. These are chronic issues that must be managed by patient education, appropriate medical care, and an understanding of ways to compensate for lost autonomic functions.

References

1. Mohrman D, Heller L. Chapter 9: Regulation of arterial pressure. *Lange cardiovascular physiology*. New York: McGraw-Hill Companies, 2006.
2. Downey J, Myers, SJ, Gonzalez, EG, et al. *The physiological basis of rehabilitation medicine*. 2nd ed. Boston: Butterworth-Heinemann, 1994.
3. Appenzeller O, Oribe E. Autonomic anatomy, histology and neurotransmission. *The autonomic nervous system: an introduction to basic and clinical concepts*. 5th ed. New York: Elsevier, 1997:2–8.
4. Bonica JJ. Autonomic innervation of the viscera in relation to nerve block. *Anesthesiology* 1968;29(4):793–813.
5. Loewy AD, Spyer KM. *Central regulation of autonomic functions*. New York: Oxford University Press, 1990.
6. Janes RD, Brandys JC, Hopkins DA, et al. Anatomy of human extrinsic cardiac nerves and ganglia. *Am J Cardiol* 1986;57(4):299–309.
7. Glenn MB, Bergman SB. Cardiovascular changes following spinal cord injury. *Top Spinal Cord Inj Rehabil* 1997;2(4):47–53.
8. Collins HL, Rodenbaugh DW, DiCarlo SE. Spinal cord injury alters cardiac electrophysiology and increases the susceptibility to ventricular arrhythmias. *Prog Brain Res* 2006;152:275–288.
9. Mohrman D, Heller L. Chapter 7: Vascular control. *Lange cardiovascular physiology*. New York: McGraw-Hill Companies, 2006.
10. Krassioukov AV, Fehlings MG. Effect of graded spinal cord compression on cardiovascular neurons in the rostro-ventro-lateral medulla. *Neuroscience* 1999;88(3):959–973.
11. Krassioukov A. Which pathways must be spared in the injured human spinal cord to retain cardiovascular control? *Prog Brain Res* 2006;152:39–47.
12. Furlan JC, Fehlings MG, Shannon P, et al. Descending vasomotor pathways in humans: correlation between axonal preservation and cardiovascular dysfunction after spinal cord injury. *J Neurotrauma* 2003;20(12):1351–1363.
13. Quinton P. Sweating and its disorders. *Annu Rev Med* 1983;34:429–452.
14. Krassioukov A, Claydon VE. The clinical problems in cardiovascular control following spinal cord injury: an overview. *Prog Brain Res* 2006;152:223–229.
15. Schramm LP. Spinal sympathetic interneurons: their identification and roles after spinal cord injury. *Prog Brain Res* 2006;152:27–37.
16. Grimm DR, De Meersman RE, Almenoff PL, et al. Sympathovagal balance of the heart in subjects with spinal cord injury. *Am J Physiol* 1997;272(2 Pt 2):H835–H842.
17. Teasell RW, Arnold JM, Krassioukov A, et al. Cardiovascular consequences of loss of supraspinal control of the sympathetic nervous system after spinal cord injury. *Arch Phys Med Rehabil* 2000;81(4):506–516.
18. Legramante JM, Raimondi G, Massaro M, et al. Positive and negative feedback mechanisms in the neural regulation of cardiovascular function in healthy and spinal cord-injured humans. *Circulation* 6 2001;103(9):1250–1255.
19. Bilello JF, Davis JW, Cunningham MA, et al. Cervical spinal cord injury and the need for cardiovascular intervention. *Arch Surg* 2003;138(10):1127–1129.
20. Tibbs PA, Young B, McAllister RG, et al. Studies of experimental cervical spinal cord transection. Part I: Hemodynamic changes after acute cervical spinal cord transection. *J Neurosurg* 1978;49(4):558–562.
21. Tibbs PA, Young B, McAllister RG Jr, et al. Studies of experimental cervical spinal cord transection. Part III: Effects of acute cervical spinal cord transection on cerebral blood flow. *J Neurosurg* 1979;50(5):633–638.
22. Tibbs PA, Young B, Todd EP, et al. Studies of experimental cervical spinal cord transection. Part IV: Effects of cervical spinal cord transection on myocardial blood flow in anesthetized dogs. *J Neurosurg* 1980;52(2):197–202.
23. Tibbs PA, Young B, Ziegler MG, et al. Studies of experimental cervical spinal cord transection. Part II: Plasma norepinephrine levels after acute cervical spinal cord transection. *J Neurosurg* 1979;50(5):629–632.
24. Guha A, Tator CH. Acute cardiovascular effects of experimental spinal cord injury. *J Trauma* 1988;28(4):481–490.
25. Bravo G, Guizar-Sahagun G, Ibarra A, et al. Cardiovascular alterations after spinal cord injury: an overview. *Curr Med Chem Cardiovasc Hematol Agents* 2004;2(2):133–148.
26. Claus-Walker J, Halstead LS. Metabolic and endocrine changes in spinal cord injury: II (section 1). Consequences of partial decentralization of the autonomic nervous system. *Arch Phys Med Rehabil* 1982;63(11):569–575.
27. Ditunno JF, Little JW, Tessler A, et al. Spinal shock revisited: a four-phase model.[see comment]. *Spinal Cord* 2004;42(7):383–395.
28. Yardley CP, Fitzsimons CL, Weaver LC. Cardiac and peripheral vascular contributions to hypotension in spinal cats. *Am J Physiol* 1989;257(5 Pt 2):H1347–H1353.
29. Hall ED, Wolf DL. Post-traumatic spinal cord ischemia: relationship to injury severity and physiological parameters. *Cent Nerv Syst Trauma* 1987;4(1):15–25.

30. Castro-Moure F, Kupsky W, Goshgarian HG. Pathophysiological classification of human spinal cord ischemia. *J Spinal Cord Med* 1997;20(1):74–87.
31. Blood pressure management after acute spinal cord injury. *Neurosurgery* 2002;50(3 Suppl):S58–S62.
32. Lehmann KG, Lane JG, Piepmeier JM, et al. Cardiovascular abnormalities accompanying acute spinal cord injury in humans: incidence, time course and severity. *J Am Coll Cardiol* 1987;10(1):46–52.
33. Mathias CJ, Christensen NJ, Frankel HL, et al. Cardiovascular control in recently injured tetraplegics in spinal shock. *QJM* 1979;48(190):273–287.
34. Management of acute spinal cord injuries in an intensive care unit or other monitored setting. *Neurosurgery* 2002;50(3 Suppl):S51–S57.
35. Tator CH, Rowed DW, Schwartz ML, et al. Management of acute spinal cord injuries. *Can J Surg* 1984;27(3):289–293.
36. Levi L, Wolf A, Belzberg H. Hemodynamic parameters in patients with acute cervical cord trauma: description, intervention, and prediction of outcome. *Neurosurgery* 1993;33(6):1007–1016; discussion 1016–1007.
37. Vale FL, Burns J, Jackson AB, et al. Combined medical and surgical treatment after acute spinal cord injury: results of a prospective pilot study to assess the merits of aggressive medical resuscitation and blood pressure management. *J Neurosurg* 1997;87(2):239–246.
38. Ball PA. Critical care of spinal cord injury. *Spine* 15 2001;26(24 Suppl):S27–S30.
39. Zach GA, Seiler W, Dollfus P. Treatment results of spinal cord injuries in the Swiss Parplegic Centre of Basle. *Paraplegia* 1976;14(1):58–65.
40. Wolf A, Levi L, Mirvis S, et al. Operative management of bilateral facet dislocation. *J Neurosurg* 1991;75(6): 883–890.
41. Ploumis A, Yadlapalli N, Fehlings MG, et al. A systematic review of the evidence supporting a role for vasopressor support in acute SCI. *Spinal Cord.* 2010;48(5):356–362.
42. Gilgoff IS, Ward SL, Hohn AR. Cardiac pacemaker in high spinal cord injury. *Arch Phys Med Rehabil* 1991;72(8): 601–603.
43. Mathias CJ. Bradycardia and cardiac arrest during tracheal suction—mechanisms in tetraplegic patients. *Eur J Intensive Care Med* 1976;2(4):147–156.
44. Zipnick RI, Scalea TM, Trooskin SZ, et al. Hemodynamic responses to penetrating spinal cord injuries [see comment]. *J Trauma* 1993;35(4):578–582; discussion 582–573.
45. Frankel HL, Mathias CJ, Spalding JM. Mechanisms of reflex cardiac arrest in tetraplegic patients. *Lancet* 1975;2(7946):1183–1185.
46. Pasnoori VR, Leesar MA. Use of aminophylline in the treatment of severe symptomatic bradycardia resistant to atropine. *Cardiology in review*. 2004;12(2):65–68.
47. Sakamoto T, Sadanaga T, Okazaki T. Sequential use of aminophylline and theophylline for the treatment of atropine-resistant bradycardia after spinal cord injury: a case report. *J Cardiol* 2007;49(2):91–96.
48. Weant KA, Kilpatrick M, Jaikumar S. Aminophylline for the treatment of symptomatic bradycardia and asystole secondary to cervical spine injury. *Neurocrit Care* 2007;7(3):250–252.
49. Whitman CB, Schroeder WS, Ploch PJ, et al. Efficacy of aminophylline for treatment of recurrent symptomatic bradycardia after spinal cord injury. *Pharmacotherapy* 2008;28(1):131–135.
50. Ruiz-Arango AF, Robinson VJB, Sharma GK. Characteristics of patients with cervical spinal injury requiring permanent pacemaker implantation. *Cardiol Rev* 2006;14(4):e8–e11.
51. Theodore J, Robin ED. Speculations on neurogenic pulmonary edema (NPE). *Am Rev Respir Dis* 1976;113(4): 405–411.
52. Karlsson AK. Autonomic dysfunction in spinal cord injury: clinical presentation of symptoms and signs. *Prog Brain Res* 2006;152:1–8.
53. Phanthumchinda K, Khaoroptham S, Kongratananan N, et al. Neurogenic pulmonary edema associated with spinal cord infarction from arteriovenous malformation. *J Med Assoc Thai* 1988;71(3):150–153.
54. Kiker JD, Woodside JR, Jelinek GE. Neurogenic pulmonary edema associated with autonomic dysreflexia. *J Urol* 1982;128(5):1038–1039.
55. Gondim FAA, Lopes ACA Jr, Oliveira GR, et al. Cardiovascular control after spinal cord injury. *Curr Vasc Pharmacol* 2004;2(1):71–79.
56. Krassioukov AV, Weaver LC. Reflex and morphological changes in spinal preganglionic neurons after cord injury in rats. *Clin Exp Hypertens* 1995;17(1–2):361–373.
57. Maiorov DN, Weaver LC, Krassioukov AV. Relationship between sympathetic activity and arterial pressure in conscious spinal rats. *Am J Physiol* 1997;272 (2 Pt 2):H625–H631.
58. Mathias CJ. Orthostatic hypotension: causes, mechanisms, and influencing factors. *Neurology* 1995;45(Suppl 5):S6–S11.
59. Nitsche B, Perschak H, Curt A, et al. Loss of circadian blood pressure variability in complete tetraplegia. *J Hum Hypertens*1996;10(5):311–317.
60. Krum H, Louis WJ, Brown DJ, et al. Diurnal blood pressure variation in quadriplegic chronic spinal cord injury patients. *Clin Sci (Colch)* 1991;80(3):271–276.
61. Jacobs PL, Mahoney ET, Robbins A, et al. Hypokinetic circulation in persons with paraplegia. *Med Sci Sports Exerc* 2002;34(9):1401–1407.
62. de Groot PC, Bleeker MW, van Kuppevelt DH, et al. Rapid and extensive arterial adaptations after spinal cord injury. *Arch Phys Med Rehabil* 2006;87(5): 688–696.
63. de Groot PC, van Dijk A, Dijk E, et al. Preserved cardiac function after chronic spinal cord injury. *Arch Phys Med Rehabil* 2006;87(9):1195–1200.
64. Nash MS, Bilsker S, Marcillo AE, et al. Reversal of adaptive left ventricular atrophy following electrically-stimulated exercise training in human tetraplegics. *Paraplegia* 1991;29(9):590–599.
65. Peronnet F, Beliveau L, Boudreau G, et al. Regional plasma catecholamine removal and release at rest and exercise in dogs. *Am J Physiol* 1988;254(4 Pt 2):R663–R672.
66. Jensen-Urstad M, Svedenhag J, Sahlin K. Effect of muscle mass on lactate formation during exercise in humans. *Eur J Appl Physiol Occup Physiol* 1994;69(3):189–195.
67. Schmid A, Huonker M, Stahl F, et al. Free plasma catecholamines in spinal cord injured persons with different injury levels at rest and during exercise. *J Auton Nerv Syst* 1998;68(1–2):96–100.

68. Levin BE, Martin BF, Natelson BH. Basal sympathoadrenal function in quadriplegic man. *J Auton Nerv Syst* 1980;2(4):327–336.
69. Schmid A, Halle M, Stutzle C, et al. Lipoproteins and free plasma catecholamines in spinal cord injured men with different injury levels. *Clin Physiol* 2000;20(4):304–310.
70. Schmid A, Huonker M, Barturen JM, et al. Catecholamines, heart rate, and oxygen uptake during exercise in persons with spinal cord injury. *J Appl Physiol* 1998;85(2):635–641.
71. Frisbie JH, Steele DJ. Postural hypotension and abnormalities of salt and water metabolism in myelopathy patients. *Spinal Cord* 1997;35(5):303–307.
72. Sclater A, Alagiakrishnan K. Orthostatic hypotension. A primary care primer for assessment and treatment. *Geriatrics* 2004;59(8):22–27.
73. Illman A, Stiller K, Williams M. The prevalence of orthostatic hypotension during physiotherapy treatment in patients with an acute spinal cord injury. *Spinal Cord* 2000;38(12):741–747.
74. Mathias CJ, Frankel HL. *Autonomic disturbance in spinal cord lesions*. Oxford, UK: Oxford Medical Publications, 1992.
75. Faghri PD, Yount JP, Pesce WJ, et al. Circulatory hypokinesis and functional electric stimulation during standing in persons with spinal cord injury. *Arch Phys Med Rehabil* 2001;82(11):1587–1595.
76. Ten Harkel AD, van Lieshout JJ, Wieling W. Effects of leg muscle pumping and tensing on orthostatic arterial pressure: a study in normal subjects and patients with autonomic failure. *Clin Sci (Colch)* 1994;87(5):553–558.
77. Jacobsen TN, Nielsen HV, Kassis E, et al. Subcutaneous and skeletal muscle vascular responses in human limbs to lower body negative pressure. *Acta Physiol Scand* 1992;144(3):247–252.
78. Houtman S, Colier WN, Oeseburg B, et al. Systemic circulation and cerebral oxygenation during head-up tilt in spinal cord injured individuals. *Spinal Cord* 2000;38(3):158–163.
79. Gonzales F, Chang JY, Banovac K, et al. Autoregulation of cerebral blood flow in patients with orthostatic hypotension after spinal cord injury. *Paraplegia* 1991;29:1–7.
80. Mathias CJ. Orthostatic hypotension and paroxysmal hypertension in humans with high spinal cord injury. *Prog Brain Res* 2006;152:231–243.
81. Schmitt JK, Koch KS, Midha M. Profound hypotension in a tetraplegic patient following angiotensin-converting enzyme inhibitor lisinopril. Case report. *Paraplegia* 1994;32(12):871–874.
82. Claydon VE, Steeves JD, Krassioukov A. Orthostatic hypotension following spinal cord injury: understanding clinical pathophysiology. *Spinal Cord* 2006;44(6):341–351.
83. Mukand J, Karlin L, Barrs K, et al. Midodrine for the management of orthostatic hypotension in patients with spinal cord injury: a case report. *Arch Phys Med Rehabil* 2001;82(5):694–696.
84. Barber DB, Rogers SJ, Fredrickson MD, et al. Midodrine hydrochloride and the treatment of orthostatic hypotension in tetraplegia: two cases and a review of the literature. *Spinal Cord* 2000;38(2):109–111.
85. Groomes TE, Huang CT. Orthostatic hypotension after spinal cord injury: treatment with fludrocortisone and ergotamine. *Arch Phys Med Rehabil* 1991;72(1):56–58.
86. Gimovsky ML, Ojeda A, Ozaki R, et al. Management of autonomic hyperreflexia associated with a low thoracic spinal cord lesion. *Am J Obstet Gynecol* 1985;153(2):223–224.
87. Thompson CE, Witham AC. Paroxysmal hypertension in spinal cord injuries. *N Engl J Med* 1948;239(8):291–294.
88. Mathias CJ, Christensen NJ, Corbett JL, et al. Plasma catecholamines during paroxysmal neurogenic hypertension in quadriplegic man. *Circ Res* 1976;39(2):204–208.
89. McGuire TJ, Kumar VN. Autonomic dysreflexia in the spinal cord-injured. What the physician should know about this medical emergency. *Postgrad Med* 1986;80(2):81–84, 89.
90. Young JS. Use of guanethidine in control of sympathetic hyperreflexia in persons with cervical and thoracic cord lesions. *Arch Phys Med Rehabil* 1963;44:204–207.
91. Lindan R, Joiner E, Freehafer AA, et al. Incidence and clinical features of autonomic dysreflexia in patients with spinal cord injury. *Paraplegia* 1980;18(5):285–292.
92. Erickson RP. Autonomic hyperreflexia: pathophysiology and medical management. *Arch Phys Med Rehabil* 1980;61(10):431–440.
93. Kurnick NB. Autonomic hyperreflexia and its control in patients with spinal cord lesions. *Ann Intern Med* 1956;44(4):678–686.
94. Ragnarsson K, Hall K, Wilmot C, et al. Pulmonary, cardiovascular, and metabolic conditions. In: spinal cord injury: *Clinical Outcomes from the Model system.* pages 79–99. Stover S, DeLisa JA, Witeneck G, eds. Gaithersburg, MD: Aspen Publishers, Inc., 1995.
95. Krassioukov AV, Furlan JC, Fehlings MG. Autonomic dysreflexia in acute spinal cord injury: an under-recognized clinical entity. *J Neurotrauma* 2003;20(8):707–716.
96. Helkowski WM, Ditunno JF Jr, Boninger M. Autonomic dysreflexia: incidence in persons with neurologically complete and incomplete tetraplegia. *J Spinal Cord Med* 2003;26(3):244–247.
97. Trop CS, Bennett CJ. The evaluation of autonomic dysreflexia. *Semin Urol* 1992;10(2):95–101.
98. Eade MN. Paroxysmal hypertension in spinal cord injuries (autonomic hyperreflexia). *N Z Med J* 1964;63:574–580.
99. Bloch RF. *Autonomic dysfuntion* In: *Management of Spinal Cord Injuries*. Baltimore Williams & Wilkins, 1986.
100. Kewalramani LS. Autonomic dysreflexia in traumatic myelopathy. *Am J Phys Med* 1980;59(1):1–21.
101. Pfitzner J. Poiseuille and his law. *Anaesthesia* 1976;31(2):273–275.
102. Karlsson AK. Autonomic dysreflexia. *Spinal Cord* 1999;37(6):383–391.
103. Yarkony GM, Katz RT, Wu YC. Seizures secondary to autonomic dysreflexia. *Arch Phys Med Rehabil* 1986;67(11):834–835.
104. Kursh ED, Freehafer A, Persky L. Complications of autonomic dysreflexia. *J Urol* 1977;118(1 Pt 1):70–72.
105. Eltorai I, Kim R, Vulpe M, et al. Fatal cerebral hemorrhage due to autonomic dysreflexia in a tetraplegic patient: case report and review. *Paraplegia* 1992;30(5):355–360.
106. Dolinak D, Balraj E. Autonomic dysreflexia and sudden death in people with traumatic spinal cord injury. *Am J Forensic Med Pathol* 2007;28(2):95–98.
107. Colachis SC III. Hypothermia associated with autonomic dysreflexia after traumatic spinal cord injury. *Am J Phys Med Rehabil* 2002;81(3):232–235.

108. Chaves CJ, Lee G. Reversible posterior leukoencephalopathy in a patient with autonomic dysreflexia: a case report. *Spinal Cord* 2008;46(11):760–761.
109. Bhambhani Y. Physiology of wheelchair racing in athletes with spinal cord injury. *Sports Med* 2002;32(1):23–51.
110. Cole TM, Kottke FJ, Olson M, et al. Alterations of cardiovascular control in high spinal myelomalacia. *Arch Phys Med Rehabil* 1967;48(7):359–368.
111. Hall PA, Young JV. Autonomic hyperreflexia in spinal cord injured patients: trigger mechanism—dressing changes of pressure sores. *J Trauma* 1983;23(12):1074–1075.
112. Sheel AW, Krassioukov AV, Inglis JT, et al. Autonomic dysreflexia during sperm retrieval in spinal cord injury: influence of lesion level and sildenafil citrate. *J Appl Physiol* 2005;99(1):53–58.
113. Ekland MB, Krassioukov AV, McBride KE, et al. Incidence of autonomic dysreflexia and silent autonomic dysreflexia in men with spinal cord injury undergoing sperm retrieval: implications for clinical practice. *J Spinal Cord Med* 2008;31(1):33–39.
114. Elliott S, Krassioukov A. Malignant autonomic dysreflexia in spinal cord injured men. *Spinal Cord* 2006;44(6):386–392.
115. Linsenmeyer TA, Campagnolo DI, Chou IH. Silent autonomic dysreflexia during voiding in men with spinal cord injuries. *J Urol* 1996;155(2):519–522.
116. Giannantoni A, Di Stasi SM, Scivoletto G, et al. Autonomic dysreflexia during urodynamics. *Spinal Cord* 1998;36(11):756–760.
117. Kirshblum SC, House JG, O'Connor KC. Silent autonomic dysreflexia during a routine bowel program in persons with traumatic spinal cord injury: a preliminary study. *Arch Phys Med Rehabil* 2002;83(12):1774–1776.
118. Furusawa K, Sugiyama H, Ikeda A, et al. Autonomic dysreflexia during a bowel program in patients with cervical spinal cord injury. *Acta Med Okayama* 2007;61(4):221–227.
119. Furusawa K, Sugiyama H, Tokuhiro A, et al. Topical anesthesia blunts the pressor response induced by bowel manipulation in subjects with cervical spinal cord injury. *Spinal Cord* 2009;47(2):144–148.
120. Lisenmeyer TA. Acute management of autonomic dysreflexia: individuals with spinal cord injury presenting to health-care facilities. *Clinical practice guidelines. Consortium for spinal cord medicine.* Washington, DC: Paralyzed Veterans Association, 2001:1–25.
121. Braddom RL, Rocco JF. Autonomic dysreflexia. A survey of current treatment. *Am J Phys Med Rehabil* 1991;70(5): 234-241.
122. Acute management of autonomic dysreflexia: adults with spinal cord injury presenting to health-care facilities. Consortium for spinal cord. *J Spinal Cord Med.* 1997;20(3):284–308.
123. Watson N. Anti-coagulant therapy in the prevention of venous thrombosis and pulmonary embolism in the spinal cord injury. *Paraplegia* 1978;16(3):265–269.
124. Waring WP, Karunas RS. Acute spinal cord injuries and the incidence of clinically occurring thromboembolic disease. *Paraplegia* 1991;29(1):8–16.
125. Myllynen P, Kammonen M, Rokkanen P, et al. Deep venous thrombosis and pulmonary embolism in patients with acute spinal cord injury: a comparison with nonparalyzed patients immobilized due to spinal fractures. *J Trauma* 1985;25(6):541–543.
126. Merli GJ, Herbison GJ, Ditunno JF, et al. Deep vein thrombosis: prophylaxis in acute spinal cord injured patients. *Arch Phys Med Rehabil* 1988;69(9):661–664.
127. Geerts WH, Code KI, Jay RM, et al. A prospective study of venous thromboembolism after major trauma. *N Engl J Med* 1994;331(24):1601–1606.
128. Clagett GP, Anderson FA Jr, Heit J, et al. Prevention of venous thromboembolism. *Chest* 1995;108 (4 Suppl):312S–334S.
129. Green D, Lee MY, Lim AC, et al. Prevention of thromboembolism after spinal cord injury using low-molecular-weight heparin. *Ann Intern Med* 1990;113(8):571–574.
130. Rossi EC, Green D, Rosen JS, et al. Sequential changes in factor VIII and platelets preceding deep vein thrombosis in patients with spinal cord injury. *Br J Haematol* 1980;45(1):143–151.
131. Merli GJ, Crabbe S, Paluzzi RG, et al. Etiology, incidence, and prevention of deep vein thrombosis in acute spinal cord injury. *Arch Phys Med Rehabil* 1993;74(11):1199–1205.
132. Mattos MA, Londrey GL, Leutz DW, et al. Color-flow duplex scanning for the surveillance and diagnosis of acute deep venous thrombosis. *J Vasc Surg* 1992;15(2):366–375; discussion 375–366.
133. Persson AV, Jones C, Zide R, et al. Use of the triplex scanner in diagnosis of deep venous thrombosis. *Arch Surg* 1989;124(5):593–596.
134. Powell M, Kirshblum S, O'Connor KC. Duplex ultrasound screening for deep vein thrombosis in spinal cord injured patients at rehabilitation admission. *Arch Phys Med Rehabil* 1999;80(9):1044–1046.
135. Kadyan V, Clinchot DM, Mitchell GL, et al. Surveillance with duplex ultrasound in traumatic spinal cord injury on initial admission to rehabilitation. *J Spinal Cord Med* 2003;26(3):231–235.
136. Kadyan V, Clinchot DM, Colachis SC. Cost-effectiveness of duplex ultrasound surveillance in spinal cord injury. *Am J Phys Med Rehabil* 2004;83(3):191–197.
137. Virchow R. Thrombose und Embolie. Matzdorff ea, transCanton, MA, 1998.
138. Frieden RA, Ahn JH, Pineda HD, et al. Venous plethysmography values in patients with spinal cord injury. *Arch Phys Med Rehabil* 1987;68(7):427–429.
139. Rouleau P, Guertin PA. Early changes in deep vein diameter and biochemical markers associated with thrombi formation after spinal cord injury in mice. *J Neurotrauma* 2007;24(8):1406–1414.
140. Frisbie JH. Fibrinogen metabolism in patients with spinal cord injury. *J Spinal Cord Med* 2006;29(5):507–510.
141. Ersoz G, Ficicilar H, Pasin M, et al. Platelet aggregation in traumatic spinal cord injury. *Spinal Cord* 1999;37(9):644–647.
142. Boudaoud L, Roussi J, Lortat-Jacob S, et al. Endothelial fibrinolytic reactivity and the risk of deep venous thrombosis after spinal cord injury. *Spinal Cord* 1997;35(3):151–157.
143. Winther K, Gleerup G, Snorrason K, et al. Platelet function and fibrinolytic activity in cervical spinal cord injured patients. *Thromb Res* 1992;65(3):469–474.
144. Rowbotham BJ, Carroll P, Whitaker AN, et al. Measurement of crosslinked fibrin derivatives—use in the diagnosis of venous thrombosis. *Thromb Haemost* 1987;57(1):59–61.

145. Bounameaux H. Low molecular weight heparins and prevention of postoperative thrombosis. *Br J Surg* 1989;76(5):524.
146. Roussi J, Bentolila S, Boudaoud L, et al. Contribution of D-Dimer determination in the exclusion of deep venous thrombosis in spinal cord injury patients. *Spinal Cord* 1999;37(8):548–552.
147. Furlan JC, Fehlings MG. Role of screening tests for deep venous thrombosis in asymptomatic adults with acute spinal cord injury: an evidence-based analysis. *Spine* 2007;32(17):1908–1916.
148. Meythaler JM, DeVivo MJ, Hayne JB. Cost-effectiveness of routine screening for proximal deep venous thrombosis in acquired brain injury patients admitted to rehabilitation. *Arch Phys Med Rehabil* 1996;77(1):1–5.
149. Green D, Rossi EC, Yao JS, et al. Deep vein thrombosis in spinal cord injury: effect of prophylaxis with calf compression, aspirin, and dipyridamole. *Paraplegia* 1982;20(4):227–234.
150. Green D, Lee MY, Ito VY, et al. Fixed- vs adjusted-dose heparin in the prophylaxis of thromboembolism in spinal cord injury. *JAMA* 1988;260(9):1255–1258.
151. Winemiller MH, Stolp-Smith KA, Silverstein MD, et al. Prevention of venous thromboembolism in patients with spinal cord injury: effects of sequential pneumatic compression and heparin. *J Spinal Cord Med* 1999;22(3):182–191.
152. Merli GJ, Crabbe S, Doyle L, et al. Mechanical plus pharmacological prophylaxis for deep vein thrombosis in acute spinal cord injury. *Paraplegia* 1992;30(8):558–562.
153. Aito S, Pieri A, D'Andrea M, et al. Primary prevention of deep venous thrombosis and pulmonary embolism in acute spinal cord injured patients. *Spinal Cord* 2002;40(6):300–303.
154. Deep K, Jigajinni MV, McLean AN, et al. Prophylaxis of thromboembolism in spinal injuries—results of enoxaparin used in 276 patients. *Spinal Cord* 2001;39(2):88–91.
155. Thumbikat P, Poonnoose PM, Balasubrahmaniam P, et al. A comparison of heparin/warfarin and enoxaparin thromboprophylaxis in spinal cord injury: the Sheffield experience. *Spinal Cord* 2002;40(8):416–420.
156. Prevention of venous thromboembolism in the acute treatment phase after spinal cord injury: a randomized, multicenter trial comparing low-dose heparin plus intermittent pneumatic compression with enoxaparin. *J Trauma* 2003;54(6):1116–1124; discussion 1125–1116.
157. Prevention of venous thromboembolism in the rehabilitation phase after spinal cord injury: prophylaxis with low-dose heparin or enoxaparin. *J Trauma* 2003;54(6):1111–1115.
158. Hebbeler SL, Marciniak CM, Crandall S, et al. Daily vs twice daily enoxaparin in the prevention of venous thromboembolic disorders during rehabilitation following acute spinal cord injury. *J Spinal Cord Med* 2004;27(3):236–240.
159. Chiou-Tan FY, Garza H, Chan KT, et al. Comparison of dalteparin and enoxaparin for deep venous thrombosis prophylaxis in patients with spinal cord injury. *Am J Phys Med Rehabil* 2003;82(9):678–685.
160. Slavik RS, Chan E, Gorman SK, et al. Dalteparin versus enoxaparin for venous thromboembolism prophylaxis in acute spinal cord injury and major orthopedic trauma patients: 'DETECT' trial. *J Trauma* 2007;62(5):1075–1081; discussion 1081.
161. Prevention of thromboembolism in spinal cord injury. Consortium for spinal cord medicine. *J Spinal Cord Med* 1997;20(3):259–283.
162. Wysowski DK, Talarico L, Bacsanyi J, Botstein P. Spinal and epidural hematoma and low-molecular-weight heparin. *N Engl J Med* 1998;338(24):1774–1775.
163. Khansarinia S, Dennis JW, Veldenz HC, Butcher JL, Hartland L. Prophylactic Greenfield filter placement in selected high-risk trauma patients. *J Vasc Surg* 1995;22(3):231–235; discussion 235–236.
164. Wojcik R, Cipolle MD, Fearen I, et al. Long-term follow-up of trauma patients with a vena caval filter. *J Trauma* 2000;49(5):839–843.
165. Giannoudis PV, Pountos I, Pape HC, et al. Safety and efficacy of vena cava filters in trauma patients. *Injury* 2007;38(1):7–18.
166. Balshi JD, Cantelmo NL, Menzoian JO. Complications of caval interruption by Greenfield filter in quadriplegics. *J Vasc Surg* 1989;9(4):558–562.
167. Maxwell RA, Chavarria-Aguilar M, Cockerham WT, et al. Routine prophylactic vena cava filtration is not indicated after acute spinal cord injury. *J Trauma* 2002;52(5):902–906.
168. Johns JS, Nguyen C, Sing RF. Vena cava filters in spinal cord injuries: evolving technology. *J Spinal Cord Med* 2006;29(3):183–190.
169. Gorman PH, Qadri SF, Rao-Patel A. Prophylactic inferior vena cava (IVC) filter placement may increase the relative risk of deep venous thrombosis after acute spinal cord injury. *J Trauma* 2009;66(3):707–712.
170. Snow V, Qaseem A, Barry P, et al. Management of venous thromboembolism: a clinical practice guideline from the American College of Physicians and the American Academy of Family Physicians. *Ann Intern Med* 2007;146(3):204–210.
171. Segal JB, Streiff MB, Hofmann LV, et al. Management of venous thromboembolism: a systematic review for a practice guideline. *Ann Intern Med* 2007;146(3): 211–222.
172. McKinley WO, Jackson AB, Cardenas DD, et al. Long-term medical complications after traumatic spinal cord injury: a regional model systems analysis. *Arch Phys Med Rehabil* 1999;80(11):1402–1410.
173. Qureshi MM, Cudkowicz ME, Zhang H, et al. Increased incidence of deep venous thrombosis in ALS. *Neurology* 2007;68(1):76–77.
174. Kim SW, Charallel JT, Park KW, et al. Prevalence of deep venous thrombosis in patients with chronic spinal cord injury. *Arch Phys Med Rehabil* 1994;75(9):965–968.
175. Sawka MN, Latzka WA, Pandolf KB. Temperature regulation during upper body exercise: able-bodied and spinal cord injured. *Med Sci Sports Exerc* 1989; 21(5 Suppl):S132–S140.
176. Wallin BG, Stjernberg L. Sympathetic activity in man after spinal cord injury. Outflow to skin below the lesion. *Brain* 1984;107(Pt 1):183–198.
177. Downey JA, Chiodi HP, Darling RC. Central temperature regulation in the spinal man. *J Appl Physiol* 1967;22(1):91–94.

CHAPTER 10 ■ RESPIRATORY MANAGEMENT OF THE SPINAL CORD–INJURED PATIENT

AKSHAT SHAH, KAZUKO SHEM, STEVE McKENNA, AND MIKE BERLLY

INTRODUCTION

Respiratory complications are the leading cause of death in persons with spinal cord injury (SCI) and present unique challenges in their care (1–5). Although much is known about pulmonary complications, there are very few studies with large sample sizes and comparison groups, and there is little evidence-based literature on the management of this important issue. Current practice principles are based largely on expert panel opinion and clinical expertise (6). Furthermore, some protocols in SCI deviate from established practices in able-bodied individuals (7). The primary concept that defines the difference between spinal cord and able-bodied patients is the "Healthy Lung Model." Most able-bodied patients with respiratory distress enter the hospital with some impairment in intrinsic lung function from trauma, scarring, inflammation, infection, etc. Isolated SCI without pulmonary trauma results in an impairment of ventilation that is, gas movement without directly affecting lung tissue.

There are primarily three key pulmonary problems in individuals with SCI: secretion management, atelectasis, and hypoventilation. Patients with tetraplegia and high paraplegia lose intercostal muscle innervations and, therefore, are dependent primarily on the diaphragm for inhalation that leads to atelectasis and hypoventilation. The loss of innervation of respiratory muscles that are used in forceful expiration required for an effective cough leads to difficulty with clearing secretions. The goals of management of pulmonary complications are related to these problems. This chapter focuses on the respiratory dysfunction and complications secondary to SCI and their diagnoses and treatment options, in the acute and chronic phases.

PHYSIOLOGY

The main muscles of inspiration are the diaphragm, the external intercostal muscles, and the accessory muscles. Normal respiration requires the coordination of muscles innervated at various levels in the spinal cord. Cervical levels 3, 4, and 5 innervate the diaphragm. Injury to the cord at or above C5 causes impairment of diaphragmatic function. In normal respiration, the diaphragm provides approximately 65% of the vital capacity (VC) in able-bodied individuals. SCI disrupts the function of these inspiratory muscles differentially based on the level of injury. Video fluoroscopy studies of the diaphragm after SCI may show asymmetrical function, which can further impair respiratory function.

The muscles least likely to be affected by SCI are the accessory muscles of respiration, which are innervated from the most superior portion of the spinal cord. The spinal accessory nerve fibers arise from the superior segment of the spinal cord, return through the foramen magnum, and then descend through the jugular foramen at the base of the skull as cranial nerve XI (8). Because the spinal accessory nerve is infrequently disrupted by SCI, many patients will have preservation of the trapezius and sternocleidomastoid muscle function. The sternocleidomastoid originates from the mastoid process of the skull and inserts into the sternum and clavicle (part of the thoracic cage). The scalene muscles are innervated by the 3rd to 8th cervical nerve roots (9). Together, the sternocleidomastoid, trapezius, and scalene muscles lift the rib cage to expand the lungs. These accessory muscles of respiration provide very little assistance during normal respiration. However, they can function to preserve respiration for an extended period of time even in patients with high cervical SCI before fatigue leads to complete respiratory failure (10). Observation of the accessory muscles working extremely hard during inspiration should be appreciated as a sign of impending respiratory failure.

The thoracic spinal cord provides innervation to the internal and external intercostal muscles. Fibers of the external intercostal muscles originate from the posterior surface of each rib to a point anterior on the subsequent rib, forming a rhomboid geometry (8). During contraction, shortening of the external intercostal muscle fibers pulls the geometry into a rectangle that lifts the rib cage to assist with forced inhalation. These muscles can be seen retracting after SCI, as they work to maintain respiratory function.

Expiration is normally passive. Expiratory muscles become important when minute ventilation increases and expulsive forces are needed for effective cough to clear secretions (11). The primary muscles of expiration are the rectus abdominus, transverses abdominus, internal and external obliques, and pectoralis major and, to a lesser extent, the internal intercostal muscles. The abdominal muscles are innervated by both the thoracic and the lumbar spinal cord (T7-L1). Complete SCI at T6 and above results in an ineffective cough with difficulty clearing secretions and mucus plugging. Because of the loss of abdominal muscle strength, the VC in tetraplegia is affected by the position of the patient, with a 15% decrease in the upright position relative to supine. When upright, the flaccid abdominal musculature places the diaphragm in a less efficient position for breathing, increasing residual volume (9,12,13). An abdominal binder substitutes for abdominal tone, by placing the diaphragm in a more efficient position, and has been shown to improve VC but may decrease other respiratory parameters (14–16).

THE ACUTE INJURY

During the first week post acute SCI, the development of respiratory failure is a major concern. A $PaCO_2$ greater than 50 mm Hg or a PaO_2 of 50 mm Hg or below define respiratory failure while on room air and/or the need for ventilator support (10). The risk of respiratory failure is directly associated with the level and completeness of cervical injury; that is, the higher and more complete the injury, the greater the risk of respiratory failure (10,17,18). Como et al. reported that 100% of patients with complete C5 and higher injuries required tracheostomy for respiratory failure (17). Of the patients with complete injuries of C6 and below, 79% received a definitive airway, and 50% required tracheostomy (17). Another study reported that all patients with C3 injuries and above required tracheostomies (19). Patients with C8 injuries and below did not require tracheostomies, while those with injuries between C4 and C7 had variable rates of tracheostomies. However, patients in the latter group with C4 and 5 injuries had rates of 60% to 80%, while rates precipitously dropped with injuries at C6 and C7 (19). Although the studies reported different rates of risk, it is clear that a high percentage of neurologically complete patients with injuries above C5 will require tracheostomies. Hassid et al. studied the rates of tracheostomies of lower cervical spine injuries from C5 to T1; 75% of these patients required definitive airway management if their lesion was complete, falling to 50% if the injury was incomplete (20). Of those patients with incomplete injuries, the risk of needing tracheostomy changed with ASIA Impairment Scale (AIS) grade: 76% of patients with cervical AIS A and B injuries, 38% of AIS C, and 23% of AIS D patients required tracheostomy (21). Other risk factors include age greater than 45 years for injuries between C4 and 7 and the presence of pneumonia and copious secretions (18,19,22). Although it is well established that cervical SCI has a high risk of respiratory complications, it should be recognized that patients with high thoracic SCI also have a relatively high risk of respiratory complications (51%) such as the need for intubation, pneumonia, and death (22).

In the emergency room, most patients with C4-C6 injuries breathe comfortably and present with normal blood gasses. However, these patients are at high risk for complications over the next 3 to 5 days (10,23). Physicians are often unfamiliar with this later compromise, highlighted when a patient is extubated soon after spinal stabilization surgery in the first few days postinjury only to be emergently reintubated within several days. While the patient was breathing adequately prior to surgery, the assumption is that the patient can be rapidly extubated postsurgery. Postoperative patients should be weaned slowly if their VC is below 15 mL/kg of ideal body weight, their cough is weak, they have a smoking history, they have premorbid illnesses, or they are older than 45 years. Prior to weaning, the patient should be afebrile, have clear lungs, a normal chest x-ray, and oxygenate well.

The approach to pulmonary management after SCI is based upon a sequence of events that occur immediately after injury in a "healthy lung" (Fig. 10.1). Respiratory dysfunction can be categorized into the following main areas: decreased inspiratory capacity, impaired cough, atelectasis and retained secretions, mucous plugging, autonomic nervous system dysfunction and secondary bronchospasm, and chest trauma.

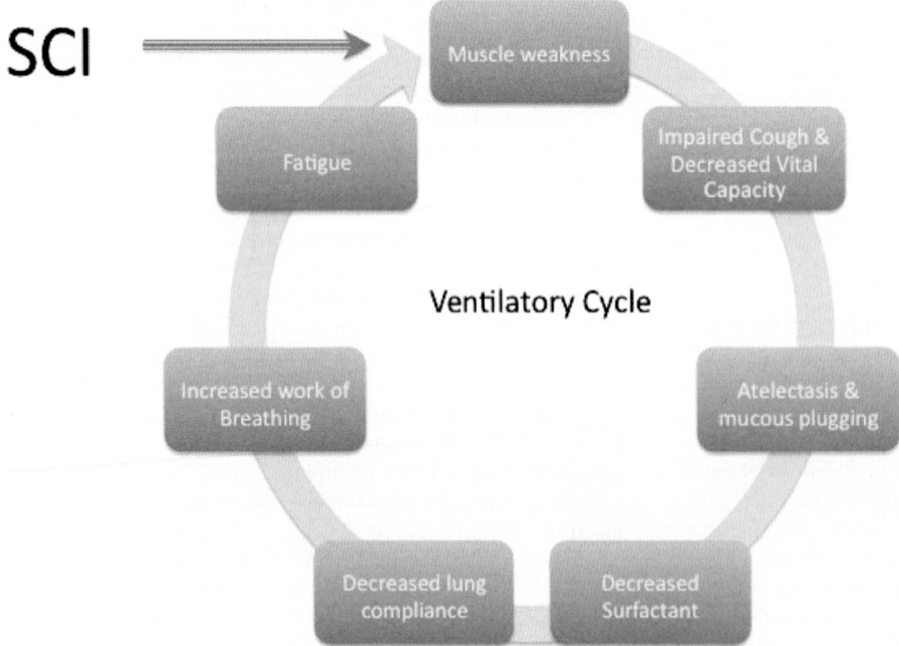

FIGURE 10.1. Progressive cycle of ventilatory dysfunction after SCI.

Muscle Weakness Resulting in Impaired Inspiratory Capacity

With injuries between C2 and 5, the more rostral the level of injury, the more pronounced inspiratory weakness becomes, ultimately leaving only various degrees of diaphragm and neck accessory muscle function available. The diaphragm and other accessory muscles of respiration may overwork and rapidly fatigue after injury. This ventilatory impairment should be monitored by VC measurements three times per day over at least the first 5 days. There are several reasons for fatigue of the muscles of respiration. During inspiration in the able-bodied individuals, the abdominal and intercostal muscles will contract, stabilizing the rib cage and placing the diaphragms in an efficient position for inhalation. During spinal shock, the intercostal and abdominal muscles are flaccid. The paralyzed intercostal muscles are drawn inward with inspiration and the paralyzed abdominal wall moves outward rather than contracting. These paradoxical movements result in a significant drop in the efficiency of breathing. The deteriorating VC correlates with diaphragm fatigue. In the obese patient, this is further exaggerated by the additional weight of the chest wall and abdomen, increasing the work and decreasing efficiency of breathing. Patients may also lose up to one motor root level within the first few days postinjury due to cord swelling or bleeding (17). For example, an individual with C4 tetraplegia on admission may become C3, which has significant implications for respiratory function (Fig. 10.1).

Muscle Weakness Resulting in Impaired Cough

Cough becomes impaired even at injuries as low as T12. With higher neurological levels, the ability to generate the force needed for an adequate cough decreases because of lack of abdominal and intercostal muscles. Once peak cough flows (PCFs) fall to less than 160 L/min, there is insufficient force to generate an effective cough (24,25). Low cough flows are associated with increased mortality and failed extubations (26).

Atelectasis

Atelectasis is the most common respiratory complication in acute SCI (9,10,27) and can lead to a cascade of complications including pneumonia and respiratory failure. Atelectasis, the state of airlessness within the lungs, is diagnosed either clinically or radiographically. In acute tetraplegia, this will occur secondary to impaired expansion of the lungs, a weak cough, and retained bronchial secretions with mucus plugs (27,28). Decreased inflation of the alveoli also leads to a significant reduction in the release of surfactant, which further contributes to atelectasis (27). Atelectasis will worsen as respiratory muscles fatigue, secretions accumulate, and lung compliance decreases. Segments of collapsed lungs no longer participate in respiratory exchange and contribute to alveolar ventilation and pulmonary perfusion mismatch. This ventilatory dysfunction represents the pivotal step in SCI patients. At this point, patients are highly susceptible to development of pneumonia and acute respiratory complications. Once these processes occur, the patient no longer fits the "healthy lung" model and must be treated according to the same principles as in able-bodied individuals with lung injury.

Retained Secretions and Development of Mucus Plugs

Hypersecretion of bronchial mucus occurs after tetraplegia, especially in individuals who smoke. Copious sputum over the first 6 days postinjury has been found to be an independent predictor of the need for ventilation (23). The secretions are abnormal in both amount and chemical content but tend to return toward normal over the subsequent months, suggesting a neuronal influence of bronchial mucus gland secretions. It has been speculated that the mucus hypersecretion is due to the loss of sympathetic control and unopposed vagal activity in the days to weeks after injury (29). Adrenergic innervation also influences the beating rate of airway cilia (12).

Patients with tetraplegia may be "drowning" in their own secretions and cannot adequately expectorate. Expiration is normally passive, but abdominal muscles are important when minute ventilation increases and expulsive forces are needed for effective cough to clear secretions (11). As the diaphragm relaxes during expiration, the flaccid chest wall moves outward, limiting the expiratory reserve volumes to less than 20% of normal (30). Since the abdominal musculature is also flaccid, forced expiration is severely compromised (30). The combination of increased bronchial secretions and an ineffective cough can lead to mucus plugs and sudden respiratory distress.

Bronchospasm

Resting airway tone is potentially increased in individuals with tetraplegia. Due to autonomic changes, bronchospasm is routinely seen in acute cervical injuries, even without a prior history of asthma (31,32). Bronchospasm can rapidly increase the work of breathing and necessitate the use of bronchodilators. In two separate studies of patients with chronic SCI, when ipratropium by inhalation was used in individuals with tetraplegia, the forced VC increased significantly from 41% to 50%, independent of history of asthma or smoking (31,33). The response was attributed to unopposed parasympathetic bronchoconstrictor activity due to loss of sympathetic innervation of the airway. Transection of the cervical spine interrupts the sympathetic nerve supply to the lungs, which originates from the upper six thoracic ganglia (34). Parasympathetic innervation, arising from the vagal nuclei of the brainstem, remains intact leading to increased airway tone.

Complications Due to Chest Trauma

The high incidence of pulmonary complications with thoracic vertebral injuries, especially pleural effusion and pneumohemothorax, may be explained by significant associated chest trauma (10,12). There may be rib fractures with flail chest, pulmonary contusions or laceration, avulsion of a bronchus, rupture of the diaphragm or esophagus, pneumothorax, hemothorax, and hemopericardium. A normal chest x-ray and arterial blood gas on initial evaluation does not necessarily exclude the presence of above injuries; therefore, a high degree of vigilance must be maintained. Avulsion of a major airway or esophageal rupture requires immediate surgical intervention. Traumatic pneumothorax or hemothorax requires tube thoracostomy.

Cotton et al. (22) found that respiratory complications occurred in 51% of patients with T1-6 SCI versus 34.5% of T7-12 SCI. The need for intubation, the risk of pneumonia, and the risk of death were significantly greater for patients with T1-6 SCI. T1-6 SCI may be associated with more respiratory complications relative to the lower thoracic injuries because of the loss of sympathetic influence on bronchial tone and weaker abdominal musculature similar to cervical SCI (35), as well as a weaker cough.

Following thoracic surgery, or chest tube placement, there is a higher likelihood for adhesions between the parietal and visceral pleura. If a patient is on a ventilator with low tidal volumes (TVs), persistent atelectasis may occur, causing weaning to be more difficult. In our clinical practice, patients with a pneumothorax can be ventilated with TVs up to 15 mL/kg of ideal body weight to prevent atelectasis and adhesions once a chest tube is placed.

PNEUMONIA

Pneumonia is an inflammatory process of the lungs that alters normal pulmonary function. The diagnosis of pneumonia in patients with SCI is complicated by the baseline prevalence of retained secretions. The incidence of atelectasis and/or pneumonia during inpatient rehabilitation has been estimated between 9.1% and 14.8% for individuals entering the model SCI systems program since 1996 (35). The risk of acquiring ventilator-associated pneumonia (VAP) increases by 1% to 3% per day of intubation (11). All patients with suspected pneumonia should have a chest radiograph. Comparison with baseline can be useful to determine development of new silhouette signs, air bronchograms, or alveolar infiltrates. In addition, the extent of pneumonia can be assessed by changes in the findings on radiograph. Controversy regarding the use of sputum cultures for the diagnosis and treatment of pneumonia has been reduced by recommendations from the American Thoracic Society and the Infectious Diseases Society of America (ATS/IDSA) guidelines for the management of adults with hospital-acquired, ventilator-associated, and health care–associated pneumonia (36). In patients suspected of acute pneumonia, blood and sputum cultures should be obtained and empiric antibiotic therapy should be initiated using local antibiograms to guide therapeutic decisions. Particular attention should be given to the coverage of Pseudomonas, resistant Staphylococcus, and extended-spectrum beta-lactamase–producing organisms (36). If clinical response is noted in 48 to 72 hours, lower respiratory tract cultures obtained bronchoscopically or nonbronchoscopically may be used to guide therapy. If clinical response is not noted, further investigation such as bronchoalveolar lavage or protected specimen brush for quantitative cultures may be required (36).

Aspiration pneumonia, which can occur frequently in individuals with SCI, is characterized by two phases of lung injury. Initially, chemical injury pneumonitis results from acute exposure of the pulmonary mucosa to aspirated material. Subsequent infection with pathogenic bacteria from the oral flora may later result in the development of mixed aerobic/anaerobic pneumonia (37,38). In a study of 187 patients with SCI admitted to rehabilitation, 22.5% were noted to have symptoms suggestive of dysphagia and 16.5% had videofluoroscopic swallow studies, confirming aspiration or need for modified diet to lower the risk of aspiration (39).

This incidence of aspiration pneumonia following SCI varies widely. Several risk factors associated with aspiration include presence of a tracheostomy, anterior approach for surgical stabilization, and ongoing mechanical ventilation (39). The reported incidence of risk of aspiration following tracheostomy varies widely from 7% to 87% (37–41). The effects of tracheostomy with other specific risk factors including an anterior spinal stabilization have been reported to result in a rate of dysphagia as high as 48%. Ventilator dependence alone was associated with a higher incidence of dysphagia, aspiration, and other long-term complications (39).

Medications

A variety of medications are used in the direct management of the respiratory system or have an impact on the respiratory system of patients following SCI. Several agents may be nebulized to assist in the clearance of tenacious secretions often seen in acute SCI. Isotonic sterile saline may assist in mobilizing thickened secretions by simple hydration. Nebulized mucolytics such as sodium bicarbonate or acetylcysteine may also be effective. Because acetylcysteine may trigger bronchospasm, it should be given with a bronchodilator such as a beta-agonist (6). "The slide test" is conducted by placing a small amount of mucus from bronchial secretions on several glass laboratory slides and applying different mucolytics to determine the optimal agent (42).

The ATS/IDSA concluded that there is a trend for reduced VAP with sucralfate, but a slightly higher rate of gastric bleeding compared with the use of Histamine-2 (H2) antagonists. If stress ulcer prophylaxis is needed, the use of either an H2 antagonist or sucralfate is acceptable (36). Gastric acid suppressive therapy with H2 blockers or proton pump inhibitors also appears to increase the risk of community-acquired pneumonia. Currently, consensus guidelines recommend 4 weeks of a proton pump inhibitor for patients with SCI (6).

Controversy exists regarding the ideal treatment of reactive airway disease. Historically, most patients with SCI have received short-term treatment with beta-agonists such as Albuterol to facilitate bronchodilation and mucus clearance. In the able-bodied population, the long-term use of short-acting beta-agonists downregulates beta receptors–inducing tolerance that has been linked to an eventual increase in asthma attacks (43–45). Moreover, use of long-acting beta-agonists has been linked to increased mortality when used without concomitant inhaled corticosteroids (46). Therefore, the use of inhaled corticosteroids with an as-needed basis use of short-acting beta-agonists as the first-line treatment of reactive airway disease has been recommended. In patients with SCI, the short-term use of bronchodilators has been repeatedly reported (31,32,47,48). However, the long-term benefits of inhaled bronchodilators, inhaled steroids, or the combination have not been studied in the SCI population. Currently, our institution chooses to treat reactive airways with short-acting bronchodilators adding inhaled steroids when tolerance to beta-agonists develops. Further studies must be undertaken to determine if long-term beta-agonists without inhaled steroids increase mortality in SCI as in the able-bodied population.

Cromolyn sodium is an inhaled anti-inflammatory agent that is rarely used in the control of asthma since the widespread acceptance of inhaled corticosteroids. Cromolyn sodium has not been studied in tetraplegia; however, theoretically, it could be beneficial as an adjunct anti-inflammatory (6). Anticholinergic agents such as metaproternol and ipratropium have been shown to increase forced expiratory volume in one second (FEV1) by at least 12% in greater than 40% in tetraplegic individuals with nonacute dyspnea (6,31,32). Long-term use of anticholinergics agents may thicken secretions and decrease production of surfactant by type II alveolar cells (6). However, trials of anticholinergics alone in able-bodied patients with reactive airway disease have shown benefit in both decreasing acute exacerbations and controlling chronic asthma (49–52). In our experience, inhaled ipratropium is effective in short-term optimization of the FEV gain; however, it can be titrated off once patients have achieved full ventilatory-free breathing to minimize long-term secretion thickening. High-dose methylprednisolone in the setting of SCI patients administered was noted to increase the risk for atelectasis and pneumonia in older patients (53).

Two classes of agents have been studied to improve endurance and contractility of respiratory muscles: anabolic steroids and methylxanthines. Oxandrolone, an anabolic steroid, given for 30 days at a dose of 20 mg/d in a study of 10 patients with chronic tetraplegia showed an increase in FVC from 2.8 to 3.0 L. Maximal inspiratory and expiratory pressures as well as subjective symptoms of dyspnea improved; however, the benefits only lasted while the drug was given (33). Methylxanthines, such as theophylline, may improve diaphragmatic contractility in able-bodied patients with chronic obstructive pulmonary disease (COPD) (54,55) but have not been studied in the SCI population (6).

ASSESSMENT

In an acute cervical or thoracic SCI, a pulmonary assessment to determine the need for immediate respiratory intervention must be done without delay. Asking the patient about shortness of breath must be part of review of systems. Physical examination should include respiratory rate, VC, continuous pulse oximetry, and observation of the pattern of breathing. The most common abnormal breathing pattern, called "paradoxical abdominal breathing," is isolated diaphragmatic breathing with chest wall retraction during inspiration (56–58). Signs of impending respiratory failure include tachypnea, progressive desaturation, and a decrease in VC to less than 15-mL/kg ideal body weight (27).

Laboratory studies should include an ABG and chest x-ray. An ABG is used to evaluate the overall impact of pulmonary dysfunction (57). Arterial oxygen tension (PaO_2) is considered the most sensitive tool for evaluation of atelectasis. Arterial carbon dioxide tension ($PaCO_2$) is used to evaluate ventilation abnormalities. After the initial ABG, noninvasive measurement of O_2 saturation and end tidal CO_2 levels can be used. The pulse oximeter can be left on continuously while the patient is confined to bed. The ABG should still be obtained for changes in clinical status or after a ventilator setting change. Chest radiographs should be obtained serially, initially to assess for chest trauma and later for atelectasis, pulmonary edema, and aspiration (27). Chest trauma may require immediate surgical intervention and ventilatory support.

VC is the best predictor of respiratory muscle fatigue. A baseline VC should be obtained upon admission and then monitored as frequently as every 8 hours for the first several days and frequently thereafter if there is a concern about deteriorating respiratory condition (28). In individuals with C5 or C6 SCI, there can be 30% to 50% reduction in predicted VC within the first week (12,58,59). Serial measurement of the VC should alert the health care providers to the patient's level of diaphragm fatigue and the impending need for intubation. Knowing the baseline and following the pattern of VC changes are essential. For example, if the admission VC was 25% of predicted value and 3 days later is 15%, immediate and aggressive respiratory therapy is required, and there is a strong likelihood that intubation or noninvasive respiratory support such as Bi-level positive airway pressure (BiPAP) may be required.

The need for respiratory support may become more urgent if the chest radiographs show atelectasis, oximetry readings deteriorate, or if the patient has comorbidities such as obesity, prior lung disease, history of smoking, positive toxicology screen, chest trauma, or copious pulmonary secretions (27). If the VC approaches 10 mL/kg of ideal body weight, immediate support (i.e., intubation) is almost always indicated. PCF is another useful tool, as it can determine the strength (and weakness) of the abdominal muscles, which, if low, will impair the ability to cough. PCF also correlates well with the ability to decannulate a patient from the ventilator (see later). Fluoroscopy is a useful tool to determine when diaphragm paralysis is suspected. If the VC is lower than one would expect for the level of injury and associated problems, fluoroscopy is indicated.

A thorough review of past medical history (PMH) should include all problems that increase the risk of pulmonary disease or the ability of the patient to withstand pulmonary complications. Relevant PMH includes review of prior lung disease including asthma, COPD, cancer, and sleep apnea. Substance abuse and specifically smoking history are very important, because smoking leads to increased secretions (6). Morbid obesity will increase the work of breathing and the risk of sleep apnea. Malnutrition will interfere with healing, increase the risk infections, and should be prevented. A patient with any significant additional medical problem will have decreased reserves to resist respiratory complications. This could be as simple as a urinary tract infection. Older age is an additional risk factor. Preventing rapid weight loss is also important in severely obese patients since it will lead to rapid muscle loss, including the muscles of respiration. Peripheral hyperalimentation should therefore be considered early in patients with high level of injuries.

TREATMENT

The aggressive management of atelectasis and secretions are the cornerstones of early treatment. Intense pulmonary toilet has been shown to improve outcomes in individuals with SCI (12,23,60). Emphasis should be on the expansion of the lungs and clearing of secretions. Expansion of the lungs can be accomplished in several different ways: including intermittent positive pressure breathing (IPPB), intrapulmonary percussive ventilation (IPV), inflation by Ambu bags, or using high TV settings on the mechanical ventilator (10). Since many individuals with SCI will require mechanical ventilation, health care providers managing individuals with SCI should be aware of the most common complications in individuals who are ventilator dependent.

Bronchospasm secondary to a past history of asthma or because of autonomic changes seen in acute injury necessitates the use initially of bronchodilators every 4 hours. The treatment should not be delayed for bronchospasm to be obvious. Our center's guidelines recommend the use of bronchodilators for all acute patients with VC of less than 65% of predicted value. Bronchodilators can be administered through IPPB, IPV, or nebulizers. For ventilated patients, the use of larger TVs, up to 20 mL/kg, has been shown to decrease atelectasis but should be used while monitoring pressures (61) (see later.)

IPPB, inflation by an Ambu bag, or incorporating sighs into the mechanical ventilation settings are different methods by which large volume expansion of lungs can occur (6,10). IPPB is a mechanical device used to deliver a positive pressure breath on triggering of the machine by the patient and is usually used with a bronchodilator. The level of pressure should be started at 10 to 15 cm H_2O and increased gradually, but it should not exceed 40 cm H_2O (6). IPPB administration of bronchodilators however may not be available as the machine is no longer in production.

IPV is another therapeutic modality used to deliver a deep breath while mobilizing retained secretions (Fig. 10.2). IPV delivers high-frequency pulsations of pressurized air at rates of 100 to 300 cycles/min (2–5 Hz) in the form of a "flutter valve." These vibrations loosen retained secretions and deliver aerosol to hydrate viscous mucus plugs. IPV can be used in combination with positive pressure ventilation through a simple interface with the ventilator circuit. A mouthpiece is used for nonventilated patients. Following IPV, the secretions will need to be cleared through either suctioning or a cough assist machine.

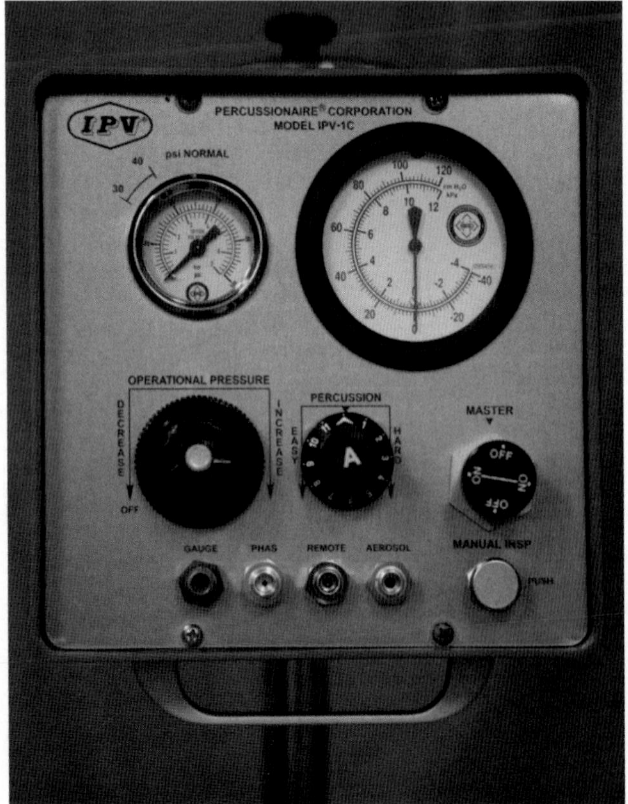

FIGURE 10.2. Intrapulmonary percussive ventilation.

EzPAP is a positive expiratory pressure system used to improve lung expansion. Flow is increased on inspiration using positive expiratory pressure provided during expiration. By expanding lungs, EzPAP improves atelectasis, secretion clearance, and oxygenation and may be used with nebulizers. Potential complications of EzPAP include increased airway resistance and the work of breathing and therefore may not be appropriate for the patient with low or deteriorating VC. Other potential complications of EzPAP include barotraumas, pneumothorax, hypocarbia, gastric distension, and air trapping. It has been studied for the treatment of bronchiectasis showing improvement in atelectasis and secretion clearance, but it has not to date been studied in SCI. Since IPPB is no longer an option in most settings, EzPAP needs to be studied as a potential substitute.

McMichan recommends early and frequent fiberoptic bronchoscopy and bronchial lavage for secretion clearance (62). However, bronchoscopy will irritate the airways causing more secretions and bleeding. Aggressive management of atelectasis and secretions by respiratory therapists dedicated to a spinal cord unit has been shown to decrease the risk of pneumonia and virtually eliminate the need for bronchoscopy (23,60).

Suctioning is needed for secretion management and optimal ventilation but is not without complications. Possible complications seen with suctioning in SCI include hypoxia, hypotension, infection, tracheal mucosa damage, vagal nerve stimulation, patient anxiety and fear, and increased bronchial mucus production (63). In an individual with concomitant brain injury, suctioning can cause an acute increase in intracranial pressure (63). Isotonic sterile saline is used during suctioning to mobilize secretions that are thickened due to dehydration (6).

Assisted coughing is used to duplicate a normal cough and can be provided through a variety of techniques. A "quad cough" is a maneuver in which a care provider performs an abdominal thrust and/or squeeze over the chest wall that is coordinated with either the patient's spontaneous breath or an assisted breath. "Quad coughing" tries to mimic a natural cough by helping to mobilize secretions from the lower portions of the lungs. An open hand, palms down, is placed below the patient's rib cage, between the xyphoid process and the umbilicus. After a deep breath is taken by the patient, or given by the ventilator or Ambu bag, a caregiver pushes upward and inward as the patient attempts to cough (Fig. 10.3). Contraindications to quad coughing include an unstable spine in traction, internal abdominal complications, chest trauma such as fractured ribs, and a recently placed vena cava filter (6,64).

The cough assist mechanical insufflation-exsufflation devise (Cough Assist; J H Emerson Co.) is effective in clearing secretions and eliminates the need for chest wall compression or invasive suctioning (Fig. 10.4) It effectively clears retained bronchopulmonary secretions, is able to bring up large mucus plugs, and reduces the risk of respiratory complications and the need for bronchoscopy (65). By decreasing the need for deep suctioning, it is less irritating to the lungs and is more

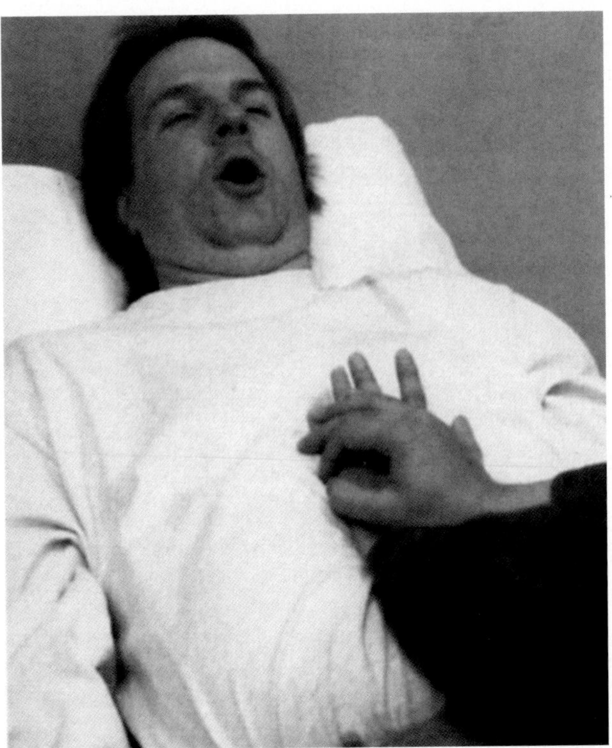

FIGURE 10.3. Picture of assisted cough technique.

comfortable to the patient (65,66).The cough assist machine achieves this by gradually applying a positive pressure to the airway and then rapidly shifting to negative pressure. The rapid shift in pressure produces a high expiratory flow from the lungs, simulating a cough. Usual insufflation-exsufflation pressures are +40 to −40 cm H_2O, generating approximately 10 L/s expiratory flows. The cough assist machine can be applied via tracheostomy, facemask, or mouthpiece. It does not produce macroscopic tissue damage, as can be seen with suctioning. It is much more effective than quad coughing and suctioning and is better tolerated by the patients when compared to endotracheal suctioning. Moreover, compared with an inline suction catheter that preferentially clears the right lung due to the vertical anatomy of the right bronchus and cannot efficiently remove plugs larger than the catheters own diameter, cougulation removes mucous plugs from both lung fields equally, despite their size. Contraindications include a history of bullous emphysema, known susceptibility to pneumothorax or pneumomediastinum, or recent barotrauma.

The uses of a Roto-rest (kinetic therapy) bed and postural drainage have been promoted to improve respiratory secretion drainage and decrease the incidence of pneumonia (60,67). Postural drainage can be used for 20 minutes each morning followed by aggressive respiratory therapy (67,68). Some institutions utilize hospital beds that rotate the patient back and forth to facilitate oscillation of ventilation perfusion zones of the lungs and increase postural drainage (Rota Rest; Kinetic Concepts Incorporated; San Antonio, Texas). In addition, early mobilization of patients to the edge of the bed, into the wheelchair, or onto a tilt table can significantly help drainage.

Chest clapping, percussion, and vibration, either with a mechanical vibration or by hand, may be used to loosen the secretions and may help drain lobes that have secretions in them. Positioning the patient so that the involved lung area is in a superior position allows gravity to help it drain. Frequently, however, in the acute SCI patient, the presence of a halo vest, the location of the patient's injury, pain, or blood pressure alterations limit the use of chest physiotherapy if the patient is placed in the Trandelenburg positions. Some beds come with automatic turning and vibration settings that can be helpful in patients for whom positioning for treatments is a problem (69).

An alert and cooperative patient is important in the optimal use of these respiratory therapy techniques. Pain management needs to be aggressive since it may interfere with the ability of the patient to take deep breaths and cooperate with the treat-

Mechanical Insufflator-Exsufflator Automatic version

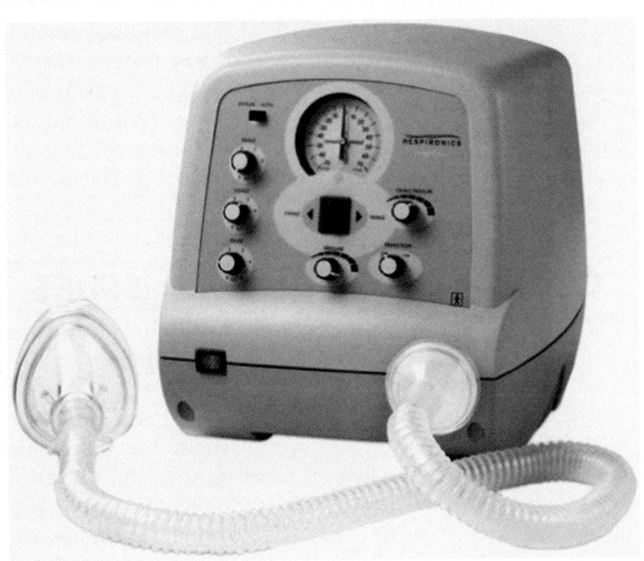

Phillips Respironics

Manual version

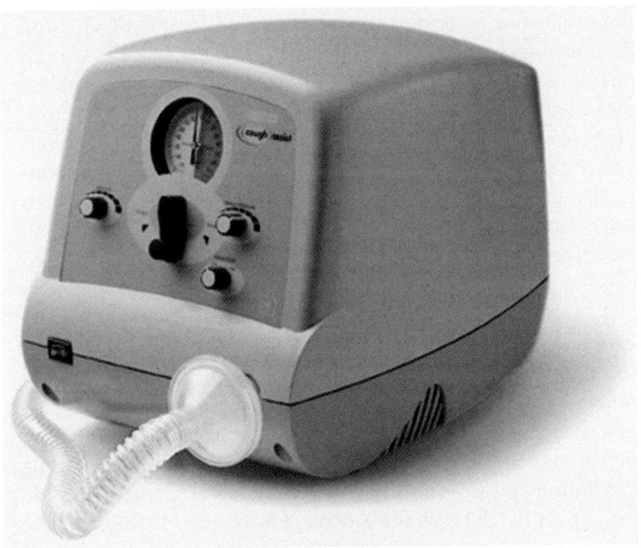

Phillips Respironics

FIGURE 10.4. Mechanical insufflator-exsufflator automatic version.

ments. In alert patients, patient-controlled analgesic (PCA) is an option. Even for individuals who are unable to press the button, family and nurses can use the PCA at the patient's request. Heavy sedation with medication should be avoided as it makes ongoing assessments difficult, that is, when the neurologic exam is deteriorating. Chemical sedation often leads to the need for more sedatives: as the sedation wears off, patients often become agitated because they are waking up confused and, as a consequence, they are given more sedatives. Instead, nursing or caregiver should be instructed to address the patient's anxiety and fear by talking to the patient, calming them down, explaining procedures, and keeping them oriented. If the patient has lost the ability to speak, alternative communication systems should be initiated as soon as possible.

Incentive Spirometry and Resistive Training

Exercises to improve respiratory function include inspiratory resistance muscle training, abdominal weight, and incentive spirometry. Respiratory muscle training has been shown to improve pulmonary function by strengthening and improving endurance of the diaphragm and accessory respiratory muscles in some studies (70,71). Incentive spirometry is a technique that uses a simple bedside device to encourage the patient to inhale as deeply as possible. The purpose is to prevent or treat atelectasis; however, there are no documented studies indicating efficacy of incentive spirometry in tetraplegic patients. Weights placed on the abdomen to help improve the strength of the muscles of respiration have a similar concept (6,69).

Intubation

Signs of impending diaphragm fatigue and respiratory failure should be closely monitored to prevent the need for emergent intubation. Indications for intubation despite aggressive noninvasive techniques include VC trending downward and less than 15-mL/kg ideal body weight, increasing oxygen requirements, increasing respiratory rate, rising PCO_2, and diminishing breath sounds in the lung fields (11,27). Como recommends semielective intubation at the first sign of respiratory distress in complete cervical SCI, especially C5 and above (17). It is wise to intubate during the daytime hours, preferably by practitioners with considerable experience under controlled circumstances rather than emergently (11,17). Studies have shown orotracheal intubation is safe in the setting of an unstable cervical spine (11). Intubation with fiberoptic endoscopy is preferred to avoid unnecessary cervical manipulation (18).Concomitant facial fractures are a relative contraindication to nasotracheal intubation. Use of succinylcholine at the time of intubation is contraindicated if the SCI occurred more than 24 hours before administration because of the risk of precipitating hyperkalemia (18). Imminent intubation may be prolonged by the use of noninvasive ventilation. BiPAP or continuous positive airway pressure (CPAP) can delay muscle fatigue and atelectasis for a while. However, it is the authors' experience that this is generally impractical. The usual need for nasogastric or orogastric tubes acutely to decompress the stomach interferes with the oral or nasal seal required to maintain assistive pressures. Patients who require respiratory assistance the most (i.e., high cervical injuries) either need intubation for urgent surgery or have Halo rings applied to traction. The Halo ring often interferes with placement of the forehead component of nasal masks. And finally, patient tolerance, an issue even when noninvasive methods are used postextubation, is extremely variable.

Timing of Tracheostomy

Prolonged nasotracheal or endotracheal intubation has been associated with complications such as subglottic stenosis and sinusitis (27). Tracheostomy is more comfortable for the patient and allows easier suctioning and pulmonary hygiene compared with nasotracheal and endotracheal intubation. Tracheostomy is easier for the patient when attempting to wean, as there is less dead space and reduced airway resistance. Tracheostomy allows the patient to get out of bed and begin rehabilitation earlier. The decision to perform a tracheostomy should not be prolonged beyond 1 to 2 weeks.

Tracheotomy does carry surgical risks including bleeding, infection, and tracheal injury. The period of time that should separate tracheostomy tube placement and anterior cervical stabilization should be no less than 1 week, preferably 2 weeks, due to increased risk of wound contamination (11). If the patient requires an anterior cervical surgery, prioritization of spinal surgery or tracheostomy based on urgency should be decided. It is recommended to start with a cuffed tracheostomy that can protect the lungs against aspiration and emesis, which allows full expansion of the lungs (27). Cuff pressures should be monitored and maintained below 25 cm H_2O to avoid tracheal injury.

There are negative aspects to tracheostomy that include increased secretion production, bacterial colonization, and difficulty with communication. Some physicians are reluctant to perform tracheotomies until several attempts at ventilator weaning and extubation have occurred, but this should be discouraged. Premature extubation in an attempt to avoid tracheostomy frequently leads to reintubation and subsequent tracheostomy. Failed attempts to extubate may prolong endotracheal intubation, increase tracheal and laryngeal trauma and infection, and prolong the patient's stay in the intensive care unit (19). The risk factors for requiring a tracheostomy include C2-4 levels, neurologically complete cervical injuries, older than 45 years of age, previous pulmonary impairment, smoking history, preexisting comorbid medical problems, and active pneumonia (19).

COMMON RESPIRATORY ISSUES

Increased Work of Breathing

Compensating for the inability to move air in and out of the lungs can be accomplished in several ways. The traditional method of invasive mechanical ventilation is still the most commonly used today, via an oral endotracheal tube or tracheostomy tube. An array of settings includes pressure limited, volume limited, synchronized, and mandatory, or intermittent mandatory ventilation (IMV). Each setting differs in either the limitation in TV delivered or pressure delivered and the degree of spontaneous breathing permitted.

Noninvasive ventilation can be delivered via a mouthpiece, nose mask, or oral seal. The same principles apply as to traditional ventilation, except that one eliminates the need for invasive tubes in the bronchopulmonary tree. However, issues of gastric distension, aspiration, patient discomfort with the masks, and leaks via open nasopharynx or oropharynx do occur (25). Recently, clinicians have begun to utilize direct electrode stimulation of the diaphragm. Electrodes can be placed laparascopically, limiting the invasive aspect while maintaining the effect of diaphragmatic contractility (72).

Ventilator Settings

Ventilator setting is among the most controversial paradigms in the respiratory treatment in SCI. The rationale is to reverse the atelectasis and mucous trapping by hyperventilating the lungs. Protocols vary but generally ventilation with TV of 15 to 20 mL/kg are routinely used in the spinal cord population (42,60,69). These large volumes have been challenged. The publication of the ARDSNet trail in 2000 outlined a significant increase in mortality in patients treated with high TV. In fact, the trial was stopped early as the low TV group (6 mL/kg) proved to be far more efficacious in preventing mortality from acute lung disease. However, these results specifically excluded patients with neuromuscular disease and included those patients with FIO_2/PaO_2 ratios lower than 300, indicating hypoxemia (7). As previously explained, patients with isolated SCI have restrictive ventilatory defects without acute lung injury or hypoxemia.

A recent study reviewed clinical practice since the ARDSNet trial and reported that most practitioners have moved toward using the lower TV paradigm (73). Interestingly though, the authors also reported that pressure rather than TV was associated with increased mortality. The odds of death increased multiplicatively with each cm H_2O increase of plateau pressure (Pplat). They concluded that although physicians used lower TVs after publication of the ARDSnet trial, plateau pressure was strongly predictive of mortality and may reflect disease severity independent of TV (73).

The conclusion seems to indicate a role for higher lung volumes in patients with SCI recognizing the need for using lung pressures as the limiting factor in ventilator settings. A strategy used at our institution is to slowly increase TV by 100 mL/d with the goal of reaching 15 to 20 mL/kg TV. Each adjustment is accompanied by appropriate changes in dead space to maintain normocapnea. Increases in volumes are held when peak pressures exceed 35 mm H_2O or when plateau pressures exceed 25 mm H_2O. The critical point is to recognize that unless interventions are made at this stage, patients have a 50% incidence of developing pneumonia (67). If pneumonia leads to any evidence of significant acute intrinsic lung injury, clinicians should strongly consider reverting back to the low lung volume model as outlined by the ARDSNet study.

Increased Atelectasis and Decreased Mucociliary Clearance

Again large volumes are used to mechanically expand closed alveoli and lung segments. Once the lungs open, the focus shifts to removal of residual trapped mucous. Nebulized Albuterol and Atrovent help to reverse any bronchospasm, and mucolytics such as *N*-acytylcysteine and sodium bicarbonate may be used to thin secretions. The techniques previously described to expand the lungs to loosen secretions and remove them may be used.

Weakened Respiratory Muscles

Like all weakened muscles, the diaphragm and accessory breathing muscles respond to a consistent strengthening and conditioning program. Sustained repetitive resistance training will over time increase the force of contraction via recruitment, hypertrophy, or neurological recovery. Conceptually, progressive weaning techniques challenge the muscles incrementally each day, preparing the body for 24 hours of voluntary breathing. The chances of fatigue and hence failure to wean are reduced by "building" up and preparing for the workload of breathing. A few studies have employed use of specialized partial rebreathers or inspiratory muscle retrainers that provide varying degree of resistance (74–76). Patients who complied with a regimented training schedule showed significant increases in respiratory values including vital capacities. However, this gain was seen in all patients who complied with a regimented program regardless of usage of "specialized mechanical trainers" (76). This would seem to indicate that repetitive exercise of the respiratory muscles is beneficial regardless of the method employed.

Neuropraxic regeneration is postulated to occur in approximately 6 weeks. As this occurs, VC may increase. Axonal regeneration of phrenic nerve for diaphragmatic function may take over 12 months (77). Therefore, delayed diaphragm recovery is possible, especially with higher cervical levels of injury (C1-4); but if diaphragmatic paralysis has persisted beyond 1 year, the chance of fully independent breathing is probably less than 5% (78).

WEANING PROTOCOLS

Ventilation Mode

The first step to weaning is to identify the method of ventilation one would begin to wean from. SIMV or CPAP mechanical ventilation is used in many medical and surgical ICUs as a preferred method of weaning. For SCI patients, a progressive-free breathing technique via t-piece can be used to optimize the aforementioned resistance training effect. Peterson et al. reported that 67% of SCI patients successfully weaned from the ventilator as compared to 34% using IMV weaning (79). Others have chosen noninvasive methods. We generally employ several of these methods depending on the level of injury, age and comorbidities, and history of tracheotomy. More recently, we have used noninvasive methods to avoid tracheotomies in acutely injured patients with endotracheal intubations. We previously stated that the use of noninvasive ventilation in an acute SCI was not adequate to avoid oral intubation; however, the use of noninvasive methods after extubation to avoid tracheostomies has been of great benefit. The main reasons for the discrepancy between successful use of noninvasive ventilation in avoiding tracheostomies but not initial oral intubation stem from the ability to extubate after reversal of atelectasis, improvement in pulmonary compliance, eliminating oxygen requirements, and improved patient participation. Whatever method a clinician chooses to use, failure to wean is usually avoided by using the method that the clinician, nurses, and respiratory therapists all agree with. Any disagreement among the health care providers often spells failure for the patient.

Tracheostomy Selection

Tracheostomy tubes are curved tubes that allow for ventilation through a tracheostomy. There are numerous manufacturers that offer multiple types and specialized options. Most patients arrive postoperatively with sutured cuffed nonfenestrated tubes in situ. The stoma may take 1 to 2 weeks to heal prior to the first change of the tube. The decision on which type of tube to choose is largely dependent on the clinical scenario and the goals anticipated for the patient (Table 10.1).

The primary goal at this stage is to allow for ventilation while establishing an environment for weaning. Therefore, the first decision centers on whether to use a cuffed or an uncuffed tracheostomy tube. A cuffed tracheostomy tube has an inflatable balloon over the distal shaft of the tube that should be inflated with either air or saline depending upon the manufacturer's specifications. Cuffed tubes maintain a barrier that helps prevent aspiration around the tube into the lungs. Patients with copious secretions or those with known aspiration may need this type of tube. Cuff deflation may also make IPV, IPPB, and cough assist machines less effective due to leakage of air around the tracheostomy. With traditional cuffed tubes, the cuffs even when deflated partially obstruct space around the tube and decrease the airway lumen when attempting to either wean or phonate through the nasopharynx. This translates into increased resistance and work of breathing. Uncuffed tubes eliminate the obstruction but add the risk of an unprotected airway during aspiration. Fenestrated tubes provide holes in the shaft proximal to the cuff allowing for greater air entry in to the nasopharynx when the tube is capped. This increases the volume of air movement leading to stronger phonation. Complications of fenestrated tubes include ineffective ventilation via air leak into the nasopharynx and increased granulation (80).

Bivona produces a silicone tracheostomy tube in which the cuff is contiguous with the body of the tube and when deflated lie flush, thus eliminating both the partial obstruction created by traditional cuffed tracheostomy tubes when weaning and the risk of aspiration with cuffless tracheostomy tubes. The Jackson tracheostomy tube is metal and cuffless. Plastic tracheostomy tubes tend to cause irritation and increased secretions, whereas metal tracheostomy tubes do not cause the same problem. However, they can only be used when positive pressure treatments are no longer required. Additionally, one cannot use a cough assist machine with a metal tracheostomy since it lacks a site for attachment.

Criteria for Weaning

There is no universal agreement as to which patients will be able to wean off the ventilator. Prognosis can be largely based on neurological level of injury (NLI), phrenic nerve conduction, diaphragmatic needle EMG recruitment, fluoroscopic diaphragm evaluation, and strength as measured by VC. NLI serves as a gross determinant of weaning prognosis. Wicks et al. studied 134 patients with ventilatory dependant tetraplegia. Approximately 80% of patients with injuries C4 and below successfully weaned by discharge, 50% weaned at a C3 level, 28% with C2 level injuries, and no patient successfully weaned with C1 injuries (81). A later study by Peterson reported that up to 83% of patients with C3 or C4 injuries could successfully wean (79). Recently though, these values have been questioned. Chiodo et al. retrospectively studied 26 subjects with ventilator-dependant tetraplegia admitted for acute rehabilitation. In their series, the wean rate was 0% of patients with C2-level injuries, 25% with C3, 77% with C4, and 50% with C5 (82). The authors concluded that pattern of diaphragmatic sparing rather than the neurological level was important in determining if patients with C4 or C5 injuries weaned (82).

Patients who achieved maximal negative inspiratory forces of greater than 40 mL H_2O and VC greater than 17 mL/kg body weight were successfully able to wean (42,60,69,82). EMG recruitment is also a useful indicator for successful weaning (82). Many hospitals without specialized SCI expertise wean based on a variety of factors including but not limited to clinical judgment, tolerance of CPAP or Pressure Support, and ABG values. As previously mentioned, most centers utilize lower TVs to ventilate and omit the variety of aggressive pulmonary toilet measures and cough assist techniques. Hence the patient with SCI is extubated in an environment that does not compensate for a baseline-decreased cough, VC, and muscle weakness. Often these patients develop worsened function and respiratory distress and may require emergent reintubation. Therefore, it is

TABLE 10.1

TRACHEOSTOMY DECISIONS

Clinical scenario	Decision	Rationale
Known aspirator/excessive secretions	Cuffed versus uncuffed	Cuff around the outside of the tube provides a barrier for materials entering lungs
Weaning via nasopharynx with tube capped	Cuffed versus uncuffed	Cuffless tubes provide greater volume for air exchange decreasing work of breathing
Phonation	Fenestrated versus nonfenestrated Cuff versus uncuffed	Fenestrations and cuffless tubes increase volume of air through vocal cords increasing strength of talking
Aspiration, weaning, and phonation	Silicone tracheostomy tubes	Cuff inflation for managed, controlled leaks Protection from potential aspiration during feeding When totally deflated, it adds no distinguishable dimension to the outer diameter of the tube's shaft

incumbent on the spinal cord practitioner to wean patients in the safest environment possible. As such patients should meet specific criteria that optimize the chances for successful weaning.

First, patients should have healthy lungs prior to the start of the weaning process. That is, any underlying pneumonia should be treated, atelectasis should be reversed, and the lungs cleared of as much mucous as possible, with a clear chest x-ray. Patients should require minimal, if any, supplemental oxygen as increased need indicates continued impairment in gas exchange. ABG values should be within normal limits, and patients should remain afebrile, hemodynamically stable, and be without any other significant medical conditions to allow the body to direct all available energies to meet the work of breathing. VC should be approximately 10 mL/kg of body weight before weaning is started (69,83). Lastly, but most importantly, patients need to be psychologically prepared, understanding, and accepting of any protocol the clinician wishes to implement. Each step must be explained fully and clear goals should be established to avoid miscommunication, disappointment, and losing faith in the program. For example, the protocol for our institution begins with a short defined time period for weaning (30 minutes) while supine in bed. Patients are told that this is the point they will stop at regardless of the desire and perceived ability to continue. They additionally will not be allowed to wean in the wheelchair at this phase. The mutual understanding allows patients to achieve a sense of success upon meeting the initial goal and physicians to maintain a sense of control during the process.

Weaning

Once the clinician has identified that the patient is appropriate for weaning, identified the method of weaning, and the type of tracheostomy tube needed, the process of weaning can begin. A sample weaning protocol utilized at our institution is listed in Table 10.2. Patients are given short trials of Voluntary breathing through the tracheostomy tube (t-tubing) to accustom them

TABLE 10.2

PROTOCOL FOR WEANING IN SCI

Criteria for weaning:

1. VITAL SIGNS: Heart rate and blood pressure should be stable. Temperature ≤ 101°F.
2. Evidence of some spontaneous respirations, an initial VC of at least 10 mL/kg ideal bodyweight. Maximum inspiratory pressure ≥ 30 cm H_2O pressure (MIP) may be used at the physician's discretion.
3. FiO_2 ON VENTILATOR: 25% maximum.
   - * PaO_2 > 75
   - * PCO_2 35–45 *No Pressure Support
   - * PH 7.35–7.45
4. CHEST X-RAY: Clear with modest manageable secretions.
5. NUTRITION: Nutritional needs should be addressed and serum K+ should be optimally >4.5 mEq/L.
6. ADVERSE MEDICATIONS: The staff must be aware of medications affecting muscle activity or VC (e.g., Demerol, Valium).
7. PSYCHOLOGICAL: The patient must be willing to participate in weaning process.
8. Medically stable for at least 24 h.

A. T-tubing schedule:

1. **Initial trial**
   - A. VC Measurements: In the supine position, VC measurement will be performed before t-tube trial, after trial, and prn.
   - B. T-PIECE: Place the patient on an aerosol mist per t-piece with the FiO_2 10% >FiO_2 required on the ventilator (as needed).
   - C. TRIAL LENGTH: Initial t-tube trial should be 30 min, under constant supervision. VC measured immediately after the trial.
   - D. OXIMETRY: Oximetry readings monitored throughout trial. If O_2 SAT is consistently <95%, increase FiO_2 by 5%, check VC. If FiO_2 total requirement is >15% of baseline FiO_2, place back on ventilator.
   - E. PARAMETERS OF AN UNSUCCESSFUL TRIAL: Place the patient back on ventilator on previous settings (FiO_2, Rate, Vt) for
     1. Deterioration of VC by 25% from starting VC
     2. Respiratory rate ≥ 25 bpm
     3. O_2 SAT ≤ 95% despite an additional increase in FiO_2 of 5%
     4. Patient anxiety/panic with weaning that cannot be lessened with psychological support
   - F. A successful trial is the absence of these parameters and a post-VC measured at ≥80% of the pre-VC.
   - G. The times and lengths of trials documented.
   - H. REST PERIODS: There should be at least a 3-h rest between t-tubing trials.

B. Increasing trials:

1. Trials may be increased by 1- to 2-h BID increments daily until the patient is t-tubing for 6-h BID as long as the VC does not decrease by 25% of baseline.
2. The patient may be t-tubed for longer periods if there is improvement or maintenance of the MIP and VC.
3. If the VC decreases by 25% from original VC, the patient should be returned to the ventilator.
4. Strongly recommended that once the patient is t-tubing for 8–10 h, further weaning occurs after therapy so that the patient may be up in the wheelchair for daily therapy.
5. When returning the patient to the ventilator after prolonged trial periods, the patient may be anxious and "fight" machine. The physician should be contacted for consideration of parameter change from SIMV to Assist/Control.

C. T-tubing up in wheelchair:

When VC > 20 mL/kg supine, may check VC sitting up in wheelchair. The patient may t-tube in wheelchair as long as sitting up VC > 15 mL/kg. A heat-and moisture exchanger (or artificial nose) may be used, with supplemental O_2 added as needed.

to the process and recondition the muscles. Each day the length of time of weaning is advanced by a set amount as long as the patient continues to meet the criteria for weaning. VC or inspiratory forces are serially measured to track improvements or deteriorations in function. Additionally, they can be used to gauge the ability of patients to tolerate transitions from weaning in bed to weaning upright in a wheelchair. Ultimately, patients are slowly conditioned to tolerate complete independence from the ventilator. They are then transitioned to physiological breathing via the nasopharynx by plugging or capping the tracheostomy tube. Caution must be used as some patients may have difficulties with secretion clearance at this phase as nasopharyngeal breathing eliminates the ability to use a tracheostomy mist that helps keep secretions thin. We recommend continuing aggressive pulmonary toilet throughout the whole protocol.

The patient is ready for decannulation when secretions are minimal and are easily brought up orally. The lungs should be free of infection for at least 1 week. The patient should be eating orally with minimal risk of aspiration. At our center, the patients have their tracheostomy plugged for at least 72 hours without complications, before we consider decannulation. A PCF of ≥160 L/min correlates with successful decannulation in persons with neuromuscular disease (25,84).

Electrical Stimulation to Improve Respiration

Up to 25% of acutely injured patients will require ventilation. The concept of electrical stimulation, initially described as phrenic nerve stimulation (PNS), dates back to the 18th century (85). Glenn and colleagues made significant technological advances that led to the development of the current phrenic nerve pacing system. Diaphragm pacing (DP) through electrical stimulation of PNS may be an option for those individuals with cervical injury above C3, which usually leaves the phrenic nerves intact. As an alternative to mechanical ventilation, phrenic nerve pacing results in a significant improvement in quality of life for these individuals who will otherwise require a mechanical ventilator 24 h/d (85). Patients with PNS report more normal breathing and better general health. Negative pressure ventilation provided by PNS compared with positive ventilation provided by mechanical ventilators might reduce barotraumas and improved cardiovascular function. With PNS, external devices such as a ventilator and tubing are eliminated. Thus, transfer from bed to chair and transportation in the community are made much less cumbersome. Benefits of pacing include elimination of fear of accidental disconnection from a ventilator and discomfort from tension on the tracheostomy tube, improved speech, improved olfactory sensation, and elimination of ventilator noise (86). PNS has also been successfully implanted in children (87).

PNS is not inexpensive and there are risks associated with the implantation of PNS. Potential candidates need to be carefully screened and specific criteria should be met (87). Eligibility criteria include (a) patient highly motivated to improve overall function, (b) supportive caregiver system, (c) medical stability, and (d) appropriate patient and caregiver expectations for the benefits of PNS. Medical contraindications include significant lung, chest wall, or primary muscle diseases. Before PNS can be implanted, phrenic nerve function needs to be assessed thoroughly. Absent or significantly reduced phrenic nerve function is a contraindication. Serial phrenic nerve conduction studies may be indicated prior to making a decision to implant the system. Lower motor neuron injury to phrenic nerves has been known to recover within 3 to 11 months after SCI at C4 and C5 levels (88). With the recovery of phrenic nerves, there is associated improvement in respiratory function, and the patients can be weaned from the ventilator. Therefore, PNS is usually not implanted until at least 12 months postinjury (86,89).

Phrenic nerve function can be assessed both by nerve conduction study (NCS) of the phrenic nerve with measurements of conduction times and amplitudes and by fluoroscopic evaluation of diaphragm during PNS (86). The amplitude may be diminished due to atrophy of the diaphragm or due to technical difficulties associated with NCS such as electrode placement and fatty tissue. Thus the amplitude is a less reliable indicator compared with conduction time. Normal mean onset latency of the phrenic nerve is 7 to 9 milliseconds in adults, but successful pacing has been accomplished in individuals with latencies up to 14 milliseconds (86). With fluoroscopic visualization, the diaphragm usually descends more than 5 cm in individuals with normal function. During electrical stimulation of the phrenic nerve, it should descend at least 3 to 4 cm in potential candidates for implantation.

Conventional phrenic nerve pacing requires thoracotomy for the placement of electrodes, which are placed on each phrenic nerve during one surgical procedure. Potential complications of electrode placement include iatrogenic injury to the phrenic nerve and infection in those patients who may be chronically colonized with pathogenic bacteria from chronic tracheostomies and urinary catheters. The electrode wires are connected to a radiofrequency receiver that is usually placed over the anterior chest wall (86). There are three commercially available PNS systems in the world: Avery Biomedical Devices, Atrotech OY, and Medimplant system, but only the Avery system is currently available in the United States. The most recently developed Mark IV transmitter by Avery Biomedical Devices allows greater flexibility for stimulus parameters and has a longer battery life.

After surgical implantation of the phrenic nerve pacemaker, a period of 2 weeks is needed for the resolution of edema and inflammation from the surgical intervention (86). The transition from mechanical ventilation to full-time PNS must be individualized, but it involves gradual conditioning of the phrenic nerve and the diaphragm over weeks. Tracheostomy should not be discontinued in case of PNS failure and for pulmonary hygiene and secretion management (90). There are reports of successful long-term PNS for more than 10 years (86). In a case series of individuals with C3-5 SCI who have sustained axonal loss of the phrenic nerve, one option of PNS using intercostal to phrenic nerve transfer at the same time the phrenic nerve pacemaker is implanted has been reported (91).

More recently, DP through electrical stimulation can be accomplished with intramuscular electrodes placed directly into the diaphragm (85,92,93). Using four laparoscopic ports, two intramuscular electrodes are implanted into each hemidiaphragm near the phrenic nerve motor points. With this method, the phrenic nerve is activated through electrical current spread through the muscular diaphragm; therefore, higher stimulus currents in the range of 24 to 25 mA are required (86). Advantages of diaphragmatic pacing over PNS include laparoscopic approach versus the traditional thoracotomy required for placement of the phrenic nerve stimulators, as well as decreased risk of iatrogenic phrenic nerve damage, lower cost, and decreased hospital length of stay. Preoperative workup is similar as that for phrenic nerve stimulators (94). The current system has electrode wires exiting the skin and has a small risk of infection. This is currently FDA approved and available at a number of sites around the world.

Electrical stimulation of the upper thoracic ventral roots to activate the inspiratory intercostal muscles is also being used. In clinical trials, ventilation volumes generated by this method were close to the volumes achieved with unilateral diaphragm stimulation but were not sufficient to maintain long-term ventilatory support (86). This method has been used in individuals with long-term tetraplegia who sustained their injuries during their childhood or adolescence (93).

Respiratory Problems in Chronic SCI

In chronic SCI, in addition to the level and severity of injury, pulmonary function is influenced by age, time since injury, lifetime smoking, obesity, and maximum inspiratory pressure (MIP) (95). Diseases of the respiratory system are now the leading cause of death following SCI (3,4,69,96,97). In recent data published from the National Spinal Cord Injury Statistical Center, respiratory complications account for 20.8% of all deaths in individuals with SCI who died from known causes. Of deaths due to respiratory diseases, 72.3% are specifically due to pneumonia (96). Model SCI System data reveal that pneumonia is the leading cause of death for each age group and all time periods postinjury. Pneumonia is by far the leading cause of death for persons with neurologically complete and incomplete tetraplegia, 24.7% of deaths for those with C1-4 injuries, and 19.7% of deaths for those with C5-8 injuries (4,97). What is even more significant is that mortality rates due to respiratory diseases have been increasing in persons with SCI, not decreasing. During the years 1988 to 1992, mortality from respiratory causes was 13.8%, while in 1993 to 1998 mortality due to respiratory causes was 22% after the first year of injury (4). After adjusting for age and sex, persons with SCI have a 36 times greater risk of death from pneumonia and persons with high-level motor complete tetraplegia have more than 150 times greater risk from pneumonia than the general population. Even after the fifth postinjury year, the mortality rate for pneumonia in SCI is 19 times normal (97).

Age, level, completeness of injury, and time since injury still remain as key predictors of survival for persons who are ventilator dependent (4). For example, the life expectancy for a 30-year-old with C1-5 ASIA SCI who is ventilator dependent is 18.6 years, but it is only 2.2 years for an 80-year-old (4). Risk factors for remaining ventilator dependent include (a) high level of neurological injury, (b) age greater than 50 years old, and (c) other associated injuries (81). Of the patients who leave the initial hospitalization still ventilator dependent, the survival rates decline over the first 5 years to 90% at 1 year, 56% at 3 years, and 33% at 5 years. Therefore, concerted efforts need to be made to wean patients from mechanical ventilation at the initial hospitalization to reduce the financial and emotional burden of care and to improve overall quality of life (81).

Morbidity and Pneumonia in Chronic SCI

Respiratory complications such as pneumonia are also a major source of morbidity and hospitalization (6,98–104). The most comprehensive data on annual rates of respiratory complications were reported by McKinley et al. utilizing Model SCI System data who found that for patients with neurologically complete injuries the probability of experiencing at least one episode of pneumonia and/or atelectasis during the preceding year was 9.9%, 9.8%, 6.4%, 4.9%, 4.1%, and 3.7% for 1, 2, 5, 10, 15, and 20 years postinjury, respectively (102). For persons with incomplete tetraplegia, the rates were slightly lower, with 3.1%, 3.8%, 3.3%, 2.2%, and 1.8% at 1, 2, 5, 10, and 15 years postinjury. For all persons, including those with paraplegia and incomplete injuries over the age of 60 years, the rates were 5.6%, 5.9%, 7.1%, 4.1%, and 3.6% at years 1, 2, 5, 10, and 15 years postinjury (102). As patients survive longer after SCI, and the mean age of new traumatic SCI increases, with greater than 10% of new injuries in persons over the age of 60 years, the ability to prevent and treat pneumonia early is extremely important. Respiratory infections in SCI are even greater in independent living centers, as Meyers et al. found the annual rate of respiratory infections (including influenza and pneumonia, but not colds) to be in the range of 18% to 25% for patients with "high-level" SCI (103). Therefore, threshold for hospitalization to treat pneumonia in this patient population needs to be significantly lower than for the able-bodied population. Hospitalization should also be considered for management of acute bronchitis.

Respiratory complications were the third most common reason for hospitalizations for people with SCI greater than 1 year and were more likely in persons with tetraplegia, AIS A, B, or C level injuries (98). A trend of increased rehospitalization was seen at 5 and 10 years after discharge, with statistically significant increase noted at 15 years postinjury. Similar to an increased incidence in respiratory infections (103), the rate of rehospitalization was significantly higher at years 1, 5, and 20 for those who resided in a skilled nursing facility (96).

Much of what we know about respiratory management and complications are in the veteran population. For example, veterans with chronic SCI averaging 20 years postinjury are twice as likely to see a physician for pneumonia compared to the general population of veterans (105). The rate of visits for acute bronchitis is 22 to 32 visits per 1,000 SCI veterans compared with an estimated rate of 18 visits per 1,000 in the general population (105). Up to 30% of veterans with SCI who presented with acute respiratory infections were hospitalized within 60 days (106). Treatment of community acquired pneumonia (CAP; defined as pneumonia not acquired in a hospital or a long-term care facility) was recently reviewed in the Veterans Administration Health care system with the finding that most SCI patients with pneumonia were admitted for treatment, with an average length of stay of 19.3 days (104). Of the patients followed, short-term mortality was 7.3% with mortality over the next 4 years being 42.1% (104). Another recent study found that CAP in the SCI population required an average length of stay of 13.5 days, with almost 9% mortality within 30 days of admission (107).

The major reason for respiratory complications in patients with SCI is generalized weakness of inspiratory and expiratory musculature (108,109).This results in a diminution in the ability to take a deep breath (VC) and an ineffective cough (decreased CPF) with the inability to clear airway secretions that result in a tendency to develop atelectasis (partial lung collapse) and more severe lower respiratory tract infections (RTIs) (e.g., pneumonia). Persons with SCI, especially tetraplegia, have difficulty generating an adequate cough as documented by their cough peak flows (CPF; the maximum flow generated during a cough performed with maximal force and started after a full inspiration) (110,111). In neurologically intact subjects, the value of CPF has been reported between 300 and 700 L/min with even higher flows in young and physically fit men (112). However, in individuals with SCI, the value of CPF can be reduced significantly. In one study, CPF in individuals with tetraplegia was 220 L/min (110). In another study performed on participants with C4-7 complete and incomplete tetraplegia, the mean CPF was 203 L/min [±52] and 238 L/min [±67], unassisted and manually assisted, respectively (111). This is extremely significant because maximum unassisted flows below 300 L/min have been demonstrated to carry a high risk of pneumonia and respiratory failure in other populations of patients with respiratory muscle weakness unless one is set up with means to increase CPF during episodes of RTI (113). Furthermore, VC and CPF can markedly decrease during RTIs, further impairing CPF when the individual needs to be able to clear secretions in order to avoid serious respiratory complications (113). Additional psychosocial considerations that should be made in the management of respiratory complications include risk for other adverse events, the availability of caregivers, and the ability to return for follow-up appointments.

In patients with chronic SCI who are not ventilator dependent, symptoms of dyspnea may affect their quality of life. Dyspnea may occur while talking, dressing, or eating, with talking being the main activity associated with dyspnea in manual wheelchair users (114). Many individuals with respiratory dysfunction secondary to SCI may not need mechanical ventilation but still require a tracheostomy: (a) to relieve obstructive breathing especially associated with sleep apnea, (b) to maintain access for pulmonary toilet, and (c) for emergency access for mechanical ventilation. To avoid complications associated with tracheostomy tubes, in individuals who need tracheostomy but who do not need mechanical ventilation may be able to use "tracheal stoma stents" (90). The benefits of tracheal stents are improvement in local comfort, secretions, and vocalization.

In Japan, long-term ventilation with noninvasive positive pressure ventilation has been used successfully in individuals with high tetraplegia (115). Other noninvasive options for ventilatory support that have been tried in individuals with tetraplegia include intermittent abdominal pressure ventilator, nasal or oral intermittent positive pressure ventilation, and glossopharyngeal breathing (GPB) (25).

Although most individuals with cervical cord injuries are weaned successfully from mechanical ventilation, there are a few individuals who may experience late-onset ventilatory failure. These individuals may present with unexplained tachypnea, dyspnea, daytime somnolence, erythrocytosis, fluctuating mental alertness, and respiratory dysfunction with increased positional influence on breathing. Possible etiologies include cervical cord compression with cervical stenosis and posttraumatic syringomyelia, progressive scoliosis or kyphosis, sleep apnea, and/or loss of diaphragmatic motor neuron associated with aging. Comprehensive evaluation is indicated to assess the change in the extent of ventilatory failure and to attempt to diagnose potentially treatable etiologies. Supportive ventilation such as CPAP, BiPAP, oxygen supplementation, tracheotomy, and mechanical ventilation may be indicated. Other possible interventions may include preventing further decline in respiratory function by discontinuing cigarette smoking, instituting a strengthening program of respiratory muscles, and teaching GPB (116).

Glossopharyngeal Breathing

GPB is a technique that involves rapidly taking small gulps, six to nine gulps of 60 to 200 mL each, using the tongue and pharyngeal muscles to project the air past the glottis into the lungs. It is a useful technique even in patients who have no diaphragmatic strength; however, it requires an intact midbrain to be successful. Many patients can learn to use this technique to increase the VC, which allows for assistance in cough, improvement in audibility of the patient's voice, and ventilator-free time in patients with otherwise minimal VC (25,69).

Influenza and Pneumococcal Vaccination

The immunological response to influenza vaccination in persons with SCI is similar to that of the able-bodied population (117). In the Veterans Administration, there has been a concerted effort to increase the rate of influenza vaccination. In the late 1990s, the reported rate of influenza vaccination in patients with SCI who are older than 65 years ranged from 13% to 26% (118). In Veterans, an intervention program, which included patient and provider education and reminders such as posters, letters, and flyers, has proven to be effective in increasing the rates of vaccination (119). Only 35.3% of veterans with SCI had not received influenza vaccination in a survey completed in 2000 (118). In 2005, the Center for Disease Control and Prevention (CDC) recommended annual influenza vaccination for SCI patients. The overall rate of influenza vaccination for the entire population of SCI patients increased to over 50% to 60% within 1 year using patient and provider reminders, letters, posters, and education (120). Influenza is still diagnosed mostly by clinical symptoms, and there is not enough scientific evidence yet to support the use of antiviral medications in SCI (121).

To date, there are no specific recommendations for pneumococcal vaccinations for individuals with SCI. However, as noted above, individuals with SCI are more likely to die from pneumonia than those in the general population, and *Streptococcus pneumoniae* is the most common pathogen of community-acquired pneumonia. In SCI, protective antibody may be present for at least 5 years after vaccination. The current CDC recommendations for a one time pneumococcal vaccination should be followed for individuals with 65 years of age or older (122). There are very little data available regarding vaccine effectiveness in young individuals in general because most individuals in that age group do not meet the current criteria for receiving the vaccine unless underlying diseases are present. However, just as with influenza vaccination, SCI may need to be considered as one of the "underlying diseases" also for the pneumococcal vaccination (123).

Sleep Apnea

The estimated prevalence of sleep disordered breathing (SDB) in SCI has been reported to be from 15% to as high as 62%, and it is more prevalent in tetraplegia compared with paraplegia (124–129). SDB is usually not apparent until 2 weeks postinjury. The prevalence peaks at 83% at 3-month postinjury in acute tetraplegia (124). Obstructive sleep apnea (OSA) is the predominant form of SDB in SCI. Suspected risk factors for SDB include (a) increased neck circumference, (b) individuals with SCI spending more time supine while asleep, (c) increase in waist circumference, (d) use of sedating medication such as benzodiazepine or baclofen, (e) unopposed parasympathetic activation of the upper airway vasculature and mucosa that may increase the extraluminal tissue pressure and decrease the upper airway diameter and patency, (f) higher level of SCI, and (g) obesity with BMI of 30 kg/m^2 (123,130). Clinical suspicion needs to be high and symptoms such as snoring, daytime somnolence, and morning headaches should be sought (116). Because of the relative high incidence of SDB in the tetraplegic population, SDB should be considered in even marginally obese individuals and in those who do not have complaints of daytime sleepiness (131). Cognitive disturbance might be a predictor of SDB (131). Snoring, which is thought to be a useful clinical marker for OSA, is common (43%) in individuals with SCI, and it is associated the most with obesity, diazepam alone or baclofen, and diazepam (132).

Monitoring with pulse oximetry can detect nocturnal arterial oxygen desaturation, but ideally, polysomnography in an accredited sleep laboratory should be performed. Substantial increase in the amount of light sleep and an absolute and relative reduction in the amount of deep and Rapid Eye Movement SIMV= Synchronized Intermittent Mandatory Ventilation REM stage sleep have been reported in individuals with high cervical injury (133). Treatment of sleep apnea includes traditional measures such as nasal CPAP, nasal Bi-PAP, and supplemental oxygen (116). Nasal CPAP is the most commonly used treatment. The most common side effects are nasal congestion and mask discomfort (130). Weight reduction and reduction of smoking and alcohol consumption should be advised (134). A 6-week program of resistive inspiratory muscle training has been shown to be effective in improving maximum inspiratory pressure (MIP) and reducing the amount of desaturation during sleep (135).

In addition to SDB, chronic alveolar hypoventilation and late-onset chronic ventilatory insufficiency can occur (133,136). Irrespective of changes in VC, hypercapnea and oxyhemoglobin desaturation increase over time for individuals with SCI (133,136). Appropriate labs should be routinely performed.

References

1. Brown R, DiMarco AF, Hoit JD, et al. Respiratory dysfunction and management in spinal cord injury. *Respir Care* 2006;51:853–868.
2. Garshick E, Kelley A, Cohen SA, et al. A prospective assessment of mortality in chronic spinal cord injury. *Spinal Cord* 2005;43:408–416.
3. DeVivo MJ, Ivie CS. Life expectancy of ventilator-dependent persons with spinal cord injuries. *Chest* 1995;108: 226–232.
4. Devivo MJ, Krause JS, Lammertse DP. Recent trends in mortality and causes of death among persons with spinal cord injury. *Arch Phys Med Rehabil* 1999;80:1411–1419.
5. Shavelle RM, DeVivo MJ, Strauss DJ, et al. Long-term survival of persons ventilator dependent after spinal cord injury. *J Spinal Cord Med* 2006;29:511–519.
6. Consortium for Spinal Cord Medicine. Respiratory management following spinal cord injury: a clinical practice guideline for health-care professionals. *J Spinal Cord Med* 2005;28:259–293.
7. The Acute Respiratory Distress Syndrome Network. Ventilation with lower tidal volumes as compared with traditional tidal volumes for acute lung injury and the acute respiratory distress syndrome. *N Engl J Med* 2000;342:1301–1308.
8. Gosling JA. *Human anatomy: color atlas and text.* 3rd ed. C.V. Mosby; 1996.
9. Winslow C, Rozovsky J. Effect of spinal cord injury on the respiratory system. *Am J Phys Med Rehabil* 2003;82:803–814.
10. Jackson AB, Groomers TE. Incidence of respiratory complications following SCI. *Arch Phys Med Rehab* 1994;75:270–275.
11. Ball PA. Critical care of spinal cord injury. *Spine* 2001;26(24 Suppl):S27–S30.
12. Slack RS SW. Respiratory dysfunction associated with traumatic injury to the central nervous system. *Clin Chest Med* 1994;15:739–749.
13. Forner JV, Llombart RL, Valledor MC. The flow-volume loop in tetraplegics. *Paraplegia* 1977;15:245–251.
14. Estenne M, DeTroyer A. Mechanism of the postural dependence of vital capacity in tetraplegic subjects. *Am Rev Respir Dis* 1987;135:367–371.
15. Maloney FP. Pulmonary function in quadriplegia: effects of a corset. *Arch Phys Med Rehabil* 1979;60:261–265.
16. Wadsworth BM, Haines TP, Cornwell PL, et al. Abdominal binder use in people with spinal cord injuries: a systematic review and meta-analysis. *Spinal Cord.* 2009;47:274–285.
17. Como JJ, Sutton ER, McCunn M, et al. Characterizing the need for mechanical ventilation following cervical spinal cord injury with neurological deficit. *J Trauma.* 2005;59:912–916.
18. Stevens RD, Bhardwaj A, Kirsch JR, et al. Critical care and perioperative management in traumatic spinal cord injury. *J Neurosurg Anesthesiol* 2003;15:215–229.
19. Harrop J, Sharan A, Scheid E, et al. Tracheostomy placement in patients with complete cervical spinal cord injuries: American Spinal Injury Association Grade A. *J Neurosurg* 2004;100:20–23.
20. Hassid V, Schinco M, Tepas J, et al. Definitive establishment of airway control is critical for optimal outcome in lower cervical spinal cord injury. *J Trauma* 2008;65:1328–1332.
21. Burns SP, Rad MY, Bryant S, et al. Long-term treatment of sleep apnea in persons with spinal cord injury. *Am J Phys Med Rehabil* 2005;84:620–626.
22. Cotton BA, Pryor JP, Chinwilla I, et al. Respiratory complications and mortality risk associated with thoracic spine injury. *J Trauma* 2005;59:1400–1409.
23. Claxton R, Wong DT, Chung F, et al. Predictors of hospital mortality and mechanical ventilation in patients with

cervical spinal cord injury. *Can J Anesthesia* 1998;45: 144–149.

24. Burns SP. Acute Respiratory Infections in Persons with Spinal Cord Injury. *Phys Med Rehabil Clin N Am* 2007;18:203–216.
25. Bach JR, Saporito LR. Criteria for extubation and tracheostomy tube removal for patients with ventilatory failure. A different approach to weaning. *Chest* 1996;110: 1566–1571.
26. Smina M, Salam A, Khamiees M, et al. Cough peak flows and extubation outcomes. *Chest* 2003;24:262–268.
27. Lanig IS, Peterson WP. The respiratory system in spinal cord injury. *Phys Med Rehabil Clin N Am* 2000;11:29–43.
28. Carter RE. Respiratory aspects of spinal cord injury management. *Paraplegia* 1987;25:262–266.
29. Bhaskar KR, Brown R, O'Sullivan DD, et al. Bronchial mucus hypersecretion in acute quadriplegia. Macromolecular yields and glycoconjugate composition. *Am Rev Resp Dis* 1991;143:640–648.
30. Lemons VR, Wagner FC Jr. Respiratory complications after cervical spinal cord injury. *Spine* 199419: 2315–2320.
31. Almenoff PL, Alexander LR, Spungen AM, et al. Bronchodilatory effects of iparatropium bromide in patients with tetraplegia. *Paraplegia* 1995;33:274–277.
32. Spungen AM, Dicpinigaitis PV, Almenoff PL, et al. Pulmonary obstruction in individuals with cervical spinal cord lesions unmasked by bronchodilator administration. *Paraplegia* 1993;31(6):404–407.
33. Spungen AM, Grimm DR, Stakhan M, et al. Treatment with anabolic agent is associated with improvement in respiratory function in persons with tetraplegia: a pilot study. *Mt Sanai J Med* 1999;66(3):201–205.
34. Gonzalez EG, Edelstein JE, et al. *Physiological basis of rehabilitation medicine.* Woburn, MA: Butterworth-Heinmemann; 2001.
35. Chen D Apple DF, Hudson LM, et al. Medical complications during acute rehabilitation following spinal cord injury current experience of the model systems. *Arch Phys Med Rehabil* 1999;80:1397–1401.
36. American Thoracic Society; Infectious Diseases Society of America. Guidelines for the management of adults with hospital-acquired, ventilator-associated, and healthcare-associated pneumonia. *Am J Respir Crit Care Med* 2005;171(4):388–416.
37. Bartlett J, Gorbach SL, Finegold S. The bacteriology of aspiration pneumonia. *Am J Med* 1974;56:202–207.
38. Bartlett J, Gorbach SL, Tally F, et al. Bacteriology and treatment of primary lung abscess. *Am Rev Respir Dis* 1974;109:510–519.
39. Kirshblum S, Johnston MV, Brown J, et al. Predictors of dysphagia after spinal cord injury. *Arch Phys Med Rehab* 1999;80(9):1101–1105.
40. DeVita MA, Spierer-Rundback L. Swallowing disorders in patients with prolonged orotracheal intubation or tracheostomy tubes. *Crit Care Med* 1990;18(12): 1328–1330.
41. Elpern EH, Scott MG, Petro L, et al. Pulmonary aspiration in mechanically ventilated patients with tracheostomies. *Chest* 1994;105(2):563–566.
42. Berlly M, Shem K. Respiratory management during the first five days after spinal cord injury. *J Spinal Cord Med* 2007;30:309–318
43. Lanes SF, Garcia Rodriguez LA, Huerta C. Respiratory medications and risk of asthma death. *Thorax* 2002;57(8):683–686.
44. Salpeter SR, Ormiston TM, Salpeter EE. Meta-analysis: respiratory tolerance to regular beta2-agonist use in patients with asthma. *Ann Intern Med* 2004;140(10): 802–813.
45. Spitzer WO, Suissa S, Ernst P, et al. The use of beta-agonists and the risk of death and near death from asthma. *N Engl J Med* 1992;326:501–506.
46. Salpeter SR, Buckley NS, Ormiston TM, et al. Meta-analysis: effect of long-acting beta-agonists on severe asthma exacerbations and asthma-related deaths. *Ann Intern Med* 2006;144:904–912.
47. Schilero GJ, Grimm D, Spungen AM, et al. Bronchodilator responses to metaproterenol sulfate among subjects with spinal cord injury. *J Rehabil Res Dev* 2004;41:59–64.
48. Grimm DR, Schilero GJ, Spungen AM, et al. Salmeterol improves pulmonary function in persons with tetraplegia. *Lung* 2006;184:335–339.
49. Gross N. Anticholinergic agents in asthma and COPD. *Eur J Pharmocol* 2006;533:36–39.
50. Summers QA, Tarala RA. Nebulized ipratropium in the treatment of acute asthma. *Chest* 1990;97:425–429.
51. Teale C, Morrison JF, Muers MF, et al. Response to nebulized ipratropium bromide and terbutaline in acute severe asthma. *Resp Med* 1992;86:215–218.
52. Westby M, Benson M, Gibson P. Anticholinergic agents for chronic asthma in adults. *Cochrane Database Syst Rev* 2004(3):CD003269.
53. Matsumoto T, Tamaki T, Kawakami M, et al. Early complications of high-dose methylprednisolone sodium succinate treatment in the follow-up of acute cervical spinal cord injury. *Spine* 2001;26:426–430.
54. Foxworth JW, Reisz GR, Knudson SM, et al. Theophylline and diaphragmatic contractility. Investigation of a dose-response relationship. *Am Rev Respir Dis* 1988;138:1532–1534.
55. Murciano D, Aubier M, Lecocguic Y, et al. Effects of theophylline on diaphragmatic strength and fatigue in patients with chronic obstructive pulmonary disease. *N Engl J Med* 1984;311:349–353.
56. McBride DQ, Rodts GE. Intensive care of patients with spinal trauma. *Neurosurg Int Care* 1994;5:755–766.
57. Sortor S. Pulmonary issues in quadriplegia. *Eur Respir Rev* 1992;2:330–334.
58. Waters RJ, Meyers PR, Adkins R, et al. Emergency, acute, and surgical management of spine trauma. *Arch Phys Med Rehabil* 1999;80:1383–1390.
59. Powell M, Kirshblum S, O'Connor KC. Duplex ultrasound screening for deep vein thrombosis in spinal cord injured patients at rehabilitation admission. *Arch Phys Med Rehabil* 1999;80:1044–1046.
60. Wallbom AS, Thomas E. *Acute ventilator management and weaning in individuals with high tetraplegia.* St. Louis, MO: Thomas Land Publishers Birmingham, AL, Inc.; 2005.
61. Peterson WP, Barbalata L, Brooks CA, et al. The effect of tidal volumes on the time to wean persons with high

tetraplegia from ventilators. *Spinal Cord* 1999;37: 284–288.

62. McMichan JC, Michel L, Westbrook PR. Pulmonary dysfunction following traumatic quadriplegia. Recognition, prevention, and treatment. *JAMA* 1980;243(6):528–531.
63. Cook N. Respiratory care in spinal cord injury with associated traumatic brain injury: bridging the gap in critical care nursing intervention. *Int Crit Care Nurs* 2003;19:143–153.
64. Kinney TB, Rose SC, Valji K, et al. Does Cervical spinal cord injury induce a higher incidence of complications after prophylactic Greenfield filter usage? *J Vasc Interv Radiol* 1996;7:907–915.
65. Gomez-Merino E, Sancho J, Marin J. Mechanical insufflation-exsufflation: pressure, volume, and flow relationships and the adequacy of the manufacturer's guidelines. *Am J Phys Med Rehabil* 2002;81:579–583.
66. Garstang SV, Kirshblum S, Wood KE. Patient preference for in-exsufflation for secretion management in spinal cord injury. *J Spinal Cord Med* 2000;23:80–85.
67. Fishburn MJ, Marino RJ, Ditunno JF. Atelectasis and pneumonia in acute spinal cord injury. *Arch Phys Med Rehabil* 1990;71:197–200.
68. Winslow C, Bode R, Felton D, et al. Impact of respiratory complications on length of stay and hospital costs in acute cervical spine injury. *Chest* 2002;121:1548–1554.
69. Peterson P, Kirshblum SC. Respiratory management in spinal cord injury. In: Kirshblum SC, Campagnolo D, DeLisa JE, eds. *Spinal cord medicine*. Philadelphia, PA: Lippincott/Williams & Wilkins; 2002:135–154.
70. Lin KH, Chuang CC, Wu HD, et al. Abdominal weight and inspiratory resistance: their immediate effects on inspiratory muscle functions during maximal voluntary breathing in chronic tetraplegic patients. *Arch Phys Med Rehabil* 1999;80:741–745.
71. Van Houtte S, Vanlandewijck Y, Gosselink R. Respiratory muscle training in persons with spinal cord injury: a systematic review. *Resp Med* 2006;100:1886–1895.
72. Delardo AF, Onders RP, Ignagni A, et al. Diaphragm electrodes in tetraplegic phrenic nerve pacing via intramuscular subjects. *Chest* 2005;127:671–678.
73. Checkley W, Brower R, Korpak A, et al. Effects of a clinical trial on mechanical ventilation practices in patients with acute lung injury. *Am J Resp Crit Care Med* 2008;177:1215–1222.
74. Gross D, Ladd HW, Riley EJ, et al. The effect of training on strength and endurance of the diaphragm in quadriplegia. *Am J Med* 1980;68:27–35.
75. Leith D, Bradley M. Ventilatory muscle strength and endurance training. *J Appl Physiol* 1976;41:508–516.
76. Liaw MY, Lin MC, Cheng P. Resistive inspiratory muscle training: its effectiveness in patients with acute complete cervical cord injury. *Arch Phys Med Rehabil* 2000;81:752–756.
77. McKinley W. Late return of diaphragm function in a ventilator-dependent patient with a high cervical tetraplegia: case report, and interactive review. *Spinal Cord* 1996;34:626–629.
78. Oo T, Watt JW, Soni BM, et al. Delayed diaphragm recovery in 12 patients after high cervical spinal cord injury. A retrospective review of the diaphragm status of 107 patients ventilated after acute spinal cord injury. *Spinal Cord* 1999;37:117–122.
79. Peterson W, Charlifue W, Gerhart A, et al. Two methods of weaning persons with quadriplegia from mechanical ventilators. *Paraplegia* 1994;32:98–103.
80. Report H. Misuse of fenestrated tracheostomy tubes [Hazard Report]. Health devices. 1978 Jan;7(3):91
81. Wicks AB, Menter RR. Long-term outlook in quadriplegic patients with initial ventilator dependency. *Chest* 1986;90:406–410.
82. Chiodo AE, Scelza W, Forchheimer M. Predictors of ventilatory weaning in individuals with high cervical spinal cord inury. *J Spinal Cord Med.* 2008;31:72–77.
83. Gardner BP, Watt JW, Krishnan KR. The artificial ventilation of acute spinal cord damaged patients: a retrospective study of forty-four patients. *Paraplegia* 1986;24:208–220.
84. Bach JR, Alba AS. Noninvasive options for ventilatory support of the traumatic high level quadriplegia patient. *Chest* 1990;98:613–619.
85. DiMarco AF, Onders RP, Ignagni A, et al. Phrenic nerve pacing via intramuscular diaphragm electrodes in tetraplegic subjects. *Chest* 2005;127:671–678.
86. DiMarco AF, Onders RP, Ignagni A, et al. Inspiratory muscle pacing in spinal cord injury: case report and clinical commentary. *J Spinal Cord Med* 2006;29:95–108.
87. Shaul DB, Danielson PD, McComb JG, et al. Thoracoscopic placement of phrenic nerve electrodes for diaphragmatic pacing in children. *J Pediatr Surg* 2002;37(7):974–978.
88. Strakowski JA, Pease W, Johnson EW. Phrenic nerve stimulation in the evaluation of ventilator-dependent individuals with C4- and C5- level spinal cord injury. *Am J Phys Med Rehabil* 2007;86:153–157.
89. Lieberman JS, Corgil G, Nayak NN, et al. Serial phrenic nerve conduction studies in candidates for diaphragm pacing. *Arch Phys Med Rehabil* 1980;61:528–531.
90. Hall AM, Watt JW. The use of tracheal stoma stents in high spinal cord injury: a patient-friendly alternative to long-term tracheostomy tubes. *Spinal Cord* 2008. Nov;46(11):753–755.
91. Krieger LM, Krieger AJ. The intercostal to phrenic nerve transfer: an effective means of reanimating the diaphragm in patients with high cervical spine injury. *Plastic Recon Surg* 2000;105:1255–1261.
92. Onders RP, Elmo M, Khansarinia S, et al. Complete worldwide operative experience in laparoscopic diaphragm pacing: results and differences in spinal cord injured patients and amyotrophic lateral sclerosis patients. *Surg Endosc* 2009;23:1433–1440. Epub 2008 Dec 6.
93. Onders RP, Elmo MJ, Ignagni AR. Diaphragm pacing stimulation system for tetraplegia in individuals injured during childhood or adolescence. *J Spinal Cord Med* 2007;30(Suppl 1):S25–S29.
94. Alshekhlee A, Onders RP, Syed TU, et al. Phrenic nerve conduction studies in spinal cord injury: applications for diaphragmatic pacing. *Muscle Nerve* 2008;38:1546–1552.
95. Jain NB, Brown R, Tun CG, et al. Determinants of forced expiratory volume in 1 second (FEV1), forced vital capacity (FVC), and FEV1/FVC in chronic spinal cord injury. *Arch Phys Med Rehabil* 2006;87:1327–1333.
96. Devivo MJ. Epidemiology of traumatic spinal cord injury. In: Kirshblum SC, Campagnolo D, DeLisa JL, eds. *Spinal*

cord medicine. Philadelphia: Lippincott/Williams & Wilkins; 2002:69–81

97. Devivo MJ, Stover SL. Long-term survival and causes of death. In: Stover SL, DeLisa JL, Whiteneck GG, eds. *Spinal cord injury: clinical outcomes from the model systems*. Gaithersburg, MD: Aspen Publishers; 1995:289–316.
98. Cardenas DD, Hoffman JM, Kirshblum S, et al. Etiology and incidence of rehospitalization after traumatic spinal cord injury: a multicenter analysis. *Arch Phys Med Rehabil* 2004;85:1757–1763.
99. Sipski ML, Richards JS. Spinal cord injury rehabilitation: state of the science. *Am J Phys Med Rehabil* 2006;85:210–342
100. Ragnarsson KT, Hall KM, Wilmot CB, et al. Management of pulmonary, cardiovascular and metabolic conditions after spinal cord injury. In: Stover SL, DeLisa JL, Whiteneck GG, eds. *Spinal cord injury: clinical outcomes for the model systems*. Gaithersberg, MD: Aspen Publishers; 1995:79–99.82.
101. McCrory DC, Samsa GP, Hamilton BP, et al. Treatment of pulmonary disease following spinal cord injury. Evid Rep Technol Assess (Summ). 2001 Jun;(27):1–4.
102. McKinley WO, Jackson AB, Cardenas DD, et al. Long-term medical complications after traumatic spinal cord injury: a regional model systems analysis. *Arch Phys Med Rehabil* 1999;80:1402–1410.
103. Meyers AB, Bisbee A, Winter M. The "Boston Model" of managed care spinal cord injury: a cross-sectional study of the outcomes of risk-based, pre-paid, managed care. *Arch Phys Med Rehabil* 1999;80:1450–1456.
104. Burns SP, Weaver FM, Parada JP, et al. Management of community-acquired pneumonia in persons with spinal cord injury. *Spinal Cord* 2004;42:450–458.
105. Smith BM, Evans CT, Kurichi JE, et al. Acute respiratory tract infection visits of veterans with spinal cord injuries and disorders: rates, trends, and risk factors. *J Spinal Cord Med* 2007;30:355–361.
106. Weaver FM, Smith B, Evans CT, et al. Outcomes of outpatient visits for acute respiratory illness in veterans with spinal cord injuries and disorders. *Am J Phys Med Rehabil* 2006;85:718–726.
107. Chang H, Evans C, Weaver F, et al. Etiology and outcomes of veterans with spinal cord injury and disorders hospitalized and community acquired pneumonia. *Arch Phys Med Rehabil* 2005;86(2):262–267.
108. Bach JR. Inappropriate weaning and late onset ventilatory failure of individuals with traumatic spinal cord injury. *Paraplegia* 1993;31:430–438.
109. Bach JR, Rajaraman R, Ballanger F, et al. Neuromuscular ventilatory insufficiency: effect of home mechanical ventilator use v oxygen therapy on pneumonia and hospitalization rates. *Am J Phys Med Rehabil* 1998;77:8–19.
110. Kirby NA, Barnerias MJ, Siebens AA. An evaluation of assisted cough in quadriparetic patients. *Arch Phys Med Rehabil* 1966;47:705–710.
111. Jaegar RJ, et al. Cough in spinal cord injured patients: comparison of three methods to produce cough. *Arch Phys Med Rehabil* 1993;74:1358–1361.
112. Leiner GC. Cough peak flow rate. *Am J Med Sci* 1966;22:121–124.
113. Gomez-Merino E, Bach JR. Duchenne muscular dystrophy: prolongation of life by noninvasive ventilation and mechanically assisted coughing. *Am J Phys Med Rehabil* 2002;81:411–415.
114. Grandas NF, Jain NB, Denckla JB, et al. Dyspnea during daily activities in chronic spinal cord injury. *Arch Phys Med Rehabil* 2005;86:1631–1635.
115. Toki A, Tamura R, Sumida M. Long-term ventilation for high-level tetraplegia: a report of 2 cases of noninvasive positive pressure ventilation. *Arch Phys Med Rehabil* 2008;89:779–783.
116. Eltorai IM, Segal J. *Emergencies in chronic spinal cord injury patients*. 3rd ed. New York, NY: Eastern Paralyzed Veterans Association; 2001
117. Trautner BW, Atmar RL, Hulstrom A, et al. Inactivated influenza vaccination for people with spinal cord injury. *Arch Phys Med Rehabil* 2004;85:1886–1889.
118. Evans CT, Legro MW, Weaver FM, et al. Influenza vaccination among veterans with spinal cord injury: Part 1. A survey of attitudes and behavior. *J Spinal Cord Med* 2003;26:204–209.
119. Weaver FM, Goldstein B, Evans CT, et al. Influenza vaccination among veterans with spinal cord injury: Part 2. Increasing vaccination rates. *J Spinal Cord Med* 2003;26:210–218.
120. Weaver FM, Smith B, LaVela S, et al. Interventions to increase influenza vaccination rates in veterans with spinal cord injuries and disorders. *J Spinal Cord Med* 2007;30:10–19.
121. Evans CT, Lavel SL, Smith B, et al. Infl uenza diagnosis and treatment in veterans with spinal cord injury. *Arch Phys Med Rehabil* 2006;87:291–293.
122. Report from the Advisory Committee on Immunization Practices (ACIP): Decision Not to Recommend Routine Vaccination of All Children Aged 2–10 Years with Quadrivalent Meningococcal Conjugate Vaccine (MCV4). *MMWR Morbid Mortal Wkly Rep*. 2008;57(17)462–465.
123. Waites KB, Canupp KC, Chen YY, et al. Revaccination of adults with spinal cord injury using the 23-valent pneumococcal polysaccharide vaccine. *J Spinal Cord Med* 2008;31:53–59.
124. Berlowitz DJ, Brown DJ, Campbell DA, et al. A longitudinal evaluation of sleep and breathing in the first year after cervical spinal cord injury. *Arch Phys Med Rehabil* 2005;86:1193–1199.
125. Burns SP, Little JW, Hussey JD, et al. Sleep apnea syndrome in chronic spinal cord injury: associated factors and treatment. *Arch Phys Med Rehabil* 2000;81: 1334–1339.
126. Flavell H, Marshall R, Thornton AT, et al. Hypoxia episodes during sleep in high tetraplegia. *Arch Phys Med Rehabil* 1992;73:623–627.
127. Klefbeck B, Sternhag M, Weinberg J, et al. Obstructive sleep apneas in relation to severity of cervical spinal cord injury. *Spinal Cord* 1998;36:621–628.
128. Leduc BE, Dagher JH, Mayer P, et al. Estimated prevalence of obstructive sleep apnea-hypopnea syndrome after cervical cord injury. *Arch Phys Med Rehabil* 2007;88:333–337.
129. Short DJ, Stradling JR, Williams SJ. Prevalence of sleep apnoea in patients over 40 years of age with spinal cord lesions. *J Neurol Neurosurg Psych* 1992;55:1032–1036.
130. Burns SP, Kapur V, Yin KS, et al. Factors associated with sleep apnea in men with spinal cord injury:

a population-based case-control study. *Spinal Cord* 2001;39:15–22.
131. Stockhammer E, Tobon A, Michel F, et al. Characteristics of sleep apnea syndrome in tetraplegic patients. *Spinal Cord* 2002;40:286–294.
132. Ayas NT, Epstein LJ, Lieberman SL, et al. Predictors of loud snoring in persons with spinal cord injury. *J Spinal Cord Med* 2001;24:30–34.
133. Bonekat HW, Anderson G, Squires J. Obstructive disordered breathing during sleep in patients with spinal cord injury. *Paraplegia* 1990;28:392–398.
134. Biering-Sørensen M, Norup PW, Jacobsen E, et al. Treatment of sleep apnoea in spinal cord injured patients. *Paraplegia* 1995;33:271–273.
135. Wang TG, Wang YH, Tang FT, et al. Resistive inspiratory muscle training in sleep-disordered breathing of traumatic tetraplegia. *Arch Phys Med Rehabil* 2002;83: 491–496.
136. Bach JR. Chronic alveolar hypoventilation as a late complication of spinal cord injury. *J Spinal Cord Med* 1995;18:255.

CHAPTER 11 ■ GASTROINTESTINAL DISORDERS

DAVID CHEN AND ALAN S. ANSCHEL

INTRODUCTION

Alterations in function of the gastrointestinal (GI) system are generally less obvious than those changes seen in other body systems following spinal cord injury (SCI). Certain aspects of GI function (e.g., gastric digestion, absorption) change very little following an SCI, while other aspects are significantly altered (e.g., bowel evacuation). However, these changes may have significant psychosocial implications and have the potential to influence the social, emotional, and physical well-being of individuals with SCI.

This chapter reviews the normal neuroanatomy, anatomy, and physiology of the GI system. In addition, the physiologic and functional changes that occur following SCI, management of the neurogenic bowel, and common GI complications that occur in persons with SCI are discussed.

NEUROLOGIC CONTROL OF THE GASTROINTESTINAL SYSTEM

Enteric Nervous System

In general, throughout the GI tract, there are five tissue layers present that make up the GI wall. The serosa is the external layer of the wall. The next two layers contain the externally placed longitudinal and internally placed circular muscle layers that are responsible for the propulsive and mixing actions of the gut. The externally placed submucosal and internally placed mucosal layers are responsible for most of the secretory activity of the gut (1).

Electrical activity within the gut transmits through gap junctions and consists of slow wave and spike potentials. Slow waves are slow changes in the resting membrane potential. Spike potentials, which are responsible for the rhythmic contractions in the GI tract, are action potentials that are 10 to 40 times as long as normal nerve fiber action potentials. Calcium-sodium channels, which take longer to open and close, are utilized in the GI tract to propagate action potentials instead of the more commonly utilized sodium-potassium channels (1).

The enteric (intrinsic) nervous system consists of the myenteric plexus and submucosal plexus. The myenteric plexus (Auerbach plexus), which is located between the longitudinal and circular muscle layers, controls motor activities such as tonic and rhythmic contractions that assist in propelling stool throughout the colon. The submucosal plexus (Meissner plexus), which is located in the submucosa, controls local intestinal secretion and absorption. The enteric nervous system can function independently but is partially influenced by the autonomic nervous system (1,2).

Neurotransmitters such as acetylcholine, norepinephrine, dopamine, cholecystokinin, and somatostatin can also influence the enteric nervous system. In general, acetylcholine is excitatory and norepinephrine is inhibitory (1).

Autonomic Nervous System

In general, the parasympathetic (PS) nervous system increases peristalsis, stimulates secretions, relaxes sphincters, and increases gut motility (3). The short postganglionic fibers of the PS nervous system secrete the neurotransmitter acetylcholine and terminate near the neurons of the myenteric plexus and submucosal plexus. The vagus nerve (cranial nerve X) supplies the PS innervation from the esophagus to the midtransverse colon. There is minimal PS innervation to the small intestine. The pelvic nerve, which originates in the lateral anterior gray columns of spinal cord segments S2-4, supplies the PS innervation from the midtransverse colon to the rectum.

In general, the sympathetic nervous system (SNS) decreases peristalsis, inhibits secretions, contracts sphincters, and decreases gut motility (3). These neurons of the SNS generally secrete the neurotransmitter norepinephrine. The preganglionic fibers originate in the intermediolateral column of the spinal cord between T5 and L2. The superior and inferior mesenteric (T9-12) and hypogastric nerves (T12-L3) contain postganglionic sympathetic neurons (Fig. 11.1).

NORMAL PHYSIOLOGY AND ANATOMY OF THE GI TRACT

Mastication

Mastication aids digestion by increasing the exposed surface area of food particles to digestive enzymes. The motor branch of cranial nerve V supplies the motor control of mastication. Saliva excreted by the parotid, submandibular, and sublingual salivary glands aids mastication. The parotid gland secretes ptyalin, an enzyme that digests starch. The submandibular and sublingual glands secrete mucin for lubrication (4).

Deglutition (Swallowing)

Normal swallowing consists of the voluntary, pharyngeal, and esophageal stages. During the voluntary stage, food is sent posteriorly into the pharynx by the upward and backward pressure of the tongue against the palate. Food moves from the pharynx to the esophagus during the involuntary pharyngeal phase. During this phase, the soft palate is pulled upward to

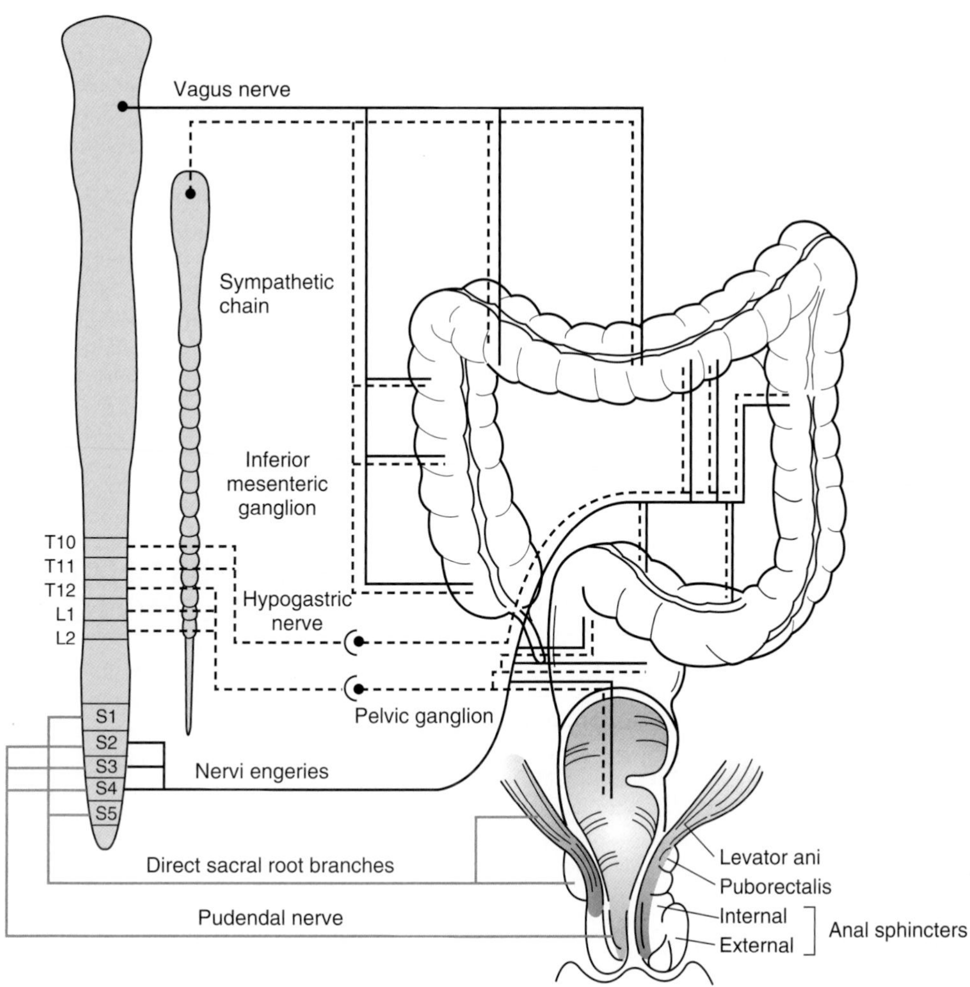

FIGURE 11.1. Innervation of the GI tract. (Reproduced from Steins SA, Bergman SB, Goetz LL. Neurogenic bowel dysfunction after spinal cord injury: clinical evaluation and rehabilitative management. *Arch Phys Med Rehabil* 1997;78:S86–S100, with permission.)

close off the nasal passages, and the palatopharyngeal folds pull together to allow only small particles that have been broken down to pass. To help prevent aspiration, the vocal cords close and the larynx is pulled anteriorly and upward, thus causing the epiglottis to close off the larynx. In addition, pharyngeal muscular peristaltic waves propel food into the esophagus. During the involuntary esophageal phase, vagally controlled peristaltic waves move food down the esophagus. When food particles reach the lower esophagus, the normally tonically constricted lower esophageal sphincter relaxes, allowing passage of esophageal contents into the stomach (4).

Stomach

The stomach's main functions are to serve as a reservoir for ingested food products, to mix food products with gastric secretions, to reduce solids to small particles, and to regulate the delivery of food products into the duodenum. When food enters the stomach, the gastric body and fundus relax, permitting increased storage capacity. The vagally controlled pacemaker potentials stimulate gastric contractions. Sympathetic input further modulates the contractions (5). Food particles are prevented from entering the duodenum by the tonically contracted pyloric sphincter. Neural signals from the distended stomach and the influences of gastrin, cholecystokinin, and secretin further influence the opening or closing of the pyloric sphincter (4).

Two types of secretory glands are located within the gastric mucosa. The oxyntic glands located in the body and fundus of the stomach secrete hydrochloric acid, pepsinogen, and intrinsic factor. Pepsinogen when combined with hydrochloric acid converts to pepsin, a proteolytic enzyme. Intrinsic factor is necessary for vitamin B_{12} absorption. The pyloric glands located in the antrum of the stomach secrete protective mucus (6).

Small Intestine, Pancreas, Liver

The main purpose of the small intestine is to digest and absorb nutrients with assistance from products made by the liver and pancreas. In the small intestine, pancreatic amylase digests carbohydrates, numerous pancreatic enzymes digest proteins, and lipase digests fats. Segmental concentric contractions controlled by the myenteric plexus mix and propel food particles through the small intestine (6).

The products secreted by the pancreas have numerous functions in normal digestion. Insulin is secreted by the islets of Langerhans. Sodium bicarbonate is secreted to neutralize the acidic stomach contents. Trypsin and chymotrypsin digest proteins, amylase digests starches, lipase digests fats, secretin stimulates bicarbonate formation, and gastrin stimulates digestive enzymes (6).

The liver produces bile acids that emulsify large fat particles, thus aiding digestion. Bile acids are subsequently stored in the gallbladder and released under the influence of cholecystokinin and autonomic nervous input (6).

Colon (Large Intestine)

The colon begins in the right lower quadrant as the cecum and is anatomically divided into the ascending, transverse, descending, and sigmoid colon. The rectum and anus mark the termination of the colon.

The primary function of the ascending colon is to absorb electrolytes and water, and the primary function of the descending colon is to store fecal material until evacuation (2). Absorbing water and electrolytes, secreting mucus for lubrication, forming the stool, and supporting the growth of symbiotic bacteria are other functions of the colon. Normal colonic transit time takes between 12 and 30 hours from the ileocecal valve to the rectum (7).

Haustrations and mass movements are two types of colonic motility. Circular muscular contractions of the colon that cause mixing of the colonic contents are called haustrations. Haustrations generally do not cause forward movement of the stool (4). Mass movements are large areas of muscular contractions that propel stool forward within the colon. These mass movements last 10 to 30 minutes and occur only a few times a day (4,8).

Reflexes of the GI Tract

The gastrocolic, colocolonic, and rectocolic reflexes generally stimulate colonic motility. The gastrocolic reflex describes the increase in colonic activity after ingestion of a meal. The mechanism for this cholinergic-mediated reflex, which is blunted by atropine, has not been well defined. The colocolonic intramural reflex is controlled by the myenteric plexus. This reflex, which occurs even when the colon is removed from the body, causes the muscles above the dilatation to constrict and those below the dilatation to relax, causing the stool to be propelled caudally. The rectocolic reflex, pelvic nerve mediated, is responsible for the colonic peristalsis that occurs in response to chemical or mechanical stimulation of the rectum or anal canal (9) (Fig. 11.1). This reflex is the basis for the use of digital stimulation and suppositories in performing the bowel program in persons with SCI.

Additional reflexes that may be involved in defecation include the rectoanal inhibitory reflex and the anorectal excitatory reflex. It is hypothesized that as stool moves into the rectum causing distention, initiation of the rectoanal inhibitory reflex leads to internal anal sphincter relaxation, rectal contraction, and the beginning of defecation. As stool passes through the anal canal, rectal contraction is maintained through the anorectal excitatory reflex as a secondary defecation reflex (10–12).

Normal Defecation

The internal and external anal sphincters control the anal canal. The internal anal sphincter is composed of involuntary smooth muscle and provides continence in the resting state by remaining tonically contracted. The external anal sphincter, innervated by the pudendal nerve (S2-4), is composed of striated muscle, provides voluntary control of defecation, and prevents incontinence along with the puborectalis during cough or Valsalva maneuver.

The sequence of events in normal defecation includes colonic contractions causing the stool to move from the colon to the rectum. Stool then distends the rectum, stretching the puborectalis muscle that causes a reflex relaxation of the internal anal sphincter (anorectal inhibitory reflex). This then causes the conscious urge to defecate, but the external anal sphincter and puborectalis muscles prevent defecation (i.e., the holding reflex). Under voluntary control, the external anal sphincter and puborectalis muscles relax, thus allowing defecation. Abdominal musculature aids defecation by increasing intra-abdominal pressure (9).

GASTROINTESTINAL CHANGES FOLLOWING SCI

Dysphagia is a common problem following a cervical SCI. This dysphagia is almost always transient and often related to soft tissue swelling especially after an anterior spinal surgery. Tracheostomies and cervical immobilizing braces such as a Halo orthosis also contribute to dysphagia (13,14). Although some individuals with tetraplegia suffer from gastroesophageal reflux, esophageal function generally remains intact after an SCI (15).

Changes in gastric motility often occur in tetraplegia but generally are not present in paraplegia (9,16). In tetraplegia, dissociation of antral and duodenal motility occurs. In addition, gastric pacemaker potentials no longer originate in the antrum in most tetraplegic individuals (17). This contributes to decreased gastric emptying often experienced by individuals with tetraplegia. It is unclear whether or not the gastrocolic reflex is functional after an SCI. A study by Connell et al. (18) documented the presence of the gastrocolic reflex, but Glick et al. (19) reported the absence of the gastrocolic reflex after SCI.

It has been suggested that increased gallbladder disease may occur in injuries above T10. Since the sympathetic supply to the gallbladder originates between T7 and T10, abnormal gallbladder motility and enterohepatic circulation may be caused by decreased sympathetic input (20).

Anal sphincter tone is directly related to the SCI level. When an SCI occurs above the conus medullaris (T12), the anal sphincter becomes spastic. Voluntary control is lost but reflex activity is intact. This situation is commonly referred to as an upper motor neuron (UMN) bowel. In lesions above T1, there is prolonged mouth to cecum transit time. In addition, SCI individuals have delayed left colon and rectal transit times as compared to controls (7). When an SCI occurs below T12, the anal sphincter is denervated and therefore flaccid. Voluntary and reflex activity is lost and is commonly referred to as a lower motor neuron (LMN) bowel (2).

Decreased colonic motility, especially of the descending colon, leading to constipation or an ileus commonly occurs after an SCI. Loss of normal autonomic control, use of narcotics, immobility, and loss of abdominal musculature all may contribute. In an individual with a UMN bowel, the spastic anal sphincter may contribute to constipation by preventing stool evacuation. In an individual with an LMN bowel, the descending colon, sigmoid colon, and rectal denervation with the resultant absence of peristalsis contribute to constipation, but often with incontinence due to the flaccid sphincter.

BOWEL MANAGEMENT FOLLOWING SPINAL CORD INJURY

The effective management of the neurogenic bowel is important to prevent potential GI complications and can have a significant influence on successful reintegration of the SCI individual to his or her home, school, or work, and for quality of life. Bowel dysfunction is considered by many individuals with SCI as a major life-limiting problem (21). More than one third of persons with SCI rated bowel and bladder issues as having the most significant effect on their lives (22). Fear of bowel accidents is a frequent cause of people with SCI not to participate in social and other outside activities.

An effective and successful bowel program implies the predictable, regular, and thorough evacuation of the bowels without the occurrence of incontinence and prevention of complications. An effective bowel management regimen takes into consideration diet and nutritional factors, use of pharmacologic agents when necessary, and a well-developed, appropriate program, which is consistent with the neurologic condition and needs of the individual. Other factors such as availability of caregiver assistance, the need and use of adaptive equipment, home accessibility, activity level and lifestyle, and return to work/school issues also must be considered. It is important to emphasize that each SCI individual is unique and that differences in bowel programs between persons should be anticipated to meet individual needs.

Pharmacologic Agents

Although commonly used in the initial establishment of a bowel program following a new SCI, the routine use of oral medications, suppositories, or other bowel preparations is not always required or necessary long term in persons with SCI to effectively manage their bowels. Through proper diet and fluid management, many individuals are able to maintain adequate stool bulk, consistency, and colonic transit without oral medications or supplements. In many instances, evacuation of the formed stool from the rectum does not require the use of specialized bowel preparations or medications. The use of pharmacologic agents should be looked upon as an adjunctive tool to facilitate an effective overall bowel program. Commonly used medications fall into four general categories: stool softeners, bulk formers, peristaltic stimulants, and contact irritants.

Stool softeners: When fluid management and dietary modifications are not effective in maintaining sufficiently soft, yet formed, stool to facilitate regular bowel movements, the use of oral medications to soften stool is often helpful. Docusate sodium (Colace) and docusate calcium (Surfak) are surface-active agents that act to emulsify fat in the GI tract and decrease the reabsorption of water in the colon, thereby increasing the water content of the stool. Keeping the stool soft, yet still formed, may help decrease the potential to develop hemorrhoids in patients who strain to have a bowel movement. It is important to recognize that appropriate fluid intake is necessary for these agents to be effective. These agents are not stimulants or laxatives and, therefore, are not specifically intended to enhance bowel or colonic transit or peristalsis. The laxative/stool softener Peri-Colace combines sennosides and docusate sodium.

Bulk formers: Bulk-forming agents act to increase the bulk of stool in the bowels by the absorption of water and expanding its volume. The increased volume or bulk of the stool in the bowel lumen distends the bowel and stimulates peristalsis. Bulk-forming agents include psyllium (Fiberall, Metamucil, Naturacil), calcium polycarbophil (FiberCon), and methylcellulose (Citrucel). Excessive use of these agents can cause diarrhea, and if adequate amounts of fluid are not taken with the agents, gastric and bowel obstruction can occur.

Peristaltic stimulants and prokinetic agents: Unlike bulk formers, peristaltic stimulants enhance bowel peristalsis and colonic transit by direct stimulation of the colonic intramural plexus.

Senna (Senokot) is a commonly used oral peristaltic stimulant in the management of neurogenic bowels in individuals with SCI. Its mechanism of action is believed to be through the stimulation of Auerbach plexus to induce peristalsis in the colon. Senna facilitates bowel movements about 6 to 12 hours after ingestion and frequently is used in establishing a bowel program in persons with UMN lesions. For an evening bowel program, senna should be taken at midday, and for a morning program, it should be taken at bedtime. Long-term complications of senna can include melanosis coli, a staining of the colonic mucosa seen on colonoscopy, and cathartic colon, which is a progressive decrease in responsiveness over time that may lead to a dilated, atonic bowel (23).

Metoclopramide (Reglan), a cholinergic agonist and dopamine antagonist, is frequently used in individuals with slow gastric emptying due to its ability to increase gastric motility and emptying, without affecting colonic activity (24,25). However, one should be aware of its extrapyramidal side effects and avoid its use in persons also taking monoamine oxidase inhibitors or antidepressants. Prokinetic agents, such as cisapride and tegaserod, previously prescribed to enhance colonic peristalsis, have been taken off the market.

Contact irritants: These agents increase peristalsis of the colon by direct irritation or stimulation of the colonic mucosa. Several agents in this category are commonly used in the bowel management of persons with SCI and may be available in a variety of forms, such as oral tablets, suppositories or liquid enemas.

Bisacodyl (Dulcolax) is one of the most commonly used contact irritants. It is available as an oral tablet, suppository, and enema. The bisacodyl suppository may have a vegetable oil base (Dulcolax) or a polyethylene glycol (PEG) base (Magic Bullet), and there are reports of decreased bowel care time with the PEG-based preparations (26,27). The PEG suppositories are water soluble and rapidly dissolve allowing for quick delivery and bioavailability of the bisacodyl to the colonic mucosa as compared to the vegetable oil–based suppositories that require the body to melt the suppository before the bisacodyl can make contact with the colonic mucosa. It has been reported that the time to flatus with PEG is substantially shorter when compared to the hydrogenated vegetable oil suppositories (12 and 31 minutes, respectively). Time to defecation with a PEG suppository is also significantly shorter as compared to the vegetable oil–based suppository (32 versus 58 minutes, respectively). Stool volume and frequency of episodes of bowel incontinence are similar with the use of either formulation. Interestingly, results in stool production, number of incontinent episodes, total time of digital stimulations, as well as time to flatus and defection were similar when comparing the PEG suppository to the Theravac SB Mini-Enema (while Theravac has been discontinued and no longer commercially available, Enemeez uses a similar formulation of docusate sodium, PEG, and glycerin) (26,28). Enemeez-Plus combines the liquid form of docusate sodium with 20 mg of benzocaine, which through its local anesthetic effect may decrease the amount of afferent stimulation that accompanies a bowel program, which is important in those persons susceptible to autonomic dysreflexia (AD). It is important to remember that for any of the contact irritant preparations to be effective, the rectal vault within the reach of the inserted finger should be clear of as much stool as possible prior to insertion of the suppository or enema, so that the active agent may readily reach the bowel wall. The oral tablet form of bisacodyl is generally reserved for those situations such as constipation and poor bowel program results and is not recommended for regular scheduled use. In refractory cases, a homeopathic product marketed as "Magic Cleanse" by the same company that manufactures the Magic Bullet can be used as an oral agent. It is administered as an oral elixir that has several ingredients including cascara sagrada, bark, prune fruit, enzymes, and other ingredients.

Glycerin suppositories are also commonly used in bowel programs in SCI persons to evacuate stool from the rectum and, in addition to being contact irritants, also act as a lubricating agent. It does not produce an effect as the bisacodyl or Enemeez but is often used during the transition of suppositories to digital stimulation alone to perform the bowel program. Carbon dioxide (CO_2) suppositories are still used in some persons with SCI to perform a bowel program. Following insertion of the suppository, a chemical reaction of the active ingredients of the suppository results in the production of CO_2, which expands the lower colon, stimulating the colonic mucosa and producing peristalsis.

Laxatives: There are many oral laxatives available on the market. Saline laxatives are salts, usually of magnesium, sodium, or potassium. These include milk of magnesia, magnesium citrate, and fleets phosphosoda. The saline laxatives act by drawing fluid into the small intestine stimulating colonic motility. Hyperosmolar laxatives, which include lactulose, sorbitol, and PEG (GoLytely, Miralax, CoLyte), are metabolized in the colon into short chain amino acids and act osmotically to draw fluid into the colonic lumen. PEG preparations are used to assist in cleansing out the bowel and do not cause electrolyte disturbances. Lactulose (Chronulac) is an agent more commonly used to prevent and treat hepatic encephalopathy that has bowel effects similar to bulk forming agents. Lactulose produces an osmotic effect in the colon itself similar to many oral laxatives without affecting stool bulk, resulting in bowel distention and peristalsis. While it can assist in helping to clean the bowel, it may cause cramping and increased flatulence.

Enemas should be used only when there is a great deal of bowel impaction despite the use of oral medications and suppositories. Persistent enema use may cause a dependency on higher volumes for stimulation. In addition, trauma and electrolyte disturbances may occur.

Diet and Nutrition

An individual's diet may significantly affect the effectiveness of his or her bowel management. When making bowel management recommendations, one should take into consideration the patient's premorbid dietary history, habits, and food intolerances.

No prospective studies have specifically addressed the issue of specific diets or the influence of special diets on the effective management of the neurogenic bowel in persons with SCI. Of the studies that have dealt with the subject of diet and its effect on bowel function, the majority have focused primarily on specific dietary components, the most common being fiber.

In able-bodied persons, increased dietary fiber is frequently recommended to promote regular bowel movements and decrease constipation. Dietary fiber is a plant component commonly found in vegetables, fruits, grains, and cereals. The role of fiber in promoting these effects is believed to occur by increasing stool water content, which increases stool bulk (weight and volume) and subsequently results in decreased intestinal transit time.

There is a common belief that high fiber intake should be uniformly recommended in persons with SCI in order to enhance regular bowel movements. However, no studies have shown convincing evidence that increased dietary fiber results in improved bowel function or better results with bowel programs in SCI persons. In fact, several studies have shown that increased fiber may have the opposite effect in SCI persons than that seen in able-bodied persons. Menardo et al. reported that persons with chronic SCI who were receiving a standard amount of daily fiber showed significantly delayed left colonic transit (7). More recently, Cameron et al. reported that a nominal increase in dietary fiber in persons with recent SCI resulted in a significant increase in rectosigmoid and colonic transit time (29). They concluded that dietary fiber did not have the same effect on bowel function in SCI persons that it is believed to have in persons with normal bowel function.

While unproven, there likely is some benefit to the inclusion of a reasonable amount of fiber in the daily diet of persons with SCI. It has been recommended that a diet should include at a minimum 15 g of fiber daily (30). The effects on stool consistency, frequency of bowel movements, and response to the bowel program should be monitored, and gradual adjustments to the amount of fiber intake should be made depending on these observations. Given the lack of evidence for its benefit and the potential for negative effects, high fiber diets (20 to 30 g daily) should probably be avoided.

Fluid intake has a significant effect on the water content of stool, and therefore, influences stool consistency. By maintaining a soft, formed consistency, the complications often seen with hard stools, such as constipation, obstruction, hemorrhoids, and anal fissures, can be prevented or minimized. There are no clearly established guidelines as to the appropriate amount of fluids that should be included in the diet of an individual with SCI to optimize bowel function and management. It has been suggested that individuals with SCI should consume 2 to 3 L of fluids daily to optimize stool consistency and facilitate effective bowel management (31). In determining the appropriate amount of fluids, however, one must take into account the method of bladder management being used, and how this may affect urine volume, the frequency that intermittent catheterization may need to be performed or altered, or a urinary drainage bag needs to be emptied, so that the potential for bladder complications is not increased.

Other dietary and nutritional factors, which should be considered in promoting effective bowel management, include avoiding foods that are known to have a propensity to produce flatulence or significantly affect stool consistency. Caffeine and foods containing large amounts of spices and fat are known to cause diarrhea in some individuals with SCI.

Establishing a Bowel Program

A bowel program is a regularly performed routine intended on effectively evacuating the bowel in a timely and predictable manner, so that unplanned evacuations and the development of other GI complications are avoided or minimized. Taking into consideration the influence of diet and nutrition, and the availability and need for appropriate medications, the primary consideration in the development and alteration of a bowel management regimen is the individual with an SCI.

The time of day that the program is performed should be consistent to facilitate predictable and complete evacuation. Factors to consider when establishing a schedule include whether the individual has a UMN versus LMN bowel, preinjury patterns or habits of elimination, lifestyle and anticipated activities (e.g., work or school schedules), home/bathroom accessibility, and availability of attendant care or caregiver assistance, if needed.

A bowel program should be initiated early during the acute care period/hospitalization following a new SCI. In doing so, common complications, such as abdominal distension, which may also cause respiratory compromise in higher level injuries, obstruction, impaction, or diarrhea, may be avoided.

The procedures used for a bowel program and the need for medications depend upon the level of neurologic injury, the extent of neurologic impairment, and its subsequent effect on bowel function. Bowel programs should optimally be performed in the sitting position (on a padded commode), allowing gravity to assist. If performing this in bed, the patient should be in the right side lying position to take advantage of gravity and the normal rectal curvature. Daily and alternate-day bowel programs are the most common among patients with chronic UMN injuries. Bowel program regimens should take less than 1 hour and typically are completed within 45 minutes. Patients who perform their bowel programs daily or every other day have significant reduction in bowel care time as compared to bowel programs performed weekly or biweekly (32).

Patients with complete spinal cord injuries above T6 are at the greatest risk for episodes of AD. It has been noted that patients can develop asymptomatic episodes of hypertension and bradycardia during routine bowel programs. In a study by Kirshblum et al., all patients enrolled in the study had an increase in systolic blood pressure (SBP) > 20 mm Hg above baseline, and 70% of patients enrolled had an SBP > 40 mm Hg above baseline (40% of patients reached an SBP > 170 mm Hg at least once during their bowel program) (33). Furusawa et al. (34) reported that hypertensive episodes during routine bowel programs were transient with vital signs returning to baseline within 5 minutes. They also noted that the greatest periods of hypertension and drops in heart rate occurred during manual removal of stool. In a follow-up study, Furusawa et al. (35) suggested that topical anorectal anesthesia with lidocaine jelly immediately before routine bowel programs may help minimize AD symptoms (i.e., headache, facial flushing, goose bumps, hypertension, and bradycardia).

Persons with incomplete neurologic impairments may retain the ability to sense rectal fullness and the need to evacuate the bowels, and also the ability to contract the external anal sphincter. In these individuals, no special measures or maneuvers may be necessary to move their bowels and evacuate appropriately.

Those with lower lumbar and sacral level injuries usually manifest areflexic bowel function (i.e., LMN bowel). This is characterized by a flaccid rectum with absence of spinal-mediated reflex activity. In these individuals, manual removal of stool from the rectum is usually required to manage the bowels. Stool softeners and bulking agents may be necessary to maintain adequate stool consistency to facilitate easy removal. Contact irritant suppositories would not be effective in these persons, due to the absence of spinal reflex activity in the rectum. In individuals with this type of bowel function, the program should initially be performed daily, and may require twice daily programs. Assistive techniques such as Valsalva maneuver, abdominal massage in a clockwise direction starting in the right lower quadrant and progressing along the course of the colon, increase in physical activity, standing, and completing the bowel program in a commode chair rather than in bed can also greatly facilitate the process. Adjustment in frequency or schedule depends on results achieved.

Individuals with higher level injuries (cervical and thoracic) usually have reflexic bowel function (UMN bowel). This type of bowel function is characterized by the presence of reflex bowel activity in the rectum due to the preservation of spinal-mediated sacral reflex activity. This type of bowel activity may not be present for the first 4 to 6 weeks postinjury, but generally appears following the period of spinal shock.

In persons with UMN lesions, the patient is often initiated on "3-2-1" program consisting of a stool softener (i.e., ducosate sodium) three times per day, two stimulants (i.e., senna) given 8 hours before the suppository, and one suppository started once bowel sounds are present. To utilize the gastrocolic reflex, patients should be instructed to perform their bowel program 20 to 30 minutes after eating. Caffeine may act as a stimulant and may be used prior to a bowel program to help facilitate fecal evacuation. Stool evacuation occurs by means of reflex activity of the rectum in response to a stimulus administered in the rectum. Initially, digital stimulation of the rectum is generally an effective stimulus. Digital stimulation is the insertion of a well-lubricated gloved finger by the individual or caregiver, or an adapted plastic device for those without adequate hand function, into the rectum and rotation of the finger or device to provide physical stimulation to the rectal wall to evacuate the stool in the rectal vault. Digital stimulation should be performed for approximately 15 to 20 seconds and should be performed every 10 to 15 minutes to check for stool that may remain in the rectal vault until there is closure around the finger by the internal sphincter or there are no results after two stimulations. Ideally the bowel program should be performed at the same time of day to facilitate "retraining" of the bowel. The bowel program should initially be performed daily and adjustments in frequency made depending on results. In many instances, persons are able to eliminate the use of contact irritants and rely only on digital stimulation to empty their bowels effectively. The use of stool softeners and bulking agents are at times necessary in individuals with reflexic bowel function to maintain adequate stool consistency to facilitate effective results with the bowel program and prevent complications such as diarrhea.

Despite similarities in neurologic injuries and bowel function, it is important to recognize that each individual is unique in their response to these GI management measures, and that there will be differences in bowel program details and frequency, medications required, and adaptive equipment needed from person to person. Periodically, the effectiveness of an individual's bowel program needs to be reevaluated, and modifications made to the regimen. It is generally recommended that if changes are made to the bowel program, the routine should be maintained for three to five bowel care cycles before deciding if the changes are effective or if further changes are necessary (30).

For individuals with a chronically ineffective bowel program, there are options available, including an enema continence catheter (antegrade and retrograde), transcolonic irrigation, or a colostomy. The enema continence catheter is a specially designed catheter that is inserted into the rectum. A balloon is inflated to hold the catheter in place and an enema is given. Once completed, the balloon is deflated and the catheter is removed; bowel contents then empty (34). The Malone procedure, an antegrade continence enema (ACE) procedure (37) uses a segment of bowel, usually the appendix, to create a tunnel into the ascending colon to administer an enema. This provides a continent, independent catheterizable stoma. Both of these procedures have been described for the pediatric population with only small reports in adults (38,39). These techniques, however, may preclude the need for a colostomy in those individuals with a persistent unsuccessful bowel program.

Transanal colonic irrigation provides another option for patients who have failed conservative bowel management using oral medications, stool softeners, rectal suppositories, digital stimulation, and dietary modifications. In patients suffering from severe colonic dysmotility who are considering surgical intervention (i.e., colostomy or an antegrade enema via an appendicostomy), a trial of transanal colonic irrigation can be considered as an alternative. Several reports including one randomized controlled trial have suggested that transanal colonic irrigation decreases frequency of constipation, fecal incontinence, and time spent on a bowel management program, and increase independence in bowel care (40–42). On average, patients used 650 mL of tap water every day or every other day with a minority of patients irrigating infrequently as once per week. Reported complications included difficulties with insertion of the rectal catheter, minor rectal bleeding, expulsion of the catheter, abdominal discomfort, leakage of irrigation fluid, and burst of rectal balloon. Transient episodes of dysreflexia were reported in a few patients with injury levels above T7. The product-related cost of the transanal irrigation is greater when compared to conservative managements with oral medications and suppositories but is less when calculated as total cost to society (irrigation decreases caregiver's costs by increasing patient's independence in their bowel care and increases their productivity by decreasing their bowel management time) (43).

A colostomy is reserved for individuals as an adjunct treatment for a pressure ulcer or if there is severe constipation with a failure of establishing an adequate and timely bowel program (9). When performed to assist with wound healing, reversing the colostomy can be performed after healing occurs. When performed otherwise in candidates who understand the limitations of the procedure (i.e., body image), colostomies enhance the quality of life and reduce the time needed for bowel care (44–46). High placement of the stoma has been reported to allow the best visualization and self-management.

GASTROINTESTINAL COMPLICATIONS FOLLOWING SCI

GI-related medical complications are common both in the acute period after a new SCI and in the long term and are a significant cause of morbidity and mortality in persons with SCI. GI disorders are the eighth leading cause of death as reported by the Model Systems SCI Program (47).

Numerous authors have reported on the high prevalence of chronic GI problems with constipation being one of the most frequently cited issues (48–52). GI-related complications are a frequent reason for rehospitalizations following injury (21), and has been reported as the sixth leading cause of rehospitalization in persons with chronic SCI (52). Some of other GI complications in persons with SCI include an acute abdomen, ileus, gastritis and ulcers, hemorrhoids, cholelithiasis, pancreatitis, and cancer.

Acute Abdomen

Acute abdominal emergencies are often a challenge to detect and diagnose in persons with SCI. During the early period following injury, it has been reported in as high as 5% of new patients (53). One cause of an acute abdomen, GI hemorrhage, has been reported in one large series to have occurred in over 3% of persons in the acute period after SCI (54).

The diagnosis and therefore management of acute abdominal conditions are made difficult by the absence of the usual signs and symptoms of abdominal pathology due to impaired sensory, motor, and reflex functions. This often results in significant delay in diagnosing the problem and initiating treatment (55). Clinical findings that may raise the suspicion for and can be helpful in identifying the occurrence of an acute abdomen in persons with SCI include constipation, abdominal spasticity, shoulder tip pain, and abdominal pain with bloating. If bowel sounds become hyperactive and then disappear, this may be suggestive of an obstruction (56,57). It is important to have an extremely high level of suspicion in evaluating these individuals. Performing lab tests, ultrasonography and/or a CT scan of the abdomen early is often helpful to confirm the diagnosis.

Ileus

An adynamic ileus is one of the most common GI complications following SCI, especially in the acute period following injury where the incidence has been reported to be as high as 8% (52,58). In one series reported by Gore et al., it was suggested that this condition was more common in complete neurologic injuries and in persons with cervical and upper thoracic level injuries (58). However, others have reported that the level of neurologic injury is not a factor when examining who is at risk for development of this condition (52).

In the acute period following SCI, an ileus frequently occurs within the first 24 to 48 hours of injury and generally resolves within 2 to 3 days of onset. This is most likely due to the loss of both sympathetic and parasympathetic activity during spinal shock. Management generally includes maintaining the patient with no oral intake (NPO) and nasogastric (NG) decompression (without suction) until bowel sounds return. In situations where an ileus persists, or is accompanied by gastric dilatation or slow emptying, the use of metoclopramide can be effective in enhancing return of GI peristalsis (59). If an ileus is prolonged, nutrition by other means is strongly recommended, so that the nutritional status of the individual is maintained. If the ileus continues or develops in the chronic period after SCI, a trial of erythromycin may be used (60). In severe cases, the use of neostigmine has been reported (61), and if severe, the patient may require surgical consultation.

In chronic SCI patients, Ogilvie syndrome (acute colonic pseudo-obstruction) is characterized by significant dilatation of the large bowel (>12 cm) in the absence of demonstrable distal intestinal obstruction. Classically the cecum is the largest site of dilation and most at risk for perforation. The pathophysiology of this syndrome is not clearly understood but is believed to be related to an imbalance between the sympathetic and PS nervous system causing impaired peristalsis of the GI tract. Patients typically will present with abdominal distention and pain or discomfort depending on the level of their injury. The workup includes lab tests and radiological imaging including CT scan of the abdomen. Gastroenterology and/or surgical consult should be undertaken.

Gastritis and Ulcers

Gastritis and the development of ulcers in persons with SCI are frequently reported complications, both in the chronic and in the acute periods following injury. Stinneford et al. reported that in their series of chronic patients, 61% reported symptoms of heartburn and in those who underwent endoscopy and motility studies, common findings included evidence of inflammation and slowly propagating, abnormal peristalsis contractions (51). The clinical development of peptic ulcer disease (PUD) in the acute or chronic period has been reported to occur in from 4% to 24% of persons with SCI (21,52,58,62,63).

The risk for the development of gastritis and ulcer disease appears to increase with higher neurologic levels and completeness of injuries (53). It has also been suggested that increased respiratory complications are a significant risk factor for PUD. The use of steroids in the acute period following SCI does not appear to be associated with an increased incidence of PUD (53).

The use of stress ulcer prophylaxis is recommended (histamine 2 blockers or proton pump inhibitors [PPIs]) usually for 4 weeks unless other risk factors are present (64). PPIs are more effective in preventing upper GI bleeding in high risk patients, however may increase the rate of *Clostridium difficile* stool infections. It has also been suggested that providing nutritional support to meet a newly SCI person's total energy requirement as early as possible decreases the risk for significant PUD (65).

Hemorrhoids

The chronic physical stimulation to the anus and rectum, which comes with the need to perform a bowel program in persons with impaired bowel function, unfortunately results in the frequent development of hemorrhoids in individuals with SCI. It has been reported that 57% of individuals more than 5 years postinjury complained of symptomatic hemorrhoids (19). Bleeding is generally the presenting symptom, but prolapse of the rectal mucosa may also occur resulting in the chronic secretion of fluid, which may result in skin breakdown in the perianal region. Smaller hemorrhoids will generally respond to hydrocortisone suppositories or creams, which should be used after completion of the bowel program. For larger hemorrhoids or prolapsed internal hemorrhoids, sclerotherapy, elastic band ligation, or a hemorroidectomy may be indicated. Rectal bleeding should not be attributed to hemorrhoids until anoscopy or a rectal examination is performed.

Cholelithiasis

It has been suggested that there is an increased risk for the development of cholelithiasis in persons with SCI. Unfortunately, the true incidence and prevalence of this GI complication in the SCI population is unclear because many individuals with gallstone disease are asymptomatic.

In one autopsy series, Apstein et al. (20) reported a 29% prevalence of gallstone disease compared to 11% in a noninjured control group. He found no difference in age, level, or duration of neurologic injury in those persons with SCI with gallstone disease compared to those without gallstones. In a larger prospective study using abdominal ultrasound, Apstein et al. (66) reported a higher prevalence of gallstones in persons with SCI (34%) versus age-matched, non-SCI controls (17%), and found the difference significantly higher in persons under age 40 years and those with neurologic levels above T10.

Although the reason for the apparent increased prevalence of cholelithiasis in SCI persons is not clearly known, theories include abnormal gallbladder motility due to impaired sympathetic innervation resulting in bile stasis, decreased intestinal transit leading to impaired enterohepatic circulation, and metabolic changes leading to abnormal biliary lipid secretion (20,66).

Due to altered sensation after SCI, the diagnosis may be more challenging. However, the majority of patients still present with traditional symptoms, often with radiation of the pain to the right shoulder (especially in persons with tetraplegia), and may still have findings such as right upper quadrant abdominal pain and tenderness (67,68). A high index of suspicion and laboratory and radiographic tests are essential in making a timely diagnosis. Consultation with a gastroenterology and surgery is recommended for further treatment recommendations.

Pancreatitis

In the differential diagnosis of an acute abdomen that develops in a person with SCI, pancreatitis should be considered. Although the incidence of pancreatitis after SCI is not known, it has been suggested that the use of high-dose steroids may predispose persons with acute SCI to development of this condition, and should be considered in individuals with unresolving ileus or recurrence of an adynamic ileus (53). Acute pancreatitis in the setting of high-level SCI may result from a combination of locally mediated sphincter of Oddi dysfunction and vagal dominant innervation of the pancreatic gland in autonomic failure (69). The clinical recognition is hampered by diminished or lost visceral sensitivity and therefore is based on laboratory investigations. Treatment of pancreatitis in the SCI individual is similar to that in the general population and includes resting the gut by maintaining the patient NPO, the use of NG suctioning to reduce gastric acids, and the correction of fluid and electrolyte imbalances. When the ileus has resolved, abdominal pain, if present, ceases, and the serum amylase or lipase has returned to near normal, gradual reintroduction of oral nutrition may begin initially with clear liquids and advancing to solid foods as tolerated.

Superior Mesenteric Artery Syndrome

Superior mesenteric artery (SMA) syndrome is seen mostly in patients with tetraplegia who present with abdominal distention, discomfort, and recurrent emesis following eating (70,71). It is caused by obstruction in the distal part of the duodenum as it passes behind the SMA and in front of the spine and aorta. It often occurs in patients who are immobilized and have lost a significant amount of weight and retroperitoneal fat. It is worse in the supine position and in patients who are in a body jacket. Upper GI series reveal an abrupt cessation of barium in the third part of the duodenum. Treatment includes sitting the patient in upright or positioning them in left sidelying after meals, nourishment to restore weight, and applying a lumbosacral corset to push the abdominal contents upward. Surgery is rarely indicated.

Cancer

It is uncertain whether or not colorectal cancer is increased after an SCI. In one study, the incidence of colorectal cancer was found to be two to six times higher than in the normal population (72), and in another study the incidence was the same as in the normal population (73). As with the non-SCI population, routine screening for colorectal cancer should be performed. Rectal exam should be performed annually for individuals older than 40 years. However, in SCI, false positives occur commonly since the individual is routinely performing a bowel program that may produce minor bleeding. Sigmoidoscopy or colonoscopy should be performed every 3 to 5 years routinely in patients over the age of 50 years (9).

CONCLUSION

Alterations in function of the GI system following SCI and their impact on bowel function can have profound effects on the individual with SCI in terms of not only the physical changes and risk of secondary GI complications but also its potential to affect quality of life. An increased understanding and knowledge of the physiologic and functional changes to the GI system, and an awareness of potential secondary complications that may occur after these injuries have improved the ability of healthcare professionals to more effectively manage and better educate patients and their families and caregivers in this area.

References

1. Guyton AC. General principles of gastrointestinal function—motility, nervous control, and blood circulation. In: Guyton AC, ed. *Textbook of medical physiology*. 8th ed. Philadelphia: W.B. Saunders, 1991:688–697.
2. Chen D, Nussbaum S. The gastrointestinal system following spinal cord injury and bowel management. In: Hammond M, ed. *Physical medicine and rehabilitation clinics of North America—spinal cord injury*. Philadelphia: W.B. Saunders, 2000:45–56.
3. Zejdlik CP. Reestablishing bowel control. In: *Management of spinal cord injury*. Boston: Jones and Bartlett Publishers, 1992:398–400.
4. Guyton AC. Transport and mixing of food in the alimentary tract. In: Guyton AC, ed. *Textbook of medical physiology*. 8th ed. Philadelphia: W.B. Saunders, 1991:698–708.
5. Malagelada J-R, Azpiroz F, Mearin F. Gastroduodenal motor function in health and disease. In: Sleisenger MH, Fordtran JS, eds. *Gastrointestinal disease*. 5th ed. Philadelphia: WB Saunders, 1993:486–508.
6. Guyton AC. Secretory functions of the alimentary tract. In: Guyton AC, ed. *Textbook of medical physiology*, 8th ed. Philadelphia: W.B. Saunders, 1991:709–725.
7. Menardo G, Bausano G, Corazziari E, et al. Large-bowel transit in paraplegic patients. *Dis Colon Rectum* 1987;30:924–928.
8. Nino-Murcia M, Stone JM, Chang PJ, et al. Colonic transit in spinal cord injured patients. *Invest Radiol* 1990;25:109–112.
9. Steins SA, Bergman SB, Goetz LL. Neurogenic bowel dysfunction after spinal cord injury: clinical evaluation and rehabilitative management. *Arch Phys Med Rehabil* 1997;78:S86–S100.
10. Denny-Brown D, Robertson EG. An investigation of the nervous control of defecation. *Brain* 1935;58:256–310.
11. Shafik A, El-Sibai O, Shafik IA. Physiologic basis of digital-rectal stimulation for bowel evacuation in patients with spinal cord injury: identification of an anorectal excitatory reflex. *J Spinal Cord Med* 2000;23: 270–275.
12. Shaflik A, Shaflik A, Ahmed I. Role of positive anorectal feedback in rectal evacuation: the concept of a second defecation reflex: the anorectal reflex. *J spinal Cord Med* 2003;26:380–383.
13. Martin RE, Neary MA, Diamant NE. Dysphagia following anterior cervical spine surgery. *Dysphagia* 1997;12:2–8.
14. Kirshblum S, Johnston M, Brown J, et al. Predictors of dysphagia after spinal cord injury. *Arch Phys Med Rehabil* 1999;80:1101–1106.

15. Singh RVP, Suys S, Villanueva PA. Prevention and treatment of medical complications. In: Benzel EC, Tator CH, eds. *Contemporary management of spinal cord injury*. Park Ridge: American Association of Neurologic Surgeons, 1995:209.
16. Rajendran SK, Reiser JR, Bauman W, et al. Gastrointestinal transit after spinal cord injury: effect of cisapride. *Am J Gastroenterol* 1992;87:1614–1617.
17. Fealey RD, Szurszewski JH, Merritt JL, et al. Effect of traumatic spinal cord transection on human upper gastrointestinal motility and gastric emptying. *Gastroenterology* 1984;87:69–75.
18. Connell AM, Frankel H, Guttmann L. The motility of the pelvic colon following complete lesions of the spinal cord. *Paraplegia* 1963;1:98–115.
19. Glick ME, Meshkinpour H, Haldeman S, et al. Colonic dysfunction in patients with spinal cord injury. *Gastroenterology* 1984;86:287–294.
20. Apstein MD, Dalecki-Chipperfield K. Spinal cord injury is a risk factor for gallstone disease. *Gastroenterology* 1987;92:966–968.
21. Stone JM, Nino-Murcia M, Wolfe VA, et al. Chronic gastrointestinal problems in spinal cord injury patients: a prospective analysis. *Am J Gastroenterology* 1990;85:1114–1119.
22. Hanson RW, Franklin MR. Sexual loss in relation to other functional losses for spinal cord injured males. *Arch Phys Med Rehabil* 1976;57:291–293.
23. Gattuso JM, Kamm MA. Adverse effects of drugs used in the management of constipation and diarrhoea. *Drug Saf* 1994;10:47–65.
24. Dowling PM. Prokinetic drugs: metoclopramide and cisapride. *Can Vet J* 1995;36:115–116.
25. Segal JL, Milne N, Brunnemann SR, et al. Metoclopramide-induced normalization of impaired gastric emptying in spinal cord injury. *Am J Gastroenterol* 1987;82:1143–1148.
26. House JG, Steins SA. Pharmacologically initiated defecation of persons with spinal cord injury: effectiveness of three agents. *Arch Phys Med Rehabil* 1997;78:1062–1065.
27. Steins SA. Reduction in bowel program duration with polyethylene glycol-based bisacodyl suppositories. *Arch Phys Med Rehabil* 1995;76:674–677.
28. Stiens SA, Luttrel W, Binard JE. Polyethylene glycol versus vegetable oil based bisacodyl suppositories to initiate side-lying bowel care: a clinical trial in persons with spinal cord injury. *Spinal Cord* 1998;36:777–781.
29. Cameron KJ, Nyulasi IB, Collier GR, et al. Assessment of the effect of increased dietary fibre intake on bowel function in patients with spinal cord injury. *Spinal Cord* 1996;34:277–283.
30. Consortium for Spinal Cord Medicine. *Neurogenic bowel management in adults with spinal cord injury*. Washington, DC: Paralyzed Veterans of America, 1998.
31. Rehabilitation Institute of Chicago. *Spinal cord injury: educational guide for individuals and families*. Chicago: Rehabilitation Institute of Chicago, 1998.
32. Kirshblum SC, Gulati M, O'Connor KC, et al. Bowel care practices in chronic spinal cord injury patients. *Arch Phys Med Rehabil* 1998;79:20–23.
33. Kirshblum SC, House JG, O'Connor KC. Silent autonomic dysreflexia during a routine bowel program in persons with traumatic spinal cord injury: a preliminary study. *Arch Phys Med Rehabil* 2002;83:1774–1776.
34. Furusawa K, Sugiyama H, Ikeda A, et al. Autonomic dysreflexia during a bowel program in patients with cervical spinal cord injury. *Acta Medica Okayama* 2007;61:221–227.
35. Furusawa K, Sugiyama H, Tokuhiro A, et al. Topical anesthesia blunts the pressor response induced by bowel manipulation in subjects with cervical spinal cord injury. *Spinal Cord* 2009;47:144–148.
36. Shandling B, Gilmore RF. The enema continence catheter in spinal bifida: successful bowel management. *J Pediatr Surg* 1987;22:271–273.
37. Malone PS, Ransley PG, Kiely EM. Preliminary report: the antegrade continence enema. *Lancet* 1990;336: 1217–1218.
38. Christensen P, Kvitzau B, Krogh K, et al. Neurogenic colorectal dysfunction-use of new antegrade and retrograde colonic wash-out methods. *Spinal Cord* 2000;38:255–261.
39. Yang CC, Stiens SA. Antegrade continence enema for the treatment of neurogenic constipation and fecal incontinence after spinal cord injury. *Arch Phys Med Rehabil* 2000;81:683–685.
40. Christensen P, Bazzocchi G, Coggrave M, et al. A randomized, controlled trial of transanal irrigation versus conservative bowel management in spinal cord injured patients. *Gastroenterology* 2006;131:738–747.
41. Christensen P, Bazzocchi G, Coggrave, M, et al. Outcome of transanal irrigation for bowel dysfunction in patients with spinal cord injury. *J Spinal Cord Med* 2008;31:560–567.
42. Faaborg PM, Christensen P, Kvitsau B, et al. Long-term outcome and safety of transanal colonic irrigation for neurogenic bowel dysfunction. *Spinal Cord* 2008;31:1–5.
43. Christensen P, Andreasen J, Ehlers L. Cost-effectiveness of transanal irrigation versus conservative bowel management for spinal cord injury patients. *Spinal Cord* 2009;47:138–143.
44. Stone JM, Wolfe VA, Nino-Murcia M,et al. Colostomy as treatment for complications of spinal cod injury. *Arch Phys Med Rehabil* 2009;71:514–518.
45. Luther SL, Nelson AL, Harrow JJ, et al. A comparison of patient outcomes and quality of life in persons with neurogenic bowel: standard bowel care program vs colostomy. *J Spinal Cord Med* 2005;28:387–393.
46. Kelly SR, Shashidharan M, Borwell B, et al. The role of intestinal stoma in patients with spinal cord injury. *Spinal Cord* 1999;37:211–214.
47. The 2007 Annual Report for the Model Spinal Cord Injury Systems. Available at: http://www.spinalcord.uab.edu/show.asp?durki=116891&site=4716&return=19775. Accessed August 5, 2009.
48. Han RR, Kim JH, Kwon BS. Chronic gastrointestinal problems and bowel dysfunction in patients with spinal cord injury. *Spinal Cord* 1998;36:485–490.
49. Kirk PM, King, RB, Temple R, et al. Long-term follow-up of bowel management after spinal cord injury. *SCI Nursing* 1997;14:56–63.
50. Menter R, Weitzenkamp D, Cooper D, et al. Bowel management outcomes in individuals with long-term spinal cord injuries. *Spinal Cord* 1997;35:608–612.

51. DeLooze, D, Van Laere M, DeMuyuck M, et al. Constipation and other chronic gastrointestinal problems in spinal cord injury patients. *Spinal Cord* 1998;36:63–66.
52. Cardenas DD, Hoffman JM, Kirshblum S, et al. Etiology and incidence of rehospitalization after traumatic spinal cord injury: a multi-center analysis. *Arch Phys Med Rehabil* 2004;85:1757–1763.
53. Berlly MH, Wilmot CB. Acute abdominal emergencies during the first four weeks after spinal cord injury. *Arch Phys Med Rehabil* 1984;65:687–690.
54. Chen D, Apple DF, Hudson LM, et al. Medical complications during acute rehabilitation following spinal cord injury—current experience of the model systems. *Arch Phys Med Rehabil* 1999;80:1397–1401.
55. Longo WE, Ballantyne GH, Modlin IM. Colorectal disease in spinal cord patients. An occult diagnosis. *Dis Colon Rectum* 1990;33:131–134.
56. Miller LS, Staas WE, Herbison GS. Abdominal problems in patients with spinal cord lesions. *Arch Phys Med Rehabil* 1975;56:405–408.
57. Juler GL, Eltorai IM. The acute abdomen in spinal cord patients. *Paraplegia* 1985;23:118–123.
58. Gore RM, Mintzer RA, Calenoff L. Gastrointestinal complication of spinal cord injury. *Spine* 1981;6:538–544.
59. Miller F, Fenzl TC. Prolonged ileus with acute spinal cord injury responding to metoclopramide. *Paraplegia* 1981;19:43–45.
60. Clanton LJ, Bender J. Refractory spinal cord injury induced gastroparesis: resolution with erythromycin lactobionate: a case report. *J Spinal Cord Med* 1999;22:236–238.
61. Trevisani GT, Hyman NH, Church JM. Safe and effective treatment of acute colonic pseudo-obstruction. *Dis Colon Rectum* 2000;43:599–603.
62. Stinneford JG, Keshavarzian A, Nemchausky BA, et al. Esophagitis and esophageal motor abnormalities in patients with chronic spinal cord injuries. *Paraplegia* 1993;31:384–392.
63. Kiwerski J. Bleeding from the alimentary canal during the management of spinal cord injury patients. *Paraplegia* 1986;24:92–96.
64. Consortium for Spinal Cord Medicine. Early acute management in adults with spinal cord injury. *Clinical practice guidelines for health-care professionals*. Washington, DC: Paralyzed Veterans of America, 2008.
65. Kuric J, Lucas CE, Ledgerwood AM, et al. Nutritional support: a prophylaxis against stress bleeding after spinal cord injury. *Paraplegia* 1989;27:140–145.
66. Apstein MD, George B, Tchakarova B. Spinal cord injury is a risk factor for cholesterol gallstone disease: a prospective study. *J Am Paraplegia Soc* 1991;14:197–198.
67. Moonka R, Stiens SA, Resnick WJ, et al. Prevalence and natural history of Gallstones in spinal cord injured persons. *J Am Coll Surg* 1999;189:274–281.
68. Tola VB, Chamberlain S, Kostyk SK, et al. Symptomatic gallstones in patients with spinal cord injury. *J Gastrointest Surg* 2000;4:642–647.
69. Nobel D, Baumberger M, Eser P, et al. Nontraumatic pancreatitis in spinal cord injury. *Spine* 2002;27:E228–E232.
70. Gore RM, Mintzer RA, Calenoff L. Gastrointestinal complications of spinal cord injury. *Spine* 1981;6:538–544.
71. Roth EJ, Fenton LI, Gaebler-Spira DJ, et al. Superior mesenteric artery syndrome in acute traumatic quadriplegia: case reports and literature review. *Arch Phys Med Rehabil* 1991;72:417–420.
72. Frisbie J, Chopra S, Foo D, et al. Colorectal carcinoma an myelopathy. *J Am Paraplegia Soc* 1984;7:33–36.
73. Stratton M, McKirgan L, Wade T, et al. Colorectal cancer in patients with previous spinal cord injury. *Dis Colon Rectum* 1996;39:965–968.

CHAPTER 12 ■ METABOLIC DISORDERS

DAVID R. GATER, JR AND AJIT B. PAI

INTRODUCTION

The word "metabolism" is derived from the Greek *metaballein*, which means to turn about, change, or alter. Metabolism can be defined as the sum of all physical and chemical processes by which living organized substance is produced and maintained (anabolism), and also the transformation by which energy is made available for use by the organism (catabolism). The neurologically intact living human body is an amazing biological machine that thinks, moves, senses, assimilates, eliminates, and coordinates its intrinsic needs with its external environment in an efficient way, subject to the complex and occasionally counterintuitive choices of its user. It is a carbon-based entity that is also subject to the laws of natural science and, as such, subscribes to the metabolic dictum "use it or lose it." Each body is uniquely assembled from a genetic code blended from its parents' genetic material to yield a complex being of coordinated cells working in concert to yield collaborative organ systems with the common basic goal of sustaining life. An additional goal unique to human beings, perhaps, is to live that life abundantly.

Inherent to human metabolism is the concept of homeostasis, in which the body tends toward metabolic stability through a series of neurohumoral feedback loops incorporating information from, yet transcending, each of the body's organ systems. More efficient than the most complex and advanced computer system known to man, the body is under constant surveillance to coordinate the supply and demands of every organ system. While local control systems exist within each organ system, the whole-body integration of metabolic information is processed in the central nervous system (CNS) primarily at the brain's subcortical level; responses are generated and conducted through neurohumoral pathways involving both the spinal cord and the endocrine system. Disruption of the CNS by a spinal cord injury (SCI), therefore, profoundly impacts whole-body metabolism and potentially every organ system. This chapter reviews the metabolic dysfunction associated with SCI as it applies to energy and bone/mineral metabolism and offers clinical recommendations for its management.

ENERGY METABOLISM

In order to appreciate the profound impact of SCI on energy metabolism, one must first understand the concept of energy balance. Simply, energy balance represents the sum total of energy intake and expenditure. In fact, energy homeostasis reflects a complex and ever dynamic relationship between relative rates of change for energy intake and energy expenditure that are subject to genetic programming, intrinsic requirements, and extrinsic demands. The hypothalamus is the control center for most, if not all, metabolic adjustments within the human body and is subject to a variety of circulating substrates, hormones, neuropeptides, and neurotransmitter signals (1). The lateral nuclei of the hypothalamus serve as the body's appetite center, stimulating the perceived need for energy substrates. In the preprandial state, that is, before a meal, this center is particularly responsive to increasing levels of cortisol and ghrelin, a gastrointestinal (GI) peptide known to stimulate appetite. Conversely, the satiation center appears to reside in the ventromedial nuclei of the hypothalamus and responds to biomarkers within the body that indicate energy excess particularly in the postprandial state, including insulin, glucose, leptin, cholecystokinin, glucagon-like peptide-1, and apolipoprotein A-IV. Summation of these numerous signals determines the extent and intensity of a person's appetite, but human appetite is also subject to external factors including emotion, food characteristics, lifestyle behaviors, and environmental cues (1). Physiological signals from the hypothalamus can be blunted or ignored in the presence of these psychological influences, leading to overfeeding or underfeeding.

Energy intake is provided through the ingestion of foodstuffs of varying caloric densities. Fats contain roughly 9 kcal/g, carbohydrates and proteins contain approximately 4 kcal/g, and alcohol contains approximately 7 kcal/g. Carbohydrates, proteins, and fats are processed in the digestive tract and immediately used for reparative and metabolic functions or are stored as future fuel sources. Only small amounts of carbohydrates are stored as glycogen in muscle (150 g) and liver (90 g), and even smaller amounts are used for immediate metabolism and repair. Excess carbohydrates are converted to fat and stored efficiently as adipose tissue. Similarly, ingested protein is digested into amino acids, and those that are not immediately incorporated into structural proteins, hormones, or enzymes are converted into adipose tissue, with the excess nitrogen excreted in the urine and feces. Dietary fat and cholesterol is readily digested and packaged into water-soluble chylomicrons, which can be transported to the liver and adipocytes for processing and storage. Adipose tissue (fat) is a specialized connective tissue comprising lipid-filled cells (adipocytes) contained within a framework of collagen fibers. The adipocyte comprises greater than 90% triglycerides, with small amounts of free fatty acids, diglycerides, cholesterol, phospholipids, monoglycerides, and minimal amounts of water and protein. While functioning as a reservoir for energy storage, adipose tissue also serves as insulation for conserving heat and as a mechanical cushion.

Fat storage (lipogenesis) occurs from the processing of primary foodstuffs during parasympathetic-mediated postprandial conditions. Fat is the most efficient way for energy to be stored within the body, with an energy density of 9 kcal/g of tissue, compared with carbohydrates or proteins (both 4 kcal/g). It is also the least heavy of the energy substrates, with a molecular density of 0.901 g/mL, compared to the density of fat-free body mass that is about 1.100 g/mL. For mobility, it makes sense to store energy as fat rather than glycogen, because for each gram of glycogen stored in the liver or muscle about 3 g of water must also be stored. Regardless of foodstuff composition, a diet high in caloric density will ultimately result in adipose accumulation when energy needs are sufficiently met. As the energy system is stressed in times of relative famine, carbohydrates and proteins are actually catabolized sooner and at higher rates than adipose tissue. Subsequently, attempts to diet for rapid weight loss often result in early loss of water, protein, and carbohydrates with relatively small amounts of adipose reduction. Since the protein stores utilized come primarily from skeletal muscle, resting metabolism is subsequently reduced following rapid weight loss, resulting in a lower rate of energy expenditure at rest and during exercise that ultimately favors accumulation of more energy storage, that is, adipose tissue. The hypothalamus is constantly monitoring energy status and requirements, including current and chronic conditions, in order to ensure it will have sufficient energy stores to meet total daily energy needs.

Total daily energy expenditure (TDEE) is comprised of three primary components: basal metabolism, TEA, and thermic effect of food in descending order of contribution. Basal metabolic rate (BMR) represents the minimal energy expenditure required to sustain life when the body is at rest and contributes roughly 60% to 75% to TDEE (2). Basal metabolism includes bone and tissue remodeling based on relative need and recent demands. The thermic effect of activity (TEA) represents additional energy (5% to 32% TDEE) required to mobilize the body, or segments of the body, through its environment (3). Larger body segments require significantly more energy to move than do smaller segments, such that TEA is significantly greater for lower extremity (LE) than upper extremity work, for example, despite working at similar heart rates. The third component of TDEE reflects the energy required to digest food and is referred to as the thermic effect of a meal (TEM). It appears to be the least variable of the contributors and only accounts for about 8% to 10% of TDEE (4).

In addition to meeting acute energy requirements, energy metabolism is also subject to anabolic and catabolic processes within the body, that is, protein assimilation or degradation involving muscle, organs, enzymes, and most life-sustaining structures. Protein structures within the body represent metabolic machinery, that is, they consume energy, whereas accumulations of fat and carbohydrate within the body are metabolically nascent. Fat-free lean mass (FFM) comprising muscle, bone, and organs contributes the majority of resting energy expenditure (REE), with skeletal muscle contributing the greatest variability depending upon its total mass (5,6). In the neurologically intact adult human, for example, the liver utilizes approximately 29% of REE, with brain contributing 19%, heart 10%, kidney 7%, skeletal muscle 18%, and 17% attributed to the remaining organ systems (7). It is not surprising, therefore, that there exists a direct linear relationship

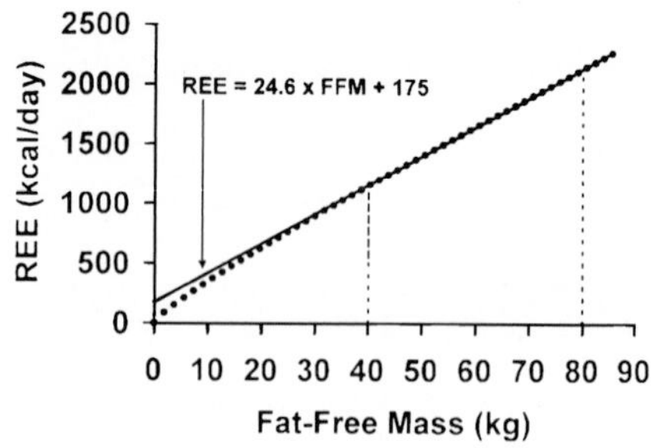

FIGURE 12.1. Relationship between FFM and REE. (From Wang Z, et al. *Am J Physiol Endocrinol Metab* 2000;279:E539–E545.)

between FFM and REE as demonstrated in Figure 12.1, such that increases in FFM are associated with proportional increases in REE (8,9).

SCI ON ENERGY METABOLISM

SCI profoundly impacts energy metabolism through its effect on the somatic nervous system, as well as the autonomic nervous system (ANS). Somatic disruption of the CNS communication with the peripheral nervous system leads to marked atrophy of the affected myotomes. Sarcopenia occurs rapidly and progressively until a new "set point" for muscle mass is established, based on the blunted or absent activation of motor units (10). Cox et al. (11) originally documented these disparities and recommended adjusting caloric intake to 22.7 kcal/kg/day for persons with chronic tetraplegia and 27.9 kcal/kg/day for those with chronic paraplegia; unfortunately, these results have yet to be replicated. Rodriguez et al. (12) demonstrated that persons with acute SCI remained in negative nitrogen balance for at least 8 weeks despite 120% caloric overfeeding and dietary protein supplementation of 2 g/kg/day; in contrast, non-SCI trauma patients achieved positive nitrogen balance within 3 weeks. The obligatory sarcopenia following paralysis was again studied by this group several years later and prompted them to recommend using indirect calorimetry rather than standardized equations to determine caloric and protein needs following acute SCI. Further, if standardized equations such as the Harris-Benedict were to be used, this group strongly discouraged using either sedentary or trauma/stress correction factors when estimating initial energy requirements (13). Subsequent investigations have further substantiated this contention (14–18). Mollinger et al. (18) demonstrated that BMR and TDEE were significantly reduced in persons with SCI compared to estimates for non-SCI individuals and appeared to be related to the neurological level of injury (NLI). Another group compared TDEE between subjects with or without SCI using a respiratory chamber and found a 22% reduction for those with SCI, which was not accounted for even after adjustments for fat-free mass (FFM), fat mass (FM), and age (17). Likewise, Buchholz et al. (15) showed a 14% reduction in BMR for persons with paraplegia compared to age- and gender-matched non-SCI controls. Bauman et al. (14) demonstrated an approximate 10% lower REE for persons with SCI compared to their monozygotic twin without SCI. The reduction in energy expenditure for this group was highly correlated with reduced muscle mass as determined by total body potassium.

Castro et al. (19) noted the cross-sectional area (CSA) of LE musculature was 45% to 80% of that of age- and weight-matched able-bodied (AB) controls 24 weeks after injury. Modlesky et al. (20) demonstrated significantly reduced fat-free soft tissue mass and a reduced proportion of skeletal muscle mass in the thighs of persons with SCI compared to AB controls. Another group recently demonstrated 37.5% less skeletal muscle mass by partial body potassium measures in the LE of persons with SCI compared to matched AB control subjects (21). Although less profound than complete SCI, subjects with incomplete SCI have also been shown to have significantly smaller (24% to 31%) average muscle CSA in affected LE muscles as compared with control subjects (22). It has recently been demonstrated in animal models that gene and protein expression of pathways associated with protein synthesis are reduced after SCI (23,24). It is widely recognized that reduced skeletal muscle contractile activity and demands will diminish anabolic hormone responses in humans as well, and so it is not surprising that anabolic hormones such as testosterone, luteinizing hormone (LH), follicle-stimulating hormone (FSH), growth hormone (hGH), and insulin-like growth factor-1 are reduced in persons with SCI compared to age- and gender-matched non-SCI individuals (25–28). When compared to age- and gender-matched non-SCI controls, 9 of 20 individuals with SCI were found to have abnormally low testosterone levels, and subjects with SCI had significantly blunted hGH responses to an arginine stimulation test compared to the non-SCI controls (25). It appears that these changes occur fairly soon after the onset of SCI, as demonstrated by Schopp et al. (26) for 92 men participating in acute SCI rehabilitation who were found to have significantly reduced testosterone levels compared to the standard physiological range. In a recent investigation, 60% of men with acute and chronic SCI were noted to have low testosterone levels that were significantly associated with less time since injury, lower hemoglobin, and higher prolactin levels (28). Kostovski et al. (27) have also recently demonstrated reduced testosterone, free testosterone, and gonadotropins (LH and FSH) in men with chronic tetraplegia compared to matched AB subjects. These findings are in concert with current understanding of the molecular mechanisms regulating muscle mass found in exercise literature (29–31). At least one study has demonstrated an improvement in motor scores following testosterone replacement, although neither muscle mass nor energy expenditure was reported, and functional independence measures scores at discharge were not significantly different than the untreated group (32). While it would appear prudent to provide testosterone replacement to achieve physiologically normal ranges of free testosterone and sustain muscle mass (33–35), such practice has yet to be scientifically validated in men with SCI.

Autonomic disruption following higher levels of SCI (above T6) also significantly impact energy metabolism (36,37). The sympathetic nervous system arises from the thoracolumbar regions of the spinal cord and is responsible for fight/flight mechanisms, which can profoundly impact resting metabolism. Relative to preinjury, persons with SCI have a parasympathetic-dominant ANS at rest and during activity, resulting in diminished circulating catecholamines, diminished cardiovascular (CV) inotropic and chronotropic responses, and neurogenic hypotension (38–42). Except for acute bouts of autonomic dysreflexia, the blunted sympathetic nervous system responses in SCI are expected to reduce whole-body metabolic demands at rest and during activities (36,37,39,42,43). Hence, significant changes in skeletal muscle mass and sympathetic blunting appear to be the primary contributing factors to lowered energy expenditure following SCI. It is important to understand, however, that body weight may remain relatively stable since sarcopenia may be masked by an off-setting accumulation of body fat in the presence of a positive energy balance. It becomes of paramount importance, therefore, to accurately distinguish between FM and FFM in the person with SCI, which requires carefully scrutinized body composition assessment techniques.

BODY COMPOSITION AND OBESITY IN SCI

The science of assessing human body composition is largely based on the dissection of three male cadavers in the mid-20th century with the subsequent determination of density for the constituent components (44). Notably, the body could be divided into FM with a known density of 0.901 g/mL and FFM with a density of 1.100 g/mL. The FFM for the cadavers (ages: 25, 35, and 46 years old) studied was further characterized as 73.8% water (density = 0.9937 g/mL), 19.4% protein (density = 1.340 g/mL), and 6.8% mineral (density = 3.038 g/mL) constituents. Body composition assessment moved forward using these values as indicators of the "Reference Body," and determination of whole-body density using Archimedes' principle of comparing a person's weight in air and underwater (hydrodensitometry) allowed equations to be developed that estimated per cent body fat (%BF) (44,45). These two-compartment models (FM and FFM) relied on the accuracy of several important assumptions, including (a) the separate densities of the body components were known and additive, (b) the densities of the constituents of the body were relatively constant from person to person, (c) the proportions of the constituents other than fat were relatively constant from person to person, and (d) the person being measured differed from the standard "Reference Body" only in the amount of body fat present (44,45). Several other techniques for determining body composition have been developed over the years and were validated against hydrodensitometry, including anthropometrics (skinfold thickness, circumference, limb/body girth, height/length), hydrometry, air displacement plethysmography, bioelectrical impedance analyses, and dual-energy x-ray absorptiometry (DXA) (46). For those populations that did not violate the initial assumptions listed above, these techniques have proven beneficial toward the science of exercise and nutritional interventions. However, utilization of these methods for persons with SCI would violate at least three of the four assumptions listed for the two-compartment model and would grossly underestimate %BF in this special population (46–48). As discussed later in this chapter, numerous studies have demonstrated diminished bone mineral content in persons with SCI, particularly in the lower extremities (LE) due to reduced longitudinal loading on skeletal mass and reductions in muscle mass (20,49–53). Similarly, total body water is reduced following SCI due to the marked reduction in muscle mass, although extracellular body water (especially interstitial) appears to be increased (54–56). In order to accurately determine body composition, therefore, in persons with SCI, these components must be judiciously measured and FFM divided into its constituents as is done with four-compartment modeling (57,58). Four-compartment modeling separately measures total body density, total body water, and bone mineral content to derive %BF (57). To date, only one study has been reported in the literature using the four-compartment model (59), but our lab has recently initiated an investigation to validate body composition assessment techniques against the criterion four-compartment model.

Body mass index (BMI) also needs to be critically evaluated when reviewing literature pertaining to obesity in SCI. BMI was introduced by the World Health Organization (WHO) in 1998 as a measure to allow international comparisons for persons with and at risk for obesity and its comorbidities. Briefly, BMI evaluates a person's weight relative to his or her height squared (kg/m^2) but does not take into account differences in body composition, particularly in special populations such as SCI where muscle, bone, and water mass are significantly diminished (60). While a BMI between 20 and 25 would be considered normal weight in non-SCI populations, several studies reporting BMI in this range for SCI have demonstrated abnormally high percentages of body fat, especially worrisome since most of those methodologies underestimate %BF in SCI (15,20,54,59,61–64). For example, in comparing SCI (paraplegia) to matched non-SCI controls, Buchholz et al. (15) reported mean BMI and %BF determined by hydrometry of 24.3 ± 6.0 kg/m^2 and 30.8%BF versus 23.5 ± 1.8 kg/m^2 and 22.8%BF, for SCI versus non-SCI controls, respectively. Modlesky et al. (20) reported a mean BMI of only 24.6 kg/m^2 for n = 8 persons with paraplegia, although they were reported to have 33.8%BF by DXA. Similarly, Jones et al. (61) demonstrated that a mean BMI of 23.1 kg/m^2 translated to 27.5%BF in n = 19 men with SCI, compared to a BMI of 24.0 kg/m^2 and 18.1%BF in age-matched controls. Another recent investigation reported that 133 men with SCI were 13% fatter (by DXA) than age-, height-, and ethnicity-matched controls without SCI. Specifically, those with paraplegia and BMI of 25.4 kg/m^2 had 34.2%BF, whereas men with tetraplegia and BMI of 25.8 kg/m^2 had 36.3% body fat (63). Our laboratory has published the only data so far in the literature utilizing four-compartment modeling to determine body fat in SCI and demonstrated normal BMI of 24.8 kg/m^2 in n = 13 lean-appearing persons with paraplegia, although they should more appropriately be diagnosed as obese (%BF > 22%) considering their 27.7% body fat (59). While these data clearly demonstrate obesity in SCI at BMI > 25 kg/m^2, it is likely that the true cutoff for obesity by BMI in this population is closer to 20 or 22 kg/m^2 (48). Recent literature would suggest that the increased adipose load experienced by persons with SCI places them at significantly greater risk for metabolic disorders than the non-SCI population.

METABOLIC SYNDROME IN SCI

The metabolic syndrome is a constellation of findings including central (truncal) obesity, dyslipidemia, hypertension, and insulin resistance with an associated proinflammatory/prothromboitc state that appears to directly promote the development of atherosclerotic CV disease (65). Recent investigations have implicated adipose tissue accumulation as the primary driver of the syndrome (65–73). The amount of adipose stored and where it is stored on a given individual are factors of genetic influence and environmental exposure, that is, the phenotypic expression of inherited potential demonstrated as a function of behavioral choices and limitations. Android (apple-shaped) obesity is associated with greater CV risk and appears to result from a genetic predisposition for some individuals to accumulate visceral (central) adipose tissue, whereas persons with a genetic predisposition for gynoid (pear-shaped) obesity more rapidly accumulate fat stores in the hips and thighs, with relatively less risk for CV consequences (74,75). An estimated heritability for obesity of between 50% and 90% falls well short of explaining the rapid increase in societal obesity over the past 20 years, suggesting that phenotypic expression of specific genomes can be drastically influenced by environmental factors (76–80). Specific factors contributing to this trend include diminished physical activity, increasingly frequent sedentary choices for leisure activity, and easy access to highly palatable, high-caloric, low-nutrient density foods in our industrialized society (80).

Previously considered benign stored energy, adipose tissue is now known to secrete a number of hormones, proinflammatory cytokines, and prothrombotic agents that mediate the metabolic syndrome and its associated morbidities (81). The pathophysiological consequences of obesity within a given individual are subject to that person's genetic sensitivity to those cytokines and hormones, as well as the volume of adipose tissue secreting these agents (82).

Hormones secreted from adipose tissue include leptin, adiponectin, and resistin, which impact appetite, energy metabolism, and insulin sensitivity. Leptin, released from adipocytes, activates areas in the paraventricular hypothalamus to suppress appetite and to stimulate basal metabolism, partly through activation of the sympathetic nervous system (83–85). Unfortunately, as adipose tissue increases in volume, it suppresses the effects of leptin, suggesting a leptin-resistance syndrome not unlike that associated with insulin resistance (86). Interestingly, adiponectin is also secreted from adipose tissue, but unlike leptin, adiponectin levels decrease with increased adiposity, indicating a type of downregulation, that is perhaps tied to increasing insulin resistance (87). Adiponectin appears to have cardioprotective effects, increasing glucose disposal and energy oxidation in the CNS and facilitating insulin at the periphery. Resistin is also derived from adipocytes and directly inhibits insulin signaling mechanisms at the receptor level in hepatic tissue, possibly through inflammatory pathways (88). Previously implicated in animal studies, its association with insulin resistance in humans appears to be through different mechanisms than in the rodent model; resistin has only been recently recognized to contribute to the metabolic syndrome and CV inflammation (89–95).

Inflammatory cytokines are a group of proinflammatory proteins that have been demonstrated to be secreted in relatively large amounts from adipocytes, particularly those found in abdominal and visceral fat (96–99). Specifically, interleukin-6 (IL-6) is a potent proinflammatory protein released from both visceral and, in lesser amounts, subcutaneous adipocytes that also stimulates the release of C-reactive protein (CRP) from the liver (100,101). Il-6 released from adipocytes has also been shown to stimulate the release of corticosteroids from the adrenal cortex, further exacerbating the hyperglycemia associated with obesity and the metabolic syndrome (102). Similarly, tumor necrosis factor-α (TNF-α) is a proinflammatory protein secreted from adipocytes that facilitates the synthesis of acute phase reactants (CRP and fibrinogen) in the liver (101,103). This group of proinflammatory agents contributes directly and indirectly to vascular endothelial cell injury and apoptosis (104). While IL-6 and TNF-α can independently contribute to low-grade vascular inflammation, the amplification of their effect through hepatic CRP production makes the latter an excellent marker for vascular inflammation and for future CV risk (104,105). Few studies have investigated the proinflammatory state of the vascular tree in SCI (106,107). Lee et al. (106) recently reported elevated CRP levels in the "high risk" range for a convenience sample of veterans with SCI, 22.6% of whom were classified with metabolic syndrome using conservative standards. Manns et al. (107) also reported CRP levels in the "high risk" range for 22 individuals with paraplegia who had mean %BF of 26.7. IL-6 and TNF- a have not yet been reported in the SCI population.

Adipocytes have been strongly associated with two powerful prothrombotic agents that increase the risk of blood clotting in the vascular tree and are associated with increased risk for CV disease. Plasminogen activator inhibitor (PAI-1) is a strong inhibitor of fibrinolysis secreted by adipocytes and has been demonstrated to be present in concentrations directly proportional to total adipose mass (108,109). Initially thought to be a mediator of insulin resistance, thrombin-activatable fibrinolysis inhibitor (TAFI) has also been directly tied to increasing levels of adipose tissue, although it appears to be secreted predominantly by the liver in response to elevated LDL cholesterol (109,110). Both PAI-1 and TAFI impair fibrinolysis and increase one's risk for thromboembolism. Since patients with acute and chronic SCI are already at higher risk for thromboembolism due to relative vascular stasis (111) and the low-grade vascular inflammation listed above, these mediators of clotting abnormalities associated with obesity would appear to amplify that risk. To date, only one study has reported PAI-1 in SCI, and although it appears to be correlated with visceral fat, it was not clear that it contributed to additional CV or thromboembolic risk (112).

Dyslipidemia results directly from the accumulation of adipose tissue. Nonesterified fatty acids are the products of adipose tissue lipolysis and are the primary source of nutrient energy in the fasted state. As adipose tissue accumulates, the accelerated release of nonesterified fatty acids from adipocytes occurs even in the face of rising insulin, which suppresses lipolysis under normal conditions. The rise of circulatory nonesterified fatty acids is associated with a marked influx into both muscle and liver. In the liver, nonesterified fatty acids accumulate and increase triglyceride concentrations, contributing to insulin resistance within the liver. Additionally, the liver becomes overwhelmed with the accumulation of nonesterified fatty acids and triglycerides, resulting in the excessive production of very low (VLDL) and low density (LDL) lipoproteins, as well as apolipoprotein B, which is the major protein of LDL (113,114). Apolipoprotein B has, in fact, been more strongly correlated with premature coronary artery disease than either total cholesterol or LDL cholesterol levels in some recent investigations (115,116). Conversely, apolipoprotein A, which is the major protein of high-density lipoprotein (HDL-c) cholesterol, is produced at a significantly lower rate and catabolized at a higher rate in the continued presence of elevated triglycerides and nonesterified fatty acids. HDL-c is also more likely to be catabolized in the presence of elevated triglyceride concentrations, which increase the synthesis of hepatic lipase (113,117,118). Local hepatic lipid metabolism changes subsequently impact the lipid profile (elevated triglycerides, elevated VLDL-c, elevated LDL-c, and reduced HDL-c) in the whole-body circulatory system, creating an atherogenic environment throughout the vascular tree (114,119). Numerous studies have demonstrated significant dyslipidemia in SCI despite relatively normal total cholesterol, with tetraplegia seemingly more affected than paraplegia (106,120–126). Of particular concern, Bauman and Spungen (127) recently reported that of 103 male veterans with tetraplegia and 119 with paraplegia, 63% had HDL-c values less than 40 mg/dL, 44% had values less than 35 mg/dL, and 19% had values less than 30 mg/dL, which would appear to confer significantly greater risk for CV disease than experienced by the non-SCI population.

Adipose tissue accumulation contributes to *insulin resistance* through a number of different mechanisms (81,128,129). Free-fatty acid accumulation with muscle and liver cells reduces the glucose concentration gradient such that passive glucose transport is diminished. Increasing levels of nonesterified fatty acids in muscle contribute to insulin resistance, presumably through serine phosphorylation of the insulin receptors caused by elevated fatty acid metabolites (e.g., fatty acyl CoA, diacylglycerol, and ceramides) within the muscle cell (129,130). Phosphorylation of the insulin receptor substrates (IRS-1 and IRS-2) inhibits their ability to activate the phosphatidylinositol 3-kinase (PI-3 kinase) cascade within the cell, which is necessary to activate GLUT1 and GLUT4 receptor translocation to the cell membrane and facilitate passage of glucose into the cell. IL-6 and TNF-α similarly increase serine phosphorylation of IRS-1 and IRS-2 (129); the net result is to reduce the activity of the insulin/PI-3 kinase cascade and subsequently increase insulin resistance. As fat acTcumulation within the liver increases (fatty liver), the resulting insulin resistance allows for enhanced gluconeogenesis and hepatic glucose output, further contributing to hyperglycemia (131). As fat accumulates within skeletal muscle, insulin resistance worsens and hyperglycemia begins to mediate the effects consistent with type 2 diabetes mellitus (DM).

Glucose intolerance has been reported in a large percentage (50% to 67%) of SCI patients and is often characterized by hyperinsulinemia in response to a glucose challenge for this population (132). Petry et al. (133) found that glycosylated hemoglobin (HbA1c) levels above 6.0 in SCI patients significantly correlated with impaired glucose tolerance or frank diabetes and recommended routine HbA1c screening for patients with SCI. Aksnes et al. (134) noted an association between whole-body insulin-mediated glucose uptake and skeletal muscle mass in tetraplegics, suggesting loss of muscle mass as the primary reason for insulin insensitivity; body fat was not considered. The hyperinsulinemia in these patients may therefore be related to body composition changes as has been reported in the general population (135,136). Bauman and Spungen (137) reported that 62% of quadriplegics with a mean duration of injury of 17 years had abnormal glucose tolerance tests, as compared to only 18% of age-matched controls with similar BMI.

Hypertension has long been associated with obesity, but recently strong evidence has emerged to provide the mechanisms associated with adipose tissue. As indicated above, proinflammatory agents associated with adipose tissue can directly injure the arterial endothelium and lead to arterial stiffness and dysfunction. Data from the Framingham study recently demonstrated that 70% of new onset essential hypertension cases were directly related to excess body fat (138). There have been several recent reviews demonstrating the relationship between obesity, particularly visceral obesity, and hypertension (139–143). As discussed earlier, visceral fat has been demonstrated to increase plasma leptin concentration, which directly increases sympathetic nervous system activity (144,145). Visceral fat also increases renin-angiotensin-aldosterone system (RAAS) activity through several mechanisms described below. TNF-α secreted by adipocytes is known to increase angiotensinogen production within the liver, which directly exerts vasoconstriction in the arterial tree. Recent evidence has shown that adipocytes can directly synthesize and secrete angiotensinogen, independent of TNF-α (146). Subsequently, the RAAS activation further contributes to aldosterone production, with concomitant sodium reabsorption and volume expansion, worsening hypertension (140). Finally, visceral obesity can cause direct mechanical compression of the kidneys, with subsequent increases in intrarenal pressures and sodium retention (145). Despite SCI neuropathophysiology, which should lead to neurogenic hypotension, we have recently reported hypertension in 22% of a large veteran cohort with SCI; 68% of the cohort had BMI > 23 kg/m^2, suggesting a relationship between hypertension and obesity may exist in this population (147). The prevalence of hypertension in veterans with SCI is not clearly known, but may be as high as 45% as recently reported by Lee et al. (148) in a smaller veteran cohort.

Despite the information provided above, in 2008, the Agency for Healthcare Research and Quality reported that "the existing evidence does not indicate that adults with SCI are at markedly greater risk for carbohydrate and lipid disorders or subsequent CV sequelae than able-bodied adults"(149). The report was limited to epidemiological investigations reported after 1990 with at least 100 subjects and to interventional studies from 1996 to 2007. The report acknowledges that the evidence is limited by relatively few studies, small sample sizes, lack of appropriate control groups, failure to adjust for known confounding variables, and variations in reported outcomes. Since the time of that report, several additional contributions to the literature have been provided, which may shed additional light on the controversy. Before discussing those studies, however, it would be prudent to review the current definitions of the metabolic syndrome.

Definitions for the metabolic syndrome have been drafted by several organizations over the past few years, including the National Cholesterol Education Project Adult Treatment Panel III (NCEP ATP III), the WHO, and the International Diabetes Federation (IDF) that are the three most commonly utilized for reporting and comparison. In 1998, the WHO definition of the metabolic syndrome focused on the central role of DM plus at least two of the following: obesity (BMI > 30 kg/m^2 or Waist-to-hip ratio > 1), dyslipidemia (TG ≥ 150 mg/dL and/or HDL-c < 35 mg/dL in men or <39 mg/dL in women), hypertension (blood pressure ≥ 140/90 mm Hg), and microalbuminuria (150). The third adult treatment panel of the National Cholesterol Education Project (ATP III) definition of the metabolic syndrome placed equal emphasis on any three of the following: obesity (waist circumference ≥ 102 cm in men, or ≥ 88 cm in women), dyslipidemia (TG ≥ 150 mg/dL and/or HDL-c < 40 mg/dL in men, <50 mg/dL in women), hypertension (BP ≥ 130/85 mm Hg), and fasting glucose > 110 mg/dL (151). Most recently, the IDF definition of metabolic syndrome has emphasized the role of central obesity (waist circumference ≥ 94 cm in men, ≥ 80 cm in women) plus any two of the following: dyslipidemia (TG ≥ 150 mg/dL or on treatment; HDL-c < 40 mg/dL for men, <50 mg/dL for women or on HDL-c treatment), hypertension (≥130 mm Hg systolic or ≥85 mm Hg diastolic, or on treatment for hypertension), fasting glucose ≥ 100 mg/dL or previously diagnosed with type 2 DM (152). Application of these definitions may be somewhat erroneous in populations with SCI whose blood pressure abnormalities would be confounded by neurogenic hypotension, and whose waist circumferences may be expanded due to abdominal muscle paralysis.

Liang et al. (153) demonstrated a similar prevalence of metabolic syndrome in 185 men with SCI compared to age- and race-matched men found in the NHANES 1999 to 2002 dataset, with lower absolute levels of total cholesterol, HDL-c, LDL-c, TG, and fasting glucose in those with SCI. Using ATP III criteria, however, Nash et al. (154) reported 34% of n = 41 persons with paraplegia had metabolic syndrome, with 29% having hypertension and 76% with HDL-c < 40 mg/dL. Also using the ATP III criteria, Maruyama et al. found that of 44 persons with SCI, 43% met the definition for metabolic syndrome. Our lab recently reported preliminary, retrospective data on 477 veterans with SCI screened for metabolic syndrome using the IDF criteria previously reported (152), but substituting BMI > 25 kg/m^2 for waist circumference to denote obesity. Within the sample, 56.5% were considered obese with BMI > 25 kg/m^2, 63.4% had HDL-c < 40 mg/dL, 48.7% had fasting blood glucose > 100 mg/dL, 56.5% had hypertension, and 44.8% met criteria as having the metabolic syndrome (155). Our contention remains that the obesity is the primary mediator of the metabolic syndrome in SCI, and that interventions should be focused on behavioral aspects of obesity management in this special population (48).

MANAGEMENT OPTIONS

Management strategies for the prevention and/or treatment of the metabolic syndrome in SCI should follow recent guidelines emphasizing antiatherogenic dietary modification and increased physical activity for weight reduction, as well as antihypertensive therapy, dysplipidemia therapy, and glucose management (156–158). The Dietary Guidelines of America (2005) have made general recommendations for adults who are at normal or overweight, with both dietary guidelines and activity recommendations, that when adhered to have been demonstrated to significantly reduce one's risk for the metabolic syndrome (159,160). Greater emphasis is placed on the ingestion of nutrient-dense foods that limit saturated and trans fats, cholesterol, added sugars, salt, and alcohol. Further, foods with a high glycemic index such as juice, soda, baked goods, candy, sweetened cereals, canned fruits with syrup and dried fruits should be avoided, as they rapidly increase insulin secretion and subsequently facilitate lipogenesis and hyperinsulinemia. Relatively low-fat (approximately 28% of total calories) diets with complex rather than simple carbohydrates have been demonstrated to promote modest, sustainable weight loss. Rapid weight loss diets are discouraged, as they promote additional muscle loss and dehydration,

TABLE 12.1

ANTIHYPERTENSIVE MEDICATIONS WITH COMORBIDITIES

Heart failure	Thiazide, BB, ACE inhibitor, ARB, ALDO antagonist
Post-MI	BB, ACE inhibitor, ALDO antagonist
High CVD risk	Thiazide, BB, ACE inhibitor, calcium channel blocker
Diabetes	Thiazide, BB, ACE inhibitor, ARB, calcium channel blocker
Chronic renal Dz	ACE inhibitor, ARB
Stroke prevention	Thiazide, ACE inhibitor

ACE, angiotensin-converting enzyme; ARB, angiotensin receptor blocker; ALDO, aldosterone; BB, beta-blocker.

resulting in further reductions of basal metabolism that typically preclude future attempts at weight maintenance and energy balance (161,162). Successful diets (those that facilitate future weight maintenance) usually promote reductions of caloric intake sufficient to allow negative energy balance of 100 to 200 kcal/day, with weight loss of approximately 1 to 2 pounds/week. Exercise will be addressed in Chapter 24 and can play an important role in obesity prevention and management. Unfortunately, most exercise studies to date involving persons with SCI have focused on outcome variables for cardiopulmonary fitness, strength, endurance, and some combination of risk factors including dyslipidemia and glucose tolerance, without emphasis on adipose reduction (163–165). Few studies have even attempted to measure changes in %BF in response to exercise, and only modest improvements have been reported for those that did using LE functional electrical stimulation (FES) (166,167).

Pharmacological interventions to reduce blood pressure (Table 12.1) and lipids (Table 12.2) are certainly appropriate within suggested guidelines (156–158), but greater emphasis on increasing HDL-c should be considered in persons with SCI (168). Finally, glucose control is strongly encouraged, but the clinician is cautioned against using solely pharmacological interventions for glucose control without employing additional behavior interventions (i.e., diet and exercise), since several investigations have reported weight gain and increased CV risk with the use of insulin analogs, sulfonylureas, biguanides, and thiazolidinediones (169–173). Increasing insulin sensitivity will undoubtedly reduce plasma (glucose) and improve glycemic control; however, the increased cellular glucose transport will subsequently facilitate fat storage, increasing one's risk for obesity and its sequelae.

TABLE 12.2

LIPID-MODIFYING MEDICATIONS

HMG CoA reductase inhibitors	Atorvastatin, fluvastatin, lovastatin, pravastatin, rosuvastatin, and simvastatin
Bile acid sequestrants	Colesevelam, cholestyramine, and colestipol—and nicotinic acid (Niacin)
Fibric acid derivatives	Gemfibrozil, fenofibrate, and clofibrate

BONE METABOLISM

As with energy metabolism, the physiology of bone metabolism is complex and incompletely understood, although science has made remarkable progress in recent years. Bone is a dynamic, mineralized connective tissue composed of a number of cell types, blood vessels, lymphatics, and nerves arranged in specific architecture to provide rigidity, shape, protection, support for body structures, and mobility. The human skeleton consists of flat bones (e.g., skull, scapula, and ilium) and long bones (e.g., humerus, femur, and tibia), which can be further characterized histologically as either cortical (compact) or trabecular (cancellous) bone. Cortical bone, found primarily in the shafts of long bones and the surfaces of flat bones, is laid down concentrically around central tubes called Haversian canals that contain blood vessels, lymphatics, nerves, and connective tissue. Concentric rings (lamellae) of bone matrix surround each Haversian canal and contain osteocyte-filled lacunae. Trabecular bone is less plentiful and forms the ends of long bones as well as the inner portions of flat bones. It contains interconnecting plates and bars called trabeculae arranged in a honeycomb appearance around the intervening marrow. The lamellae of trabecular bone has collagen fibers arranged in parallel fashion such as is found in vertebral bodies that can withstand great compressive forces, while the lamellae of cortical bone is arranged concentrically. In general, each bone is comprised of an outer layer of cortical bone surrounding the underlying trabecular bone and the medullary cavity. The outer membrane of cortical bone (periosteum) is comprised of two fibrous layers, the innermost of which has osteogenic capacity for growth through a process called periosteal apposition. The inner surface of cortical bone is referred to as the endosteum, where most bone resorption occurs. It is notable that both periosteum and endosteum contain bone-building and bone-resorption cell types, as well as their progenitors.

Bone is maintained by a process called remodeling, which helps regenerate the entire skeletal structure every 10 years (174). A balance between bone anabolism and catabolism enables bones to stay strong and support the soft tissues of the body, relative to its demonstrated needs. Osteoblasts (and their mature form, osteocytes) originate from mesenchymal cells and create new bone. Conversely, osteoclasts are responsible for bone resorption and are derived from hematopoietic cells. The roles of these cells are not mutually exclusive; they must work in conjunction during the process of remodeling. To activate osteoclastic activity, a receptor activator of NF-κB ligand (RANKL) is expressed on the surface of osteoblasts that binds with its receptor RANK, which is on the surface of osteoclasts and their precursors (175). RANKL is also neutralized by the receptor osteoprotegerin (OPG), which is produced by osteoblasts. The interaction between RANKL, RANK, and OPG has been determined to be fundamental to the development and activation of osteoclasts (176).

The combination of osteoblasts, osteoclasts, osteocytes, capillaries, nerves, and connective tissue creates the basic multicellular unit of bone (177). In bone remodeling, osteoclasts remove old bone by acidification and proteolytic digestion, while osteoblasts continuously secrete osteoid that will

TABLE 12.3

HORMONES INFLUENCING BONE AND CALCIUM METABOLISM

Hormone	Function	Effect of SCI
Vitamin D	Ca^{2+} absorption in gut	Reduced calcitriol
PTH	Stimulates osteoclasts Increases Ca^{2+} resorption in kidney Stimulates calcitriol formation	Early hypoparathyroidism followed by late hyperparathyroidism
Calcitonin	Inhibits osteoclast activity Increases renal tubular excretion of Ca^{2+}	
Testosterone		Reduced testosterone
Estrogen		Reduced estrogen

eventually form new bone (174). During bone formation, a few osteoblasts are left behind in the osteoid matrix and are subsequently called osteocytes. They serve as mechanosensory cells that respond to mechanical load signals (178–180). Loading of bones increases osteoblastic activity and decreases osteoclastic activity along periosteal surfaces in order to strengthen bone (178,181,182). Of note, increased remodeling from a higher rate of osteoblastogenesis and osteoclastogenesis can lead to acceleration of bone mineral loss as resorption is faster than bone formation (174).

Bone remodeling is influenced by mechanical loading, hormonal milieu, and neural modulation. Increased stress and strain, and particularly longitudinal loading, cause focal acquisition of bone in accord with Wolff law (183). Hormones that influence bone and calcium metabolism include primarily vitamin D, parathyroid hormone (PTH), and calcitonin, as well as testosterone, estrogen, hGH, and glucocorticoids (Table 12.3). As with energy metabolism, the body is continuously monitoring regional bone requirements and weighing those against the body's need for free calcium, which is essential for blood coagulation, skeletal muscle contraction, and nerve function. Ninety-nine percent of calcium is stored in bone, a small portion is present within cells, and of the remaining calcium in the plasma, a portion is bound to proteins. In addition to calcium stored in bone, intracellular and extracellular calcium is replenished by dietary calcium from the GI tract and by reabsorption of filtered calcium in the kidneys.

Vitamin D is a fat-soluble vitamin that is naturally present in few foods, added to others, and available as a food supplement. It is produced endogenously when ultraviolet rays from the sun trigger synthesis in the skin. Vitamin D is hydroxylated by the liver to 25-hydroxyvitamin D (calcidiol), and again at the kidney to 1,25-dihydroxyvitamin D (calcitriol), which is the active hormone responsible for calcium absorption in the gut. When plasma calcium levels are high, the production of calcitriol is reduced and less dietary calcium is absorbed from the gut. Conversely, when plasma calcium levels are low, calcitriol production is increased, resulting in increased dietary calcium absorption. PTH is secreted by the chief cells of the parathyroid glands in response to reduced plasma ionized calcium concentrations. PTH has three actions by which it increases plasma calcium. First, it stimulates osteoclastic activity to cause bone resorption and increase plasma calcium. PTH also increases reabsorption of calcium at the distal tubules of the kidney, which also increases plasma calcium. Finally, PTH stimulates the formation of calcitriol in the kidneys, which subsequently increases dietary calcium absorption from the gut. Conversely, elevated plasma calcium concentration inhibits the secretion of PTH by way of a negative feedback loop, ultimately reducing calcium reabsorption at the kidneys and gut, and reducing bone resorption. Calcitonin is secreted from the parafollicular (clear or C) cells of the thyroid gland in response to elevated plasma calcium levels. Calcitonin directly inhibits osteoclast activity to reduce bone resorption and also increases renal tubular excretion of calcium to reduce plasma calcium concentration. HGH, testosterone, and estrogen all appear to facilitate bone formation (184–188), whereas glucocorticoids clearly contribute to bone resorption (189–191).

SCI ON BONE METABOLISM

After SCI, multiple mechanisms contribute to bone loss, including mechanical, hormonal, and neural changes that ultimately favor bone reabsorption (178). The primary mechanism for bone loss appears to be the reduction in mechanical loading on bone. Paralysis of skeletal musculature below the level of SCI prevents the usual application of external forces (muscle contraction and gravitational loading) required to prevent bone resorption, due to withdrawal of stress and strain upon bone as modeled by Wolff law (183). In vitro and in vivo studies have shown unloading bone to increase osteoclast number and surface activity (192,193). Minaire et al. (194) showed an increase in bone resorption due to increased number and activity of osteoclasts to be the major culprit in bone loss. Similar findings have been demonstrated in humans, unrelated to SCI (195,196). Bone loss after SCI occurs in the LE in paraplegia as well as tetraplegia, whereas bone loss in the upper extremities (UE) appears relegated to SCI above T1 (197–204). UE bone loss attributed solely to tetraplegia lends further credence to the importance of mechanical loading, since the relative increased use of UE for persons with paraplegia is correlated with normal or above normal UE bone mass (53,201,203). Multiple studies have surmised that bone resorption peaks between 10 and 16 weeks post-SCI, that is, during the period of relative bed rest and initial rehabilitation, with markers of bone resorption staying elevated after 1 year postinjury (49,50,205–207). Bone markers indicating resorption include hydroxyproline, deoxyproline, pyridinoline, deoxypyridinoline, type 1 collagen C-telopeptide, and N-telopeptide, and their relative concentrations are highly correlated with total bone loss (49,200,206,208,209). During the early post-SCI period, the receptor activator of NF-6B ligand (RANKL) expression is increased in rats, with an increased ratio of RANKL to OPG after SCI (210). The increased RANKL: OPG ratio can lead to osteoclastogenesis, which will inevitably contribute to bone loss. Additionally, Morse et al. (211) found that severe cervical injury is associated with decreased circulating OPG levels, which would further increase the RANKL: OPG ratio.

Hormonal alterations after SCI may also impact bone resorption. It is typically reported that the Vitamin D-PTH axis is depressed in individuals after immobilization (212). Several studies have examined Vitamin D levels (calcidiol vs. calcitriol) after SCI, with conflicting reports of deficiency (213–215). One study demonstrated low levels of calcidiol, but elevated calcitriol in persons with SCI compared to non-SCI controls (213). Vaziri et al. (215) conversely reported reduced calcitriol and PTH in persons with chronic SCI when compared to AB controls; with deficiencies more pronounced in tetraplegia than paraplegia. These conflicting reports may be attributed to differences in race, diet, activity, and sunlight exposure. Interestingly, Bauman et al. (216) demonstrated that low or normal vitamin D levels were relatively refractory to vitamin D administration and calcium supplementation over periods of 2 weeks, and 12 months, respectively, with no significant change in serum calcium concentration. Nonetheless, a more recent investigation of patients with motor complete SCI demonstrated significant improvements in LE bone mineral density (BMD) determined by DXA following 6, 12, 18, and 24 months administration of a vitamin D analog (1-alpha-hydroxyvitamin D(2)) compared to placebo (214). Many studies have shown an acute and chronic reduction of PTH following SCI, with suppression starting as early as 3 weeks and lasting greater than 5 years (206,208,215). In addition, the degree of impairment appears to impact the level of suppression; a complete injury appears to have greater changes from baseline of PTH than an incomplete injury (217). This disturbance of PTH actually reverses in the years following SCI; at times, by year 9 postinjury, there is a secondary hyperparathyroidism (178,213,218). However, another study demonstrated that PTH continues to remain subbaseline chronically for persons with SCI compared to non-SCI controls (215).

Sex steroids impact bone metabolism after SCI through a number of complex mechanisms. SCI appears to have a profound impact on the hypothalamic-pituitary-gonadal axis, with a marked reduction in anabolic potential as reported earlier (25–27,219). In men with SCI, total testosterone and the free androgen index were significantly lower as compared to AB controls (220). In 2007, Celik et al. (221) corroborated this finding by reporting a negative androgen status present especially in the first year after injury. In women with SCI, estrogen levels are also significantly lower than controls (178,222). It has been noted in mice that the deficiency of sex steroids increases the production of osteoclasts and osteoblasts resulting in an increase of bone remodeling (174,223–225). Of note, however, in 17 ambulatory women, premenopaus and postmenopause, compared to 20 premenopausal and postmenopausal women with SCI, trabecular bone of the distal femur and proximal tibia was compared and mechanical unloading was determined to be of greater importance than estrogen loss on bone architecture in middle-aged women (226).

Neuronal changes may also have a profound impact on bone resorption after SCI (192,193). Both sympathetic and sensory nerve fibers are present in skeletal periosteum, bone marrow, and mineralized bone, forming dense parallel networks around blood vessels adjacent to bone trabeculae (227,228). In rats, chemical sympathectomy decreased the numbers of both preosteoclasts and osteoclasts, leading to a net bone resorption (229). Recent investigations, however, have demonstrated that sympathetic stimulation increases osteoclastic activity and reduces osteoblastic activity in animal models (230–232). Togari et al. (231) demonstrated that both human osteoblastic cells and osteoclastic cells are equipped with adrenergic receptors and neuropeptide receptors. It has also been shown that beta-adrenergic agonists directly stimulate bone resorption via matured osteoclasts (230). Further, severe and localized osteoporosis is attributed to the high sympathetic tone in a localized region for patients with complex regional pain syndrome type I (232). It would appear counterintuitive, therefore, that sympathetic blunting associated with SCI would precipitate bone resorption. Several explanations should be considered. First, mechanical unloading of bone may impact adrenergic receptors in bone, as Kondo et al. (192) demonstrated unloading inhibits osteoblasts and stimulates osteoclasts via sympathetic nervous system activation, which could be suppressed by beta blockade. Secondly, blunted sympathetic activity may significantly reduce vascular perfusion of bone, leading to relative stasis and local hyperpressure, accelerating bone resorption (233). Finally, intermittent recurrent bouts of autonomic dysreflexia might significantly influence adrenergic tone to the extent that osteoclastic activity exceeds that of osteoblasts, further contributing to bone loss.

IMMOBILIZATION HYPERCALCEMIA

Calcium levels increase within 10 days after SCI and peak between 1 and 6 months (234–237). These changes are further exacerbated by decreased renal function, which may be associated with impairment of renal reabsorption of calcium (178,236). It has also been suggested that calcium uptake in the GI tract is impaired following SCI (238). Both hypercalcemia and hypercalciuria are seen as a result of changes in calcium homeostasis following SCI. Immobilization hypercalcemia (IH) occurs in 10% to 23% of persons with SCI and often affects adolescents and young adult males, likely related to rapid bone turnover during growth (235). Other risk factors for hypercalcemia following SCI include complete neurologic injuries, high cervical levels, dehydration, and prolonged periods of immobilization (235). Symptoms of IH are often insidious and include nausea, vomiting, polydipsia, polyuria, and lethargy; rarely seen are severe muscle wasting and cachexia (236). In those patients with hypercalciuria, a negative calcium balance actually precludes restriction of dietary calcium (236). Stewart et al. (212) showed that an increase in dietary calcium did not increase levels of urinary or serum calcium. Another group found there to be a difference in calcium balance before and after 6 months post-SCI, with a transformation from negative to positive balance associated with longer durations of injury (239).

Hansen et al. (240) examined the incidence of urinary calculi in 236 individuals with SCI who were injured between 1956 and 1990; at follow-up, 20% had at least one episode of renal calculi and 14% had at least one episode of bladder calculi. Despite the high rate of urinary calculi in persons with SCI, Kohli and Lamid (241) found no correlation between serum calcium levels and urinary stones. Nonetheless, IH remains a risk factor for urolithiasis in the acute setting after SCI, and therefore treatment for asymptomatic hypercalcemia is often recommended (242).

Diagnosis of IH can be made based on historical factors and a basic metabolic panel. A serum calcium level should be evaluated, with correction for a low serum albumin if present; ionized calcium should also be measured. If the patient does not have risk factors, PTH, thyroid studies, and vitamin D levels should be checked. PTH levels should be low in hypercalcemia due to SCI; however, if elevated, primary hyperparathyroidism must be investigated.

Initial treatment for IH should include early mobilization and intravenous (IV) hydration with normal saline (100 to 150 mL/hour as tolerated) to increase glomerular filtration and increase calcium excretion. Furosamide may be used after hydration to protect against volume overload and to inhibit calcium reabsorption by the kidney. Thiazide diuretics are contraindicated due to their calcium-sparing properties. Foley catheter placement will likely be required for fluid management. As calcitriol levels are low, intestinal absorption of calcium is suppressed; therefore, restriction of dietary calcium is unnecessary. During the acute phase, vitamin C restriction may reduce the formation of calcium oxalate stones. In the acute rehabilitation phase, such treatment could limit therapies, however, and a single dose of pamidronate (30 to 90 mg) administered IV over 4 to 24 hours should be considered as the treatment of choice due to its rapid onset of action (243–245). Pamidronate and other second-generation, nitrogen-containing bisphosphonates are potent inhibitors of osteoclastic activity and rapidly slow bone resorption even under conditions of mechanical unloading (246,247). Serum calcium reduction is seen within 3 days with treatment and symptoms resolve as calcium is lowered; serum calcium falls to a nadir within 7 days and may remain normal for several weeks or longer. Some individuals may require repeat treatment, so continued monitoring of ionized calcium levels following treatment is recommended. Standing has been reported to decrease hypercalciuria in the early phase of management (248,249). Other medications that have been used to treat IH with varying degrees of success include calcitonin, etidronate, and glucocorticoids (250) (Table 12.4).

TABLE 12.4

CLINICAL REVIEW OF IMMOBILIZATION HYPERCALCEMIA

Etiology	Impairment of calcium homeostasis
Epidemiology	10%–23% of individuals with SCI
Course	Onset 10 d, peak 1–6 mo
Risk factors	Adolescents or young adult males Complete neurologic lesion High cervical level Dehydration Prolonged immobilization
Symptoms	Nausea Vomiting Polydipsia Polyuria Lethargy Muscle wasting (rare) Cachexia (rare)
Diagnosis	History Basic metabolic panel
Treatment	Primary Early mobilization IV hydration Foley catheter placement Pamidronate IV (single dose) Secondary Furosemide (possible) Vitamin C Tertiary Calcitonin Etidronate Glucocorticoids
Follow-up	Serum Ca^{2+} reduction in 3 days Resolution of symptoms with Ca^{2+} reduction Serum Ca^{2+} nadir in 7 days
Complications	Urolithiasis

HETEROTOPIC OSSIFICATION

Heterotopic ossification (HO) is most commonly seen in acute SCI, characterized by the formation of extra-osseous lamellar bone in soft tissue surrounding peripheral joints below the level of neurological injury, most commonly at the hips, knees, or shoulders, although reports of elbow involvement have also been reported (251–256). While the exact mechanism underlying the development of HO after SCI is incompletely understood, prevailing theory suggests that a combination of proprioceptive dysfunction related to CNS disruption, IH, local inflammatory changes 2 degrees to trauma, spasticity, and humoral factors may lead to the migration of mesenchymal osteoprogenitor cells into the joint space (251,252,257,258). At least two processes have an important role in the genesis of HO after SCI; the activation of pluripotential mesenchymal cells in the soft tissue and the local production of bone morphogenic protein(s) (BMP) (259). Mesenchymal cells in muscle may switch their differentiation from fibroprogenitor to osteoprogenitor pathway under the influence of BMP, and then further proliferate and differentiate into bone-forming cells. The specific factors involved in triggering the activation of mesenchymal cells in muscle and local induction of BMP expression are still unknown. Biochemical analysis of the organic matrix of HO has demonstrated its similarity to newly formed bone, which has not yet completely mineralized (260). Histology of HO is similar to normotopic mature bone with well-developed cortical and trabecular structures as well as bone (261). In the early stage of HO development, the central area contains undifferentiated mesenchymal cells surrounded with a more dense cellular zone that gradually undergoes mineralization (262,263). The process of maturation of HO has a centripetal pattern, where bone formation starts at the periphery and progresses to the central part of the lesion. In the process of HO formation, both membranous and endochondral ossifications are present, but usually membranous type predominates (Fig. 12.2).

Although the incidence of HO in SCI has been reported as high as 53% early after injury, the incidence of clinically significant HO (with diminished ROM that interferes with function) is closer to 10% to 20%, with 5% to 8% progressing to ankylosis (253–255). Risk factors for HO following SCI include male gender, older age, complete neurologic injuries, deep vein thrombosis (DVT), spasticity, and pressure ulcer (264,265). In children, the risk of HO is lower.

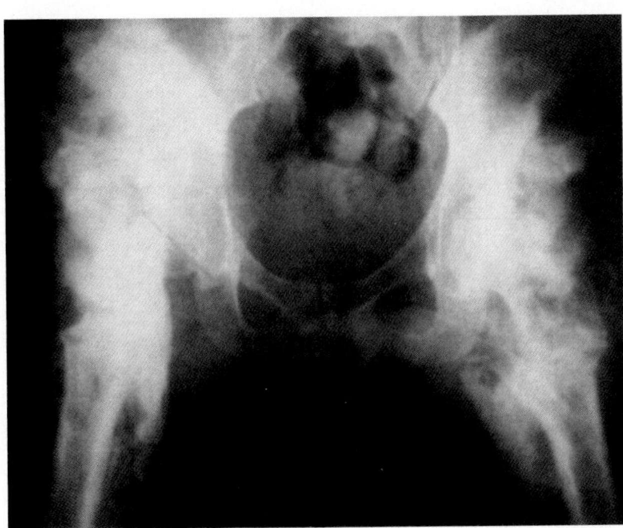

FIGURE 12.2. Heterotopic ossification around both hips in a person with paraplegia with bilateral hip joint ankylosis by AP radiograph.

In approximately 90% of patients with SCI, HO develops around the hip. Less frequent locations include the knee, elbow, and shoulder. In the hip, HO is found most commonly on the anteromedial aspect of the joint. In the knee, it is usually around the medial epicondyle of the femur. HO is rare in the small joints of the hand and foot. Ossification is extra-articular and always found below the level of SCI.

In the early stage of HO, fever is one of the first symptoms, usually higher at night and as high as 103°F, however is not always present. Several days later joint swelling occurs that limits range of motion. The patients with a preserved sensory function may have pain in the affected region. When the hip is involved, the entire thigh and knee may show edema. Some patients develop a knee effusion. HO most commonly develops between one to 6 months after injury with peak incidence at 2 months. Complications of the HO can include loss of ability to sit secondary to reduced ROM, chronic pain, development of pressure ulcers, deep venous thrombosis (DVT), increase in spasticity, and in severe cases, adjacent neurovascular structures may be compromised leading to distal extremity swelling and nerve entrapment (266). HO may occur several years after the initial SCI associated with a newly acquired pressure ulcer, DVT, or fracture (251,253,254). The appearance of HO late after SCI is associated with a benign course and preservation of joint function (267).

Differential diagnosis for this clinical presentation includes a DVT, fracture of the LE, impending pressure ulcer, septic arthritis, and cellulitis. Since DVT and pressure ulcer may coexist with HO, one should always consider a combination of disorders occurring at the same time.

Alkaline phosphatase (ALP) is a nonspecific marker but may be the least expensive and earliest laboratory indicator of HO, with elevations present within 2 to 3 weeks after HO initiation. Although ALP usually rises reflecting osteoblastic activity during the formation of HO, in many patients it is not elevated. ALP is also limited because of other causes for it to be elevated, that is, skeletal injuries, surgery, and abdominal issues post-SCI. ALP levels do not correlate with degree of bone activity and should not be used to predict HO severity or maturity. Additional nonspecific biomarkers include CRP, erythrocyte sedimentation rate (can be as high as 100 mm/hour), and creatine phosphokinase (CPK) due to damage of surrounding muscle tissue, as well as hydroxyproline and prostaglandin E2 (PGE2) excretion in 24-hour urine collections (251, 253).

The gold standard for diagnosis is three-phase bone scan (bone scintigraphy). Technetium 99m labeled diphosphonate is used as radionucleotide, which has a high affinity for newly developing bone. The phases of this scan include dynamic blood flow phase, static blood pool phase, and static bone/ossification phase. Evidence of HO on 3-phase bone scan can be seen as early as 2 to 3 weeks after injury on the first two phases that demonstrate hyperemia and blood pooling (251,253,254,268,269). The third phase shows positive uptake approximately 2 to 4 weeks later. Plain radiographs may lag behind another few weeks (average 3 weeks) to show some findings and may take 2 to 3 months to show periarticular bone formation; thus, they are not sensitive for early diagnosis of HO.

Ultrasonography can be used to diagnose HO in its early stage and reveals an echogenic peripheral zone and echolucent center (263). When HO develops in muscle, the characteristic findings are a reduction of normal lamellar pattern of muscle fibers and an irregular echogenic tissue pattern, indicating muscle infiltration with liquid mass. During the process of HO maturation, more calcified tissue can be identified on ultrasonography, first at the periphery of the lesion and later in the central part. Serial studies of patients with HO showed that within 2 weeks, the echolucent zone developed echogenic bands, indicating an increase of calcification of the tissue. At this stage, the first signs of bone formation can be also appreciated radiographically. The sonographic evaluation showed a maturation of HO similar to "zone phenomenon" seen in myositis ossificans (270,271).

Magnetic resonance imaging (MRI) can also be helpful in diagnosing HO early, while computed tomography (CT) is useful to determine bone volume for planned surgical resection. CT is not helpful in making the early diagnosis of HO.

To determine the maturity of HO, bone scintigraphy is the best method, with a serial decrease or a steady-state uptake ratio being a reliable indicator of maturity. The value of this test in preoperative evaluation is limited, however, due to frequent finding of considerable activity of HO even after a few years. The quantitative assessment of radioactive uptake at the site of HO, which is not routinely obtained, offers more precise preoperative measure of HO maturation (272).

The extent of tissue involvement by HO varies. In some patients, only a small amount of bone develops around the joint usually not causing joint dysfunction, while in others, a massive ossification can be found with bony bridges between proximal and distal region of joint, resulting in severe functional limitations or ankylosis of the joint (Fig. 12.3).

Several classifications for HO are available that are predominantly based on radiographic findings. The Brooker classification, mostly used for patients after hip replacement, utilizes 4 classes and is only applied for HO around the hip (273). Another classification by Finerman and Stover (274) describes five different grades for HO around the hip and is also based on radiographic evaluation. Garland et al. (275) proposed a radiographic classification for preoperative grading of the extent of bone formation in soft tissue. In this classification, there are five groups: 1, minimal; 2, mild; 3, moderate; 4, severe; and 5, ankylosis. This classification can

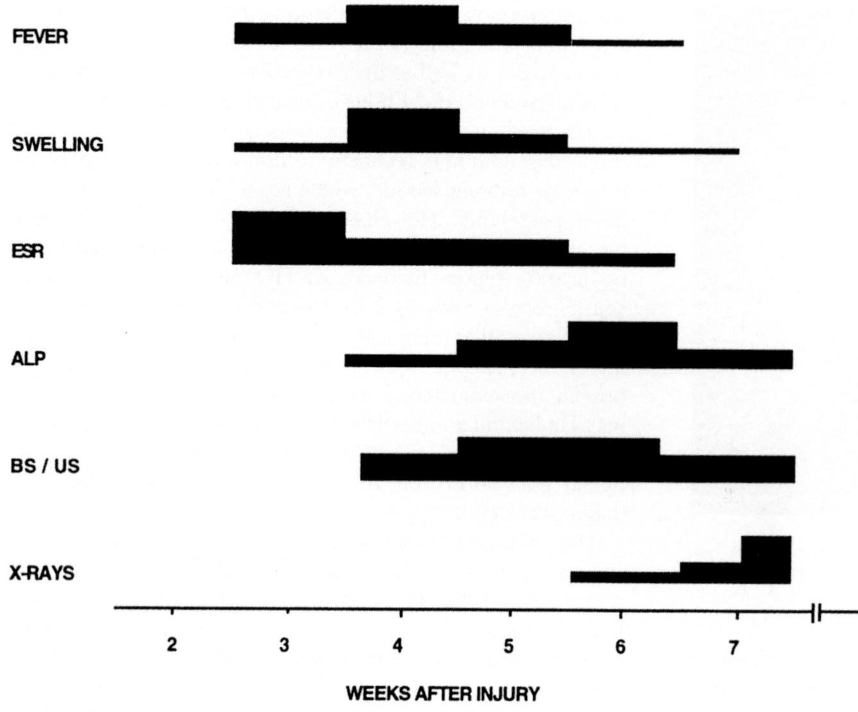

FIGURE 12.3. Time course of clinical findings associated with heterotopic ossification after SCI. Erythrocyte sedimentation rate (ESR), serum alkaline phosphatase (ALP), bone scintigraphy (BS), ultrasound (US).

be used for any location of HO. There are no classifications that combine functional impairment and radiographic findings that may be important in the decision-making process for further therapy.

On the basis of radiographic findings and clinical course, Garland and Orwin (275) proposed two classes of HO. Class I is patients with radiographic progression of HO and elevated serum ALP for five to 6 months; HO thereafter becomes inert. Class II is characterized by a radiographic progression of HO with a persistent activity on the bone scan for an extended period of time. Some of the patients in class II ultimately require surgery.

There is no definitive protocol for prophylaxis against the formation of HO. Stover et al. (276) studied prospectively a dose of etidronate 20 mg/kg/day for 2 weeks, followed by 10 mg/kg/day for 10 weeks initiated 20 to 121 days postinjury. When treatment was completed, the HO in the treatment group was significantly less compared with the placebo group. Ossification did occur after the etidronate was discontinued, with both groups having equal incidence of HO, however, with less functional deficits in the treated group. Limitations of this study, however, include that only radiography was used to monitor the degree of HO.

Prophylaxis of HO in SCI patients has been studied with varying degrees of success using other therapeutic options (269–272,277–280). NSAID use in patients with SCI (i.e., indomethacin at 75 mg daily for 3 weeks within 5 weeks of injury) was reported to develop less HO formation as compared with placebo (277). Cox-2 inhibitors have also been shown to be helpful (278). Warfarin may also be an effective agent by inhibiting the formation of osteocalcin (281). Despite the available therapeutic options, prophylaxis is still not routinely used because of the relatively low incidence of morbidity and the potential interference with bone healing postsurgery (265,282).

Since there is no definitive effective prevention of HO after SCI, the goal is to diagnose and treat HO in the initial stage of development prior to formation of mineralized tissue. Treatment options include ROM with gentle stretching after the acute inflammatory period is over (1 to 2 weeks), bisphosphonates, NSAIDS (e.g., indomethacin) if not contraindicated, as well as possible radiation therapy and surgical excision (283).

There is debate as to whether ROM has an impact on the formation or worsening of HO once it is present. Animal models have shown that new bone formation may occur following ROM, stretching, and forceful manipulation, which may cause soft tissue bleeding (284). However, there is limited documentation substantiating this relationship in the SCI population (270). Since most persons with SCI undergo stretching as part of their rehabilitation, if this was a source of HO formation, one would expect a higher incidence of HO and affecting more joints in the same individual than is currently documented. Once HO is diagnosed, it is controversial if an aggressive ROM program will induce additional tissue microtrauma, which may lead to an increased formation of HO (285). Careful and gentle mobilization of the affected joints is recommended to prevent further loss of ROM and does not appear to accelerate HO formation (286). Aggressive ROM (beyond the initial end-point) especially during the acute inflammatory phase is not recommended and should wait until the acute inflammatory signs have subsided; similarly, FES is relatively contraindicated during the acute phase (285). The ultimate goal is to maintain functional ROM for the individual.

Treatment with bisphosphonates has been shown to decrease the rate of new bone formation in patients with HO; however, it has no effect on bone that has already been deposited. Disodium etidronate inhibits osteoclastic activity and conversion of calcium phosphate to hydroxyapatite. This drug blocks the late phase of bone formation, the stage of mineralization, preventing the conversion of amorphous calcium phosphate to hydroxyapatite. Etidronate has no effect on the early phase of ossification when nonossified bone matrix is produced by osteoblasts. It was found that etidronate has in addition to its inhibitory effect on mineralization, an anti-inflammatory effect, by reducing the production of cytokines (287). Clinically, this effect is seen as a rapid reduction of soft tissue swelling after initiation of therapy. The protocol initially designed for prophylaxis of HO by Stover et al. (276) in 1976 was subsequently adopted for the treatment of HO. This recommendation was to start with an oral dose of etidronate of 20 mg/kg/day for 2 weeks, followed by a dose of 10 mg/kg/day for total of 3 months. Newer therapeutic protocols have been recommended using higher doses of etidronate for an extended period of time to prevent rebound formation of HO.

The current recommendation is for oral administration of etidronate 20 mg/kg/day for 6 months if the CPK level is elevated at the time of diagnosis or 20 mg/kg/day for 3 months, followed by 10 mg/kg/day for an additional 3 months if the initial CPK level is normal (288). With this regimen, there is faster resolution of edema with less rebound formation after the medication was discontinued. If CPK is elevated, or CRP > 8, some recommend addition of a NSAIDs until the CRP < 2 or CPK normalizes. The most common side effect of etidronate is GI, including nausea and vomiting in 10% to 20% of patients. Administering the medication in divided doses 1 to 2 hours before meals improves this problem. Clinical trials with newer generation bisphosphonates are ongoing. Although IV administration of etidronate reportedly led to quicker resolution of edema with less rebound formation after the medication was discontinued (289), this formulation is no longer available. NSAIDs have been studied in the treatment of HO (277,278), although often limited in use because of the GI complications especially in the initial periods post-SCI.

Radiation therapy has been described for patients with early HO formation (290). Different dosages of radiation were used to the hip; from single dose 8 Gy irradiation up to 20 Gy in total from multiple doses. Radiation therapy was effective as a primary treatment for early HO, as most patients showed no progression of their HO, with no adverse effects noted. There were also no differences in the fractionated regimen as compared with the single dose treatment. The long-term risks, however, were not studied. Given the possibility of long-term complications, radiation treatment is usually not utilized as a primary treatment (see below).

Surgical excision should be reserved for patients with severely limited ROM that causes functional limitations (5% to 8%). Surgical indications for resection are to improve mobility and activity of daily living (275,286) and prevent or treat medical complications such as pressure ulcers or neurovascular compression (291). The main reasons for resection of HO around the hips and knees are limitations in sitting, positioning, and dressing. Surgical indications for removal of HO around the elbow and shoulder are for improvements in feeding, hygiene, dressing, and for clinical evidence of progressive ulnar nerve compression (292,293). Most clinicians recommend waiting until after the ectopic bone is mature by bone scan, which may take up to12 to 18 months to occur. For clear indications, the surgery can be performed earlier (293). MRI or CT scan determines preoperative localization of HO.

Various surgical approaches have been utilized for the resection of HO. Wedge resection is the most common procedure; however, the bone resection is frequently associated with a significant blood loss. Other complications include wound infection, neurologic or vascular injury, and recurrence of the HO. After resection, it is beneficial to start gentle ROM at 72 hours postoperatively and wait 1 to 2 weeks until soft tissue swelling subsides until active physical therapy is commenced (275,279). Etidronate (20 mg/kg for 3 to 6 months) may be used as single or combination adjuvant therapy with NSAIDs (275,294). Radiation therapy has been recommended as a secondary therapeutic modality following surgical removal of HO. Different radiation protocols have been used. Van Kuijk et al. (295) described three patients who developed an osteonecrosis after surgery for HO, followed by a single low dose of radiation and use of a NSAID. While radiation decreases the degree of recurrence of HO, complications include delayed wound healing, osteonecrosis, and the risk of developing sarcoma (253,295). Further study in this area is needed.

Recurrence of HO after resection is common (251,253,282,294,296), but one should measure the success of the surgery by the functional improvement, that is, wheelchair sitting, grooming, hygiene, feeding, and mobility capabilities. A proper wheelchair seating evaluation should take place after surgery of HO about the hip, to protect the skin and improve the sitting posture of the patients (Table 12.5).

OTHER FACTORS AFFECTING BONE METABOLISM

As noted earlier in this chapter, adiposity is markedly elevated in individuals with SCI, and a number of proinflammatory cytokines are secreted from adipose tissue, including IL-1, IL-6, and TNF-α, as well as the hormone, leptin (96–100,103). Multiple cytokines have been considered to be involved in the increase in bone loss after SCI, including IL-1, IL-6, and TNF-α, which appear to stimulate osteoclast formation (297). In 1998, Demulder et al. (298) examined conditioned media of iliac bone marrow from individuals with paraplegia and noted that IL-6 levels found in the conditioned media were significantly higher than those in sternal conditioned media. Also noted, the iliac conditioned media increased osteoclast-like cell formation in normal bone marrow. When addition of an anti–IL-6 monoclonal antibody was added to the cultures, there was a decrease in osteoclast-like cells. Research also shows both estrogen and androgen to suppress production of IL-6; thus, a decrease in sex steroids would contribute to an increase of IL-6 and bone resorption (174,299). IL-1 and TNF-α similarly increase bone resorption by enhancing RANKL-mediated stimulation of osteoclasts; TNF-α also enhances mobilization of osteoclast progenitors from bone marrow and inhibits osteoblastic activity (300–302). Maruyama et al. (112) demonstrated that adipose tissue is positively associated with leptin, which may play a central role in the regulation of the sympathetic nervous systems control over bone resorption (303).

DIAGNOSING OSTEOPOROSIS IN SCI

Diagnosis of osteoporosis in SCI is similar to the AB population. Currently, there are no guidelines regarding when to obtain bone densitometry; however, DXA remains the gold

TABLE 12.5

CLINICAL REVIEW OF HETEROTOPIC OSSIFICATION

Epidemiology	Clinically significant 10%–20%
Course	Onset 1–6 mo, peak 2 mo
Risk factors	Male gender
	Older age
	Complete neurologic injury
	DVT
	Spasticity
	Pressure ulcer
Symptoms	Painful (if sensate)
	Limited ROM
	Localized swelling
	+/– Erythema
	+/– Warmth
Diagnosis	Biomarkers
	Serum ALP
	CRP
	ESR
	CPK
	Hydroxyproline (urine)
	PGE2 (urine)
	Nuclear medicine
	Three-phase bone scan
	Imaging
	Plain radiographs
	MRI
	Ultrasonography
	CT
Treatment	Pharmacologic
	Disodium etidronate
	Normal CPK
	20 mg/kg/d × 3 mo followed by 10 mg/kg/d × 3 mo
	Elevated CPK
	20mg/kg/d × 6 mo
	NSIADs if elevated CRP
	Surgical
	Wedge resection
Follow-up	Postsurgical
	NSAIDs, bisphosphonates, and/or radiation therapy
Complications	Limited ROM causing functional impairment, skin breakdown from change in pressure

standard to measure BMD, although quantitative CT is being considered as an expensive but more valid and reliable alternative. In the AB population, T-score > –1.0 places individuals in the low risk category, with recommendations to use calcium and vitamin D supplements along with exercise and to repeat DXA in 2 to 5 years (304). Individuals with T-score between –1.0 and –2.5 are considered osteopenic and at high risk for osteoporosis, while T-score < –2.5 is considered indicative of osteoporosis. Recommendations for treatment of osteoporosis in the AB population include the use of calcium, vitamin D, exercise, and antiresorptive therapy, with repeat DXA in 1 to 2 years. In women aged greater than 65 years, universal screening has been shown to be cost-effective (305); however, there are no data addressing screening for osteoporosis in the SCI population. In addition to DXA, serum values of ionized calcium, calcitriol, and PTH can be monitored. Plain radiographs may be helpful in diagnosing occult fractures.

Lazo et al. (306) reported in 2001, out of 41 men with SCI, 61% met WHO criteria for osteoporosis, 19.5% for osteopenia, and 19.5% were considered normal via DXA. Individuals with SCI and osteoporosis are at increased risk of fracture, and the incidence of LE fracture after SCI has been reported as high as 34% (306). The risk of low energy fractures in the LE of individuals with SCI is approximately twice that of the normal population (307). These fractures can occur during simple tasks such as transferring from bed to chair or turning in bed (308).

The relationship between the WHO classification (developed for postmenopausal women) and fracture risk in person with SCI is unknown. The distal femur and proximal tibia have been proposed as sites for BMD measurements in SCI since they are the most common sites of fracture after SCI (309). Hip BMD only moderately correlates with distal femur BMD and only marginally with proximal tibia BMD.

Garland et al. (310) reported that patients who experience pathologic fractures of their LEs have lost 50% of the BMD of their knees (relative to able-bodied group) and that the fracture threshold of the knee is 0.6 g/cm^2. A study utilizing quantitative CT, which calculates volumetric densities, reported a fracture threshold of approximately 110 mg/cm^3 in the distal femur and 70 mg/cm^3 in the distal tibia (311). Below these levels, fracture due to minor trauma is common. In 2008, Morse noted a study of 315 veterans with SCI, in which 2.6% of hospital admissions were for fracture treatment (312). Risk factors for osteoporosis in SCI include completeness of injury, increased BMI, sex steroid deficiency, chronic glucocorticoid excess, alcoholism, hypercalciuria, and cigarette smoking (310,313,314). Multiple studies have looked at BMD following SCI, and it has been shown that BMD starts to decline as early as 6 weeks postinjury with a continual increase in bone resorption over the next few weeks to 1 year (49,50,205–207,233). Bone loss, however, continues for years postinjury. Trabecular bone after a few years of loss levels off, whereas the cortical bone sites appear to decrease progressively beyond 10 after SCI (308). In 2006, Bauman et al. (315) found a significant correlation between leg lean mass loss and leg BMD loss in veterans with SCI. Bone loss is seen below the NLI with most changes occurring in the LE (49,198,306,316). Long bones appear most susceptible in individuals with SCI, as compared to the vertebral bodies in the general population. Multiple studies have shown that the trabecular-rich zones in long bones are primarily affected, notably the distal femur and proximal tibia (197,198,200). One study showed that during the first year of injury, there is a decline in bone mineral content of 4% per month in trabecular bone and 2% per month in compact bone (317).

There has been a lack of consensus with regard to bone mass of the L-spine in persons with chronic SCI. Despite the presence of risk factors for osteoporosis of the spine, as in the periphery, prior studies employing stand DXA imaging techniques alone have consistently reported an absence of vertebral bone loss, or, in some reports, even increased vertebral bone mass (318–320). Various explanations have been proposed to explain this, including continued application of gravity-related forces, the effects of prolonged seated posture, and a different mechanical function of the spine than that of the limbs. Recently, reports have challenged this notion that the vertebral bodies are spared bone loss after paralysis, suggesting that the absence of osteoporosis of the spine is a spurious finding of the DXA testing (due to the presence of osteophytes, vascular calcification, microcompression fractures, and other skeletal abnormalities in persons with SCI), and that in fact osteoporosis occurs in the spine below the level of the injury as well (321–323). In testing the lumbar spine (in chronic SCI), as measured by quantitative CT scan, individuals with chronic SCI have significant loss of spine bone mass, as they do of the extremities below the level of lesion (318,321,324). Therefore, individuals with chronic SCI who have moderate to severe DJD have bone loss of the L-spine that may be underestimated by DXA, reducing the clinicians' awareness of the risk of fracture. Therefore, relying solely on AP, DXA measurement of vertebral body density should be avoided. Quantitative CT or possibly, as suggested in the literature, lateral or midlateral DXA of the spine, if the technical capacity is available to perform this measurement, are the preferred methods of imaging of the lumbar spine in individuals with degenerative changes (321).

MANAGEMENT STRATEGIES

Since mechanical unloading appears to be a primary mechanism of bone resorption after SCI, loading bones with standing frame or tilt table, mechanically aided walking, FES, exercise, or ultrasound would appear to be viable options for intervention. Recently, an excellent review was published on the nonpharmacological treatments and prevention of bone loss in the acute and chronic phases after SCI (325).

The studies on weight bearing in the early period post injury are conflicting. Ben et al. (326) assessed the impact of tilt table standing 30 minutes, three times weekly for 12 weeks in 20 individuals with paraplegia and found no significant changes in femur BMD as determined by DXA. Although other studies have found statistically significant reductions in bone loss after passive standing (248, 325), it remains unclear that the intervention is of clinical significance, since BMD continued to decrease to levels in the severely osteoporotic range (327,328). In the chronic phase, there is little evidence for any gain in BMD after the first year of injury (325). Passive standing alone appears inadequate to prevent LE osteoporosis after SCI, and if weight bearing intervention is considered, it should be more aggressive and intervene in the early period after injury (325).

Two studies in humans have evaluated the use of whole-body vibration on BMD, both have shown significant increases in BMD with prolonged use of whole-body vibration (329,330). However, there are currently no studies in the literature evaluating the benefit of vibration therapy for persons with SCI.

In the AB population, physical exercise has a positive effect on BMD (268–270). However, little research has been completed in the SCI population. In a cross-sectional study, Jones et al. (331) demonstrated significantly lower BMD in the LE but not UE of active individuals with SCI (greater than 60 minutes of UE exercise per week) compared to AB controls. Limited ambulation associated with FES-assisted gait (Parastep 1) also failed to significantly alter LE BMD after 32 training sessions (332). In 2006, Giangregorio et al. (333) evaluated 14 individuals with incomplete SCI using body weight supported treadmill training (BWSTT) 3×week for 48 weeks with no significant changes in LE BMD or biochemical markers found. Of note, Kaplan et al. (239) showed early ambulation, decreased hypercalciuria, and modified calcium balance in a positive direction in a small number of subjects with paraplegia, but BMD was not assessed.

Electrical stimulation in the early period postinjury may impact bone loss with stimulation 5 days/week (325). In the chronic phase, the studies are conflicting, but those studies that show improvement seem to be those with longer periods of training (i.e., 12 months) and high frequency (i.e., 5 days/week) (334–337). The challenge is to provide sufficient mechanical stimulus without increasing the risk of fracture. The positive effect of electrical stimulation on bone only remains if the stimulus is continued and in sufficient amounts. Therefore, the recommendation is that ES should be used at least 2 to 3×/week, and continued for the long term if the bone mass is not to decline further.

Multiple studies have evaluated BMD of the femoral neck after FES and showed no significant changes (338–339). One study showed a statistically significant increase of BMD at the distal femur for those subjects able to achieve a threshold power output of 18 watts with FES, but the clinical significance remains unclear; PTH and serum osteocalcin increased 75% above baseline over the 6 months of training despite unchanged urinary calcium and hydroxyproline, suggesting an increase in bone turnover without concomitant resorptive activity (334). Mohr et al. (335) evaluated 10 individuals with SCI after 12 months of FES upright cycling 30 minutes/day, 3 days/week, followed by 6 months with only one weekly training session. DXA showed a statistically significant increase in the BMD of the proximal tibia, but not femoral neck, and after the 6 months of reduced training no difference was observed between groups. Two other studies show variable increases in lumbar spine, proximal tibia, and distal femur BMD after use of FES; however, there are no consistent data as to the length of time required to elicit a significant effect on the LE (336,340). FES seems to have an impact on bone density in the LE; however, continued use over a prolonged period of time may be necessary for true benefit.

Studies evaluated the influence of spasticity on BMD, and the results are inconsistent (325). Although some studies found higher BMD in persons with greater spasticity (203,311), the available studies are generally of low level of evidence and do not support the hypothesis that spasticity maintains BMD in SCI.

In the non-SCI population, supplementation of calcium and vitamin D is recommended for individuals who have or are at high risk for osteoporosis (T-score between −1.0 and −2.5); current recommendations advise 1 to 2 g/day of calcium along with 400 to 2,000 U/day of Vitamin D (304). Despite evidence cited above, there are currently no specific recommendations for calcium or Vitamin D supplementation in the SCI population, beyond those offered to the general public. A fear that calcium supplementation will increase hypercalcemia and hypercalciuria leading to urolithiasis has been proved incorrect by Stewart et al. (212).

Hormone replacement therapy (HRT) has fallen out of favor as prevention of osteoporosis in the AB population after the Women's Health Initiative's findings of increased risk of CV disease and breast cancer. However, there is one study that examined the use of HRT in women with SCI (341). Of 11 women with SCI who were using HRT, six were started for menopausal symptoms and five for osteoporosis prevention. Eleven other women were at one point in time on HRT, but had since discontinued use. Of those who discontinued use, two were diagnosed with breast cancer, three did not experience the desired effects, four experienced side effects, and two stopped based on personal choice. With increasing evidence that individuals with SCI are at high risk for CV disease, especially venous thromboembolism, the risk-benefit profile for using HRT in SCI appears suboptimal.

Bisphosphonates act by preferentially binding to bone at sites of active osteoclastic bone resorption, where they are taken up by the osteoclast and inhibit resorption (342). Of note, the presence of a nitrogen or amino group in second-generation bisphosphonates increases the antiresorptive potency by 100 to 10,000 relative to etidronate (246). Zoledronate is the most potent inhibitor of bone resorption (10,000-fold greater than etidronate), followed by risedronate (2,000-fold), ibandronate (1,000-fold) alendronate (500-fold), and pamidronate (100-fold). New preparations of once-weekly (alendronate and risedronate) or monthly (ibadronate and risedronate) administered oral medications have markedly improved compliance. Intravenous preparations of pamidronate (monthly), ibandronate (quarterly), and zoledronate (once yearly) have reduced administrative frequency even moreso, although the incidence of flu-like side effects is greater for the IV preparations. All of the second-generation bisphosphonates have been shown to increase bone mass in the spine and hip as well as decrease bone resorption; thus, they have been approved for prevention and treatment of osteoporosis (343,344). Moran de Brito et al. (345) randomly assigned 19 individuals with SCI to control (1 g calcium daily) or experimental groups (1 g calcium and 10 mg alendronate daily) over a 6-month period and found significant difference of only two of twelve parameters on whole-body DXA. Bauman et al. (346) randomized 11 subjects in a prospective placebo-controlled trial to either intravenous pamidronate (n = 6) or normal saline (n = 5) administered at 1, 2, 3, 6, 9, and 12 months over the course of the investigation; pamidronate failed to prevent clinically significant bone loss. In 2007, Gilchrist et al. (347) evaluated oral alendronate administration in a prospective, double-blind, randomized, placebo-controlled study in which 31 subjects received either 70 mg/week of alendronate or placebo administered within 10 days of injury and continued for 12 months. After 1 year, those subjects receiving alendronate demonstrated 5.3% less whole-body BMD change and 17.6% less decrease in total hip BMD. Other studies have also shown some benefit and would appear to support the use of bisphosphonates after SCI (209,348,349); however, the optimal timing, duration, and long-term side effects of these medications for use in the SCI population have yet to be determined (350). A recent systematic review concluded, "given the generally low internal validity of studies, poor statistical power, lack of clinically relevant outcomes, and uncertain generalizability, interpretation of findings is guarded. The minimal evidence currently available does not provide adequate justification for routine use of bisphosphonates therapy for prevention or treatment of BMD loss after SCI" (350).

Calcitonin inhibits bone metabolism and can increase bone mass. It inhibits osteoclast activity and prevents osteoclastogenesis (304,351). In the AB population, calcitonin has been shown to decrease the risk of new vertebral fractures in postmenopausal women with osteoporosis (352). Hypercalcemia from immobilization has been shown to be reduced with concurrent treatment with calcitonin and etidronate (250). However, no studies have looked at BMD or risk of fracture after calcitonin administration in the SCI population.

As with energy metabolism, research in the area of bone metabolism in persons with SCI appears ripe for investigation. The pathophysiology and mechanisms of disease need to be further clarified, as well as the potential risks and benefits of long-term treatment. Randomized, controlled trials (RCT) with carefully selected interventions and outcome measures need to be conducted in order to fully appreciate mechanisms and treatment options for this population at high risk for osteoporosis and its subsequent comorbidities.

References

1. Schwartz MW, Woods SC, Porte D, et al. Central nervous system control of food intake. *Nature* 2000;404(6778):661–671.
2. Shetty PS, Henry CJK, Black AE, et al. Energy requirements of adults: An update on basal metabolic rates (BMRs) and physical activity levels (PALs). *Eur J Clin Nutr* 1996;50:S11–S23.
3. Westerterp MR. Physical activity as determinant of daily energy expenditure. *Physiol Behav* 2008;93(4–5):1039–1043.
4. Segal KR, Presta E, Gutin B. Thermic effect of food during graded-exercise in normal weight and obese men. *Am J Clin Nutr* 1984;40(5):995–1000.
5. Illner K, Brinkmann G, Heller M, et al. Metabolically active components of fat free mass and resting energy expenditure in nonobese adults. *Am J Physiol Endocrinol Metab* 2000;278(2):E308–E315.
6. Sparti A, DeLany JP, de la Bretonne JA, et al. Relationship between resting metabolic rate and the composition of the fat-free mass. *Metabolism* 1997;46(10):1225–1230.
7. Ross Conference on Medical R, Ross L. *Assessment of energy metabolism in health and disease: Report of the First Ross Conference on Medical Research*. Columbus, Ohio: Ross Laboratories; 1980.
8. Wang ZM, Heshka S, Gallagher D, et al. Resting energy expenditure-fat-free mass relationship: new insights provided by body composition modeling. *Am J Physiol Endocrinol Metab* 2000;279(3):E539–E545.
9. Nielsen S, Hensrud DD, Romanski S, et al. Body composition and resting energy expenditure in humans: role of fat, fat-free mass and extracellular fluid. *Int J Obesity* 2000;24(9):1153–1157.
10. Zhang P, Chen XP, Fan M. Signaling mechanisms involved in disuse muscle atrophy. *Med Hypotheses* 2007;69(2):310–321.
11. Cox SAR, Weiss SM, Posuniak EA, et al. Energy-expenditure after spinal-cord injury - an evaluation of stable rehabilitating patients. *J Trauma-Injury Infect Crit Care* 1985;25(5):419–423.
12. Rodriguez DJ, Clevenger FW, Osler TM, et al. Obligatory negative nitrogen-balance following spinal-cord injury. *J Parenter Enteral Nutr* 1991;15(3):319–322.
13. Rodriguez DJ, Benzel EC, Clevenger FW. The metabolic response to spinal cord injury. *Spinal Cord* 1997;35(9):599–604.
14. Bauman WA, Spungen AM, Wang J, et al. The relationship between energy expenditure and lean tissue in

monozygotic twins discordant for spinal cord injury. *J Rehabil Res Dev* 2004;41(1):1–8.
15. Buchholz AC, McGillivray CF, Pencharz PB. Differences in resting metabolic rate between paraplegic and able-bodied subjects are explained by differences in body composition. *Am J Clin Nutr* 2003;77(2):371–378.
16. Buchholz AC, Pencharz PB. Energy expenditure in chronic spinal cord injury. *Curr Opin Clin Nutr Metab Care* 2004;7(6):635–639.
17. Monroe MB, Tataranni PA, Pratley R, et al. Lower daily energy expenditure as measured by a respiratory chamber in subjects with spinal cord injury compared with control subjects. *Am J Clin Nutr* 1998;68(6):1223–1227.
18. Mollinger LA, Sparr GB, El Ghatet AZ. Daily energy expenditure and basal metabolic rates of patients with sponak cord injury. *Arch Phys Med Rehabil* 1999;66:420–426.
19. Castro MJ, Apple DF, Hillegass EA, et al. Influence of complete spinal cord injury on skeletal muscle cross-sectional area within the first 6 months of injury. *Eur J Appl Physiol* 1999;80(4):373–378.
20. Modlesky CM, Bickel CS, Slade JM, et al. Assessment of skeletal muscle mass in men with spinal cord injury using dual-energy X-ray absorptiometry and magnetic resonance imaging. *J Appl Physiol* 2004;96(2):561–565.
21. Wielopolski L, Ramirez LM, Spungen AM, et al. Measuring partial body potassium in the legs of patients with spinal cord injury: a new approach. *J Appl Physiol* 2009;106(1):268–273.
22. Shah PK, Stevens JE, Gregory CM, et al. Lower-extremity muscle cross-sectional area after incomplete spinal cord injury. *Arch Phys Med Rehabil* 2006;87(6):772–778.
23. Drummond MJ, Glynn EL, Lujan HL, et al. Gene and protein expression associated with protein synthesis and breakdown in paraplegic skeletal muscle. *Muscle Nerve* 2008;37(4):505–513.
24. Dreyer HC, Glynn EL, Lujan HL, et al. Chronic paraplegia-induced muscle atrophy downregulates the mTOR/S6K1 signaling pathway. *J Appl Physiol* 2008;104(1):27–33.
25. Tsitouras PD, Zhong YG, Spungen AM, et al. Serum testosterone and growth-hormone insulin-like growth-factor-i in adults with spinal-cord injury. *Horm Metab Res* 1995;27(6):287–292.
26. Schopp LH, Clark M, Mazurek MO, et al. Testosterone levels among men with spinal cord injury admitted to inpatient rehabilitation. *Am J Phys Med Rehabil* 2006;85(8):678–684.
27. Kostovski E, Iversen PO, Birkeland K, et al. Decreased levels of testosterone and gonadotrophins in men with long-standing tetraplegia. *Spinal Cord* 2008;46(8):559–564.
28. Clark MJ, Schopp LH, Mazurek MO, et al. Testosterone levels among men with spinal cord injury - Relationship between time since injury and laboratory values. *Am J Phys Med Rehabil* 2008;87(9):758–764.
29. Rasmussen BB, Richter EA. The balancing act between the cellular processes of protein synthesis and breakdown: Exercise as a model to understand the molecular mechanisms regulating muscle mass. *J Appl Physiol* 2009;106(4):1365–1366.
30. Drummond MJ, Dreyer HC, Fry CS, et al. Nutritional and contractile regulation of human skeletal muscle protein synthesis and mTORC1 signaling. *J Appl Physiol* 2009;106(4):1374–1384.
31. Miyazaki M, Esser KA. Cellular mechanisms regulating protein synthesis and skeletal muscle hypertrophy in animals. *J Appl Physiol* 2009;106(4):1367–1373.
32. Celik B. Testosterone replacement therapy and motor function in men with spinal cord injury. *Am J Phys Med Rehabil* 2008;87(12):1054–1055.
33. Arver S, Lehtihet M. Current guidelines for the diagnosis of testosterone deficiency. In: *Advances in the management of testosterone deficiency*. vol. 37, 2009:5–20.
34. Gooren LJG. Advances in testosterone replacement therapy. In: *Advances in the management of testosterone deficiency*. vol. 37, 2009:32–51.
35. Bhasin S, Cunningham GR, Hayes FJ, et al. Testosterone therapy in adult men with androgen deficiency syndromes: An endocrine society clinical practice guideline. *J Clin Endocrinol Metab* 2006;91(6):1995–2010.
36. Yilmaz B, Yasar E, Goktepe S, et al. Basal metabolic rate and autonomic nervous system dysfunction in men with spinal cord injury. *Obesity* 2007;15(11):2683–2687.
37. Jeon JY, Steadward RD, Wheeler GD, et al. Intact sympathetic nervous system is required for leptin effects on resting metabolic rate in people with spinal cord injury. *J Clin Endocrinol Metab* 2003;88(1):402–407.
38. Brown R, Macefield VG. Assessing the capacity of the sympathetic nervous system to respond to a cardiovascular challenge in human spinal cord injury. *Spinal Cord* 2008;46(10):666–672.
39. Lucin KM, Sanders VM, Jones TB, et al. Alterations in sympathetic nervous system and hypothalamic-pituitary-adrenal axis function after experimental spinal cord injury. *J Neurochem* 2005;94:44–44.
40. Houtman S, Oeseburg B, Hughson RL, et al. Sympathetic nervous system activity and cardiovascular homeostasis during head-up tilt in patients with spinal cord injuries. *Clin Auton Res* 2000;10(4):207–212.
41. Steinberg LL, Lauro FAA, Sposito MMM, et al. Catecholamine response to exercise in individuals with different levels of paraplegia. *Braz J Med Biol Res* 2000;33(8):913–918.
42. Claydon VE, Krassioukov AV. Orthostatic hypotension and autonomic pathways after spinal cord injury. *J Neurotrauma* 2006;23(12):1713–1725.
43. Webber J, Macdonald IA. Signalling in body-weight homeostasis: neuroendocrine efferent signals. *Proc Nutr Soc* 2000;59(3):397–404.
44. Brozek J, Grande F, Andersson JT. Densiometric analysis of body composition: revision of some quantitative assumptions. *Ann NY Acad Sci* 1963;110:113–130.
45. Siri W. Body composition from fluid spaces and density: analysis of methods. In: Brozek J, Henschel A, eds. *Techniques for measuring body composition*. 1 ed. Washington D.C.: National Academy of Sciences, 1961:223–224.
46. Gater D, Clasey J. Body composition assessment in spinal cord injury clinical trials. *Top Spinal Cord Inj Rehabil* 2006;11(3):36–49.
47. Clasey JL, Gater DR. Body composition assessment in adults with spinal cord injury. *Top Spinal Cord Inj Rehabil* 2007;12(4):8–19.
48. Gater DR. Obesity after spinal cord injury. *Phys Med Rehabil Clin North Am* 2007;18(2):331–351.

49. Maimoun L, Couret I, Micallef JP, et al. Use of bone biochemical markers with dual-energy X-ray absorptiometry for early determination of bone loss in persons with spinal cord injury. *Metab-Clin Exp* 2002;51(8):958–963.
50. Maimoun L, Couret I, Mariano-Goulart D, et al. Changes in osteoprotegerin/RANKL system, bone mineral density, and bone biochemicals markers in patients with recent spinal cord injury. *Calcif Tissue Int* 2005;76(6):404–411.
51. de Bruin ED, Vanwanseele B, Dambacher MA, et al. Long-term changes in the tibia and radius bone mineral density following spinal cord injury. *Spinal Cord* 2005;43(2):96–101.
52. Zehnder Y, Luthi M, Michel D, et al. Long-term changes in bone metabolism, bone mineral density, quantitative ultrasound parameters, and fracture incidence after spinal cord injury: a cross-sectional observational study in 100 paraplegic men. *Osteoporos Int* 2004;15(3):180–189.
53. Clasey JL, Janowiak AL, Gater DR. Relationship between regional bone density measurements and the time since injury in adults with spinal cord injuries. *Arch Phys Med Rehabil* 2004;85(1):59–64.
54. Buchholz AC, McGillivray CF, Pencharz PB. The use of bioelectric impedance analysis to measure fluid compartments in subjects with chronic paraplegia. *Arch Phys Med Rehabil* 2003;84(6):854–861.
55. Cardus D, McTaggart WG. Body composition in spinal cord injury. *Arch Phys Med Rehabil* 1985;66:257–259.
56. Nuhlicek DNR, Spurr GB, Barboriak JJ, et al. Body-composition of patients with spinal-cord injury. *Eur J Clin Nutr* 1988;42(9):765–773.
57. Heymsfield SB, Lichtman S, Baumgartner RN, et al. Body-composition of humans - comparison of 2 improved 4-compartment models that differ in expense, technical complexity, and radiation exposure. *Am J Clin Nutr* 1990;52(1):52–58.
58. Heyward VH. ASEP methods recommendation: body composition assessment. *J Exerc Physiol Online* 2001;4(4):1–12.
59. Clasey JL, Gater DR. A comparison of hydrostatic weighing and air displacement plethysmography in adults with spinal cord injuries. *Arch Phys Med Rehabil* 2005;86(11):2106–2113.
60. Gater DR. Pathophysiology of obesity after spinal cord injury. *Top Spinal Cord Inj Rehabil* 2007;12(4):20–34.
61. Jones LM, Legge M, Goulding A. Healthy body mass index values often underestimate body fat in men with spinal cord injury. *Arch Phys Med Rehabil* 2003;84(7):1068–1071.
62. Maggioni M, Bertoli S, Margonato V, et al. Body composition assessment in spinal cord injury subjects. *Acta Diabetologica* 2003;40:S183–S186.
63. Spungen AM, Adkins RH, Stewart CA, et al. Factors influencing body composition in persons with spinal cord injury: a cross-sectional study. *J Appl Physiol* 2003;95(6):2398–2407.
64. Spungen AM, Wang J, Pierson RN, et al. Soft tissue body composition differences in monozygotic twins discordant for spinal cord injury. *J Appl Physiol* 2000;88(4):1310–1315.
65. Grundy SM. Metabolic syndrome pandemic. *Arterioscler Thromb Vasc Biol* 2008;28(4):629–636.
66. de Ferranti S, Mozaffarian D. The perfect storm: Obesity, adipocyte dysfunction, and metabolic consequences. *Clin Chem* 2008;54(6):945–955.
67. Antuna-Puente B, Feve B, Fellahi S, et al. Adipokines: The missing link between insulin resistance and obesity. *Diabetes Metab* 2008;34(1):2–11.
68. Borch KH, Braekkan SK, Mathiesen EB, et al. Abdominal obesity is essential for the risk of venous thromboembolism in the metabolic syndrome: the Tromso study. *J Thromb Haemost* 2009;7(5):739–745.
69. Lind L, Ingelsson E, Sundstrom J, et al. The impact of obesity and the metabolic syndrome on the risk of cardiovascular morbidity and mortality in middle-aged men. *Circulation* 2009;19(10):E302–E302.
70. Nita C, Hancu N, Rusu A, et al. Hypertensive waist: first step of the screening for metabolic syndrome. *Metab Syndr Relat Disord* 2009;7(2):105–109.
71. Oda E. The metabolic syndrome as a concept of adipose tissue disease. *Hypertens Res* 2008;31(7):1283–1291.
72. Ordovas JM, Corella D. Metabolic syndrome pathophysiology: the role of adipose tissue. *Kidney Int* 2008;74:S10–S14.
73. Wild SH, Byrne CD, Tzoulaki I, et al. Metabolic syndrome, haemostatic and inflammatory markers, cerebrovascular and peripheral arterial disease: The Edinburgh Artery Study. *Atherosclerosis* 2009;203(2):604–609.
74. Terry RB, Page WF, Haskell WL. Waist hip ratio, body-mass index and premature cardiovascular-disease mortality in United-States-Army Veterans during a 23-year follow-up-Study. *Int J Obes* 1992;16(6):417–423.
75. Terry RB, Stefanick ML, Haskell WL, et al. Contributions of regional adipose-tissue depots to plasma-lipoprotein concentrations in overweight men and women-possible protective effects of thigh fat. *Metab-Clin Exp* 1991;40(7): 733–740.
76. Brockmann GA, Tsaih SW, Neuschl C, et al. Genetic factors contributing to obesity and body weight can act through mechanisms affecting muscle weight, fat weight, or both. *Physiol Genom* 2009;36(2):114–126.
77. Sanders SS. PCSK1 variants: genetic risk factors for obesity. *Clin Genet* 2009;75(4):318–319.
78. Gianotti TF, Sookoian S, Gemma C, et al. Study of genetic variation in the STAT3 on obesity and insulin resistance in male adults. *Obesity* 2008;16(7):1702–1707.
79. Hill JO, Wyatt HR, Reed GW, et al. Obesity and the environment: Where do we go from here? *Science* 2003;299(5608):853–855.
80. Hill JO, Peters JC. Environmental contributions to the obesity epidemic. *Science* 1998;280(5368):1371–1374.
81. Grundy SM. A changing paradigm for prevention of cardiovascular disease: emergence of the metabolic syndrome as a multiplex risk factor. *Eur Heart J Suppl* 2008;10(B):B16–B23.
82. Barness LA, Opitz JM, Gilbert-Barness E. Obesity: Genetic, molecular, and environmental aspects. *Am J Med Genet Part A* 2007;143A(24):3016–3034.
83. Koerner A, Kratzsch J, Kiess W. Adipocytokines: leptin–the classical, resistin–the controversical, adiponectin–the promising, and more to come. *Best Pract Res Clin Endocrinol Metab* 2005;19(4):525–546.

84. Bjorbaek C, Kahn BB. Leptin signaling in the central nervous system and the periphery. *Recent Prog Horm Res* 2004;59(1):305–331.
85. Elmquist JK. Hypothalamic pathways underlying the endocrine, autonomic, and behavioral effects of leptin. *Physiol Behav* 2001;74(4–5):703–708.
86. Seeley RJ, D'Alessio DA, Woods SC. Fat hormones pull their weight in the CNS. *Nat Med* 2004;10(5):454–455.
87. Bodary PF, Eitzman DT. Adiponectin: Vascular protection from the fat? *Arterioscler Thromb Vasc Biol* 2006;26(2):235–236.
88. Rajala MW, Obici S, Scherer PE, et al. Adipose-derived resistin and gut-derived resistin-like molecule-{beta} selectively impair insulin action on glucose production. *J Clin Invest* 2003;111(2):225–230.
89. Chen BH, Song YQ, Ding EL, et al. Circulating levels of resistin and risk of type 2 diabetes in men and women: results from two prospective cohorts. *Diabetes Care* 2009;32(2):329–334.
90. Burnett MS, Devaney JM, Adenika RJ, et al. Cross-Sectional associations of resistin, coronary heart disease, and insulin resistance. *J Clin Endocrinol Metab* 2006;91(1):64–68.
91. Barnes KM, Miner JL. Role of resistin in insulin sensitivity in rodents and humans. *Curr Protein Pept Sci* 2009;10(1):96–107.
92. Li FP, He J, Li ZZ, et al. Effects of resistin expression on glucose metabolism and hepatic insulin resistance. *Endocrine* 2009;35(2):243–251.
93. Frankel DS, Vasan RS, D'Agostino RB, et al. Resistin, adiponectin, and risk of heart failure: The Framingham Offspring Study. *J Am Coll Cardiol* 2009;53(9):754–762.
94. de Luis DA, Sagrado MG, Conde R, et al. Relation of resistin levels with cardiovascular risk factors and insulin resistance in non-diabetes obese patients. *Diab Res Clin Pract* 2009;84(2):174–178.
95. Kuzmicki M, Telejko B, Szamatowicz J, et al. High resistin and interleukin-6 levels are associated with gestational diabetes mellitus. *Gynecol Endocrinol* 2009;25(4):258–263.
96. Naharci MI. The metabolic syndrome is associated with circulating adipokines in older adults across a wide range of adiposity. *J Gerontol Ser A-Biol Sci Med Sci* 2009;64(4):503–503.
97. Matsuzawa Y. White adipose tissue and cardiovascular disease. *Best Pract Res Clin Endocrinol Metab* 2005;19(4):637–647.
98. Malavazos AE, Corsi MM, Ermetici F, et al. Proinflammatory cytokines and cardiac abnormalities in uncomplicated obesity: Relationship with abdominal fat deposition. *Nutr Metab Cardiovasc Dis* 2007;17(4):294–302.
99. You TJ, Nicklas BJ, Ding JZ, et al. The metabolic syndrome is associated with circulating adipokines in older adults across a wide range of adiposity. *J Gerontol Ser A-Biol Sci Med Sci* 2008;63(4):414–419.
100. Fried SK, Bunkin DA, Greenberg AS. Omental and subcutaneous adipose tissues of obese subjects release interleukin-6: depot difference and regulation by glucocorticoid. *J Clin Endocrinol Metab* 1998;83(3):847–850.
101. Kern PA, Ranganathan S, Li CL, et al. Adipose tissue tumor necrosis factor and interleukin-6 expression in human obesity and insulin resistance. *Am J Physiol-Endocrinol Metab* 2001;280(5):E745–E751.
102. Weber MM, Michl P, Auernhammer CJ, et al. Interleukin-3 and Interleukin-6 stimulate cortisol secretion from adult human adrenocortical cells. *Endocrinology* 1997;138(5):2207.
103. Kern PA, Saghizadeh M, Ong JM, et al. The expression of tumor-necrosis-factor in human adipose-tissue - regulation by obesity, weight-loss, and relationship to lipoprotein-lipase. *J Clin Inv* 1995;95(5):2111–2119.
104. Blake GJ, Ridker PM. Novel clinical markers of vascular wall inflammation. *Circ Res* 2001;89(9):763–771.
105. Pai JK, Pischon T, Ma J, et al. Inflammatory markers and the risk of coronary heart disease in men and women. *N Engl J Med* 2004;351(25):2599–2610.
106. Lee MY, Myers J, Hayes A, et al. C-reactive protein, metabolic syndrome, and insulin resistance in individuals with spinal cord injury. *J Spinal Cord Med* 2005;28(1):20–25.
107. Manns PJ, McCubbin JA, Williams DP. Fitness, inflammation, and the metabolic syndrome in men with paraplegia. *Arch Phys Med Rehabil* 2005;86(6):1176–1181.
108. Mavri A, Stegnar M, Krebs M, et al. Impact of adipose tissue on plasma plasminogen activator inhibitor-1 in dieting obese women. *Arterioscler Thromb Vasc Biol* 1999;19(6):1582–1587.
109. Aso Y, Wakabayashi S, Yamamoto R, et al. Metabolic syndrome accompanied by hypercholesterolemia is strongly associated with proinflammatory state and impairment of fibrinolysis in patients with type 2 diabetes: synergistic effects of plasminogen activator inhibitor-1 and thrombin-activatable fibrinolysis inhibitor *Diabetes Care* 2005;28(9):2211–2216.
110. Aubert H, Frere C, Aillaud MF, et al. Weak and non-independent association between plasma TAFI antigen levels and the insulin resistance syndrome. *J Thromb Haemost* 2003;1(4):791–797.
111. Teasell RW, Hsieh JT, Aubut JAL, et al. Venous thromboembolism after spinal cord injury. *Arch Phys Med Rehabil* 2009;90(2):232–245.
112. Maruyama Y, Mizuguchi M, Yaginuma T, et al. Serum leptin, abdominal obesity and the metabolic syndrome in individuals with chronic spinal cord injury. *Spinal Cord* 2008;46(7):494–499.
113. Kolovou GD, Anagnostopoulou KK, Cokkinos DV. Pathophysiology of dyslipidaemia in the metabolic syndrome. *Postgrad Med J* 2005;81(956):358–366.
114. Raal FJ. Pathogenesis and management of the dyslipidemia of the metabolic syndrome. *Metab Syndr Relat Disord* 2009;7(2):83–88.
115. Kwiterovich J, Peter O, Coresh J, et al. Prevalence of hyperapobetalipoproteinemia and other lipoprotein phenotypes in men (aged ≤ 50 years) and women (≤60 years) with coronary artery disease. *Am J Cardiol* 1993;71(8):631–639.
116. Pischon T, Girman CJ, Sacks FM, et al. Non-high-density lipoprotein cholesterol and apolipoprotein B in the prediction of coronary heart disease in men. *Circulation* 2005;112(22):3375–3383.

117. Rashid S, Patterson BW, Lewis GF. What have we learned about HDL metabolism from kinetics studies in humans? *J Lipid Res* 2006;47(8):1631–1642.
118. Rashid S, Genest J. Effect of obesity on high-density lipoprotein metabolism. *Obesity* 2007;15(12):2875–2888.
119. Verges B. New insight into the pathophysiology of lipid abnormalities in type 2 diabetes. *Diabetes Metab* 2005;31(5):429–439.
120. Schmid A, Halle M, Stutzle C, et al. Lipoproteins and free plasma catecholamines in spinal cord injured men with different injury levels. *Clin Physiol* 2000;20(4):304–310.
121. Demirel S, Demirel G, Tukek T, et al. Risk factors for coronary heart disease in patients with spinal cord injury in Turkey. *Spinal Cord* 2001;39(3):134–138.
122. Bauman WA, Spungen AM, Adkins RH, et al. Metabolic and endocrine changes in persons aging with spinal cord injury. *Assist Technol* 1999;11(2):88–96.
123. Dallmeijer AJ, van der Woude LHV, van Kamp GJ, et al. Changes in lipid, lipoprotein and apolipoprotein profiles in persons with spinal cord injuries during the first 2 years post-injury. *Spinal Cord* 1999;37(2):96–102.
124. Moussavi RM, Ribas-Cardus F, Rintala DH, et al. Dietary and serum lipids in individuals with spinal cord injury living in the community. *J Rehabil Res Dev* 2001;38(2):225–233.
125. Ozgurtas T, Alaca R, Gulec M, et al. Do spinal cord injuries adversely affect serum lipoprotein profiles? *Mil Med* 2003;168(7):545–547.
126. Vidal J, Javierre C, Curia FJ, et al. Long-term evolution of blood lipid profiles and glycemic levels in patients after spinal cord injury. *Spinal Cord* 2003;41(3):178–181.
127. Bauman W, Spungen A. Risk assessment for coronary heart disease in a veteran population with spinal cord injury. *Top Spinal Cord Inj Rehabil* 2007;12(4):35–53.
128. Bhattacharya S, Dey D, Roy SS. Molecular mechanism of insulin resistance. *J Biosci* 2007;32(2):405–413.
129. Gallagher EJ, LeRoith D, Karnieli E. The metabolic syndrome - from insulin resistance to obesity and diabetes. *Endocrinol Metab Clin North Am* 2008;37(3):559.
130. Shulman GI. Cellular mechanisms of insulin resistance. *J Clin Invest* 2000;106(2):171–176.
131. Grundy SM. Obesity, metabolic syndrome, and cardiovascular disease. *J Clin Endocrinol Metab* 2004;89(6):2595–2600.
132. Duckworth WC, Jallepalli P, Solomon SS. Glucose intolerance in spinal cord injury. *Arch Phys Med Rehabil* 1983;64:107–110.
133. Petry C, Rothstein JL, Bauman WA. Hemoglobin A1c as a predictor of glucose intolerance in spinal cord injury. *J Am Paraplegia Soc* 1993;16(1):56.
134. Aksnes AK, Hjeltnes N, Wahlstrom EO, et al. Intact glucose transport in morphologically altered denervated skeletal muscle from quadriplegic patients. *Am J Physiol-Endocrinol Metab* 1996;34(3):E593–E600.
135. Szczypaczewsa M, Nazar K, Kaciuba-Uscilko H. Glucose tolerance and insulin response to glucose load in body builders. *Int J Sports Med* 1989;10:34–47.
136. Yki-Jarvinen H, Koivisto VA, Taskinen M, et al. Glucose tolerance, plasma lipoproteins and tissue lipoprotein lipase activities in body builders. *Eur J Appl Physiol Occup Med* 1984;53:253–259.
137. Bauman WA, Spungen AM. Disorders of carbohydrate and lipid-metabolism in veterans with paraplegia or quadriplegia - a model of premature aging. *Metab-Clin Exp* 1994;43(6):749–756.
138. Vasan RS, Larson MG, Leip EP, et al. Assessment of frequency of progression to hypertension in non-hypertensive participants in the Framingham Heart Study: a cohort study. *The Lancet* 2001;358(9294):1682–1686.
139. Bogaert YE, Linas S. The role of obesity in the pathogenesis of hypertension. *Nat Clin Pract Nephrol* 2009;5(2):101–111.
140. Castro JP, El-Atat FA, McFarlane SI, et al. Cardiometabolic syndrome: Pathophysiology and treatment. *Curr Hypertens Rep* 2003;5(5):393–401.
141. Kurukulasuriya LR, Stas S, Lastra G, et al. Hypertension in obesity. *Endocrinol Metab Clin North Am* 2008;37(3):647.
142. Singer GM, Setaro JF. Secondary hypertension: obesity and the metabolic syndrome. *J Clin Hypertens* 2008;10(7):567–574.
143. Yanai H, Tomono Y, Ito K, et al. The underlying mechanisms for development of hypertension in the metabolic syndrome. *Nutr J* 2008;7.
144. Huang Z, Willett WC, Manson JE, et al. Body weight, weight change, and risk for hypertension in women. *Ann Intern Med* 1998;128(2):81–88.
145. Wofford MR, Hall JE. Pathophysiology and treatment of obesity hypertension. *Curr Pharm Des* 2004;10(29):3621–3637.
146. Engeli S, Negrel R, Sharma AM. Physiology and pathophysiology of the adipose tissue renin-angiotensin system. *Hypertension* 2000;35(6):1270–1277.
147. LaVela SL, Weaver FM, Goldstein B, et al. Diabetes mellitus in individuals with spinal cord injury or disorder. *J Spinal Cord Med* 2006;29(4):387–395.
148. Lee MY, Myers J, Abella J, et al. Homocysteine and hypertension in persons with spinal cord injury. *Spinal Cord* 2006;44(8):474–479.
149. Wilt T, Carlson F, Goldish G, et al. Carbohydrate & lipid disorders & relevant considerations in persons with spinal cord injury. Evidence Report/Technology Assessment No. 163 (Prepared by the Minnesota Evidence-based Practice Center under Contract No. 290-02-0009.). In AHRQ Publication No. 08-E005. Rockville, MD: Agency for Healthcare Research and Quality; January 2008.
150. Alberti K, Zimmet PZ. Definition, diagnosis and classification of diabetes mellitus and its complications part 1: Diagnosis and classification of diabetes mellitus - Provisional report of a WHO consultation. *Diabetic Med* 1998;15(7):539–553.
151. Third Report of the National Cholesterol Education Program (NCEP) Expert Panel on Detection, Evaluation, and Treatment of High Blood Cholesterol in Adults (Adult Treatment Panel III) Final Report. *Circulation* 2002;106(25):3143.
152. Holt RIG. International Diabetes Federation redefines the metabolic syndrome. *Diabetes Obes Metab* 2005;7(5):618.

153. Liang H, Chen D, Wang Y, et al. Different risk factor patterns for metabolic syndrome in men with spinal cord injury compared with able-bodied men despite similar prevalence rates. *Arch Phys Med Rehabil* 2007;88(9):1198–1204.
154. Nash MS, Mendez AJ. A guideline-driven assessment of need for cardiovascular disease risk intervention in persons with chronic paraplegia. *Arch Phys Med Rehabil* 2007;88(6):751–757.
155. Castillo C, Miller J, Moore J, et al. Metabolic syndrome in veterans with spinal cord injury. *J Spinal Cord Med* 2007;30(4):403.
156. Rosenzweig JL, Ferrannini E, Grundy SM, et al. Primary prevention of cardiovascular disease and type 2 diabetes in patients at metabolic risk: An endocrine society clinical practice guideline. *J Clin Endocrinol Metab* 2008;93(10):3671–3689.
157. Bianchi C, Penno G, Daniele G, et al. Optimizing management of metabolic syndrome to reduce risk: focus on life-style. *Intern Emerg Med* 2008;3(2):87–98.
158. Despres JP, Arsenault BJ, Poirier P. Management of the atherogenic dyslipidemia of insulin resistance/metabolic syndrome: making visceral obesity/ectopic fat a new therapeutic target. *Med Clin North Am* 2008;92 (Suppl 1):11–26.
159. Fogli-Cawley JJ, Dwyer JT, Saltzman E, et al. The 2005 Dietary Guidelines for Americans and risk of the metabolic syndrome. *Am J Clin Nutr* 2007;86(4):1193–1201.
160. Fogli-Cawley JJ, Dwyer JT, Saltzman E, et al. The 2005 Dietary Guidelines for Americans and insulin resistance in the Framingham Offspring Cohort. *Diabetes Care* 2007;30(4):817–822.
161. Tsai AG, Wadden TA. The evolution of very-low-calorie diets: An update and meta-analysis. *Obesity* 2006;14(8):1283–1293.
162. Wadden TA, Foster GD, Letizia KA. One-year behavioral treatment of obesity - comparison of moderate and severe caloric restriction and the effects of weight maintenance therapy. *J Consulting Clin Psychol* 1994;62(1):165–171.
163. Gater D. Spinal cord injury. In: JK Ehrman, PM Gordon, PS Visich, SJ Keteyian, eds. *Clinical exercise physiology*. 2 ed. Champaign, IL: Human Kinetics, 2009:523–542.
164. Nash MA, Gater DR. Exercise to reduce obesity in spinal cord injury. *Top Spinal Cord Inj Rehabil* 2007;12(4): 76–93.
165. Gater D. Exercise and fitness with spinal cord injury. In: SA Sisto, E Druin, MM Sliwinski, eds. *Spinal cord injuries: management and rehabilitation*. St. Louis, MO: Mosby Elsevier, 2009:430–454.
166. Hjeltnes N, Aksnes AK, Birkeland KI, et al. Improved body composition after 8 wk of electrically stimulated leg cycling in tetraplegic patients. *Am J Physiol-Regul Integr Comp Physiol* 1997;42(3):R1072–R1079.
167. Bauman WA, Spungen AM. Body composition changes and anabolic hormone considerations with advancing age and in persons with spinal cord injury. *Wounds-A Compendium Clin Res Pract* 2001;13(4):22D–31D.
168. Bauman WA, Spungen AM. Coronary heart disease in individuals with spinal cord injury: assessment of risk factors. *Spinal Cord* 2008;46(7):466–476.
169. Srinivasan BT, Jarvis J, Khunti K, et al. Recent advances in the management of type 2 diabetes mellitus: a review. *Postgrad Med J* 2008;84(996):524–531.
170. Bagg W, Plank LD, Gamble G, et al. The effects of intensive glycaemic control on body composition in patients with type 2 diabetes. *Diabetes Obes Metab* 2001;3(6):410–416.
171. Fonseca VA, Kulkarni KD. Management of type 2 diabetes: Oral agents, insulin, and injectables. *J Am Diet Assoc* 2008;108(4):S29–S33.
172. Krentz AJ. Management of type 2 diabetes in the obese patient: current concerns and emerging therapies. *Curr Med Res Opin* 2008;24(2):401–417.
173. Home P, Pocock S, Beck-Nielsen H, et al. Rosiglitazone evaluated for cardiovascular outcomes in oral agent combination therapy for type 2 diabetes (RECORD): a multicentre, randomised, open-label trial. *The Lancet* 2009, doi:10.1016/S0140-6736(09)60953–3.
174. Manolagas SC. Birth and death of bone cells: basic regulatory mechanisms and implications for the pathogenesis and treatment of osteoporosis. *Endocr Rev* 2000;21(2):115–137.
175. Hsu H, Lacey DL, Dunstan CR, et al. Tumor necrosis factor receptor family member RANK mediates osteoclast differentiation and activation induced by osteoprotegerin ligand. *Proc Natl Acad Sci USA* 1999;96(7):3540–3545.
176. Simonet WS, Lacey DL, Dunstan CR, et al. Osteoprotegerin: a novel secreted protein involved in the regulation of bone density. *Cell* 1997;89(2):309–319.
177. Parfitt AM. Osteonal and hemi-osteonal remodeling: the spatial and temporal framework for signal traffic in adult human bone. *J Cell Biochem* 1994;55(3):273–286.
178. Jiang SD, Jiang LS, Dai LY. Mechanisms of osteoporosis in spinal cord injury. *Clin Endocrinol (Oxf)* 2006;65(5):555–565.
179. Cowin SC, Moss-Salentijn L, Moss ML. Candidates for the mechanosensory system in bone. *J Biomech Eng* 1991;113(2):191–197.
180. Doty SB. Morphological evidence of gap junctions between bone cells. *Calcif Tissue Int* 1981;33(5):509–512.
181. Santos A, Bakker AD, Klein-Nulend J. The role of osteocytes in bone mechanotransduction. *Osteoporos Int* 2009;20(6):1027–1031.
182. Papachroni KK, Karatzas DN, Papavassiliou KA, et al. Mechanotransduction in osteoblast regulation and bone disease. *Trends Mol Med* 2009;15(5):208–216.
183. Wolff J. *Das Gesetz der Transformation der Knochen*. Berlin: Ahirshwald, 1892.
184. De Souza MJ, West SL, Jamal SA, et al. The presence of both an energy deficiency and estrogen deficiency exacerbate alterations of bone metabolism in exercising women. *Bone* 2008;43(1):140–148.
185. Christmas C, O'Connor KG, Harman SM, et al. Growth hormone and sex steroid effects on bone metabolism and bone mineral density in healthy aged women and men. *J Gerontol Ser A-Biol Sci Med Sci* 2002;57(1):M12–M18.
186. Fohr B, Schulz A, Battmann A. Sex steroids and bone metabolism: Comparison of in vitro effects of 17 beta-estradiol and testosterone on human osteosarcoma cell

lines of various gender and differentiation. *Exp Clin Endocrinol Diabetes* 2000;108(6):414–423.
187. Isidori AM, Giannetta E, Greco EA, et al. Effects of testosterone on body composition, bone metabolism and serum lipid profile in middle-aged men: a meta-analysis. *Clin Endocrinol* 2005;63(3):280–293.
188. Kim H, Park H, Choi H, et al. The effects of low dose estrogen therapy on the bone mineral densities and bone metabolism of menopausal women. *J Bone Miner Res* 2008;23:S472–S472.
189. Kuroki Y, Kaji H, Kawano S, et al. Short-term effects of glucocorticoid therapy on biochemical markers of bone metabolism in Japanese patients: a prospective study. *J Bone Miner Metab* 2008;26(3):271–278.
190. Chan MHM, Chan PKS, Griffith JF, et al. Steroid-induced osteonecrosis in severe acute respiratory syndrome: a retrospective analysis of biochemical markers of bone metabolism and corticosteroid therapy. *Pathology* 2006;38(3):229–235.
191. Sobhani A, Moradi F, Moradi F, et al. Estimation of glucocorticoid effects on bone metabolism markers and bone mineral density in rats. *Bone* 2004;34:S43–S44.
192. Kondo H, Nifuji A, Takeda S, et al. Unloading induces osteoblastic cell suppression and osteoclastic cell activation to lead to bone loss via sympathetic nervous system. *J Biol Chem* 2005;280(34):30192–30200.
193. Meyers VE, Zayzafoon M, Douglas JT, et al. RhoA and cytoskeletal disruption mediate reduced osteoblastogenesis and enhanced adipogenesis of human mesenchymal stem cells in modeled microgravity. *J Bone Miner Res* 2005;20(10):1858–1866.
194. Minaire P, Neunier P, Edouard C, et al. Quantitative histological data on disuse osteoporosis: comparison with biological data. *Calcif Tissue Res* 1974;17(1):57–73.
195. Zerwekh J, Ruml L, Gottschalk F, et al. The effects of twelve weeks of bed rest on bone histology, biochemical markers of bone turnover, and calcium homeostasis in eleven normal subjects. *J Bone Miner Res* 1998;13:1594–1601.
196. Vico L, Collet P, Thomas T, et al. Effects of long-term microgravity exposure on cancellous and cortical weight-bearing bones of cosmonauts *The Lancet* 2000;355(9215):1607–1611.
197. Biering-Sorensen F, Bohr HH, Schaadt OP. Longitudinal study of bone mineral content in the lumbar spine, the forearm and the lower extremities after spinal cord injury. *Eur J Clin Invest* 1990;20(3):330–335.
198. Garland DE, Stewart CA, Adkins RH, et al. Osteoporosis after spinal cord injury. *J Orthop Res* 1992;10(3):371–378.
199. Garland DE, Adkins RH, Stewart CA. Five-year longitudinal bone evaluations in individuals with chronic complete spinal cord injury. *J Spinal Cord Med* 2008;31(5):543–550.
200. Dauty M, Perrouin Verbe B, Maugars Y, et al. Supralesional and sublesional bone mineral density in spinal cord-injured patients. *Bone* 2000;27(2):305–309.
201. Frey-Rindova P, de Bruin ED, Stussi E, et al. Bone mineral density in upper and lower extremities during 12 months after spinal cord injury measured by peripheral quantitative computed tomography. *Spinal Cord* 2000;38(1):26–32.
202. Tsuzuku S, Ikegami Y, Yabe K. Bone mineral density differences between paraplegic and quadriplegic patients: a cross-sectional study. *Spinal Cord* 1999;37(5):358–361.
203. Demirel G, Yilmaz H, Paker N, et al. Osteoporosis after spinal cord injury. *Spinal Cord* 1998;36(12):822–825.
204. Finsen V, Indredavik B, Fougner KJ. Bone-mineral and hormone status in paraplegics. *Paraplegia* 1992;30(5):343–347.
205. Maimoun L, Fattal C, Micallef JP, et al. Bone loss in spinal cord-injured patients: from physiopathology to therapy. *Spinal Cord* 2006;44(4):203–210.
206. Roberts D, Lee W, Cuneo RC, et al. Longitudinal study of bone turnover after acute spinal cord injury. *J Clin Endocrinol Metab* 1998;83(2):415–422.
207. Uebelhart D, Hartmann D, Vuagnat H, et al. Early modifications of biochemical markers of bone metabolism in spinal cord injury patients. A preliminary study. *Scand J Rehabil Med* 1994;26(4):197–202.
208. Pietschmann P, Pils P, Woloszczuk W, et al. Increased serum osteocalcin levels in patients with paraplegia. *Paraplegia* 1992;30(3):204–209.
209. Zehnder Y, Risi S, Michel D, et al. Prevention of bone loss in paraplegics over 2 years with alendronate. *J Bone Miner Res* 2004;19(7):1067–1074.
210. Jiang SD, Jiang LS, Dai LY. Effects of spinal cord injury on osteoblastogenesis, osteoclastogenesis and gene expression profiling in osteoblasts in young rats. *Osteoporos Int* 2007;18(3):339–349.
211. Morse LR, Nguyen HP, Jain N, et al. Age and motor score predict osteoprotegerin level in chronic spinal cord injury. *J Musculoskelet Neuronal Interact* 2008;8(1):50–57.
212. Stewart AF, Adler M, Byers CM, et al. Calcium homeostasis in immobilization: an example of resorptive hypercalciuria. *N Engl J Med* 1982;306(19):1136–1140.
213. Bauman WA, Zhong YG, Schwartz E. Vitamin D deficiency in veterans with chronic spinal cord injury. *Metabolism* 1995;44(12):1612–1616.
214. Bauman WA, Spungen AM, Morrison N, et al. Effect of a vitamin D analog on leg bone mineral density in patients with chronic spinal cord injury. *J Rehabil Res Dev* 2005;42(5):625–634.
215. Vaziri ND, Pandian MR, Segal JL, et al. Vitamin D, parathormone, and calcitonin profiles in persons with long-standing spinal cord injury. *Arch Phys Med Rehabil* 1994;75(7):766–769.
216. Bauman WA, Morrison NG, Spungen AM. Vitamin D replacement therapy in persons with spinal cord injury. *J Spinal Cord Med* 2005;28(3):203–207.
217. Mechanick JI, Pomerantz F, Flanagan S, et al. Parathyroid hormone suppression in spinal cord injury patients is associated with the degree of neurologic impairment and not the level of injury. *Arch Phys Med Rehabil* 1997;78(7):692–696.
218. Bauman WA, Spungen AM. Metabolic changes in persons after spinal cord injury. *Phys Med Rehabil Clin N Am* 2000;11(1):109–140.
219. Naftchi NE, Viau AT, Sell GH, et al. Pituitary-testicular axis dysfunction in spinal cord injury. *Arch Phys Med Rehabil* 1980;61(9):402–405.
220. Maimoun L, Lumbroso S, Paris F, et al. The role of androgens or growth factors in the bone resorption

process in recent spinal cord injured patients: a cross-sectional study. *Spinal Cord* 2006;44(12):791–797.
221. Celik B, Sahin A, Caglar N, et al. Sex hormone levels and functional outcomes: a controlled study of patients with spinal cord injury compared with healthy subjects. *Am J Phys Med Rehabil/Assoc Acad Physiatrists* 2007;86(10):784–790.
222. Rosenquist RC. Evaluation of 17-ketosteroid, estrogen and gonadotrophin excretion in patients with spinal cord injury. *Am J Med* 1950;8(4):534–535.
223. Jilka RL. Cytokines, bone remodeling, and estrogen deficiency: a 1998 update. *Bone* 1998;23(2):75–81.
224. Manolagas SC, Jilka RL. Bone marrow, cytokines, and bone remodeling. Emerging insights into the pathophysiology of osteoporosis. *N Engl J Med* 1995;332(5):305–311.
225. Pacifici R. Cytokines, estrogen, and postmenopausal osteoporosis–the second decade. *Endocrinology* 1998;139(6):2659–2661.
226. Slade JM, Bickel CS, Modlesky CM, et al. Trabecular bone is more deteriorated in spinal cord injured versus estrogen-free postmenopausal women. *Osteoporos Int* 2005;16(3):263–272.
227. Levasseur R, Sabatier JP, Potrel-Burgot C, et al. Sympathetic nervous system as transmitter of mechanical loading in bone. *Joint Bone Spine* 2003;70(6):515–519.
228. Serre CM, Farlay D, Delmas PD, et al. Evidence for a dense and intimate innervation of the bone tissue, including glutamate-containing fibers. *Bone* 1999;25(6):623–629.
229. Cherruau M, Morvan FO, Schirar A, et al. Chemical sympathectomy-induced changes in TH-, VIP-, and CGRP-immunoreactive fibers in the rat mandible periosteum: influence on bone resorption. *J Cell Physiol* 2003;194(3):341–348.
230. Arai M, Nagasawa T, Koshihara Y, et al. Effects of beta-adrenergic agonists on bone-resorbing activity in human osteoclast-like cells. *Biochim Biophys Acta* 2003;1640(2–3):137–142.
231. Togari A. Adrenergic regulation of bone metabolism: possible involvement of sympathetic innervation of osteoblastic and osteoclastic cells. *Microsc Res Tech* 2002;58(2):77–84.
232. Schlienger RG, Kraenzlin ME, Jick SS, et al. Use of beta-blockers and risk of fractures. *JAMA* 2004;292(11):1326–1332.
233. Chantraine A, Nusgens B, Lapiere CM. Bone remodeling during the development of osteoporosis in paraplegia. *Calcif Tissue Int* 1986;38(6):323–327.
234. Claus-Walker J, Campos RJ, Carter RE, et al. Calcium excretion in quadriplegia. *Arch Phys Med Rehabil* 1972;53(1):14–20.
235. Maynard FM. Immobilization hypercalcemia following spinal cord injury. *Arch Phys Med Rehabil* 1986;67(1):41–44.
236. Maynard FM, Imai K. Immobilization hypercalcemia in spinal cord injury. *Arch Phys Med Rehabil* 1977;58(1):16–24.
237. Naftchi NE, Viau AT, Sell GH, et al. Mineral metabolism in spinal cord injury. *Arch Phys Med Rehabil* 1980;61(3):139–142.
238. Zhou XJ, Vaziri ND, Segal JL, et al. Effects of chronic spinal cord injury and pressure ulcer on 25(OH)-vitamin D levels. *J Am Paraplegia Soc* 1993;16(1):9–13.
239. Kaplan PE, Gandhavadi B, Richards L, et al. Calcium balance in paraplegic patients: influence of injury duration and ambulation. *Arch Phys Med Rehabil* 1978;59(10):447–450.
240. Hansen RB, Biering-Sorensen F, Kristensen JK. Urinary calculi following traumatic spinal cord injury. *Scand J Urol Nephrol* 2007;41(2):115–119.
241. Kohli A, Lamid S. Risk factors for renal stone formation in patients with spinal cord injury. *Br J Urol* 1986;58(6):588–591.
242. Ost MC, Lee BR. Urolithiasis in patients with spinal cord injuries: risk factors, management, and outcomes. *Curr Opin Urol* 2006;16(2):93–99.
243. Massagli TL, Cardenas DD. Immobilization hypercalcemia treatment with pamidronate disodium after spinal cord injury. *Arch Phys Med Rehabil* 1999;80(9):998–1000.
244. Labossiere R, Hintzke C, Ileana S. Hypercalcemia of Immobilization. *J Am Med Dir Assoc* 2009;10(4):284–285.
245. Kedlaya D, Brandstater ME, Lee JK. Immobilization hypercalcemia in incomplete paraplegia: Successful treatment with pamidronate. *Arch Phys Med Rehabil* 1998;79(2):222–225.
246. Drake MT, Clarke BL, Khosla S. Bisphosphonates: Mechanism of action and role in clinical practice. *Mayo Clinic Proc* 2008;83(9):1032–1045.
247. Rogers MJ, Roelofs AJ, Coxon FP. Molecular mechanisms of bisphosphonate action: insight into structure-function relationships. *Clin Exp Metastasis* 2008;25:27–28.
248. de Bruin ED, Frey-Rindova P, Herzog RE, et al. Changes of tibia bone properties after spinal cord injury: Effects of early intervention. *Arch Phys Med Rehabil* 1999;80(2):214–220.
249. Kaplan PE, Roden W, Gilbert E, et al. Reduction of hypercalciuria in tetraplegia after weight-bearing and strengthening exercises. *Paraplegia* 1981;19(5):289–293.
250. Meythaler JM, Tuel SM, Cross LL. Successful treatment of immobilization hypercalcemia using calcitonin and etidronate. *Arch Phys Med Rehabil* 1993;74(3):316–319.
251. Bossche LV, Vanderstraeten G. Heterotopic ossification: A review. *J Rehabil Med* 2005;37(3):129–136.
252. Pape HC, Marsh S, Morley JR, et al. Current concepts in the development of heterotopic ossification. *J Bone Jt Surg-Brit Vol* 2004;86B(6):783–787.
253. van Kuijk AA, Geurts ACH, van Kuppevelt HJM. Neurogenic heterotopic ossification in spinal cord injury. *Spinal Cord* 2002;40(7):313–326.
254. Garland DE. A clinical perspective on common forms of acquired heterotopic ossification. *Clin Orthop Relat Res* 1991;(263):13–29.
255. Bravopayno P, Esclarin A, Arzoz T, et al. Incidence and risk-factors in the appearance of heterotopic ossification in spinal-cord injury. *Paraplegia* 1992;30(10):740–745.
256. Wittenberg RH, Peschke U, Botel U. Heterotopic ossification after spinal-cord injury - epidemiology and risk-factors. *J Bone Jt Surg-Brit Vol* 1992;74(2):215–218.

257. da Paz AC, Artal FJC, Kalil RK. The function of proprioceptors in bone organization: A possible explanation for neurogenic heterotopic ossification in patients with neurological damage. *Med Hypotheses* 2007;68(1):67–73.
258. Estrores IM, Harrington A, Banovac K. C-reaction protein and erythrocyte sedimentation rate in patients with heterotopic ossification after spinal cord injury. *J Spinal Cord Med* 2004;27(5):434–437.
259. Gonda K, Nakaoka T, Yoshimura K, et al. Heterotopic ossification of degenerating rat skeletal muscle induced by adenovirus-mediated transfer of bone morphogenetic protein-2 gene. *J Bone Miner Res* 2000;15(6):1056–1065.
260. Chantraine A, Nusgens B, Lapiere CM. Biochemical-analysis of heterotopic ossification in spinal-cord injury patients. *Paraplegia* 1995;33(7):398–401.
261. Hardy A, Dickson J. Pathological ossification in traumatic paraplegia. *J Bone Jt Surg-Am Vol* 1963;45B:76–87.
262. Rossier A, Bussat P, Infabte F. Current facts on para-osteoarthropathy (POA). *Paraplegia* 1973;11:36–78.
263. Cassar-Pullicino V, McClelland M, Badwan D, et al. Sonographic diagnosis of heterotopic bone formation in spinal cord patients. *Paraplegia* 1993;31(1):40–50.
264. Banovac K, Gonzalez F. Evaluation and management of heterotopic ossification in patients with spinal cord injury. *Spinal Cord* 1997;35(3):158–162.
265. Subbarao JV, Garrison SJ. Heterotopic ossification: diagnosis and management, current concepts and controversies. *J Spinal Cord Med* 1999;22(4):273–283.
266. Colachis SC, Clinchot DM, Venesy D. Neurovascular complications of heterotopic ossification following spinal-cord injury. *Paraplegia* 1993;31(1):51–57.
267. Sherman AL, Williams J, Patrick L, et al. The value of serum creatine kinase in early diagnosis of heterotopic ossification. *J Spinal Cord Med* 2003;26(3):227–230.
268. Shehab D, Elgazzar AH, Collier BD. Heterotopic ossification. *J Nucl Med* 2002;43(3):346–353.
269. Svircev JN, Wallbom AS. False-negative triple-phase bone scans in spinal cord injury to detect clinically suspect heterotopic ossification: A case series. *J Spinal Cord Med* 2008;31(2):194–196.
270. Snoecx M, Demuynck M, Vanlaere M. Association between muscle trauma and heterotopic ossification in spinal-cord injured patients—reflections on their causal relationship and the diagnostic-value of ultrasonography. *Paraplegia* 1995;33(8):464–468.
271. Thomas EA, Cassarpullicino VN, McCall IW. The role of ultrasound in the early diagnosis and management of heterotopic bone-formation. *Clin Radiol* 1991;43(3):190–196.
272. Kim SW, Wu SY, Kim RC. Computerized quantitative radionuclide assessment of heterotopic ossification in spinal-cord injury patients. *Paraplegia* 1992;30(11):803–807.
273. Brooker AF, Bowerman JW, Robinson RA, et al. Ectopic ossification following total hip-replacement - incidence and a method of classification. *J Bone Jt Surg-Am Vol* 1973;A 55(8):1629–1632.
274. Finerman GAM, Stover SL. Heterotopic ossification following hip-replacement or spinal-cord injury—2 clinical-studies with EHDP. *Metab Bone Dis Relat Res* 1981;3(4–5):337–342.
275. Garland DE, Orwin JF. Resection of heterotopic ossification in patients with spinal-cord injuries. Clin Orthop Relat *Res* 1989;(242):169–176.
276. Stover SL, Hahn H, Miller J. Disodium etidronate in the prevention of heterotopic ossification following spinal cord injury (preliminary report). *Paraplegia* 1976;14:146–156.
277. Banovac K, Williams JM, Patrick LD, et al. Prevention of heterotopic ossification after spinal cord injury with indomethacin. *Spinal Cord* 2001;39(7):370–374.
278. Banovac K, Williams JM, Patrick LD, et al. Prevention of heterotopic ossification after spinal cord injury with COX-2 selective inhibitor (rofecoxib). *Spinal Cord* 2004;42(12):707–710.
279. Biering-Sorensen F, Tondevold E. Indomethacin and disodium etidronate for the prevention of recurrence of heterotopic ossification after surgical resection—2 case-reports. *Paraplegia* 1993;31(8):513–515.
280. Cullen N, Perera J. Heterotopic ossification: pharmacologic options. *J Head Trauma Rehabil* 2009;24(1):69–71.
281. Buschbacher R, McKinley W, Buschbacher L, et al. Warfarin in prevention of heterotopic ossification. *Am J Phys Med Rehabil* 1992;71(2):86–91.
282. Jamil F, Subbarao JV, Banaovac K, et al. Management of immature heterotopic ossification (HO) of the hip. *Spinal Cord* 2002;40(8):388–395.
283. Haran M, Bhuta T, Lee B. Pharmacological interventions for treating acute heterotopic ossification. In: *Cochrane Database of Systematic Reviews* 2004.
284. Michelsson JE, Rauschning W. Pathogenesis of experimental heterotopic bone-formation following temporary forcible exercising of immobilized limbs. *Clin Orthop Relat Res* 1983;(176):265–272.
285. Crawford C, Varghese G, Mani MM, et al. Heterotopic ossification: Are range of motion exercises contraindicated? J *Burn Care Rehabil* 1986;7:323–327.
286. Subbarao JV, Nemchausky B, Gratzer M. Resection of heterotopic ossification and Didronel therapy—Regaining wheelchar independence in the spinal cord injured patient. *J Am Paraplegia Soc* 1987;10:3–7.
287. Mahy PR, Urist MR. Experimental heterotopic bone-formation induced by bone morphogenetic protein and recombinant human interleukin-1b. *Clin Orthop Relat Res* 1988;(237):236–244.
288. Banovac K, Sherman AL, Estrores IM, et al. Prevention and treatment of heterotopic ossification after spinal cord injury. *J Spinal Cord Med* 2004;27(4):376–382.
289. Banovac K, Gonzalez F, Wade N, et al. Intravenous disodium etidronate therapy in spinal-cord injury patients with heterotopic ossification. *Paraplegia* 1993;31(10):660–666.
290. Sautter-Bihl ML, Liebermeister E, Nanassy A. Radiotherapy as a local treatment option for heterotopic ossifications in patients with spinal cord injury. *Spinal Cord* 2000;38(1):33–36.
291. Wainapel SF, Rao PU, Schepsis AA. Ulnar nerve compression by heterotopic ossification in a head-injured patient. *Arch Phys Med Rehabil* 1985;66(8):512–514.
292. Banaovac K, Renfree K, Hornicek F. Heterotopic ossification after brain and spinal cord injury. *Crit Rev Phys Rehabil Med* 1998;10:223–256.

293. McAuliffe JA, Wolfson AH. Early excision of heterotopic ossification about the elbow followed by radiation therapy. *J Bone Jt Surg-Am Vol* 1997;79A(5):749–755.
294. Freebourn TM, Barber DB, Able AC. The treatment of immature heterotopic ossification in spinal cord injury with combination surgery, radiation therapy and NSAID. *Spinal Cord* 1999;37(1):50–53.
295. van Kuijk AA, van Kuppevelt HJM, van der Schaaf DB. Osteonecrosis after treatment for heterotopic ossification in spinal cord injury with the combination of surgery, irradiation, and an NSAID. *Spinal Cord* 2000;38(5):319–324.
296. Meiners T, Abel R, Bohm V, et al. Resection of heterotopic ossification of the hip in spinal cord injured patients. *Spinal Cord* 1997;35(7):443–445.
297. Datta HK, Ng WF, Walker JA, et al. The cell biology of bone metabolism. *J Clin Pathol* 2008;61(5):577–587.
298. Demulder A, Guns M, Ismail A, et al. Increased osteoclast-like cells formation in long-term bone marrow cultures from patients with a spinal cord injury. *Calcif Tissue Int* 1998;63(5):396–400.
299. Manolagas SC. The role of IL-6 type cytokines and their receptors in bone. *Ann NY Acad Sci* 1998;840:194–204.
300. Lam J, Takeshita S, Barker JE, et al. TNF-alpha induces osteoclastogenesis by direct stimulation of macrophages exposed to permissive levels of RANK ligand. *J Clin Invest* 2000;106(12):1481–1488.
301. Kim N, Kadono Y, Takami M, et al. Osteoclast differentiation independent of the TRANCE-RANK-TRAF6 axis. *J Exp Med* 2005;202(5):589–595.
302. Jimi E, Nakamura I, Ikebe T, et al. Activation of NF-kappa B is involved in the survival of osteoclasts promoted by interleukin-1. *J Biol Chem* 1998;273(15):8799–8805.
303. Takeda S, Karsenty G. Molecular bases of the sympathetic regulation of bone mass. *Bone* 2008;42(5):837–840.
304. Lorenzo J, Canalis E, Raisz L. Metabolic bone disease. In: Williams RH, Kronenberg H, eds. *Williams textbook of endocrinology*. 11th ed. Philadelphia: Saunders/Elsevier, 2008:xix, 1911.
305. Lewiecki EM, Watts NB, McClung MR, et al. Official positions of the international society for clinical densitometry. *J Clin Endocrinol Metab* 2004;89(8):3651–3655.
306. Lazo MG, Shirazi P, Sam M, et al. Osteoporosis and risk of fracture in men with spinal cord injury. *Spinal Cord* 2001;39(4):208–214.
307. Vestergaard P, Krogh K, Rejnmark L, et al. Fracture rates and risk factors for fractures in patients with spinal cord injury. *Spinal Cord* 1998;36(11):790–796.
308. Giangregorio L, McCartney N. Bone loss and muscle atrophy in spinal cord injury: epidemiology, fracture prediction, and rehabilitation strategies. *J Spinal Cord Med* 2006;29(5):489–500.
309. Shields RK, Schlechte J, Dudley-Javoroski S, et al. Bone mineral density after spinal cord injury: A reliable method for knee measurement. *Arch Phys Med Rehabil* 2005;86(10):1969–1973.
310. Garland DE, Adkins RH, Kushwaha V, et al. Risk factors for osteoporosis at the knee in the spinal cord injury population. *J Spinal Cord Med* 2004;27(3):202–206.
311. Eser P, Frotzler A, Zehnder Y, et al. Fracture threshold in the femur and tibia of people with spinal cord injury as determined by peripheral quantitative computed tomography. *Arch Phys Med Rehabil* 2005;86(3):498–504.
312. Morse LR, Battaglino RA, Stolzmann KL, et al. Osteoporotic fractures and hospitalization risk in chronic spinal cord injury. *Osteoporos Int* 2009; 20(3):385–392.
313. Reid IR. Glucocorticoid effects on bone. *J Clin Endocrinol Metab* 1998;83(6):1860–1862.
314. Cummings SR, Nevitt MC, Browner WS, et al. Risk factors for hip fracture in white women. Study of Osteoporotic Fractures Research Group. *N Engl J Med* 1995;332(12):767–773.
315. Bauman WA, Spungen AM, Wang J, et al. Relationship of fat mass and serum estradiol with lower extremity bone in persons with chronic spinal cord injury. *Am J Physiol Endocrinol Metab* 2006;290(6):E1098–E1103.
316. Uebelhart D, Demiaux-Domenech B, Roth M, et al. Bone metabolism in spinal cord injured individuals and in others who have prolonged immobilisation. A review. *Paraplegia* 1995;33(11):669–673.
317. Wilmet E, Ismail AA, Heilporn A, et al. Longitudinal study of the bone mineral content and of soft tissue composition after spinal cord section. *Paraplegia* 1995;33(11):674–677.
318. Bauman WA, Spungen AM, Wang J, et al. Continuous loss of bone during chronic immobilization: A monozygotic twin study. *Osteoporos Int* 1999;10(2):123–127.
319. Yu W, Gluer CC, Fuerst T, et al. Influence of degenerative joint disease on spinal bone-mineral measurements in postmenopausal women. *Calcif Tissue Int* 1995;57(3):169–174.
320. Riggs BL, Wahner HW, Seeman E, et al. Changes in bone-mineral density of the proximal femur and spine with aging-differeneces between the post-menopausal and senile osteoporosis syndromes. *J Clin Investig* 1982;70(4):716–723.
321. Bauman WA, Schwartz E, Song ISY, et al. Dual-energy X-ray absorptiometry overestimates bone mineral density of the lumbar spine in persons with spinal cord injury. *Spinal Cord* 2009;47(8):628–633.
322. Jaovisidha S, Sartoris DJ, Martin EME, et al. Influence of spondylopathy on bone densitometry using dual energy X-ray absorptiometry. *Calcif Tissue Int* 1997;60(5):424–429.
323. Liu CC, Theodorou DJ, Theodorou SJ, et al. Quantitative computed tomography in the evaluation of spinal osteoporosis following spinal cord injury. *Osteoporos Int* 2000;11(10):889–896.
324. Biering-Sorensen F, Bohr H, Schaadt O. Bone mineral content of the lumbar spine and lower extremities years after spinal cord lesion. *Paraplegia* 1988;26:293–301.
325. Biering-Sorensen F, Hansen B, Lee BSB. Non-pharmacological treatment and prevention of bone loss after spinal cord injury: a systematic review. *Spinal Cord* 2009;47(7):508–518.
326. Ben M, Harvey L, Denis S, et al. Does 12 weeks of regular standing prevent loss of ankle mobility and bone mineral density in people with recent spinal cord injuries? *Aust J Physiother* 2005;51(4):251–256.

327. Aleekna V, Tamulaitiene M, Sinevicius T, et al. Effect of weight-bearing activities on bone mineral density in spinal cord injured patients during the period of the first two years. *Spinal Cord* 2008;46(11):727–732.
328. Goemaere S, Van Laere M, De Neve P, et al. Bone mineral status in paraplegic patients who do or do not perform standing. *Osteoporos Int* 1994;4(3):138–143.
329. Gusi N, Raimundo A, Leal A. Low-frequency vibratory exercise reduces the risk of bone fracture more than walking: a randomized controlled trial. *BMC Musculoskelet Disord* 2006;7:92.
330. Verschueren SM, Roelants M, Delecluse C, et al. Effect of 6-month whole body vibration training on hip density, muscle strength, and postural control in postmenopausal women: a randomized controlled pilot study. *J Bone Miner Res* 2004;19(3):352–359.
331. Jones LM, Legge M, Goulding A. Intensive exercise may preserve bone mass of the upper limbs in spinal cord injured males but does not retard demineralisation of the lower body. *Spinal Cord* 2002;40(5):230–235.
332. Needham-Shropshire BM, Broton JG, Klose KJ, et al. Evaluation of a training program for persons with SCI paraplegia using the Parastep 1 ambulation system: part 3. Lack of effect on bone mineral density. *Arch Phys Med Rehabil* 1997;78(8):799–803.
333. Giangregorio LM, Webber CE, Phillips SM, et al. Can body weight supported treadmill training increase bone mass and reverse muscle atrophy in individuals with chronic incomplete spinal cord injury? *Appl Physiol Nutr Metab* 2006;31(3):283–291.
334. Bloomfield SA, Mysiw WJ, Jackson RD. Bone mass and endocrine adaptations to training in spinal cord injured individuals. *Bone* 1996;19(1):61–68.
335. Mohr T, Podenphant J, Biering-Sorensen F, et al. Increased bone mineral density after prolonged electrically induced cycle training of paralyzed limbs in spinal cord injured man. *Calcif Tissue Int* 1997;61(1):22–25.
336. Chen SC, Lai CH, Chan WP, et al. Increases in bone mineral density after functional electrical stimulation cycling exercises in spinal cord injured patients. *Disabil Rehabil* 2005;27(22):1337–1341.
337. Belanger M, Stein RB, Wheeler GD, et al. Electrical stimulation: Can it increase muscle strength and reverse osteopenia in spinal cord injured individuals? *Arch Phys Med Rehabil* 2000;81(8):1090–1098.
338. BeDell KK, Scremin AM, Perell KL, et al. Effects of functional electrical stimulation-induced lower extremity cycling on bone density of spinal cord-injured patients. *Am J Phys Med Rehabil* 1996;75(1):29–34.
339. Leeds EM, Klose KJ, Ganz W, et al. Bone mineral density after bicycle ergometry training. *Arch Phys Med Rehabil* 1990;71(3):207–209.
340. Clark JM, Jelbart M, Rischbieth H, et al. Physiological effects of lower extremity functional electrical stimulation in early spinal cord injury: lack of efficacy to prevent bone loss. *Spinal Cord* 2007;45(1):78–85.
341. Khong S, Savic G, Gardner BP, et al. Hormone replacement therapy in women with spinal cord injury - a survey with literature review. *Spinal Cord* 2005;43(2):67–73.
342. Leu CT, Luegmayr E, Freedman LP, et al. Relative binding affinities of bisphosphonates for human bone and relationship to antiresorptive efficacy. *Bone* 2006;38(5):628–636.
343. Harris ST, Watts NB, Genant HK, et al. Effects of risedronate treatment on vertebral and nonvertebral fractures in women with postmenopausal osteoporosis: a randomized controlled trial. Vertebral Efficacy With Risedronate Therapy (VERT) Study Group. *JAMA* 1999;282(14):1344–1352.
344. McClung MR, Geusens P, Miller PD, et al. Effect of risedronate on the risk of hip fracture in elderly women. Hip Intervention Program Study Group. *N Engl J Med* 2001;344(5):333–340.
345. Moran de Brito CM, Battistella LR, Saito ET, et al. Effect of alendronate on bone mineral density in spinal cord injury patients: a pilot study. *Spinal Cord* 2005;43(6):341–348.
346. Bauman WA, Wecht JM, Kirshblum S, et al. Effect of pamidronate administration on bone in patients with acute spinal cord injury. *J Rehabil Res Dev* 2005;42(3):305–313.
347. Gilchrist NL, Frampton CM, Acland RH, et al. Alendronate prevents bone loss in patients with acute spinal cord injury: a randomized, double-blind, placebo-controlled study. *J Clin Endocrinol Metab* 2007;92(4):1385–1390.
348. Minaire P, Depassio J, Berard E, et al. Effects of clodronate on immobilization bone loss. *Bone* 1987;8(Suppl 1):S63–S68.
349. Nance PW, Schryvers O, Leslie W, et al. Intravenous pamidronate attenuates bone density loss after acute spinal cord injury. *Arch Phys Med Rehabil* 1999;80(3):243–251.
350. Bryson JE, Gourlay ML. Bisphosphonate use in acute and chronic spinal cord injury: a systematic review. *J Spinal Cord Med* 2009;32(3):215–225.
351. Chambers TJ, Magnus CJ. Calcitonin alters behaviour of isolated osteoclasts. *J Pathol* 1982;136(1):27–39.
352. Chesnut CH, Silverman S, Andriano K, et al. A randomized trial of nasal spray salmon calcitonin in postmenopausal women with established osteoporosis: the prevent recurrence of osteoporotic fractures study. PROOF Study Group. *Am J Med* 2000;109(4):267–276.

CHAPTER 13 ■ NEUROGENIC BLADDER FOLLOWING SPINAL CORD INJURY

TODD A. LINSENMEYER

INTRODUCTION

Voiding dysfunction is commonly encountered in those with spinal cord disorders. These problems not only result in increased urinary tract infections (UTIs), bladder stones, and other lower urinary tract morbidity but also can potentially lead to kidney complications including renal deterioration. Therefore, timely identification of the type of voiding dysfunction, proper decision on the type of bladder management, and follow-up are important.

ANATOMY AND PHYSIOLOGY OF THE UPPER AND LOWER URINARY TRACTS

Discussions often focus on a person's "neurogenic bladder." However, it is important to remember that changes in the lower tracts, such as poor drainage or high bladder pressures, often have a direct impact on the kidneys. The urinary tract is divided into the upper and lower urinary tracts. The upper tracts are composed of the kidneys and ureters. The lower urinary tracts are composed of the bladder and urethra.

Upper Urinary Tracts

The kidney consists of two parts: the renal parenchyma and collecting system. The renal parenchyma secretes, concentrates, and excretes urine into the collecting system. In this collecting system, urine drains from multiple renal calyces into a renal pelvis. The place where the renal pelvis narrows and becomes the ureter is known as the ureteropelvic junction (1). This is of clinical significance since congenital narrowing or kidney stones can cause obstruction of the kidneys.

In the adult, the ureter is approximately 30 cm in length. In addition to the ureteropelvic junction, there are two other areas of physiologic narrowing that take on clinical significance with respect to possible obstruction from stones: the lower part of the ureter, where the iliac artery crosses over the ureter, and the ureterovesical junction (2,3). The ureterovesical junction is where the ureters traverse obliquely between the muscular and submucosal layers of the bladder wall for a distance of 1 to 2 cm before opening into the bladder. This submucosal tunnel is designed to allow urine flow into the bladder but prevents reflux backward up into the ureter. Any increase in intravesical pressure simultaneously compresses the submucosal ureter and effectively creates a one-way valve (4). Presence of ureteral muscle in the submucosal segment also has been shown to be important in preventing reflux (5). Unfortunately, this same configuration can inhibit drainage from the kidneys, if there are sustained high intravesical pressures.

Lower Urinary Tracts

Anatomically, the bladder is divided into the detrusor and the trigone. The detrusor is composed of smooth muscle bundles that freely crisscross and interlace with each other. Near the bladder neck, the muscle fibers assume three distinct layers. The circular arrangement of the smooth muscles at the bladder neck allows them to act as a functional sphincter. The trigone is located at the inferior base of the bladder and extends from the ureteral orifices to the bladder neck. The deep trigone is continuous with the detrusor smooth muscle; the superficial trigone is an extension of the ureteral musculature (4).

There is no clear demarcation of the musculature of the bladder neck and the beginning of the urethra in a man or woman. In the woman, the urethra contains an inner longitudinal and outer semicircular layer of smooth muscle. The circular muscle layer exerts a sphincteric effect along the entire length of the urethra, which is approximately 4 cm long (Fig. 13.1). In the man, the penis is made up of two corpora cavernosa that contain the spongy erectile tissue, and a corpora spongiosum that surrounds the urethra. The male urethra is divided into the posterior or prostatic urethra, extending from the bladder neck to the urogenital diaphragm, and the anterior urethra, which extends to the meatus. The junction between the anterior and posterior urethra is known as the membranous urethra.

Urinary Urethral Sphincters

Traditionally, the urethra has been thought to have two distinct sphincters: the internal and the external, or rhabdosphincter. The internal sphincter is not a true anatomic sphincter. Instead, in both men and women, the term refers to the junction of the bladder neck and proximal urethra, formed from the circular arrangement of connective tissue and smooth muscle fibers that extend from the bladder. This area is considered to be a functional sphincter because there is a progressive increase in tone with bladder filling so that the urethral pressure is greater than the intravesical pressure. These smooth muscle fibers also extend submucosally down the urethra and lie above the external rhabdosphincter (6).

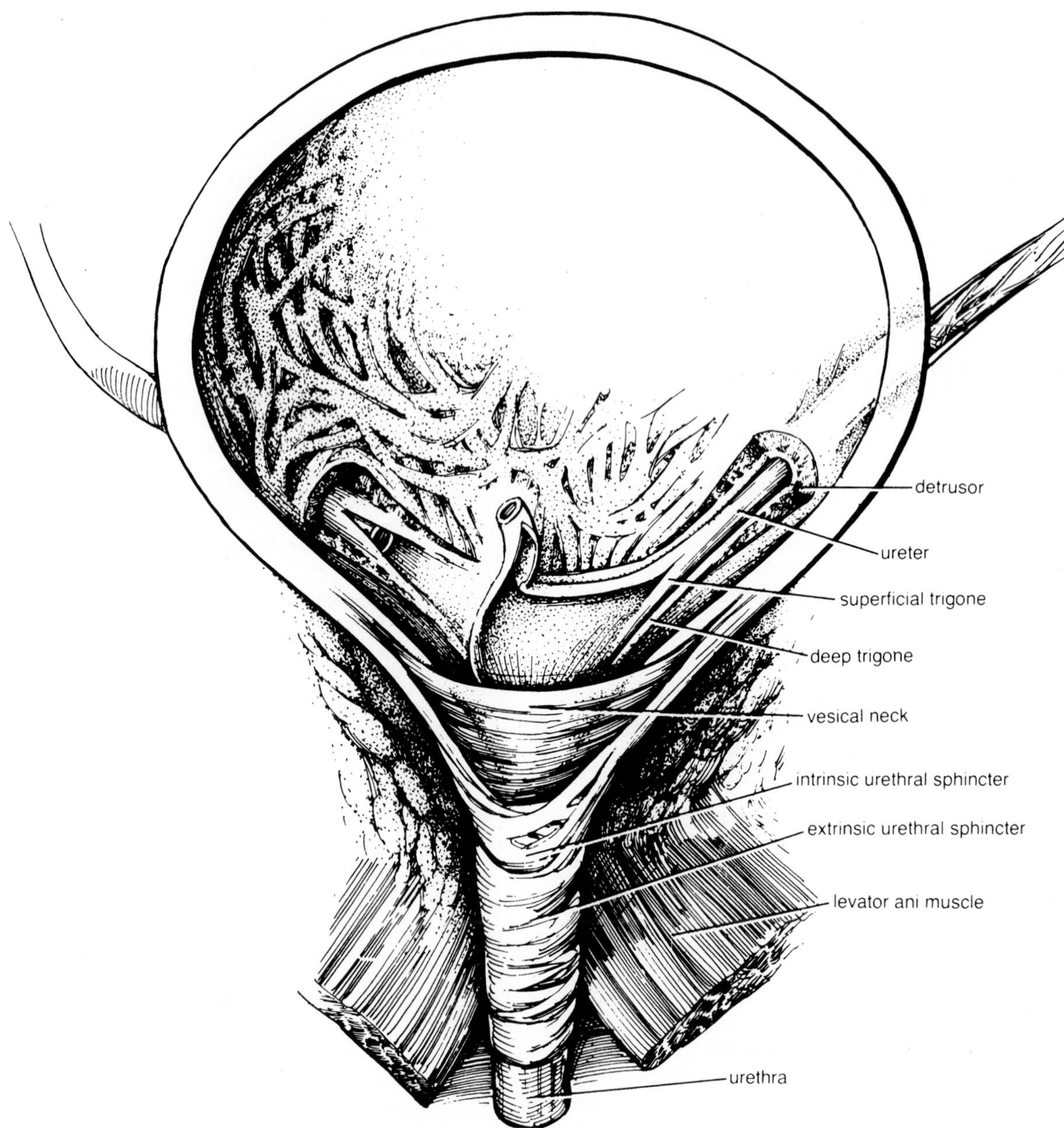

FIGURE 13.1. Anatomy of the bladder and related structures in the women. Note that there is no clear demarcation between the bladder neck and the sphincter mechanism. (From Hinman F Jr. Bladder repair: In: Hinman F Jr, ed. *Urological surgery*. Philadelphia, PA: WB Saunders, 1989, 433, with permission.)

In the man, the external or urethral rhabdosphincter often is diagrammatically illustrated as a thin circular band of striated muscle forming a diaphragm just distal to the prostatic urethra (i.e., membranous urethra). In an anatomic study, however, Myers et al. (7) reconfirmed earlier studies showing that the urethral external striated sphincter does not form a circular band but has fibers that run up to the base of the bladder. The bulk of the fibers are found at the membranous urethra (8). This sphincter is under voluntary control. The striated muscular fibers in both the man and woman are thought to have a significant proportion of slow-twitch fibers with the capacity for steady tonic compression of the urethra. In the woman, striated skeletal muscle fibers circle the upper two thirds of the urethra (8).

Normal Urine Transport from the Kidneys to the Bladder

Urine transport is the result of both passive and active forces. Passive forces are created by the filtration pressure of the kidneys. The normal proximal tubular pressure is 14 mm Hg and the renal pelvis pressure is 6.5 mm Hg, which slightly exceeds resting ureteral and bladder pressures. Active forces are due to peristalsis of the calyces, renal pelvis, and ureter. Peristalsis begins with the electrical activity of pacemaker cells at the proximal portion of the urinary collecting tract (9).

For the ureter to efficiently propel the bolus of urine, the contraction wave must completely coapt the ureteral walls (6).

Ureteral dilatation for any reason results in inefficient propulsion of the urine bolus, and this can delay drainage proximal to that point. This can result in further dilatation and over time lead to hydronephrosis.

NEUROANATOMY OF THE LOWER URINARY TRACT

Bladder storage and emptying are functions of interactions between the peripheral parasympathetic (PS), sympathetic, and somatic innervation of the lower urinary tract. Additionally, there is modulation from the central nervous system (CNS). Slight alterations in storage or emptying have significant clinical implications not only because of potential morbidity but also because of the social embarrassment of urinary incontinence, no matter how infrequently it occurs.

Bladder Neuroanatomy: Efferent System

The PS efferent supply originates from a distinct detrusor nucleus located in the intermediolateral gray matter of the sacral cord at S2–S4 (Fig. 13.2). Sacral efferents emerge as preganglionic fibers in the ventral roots (VRs) and travel through the pelvic nerves to ganglia immediately adjacent to or within the detrusor muscle to provide excitatory input to the bladder. After impulses arrive at the PS ganglia, they travel through short postganglionics to the smooth muscle cholinergic receptors. These receptors, called cholinergic because the primary postganglionic neurotransmitter is acetylcholine, are distributed throughout the bladder. Stimulation causes a bladder contraction (10,11).

The sympathetic efferent nerve supply to the bladder and urethra begins in the intermediolateral gray column from T11 through L2 and provides inhibitory input to the bladder. Sympathetic impulses travel a relatively short distance to the lumbar sympathetic paravertebral ganglia. From here, the sympathetic impulses travel along long postganglionic nerves in the hypogastric nerves to synapse at alpha- and beta-adrenergic receptors within the bladder and urethra. The primary postganglionic neurotransmitter for the sympathetic system is norepinephrine. Variations in this anatomic arrangement do occur; sympathetic ganglia sometimes also are located near the bladder, and sympathetic efferent fibers may travel along the pelvic as well as the hypogastric nerves (Fig. 13.2) (10,11).

Sympathetic stimulation facilitates bladder storage because of the strategic location of the adrenergic receptors (Fig. 13.3). Beta-adrenergic receptors predominate in the superior portion (i.e., body) of the bladder. Stimulation of beta receptors causes smooth muscle relaxation. Alpha receptors have a higher density near the base of the bladder and prostatic urethra; stimulation of these receptors causes smooth muscle contractions and therefore increases the outlet resistance of the bladder and prostatic urethra (10–12).

After SCI, several changes occur to the bladder receptors, which alter bladder function. There is evidence that when smooth muscle is denervated, its sensitivity to a given amount of neurotransmitter increases (i.e., denervation supersensitivity). Therefore, smaller doses of various pharmacologic agents would be expected to have a much more pronounced effect in those with SCI as compared to those with nonneurogenic bladders (13). A change in receptor location and density may also occur. Norlen et al. (14) found that after complete denervation there was a change from a beta-receptor predominance to an alpha-receptor predominance. Since alpha receptors cause contraction of smooth muscle, a change in receptors may be one reason for some individuals to have poor compliance of the bladder after SCI.

Animal studies have revealed that while the previously described long postganglionic neurons exist, there are ganglia close to the bladder and urethra in which there are both cholinergic and adrenergic fibers. This has been termed the urogenital short neuron system. These ganglia are composed of three cell types: adrenergic neurons, cholinergic neurons, and small intensely fluorescent (SIF) cells. The SIF cells are believed to be responsible for this interganglionic modulation of the adrenergic and cholinergic neurons. Further work is needed to define this system in humans (15).

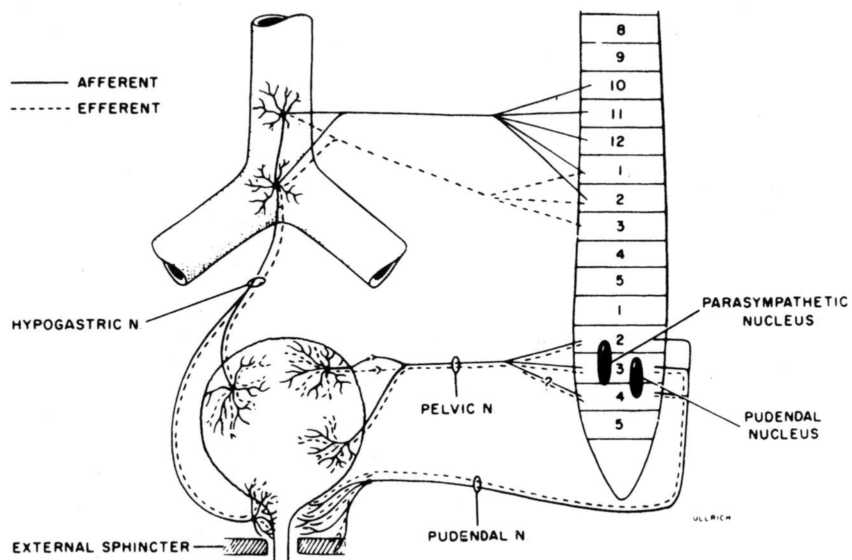

FIGURE 13.2. Peripheral innervation of the bladder and urethra. Sympathetic stimulation responsible for storage travels through the hypogastric plexus. PS stimulation causing bladder contractions travels through the pelvic nerve. (From Blaivas JG. Management of bladder dysfunction in multiple sclerosis. *Neurology* 1980;30:73, with permission.)

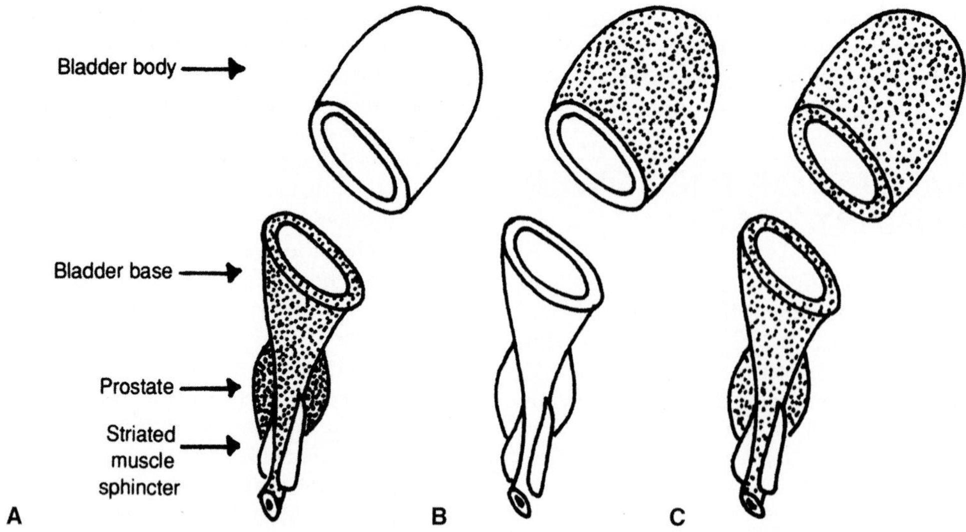

FIGURE 13.3. Location of bladder receptors. Bladder storage is maintained by simultaneous sympathetic adrenergic receptors (contraction) (**A**) and beta-adrenergic receptor (relaxation stimulation) (**B**). Bladder emptying occurs with parasympathetic cholinergic receptor stimulation(**C**). (Illustration by Carol Taylor.)

Afferent System

The most important afferents that stimulate voiding are those that pass to the sacral cord via the pelvic nerves. These afferents include two types of afferents: small myelinated A-delta and unmyelinated (C) fibers. The small myelinated A-delta fibers respond in a graded fashion to bladder distention and are essential for normal voiding. The unmyelinated (C) fibers have been termed "silent C-fibers" because they do not respond to bladder distention and therefore are not essential for normal voiding. However, these "silent C-fibers" do exhibit spontaneous firing when they are activated by chemical or cold temperature irritation at the bladder wall. Additionally, the unmyelinated (C) fibers, rather than A-delta afferents, have been found to "wake up" and respond to distention and stimulate bladder contractions in animals with suprasacral SCI.

Increased C-fiber afferent activity after SCI has been experimentally demonstrated by systemic administration of capsaicin, a neurotoxin that is known to disrupt the function of C-fiber afferents. In non-SCI animals (with A-delta afferents), there was no blockage of bladder contractions with bladder distention. However, in SCI animals, capsaicin completely blocked rhythmic bladder contractions induced with bladder distention. These findings have important potential therapeutic implications. To date, there has been some success at blocking uninhibited contractions with the use of intravesical capsaicin, and preliminary results with another C-fiber neurotoxin, resiniferatoxin (RTX), are promising (16). RTX is 1,000 times as potent as capsaicin and has such a fast onset of action that its intravesical instillation does not cause bladder discomfort that is often associated with intravesical capsaicin instillation (16).

Bladder Neurotransmitters

It is known that there are additional transmitters besides acetylcholine and norepinephrine, including nitric oxide, vasoactive intestinal polypeptide (VIP), endogenous opioid peptides, and neuropeptide Y. These transmitters may work on their own or help modulate the classic neurotransmitters. Nitric oxide and VIP have smooth muscle relaxant effects. The large number of receptors helps to explain the concept of "atropine resistance." It has been found that a single neurotransmitter-blocking agent such as atropine fails to suppress 100% of the bladder or urethral activity (13,17). This explains why a combination of agents may be more effective than a higher dose of a single agent.

Urethral Sphincter Innervation

The external urethral sphincter (EUS) classically has been described as having somatic innervation allowing the sphincter to be closed at will. Somatic efferents originate from a pudendal nucleus of sacral segments from S1–S4. Somatic efferents then travel through the pudendal nerve to the neuromuscular junction of the striated muscle fibers in the EUS.

The internal urethral sphincter has been described as being under control of the autonomic system. This area has a large number of sympathetic alpha receptors, which cause closure when stimulated. Animal studies have revealed that nitric oxide is an important neurotransmitter-mediating relaxation of the urethral smooth muscle (7,17).

The distinction between the internal and external sphincter is, however, becoming less clear. Elbadawi and Schenk (18) reported histochemical evidence of a triple innervation pattern of the external sphincter in five mammalian species, with dual sympathetic and PS autonomic components superimposed on the somatic component. Sundin and Dahlstrom (19) demonstrated sprouting and increasing adrenergic terminals after PS denervation in cats. Crowe et al. (20) reported a substantial invasion of adrenergic nerve fibers in smooth and striated muscle in the urethra in SCI patients with lower motor neuron lesions.

Influences of the Central Nervous System on the Lower Urinary Tract

Facilitation and inhibition of the autonomic nervous system is under control of the CNS. There are several theories of how this occurs. Denny-Brown and Robertson (21) suggested that micturition was primarily due to a sacral micturition reflex. According to their theory, descending nervous system pathways modulate this micturition reflex (21). Barrington, Bradley, and de Groat thought that facilitative impulses to the bladder originated from a region of the anterior pons termed "Barrington's center" (17,22,23).

De Groat et al. (17) additionally stressed the importance of the sympathetic nervous system in facilitating urine storage. Carlsson (24) provided evidence that this pontine mesencephalic area also plays a role in coordinating detrusor and sphincter activity. Stimulation of Barrington's center significantly decreased electromyographic (EMG) activity in the periurethral striated sphincter while causing a bladder contraction. In humans, this center is felt to be responsible for causing sphincter relaxation, which in turn initiates a bladder contraction. Detrusor sphincter dyssynergia (DSD), intermittent contractions of the sphincter during a bladder contraction, occurs without coordination from this center.

Transection experiments in cats suggest that the net effect of the cerebral cortex on micturition is inhibitory. This also is true for the basal ganglia and corresponds to clinical findings of detrusor hyperreflexia in those with basal ganglia dysfunction (e.g., Parkinson disease). The cerebellum is thought to maintain tone in the pelvis floor musculature and influence coordination between periurethral striated muscle relaxation and bladder emptying (14,24).

NORMAL VOIDING PHYSIOLOGY

Micturition should be considered as having two phases: the filling (storage) phase and emptying (voiding) phase. The filling phase occurs when a person is not trying to void. The emptying phase is defined as when a person is attempting to or told to void.

During filling, there should be very little rise in bladder pressure. As filling continues, low intravesical pressure is maintained by a progressive increase in sympathetic stimulation of the beta receptors located in the body of the bladder that cause relaxation, and stimulation of the alpha receptors located at the base of the bladder and urethra that causes contraction. Sympathetic stimulation also inhibits excitatory PS ganglionic transmission, which helps suppress bladder contractions. During the filling phase, there is a progressive increase in urethral sphincter EMG activity (25). Increased urethral sphincter activity also reflexly inhibits bladder contractions. When a bladder is full and has normal compliance, intravesical pressures are between 0 and 6 cm H_2O and should not rise above 15 cm H_2O. Filling continued past the limit of the viscoelastic properties of the bladder results in a steady progressive rise in intravesical pressure (26). This part of the filling curve usually is not seen in a person with normal bladder function, because this much filling would cause significant discomfort and not be tolerated.

When a patient is told to void (voiding or emptying phase), there should be cessation of urethral sphincter EMG activity and a drop in urethral sphincter pressure and funneling of the bladder neck. There is no longer reflex inhibition to the sacral micturition center from the sphincter mechanism. This is followed by a detrusor contraction. The urethral sphincter should remain open throughout voiding, and there should be no rise in intraabdominal pressure during voiding. In younger individuals, there should be no postvoid residual (PVR), although PVRs may increase with aging (see later).

CLASSIFICATION OF VOIDING DYSFUNCTION

There have been a wide variety of classifications to describe voiding dysfunctions. These classifications have been based on neurologic lesion (e.g., Bors-Comarr, Bradley), urodynamic findings (e.g., Lapides), functional classification (e.g., Wein), and combination of bladder and urethral function based on urodynamics (e.g., International Continence Society) (27–31). The International Continence Society classification: The Standardisation of Terminology of Lower Urinary Tract Function: Report from the Standardisation Sub-committee of the International Continence Society has become widely accepted by those working with voiding dysfunctions. It provides both a standardization of terminology describing bladder and urethral function and a detailed description of each of these terms (31). A urodynamic basic SCI data set has recently been developed that should be helpful in collecting information in a standardized way regarding urodynamic bladder and sphincter function in those with SCI (32).

Suprapontine Lesions

Any suprapontine lesion may affect voiding. Lesions may result from cerebrovascular disease, hydrocephalus, intracranial neoplasms, traumatic brain injury, Parkinson disease, and multiple sclerosis (MS). It should be noted that MS is unique among the suprapontine lesions because it also affects the white matter of the spinal cord and often has a relapsing and remitting nature. The expected urodynamic finding following a suprapontine lesion is detrusor hyperreflexia without DSD. Normally, the sphincter should remain relaxed during the bladder contraction. DSD occurs when the sphincter intermittently tightens during the contraction. It is important to note that voiding dysfunctions may be very different from expectations due to various factors such as medications, prostate obstruction, and possible normal bladder function but poor cognition.

Suprasacral Spinal Cord Lesions

Traumatic SCI is the most common suprasacral lesion affecting voiding. Other suprasacral lesions include transverse myelitis, MS, and primary or metastatic spinal cord tumor. Patients with suprasacral spinal cord lesions would be expected to have detrusor hyperreflexia with DSD. However, due to partial lesions, occult lesions of the sacral cord, or persistent spinal shock, this is not always the case (33).

Traumatic suprasacral SCI results in an initial period of spinal shock, in which there is hyporeflexia of the somatic system below the level of injury and detrusor areflexia. During this phase, the bladder has no contractions even with various maneuvers such as the "ice water filling" test, bethanechol supersensitivity testing, or suprapubic (SP) tapping. The neurophysiology for spinal shock and its recovery is not known. Recovery of bladder function usually follows recovery of skeletal muscle reflexes. Uninhibited bladder contractions gradually return after 6 to 8 weeks (34).

Clinically, a person with a traumatic suprasacral SCI may begin having episodes of urinary incontinence, and various visceral sensations, such as tingling, flushing, increased lower extremity spasms, or autonomic dysreflexia (AD) with the onset of uninhibited contractions. As uninhibited bladder contractions become stronger, the PVRs decrease. Rudy et al. (35) reported that voiding function appears optimal at 12 weeks postinjury. However, detrusor hyperreflexia has been reported to have a delayed onset up to 22 months postinjury (36). Eventually, all of these patients did develop uninhibited contractions. Comarr (27) considered the bladder "balanced" when PVRs were less than 20% of the total bladder capacity in those with detrusor hyperreflexia. Graham (37) reports that 50% to 70% of patients will develop balanced bladders without therapy. Unfortunately, high intravesical voiding pressures usually are required for the development of a balanced bladder. These high pressures, however, may cause renal deterioration (see Hydronephrosis; Vesicoureteral Reflux).

Traditionally, it has been thought that there is decreased activity of the EUS during acute spinal shock. However, Downie and Awad (38) noted in dogs that with surgical transection between T2 and T8, there was no change in the activity of the periurethral striated musculature despite detrusor areflexia. In humans, Nanninga and Meyer (39) found that in 44 patients in spinal shock with suprasacral lesions, all had a positive bulbocavernosus reflex and 30 of 32 had sphincter activity despite detrusor areflexia within 72 hours of injury. Koyanagi et al. (40) noted that external sphincter electrical activity was not affected during acute spinal shock but was likely to increase after recovery from spinal shock. This increase was more marked in those with high suprasacral lesions compared with low suprasacral lesions.

Detrusor external sphincter dyssynergia (DESD) also commonly occurs following suprasacral lesions. DESD is defined as intermittent or complete failure of relaxation of the urinary sphincter during a bladder contraction and voiding. This diagnosis should not be made during the filling phase if the sphincter fails to relax when there is no bladder contraction. Blaivas et al. (41) noted that it occurred in 96% of patients with suprasacral lesions and found several different patterns of DESD. Rudy et al. proposed that DESD is an exaggerated continence reflex. The continence reflex is the normal phenomenon of increasing urethral sphincter activity with bladder filling. They believed that the patterns described by Blaivas et al. represented variations of the single continence reflex (35).

In addition to the DESD, internal sphincter dyssynergia also has been reported, often occurring at the same time as DESD.

Sacral Lesions

There are a variety of lesions that may affect the sacral cord or roots. These include spinal trauma, herniated lumbar disc, primary or metastatic tumors, myelodysplasia, arteriovenous malformation, lumbar stenosis, and inflammatory process (e.g., arachnoiditis). In Pavlakis et al. series, trauma was responsible for conus and cauda equina lesions over 50% of the time. The next most common cause was L4-5 or L5-S1 intervertebral disc protrusion (42). The incidence of lumbar disc prolapse causing cauda equina syndrome is between 1% and 15% (42). Damage to the sacral cord or roots generally results in a highly compliant acontractile bladder; however, particularly in patients with partial injuries, the areflexia may be accompanied by decreased bladder compliance resulting in progressive increases in intravesical pressure with filling (43). The exact mechanism by which sacral PS decentralization of the bladder causes decreased compliance is unknown (44,45).

It has been noted that the external sphincter is not affected to the same extent as the detrusor. This is due to the fact that the pelvic nerve innervation to the bladder usually arises one segment higher than the pudendal nerve innervation to the sphincter (45). The nuclei also are located in different portions of the sacral cord, with the detrusor nuclei located in the intermediolateral cell column, and the pudendal nuclei located in the ventral gray matter. This combination of detrusor areflexia and an intact sphincter helps contribute to bladder overdistention and decompensation.

Peripheral Lesions

There are multiple etiologies for peripheral lesions that could affect voiding. The most common lesion is a peripheral neuropathy secondary to diabetes mellitus. Other peripheral neuropathies that have been associated with voiding dysfunction include chronic alcoholism, herpes zoster, Guillain-Barre Syndrome (GBS), and pelvic surgery (46,47). A sensory neuropathy is the most frequent finding in diabetes. Urodynamic findings, including decreased bladder sensation, chronic bladder overdistention, increased PVRs, and possible bladder decompensation, may result from bladder overdistension due to decreased sensation of fullness. Andersen and Bradley (48) reported that in their series, mean bladder capacity was 635 mL, with a range of 200 to 1150 mL. An autonomic neuropathy also may be responsible for decreased bladder contractility. GBS and herpes zoster are predominantly motor neuropathies. Transient voiding symptoms, predominantly urinary retention, have been reported to occur in 0% to 40% of patients and are thought to be due to involvement of the autonomic sacral PS nerves. Detrusor hyperreflexia occasionally has been found in those with GBS (49). Voiding dysfunctions resulting from pelvic surgery or pelvic trauma usually involve both motor and sensory innervation of the bladder (42).

COMPREHENSIVE EVALUATION OF VOIDING DYSFUNCTION

Neurourologic History

A thorough patient history is required to identify the neurologic diagnosis, and associated medical problems. The urologic history should include the present bladder management (type, problems, acceptance), fluid intake and output, and voiding complaints such as urgency, frequency, hesitancy, dysuria, incontinence, and AD. While symptoms can help to determine what is bothering a person, whether or not a person is out of spinal shock, and problems with bladder management, it is important not to initiate treatment based on symptoms. Symptoms often correlate poorly with actual bladder and sphincter function. Similar symptoms may occur from abnormal bladder function, abnormal sphincter function or a combination of both. Therefore, urodynamics is necessary to objectively evaluate voiding dysfunction following SCI (50).

Significant past medical history and social history includes surgery or medications that may affect voiding, allergies, smoking and drinking history, other medical problems, lifestyle/sexuality, and living environment. The functional history is of particular significance for voiding dysfunction. One should ask about hand function, dressing skills, sitting balance, ability to perform transfers, and ability to ambulate. These factors are important considerations when developing bladder management strategies.

Neurourologic Physical Examination

The neurourologic physical examination will not give objective evidence about the bladder and sphincter function. It will, however, suggest potential contributory causes of a voiding dysfunction. The neurourologic physical examination should focus on the abdomen, external genitalia, and perineal skin. When performing the rectal examination, it is important to note that it is not the overall size of the prostate but the amount of prostate growing inward that causes obstruction. Therefore, urodynamic study rather than rectal examination is needed to diagnose outflow obstruction objectively. In woman, one should examine for the location of the urethral meatus, and whether or not there is a cystocele or rectocele.

The sensory examination should focus on determining the level of injury in those with SCI. Especially important is establishing if the level of injury is above T6, which would make the patient prone to AD. Sacral sensation evaluates the afferent limb (i.e., pudendal nerve) of the sacral micturition center.

The motor examination helps to establish the level of injury and degree of completeness in those with SCI. Hand function should be assessed to determine the ability to undress or possibly perform intermittent catheterization (IC). The degree of spasticity and sitting and standing balance should be evaluated. Anal sphincter tone also should be evaluated. Decreased or absent tone suggests a sacral or peripheral nerve lesion, whereas increased tone suggests a suprasacral lesion. Voluntary contraction of the anal sphincter tests sacral innervation, suprasacral integrity, and the ability to understand commands.

Cutaneous reflexes that are helpful to the neurourologic examination are the cremasteric (L1-2), bulbocavernosus (S2-4), and anal reflex (S2-4). Absence of these cutaneous reflexes suggests pyramidal tract disease or a peripheral lesion. The bulbocavernosus reflex is a useful test to evaluate the sacral reflex arc. However, it may be unreliable. A false negative often results from a person being nervous and already having his or her anal sphincter clamped down at the time of the examination. A false negative often is due to a person being nervous and already having their anal sphincter clamped down at the time of the examination. Muscle stretch reflexes also should be evaluated. A sudden increase in spasticity may be an indication of a UTI.

Laboratory Evaluation

It is best to obtain a baseline urine for culture and sensitivity. A serum creatinine is not as helpful as a 24-hour creatinine clearance because there has to be a significant amount of kidney damage occurring prior to there being changes in the serum creatinine.

Urologic Assessment of the Upper and Lower Urinary Tract—Overview

Individuals with SCI, particularly those with the potential of poor bladder wall compliance or high intravesical voiding pressures, need constant surveillance of the upper tracts as well as lower tracts. The American Paraplegia Society has developed recommendations for the urologic evaluations of those with SCI (51). There are several tests to evaluate the upper and lower tracts. These will be discussed in the next section.

While there is strong consensus that upper and lower tract evaluations are necessary, there is not universal agreement on how often testing should be performed. There is evidence that bladder function continues to change even after 20 years postinjury, suggesting that yearly evaluations should be considered (52). People with an indwelling SP or Foley catheter, however, often will undergo yearly cystoscopy to rule out stones and bladder tumors.

Specific Upper and Lower Tract Tests

Tests designed to evaluate the upper tracts include an intravenous pyelogram (IVP), renal ultrasound, 24-hour urine creatinine clearance, and quantitative mercaptoacetyltriglycine (MAG) 3 renal scan and computerized tomography (CT). When ordering a test, one must consider if the information is needed about the function of the upper tracts or about the anatomy of the upper tracts. For example, a renal scan is better than a renal ultrasound for screening a person who clinically is doing well. If a renal ultrasound is used as a screening test for renal function, no problems will be detected until there are anatomical changes, such as hydronephrosis. However, a renal scan would detect stasis of the upper tracts long before hydronephrosis developed, but likely not detect a small kidney stone if a person was having hematuria. However, each test has certain advantages and disadvantages over other tests that should be taken into account. For example, if a person develops recurrent Proteus UTIs, he or she may require in addition to a functional study, a more detailed anatomical evaluation of the upper and lower tracts looking for potential stones.

A 24-hour urine creatinine clearance and quantitative MAG 3 renal scan evaluate upper tract function, whereas renal ultrasound and CT are used to evaluate upper tract anatomical features. An IVP evaluates both function and anatomy.

The quantitative MAG 3 radioisotope renal scan is used to monitor renal function and drainage. It has been found to be a safe and effective modality in those with SCI (53). Attempts should be made to obtain the glomerular filtration rate (GFR) or effective renal plasma flow (ERPF). A 20% decline in ERPF or slow drainage of the tracer from the upper tracts was found to influence the diagnostic and treatment in SCI patients (54). If the nuclear medicine department does not have the capability to obtain a GFR or an ERPF, a renal scan and a 24-hour urine creatinine clearance can be used to quantitatively follow year-to-year renal function. Serum creatinine is not helpful for monitoring yearly kidney function because it may remain normal despite moderate to severe renal deterioration (55).

The IVP traditionally has been used to visualize kidneys and ureters but has largely been replaced by ultrasound and renal scan. Reasons for not using IVPs to screen patients include potential allergic reactions, radiation exposure, and patient inconvenience (i.e. the laxative preparation required the night before the test) (56).

As previously discussed, the kidney ultrasound is helpful for detecting hydronephrosis and kidney stones. The major advantages of ultrasound are that it is noninvasive and does not involve any contrast agents. The major disadvantages of ultrasound are that it is user dependent and does not show renal function (57).

If further anatomic definition is needed to evaluate for stones or tumors, CT should be considered. It has largely replaced IVPs in most institutions. In a prospective study of nonenhanced helical CT scans versus IVP, CT correctly identified 36 of 37 ureteral stones with one false positive. CT had a sensitivity of 97%, specificity of 96%, and accuracy of 97% at detecting ureteric stones. This was double that of IVP (58).

Tests to evaluate the lower tracts include cystogram, cystoscopy, and urodynamics. Because each of these involves instrumentation, it is best to obtain a urine culture and sensitivity test (C&S), and give antibiotics if positive before the testing. There is frequently increased bladder overactivity and the potential of bacteriemia if the bladder becomes over distended. Even if there is no active infection, bacteria bladder colonization carries the risk of bacteriemia.

Indications for cystoscopy in those with spinal cord dysfunction include hematuria, recurrent symptomatic UTIs, recurrent asymptomatic bacteriuria with a stone-forming organism (i.e., *Proteus mirabilis*), an episode of genitourinary sepsis, urinary retention or incontinence, pieces of eggshell calculi obtained when irrigating a catheter, and long-term indwelling catheter. Cystoscopy also is indicated when one is removing an indwelling Foley catheter that has been in place for more than 3 to 4 weeks or changing to a different type of management, such as an IC or a balanced bladder. Cystoscopy can reveal a pubic hair or eggshell calculus that may be missed on radiography and serve as a nidus for bladder stones.

Urodynamic Evaluation

Urodynamics provides objective information on voiding function. Urodynamics in general terms is defined as the study of normal and abnormal factors in the storage, transport, and emptying of urine from the bladder and urethra by any appropriate method (31). When deciding on an appropriate urodynamic test, one needs to consider whether information is needed about the filling phase, emptying phase, or both phases of micturition.

The most common indications for an urodynamics evaluation include recurrent UTIs in a patient with neurogenic bladder, urinary incontinence, urinary frequency, large PVRs (i.e., retention), deterioration of the upper tracts, monitoring of voiding pressures, and evaluation and monitoring of pharmacotherapy. The physician's presence is important to help direct the urodynamics study. Typical decisions include how much water to put in the bladder, whether to repeat the study, and whether to have the patient sit or stand to void. Observing the patient during urodynamics also will help in getting an idea of factors that might influence the test, such as patient anxiety or inability to understand when told to void.

Blood pressure monitoring is particularly important in SCI patients prone to AD. Urodynamics is extremely helpful for detecting AD in men with SCI at T6. AD may occur with bladder distention or more commonly when bladder distention provokes an uninhibited contraction. This causes the sphincter to contract that causes a significant rise in blood pressure and other symptoms of AD. However, 43% of the men with SCI at T6 and above may have "silent dysreflexia" (elevated BP without any symptoms) during voiding. This would not be detected without urodynamics and simultaneous blood pressure monitoring (59).

In order to have an accurate urodynamic evaluation, it is important that a person does not have a UTI. Bladder wall inflammation is likely to cause the bladder to lose some of its compliance resulting in a smaller bladder capacity than normal. The inflammation is also likely to trigger uninhibited contractions and cause the bladder to be more overactive than usual. A recent prospective study found that 9.7% of SCI individuals, who had asymptomatic bacteriuria, developed a symptomatic UTI posttesting. Nearly 40% of SCI individuals with sterile urine developed asymptomatic bacteriuria post testing (60).

It would be expected that one or two doses of an antibiotic would clear the bacteria from the urinary tract and reduce the risk of an infection. However, it has been our practice to obtain a urine culture and sensitivity 1 to 2 weeks prior to the test. Those with pyuria or a symptomatic UTI are treated for 5 days prior to testing with the goal not only to eradicate the bacteria in the bladder but also to give adequate time to reduce inflammation of the bladder wall. Those with sterile urine or asymptomatic bacteriuria are given one or two doses of an antibiotic prior to testing. This is different from prophylactic antibiotic administration, in which an antibiotic is given just prior to instrumentation to prevent bacteriemia or infection.

Evaluation of Bladder Filling (Storage Phase)

The simplest type of bladder test to evaluate bladder filling is known as a bedside cystometrogram. This test is performed by attaching a cylinder such as 50 mL filling syringe without the plunger to a Foley catheter. Water is then slowly poured into the cylinder and allowed to drain by gravity into the bladder. The blood pressure and volume of fluid going into the bladder is recorded. The Foley is sometimes attached by means of a Y-connector to a manometer, which is used to measure the actual rise in water pressure. The filling is stopped when a person's blood pressure starts to rise (i.e., AD), no more fluid drains into the bladder or starts to rise back up the cylinder, or a person reports feeling full. This test can be used to evaluate sensation (whether or not a person is aware of the bladder being filled), stability (whether or not there is a rise in the column of water signifying a bladder contraction), and capacity (the volume at which the bladder contraction occurs). It can also be used as a screening test to determine if an SCI patient has come out of spinal shock. There are several limitations to the bedside cystometrogram, however. It is difficult to determine if small rises in the water column result from intraabdominal pressure (i.e., straining) or a bladder contraction. An iatrogenic bladder contraction can be elicited if the tip of the Foley catheter rubs against the trigone pressure sensors, which can then trigger bladder contractions. Most important, the voiding phase cannot be evaluated (61).

The carbon dioxide urodynamics has been largely replaced with water-fill urodynamics. Although the gas is cleaner and neater to use than water, the major disadvantage is that the voiding phase of micturition cannot be evaluated. Therefore, this test is of little use when trying to evaluate bladder and sphincter function during emptying.

Evaluation of Bladder Emptying

The easiest screening test to evaluate bladder emptying is a PVR. The PVR can be determined with catheterization or bladder ultrasound. A younger person should have no PVR; however, an elderly person with no voiding symptoms may have a PVR of 100 to 150 mL; however, it should not be used to characterize the specific type of voiding dysfunction. For example, a PVR may be normal despite significant outflow obstruction (e.g., benign prostate hypertrophy, sphincter-detrusor dyssynergia) as a result of a compensatory increase in the strength of detrusor contractions or of absent bladder contractions in the presence of increasing intraabdominal pressure (e.g., Valsalva maneuver, Crede maneuver). Caution also has to be taken in interpreting a large PVR. It may be abnormal because it was not taken immediately after voiding, because of poor patient understanding, or because of an abnormal voiding situation (e.g., the patient was given a bedpan at 3:00 A.M.).

The gold standard to evaluate bladder function is a multichannel water-fill urodynamic study because it measures both the filling and the emptying phase of micturition. Multichannel refers to the fact that each of the various urodynamics parameters is measured as a separate channel such as detrusor pressure, abdominal pressure, and flow rate. Urodynamic studies also may incorporate urethral pressure recordings, urethral sphincter or anal sphincter EMG, videofluoroscopy, and the use of various pharmacologic agents, such as bethanechol.

Pharmacological Testing. Pharmacologic testing is occasionally performed in conjunction with urodynamics testing. Lapides et al. popularized the bethanechol supersensitivity test to determine if a bladder was denervated (thereby having neurotransmitter supersensitivity). A 15-cm rise in pressure after subcutaneous bethanechol is given is considered positive for denervation (62). Wheeler et al. (63) have pointed out that false-positive tests may be due to UTIs, psychogenic stress, and azotemia. Therefore, this test should be interpreted in light of the rest of the neurologic examination.

Multichannel Water-Fill Urodynamic Study. A water-fill urodynamic study evaluates two distinct phases of bladder function. The first is the filling (storage) phase, during which water is being infused into the bladder. Urodynamic parameters that can be evaluated during this phase include bladder sensation, bladder capacity, bladder wall compliance, and bladder stability (whether or not there are uninhibited contractions). The second portion of the study is the voiding (emptying) phase. The voiding phase is considered to begin when a person is told to void. In those who have neurogenic bladders and reflexly void, the voiding phase is considered to begin when the person has an uninhibited contraction and voiding begins. Urodynamic parameters that can be evaluated during the voiding phase include opening or leak-point pressure (bladder pressure at which voiding begins), maximum voiding pressure, urethral sphincter activity (EMG or actual pressure), flow rate, voided volume, and PVR. In those who have the potential for AD, changes in blood pressure before, during, and after voiding should be evaluated.

A person should have no bladder sensation when the bladder is empty. During the filling phase, the first sensation of fullness (e.g., when a person would begin to think about catheterizing himself or herself) usually occurs with 100 to 200 mL within the bladder. The sensation of fullness (e.g., when a person would definitely catheterize himself or herself) occurs around 300 to 400 mL, and the onset of urgency usually occurs between 400 and 500 mL. There is, however, variability in bladder capacity, which ranges between 400 and 750 mL in adults. There should be little to no rise in the intravesical pressure, which indicates normal bladder wall compliance. Additionally, there should be no involuntary bladder contractions during this part of the study (Fig. 13.4).

During the voiding phase, the detrusor pressures usually are less than 30 cm H_2O in women and between 30 and 50 cm H_2O in men. A normal maximum flow rate is 15 to 20 mL/s and should not be less than 10 mL/s in any age group. A small volume in the bladder (less than 150 mL) can cause the flow rate to be somewhat slower. The flow usually has a bell-shaped curve, progressively increasing to its maximum rate and then decreasing. The urethral sphincter should remain open throughout voiding, and there should be no rises in intraabdominal pressure during voiding. As previously discussed, there should be no PVR, although PVRs increase with age (Fig. 13.4).

A single elevated PVR during urodynamics should be interpreted with caution because the patient may be nervous and voluntarily stop the urine stream. Several catheterized or ultrasound PVR tests should be done to confirm an increased urodynamic PVR. Urodynamics are able to characterize specific types of voiding patterns (Figs. 13.5 and 13.6) (61).

Special Considerations in Children

At one time, urodynamic evaluation was delayed until a child was school aged and definitive corrective surgery was to be performed. However, reflux and renal deterioration often occur during the first 3 years of life. McGuire et al. (64) reported that there was a high incidence of renal deterioration in patients with urethral leak-point pressures greater than 40 cm H_2O. Therefore, it is recommended that all myelodysplastic newborn children be evaluated as soon as possible (65).

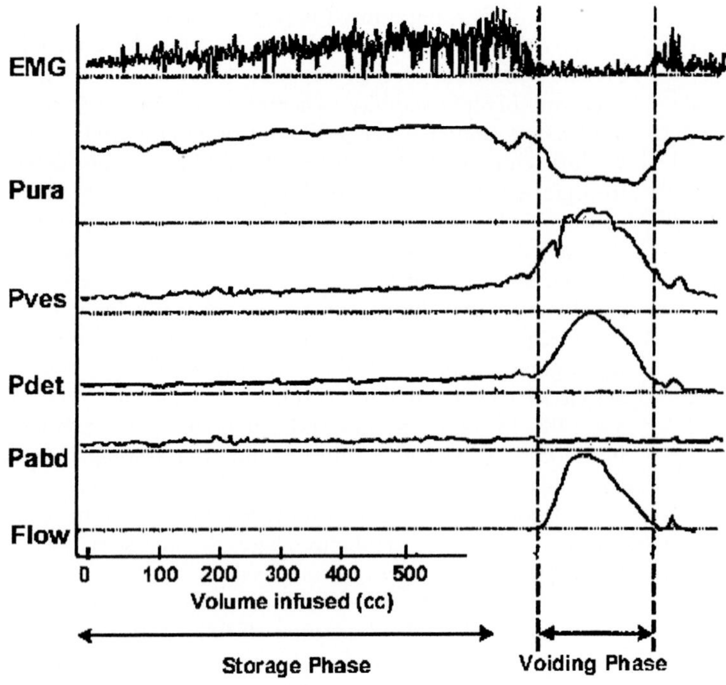

FIGURE 13.4. Normal urodynamic pattern. There is relaxation of the sphincter (Pura) followed by a bladder contraction (Pves and Pdet). There is a smooth bell-shaped urine flow.

It is difficult to obtain high-quality water-fill urodynamic studies on children younger than 4 or 5 years old. In younger children, it sometimes is necessary to use sedation or general anesthesia. It is important that children feel comfortable with the physician, nurses, and test. As a general principle, the amount of additional information gained from insertion of EMG needles usually is not enough to warrant the risk of obtaining poor urodynamics results from a crying, fearful child. This is especially true if it is anticipated that the child will come back for follow-up studies.

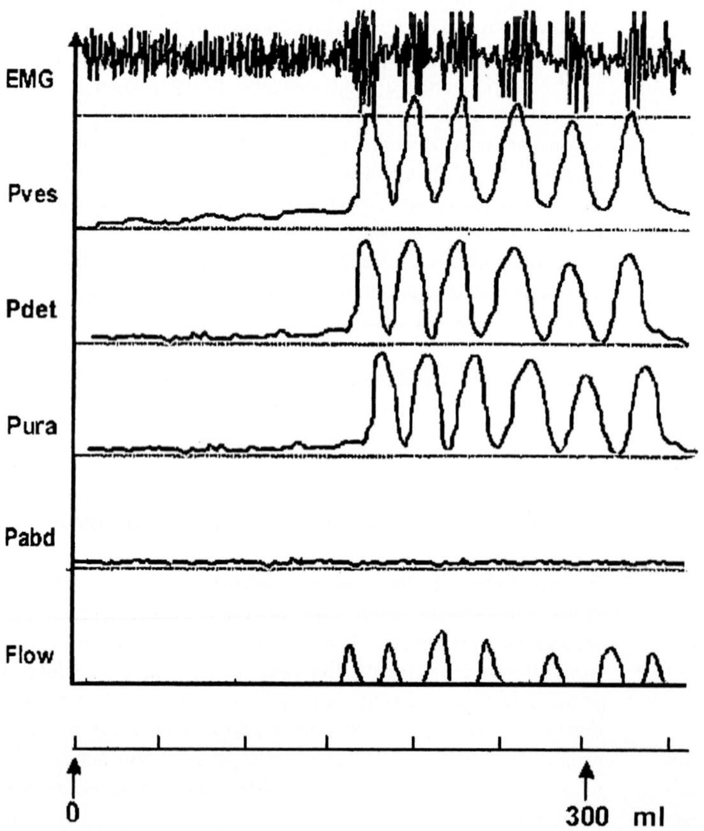

FIGURE 13.5. Urodynamics representing DSD. Note: sphincter, detrusor, and vesicle are contracting at similar times. Failure of relaxation of urethra when bladders (detrusor and vesicle) are contracting results in an intermittent urinary stream.

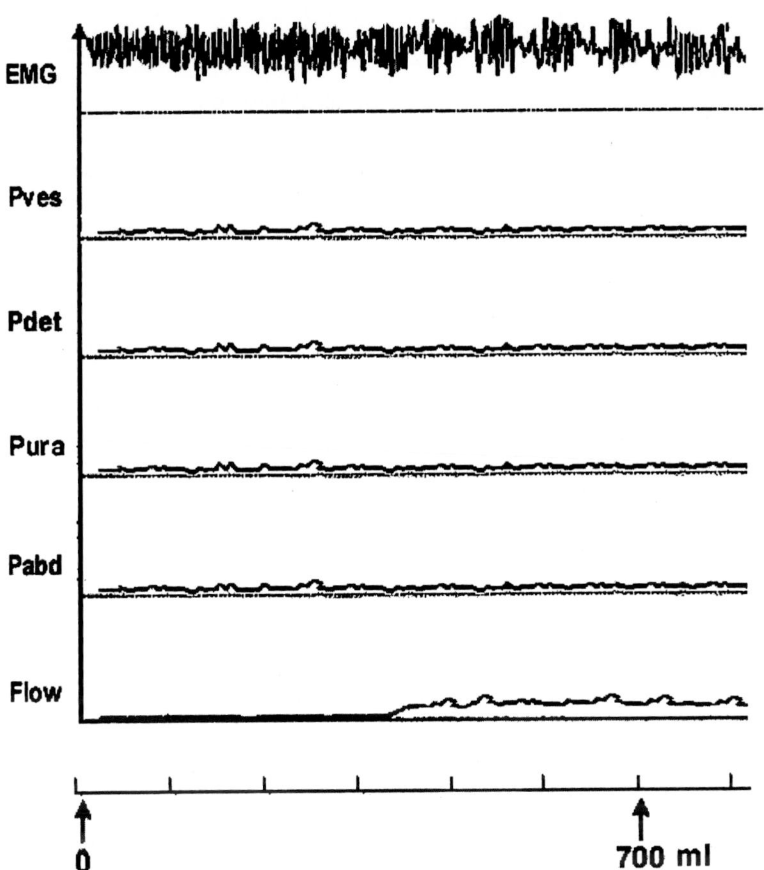

FIGURE 13.6. Urodynamics represent areflexic bladder. Note: no contractions. There may be a weak urinary stream (overflow) as the bladder becomes distended.

MANAGEMENT OF VOIDING DYSFUNCTIONS

Management of voiding dysfunctions varies depending on the type of bladder and sphincter function that a person has following SCI. This section is divided into two broad categories, suprasacral and sacral injuries. For purposes of this discussion, it will be assumed that those with suprasacral injuries have an overactive detrusor and sphincter dyssynergia while those with a sacral injury have no bladder contractions but may or may not have an underactive sphincter. It is important to realize that in reality that a person with a neurologically complete injury has varying degrees of "completeness" of injury and varying of bladder and sphincter function. Even those with the same level of injury and completeness of injury have different degrees of detrusor overactivity and sphincter dyssynergia. In addition, a person may have a combined suprasacral and sacral injury or changes in bladder or sphincter function over time. Therefore, a urodynamic evaluation is essential to characterize an individual's voiding dysfunction (50,51).

Within each of these categories, pharmacological, surgical, and supportive treatment options are discussed. As previously noted, the difference between the internal and external sphincter is becoming less distinct. Therefore, in the following discussion, "sphincter" will refer to the "sphincter mechanism," which in turn refers to both the internal and external sphincter. One must remember that bladder and sphincter function frequently changes over time.

In addition to knowing the type of bladder and sphincter function that has resulted following an SCI, a number of goals should be kept in mind. These goals include prevention of upper tract complications (e.g., deterioration of renal function, hydronephrosis, renal calculi, pyelonephritis), prevention of lower tract complications (e.g., cystitis, bladder stones, vesicoureteral reflux), and developing a realistic bladder management program that will allow a person to reintegrate most easily back into the community.

Bladder Management Following Initial SCI

Spinal shock—Immediately following SCI, a person's bladder is in spinal shock and does not have any bladder contractions. In those with suprasacral injuries, there is frequently a lack of uninhibited bladder contractions for several months, although contractions may begin as early as 2 weeks to as long as 2 years postinjury.

When a person is first admitted to the hospital with an acute SCI, there are usually a number of significant medical problems with large fluctuations in urine output in response to intravenous fluids and posttraumatic changes in fluid balances. During this time, it is best to manage the person's bladder with an indwelling catheter (Fig. 13.7). Once the patient is no longer receiving intravenous fluid, has a fluid output of less than 100 per hour, and does not have problems with orthostatic hypotension, IC can be started. IC is best started at a frequency of every 4 hours. The goal is to keep catheterization volumes from exceeding 500 mL. This can usually be accomplished by encouraging patients to have a daily 2-L fluid restriction. Sterile IC is frequently used in an inpatient setting to help decrease the spread of nosocomial infections. This can be accomplished using a sterile catheter and sterile catheter

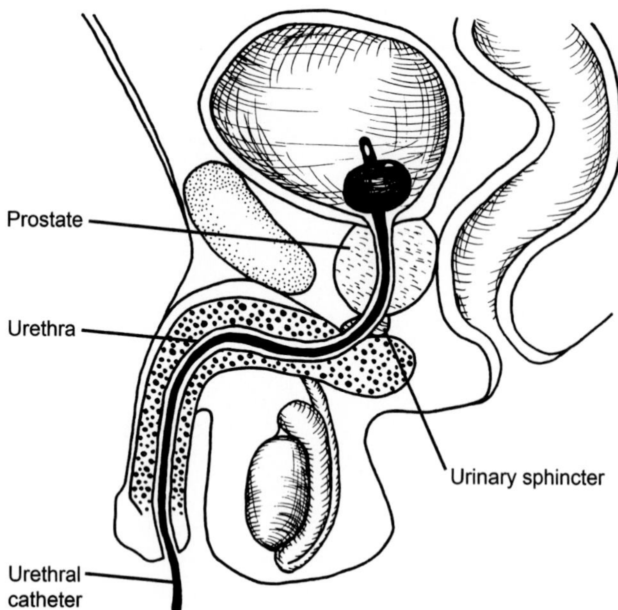

FIGURE 13.7. Example of an indwelling urethral catheter. The inflated balloon keeps the catheter in place. (Illustration by Janna Linsenmeyer.)

tray or self-contained catheter in a bag. The advantage to the self-contained catheter system is that the urine is contained in a closed system.

Out of spinal shock: When individuals with a suprasacral injury come out of spinal shock, they begin having uninhibited bladder contractions. This is called an overactive bladder. Several options are then available. Men can decide if they would like to suppress the uninhibited contractions and perform IC or whether they would like to reflexly void. Women do not have the option of reflex voiding without needing to use diapers since there is no good external collecting device for woman. Those with sacral injuries may also have incontinence but this is usually from overflow or decreased bladder wall compliance rather than from having an overactive bladder.

INCONTINENCE DUE TO THE BLADDER

Behavioral Treatment Options

Suprasacral Injuries

Individuals with incontinence caused by the bladder overactivity benefit from a scheduled (timed) voiding regimen. They are taught to catheterize or trigger a bladder contraction with SP bladder tapping prior to having their bladder reach its full capacity because uninhibited contractions often become more forceful and frequent as the bladder is reaching its full capacity. Once the contraction begins, it is very difficult to get undressed and to the bathroom in time.

Sacral Injuries

A scheduled (timed) voiding regimen is also helpful for those with sacral injuries. In this case, it is not to prevent bladder contractions from a distended bladder but to prevent overflow.

Pharmacologic Treatment Options

Suprasacral Injuries

Pharmacologic treatment is often required in addition to timed voiding in patients with incontinence caused by detrusor overactivity. An exception is a person who uses reflex voiding. In this case, the management would be directed at the sphincter.

There are currently a wide variety of medications available to quiet the bladder, which has anticholinergic effects. If a person does not tolerate one type of anticholinergic, he or she may tolerate another type. The primary action of these medications is to block acetylcholine receptors competitively at the postganglionic autonomic receptor sites. Some agents, such as oxybutynin, also have a localized smooth-muscle antispasmodic effect distal to the cholinergic receptor site and a local anesthetic effect on the bladder wall (66). Some of the more common potential side effects of anticholinergic medications include dry mouth, pupillary dilatation and blurred vision, tachycardia, drowsiness, and constipation. Dry mouth is particularly a problem for individuals on IC since they have to limit their fluid intake. Constipation is a problem for many individuals with SCI because of their neurogenic bowel, and can be a cause for AD in susceptible patients.

Newer anticholinergic agents have been developed to be more selective to the bladder receptors, have a sustained release (SR), or in the form of a topical patch. These have been developed in an attempt to lessen anticholinergic side effects, particularly dry mouth and constipation. For the SR formulations, it has not been shown whether these agents maintain their effectiveness for an entire 24-hour period, which is an important issue as those with SCI at or above T6 who have the potential to develop AD if their medications "wear off" and they begin to develop uninhibited contractions. In those with neurogenic bladders, the object is frequently to completely shut down the bladder and cause retention so that IC can be performed. Therefore, those with neurogenic detrusor overactivity often require more than the "standard" doses used for able-bodied individuals.

Tricyclic antidepressants sometimes are used alone or in combination with anticholinergic agents. These medications are thought to have a peripheral anticholinergic effect and a central effect. They have been found to suppress uninhibited bladder contractions, increase bladder capacity, and increase urethral resistance (67). There have been several reports of severe AD in SCI patients secondary to overdistention of the bladder with urine. Therefore, caution should be taken in giving these medications that depend on uninhibited contractions to void (reflex voiders).

Intravesical medications are gaining interest because oral anticholinergic medications have a number of side effects. The major advantage of intravesical medications is that there are minimal to no systemic side effects due to less systemic absorption from the bladder wall.

Intravesical lidocaine has been shown to be effective at suppressing uninhibited bladder contractions in those with overactive bladders (68). Although it has a rapid onset of action, it does not have a long duration of action. Therefore, this medication is best reserved for use in acute problems. For more long-term suppression of uninhibited bladder contractions, oxybutynin can be used for intravesical instillation (69). It not only has an anticholinergic effect but also a topical anesthetic effect. This medication is effective at suppressing uninhibited bladder contractions, but has the disadvantage of being effective for only 4 to 6 hours. We have found 5 to 10 mg dissolved in 15 to 30 mL of normal saline instilled into the bladder three to four times a day to be effective in most individuals. Since instilling intravesical oxybutynin may not be possible if a person is not at home during the day, we suggest a person substitute a lower dose of oral oxybutynin if it is inconvenient to perform intravesical instillation. One study using this dose noted in the seven men studied that there was improvement in body image and enhanced sexuality because of the significant improvement in incontinence (70). Another investigator examined 32 patients, comparing standard dosages of intravesical oxybutynin (0.3 mg/kg body weight per day) with increasing dosages in steps of 0.2 mg/kg body weight up to 0.9 mg/kg body weight per day. Twenty-one of thirty-two (66%) patients became continent with the standard dose. Seven of the eleven failures at the lower dose became continent with a median dose of 0.7 mg/kg body weight for an overall success rate of 28 of 32 (87%). Four of the eleven had no improvement, and 2 of the 11 patients had side effects with a dosage of 0.9 mg/kg body weight per day (71).

The fact that two patients had side effects at high doses suggests that there is some systemic absorption of intravesical oxybutynin. There is no commercial preparation for intravesical oxybutynin instillation. Therefore, a person has to dissolve the medication in sterile saline and instill it at 4- to 6-hour intervals. A large number of individuals abandon this because it is so labor intensive. Intravesical instillations may, however, assume a more important role of helping to control uninhibited contractions with the development of longer acting agents. Of particular interest is afferent C-fiber neurotoxins. The prototype medication is capsaicin, which is effective at suppressing uninhibited contractions for several months at a time. In a double-blind placebo-controlled study in 20 patients with spinal cord lesions, bladder capacity increased from 169±68 to 299±96 mL, and maximum detrusor pressure decreased from 77±24 to 53±27 when given an intravesical instillation capsaicin (72). Unfortunately, capsaicin frequently causes discomfort or SP pain, urgency, hematuria, and AD, which can last to up to 2 weeks post instillation.

A newer afferent C-fiber neurotoxin, resiniferatoxin toxin (RTX), has been investigated. It is 1,000 times stronger than capsaicin and is longer acting. It has an extremely rapid onset of action at desensitizing the C-fiber afferent neurons, which causes minimal discomfort when it is instilled. In a study, 14 patients with detrusor hyperreflexia were instilled with 100 mL (or the bladder capacity if lower than that volume) of 50 to 100 nm resiniferatoxin in 10% alcohol in saline through a catheter into the bladder. Treatment improved or abolished incontinence in 9 of 12 (75%) patients. Mean cystometric capacity increased from 182 to 330 mL. Maximal detrusor pressure was not modified by treatment. The effects were long lasting, up to 12 months in seven patients (73). In another prospective study, the RTX group had significant improvements compared to the placebo group with respect to the volume to first involuntary detrusor contraction (184±93 mL versus 115±61 mL (p = 0.03)) and maximal cystometric capacity (314±135 mL versus 204±92 mL (p = 0.02)) (74). RTX is superior to capsaicin at improving bladder capacity and the uninhibited detrusor contraction threshold, as well as not having the inflammatory side effects of capsaicin (75). It is our understanding that multicenter trials evaluating RTX in the United States are currently halted secondary to funding issues.

A newer modality that has been reported in individuals with SCI is the use of botulinum toxin injected into the bladder wall (76). Botulinum toxin inhibits acetylcholine release at the neuromuscular junction, which in turn blocks neuromuscular contraction and relaxes muscles that are either spastic or overactive. Doses ranging between 100 and 300 units have been confirmed by cystometry to suppress an overactive detrusor. Because it may take 1 to 4 weeks to completely deplete the acetylcholine at the neuromuscular junction, effects at quieting the bladder may be delayed. Since there is reinnervation and sprouting at the neuromuscular junctions, the effects wear off after 3 to 6 months so the injections usually need to be repeated. In addition to its known inhibitory effect on presynaptic release of acetylcholine by motor terminals, there is increasing evidence that botulinum A toxin may also affect sensory fibers. Following botulinum injections, sensory receptors P2X3 and TRPV1 were found to be decreased in biopsies 38 patients (22 with neurogenic detrusor overactivity, 16 with idiopathic detrusor overactivity) (77). A recent systematic review confirmed that botulinum toxin injections into the detrusor provide a clinically significant improvement in adults with neurogenic detrusor overactivity and incontinence refractory to other pharmacological therapy. The review points out that more studies are needed to evaluate issues such as the optimal dose, number and location of injections, and duration of effect (78). The panel for the SCI Consortium Bladder Management Guidelines lists botulinum toxin injections into the bladder (detrusor) muscle as an option for those with SCI on IC with detrusor overactivity. It is noted to consider avoiding the concurrent use of an aminoglycoside since it may potentiate the botulinum toxin (79).

In summary, there are a wide variety of pharmacologic agents that may be used by themselves or in conjunction with treatment modalities. A number of these are still undergoing investigation or used as "off label," as individuals with "neurogenic bladders" are frequently excluded from initial trials. It is important to review any relevant updates on pharmacological treatments (66–68), and when using any of the pharmacologic options, potential side effects and contraindications must be weighed against potential benefits.

Sacral Injuries

Since those with sacral injuries do not have overactive bladders, causes other than an overactive bladder should be investigated rather than only prescribing pharmacological agents to quiet the bladder.

Nonsurgical Treatment of Urinary Incontinence

Suprasacral Injuries

Intermittent Catheterization (IC): Guttman and Frankel popularized sterile IC for SCI patients in the 1960s. They reported that in 476 SCI patients monitored over 11 years on sterile IC, only 7.4% developed hydronephrosis, 4.4% had vesicoureteral reflux, 1.7% developed kidney stones, and 0.6% developed bladder stones (80). In the mid-1970s, Lapides et al. reported on the effectiveness of IC using clean technique in those with SCI. They attributed the success of IC to keeping the bladder from getting overdistended. One reason was the ease of performing clean IC compared with sterile technique, so that patients were more likely to catheterize themselves and prevent bladder overdistention than with sterile technique (81). Maynard and Glass (82) reported that 80% of patients on IC monitored for 60 months continued on IC, suggesting low morbidity and high patient acceptance.

The important principles of IC are to restrict fluids to 2 L a day and to catheterize frequently enough to keep the bladder from becoming overdistended (less than 500 mL) as this is a major cause of bladder infections.

The SCI Consortium on bladder management recommends avoiding IC in individuals who have one or more of the following: (1) inability to catheterize themselves or a caregiver who is unable to perform catheterization; (2) abnormal urethral anatomy such as stricture, false passages, and bladder neck obstruction; (3) bladder capacity < 200 mL; (4) poor cognition, little motivation, inability or unwillingness to adhere to the catheterization time schedule or the fluid intake regimen; (5) adverse reaction toward having to pass the catheter into the genital area multiple times a day; or (6) tendency to develop AD with bladder filling despite treatment (79).

Those with suprasacral injuries who perform IC usually require the addition of a pharmacological agent (see above section). This is not only to keep from having urinary incontinence but also to maintain a quiet bladder in order to maintain drainage from the upper tracts.

Use of prophylactic antibiotics is discouraged for most individuals on IC. Antibacterial prophylaxis has been shown to significantly reduce the probability of laboratory infection but not the probability of clinical infection, although a trend was noted toward fewer clinical infections. Maynard and Glass (82) reported no significant reduction was noted in the probability of clinical infection in subgroups treated promptly for laboratory infection. Of concern is that chronic use of prophylactic antibiotics will allow the bladder to become colonized with more resistant bacteria. In addition, it may be difficult to identify the type of bacteria in a person on prophylactic antibiotics who presents with a symptomatic infection. Prophylactic antibiotics have the potential to inhibit bacterial growth in the collected refrigerated urine sample even when the organisms are resistant to the prophylactic antibiotics.

Indwelling Urethral Catheterization: (Fig. 13.7) With shorter lengths of hospital stays, many people with SCI are discharged from the hospital while their bladder is still in "spinal shock." It has been recommended that indwelling catheterization be considered for individuals with SCI who have one or more of the following: (1) poor hand skills, (2) high fluid intake, (3) cognitive impairment or active substance abuse, (4) elevated detrusor pressures, (5) lack of success with other less-invasive bladder management methods, (6) need for temporary management of vesicoureteral reflux, and/or (7) limited assistance from a caregiver, making another type of bladder management not feasible (79).

A major advantage of having an indwelling catheter is the ability to have more independence. In SCI individuals discharged home on IC, the most common reason for switching to an indwelling catheter is the inability at being independent at performing IC. One study showed that 80% of those with tetraplegia prefer an indwelling catheter for social and practical methods (83). Because there is no satisfactory external collecting device for women, an indwelling catheter is particularly useful in women with poor hand function who have urinary retention and/or urinary incontinence.

A common misconception is that the indwelling catheter causes a person to develop a "lazy bladder" or forget how to void. The opposite is actually true. The indwelling catheter increases a person's bladder tone by preventing the bladder from getting chronic overdistention that is responsible for decreasing bladder contractility. For individuals who do not have a neurogenic bladder, medically justified reasons for an indwelling catheter to be in place for more than 14 days have been published (84).

Principles of daily management of an indwelling urethral catheter include encouraging a normal fluid intake unless there is a medical reason for fluid restriction; keeping the catheter taped up to the abdomen of men when they are laying down to decrease the risk of a hypospadias due to downward pulling off the catheter during an erection; daily cleaning the urethral meatus of incrustations with soap and water; preventing reflux of urine into the bladder by not raising the drainage bag above the level of the bladder; and allowing effective urine drainage into the leg bag by not allowing the leg bag get more than half full. Changing the Foley catheter every 2 to 4 weeks helps to prevent stones (encrustations) from forming on the external and internal surfaces of the catheter. These stones can block the catheter or can serve as a foreign body for the development of larger stones. In those with frequent encrustations, weekly catheter changes may be helpful. Catheter size should be limited to 14 to 16 Fr. especially in women. Larger diameter catheters may cause urethral dilatation (stretching). Health care providers will sometimes insert progressively larger diameter catheters in women who are complaining about leaking around their catheter. The larger catheter helps for a short time until the urethra has the chance to stretch to its new size; and then the leaking returns. Therefore, in women who are leaking around the catheter, it is important to identify and treat the cause rather than increasing the catheter size. Common causes of leakage include overfull leg bags or kinked tubing causing a functional obstruction, UTI, blockage from bladder stones, or detrusor overactivity. In those with detrusor overactivity, especially with suprasacral SCI, the bladder wall can develop hypertonicity from the catheter rubbing against the bladder wall provoking uninhibited bladder contractions. This can in turn cause a functional obstruction at the ureteral orifices resulting in decreased drainage from the upper tracts. Another result of uninhibited contractions is AD. Periodic monitoring with urodynamics and the use of appropriate medications should be strongly considered in these cases. With regard to prophylactic antibiotics, they are not recommended for a patient with an indwelling catheter because of the risk of developing resistant organisms (79).

Before removing an indwelling Foley catheter, we believe it is best to obtain urine culture and sensitivity tests, and to treat the patient with a culture-specific appropriate antibiotic prior to the catheter removal. This is to decrease the risk of bacteremia if the patient is unable to void and develops a distended bladder. If a Foley catheter has been in place for 4 to 6 weeks before switching a patient over to IC, cystoscopy is recommended to remove eggshell calculi and debris that may have collected in the bladder and have the potential of becoming a nidus for large bladder stones.

A concern regarding the use of an indwelling catheter has been that there are more risks using an indwelling Foley catheter compared with IC. Risks that have been described in retrospective reviews include upper tract deterioration, bladder stones, hematuria, bacteremia (especially if the catheter becomes obstructed), meatal erosions, penile scrotal fistulas and epididymitis (85,86). However, it is important to note that in these chart reviews, it is difficult to know if the indwelling catheter was inserted because of the complication or caused the complication. In a review of 58 indwelling catheter studies, it was also noted that in many of the older studies reporting upper tract hydronephrosis and renal deterioration that individuals were not on anticholinergic medication (86). It is now recognized that it is very important to relax the bladder wall in order to allow drainage form the kidneys into the bladder (79). After reviewing the literature, the authors concluded that in which patients were managed with anticholinergics, frequent catheter changes and bladder washing, and volume maintenance procedures demonstrated similar morbidity profiles to clean IC (86).

A recent prospective study revealed that in those with an SCI, there is a gradual decline in renal function no matter what type of bladder management is used. Those with indwelling catheters did better than those on IC (87). Another study retrospectively evaluated 32 patients with SCI with an indwelling catheter and 25 with SCI without a catheter. There was a statistically higher incidence of bladder stones in those with an indwelling catheter, but no overall statistically significant difference in upper tract or lower tract complications between the two groups. The authors suggested that the decision to manage a person with tetraplegia should not be based on relative risks of complications of renal deterioration. Rather, the decision to avoid an indwelling catheter should reflect patient comfort, convenience, and quality of life (88).

It has also been reported in retrospective studies that the risk of bladder cancer in those with SCI is increased in those using indwelling catheters compared with those who were not. The risk has been reported to occur after 10 years of an indwelling catheter (89). However, this comes to question in a recent study that evaluated the characteristics of bladder cancers in those with SCI. In this study, over 50% of the patients diagnosed with bladder cancer did not have an indwelling catheter. The mean length of management was 33.3 years for urethral catheters, 37.4 years for external catheters, and 24.5 years for IC. The study concludes that the neurogenic bladder, not an indwelling catheter, is a risk factor for bladder cancer. Squamous cell cancer is more common in those with neurogenic bladder. In the above study, 46.9% were squamous cell cancer, 31.3% were transitional cell cancer, 9.4% were adeno carcinoma, and 12.5% were mixed squamous cell and transitional cell cancer (90). While squamous cell carcinoma is more common in those with SCI, it should also be noted that squamous cell cancer is rare. Therefore, even though there is a greater incidence in those with SCI, the number of individuals who develop squamous cell bladder cancer is actually low (90). In a recent study, the age-standardized incidence of bladder cancer in SCI patients was 30/100,000. This was the same incidence for the general population in the area the study was conducted (91). The SCI Consortium Bladder Management guidelines recommend that those with indwelling catheters have more frequent cystoscopic examinations than those who do not have in an indwelling catheter (79). Since bladder stones are much more likely in those with indwelling catheters compared to methods without an indwelling catheter, it is particularly important to perform cystoscopy to evaluate and remove bladder stones; however, any questionable areas of the bladder can be biopsied at the same time. In those with indwelling catheters, we generally perform yearly cystoscopy of the bladder and more frequently if a person has recurrent bladder stones. (Also see Complications—Bladder Cancer section.)

Indwelling Suprapubic SP Catheterization: (Fig. 13.8) If an indwelling catheter is to be used as a long-term bladder management option, individuals may have to switch to a SP catheter. SP catheters have a number of advantages to indwelling catheters because they pass directly into the bladder and not through the urethra. The SCI Consortium guidelines recommend that SP catheters be considered for individuals with: urethral abnormalities, such as stricture, false passages, bladder neck obstruction, or urethral fistula; urethral discomfort; recurrent urethral catheter obstruction; difficulty with urethral catheter insertion; perineal skin breakdown as a result of urine; leakage secondary to urethral incompetence; psychological

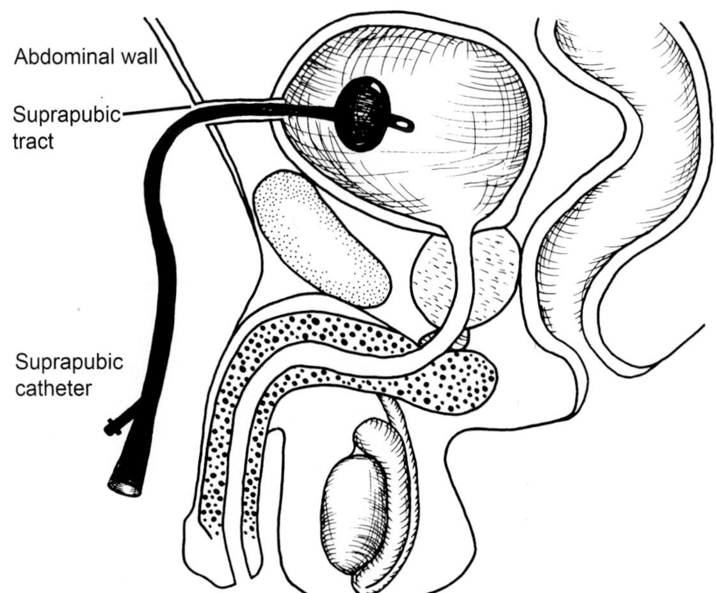

FIGURE 13.8. Example of an indwelling SP catheter. The catheter passes through the lower abdomen directly into the bladder. A tract forms between the skin and the bladder so that the catheter can easily be removed. (Illustration by Janna Linsenmeyer.)

considerations such as body image or personal preference; a desire to improve sexual genital function; and/or prostatitis, urethritis, or epididymo-orchitis (79). SP catheterization is a valuable option of urinary management for tetraplegic patients (85,86,88,92), and with the exception for bladder stones, the results of SP catheterization are comparable to paraplegic SCI patients managed with IC (88).

The principles of management of an SP catheter are the same as an indwelling urethral catheter with the exception that a 22- to 26-Fr catheter is used. The larger catheter is less likely to become kinked or obstructed. This in turn decreases the risk of bladder overdistention and subsequent AD (in those injuries at T6 or above), UTI, or possible sepsis. A SP catheter is also considered to be safer than an indwelling Foley catheter because it decreases the risk of epididymitis, urethral stricture disease, and urethral irritation (79).

Reflex Voiding: Another method of management that can be used in those with an intact sacral micturition reflex is reflex (spontaneous) voiding. This type of voiding is usually used in men rather than women since a condom catheter attached to a leg bag is used to collect the urine. Rarely, a woman will reflexively void into a diaper. Reflex voiding occurs because a spontaneous uninhibited contraction occurs when the bladder reaches a certain bladder. However, the volume that "triggers" the uninhibited bladder contraction is different for each person. One advantage to an external condom catheter and a leg bag is that it does not require good hand function. A caregiver can place on the condom catheter in the morning and not have to change it until the next day. Some assistance is needed, however, because the leg bag holds up to 1,000 mL, however should be emptied when it is half full to keep back pressure up into the bladder from occurring. Another advantage is that there is no limit on fluid intake, in contrast to those who use IC as their method of bladder management. Major disadvantages are potential penile skin breakdown and having to wear an external condom catheter and leg bag and possibly a slightly increased risk of bladder infections compared with IC.

Because men who reflexly void usually have DSD, various treatments for the sphincter are often necessary. These include alpha blockers, urethral stents, botulinum toxin injections into the sphincter, and sphincterotomy (79). These options will be discussed in more detail in the section titled "Urinary Retention due to the Sphincter." Those with reflex voiding need to have their upper tracts and lower tracts monitored. Although there is agreement that elevated voiding pressures cause upper tract problems, there is no consensus as to what voiding pressure will cause this damage (93–95). Another study revealed that the most important voiding parameter causing upper tract stasis in those who reflexly void was the duration of the bladder contraction (96). Problems in persons who reflexively void include AD, recurrent bladder infections, vesicoureteral reflux, kidney or bladder stones, kidney infection, or deterioration in bladder (progressively higher PVRs) or renal function.

Sacral Injuries

It is unusual to use an indwelling catheter or IC program, in sacral injuries because of incontinence due to an overactive bladder. Sometimes these modalities are used if there is a combined problem such as poor bladder wall compliance combined with an underactive sphincter.

Surgical Treatment Options—Incontinence Due to the Bladder

Suprasacral Injuries

Bladder Augmentation: Surgical treatment is sometimes needed to improve bladder capacity in adult patients who are incontinent and want to perform IC. The SCI Consortium guideline recommended that bladder augmentation be considered for individuals with SCI who have intractable involuntary bladder contractions causing incontinence; the ability and motivation to perform IC; the desire to convert from reflex voiding to an IC program; or high risk for upper tract deterioration secondary to hydronephrosis and/or ureterovesical reflux as a result of high pressure DSD (79). It also recommended to consider avoiding bladder augmentation in SCI individuals with inflammatory bowel disease, pelvic irradiation, severe abdominal adhesions from previous surgery, and compromised renal function (79).

An extensive preoperative evaluation is important. The history should include questions about any GI problems. Urodynamics should be performed to evaluate bladder and sphincter function. Various treatments may be needed to treat the sphincter if there is a low leak-point pressure. Laboratory work should include liver and renal function. To help reduce the risk of significant acidosis and metabolic abnormalities, bladder augmentation is best reserved for those with serum creatinine less than 2.0 mg/dL. A cystogram should be performed to evaluate for vesicoureteral reflux. Ureteral reimplantation may be considered if there is significant reflux. Upper tract evaluation is also important, both to rule out any problems and also to serve as a baseline for follow-up post augmentation (97).

There are a number of different techniques of bladder augmentation in which different segments of bowel can be used. The most common type of bladder augmentation is the clam cystoplasty. This procedure involves isolating a piece of intestine being careful to keep it attached to its mesentery, detubularizing it and sewing it onto the bladder which is first partially bivalved. Various bowel segments can be used and depend on the surgeons preference.

There are predictable metabolic abnormalities depending on the segment being used. The stomach mucosa has secretory epithelium with little resorptive function. Gastric mucosa secretes hydrochloric acid in conjunction with systemic bicarbonate release. Therefore, hypochloremic metabolic alkalosis can result if the stomach is being used, particularly if there is poor renal function. However, the stomach has the least absorptive properties and best if one is concerned about metabolic acidosis from reabsorption of urinary solutes through the bowel wall. However, this is technically more difficult than an intestinal segment closer to the bladder.

The jejunal mucosa is different from the ileum and large intestine in that it secretes sodium and chloride and may result in hyponatremia, hypochloremia, and hyperkalemia. This segment is most likely to result in metabolic abnormalities and rarely used in diversions. The ileum and colon have similar transport mechanisms. Ammonia and chloride are reabsorbed, which can lead to hyperchloremic metabolic acidosis (98).

The most frequent changes that occur include an increase in mucus in the urine, possible metabolic changes, abnormal drug absorption (especially those that are absorbed by the GI tract and excreted unchanged by the kidneys such as dilantin and certain antibiotics), osteomalacia from chronic acidosis and stones, and hyperchloremic metabolic acidosis. Long-term consequences of bowel attached to bladder are unknown. There have also been case reports of cancer including adenocarcinomas, undifferentiated carcinomas, sarcomas, and transitional cell carcinomas, in those with bladder augmentations, ileal conduits, and colon conduits (99,100).

Mast et al. (101) reported a 70% success rate at stopping incontinence (mean length of follow-up: 1½ years) and this was increased to 85% with the addition of an artificial sphincter in those with low sphincter resistance. Complications included recurrent UTI (59%) and stone formation (22%). Due to complications, however, further surgery was required for 44% of the patients. Another study evaluated clinical outcome and quality of life after enterocystoplasty in 18 patients with neurogenic bladders and three with contracted bladders due to radiation cystitis. Enterocystoplasty was performed using a 40-cm segment of terminal ileum. Their mean bladder capacities improved from 165 mL preoperatively to 760 mL postoperatively. At a mean of 36 months, 90% had acceptable continence rates and 95% reported improved quality of life (102).

Another method of surgically increasing bladder size without mucus formation and use of a bowel segment is a bladder autoaugmentation, also called a detrusor myomectomy. Through an abdominal approach, the bladder muscle is stripped away from the inner mucosal lining. Without this muscle lining, the bladder mucosa gradually stretches to become a large diverticulum, thus increasing bladder capacity. Autoaugmentation has the advantage of not causing metabolic and absorption problems as described above for bladder augmentation using a bowel segment. However, this procedure is often technically difficult, particularly in those with a neurogenic bladder who frequently have a small, a heavily trabeculated bladder and also offers only an approximate 25% increase in bladder capacity. The capacity does not immediately increase, rather gradually increases over time.

One investigator reported on bladder autoaugmentation of 50 men with neurogenic bladders. Bladder capacity increased over a period of 1 to 6 months. One patient had a bladder rupture and two reported to have "failed" due to psychological reasons (103).

More recently engineered bladder tissue, created with autologous bladder cells, has been seeded on collagen–polyglycolic acid scaffolds. The scaffold has then been sewed onto a person's own bladder in order to enlarge the bladder (104).

Urinary diversions: Another method of management is urinary diversion. Although there are many types of diversions, they can be grouped into two types: standard (noncontinent) and continent diversion (Fig. 13.9). Preoperative workup should be the same as that for bladder augmentation.

Noncontinent urinary diversion may be used as an alternative to augmentation cystoplasty or continent diversion when hand function does not permit self-catheterization. The most common standard noncontinent diversion is an ileal conduit. Ten to 15 cm of ileum, along with its mesentery, is isolated from the ileum. The isolated segment of ileum is closed off at one end, and the other end is brought out through the abdominal wall and everted as a nipple stoma. The ureters are implanted onto the side of the ureters.

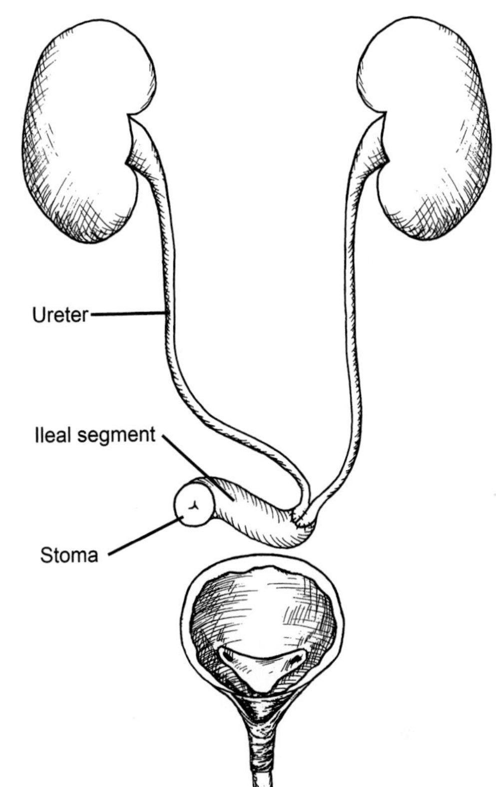

FIGURE 13.9. Example of a noncontinent urinary diversion in which the ureters are attached to a piece of ileum. One end of the ileum is attached to the skin and a stoma is created (noncontinent stoma). This type of stoma continuously drains urine into a collecting bag. The stoma can also be formed in a way that urine will not leak out (continent stoma) and requires IC in order to drain the urine from the ileal pouch. (Illustration by Janna Linsenmeyer.)

The SCI Consortium bladder management guideline recommended that urinary diversion be considered for individuals with SCI who have (1) lower urinary complications secondary to indwelling catheters, (2) urethrocutaneous fistulas, (3) perineal pressure ulcers, (4) urethral destruction in females, (5) hydronephrosis secondary to a thickened bladder wall, (6) hydronephrosis secondary to vesicoureteral reflux or failed reimplant, or (7) bladder malignancy requiring a cystectomy.

The most common reason for noncontinent urinary diversions in those with SCI is to divert the urinary stream away from the perineum because impaired healing of a pressure ulcers because of urinary incontinence, a urethral stricture or fistula. The guidelines recommend caution considering urinary diversions in SCI individuals who are too debilitated to undergo a major surgical procedure; have one of the following conditions: inflammatory bowel disease, pelvic irradiation, severe abdominal adhesions from previous surgery; or compromised renal function (79).

Continent diversions may be used in those who need to have their urinary stream diverted, but who have adequate hand function to perform IC. Continent diversions are divided into two types. The first are orthotopic diversions, in which the bowel reservoir is anastomosed to the urethra, and the second is a continent catheterizable pouch (100).

Orthotopic diversions are much like bladder augmentations and used to increase bladder capacity. Because they are attached to the urethra, people can catheterize themselves through their urethra in the same manner that they would if they were catheterizing their bladder. Continent catheterizable pouches have the advantage that the stoma can be placed in a location that makes catheterization easier. For example, the stoma can be created within the umbilicus, so that a person does not have to undress to catheterize himself or herself. The most difficult part of the continent diversion is the creation of a continent mechanism.

The SCI Consortium panel recommended that a continent urinary diversion be considered in individuals with SCI; in whom it is not feasible to augment the native bladder; who cannot access their native urethra because of congenital abnormalities; who have spasticity (making it difficult to catheterize their urethra), obesity, contracture, or tetraplegia, or who require closure of an incompetent bladder neck; females with tetraplegia in whom a chronic indwelling catheter has caused urethral erosion; males with SCI with unsalvageable bladders secondary to urethral fistula and sacral pressure ulcers; and individuals with bladder cancer requiring cystectomy (79).

The most commonly used bowel segment for this is the ileocecal valve. The right colon with or without a segment of small bowel to increase volume is used for the pouch, and the terminal ileum is used to create the catheterizable limb (97,100).

Postoperatively patients need to catheterize their pouch frequently to prevent rupture. Because there is an increase in mucus, patients are taught how to irrigate their pouch with water or normal saline. Irrigations can be decreased over time, but irrigation is recommended at least once a month as there may be malabsorption of bile salts because of the use of the ileal cecal valve. This increase in bile salts in the colon may cause diarrhea. This is best treated with oral administration of cholestyramine (105).

Long-term follow-up of bladder augmentations and urinary diversions includes regular monitoring of the upper tracts and careful monitoring of blood chemistries and renal function. Cystoscopy is used to monitor for stones or tumors (97,100).

Surgical methods also have been designed to interrupt innervation to the bladder. This can be performed centrally (e.g., subarachnoid block, cordectomy), peripherally (e.g., anterior or anteroposterior rhizotomy), or perivesically (e.g., extensive mobilization of the bladder) (106–108). Although there usually is a successful short-term outcome, decreased compliance or detrusor hyperreflexia may return. This may result from an increased sensitivity of receptors following decentralization (17). Impotence usually occurs after these procedures.

Neurostimulation: Electrical stimulation has a number of uses in treating those with voiding dysfunction. It has been used both to facilitate storage by decreasing uninhibited bladder contractions and also to improve voiding by helping to trigger uninhibited contractions. Methods to inhibit bladder contractions have had its widest use in able-bodied individuals with overactive bladders. Ohlsson and Frankenberg-Sommar (109) reported an average 49% increase in bladder capacity by stimulation of the pudendal nerve with anal and vaginal electrode plugs. Tanago (110) has reported success at selective sacral root stimulation to increase sphincter tone, which in turn suppresses detrusor activity.

In those with neurogenic bladders, investigators continue to try to improve voiding through the use of neurostimulation. Techniques include placing electrodes on the bladder itself, the pelvic nerves, conus medullaris, sacral nerves, and the sacral anterior roots. Of these, sacral anterior root stimulation has been most successful.

Brindley et al. (111) developed an anterior root stimulator that produces micturition by stimulating the sacral nerve roots. The largest experience is with surgically implanted Finetech-Brindley sacral afferent stimulator, in which there have been an estimated 800 implants over 15 years.

Sacral stimulation is not indicated unless an individual has an intact sacral reflex arc and a bladder capable of having bladder contractions (79). Stimulation of the sacral afferent nerves causes reflex activation of the efferent nerves to the sphincter. However, this reflex accommodates, so that fatigue of the sphincter occurs and the pressure generated in the urethra is overcome by the bladder contraction. A posterior rhizotomy is often performed at the same time as the sacral implant to abolish uninhibited bladder contractions, abolish contractions of the sphincter, and improve bladder wall compliance. The disadvantage of the posterior rhizotomy is the loss of reflex erections and reflex ejaculations, loss of perineal sensation, and loss of reflex bladder contractions (79,112). Van-Kerrebroeck reviewed the worldwide experience with the Finetech-Brindley sacral stimulator. In 184 cases, of which 170 were using the stimulator, 95% had PVRs less than 60 mL. There was no deterioration of the upper tracts. Two thirds of men reported stimulated erections, but only one third used these for coitus (113). Sacral stimulators are available in Europe. The FDA is currently reviewing a sacral stimulator similar to the Brindley-Finetech stimulator to be used in the United States. The Brindley stimulator is available in Europe.

Sacral Injuries

Other than enlarging the bladder because of detrusor overactivity, bladder augmentation or urinary diversion may be used for any of the indications listed above. Neurostimulation has not been used in SCI individuals with sacral injuries since they would not be expected to have an intact sacral reflex arc or bladder contractions (79).

THERAPY FOR INCONTINENCE DUE TO THE SPHINCTER

Urinary incontinence due to the sphincter may occur in those with sacral and cauda equina injuries. While uncommon, it may occur with suprasacral SCI. This is usually from an iatrogenic cause such as in those who are on alpha blockers, have had botulinum injections into the sphincter, urethral stent, sphincterotomy or females who have an overstretched urethra from a chronic large caliber urethral catheter (79). Urinary incontinence may also occur from a preexisting weak sphincter or urethral prolapse in elderly females who develop a suprasacral SCI. Urethral damage from being overstretched by a long-term large diameter urethral catheter may cause leakage around the catheter. One must also consider that leakage around a catheter is due to an obstructed catheter or overactive detrusor. Treatment for urinary incontinence due to the sphincter may be needed in those with SCI injuries if they have had prior treatment of their sphincter and want to switch to a different type of bladder management. An example would be a person who has had a sphincterotomy and wants to switch to IC or a SP catheter. Care needs to be taken trying to increase the sphincter tone in a person with a suprasacral SCI because of exacerbation of detrusor sphincter.

Behavioral Treatment Options

Suprasacral Injuries

Timed voiding sometimes is helpful in patients with mild to moderate incontinence who have normal bladder function but an underactive urethral sphincter mechanism. The object is for the patient to void before the bladder reaches full capacity. At full capacity, intravesical pressure is more likely to overcome the urethral pressure, resulting in leakage.

Pelvic floor (i.e., Kegel) exercises also may be tried in neurologically intact patients with mild to moderate stress incontinence caused by the sphincter (114). However, those with suprasacral SCI generally have difficulty voluntarily contracting their urinary sphincter. While there are no publications, there is a concern that contracting the urinary sphincter during a bladder contraction could have similar effects to DSD with the potential back pressure to the kidneys or in those with injuries at T6 and above could provoke AD.

Sacral Injuries

The above-mentioned strategies may also be effective for those with sacral injuries. As with those with suprasacral injuries, Kegel exercises usually have limited success due to the inability to voluntarily contract the sphincter.

Pharmacologic Treatment Options

Suprasacral Injuries

Alpha-adrenergic agonists may be useful at improving minimal to moderate stress incontinence caused by a weak sphincter (usually from iatrogenic causes) by stimulating the alpha receptors at the bladder neck and sphincter mechanism, thereby increasing the sphincter tone. Wyndaele (115) has reported success at decreasing urinary leakage around the Foley catheter in incomplete SCI women with patulous urethras. Ephedrine and phenylpropanolamine were two commonly used agents. Ephedrine causes a release of norepinephrine as well as directly stimulating alpha and beta receptors. Phenylpropanolamine is pharmacologically similar to ephedrine but provides less CNS stimulation (116). Phenylpropanolamine is rarely used because of reports that it may result in an increase in the risk of hemorrhagic stroke, especially in women (117).

In general, alpha agonists should be used with caution in those with suprasacral SCI because many of these individuals have overactive bladders. Increasing outlet resistance in these individuals may result in back pressure to the kidneys and in those with injuries at T6 and above may cause AD. Before medications or other treatment options are used, it is essential that detrusor overactivity or poor bladder compliance be ruled out with urodynamics and treated if present prior to the use of alpha agonists. Potential side effects and contraindications need to be weighed against potential benefits of using any agents to treat incontinence caused by the sphincter (116,117).

Bulking agents may be injected submucosally around the sphincter mechanism and bladder neck to increase urethral resistance. Periurethral collagen injection therapy is FDA approval for those with intrinsic urethral sphincter deficiency. Clinical trials have focused primarily on non-SCI individuals, but may be useful in SCI individuals who have decreased sphincter tone. In a review, silicone particles and carbon spheres gave improvement at 12 months equivalent to collagen. A comparison of paraurethral and transurethral methods of delivery of the bulking agent found similar outcome but with a higher rate of early complications in the paraurethral group. Two or three injections are likely to be required to achieve a satisfactory result (118). As with pharmacological agents, bulking agents should not be used in persons with significant detrusor overactivity or poor bladder wall compliance because obstructing the urethra has the potential to cause back pressure into the kidneys. Urodynamic evaluation is important in these individuals.

Significant progress has been made using a person's own stem cells injected into the urethra for those with weak urinary sphincters and stress urinary incontinence (SUI). One study showed the efficacy and safety of transferring autologous myoblasts and fibroblasts in the treatment of female SUI, after a follow-up of 1 year (119).

Sacral Injuries

The interventions for incontinence due to the sphincter discussed above are also applicable to those with sacral injuries. In fact, there is more use of these treatments in this group since incontinence due to the sphincter is much more likely due to sacral injuries.

Surgical Treatment Options

Suprasacral Injuries

In patients with or without a suprasacral injury, a selective injury affecting just the sphincter mechanism, such as post-prostatectomy or pelvic fracture, a surgical implantation of an artificial urethral sphincter may be considered. It has been recommended that surgery should be delayed at least 6 months to 1 year to make sure there is no spontaneous return of sphincter function. Artificial sphincters are used infrequently in the adult SCI population, because they potentially can cause upper tract damage in those with detrusor overactivity and high intravesical pressure. In addition, there is an increased risk of prosthesis infection or erosion of the cuff in SCI patients because of frequent episodes of bacteriuria. Light and Scott (120) reported that 24% of their SCI patients developed infection requiring removal of the device.

For women with stress incontinence caused by the sphincter, or intrinsic sphincter damage, such as from a long-term indwelling catheter, a variety of surgeries have been developed to anatomically improve the urethral support and position. These procedures can be performed transabdominally, transvaginally, and even without surgical incisions. One- to three-year follow-up success rates have been reported to be 57% to 91% (121). A potential problem is that the operation works too well and causes retention. Patients therefore should be aware of the possibility of needing to perform postoperative IC.

Other surgical options for those with intrinsic sphincter damage include surgical closure of the bladder neck followed by urinary diversion with an abdominal stoma that can be catheterized or the insertion of a SP tube.

Sacral Injuries

The interventions for incontinence due to the sphincter discussed above are also applicable to those with sacral injuries.

Supportive Treatment Options

Supportive options for incontinence due to the sphincter are also available for those with suprasacral and sacral SCI. Specifically, these include diapers, external condom catheters, and indwelling catheters. Diapers and external condom catheters should not be used for those with large PVRs since they do not improve bladder emptying.

THERAPY FOR RETENTION DUE TO THE BLADDER

Behavioral Treatment Options

Suprasacral Injuries

In patients with weak uninhibited bladder contractions, SP bladder tapping may be used to trigger a contraction (122). The person is instructed to tap for 15 to 20 seconds. Voiding sometimes occurs the tapping and sometimes shortly afterwards. The procedure is repeated until no further voiding occurs. It is recommended that the person taps their bladder at least 3 to 4 times daily. Individuals with injuries at T6 and above should be aware that bladder contractions and sphincter contractions Detrusor sphincter dyssynergia provoked by bladder tapping (DSD), may cause autonomic dysreflexia (AD). Therefore, treatment to relax the sphincter is frequently needed.

Sacral Injuries

Timed voiding combined with increasing intravesical pressure either manually (i.e., Crede maneuver) or through increased intraabdominal pressure (i.e., Valsalva voiding) may allow bladder emptying in those with no bladder contractions.

Crede refers to pushing down with a closed fist in the SP area with enough force to express urine from the bladder. Valsalva refers to bearing down with intra-abdominal pressure with enough force to push urine out of the bladder. The SCI Consortium guidelines recommend that one should consider not using Crede and Valsalva as a primary method of bladder management in those with SCI. If these maneuvers are to be used, it is best reserved for those who are unable to perform IC and have decreased urethral sphincter activity, such as elderly women or SCI men with lower motor lesions and sphincterotomy (79).

Crede and Valsalva maneuvers may cause exacerbation of hemorrhoids, rectal prolapse, or hernia. Increasing intraabdominal pressure in those with sphincter–detrusor dyssynergia often worsens the dyssynergia (79,123). Vesicoureteral reflux is of particular concern with these types of voiding since the pressure in the bladder is transmitted directly up to the kidneys (79).

Pharmacologic Treatment Options

Suprasacral Injuries

Bethanechol chloride, which provides relatively selective stimulation of the bladder and bowel and is resistant to rapid hydrolysis by acetylcholinesterase, is used to augment bladder contractions. A review of the literature shows that bethanechol is most useful in patients with bladder hypocontractility and coordinated sphincter function (124). Light and Scott (125) reported that it failed to induce bladder contractions in SCI patients with detrusor areflexia. Sporer et al. (126) found that bethanechol increased external sphincter pressures by 10 to 20 cm H_2O in SCI men. Therefore, it should not be used in those with sphincter-detrusor dyssynergia. It also is contraindicated in patients with bladder outlet obstruction. Potential side effects and contraindications must be weighed against potential benefits when pharmacologic agents are used to improve emptying (127).

Two investigational agents to improve bladder emptying are prostaglandins and narcotic antagonists. One study found that intravesical prostaglandin F2a was noted to increase detrusor pressures in SCI patients with suprasacral lesions (128). Narcotic antagonists are thought to block enkephalins, which are believed to inhibit the sacral micturition reflex (129).

Sacral Injuries

Bethanechol chloride and other cholinergic agents have not been found to be effective in those who do not have bladder contractions. In these individuals, the bladder may exhibit a slight increase in tone but no coordinated bladder contraction. This may make voiding more difficult if it stimulates the cholinergic receptors around the bladder neck and sphincter mechanism (124,126).

Surgical Treatment Options

Suprasacral Injuries

There have been reports of surgically reducing the size of the bladder to decrease the PVR; however, there is no effective way surgically to augment bladder contractions by operating on the bladder itself. There is a study describing the establishment of a skin-CNS-bladder reflex. This was performed in children with spina bifida who had detrusor overactivity or detrusor areflexia. The children underwent a laminectomy and a lumbar VR to S3 VR microanastomosis. The L5 dorsal root was left intact as the afferent branch of the somatic autonomic reflex pathway after axonal regeneration. Scratching the skin over the L5 dermatome was used to produce cutaneous afferent signals to trigger the new micturition reflex arc. Of the 14 patients with areflexic bladder, 12 (86%) showed improvement, with an increase in bladder capacity and mean maximum detrusor pressure. In those with detrusor overactivity, urodynamic studies were revealed a change from detrusor hyperreflexia with DESD and high detrusor pressure to nearly normal storage and synergic voiding. Changes were not noted until 8 to 12 months post surgery (130). Cloning and tissue engineering may be helpful in the future (131).

Sacral Injuries

Attempts at improving bladder emptying by performing a sphincterotomy in SCI men with urinary retention and detrusor areflexia have been reported. However, this is generally not recommended because there is a high failure rate at decreasing PVRs if the bladder does not have bladder contractions (132). There was a report of successfully maintaining voiding in 20 individuals with acontractile bladders who were dependent on IC by wrapping the latissimus dorsi muscle around the bladder, for a number of years without deterioration of upper tract function (133).

Supportive Treatment Options

A successful method for management of urinary retention caused by the bladder in those with hand function in those with suprasacral and sacral injuries is IC. In those who are unable to perform IC, an alternative is an indwelling urethral or SP catheter. Principles of management have been previously discussed. Diapers or external condom catheters are sometimes used in those who perform Crede or Valsalva voiding.

THERAPY FOR RETENTION DUE TO THE OUTLET OR SPHINCTER

Behavioral Treatment Options

Suprasacral Injuries

Timed voiding and biofeedback methods have not been reported as successful methods of treatment in patients with neurogenic DSD. Biofeedback has been reported to be successful in patients with voluntary pseudosphincter-detrusor dyssynergia. These patients, who often are children, voluntarily tighten their sphincters during voiding, resulting in large PVRs and UTIs (134).

In SCI patients with neurogenic detrusor overactivity and DSD, anal stretching or scissoring and SP bladder tapping have been reported as approaches that temporarily interrupt the dyssynergia and allow voiding (135).

Sacral Injuries

These individuals may have failure to relax the sphincter due to increased tone but since they do not have bladder contractions, they do not have true DSD. Therefore, behavior therapies directed at DSD are not effective in these individuals.

Pharmacologic Treatment Options

Suprasacral Injuries

In men with a suprasacral SCI and an intact sacral micturition reflex, reflex voiding into a condom catheter is sometimes used. However, upper tract damage or elevated PVRs can occur secondary to DSD. Alpha-adrenergic blocking agents have been shown to be effective at improving bladder emptying in patients with sphincter-detrusor dyssynergia and prostate outlet obstruction (136–138). In those with prostate outlet obstruction, alpha-adrenergic blocking agents are effective because the prostate smooth muscle is mediated by α-adrenergic stimulation.

Alpha-blocking agents may improve voiding in patients with sphincter dyssynergia secondary to an SCI due to several factors. After denervation, a supersensitivity of the urethra to α-adrenergic stimulation can occur. In addition, there may be a conversion of the usual β receptors to alpha receptors (24,26). Scott and Morrow (139) found that phenoxybenzamine worked well at decreasing residual urine volume in patients with suprasacral SCI and AD, but had variable effect on those without dysreflexia. An added benefit of α blockers is their ability to blunt AD (139,140). When deciding which alpha-blocker to use, it is important to know that the manufacturer of phenoxybenzamine has indicated a dose-related incidence of gastrointestinal tumors in rats. There have been no cases of gastrointestinal tumors linked to phenoxybenzamine in humans in more than 30 years of use (141); however, the potential medicolegal issues of long-term use of phenoxybenzamine in young SCI patients should be considered.

It is recommended to avoid alpha blockers in individuals who have symptomatic hypotension or are at great risk for orthostasis. Initiation should be at night, when supine, especially for individuals with high-level injuries. It is also recommended to use phosphodiesterase inhibitors with caution in individuals with a high-level SCI who are on alpha-blockers (79).

Three drugs that have been used for striated external sphincter relaxation are baclofen, diazepam, and dantrolene. In our experience, these agents are not as effective as α-blocking agents and should not be used as the drugs of choice for external sphincter relaxation. However, the author has noted on urodynamic studies that when baclofen is being tapered in individuals with SCI, they have an increase in DSD.

Botulinum toxin injections into the sphincter mechanism have also been used as a treatment for DSD (142). When botulinum toxin is injected into the urethral sphincter or bladder wall, it inhibits acetylcholine release at the neuromuscular junction, which in turn blocks neuromuscular contraction and relaxes muscles that are either spastic or overactive. It can, therefore, relax sphincter spasticity in those with DSD. Because over time, reinnervation of the neuromuscular junction occurs, botulinum toxin frequently loses its effectiveness after 3 to 6 months. Therefore, reinjections usually are necessary. There is no limit to the number of reinjections that may be required. In one study, botulinum toxin was injected into 24 individuals with DSD, 21 had significantly reduced urethral pressures with a concomitant decrease in PVR volumes (143). Botulinum toxin injections are especially useful in SCI individuals who have symptomatic hypotension, have adverse effects to alpha blockers, or have difficulty with compliance at taking medications. These injections should be avoided in SCI individuals who have a neuromuscular disease, a known allergy to or previous adverse effect from botulinum toxin, or are currently on an aminoglycoside (79).

Sacral Injuries

Alpha blockers may also be effective in those with sacral injuries. There is less concern about hypotension since most of these individuals do not have low base line blood pressures. In addition, botulinum toxin injected directly into the sphincter mechanism and oral agents such as baclofen, diazepam, and dantrolene, which relax the striated external sphincter, may be of benefit. As with all pharmacological agents, it is important to be familiar with any updates. Potential side effects and contraindications must be weighed against potential benefits when using these agents to improve emptying.

Surgical Treatment Options

Suprasacral Injuries

Urethral Stents, a stainless steel woven mesh stent (e.g., Urolume Endourethral Wallstent, American Medical Systems), can be used to treat sphincter dyssynergia. The stent maintains the sphincter mechanism open. Because the sphincter is not cut, the procedure is potentially reversible with removal of the stent. The stent becomes covered by epithelium in 3 to 6 months, preventing calcium encrustations. A multicenter study of 153 men with SCI revealed a significant decrease in voiding pressures and PVR volumes up to 2 years. Hydronephrosis resolved in 22 of 28 patients (78.6%) and there was no loss of erectile function. The most common complications included mild postoperative hematuria (10 patients), penile edema (2 patients), stent removal (usually caused by stent migration), and subsequent operation for bladder neck obstruction in 13 patients (144). In a 12-year follow-up study, five of the seven SCI men with urethral stents developed bladder neck dyssynergia of varying degrees, as shown on VCMG; all were successfully treated with bladder neck incision. There were no problems with stent migration, urethral erosion, erectile dysfunction, or AD (145).

Transurethral Sphincterotomy (TURS): TURS is a well-established treatment for SCI men with sphincter-detrusor dyssynergia. Indications include vesicoureteral reflux, high residuals with severe AD or recurrent UTIs, upper tract changes with sustained high intravesical pressures, and poor compliance or side effects from medications being used to relax the outlet (146,147). Perkash reported a more than 90% success rate at relief of dysreflexic symptoms, decrease in residual urine, decrease in infected urine, and significant radiologic improvement. He stressed the importance of extending the incision to the bladder neck (146). The SCI Consortium guidelines recommend that one should consider TURS to treat DSD in males with SCI who want to use reflex voiding and who are unable to perform IC; have a repeated history of AD with a noncompliant bladder; experience difficult catheterization due to false passages in the urethra or secondary bladder neck obstruction; vesicoureteral reflex; stone disease; prostate-ejaculatory reflux with the potential for repeated epididymo-orchitis; experience failure with or intolerance to anticholinergic medications for IC; and/or experience failure with or intolerance to alpha blockers with reflex voiding (79). TURS should be avoided in males with a small retractable penis unable to hold an external collecting device unless a penile implant is planned following the procedure.

Complications of a sphincterotomy may include intraoperative and perioperative bleeding, urethral stricture, erectile, and ejaculatory dysfunction. The major concerns of most SCI patients are that the procedure is irreversible, it is a surgical procedure, and they will have to wear a leg bag. The risk of bleeding from the procedure has been largely eliminated with the use of Nd:YAG contact laser sphincterotomy (79).

Longitudinal studies have shown a 30% to 60% sphincterotomy failure rate. This has been attributed to a variety of causes, such as poor patient selection (i.e., those with detrusor areflexia or bladder contractions less than 30 cm H_2O), recurrent DSD, failure to recognize the need for a concomitant procedure (such as bladder neck incision or prostate resection), or new onset detrusor hypocontractility (147). It is therefore important not only to evaluate the bladder with urodynamics but also to advise individuals there is a strong possibility that the procedure will need to be repeated.

Sacral Injuries

Surgical methods such as a urethral stent or sphincterotomy are usually unsuccessful due continuing to have large PVRs after the procedure is done (147).

Supportive Treatment Options

Supportive treatment options for urinary retention due to the sphincter either from suprasacral or from sacral injuries are the same as those for retention caused by the bladder—specifically, IC or indwelling catheters. Occasionally, a person has so much sphincter spasticity that it is difficult to pass a catheter. Instillation of lidocaine jelly down the urethra 5 minutes before catheterization, administration of α-adrenergic blockers, or use of a coudé catheter facilitate catheterization.

PEDIATRIC CONSIDERATIONS OF NEUROGENIC BLADDER MANAGEMENT

The same behavioral and pharmacologic principles discussed under the general management section apply for children. The age of the child and decreased dosages of medications need to be considered. Similarly, the same surgical procedures discussed under management can be used in children. In the past, children with vesicoureteral reflux were treated with urinary diversion, but due to long-term complications of urinary diversion and the excellent success of IC and ureteral reimplantation, this is rarely used today. Surgical procedures for children with severe incontinence include an anterior fascial sling around the urethra, and artificial urinary sphincter (120,121,148). There have been reports of 90% long-term success rates with the use of the artificial sphincter in children (148). The Kropp procedure, in which a new urethra is formed from a portion of bladder and tunneled submucosally in the trigone, has been described and may be a good alternative to an artificial urinary sphincter (149).

Clean IC has been shown to be effective treatment for children with failure to empty (150,151). It is important that children are monitored and be treated for detrusor overactivity. In one study, prophylactic use of oxybutynin and IC in newborns with myelodysplasia was found to maintain normal renal function and drainage in 92% of the children over the 5 years they were followed compared to 52% who were treated expectantly. There were no adverse effects noted from IC (150).

COMPLICATIONS OF VOIDING DYSFUNCTIONS

Urinary Tract Infections

Bacteriuria is a common problem in patients with voiding dysfunctions. Lloyd et al. followed 181 new SCI patients discharged from an acute SCI center initially with sterile urine and on a variety of bladder management programs for 1 year. At 1 year, 66.7% to 100% had at least one episode of bacteriuria depending on their bladder management program (152). Maynard and Diokno (153) reported on 50 new SCI inpatients on IC and found 88% had one or more episodes of bacteriuria (i.e., any bacteria present). Asymptomatic bacteriuria has been found to be present in 10% to 25% of community-dwelling and 25% to 40% of nursing home patients over 65 years of age (154). These numbers would be expected to be at least as high, if not higher, in those with a voiding disorder.

Traditionally, a UTI was defined as greater than 100,000 organisms in a midstream urine sample (155). The probability increased from 80% to 90% if this was found in two separate specimens. There is increasing controversy, however, about what is the true definition of a UTI. This is based on studies showing that symptomatic patients often have less than 100,000 organisms, uncertainty about the significance of asymptomatic bacteriuria and the presence or absence of pyuria, and the potential impact of other factors such as high voiding pressures, frequency of voiding, and PVRs. It has been found that 30% of able-bodied women with acute dysuria had less than 10,000 coliforms/mL and many had less than 200 per mL (156,157).

In SCI patients, Rhame and Perkash (158) reported that any specimen greater than 1,000 coliforms/mL was significant. Donovan and associates proposed that the appearance of any count of the same organism for two consecutive days was significant (159). The National Institute on Disability and Rehabilitation Research (NIDRR) UTI consensus conference based on the definition of significant bacteria on the method of urine collection and the colony count. Significant bacteria do not necessarily mean an infection, rather confidence that the bacteria cultured were from the bladder and not contamination. NIDRR defined significant bacterial counts for those on IC to be $> 10^2$ (colony forming units) cfu/mL, for those who did not use catheterization to be $>10^4$ cfu/mL, and for those who used an indwelling catheter any detectable pathogens (160). There is controversy as to whether significant bacteriuria should be regarded as a UTI or colonization.

With regard to pyuria, Stamm found that 96% of patients with symptomatic infections had ≥10 leukocytes/mm^3 (157). Deresinski et al. (161) reported that 79% of 70 SCI patients with symptoms and bacteriuria also had pyuria; however, 46% of asymptomatic patients also had significant pyuria. Anderson and Hsieh-ma (162) also found that gram-negative bacteria caused significant pyuria, but that this was not true of *Staphylococcus epidermidis* or *Streptococcus faecalis* even in high numbers.

Signs and symptoms of a UTI involving the lower tract may include dysuria, frequency, urinary incontinence, and hematuria. Unless a person has had acute retention or urologic instrumentation, fever is less likely when the lower urinary tract is involved. Whereas many SCI patients have decreased or no bladder sensation, a lower UTI often will cause cloudy, strong-smelling urine, increased abdominal or lower extremity spasticity, new onset of urinary incontinence, occasionally retention from increased DSD, or AD in those with a lesion above T6.

Patients with an acute upper tract involvement may present with any of the above signs and symptoms. They also usually will have fever and chills and an elevated serum white blood cell count. Those with sensation usually complain of costal vertebral angle tenderness. It should be noted that in the elderly, signs and symptoms may be much more subtle and patients may present simply with confusion or lethargy. UTIs should be considered in the differential diagnosis of new cognitive changes in a head-injured patient.

Treatment of Asymptomatic Urinary Tract Infection

Guidelines for treatment have been difficult to establish for asymptomatic bacteriuria because of controversy on whether this represents colonization rather than an infection. Ideally, the urine should be sterile; however, the side effects of antibiotics and development of resistant organisms need to be taken into account. Kass et al. (163) followed 225 children on CIC for 10 years and reported that in the absence of vesicoureteral reflux, bacilluria proved innocuous, with only 2.6% of subjects developing fresh renal damage. In high-grade reflux, however, 60% developed pyelonephritis. Lewis et al. followed 52 acute SCI patients during their initial hospitalization. Seventy-eight percent of patients had greater than 100,000 organisms, but only 13% had symptoms and required antimicrobial therapy over 6 months. Of interest is that 35% of cultures changed weekly from positive to negative, negative to positive, or one organism to another, necessitating a short course of antibiotics (164).

An accurate characterization of voiding dysfunction such as voiding pressure, bladder compliance, and PVRs, along with accurate characterization of level and completeness of injury often are lacking in various studies discussing UTIs in SCI patients. It is hoped that prospective evaluations considering these factors in relation to factors such as bacteriuria, pyuria, upper and lower tract anatomy, virulence of organisms, and types of bladder management will allow guidelines to be formulated for the treatment of asymptomatic bacteriuria. There is general agreement that asymptomatic bacteriuria in a patient with an indwelling Foley catheter should not be treated. Attempts should be made to eradicate asymptomatic bacteriuria in those with high-grade reflux, before urologic instrumentation, in hydronephrosis, or in the presence of urea-splitting organisms.

Treatment of Symptomatic Urinary Tract Infections

Once a urine culture has been obtained, empiric oral antibiotic treatment can be started for patients with minimal symptoms while waiting for the culture results. Patients usually do well with a 7-day course of antibiotics. In those with high fevers, dehydration, or AD, more aggressive therapy should be instituted. Hospitalization should be considered to closely monitor, hydrate, and give broad-spectrum antibiotics while waiting for the culture results and for the fever to defervescence. It is important to have an indwelling Foley catheter in place during intravenous or oral fluid hydration to keep the bladder decompressed. The author believes that it also is beneficial to give an anticholinergic medication while the Foley catheter is in place; this will decrease the intrinsic pressure within the detrusor, allowing relaxation of the ureterovesical junction and improving drainage of the kidneys. Tempkin et al. (165) showed on renal scans that there was improved drainage of the upper tracts in SCI patients given anticholinergics. Patients with significant fever should be considered to have upper tract involvement (i.e., pyelonephritis) and therefore be continued on 2 to 3 weeks of oral antibiotics after the fever has resolved. In addition, these patients should undergo a urology evaluation for the cause of urosepsis. Acutely, this should consist of a plain abdominal radiograph to rule out an obvious stone, followed by a renal ultrasound. If there is a question of a stone, hydronephrosis, or persistent fever, an abdominal/pelvic CT scan will often be diagnostic. Once the patient has been treated, it is often necessary to undergo a cystogram to evaluate for reflux, a cystoscopy to evaluate the bladder outlet and bladder, and urodynamics to evaluate voiding function.

Complications of Urinary Tract Infections

In addition to acute lower tract (i.e., cystitis) and upper UTIs (i.e., pyelonephritis), the physician should be aware of other potential problems. Those from lower UTIs include epididymitis, prostatic or scrotal abscess, sepsis, or an ascending infection to the upper tracts. Complications that may occur include chronic pyelonephritis, renal scarring, progressive renal deterioration, renal calculi if there is a urea-splitting organism such as Proteus, papillary necrosis, renal or retroperitoneal abscess, or bacteremia and sepsis.

Role of Prophylactic Antibiotics

There is controversy over the role of prophylactic antibiotics (153,166–168). Anderson (166) reported a statistically significant difference in bacteriuria in SCI inpatients on a combination of oral nitrofurantoin and neomycin/polymyxin B solution compared with controls. Merritt et al. (167) reported a statistically significant decrease in bacteriuria with methenamine salt or cotrimoxazole compared with controls at 3 to 9 months, but not at greater than 15 months. It has been found that antibiotic prophylaxis significantly reduces the probability of a laboratory infection, but not the probability of a clinical infection (153). Kuhlemeier et al. (168) evaluated vitamin C and a number of antimicrobial agents as prophylactic agents and found no beneficial effect in SCI patients compared with controls. These studies seem to show that prophylactic agents do not have a long-term effect in decreasing bacteriuria compared with controls. The role of prophylactic antibiotics in patients with recurrent clinical infections, anatomic abnormalities such as vesicoureteral reflux, or hydronephrosis is not known. Prophylactic antibiotics should be considered prior to urologic testing requiring instrumentation, particularly those with bacteriuria.

BLADDER CANCER

Kaufman et al. reported that five of six patients with squamous cell cancer had an indwelling Foley catheter in place for more than 15 to 30 years (average 21 years). Although only two of six had an obvious tumor on cystoscopy, three had gross hematuria, one had known invasive squamous cell cancer of the urethra, and only one had no signs or symptoms. Hematuria is often a presenting sign. Therefore, hematuria should be investigated especially in the absence of a symptomatic UTI (89).

In a recent study, Kalisvaart evaluated the risk factors and characteristics of bladder cancer in SCI patients by reviewing SCI patients between January 1983 and January 2007. Out of a total of 1,319 patients, 32 patients had bladder cancer. The most common histological type was squamous cell cancer (46.9%), followed by transitional cell cancer (31.3). The study suggested that it was the neurogenic bladder, not the indwelling catheter that was a risk factor for bladder cancer since 44% had a urethral catheter (mean of 33.3 years), 48% had external catheters (mean of 37.4 years), and 8% performed IC (mean of 24.5 years). Forty-two percent of the cancers were detected on screening cystoscopy. The authors conclude that urologists should consider diligent, long-term screening of all patients with SCI, not just those with indwelling catheters (90). (Also see *Nonsurgical Treatment of Urinary Incontinence Suprasacral Injuries* discussing indwelling catheters.)

There is no consensus concerning a surveillance protocol. It is recommended that those with indwelling catheters undergo cystoscopy more often than those without catheters (79). We perform yearly cystoscopy in those with indwelling catheters. While the risk of bladder cancer is small, there is higher risk of bladder stones in those with indwelling catheters. We perform cystoscopy on an annual basis on all SCI patients after 10 years of injury. This is done more frequently if a person is having a urological problem such as recurrent UTIs (see Urinary Lithiasis below).

HYDRONEPHROSIS

Ureteral dilation for any reason results in inefficient propulsion of the urine bolus due to inability of the walls to coapt completely, as well as in decreased intraluminal pressure due to the increased ureteral diameter. Over time, this may result in further distention of the ureter with eventual hydronephrosis (6,169). There are several causes for ureteral dilation. It can occur transiently from a brisk diuresis effectively overloading the ureters, not allowing enough time for individual boluses to travel down the ureter. Another cause may be a mechanical obstruction such as stone or stricture. Those with poor bladder wall compliance, DSD, or outlet obstruction may develop a functional obstruction due to high intravesical pressures. The elevated intravesical pressure increases the tension within the bladder wall, which in turn constricts the submucosal ureter as well as increasing the hydrostatic force within the bladder. Ureteral dilation will occur if ureteral peristalsis is unable to overcome these increased pressures (169,170).

McGuire et al. (64) reported that 81% of myelodysplastic children with leak-point pressures greater than 40 cm H_2O developed upper urinary tract changes, whereas only 11% with leak-point pressures below 40 cm H_2O developed upper tract changes. Hydrostatic forces in the ureter and kidneys also may be increased by vesicoureteral reflux blocking the downward egress of urine, which in turn may lead to hydronephrosis. Teague and Boyarski (171) have identified another potential cause of ureteral dilation. They found that Citrobacter sp. and *Escherichia coli* from human urine cultures injected into the lumen of dog ureters produced marked suppression of peristalsis and ureteral dilation lasting up to 2 hours.

VESICOURETERAL REFLUX

Price and Kottke (172) reported in an 8-year study that vesicoureteral reflux was one of the factors frequently associated with renal deterioration after SCI. Fellows and Silver (173) found that there was a definite association of the degree of reflux and renal damage. Vesicoureteral reflux in children has been associated with a congenital shortening or absence of the submucosal ureter, absence of ureteral muscle in the submucosal segment, or association with a paraureteral (Hutch) diverticulum of the bladder (174). In people with neurogenic voiding dysfunctions, it has been thought that high bladder pressures, recurrent UTIs, and possible changes in the oblique course of the submucosal ureter as the bladder becomes thickened result in vesicoureteral reflux. However, in a review of cystoscopic findings and in SCI individuals with and without reflux, it was found that those with reflux had a congenital posterior placed ureteral orifice (175).

Renal deterioration from reflux is thought to be secondary to recurrent pyelonephritis resulting in renal scars as well as back pressure hydronephrosis.

The mainstay of treatment in those with reflux and voiding dysfunction is to lower intravesical pressures and eradicate infections. One study found that conservative treatment with an indwelling catheter resulted in complete remission in 57.5% of individuals and a decrease in VUR in another 23.7% (176). Ureteral reimplants are technically difficult to perform in a trabeculated bladder and have not been uniformly successful.

URINARY LITHIASIS

Renal Calculi

Approximately 8% of patients with SCI develop renal calculi (177). It has been reported that 98% of renal calculi in those with SCI are composed either of calcium phosphate or of magnesium ammonium phosphate (also known as struvite). These stones are typically associated with UTIs (178). Bacteria develop a biofilm made up of sheets of organisms that secrete an extracellular matrix of bacterial glycocalyces and host proteins. The growth of this biofilm develops in a well-defined sequence. Bacteria first attach to the urothelium. This is facilitated by urease-producing bacteria, especially *P. mirabilis*, which is a urease inhibitor. This causes an increase in ammonia break down products, which alkalinizes the urine and irritates the urothelium, facilitating further bacterial adherence to the urothelium. Eventually urinary crystals such as struvite and apatite are incorporated into this biofilm, which leads to encrustation and stone development. This process is also accelerated by urease-producing bacteria, since urease alkalinizes the urine and promotes crystallization of struvite and apatite (179).

Kuhlemeier et al. (180) found that renal calculi were the single most important cause of renal deterioration. Without treatment, a patient with a staghorn calculus has a 50% chance of losing the involved kidney (181). DeVivo and Fine (177) found that SCI patients with calculi were more likely to have neurologically complete tetraplegia, have Klebsiella or Serratia infections, a history of bladder calculi, and high serum calcium values. Another study reviewing 1,669 patients with SCI between 1982 and 1996 reported the incidence of struvite stones was 1.5%; 67% of these patients had complete SCI, 5% had lesions of the cervical cord, and 53% developed their first stone greater than 10 years after injury. Only 22% had kidney stones within the first 2 years postinjury. It was noted that those with kidney stones had a higher incidence of indwelling catheters (49%), bladder stones (52%), and vesicoureteral reflux (28%) (182). Patients who present with persistent Proteus infections should be monitored for renal calculi. Urea-splitting organisms form alkaline urine that in turn causes supersaturation and crystallization of magnesium ammonium phosphate.

Previously, a surgical pyelolithotomy or nephrolithotomy was performed to remove these stones. Newer techniques, including percutaneous nephrolithotomy (PNL) and extracorporeal shock wave lithotripsy (ESWL), have largely replaced open surgical procedures (183). When PNL was compared to ESWL in treating struvite staghorn calculi, the overall stone free rate was 84.2% compared to 51.2% for ESWL treatment (184). The current AUA Nephrolithiasis Guideline recommends that PNL followed by ESWL or repeat PNL should be used for most patients, with PNL being the first part of combination therapy (185). Any of these procedures needs to be combined with sterilization of the urinary tract of urea-splitting organisms. Failure to eradicate the stone-forming organisms, usually because of incomplete removal of the kidney stone, will usually result in a recurrent kidney stone. Acetohydroxamic acid is a urease inhibitor. It works by decreasing ammonia levels and pH in the urine. Acetohydroxamic acid has been found to cause partial dissolution of struvite stones. With regard to being used as a prophylactic agent, limitations are reported side effects and high cost (186).

Bladder Calculi

Bladder stones are the second most common urinary complication after UTIs. Overall, 36% of those with SCI develop bladder stones over 8 years. These usually occur in those with indwelling catheters. The stone composition is similar to kidney stones since these stones are also formed by urease-producing organisms (187). It has been shown that bladder stone detection is unreliable using abdominal x-ray. Bladder stone detection by abdominal x-ray was only 28.6% for struvite stones and 41.9% for calcium phosphate stones (188). Ultrasound is not recommended as a modality of screening for bladder stones because it involves having to distend the bladder that may result in urinary sepsis. In those with injuries at T6 and above, bladder distention may result in AD. However, finding stone encrustation on the end of a catheter when it is removed was found to predict the presence of stones within the bladder 86% of the time (189). Cystoscopy is recommended in those with catheter encrustation, recurrent Proteus UTIs, indwelling catheter, or other reasons to suspect bladder stones not only because cystoscopy can be used for the diagnosis but also for the removal of the stones.

RENAL DETERIORATION

Renal failure previously was the leading cause of death following SCI. The death rate from renal causes was reported in the 1960s as between 37% and 76%. The use of IC and sphincterotomy has markedly reduced death from renal causes. Price and Kottke (172) followed 280 patients for 8 years and reported 78% had good function, 13% mild deterioration, 4% moderate deterioration, and 5% severe deterioration. Factors most frequently associated with renal deterioration were vesicoureteral reflux, renal calculi, recurrent pyelonephritis, and recurrent pressure ulcers. Kuhlemeier et al. evaluated 519 SCI patients with renal scans for up to 10 years. They found that factors associated with a statistically significant decreased ERPF were quadriplegia, renal stones, female patients over 30 years of age, and a history of chills and fever presumably due to acute UTIs. Renal calculi were the most important cause. Factors not found to be statistically significant included years since injury, presence of severe pressure ulcers, bladder calculi, bacteriuria without reflux, and completeness of injury (55).

RENAL AMYLOIDOSIS

Amyloidosis has been reported, albeit rarely, in patients with SCI. It has been hypothesized that this is due to the triad of three inflammatory processes, specifically pyelonephritis, pressure ulcers, and osteomyelitis. It has been suggested that amyloidosis is associated with the total mass of the inflammation rather than a single focus (190).

Amyloidosis may affect a number of organs and the clinical findings vary with the organ involved. If the liver and spleen are involved, these organs will usually be palpable. When the kidneys are involved, albuminuria has been reported as a consistent sign. Hypoproteinemia, hyline and granular casts, and azotemia are late findings of renal involvement (191). It is interesting to note that most of the publications are from 30 or more years ago. This may represent improved methods to treat the inflammatory conditions causing these disorders.

References

1. Grant JCB. *An atlas of anatomy*. 6th ed. Baltimore, MD: Williams & Wilkins, 1972:181–189.
2. Olsson CA. Anatomy of the upper urinary tract. In: Walsh PC, Gittes RF, Perlmutter AD, et al., eds. *Campbell's urology*. 5th ed. Philadelphia, PA: WB Saunders, 1986:12–29.
3. Kaye KW, Goldberg ME. Applied anatomy of the kidneys and ureters. *Urol Clin North Am* 1982;9:3–13.
4. Tanago EA. Anatomy of the lower urinary tract. In: Walsh PC, Gittes RF, Perlmutter AD, et al., eds. *Campbell's urology*. 5th ed. Philadelphia, PA: WB Saunders, 1986:46–61.
5. Stephens FD, Lenaghan D. The anatomical basis and dynamics of vesicoureteral reflux. *J Urol* 1962;87: 669–680.
6. Griffiths DJ, Notschaele C. Mechanics of urine transport in the upper urinary tract: 1. the dynamics of the isolated bolus. *Neurourol Urodyn* 1983;2:155–166.
7. Myers RP, Goellner JR, Cahill DR. Prostate shape, external striated urethral sphincter and radical prostatectomy: the apical dissection. *J Urol* 1987;138:543–547.
8. Delancey JO. Structure and function of the continence mechanism relative to stress incontinence. In: Leach GE, Paulson DF, eds. *Problems in urology: Female urology*, vol. 1. Philadelphia, PA: JB Lippincott, 1991:1–9.
9. Gosling JA, Dixon JS. Species variation in the location of upper urinary tract pacemaker cells. *Invest Urol* 1974;11:418–423.
10. Fletcher TF, Bradley WE. Neuroanatomy of the bladder-urethra. *J Urol* 1978;119:153–160.
11. Benson GS, McConnell JA, Wood JG. Adrenergic innervation of the human bladder body. *J Urol* 1979;122: 189–191.
12. Elbadawi A. Autonomic muscular innervation of the vesical outlet and its role in micturition. In: Hinman F Jr, ed. *Benign prostatic hypertrophy*. New York, NY: Springer Verlag, 1983:330–348.
13. Burnstock G. The changing face of autonomic neurotransmission. *Acta Physiol Scand* 1986;126:67–91.
14. Norlen L, Dahlstrom A, Sundin T, et al. The adrenergic innervation and adrenergic receptor activity of the feline urinary bladder and urethra in the normal state and after hypogastric and/or parasympathetic denervation. *Scand J Urol Nephrol* 1976;10:177–184.
15. Elbadawi A. Ultrastructure of vesicourethral innervation: III. axoaxonal synapses between postganglionic cholinergic axons and probably SIF-cell derived processes in feline lissosphincter. *J Urol* 1985;133:524–528.
16. Chancellor MB, De Groat WC. Intravesical capsaicin and resiniferatoxin therapy. *J Urol* 1999;162: 3–11.
17. de Groat, WC. Mechanism underlying the recovery of lower urinary tract function following spinal cord injury. *Paraplegia* 1995;33:493–505.
18. Elbadawi A, Schenk EA. A new theory of the innervation of bladder musculature: part 4. Innervation of the vesicourethral junction and external urethral sphincter. *J Urol* 1974;111:613–615.
19. Sundin T, Dahlstrom A. The sympathetic innervation of the urinary bladder and urethra in the normal state and after parasympathetic denervation at the spinal root level. *Scand J Urol Nephrol* 1973;7:131–149.
20. Crowe R, Burnstock G, Light JK. Adrenergic innervation of the striated muscle of the intrinsic external urethral sphincter from patients with lower motor spinal cord lesion. *J Urol* 1989;141:47–49.
21. Denny-Brown D, Robertson EG. On the physiology of micturition. *Brain* 1933;56:149–190.
22. Barrington FJF. The relation of the hindbrain to micturition. *Brain* 1921;44:23–53.
23. Bradley WE. Physiology of the urinary bladder. In: Walsh PC, Gittes RF, Perlmutter AD, et al., eds. *Campbell's urology*. 5th ed. Philadelphia, PA: WB Saunders, 1986: 129–185.
24. Carlsson CA. The supraspinal control of the urinary bladder. *Acta Pharmacol Toxicol* 1978;43A(Suppl II):8–12.
25. Bradley WE, Teague CT. Spinal cord organization of micturitional reflex afferents. *Exp Neurol* 1968;22:504–516.
26. Barrett DM, Wein AJ. Voiding dysfunction: diagnosis, classification and management. In: Gillenwater JY, Grayhack JT, Howards SS, et al., eds. *Adult and pediatric urology*. 2nd ed. St Louis, MO: Mosby Year Book, 1991:1001–1099.
27. Comarr AE. Diagnosis of the traumatic cord bladder. In: Boyarsky S, ed. *The neurogenic bladder*. Baltimore, MD: Williams & Wilkins, 1967:147–152.
28. Bradley WE, Chou S, Markland C. Classifying neurologic dysfunction of the urinary bladder. In: Boyarsky S, ed. *The neurogenic bladder*. Baltimore, MD: Williams & Wilkins, 1967:139–146.
29. Lapides J. Neuromuscular vesical and ureteral dysfunction. In: Campbell MF, Harrison JH, eds. *Urology*. 3rd ed. Philadelphia, PA: WB Saunders, 1970:1343–1379.

30. Wein AJ. Classification of neurogenic voiding dysfunction. *J Urol* 1981;125:605–609.
31. Abrams P, Cardozo L, Fall M, et al. The Standardisation of Terminology of Lower Urinary Tract Function: Report from the Standardisation Sub-committee of the International Continence Society. *Neurourol Urodyn* 2002;21:167–178.
32. Biering-Sørensen F, Craggs M, Kennelly M, et al. International Urodynamic Basic Spinal Cord Injury Data Set. *Spinal cord.* advance online publication, January 29, 2008; doi:10.1038/sj.sc.3102174.
33. Kaplan SA, Chancellor MB, Blaivas JG. Bladder and sphincter behavior in patients with spinal cord lesions. *J Urol* 1991;146:113–117.
34. Yalla SV, Fam BA. Spinal cord injury. In: Krane RJ, Siroky MB, eds. *Clinical neuro-urology*. 2nd ed. Boston, MA: Little, Brown & Co, 1991:319–331.
35. Rudy DC, Awad SA, Downie JW. External sphincter dyssynergia: an abnormal continence reflex. *J Urol* 140:105–110.
36. Light JK, Faganel J, Beric A. Detrusor areflexia in suprasacral spinal cord injuries. *J Urol* 1985;134:295–297.
37. Graham SD. Present urological treatment of spinal cord injury patients. *J Urol* 1981;126:1–4.
38. Downie JW, Awad SA. The state of urethral musculature during the detrusor areflexia after spinal cord transection. *Inv Urol* 1979;17:55–59.
39. Nanninga JB, Meyer P. Urethral sphincter activity following acute spinal cord injury. *J Urol* 1980;123: 528–530.
40. Koyanagi T, Arikado K, Takamatsu T, et al. Experience with electromyography of the external urethral sphincter in spinal cord injury patients. *J Urol* 1982;127:272–276.
41. Blaivas JG, Sinha HP, Zayed AAH, Labib KB. Detrusor-external sphincter dyssynergia. *J Urol* 1981;125: 542–544.
42. Pavlakis AJ, Siroky MB, Goldstein I, et al. Neurourologic findings in conus medullaris and cauda equina injury. *Arch Neurol* 1983;40:570–573.
43. Sharr MM, Carfield JC, Jenkins JD. Lumbar spondylosis and neuropathic bladder investigations of 73 patients with chronic urinary symptoms. *Br Med J* 1976;1:645.
44. Hackler RH, Hall MK, Zampieri TA. Bladder hypocompliance in the spinal cord injury population. *J Urol* 1989;141:1390–1393.
45. Sislow JG, Mayo ME. Reduction in human bladder wall compliance following decentralization. *J Urol* 1990;144:945–947.
46. Appell RA, Whiteside HV. Diabetes and other peripheral neuropathies affecting lower urinary tract function. In: Krane RJ, Siroky MG, eds. *Clinical neuro-urology*. 2nd ed. Boston, MA: Little, Brown & Co, 1991:365–373.
47. Bradley WE. Autonomic neuropathy and the genitourinary system. *J Urol* 1978;119:299–302.
48. Andersen JT, Bradley WE. Abnormalities of bladder innervation in diabetes mellitus. *Urology* 1976;7:442–448.
49. Wheeler JS Jr, Siroky MB, Pavlakis A, et al. The urodynamic aspects of the Guillain-Barre syndrome. *J Urol* 1984;131:917–919.
50. Wyndaele JJ. Correlation between clinical neurological data and urodynamic function in spinal cord injured patients. *Spinal Cord* 1997;35:213–216.
51. Linsenmeyer TA, Culkin D. APS Recommendations for the urological evaluation of patients with spinal cord injury. *J Spinal Cord Med* 1999;22(2):139–142.
52. Linsenmeyer TA, Chou F, Millis S, et al. Long-term change in bladder function following SCI. *J Spinal Cord Med* 2001;24:196(abst).
53. Bih LI, Changlai SP, Ho CC, et al. Application of radioisotope renography with technetium-99m mercaptoacetyltriglycine on patients with spinal cord injuries. *Arch Phys Med Rehabil* 1994;75:982–986.
54. Phillips JR, Jadvar H, Sullivan G, et al. Effect of radionuclide renograms on treatment of patients with spinal cord injuries. *AJR Am J Roentgenol* 1997;169:1045–1047.
55. Kuhlemeier KV, McEachran AB, Lloyd LK, et al. Serum creatinine as an indicator of renal function after spinal cord injury. *Arch Phys Med Rehabil* 1984;65: 694–697.
56. Rao KG, Hackler RH, Woodlief RM, et al. Real time renal sonography in spinal cord injury patients: prospective comparison with excretory urography. *J Urol* 1986;135:72–77.
57. Tsai SJ, Ting H, Ho CC, et al. Use of sonography and radioisotope renography to diagnose hydronephrosis in patients with spinal cord injury. *Arch Phys Med Rehabil* 2001;82:103–106.
58. Liu W, Esler SJ, Kenny BJ, et al. Low-dose nonenhanced helical CT of renal colic: assessment of ureteric stone detection and measurement of effective dose equivalent. *Radiology* 2000;215:51–54.
59. Linsenmeyer TA, Campagnolo DI, Chou I. Silent autonomic dysreflexia during voiding in men with SCI. *J Urol* 1996;155:519–522.
60. Pannek J, Nehiba M. Morbidity of urodynamic testing in patients with spinal cord injury: is antibiotic prophylaxis necessary? *Spinal Cord* 2007;45:771–774.
61. Khanna OP. Cystometry: water. In: Barrett DM, Wein AJ, eds. *Controversies in neuro-urology*. New York, NY: Churchill-Livingston, 1984:11–12.
62. Lapides J, Friend CR, Ajemian EP, et al. A new Test for neurogenic bladder. *J Urol* 1962;88:245–247.
63. Wheeler JS Jr, Culkin DJ, Canning JR. Positive bethanechol supersensitivity test in neurologically normal patients. *Urology* 1988:31:89–99.
64. McGuire EJ, Woodside JR, Borden TA, et al. Prognostic value of urodynamic testing in myelodysplastic patients. *Problems Urol* 1981;126:205–209.
65. Bauer SB. Urologic management of the myelodysplastic child. *Probl Urol* 1989;3:86–101.
66. Brown JH. Atropine, scopolamine and related antimuscarinic drugs. In: Gilman AG, Rall TW, Nies AS, et al., eds. *Goodman and Gilman's the pharmacologic basis of therapeutics*. 8th ed. New York, NY: Pergamon Press, 1990:150–165.
67. Baldessarini RJ. Drugs and the treatment of psychiatric disorders. In: Gillman AG, Rall TW, Nies AS, et al., eds. *Goodman and Gilman's the pharmacologic basis of therapeutics*. 8th ed. New York, NY: Pergamon Press, 1990:383–435.
68. Yokoyama O, Komatsu K, Kodama K, et al. Diagnostic value of intravesical lidocaine for overactive bladders. *J Urol* 2000;164(2):340–343.

69. Brendler CB, Radebaugh LC, Mohler JL. Topical oxybutynin chloride for relaxation of dysfunctional bladder. *J Urol* 1989;141:1350–1352.
70. Vaidyananthan S, Soni BM, Brown E, et al. Effect of intermittent urethral catheterization and oxybutynin bladder instillation on urinary continence status and quality of life in a selected group of spinal cord injured patients with neuropathic bladder dysfunction. *Spinal Cord* 1998;36:409–414.
71. Haferkamp A, Saehhler G, Gerner HJ, et al. Dosage escalation of intravesical oxybutynin in the treatment of neurogenic bladder patients. *J Spinal Cord* 2000;38:250–254.
72. de Seze M, Wiart L, Joseph PA, et al. Capsaicin and neurogenic detrusor hyperreflexia: a double-blind placebo-controlled study in 20 patients with spinal cord lesions. *Neurourol Urodyn* 1998;17:513–523.
73. Silva C, Rio M, Cruz F. desensitization of bladder sensory fibers by intravesical resiniferatoxin, a capsaicin analog: long-term results for the treatment of detrusor hyperreflexia. *Eur Urol* 2000;38:444–452.
74. Silva C, Silva J, Ribeiro MJ, et al. Urodynamic effect of intravesical resiniferatoxin in patients with neurogenic detrusor overactivity of spinal origin: results of a double-blind randomized placebo-controlled trial. *Eur Urol* 2005;48:650–655.
75. Giannantoni A, Di Satasi SM, Stephen RL, et al. Intravesical capsaicin versus resiniferatoxin in patients with detrusor hyperreflexia: a prospective randomized study. *J Urol* 2002;167:1710–1714.
76. Schurch B, Stohrer M, Kramer G, et al. Botulinum-A toxin for treating detrusor hyperreflexia in spinal cord injured patients: a new alternative to anticholinergic drugs? Preliminary results. *J Urol* 2000;164:692–697.
77. Apostolidis A, Popat R, Yiangou Y, et al. Decreased sensory receptors P2X3 and TRPV1 in suburothelial nerve fibers following intradetrusor injections of botulinum toxin for human detrusor overactivity. *J Urol* 2005;174:977–982.
78. Karsenty G, Denys P, Amarenco G, et al. Botulinum toxin A (Botox) intradetrusor injections in adults with neurogenic detrusor overactivity/neurogenic overactivc bladder: a systematic literature review. *Eur Urol* 2008;53:275–287.
79. Consortium for Spinal Cord Medicine. Bladder management for adults with spinal cord injury: a clinical practice guideline for health-care providers. *J Spinal Cord Med* 2006;29:527–573.
80. Guttmann L, Frankel H. The value of intermittent catheterization in the early management of traumatic paraplegia and tetraplegia. *Paraplegia* 1966/1967;4:63–84.
81. Lapides J, Diokno AC, Silber SJ, Lowe BS. Clean, intermittent self catheterization in treatment of urinary tract disease. *J Urol* 1972;107:458–461.
82. Maynard FM, Glass J. Management of the neuropathic bladder by clean intermittent catheterisation: 5 year outcomes. *Paraplegia* 1987;25:106–110.
83. Yavuzer, Gok H, Tuncer W, et al. Compliance with bladder management in spinal cord injury patients. *Spinal Cord* 2000;38:762–765.
84. CMS Manual SYSTEM PB 100-07 State Operations Providers Certification Department of Health and Human Services (DHHS) Centers for Medicare and Medicaid Services (CMS) June 28 2005. page 17
85. Weld KJ, Dmochowski RR. Effect of Bladder management on urological complications in Spinal cord injured patients. *J Urol* 2000;163:768–772.
86. Feifer A, Corcos J. Contemporary role of suprapubic cystostomy in treatment of neuropathic bladder dysfunction in spinal cord injured patients. *Neurourol Urodyn* 2008;27:475–479.
87. Drake MJ, Cortina-Borja M, Savic G, et al. Prospective evaluation of urological effects of aging in chronic spinal cord injury by method of bladder management. *Neurourol Urodyn* 2005;24:111–116.
88. Dewire DM, Owens RS, Anderson GA, et al. A comparison of the urological complications associated with long term management of quadriplegics with and without chronic indwelling urinary catheters. *J Urol* 1992;147:1060–1072.
89. Kaufman JM, Fam B, Jacobs SC, et al. Bladder cancer and squamous metaplasia in spinal cord injury patients. *J Urol* 1977;118:967–971.
90. Kalisvaart JF, Katsumi HK, Ronningen LD, et al. Bladder cancer in spinal cord injury patients. *Spinal Cord Med* 2010;48:257–261.
91. Subramonian K, Cartwright RA, Harnden P, Harrison SC, Bladder cancer in patients with spinal cord injuries. *BJU Int* 2004;93(6):739–743.
92. Mitsui T, Minami K, Furuno T, et al. Is suprapubic cystostomy an optimal urinary management in high quadriplegics? A comparative study of suprapubic cystostomy and clean intermittent catheterization. *Eur Urol* 2000;38:434–438.
93. Kim YH, Katten MW, Boone TB. Bladder leak point pressure: the measure for sphincterotomy success in spinal cord injured patients with external detrusor-sphincter dyssynergia. *J Urol* 1998;159:493–497.
94. Killorin W, Gray M, Bennet JK, et al. The value of urodynamics and bladder management in predicting upper urinary tract complications in male spinal cord injury patients. *Paraplegia* 1992;30:437–441.
95. Gerridzen RG, Thijssen AM, Dehoux E. Risk factors for upper tract deterioration in chronic spinal cord injury patients. *J Urol* 1992;147:416–418.
96. Linsenmeyer TA, Bagaria SP, Gendron B. The impact of urodynamic parameters on the upper tracts of spinal cord injured men who void reflexly. *J Spinal Cord Med* 1998;21:15–20.
97. Gray GJ, Yang C. Surgical procedures of the bladder after spinal cord injuries. *Top Spinal Cord Med* 2000;11:61–69.
98. MacDougal WS. Metabolic and neuromechanical problems of urinary intestinal diversions. In Walsh PC, Retik AB, Vaughan ED, Wein AJ, eds. *Campbells urology*. 8th ed. Philadelphia, PA: WB Saunders Co., 2002;3777–3783.
99. Golomb J, Klutke CG, Lewin KJ, et al. Bladder neoplasms associated with augmentation cystoplasty: report of 2 cases and literature review. *J Urol* 1989;142:377–380.
100. Stein JP, Skinner D. Techniques of orthotopic bladder substitutes. In: Walsh PC, Retik AB, Vaughan ED, et al., eds. *Campbells urology*, 8th ed, Philadelphia, PA: WB Saunders Co., 2002:3849–3851.
101. Mast P, Hoebeke P, Wyndaele JJ, et al. Experience with augmentation cystoplasty: a review. *Paraplegia* 1995;33:560–564.

102. Kuo HC. Clinical outcomes and quality of life after enterocystoplasty for contracted bladders. *Urol Int* 1997;58:160–165.
103. Stohrer M, Kramer G, Gopel M, et al. Bladder autoaugmentation in adult patients with neurogenic voiding dysfunction. *Spinal Cord* 1997;35:456–462.
104. Atala A, Bauer SB, Soker S, et al. Tissue-engineered autologous bladders for patients needing cystoplasty. *Lancet* 2006;367:1241–1246.
105. Anderson B, Mitchell M. Management of electrolyte disturbances following urinary diversion and bladder augmentation. *AUA News* 2000;5:1–7.
106. Misak SJ, Bunts RC, Ulmer JL, Eagles WM. Nerve interruption procedures in the urologic management of paraplegic patients. *J Urol* 1962;88:392.
107. Leach GE, Goldman D, Raz S. Surgical treatment of detrusor hyperreflexia. In: Raz S, ed. *Female urology*. Philadelphia, PA: WB Saunders, 1983:326–334.
108. Hodgkinson CP, Drukker BH. Infravesical nerve resection for detrusor dyssynergia: the Ingelman-Sundberg operation. *Acta Obstet Gynecol Scand* 1977;56: 401–408.
109. Ohlsson BL, Frankenberg-Sommar S. Effects of external and direct pudendal nerve 110 maximal electrical stimulation in the treatment of the uninhibited overactive bladder. *Br J Urol* 1989;64:374–380.
110. Tanago EA. Concepts of neuromodulation. *Neurourol Urodyn* 1993;12:497–498.
111. Brindley GS, Polkey CE, Rushton DN. Sacral anterior root stimulator for bladder control in paraplegia. *Paraplegia* 1982;20:365–381.
112. Creasey GH, Bodner DR. Review of sacral electrical stimulation in the management of the neurogenic bladder. *NeuroRehabilitation* 1994;4:266–274.
113. Van Kerrebroeck PEV. World wide experience with the Finetech-Brindley sacral anterior root stimulator. *Neurourol Urodyn* 1993;12:497–503.
114. Kegel AH. Progressive resistance exercises in the functional restoration of the perineal muscles. *Am J Obstet Gynecol* 1948;56:238–248.
115. Wyndaele JJ. Pharmacotherapy for urinary bladder dysfunction in spinal cord injury patients. *Paraplegia* 1990;28:146–150.
116. Hoffman BB, Lefkowitz RJ. Catecholamines and sympathomimetic drugs. In: Gillman AG, Rall TW, Nies AS, et al., eds. *Goodman and Gilman's the pharmacological basis of therapeutics*. 8th ed. New York, NY: Pergamon Press, 1990:187–220.
117. Kernan WN, Viscoli CM, Brass LM, et al. Phenylpropanolamine and the risk of hemorrhagic stroke. *N Engl J Med* 2000;343:1826.
118. Pickard R, Reaper J, Wyness L, et al. Periurethral injection therapy for urinary incontinence in women. *Cochrane Database Syst Rev*. 2003;(2):CD003881.
119. Mitterberger M, Marksteiner R, Margreiter E, et al. Autologous myoblasts and fibroblasts for female stress incontinence: a 1-year follow-up in 123 patients. *BJU Int* 2007;100:1081–1085.
120. Light JK, Scott FB. Use of the artificial urinary sphincter in spinal cord injury patients. *J Urol* 1983;130: 1127–1129.
121. Kelly MJ, Leach GE. Long term results of bladder neck suspension procedures. *Probl Urol* 1991;5:94–105.
122. Opitz JL. Treatment of voiding dysfunction in spinal cord injured patients: bladder retraining. In: Barrett DM, Wein AJ, eds. *Controversies in neuro-urology*. New York, NY: Churchill-Livingston, 1984:437–451.
123. Barbalias GA, Klauber GT, Blaivas JG. Critical evaluation of the Crede maneuver: a urodynamic study of 207 patients. *J Urol* 1983;130:720–723.
124. Finkbeiner AE. Is bethanechol chloride clinically effective in promoting bladder emptying? A literature review. *J Urol* 1985;134:443–449.
125. Light KJ, Scott FB. Bethanechol chloride and the traumatic cord bladder. *J Urol* 1982;128:85–87.
126. Sporer A, Leyson JFJ, Martin BF. Effects of bethanechol chloride on the external urethral sphincter in spinal cord injury patients. *J Urol* 1978;120:62–66.
127. Taylor P. Cholinergic agonists. In: Gilman AC, Rall TW, Nies AS, et al., eds. *Goodman and Gilman's the pharmacological basis of therapeutics*. 8th ed. New York, NY: Pergamon Press, 1990:122–130.
128. Vaidyanathan S, Rao MS, Mapa MK, et al. Study of intravesical instillation of 1A(*s*)-15 methy prostaglandin F_2 in patients with neurogenic bladder dysfunction. *J Urol* 1981;126:81–85.
129. Booth AM, Hisamitsu T, Kawatani M, et al. Regulation of urinary bladder capacity by endogenous opioid peptides. *J Urol* 1985;133:339–342.
130. Xiao C, Du M, Li B, et al. An artificial somatic-autonomic reflex pathway procedure for bladder control in children with spina bifida. *J Urol* 2005;173(6):2112–2116.
131. Wood D. Southgate current status of tissue engineering in urology. *Curr Opin Urol* 2008;18(6):564–569.
132. Lockhart JL, Vorstman B, Weinstein D, et al. Sphincterotomy failure in neurogenic bladder disease. *J Urol* 1986;135:86–89.
133. Ninkovic M, Stenzl A, Schwabegger A, et al. Free neurovascular transfer of latisstmus dorsi muscle for the treatment of bladder acontractility: II. Clinical results. *J Urol* 2003;169(4):1379–1383.
134. Maizels M, King LR, Firlit CR. Urodynamic biofeedback: a new approach to treat vesical sphincter dyssynergia. *J Urol* 1979;122:205–209.
135. Kiviat MD, Zimmermann TA, Donovan WH. Sphincter stretch: new technique resulting in continence and complete voiding in paraplegics. *J Urol* 1975;114:895–897.
136. Lepor H. Alpha blockers for the treatment of benign prostatic hypertrophy. *Probl Urol* 1991;5:419–429.
137. Scott MB, Morrow JW. Phenoxybenzamine in neurogenic bladder dysfunction after spinal cord injury: I. Voiding dysfunction. *J Urol* 1978;119:480–482.
138. Lepor H, Gup DI, Baumann M, et al. Laboratory assessment of terazosin and alpha 1 blockade in prostatic hyperplasia. *Urology* 1988;32(Suppl 6):21–26.
139. Scott MB, Morrow JW. Phenoxybenzamine in neurogenic bladder dysfunction after spinal cord injury: II. Autonomic dysreflexia. *J Urol* 1978;119:483–484.
140. Hoffman BB, Lefkowitz RJ. Adrenergic receptor antagonists. In: Gilman AG, Rall TW, Nies AS, et al., eds. *Goodman and Gilman's the pharmacological basis of therapeutics*. 8th ed. New York, NY: Pergamon Press, 1990:221–243.
141. Wein AJ. Prazosin in the treatment of prostatic obstruction: a placebo controlled study (editorial comment). *J Urol* 1989;141:693.

142. Dykstra DD, Sidi AA, Scott AB, et al. Effects of botulinum A toxin on detrusor sphincter dyssynergia in spinal cord injury patients. *J Urol* 1988;139:919–922.
143. Schurch B, Hauri B, Rodic A, et al. Botulinum-A toxin as a treatment of detrusor sphincter dyssynergia: a prospective study in 24 spinal cord injury patients. *J Urol* 1996;155:1023–1029.
144. Chancellor MB, Rivas DA, Linsenmeyer T, et al. Multicenter trial in North America of Urolume urinary sphincter prosthesis. *J Urol* 1994;152:924–930.
145. Hamid R, Arya M, Patel HR, et al. The mesh wallstent in the treatment of detrusor external sphincter dyssynergia in men with spinal cord injury: a 12-year follow-up. *BJU Int* 2003;91:51–53.
146. Perkash I. Modified approach to sphincterotomy in spinal cord injury patients. *Paraplegia* 1976;13:247–260.
147. Yang CC, Mayo ME. External sphincterotomy; long term follow up. *Neurourol Urodyn* 1995;14:25–31.
148. Bosco PJ, Bauer SB, Colodny AH, et al. The long term results of artificial sphincters in children. *J Urol* 1991;146:396–399.
149. Parres JA, Kropp KA. Urodynamic evaluation of the continence mechanism following urethral lengthening: reimplantation and enterocystoplasty. *J Urol* 1991;146:535–538.
150. Nabet G, Kasabian MD; Stuart B, et al. The prophylactic value of clean intermittent catheterization and anticholinergic medication in newborns and infants with myelodysplasia at risk of developing urinary tract deterioration. *Am J Dis Child* 1992;146:840–843..
151. Enrile BG, Crooks KK. Clean intermittent catheterization in children with myelodysplasia. *Clin Pediatr* 1980;19:743–745.
152. Lloyd LK, Kuhlemeier KV, Fine PR, et al. Initial bladder management in spinal cord injury: does it make a difference? *J Urol* 1986;135:523–527.
153. Maynard FM, Diokno AC. Urinary infection and complications during clean intermittent catheterization following spinal cord injury. *J Urol* 1984;132:943–946.
154. Romano JM, Kaye D. UTI in the elderly: common yet atypical. *Geriatrics* 1981;36:113–120.
155. Kass EH. The role of asymptomatic bacteriuria in the pathogenesis of pyelonephritis. In: Quinn EL, Kass EH, eds. *Biology of pyelonephritis*. Boston, MA: Little, Brown & Co, 1960:399–418.
156. Stamey TA. Recurrent urinary tract infections in female patients: an overview of management and treatment. *Rev Infect Dis* 1987; 9(Suppl 2):S195–S210.
157. Stamm WE, Counts GW, Running KR, et al. Diagnosis of coliform infection in acutely dysuric women. *N Engl J Med* 1982;307:463–468.
158. Rhame FS, Perkash I. Urinary tract infections occurring in recent spinal cord injury patients on intermittent catheterization. *J Urol* 1979;122:669–673.
159. Donovan WH, Stolov WC, Clowers DE, et al. Bacteriuria during intermittent catheterization following spinal cord injury. *Arch Phys Med Rehabil* 1978;59:351–357.
160. National Institute on Disabilities and Rehabilitation Research. The prevention and management of urinary tract infections among people with spinal cord injuries; Consensus Conference Statement. January 27–29, 1992. *J Am Paraplegia Soc* 1992;15:194–204.
161. Deresinski SC, Perkash I. Urinary tract infections in male spinal cord injured patients: part 2. Diagnostic value of symptoms and of quantitative urinalysis. *J Am Paraplegia Soc* 1985;8:7–10.
162. Anderson RU, Hsieh-ma ST. Association of bacteriuria and pyuria during intermittent catheterization after spinal cord injury. *J Urol* 1983;130:299–301.
163. Kass EJ, Koff SA, Diokno AC, et al. The significance of bacilluria in children on long term intermittent catheterization. *J Urol* 1981;126:223–225.
164. Lewis RI, Carrion HM, Lockhart JL, et al. Significance of asymptomatic bacteriuria in neurogenic bladder disease. *Urology* 1984;23:343–347.
165. Tempkin A, Sullivan G, Paldi J, et al. Radioisotope renography in spinal cord injury. *J Urol* 1985;133:228–230.
166. Anderson RU. Non sterile intermittent catheterization with antibiotic prophylaxis in the acute spinal cord injured male patient. *J Urol* 1980;124:392–394.
167. Merritt JLM, Erickson RP, Opitz JL. Bacteriuria during follow up in patients with spinal cord injury: Part II. efficacy of antimicrobial suppressants. *Arch Phys Med Rehabil* 1982;63:413–415.
168. Kuhlemeier KV, Stover SL, Lloyd LK. Prophylactic antibacterial therapy for preventing urinary tract infections in spinal cord injury patients. *J Urol* 1985;134:514–517.
169. Gillenwater JY. Hydronephrosis. In: Gillenwater JY, Grayhack JT, Howards SS, et al., eds. *Adult and pediatric urology*. 2nd ed. St. Louis, MO: Mosby Year Book, 1991:789–813.
170. Staskin DR. Hydroureteronephrosis after spinal cord injury. *Urol Clin North Am* 1991;18:309–316.
171. Teague N, Boyarsky S. Further effects of coliform bacteria on ureteral peristalsis. *J Urol* 1968;99:720–724.
172. Price M, Kottke FJ. Renal function in patients with spinal cord injury: the eighth year of a ten year continuing study. *Arch Phys Med Rehabil* 1975;56:76–79.
173. Fellows GJ, Silver JR. Long term follow up of paraplegic patients with vesico-ureteric reflux. *Paraplegia* 1976;14:130–134.
174. Winberg J. Urinary tract infections in infants and children. In: Walsh PC, Gittes RF, Perlmutter AD, et al., eds. *Campbell's urology*. 5th ed. Philadelphia, PA: WB Saunders, 1986:848–867.
175. Linsenmeyer TA, House JG, Mills SR. The role of abnormal congenitally displaced ureteral orifices in causing reflux following spinal cord injury, *J Spinal Cord Med* 2004;27(2):116–119.
176. Ponce Diaz-Reixa J, Sanchez Rod riguez-Losada J, Alvarez Castello L, et al. Vesicoureteral reflex in spinal cord injured patients. Treatment results and stastical analysis. *Actas Urol Esp* 2007;31(4):366–371.
177. DeVivo MJ, Fine PR. Predicting renal calculus occurrence in spinal cord injury patients. *Arch Phys Med Rehabil* 1986;67:722–725.
178. Burr RG. Urinary calculi composition in patients with spinal cord lesions. *Arch Phys Med Rehabil* 1978;59:84–87.
179. Griffith DP, Osborne CA. Infection(urease) stones. *Miner Electrolyte Metab* 1987;13:278–285.
180. Kuhlemeier KV, Lloyd LK, Stover SL. Long term followup of renal function after spinal cord injury. *J Urol* 1985;134:510–513.

181. Singh M, Chapman R, Tresidder GC, et al. Fate of unoperated staghorn calculus. *Br J Urol* 1973;45:581–585.
182. Donnellan SM, Bolton DM. The impact of contemporary bladder management techniques on struvite calculi associated with spinal cord injury. *BJU Int* 1999;84(3): 280–285.
183. Irwin PP, Evans C, Chawla JC, et al. Stone surgery in the spinal patient. *Paraplegia* 1991;29:161–166.
184. Lam HS, Lingman JE, Barron M, et al. Staghorn calculi:analysis of treatment results between initial pericutaneous nephrolithotomy and extra corporeal shock lithotripsy momotherapy with reference to stone surface area. *J Urol* 1992;147:1219–1225.
185. Preminger GM, Assimos DG, Lingeman JE, et al. AUA Nephrolithiasis Guideline Panel. AUA guideline on management of staghorn calculi: diagnosis and treatment recommendations. *J Urol* 2005;173:1991–2000.
186. Peterson CM. Partial dissolution of struvite calculus with oral acetohydroxamic acid. *Urology* 1983;22: 410–412.
187. DeVivo MJ, Fine PR, Cutter GR, et al. The risk of bladder calculi in patients with spinal cord injuries. *Arch Intern Med* 1985;145:428–430.
188. Linsenmeyer MA, Linsenmeyer TA. Accuracy of detecting bladder stones bases on abdominal x ray. *J Spinal Cord Med* 2004;27:438–442.
189. Linsenmeyer MA, Linsenmeyer TA. Accuracy of predicting bladder stones based on catheter encrustation in individuals with spinal cord injury. *J Spinal Cord Med* 2006;29:402–405.
190. Newman W, Jacobson AS. Paraplegia and secondary amyloidosis. Report of six cases. *Am J Med* 1953;15:216–222.
191. Thompson C, Rice M. Secondary amyloidosis in spinal cord injury. *Ann Internal Med* 1949;31(6):1057–1065.
192. Cengiz K. Uncommon Aetiology in renal amyloidosis. *Acta Clinica Belgica* 2005;59:109–113.
193. Lindermann RD, Scheer RLM, Raisz LG. Renal Amyloidosis. *Ann Internal Med* 1961;54:883.
194. Dikman HS, Kahn T, Gribetz D, et al. Resolution of renal amyloidosis. *Am J Med* 1977;63:430–433.

CHAPTER 14 ■ PRESSURE ULCERS AND SPINAL CORD INJURY

STEVEN KIRSHBLUM, KEVIN O'CONNOR, AND CONCHITA Q. RADER

INTRODUCTION

Despite advances in health care, pressure ulcers (PrUs) remain one of the most common and serious complications of spinal cord injury (SCI). Persons with SCI are vulnerable immediately after injury affecting initial rehabilitation and throughout their lifetime. PrUs can interfere with mobility and community reintegration, can lead to a loss of independence and more serious medical complications, and result in profound psychosocial consequences that may impact quality of life (1,2). It has been estimated that PrUs can account for approximately one fourth of the cost of care for individuals with SCI. It is therefore of paramount importance that health care providers who serve this population understand the pathophysiology, prevention, and management principles of PrUs.

PATHOPHYSIOLOGY

The National Pressure Ulcer Advisory Panel (NPUAP) defines a PrU as a localized injury to the skin and/or underlying tissue usually over a bony prominence, as a result of pressure or pressure in combination with shear and/or friction (3,4). A number of contributing or confounding factors are also associated with PrUs; the significance of these factors is yet to be elucidated. Other terms used include decubitus ulcers, ischemic ulcers, bed sores, or skin sores, although the preferred term is PrUs.

The primary factors leading to PrUs include pressure (applied for a prolonged period of time over bony prominences) and shear. External pressure in excess of capillary closing pressure for a period of time will produce ischemia in underlying tissue that can ultimately lead to tissue necrosis (5–7). This pressure, first quantified by Landis to be 32 mm Hg (8), has been used as the standard for judging efficacy. However, more recent studies have shown that lower pressures can occlude capillaries in elderly and debilitated individuals, and the capillary closing pressure can vary widely over different sites of the body (9,10).

There are three other contributing factors for PrU development: intensity, duration, and tissue tolerance. There is an inverse relationship between pressure and the duration of the pressure necessary to cause ulceration (11). Intense pressure applied for a short duration can be as damaging as lower intensity pressure for extended periods (12,13). In order to prevent PrUs, pressure must be relieved frequently as well as reduced at the surface-skin interface. Based on these studies, the clinical practice of weight shifting while sitting and the use of 2-hour bed-turning regimen to provide pressure relief are utilized (14,15). If pressure is relieved by shifting the body's weight, blood flows back into the tissue again, and the area becomes hyperemic. This phenomenon is called reactive hyperemia, because a bright red flush appears as the body attempts to flood the starved tissue with oxygen. This protective mechanism of local vasodilatation is a naturally occurring compensatory response to temporary ischemia. If the pressure-time threshold has been exceeded, damage continues to occur even after relief of the pressure (16).

The concept of tissue tolerance was initially described by Husain (17) and further studied by others (18,19), who found that muscle tissue is much more sensitive to the effects of pressure than is skin. When pressure is placed on a body surface, the greatest pressure is to the tissues overlying the bone. The pressure is distributed in a cone-like fashion, with the base of the cone on the underlying body surface. Ulcer presentations often reflect this concept when they appear with a small skin defect and a larger area at the base of a deep ulcer (1). When muscle is damaged without skin breakdown, a second application of less pressure and less time is needed to result in an ulcer. Clinically, at the first sign of skin impairment or blanchable hyperemia, pressure must be relieved to allow for tissue recovery.

Shear, the other primary cause of PrUs, is the application of force tangential to the skin surface and occurs when the skin remains stationary and the underlying tissue shifts (Fig. 14.1). Reichel (20) found that shearing forces cause the perforating arteries to become angulated disrupting the supply of blood. Shear, combined with pressure, can lower the threshold for skin ulceration sixfold (21). In its mildest form, shear causes skin tears, abrasions limited to the epidermal and dermal layers. Skin tears can result from varied activities, including grasping an extremity, transferring, bathing, and dressing (22). Common other causes of shearing include sitting in the semi-recumbent position, spasticity, and sliding rather than lifting during transfers.

Other Risk Factors

Pressure ulcer formation is a complex process that is still not fully understood. While the amount, duration, and frequency of the applied pressure, the soft tissue's response to loading, and the role of shear and/or friction are considered causative, individual patient characteristics may also influence their

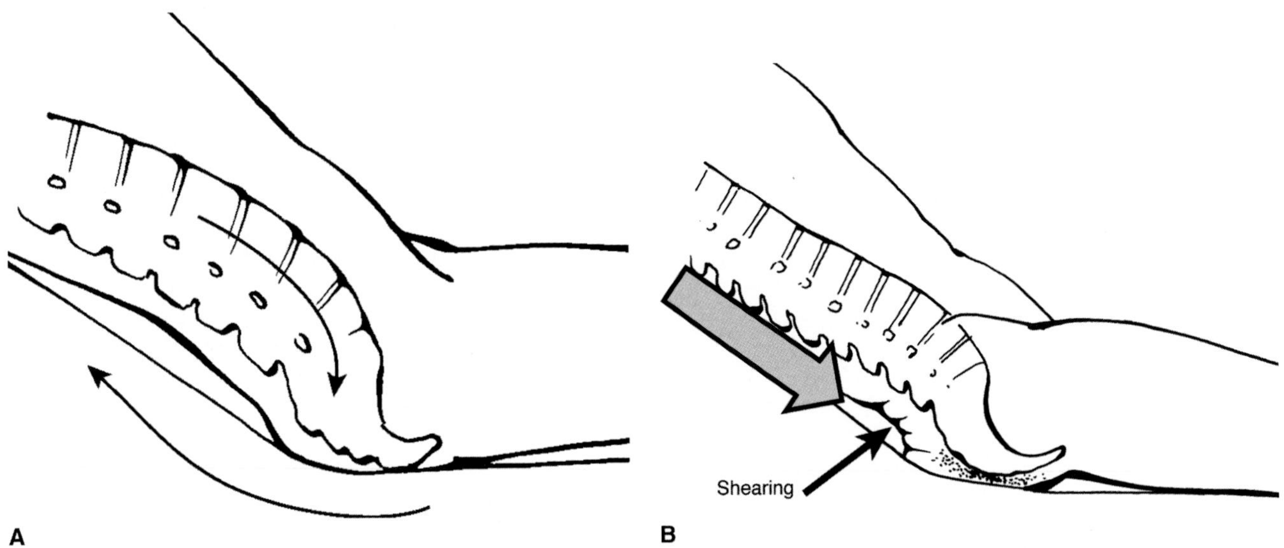

FIGURE 14.1 Illustration of shear. Shear is the application of force tangential to the skin surface and occurs when the skin remains stationary and the underlying tissue shifts (**A**). Shearing forces cause the perforating arteries to become angulated, disrupting the supply of blood (**B**).

development and healing. There is a large body of literature associating the development of PrUs with certain demographic characteristics, those associated with SCI itself, other medical and psychosocial variables.

The SCI patient is at greater risk for PrU formation than the able-bodied population because of their impaired sensation and associated loss of mobility, with potential for incontinence secondary to neurogenic bladder and bowel (23,24). SCI itself is associated with unique changes that contribute to the pathophysiology of PrUs. For example, patients with SCI have alterations in the skin collagen that is responsible for the skin's tensile strength, which contributes to its increased susceptibility to PrU development. Specifically, the activity of lysyl hydroxylase, an enzyme involved in the biosynthesis of collagen, is lower from biopsies below the level of the injury than above the level of injury and in non-SCI controls (25). In addition, there is an increased urinary excretion of the metabolite glucosyl galactosyl hydroxylysine immediately after traumatic SCI (26). Alterations in the autonomic nervous system following SCI may also affect PrU development and healing. There may be a decrease in the density of adrenergic receptors in the skin below the level of injury for SCI patients that may cause an abnormal vascular response (27,28). Patients with SCI have been shown to have a slower reflow rate after pressure is removed, and this vascular response may predispose to ulcer formation through lower tissue oxygenation and lower nutrient availability (29). Lastly, persons with SCI have higher sitting pressures than controls, most likely because of atrophied muscle tissue over bony prominences (30).

Demographic variables studied include age, gender, ethnicity, marital status, employment status, and educational achievement (1,31–34). Intrinsic variables associated with the injury itself such as level of the paralysis, completeness of the injury, longer duration of SCI, and degree of functional independence are considered risk factors (1,34,35). Having a PrU itself is a significant risk factor for developing future ulcers (1,32,36). Psychosocial variables associated with the development of PrUs include male gender, use of tobacco and alcohol, and poor nutrition (37,38).

Marital status may be a moderate factor, with being married possibly a protective factor (33–35,39,40). Some studies report psychosocial factors not being associated with PrUs in SCI that include age at onset, quality of life, depression, satisfaction with social support, and social integration (34,35,41,42) while others have reported some association (37,38). In preliminary studies, race was associated with having a PrU, more severe grades of ulcers, and having surgery for repair after SCI (43–46). In a subsequent multivariate analysis, the relationship of having a PrU and surgery was mediated by income and education rather than race alone (47). Other studies report that low educational achievement level is linked with PrU prevalence in cross-sectional studies and a risk factor in a cohort study, with a moderate level of evidence (34). Unemployment is linked to PrU prevalence in several cross-sectional studies.

Cardiac disease, diabetes mellitus, vascular disease, immune deficiencies, collagen vascular diseases, malignancies, psychosis, and pulmonary disease are all factors that are associated with PrU development and may contribute to poor wound healing (48). Diabetes mellitus has also been found to be a major contributor to nonhealing or delayed healing of wounds.

INCIDENCE AND PREVALENCE

It has been estimated that 50% to 80% of persons with SCI will, at some time after their injury, develop a PrU (2, 31,32,39,43). During the acute stage after injury, including acute hospitalization and initial rehabilitation, approximately one third (21% to 40%) of patients develop a PrU (1,31,49–53). The incidence may be lower for patients who are cared for at an acute center specializing in SCI prior to transfer and rehabilitation (54).

The incidence of PrUs seems to be steady for the first few years after injury then increases with the duration of the SCI (35,39,55). Fuhrer et al. (31) noted that in community dwelling persons with SCI, less extensive PrUs, stages I and II, comprise about 75% of the total number of ulcers observed, leaving 25% as more severe or stage III and IV ulcers. McKinley et al. (35) identified PrUs as the most common secondary complication all years after injury and increased prevalence was associated with greater number of years after injury. The annual prevalence of PrUs in SCI has been reported to be 31% to 52% with 31% to 79% of the population troubled with recurrent ulcers (1,35,56–61).

Diseases of the skin, including PrUs, were found to be the second most common overall cause of rehospitalization of persons with SCI, for all years cumulative from year 1 to 20, behind diseases of the genitourinary system (62). Cardenas et al. (62) reported that those with AIS A, B, or C paraplegia were more likely to be rehospitalized with skin issues than those with any level of tetraplegia or AIS D paraplegia. Approximately 8% of those who develop PrUs will die from related complications (63).

STAGING/GRADING

An adequate description of the PrU allows for communication among team members as well as following interventions in wound healing for both clinical outcomes and research purposes. PrUs are usually classified as stages including macroscopic and morphological criteria, specifically based on erythema of the skin and depth of the ulcer. The staging system most commonly used is based upon the NPUAP Consensus Development Conference, initially developed in 1989 and revised in 2007, which incorporated several of the most commonly used staging systems (3,4) (Table 14.1 and Fig. 14.2).

There are some limitations, however, of PrU staging. For example, a stage I ulcer may be superficial or it may sometimes be mistaken as a sign of suspected deep tissue injury. In addition, stage I ulcers are not always reliably assessed, particularly in patients with darkly pigmented skin. It may take weeks before the actual size and depth of the ulcer is known (64). When an eschar is present, a PrU cannot be accurately staged until the eschar is removed. It is also difficult to assess PrUs in patients with casts, support stockings, or other orthopaedic devices. Lastly, PrUs do not necessarily progress from stage I to IV or heal from stage IV to I.

Numerous techniques have been described to measure the size and depth of an ulcer. Generally, the ulcer is measured at its maximum dimensions and it is then diagrammed, traced, or photographed (65). A quick and easy way is to document length, width, and depth using a ruler, tape measure, or caliper. Another method is to obtain an estimate of the wound area by measuring the wound length (L) and width (W) and to multiply them. The major drawback of using length and width is that wounds may have the same linear dimensions, but could be of different shapes and areas. A two-dimensional method involves approximating the periphery of a wound with a rectangle or an ellipse, then calculating the area from its linear dimensions (length and width), using the Kundin formula (66).

Planimetry measures the wound surface area (length × width) and relative depth. The most common method of performing wound planimetry includes the use of a simple ruler or tracing grids. The wound boundary is marked on the tracing grid with a special marking pen, then the area of the wound is

TABLE 14.1

NPUAP UPDATED PRESSURE ULCER STAGING SYSTEM

Stage	Description
Unstageable: depth unknown	Full-thickness tissue loss in which the base of the ulcer is covered by slough (yellow, tan, gray, green, or brown) and/or eschar (tan, brown, or black) in the wound bed.
Suspected deep tissue injury	Purple or maroon localized area of discolored intact skin or blood-filled blister due to damage of underlying soft tissue from pressure and/or shear. The area may be preceded by tissue that is painful, firm, mushy, boggy, warmer, or cooler as compared to adjacent tissue. Deep tissue injury may be difficult to identify in patients with dark skin tones. Evolution may include a thin blister over a dark wound bed. The wound may further evolve and become covered by thin eschar. Evolution may be rapid, exposing additional layers of tissue even with optimal treatment.
Stage I	Intact skin with nonblanchable redness of a localized area usually over a bony prominence. Darkly pigmented skin may not have visible blanching; its color may differ from the surrounding area.
Stage II	Partial-thickness loss of dermis presenting as a shallow open ulcer with a red pink wound bed, without slough. May also present as an intact or open/ruptured serum-filled blister.
Stage III	Full-thickness tissue loss. Subcutaneous fat may be visible but bone, tendon, or muscles are not exposed. Slough may be present but does not obscure the depth of tissue loss. May include undermining and tunneling.
Stage IV	Full-thickness tissue loss with exposed bone, tendon, or muscle. Slough or eschar may be present on some parts of the wound bed. Often includes undermining and tunneling.

National Pressure Ulcer Advisory Panel. Pressure Ulcer Stages Revised by NPUAP. NPUAP, 2007.

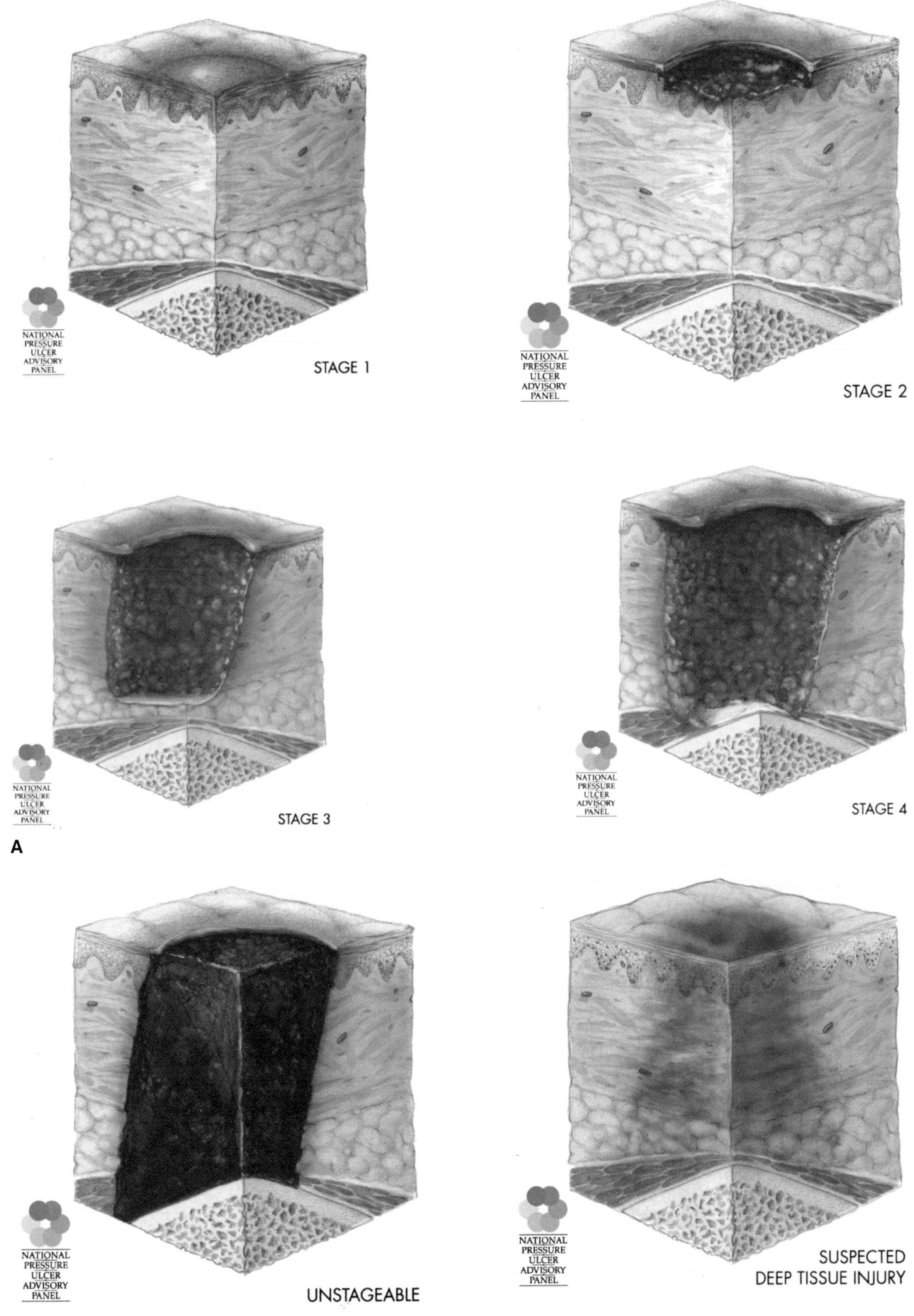

FIGURE 14.2 Pressure ulcers. (**A**) Stage 1 through 4. (**B**) Unstageable.

estimated either manually, where the number of small squares within the boundary is counted and multiplied by the area of one square to yield the area of the wound, or digitally, where the wound area is automatically calculated by placing the transparency over a device and the wound shape is retraced using a stylus (67).

Three-dimensional assessment is performed through a stereographic system, where the wound area and volume are calculated and the geometry of the wound is reconstructed using digital photography (68). Some researchers have combined standard photography with transparency tracings (69). Lastly, another method of quantitatively assessing deeper structures is through high-resolution ultrasound scanning, which permits the quantitative assessment of structural changes of deeper structures in closed and open wounds (70).

COSTS

Despite the attention given to preventive strategies, PrUs remain common among persons with acute and chronic SCI. PrUs are responsible for physical, social, and vocational losses as well as a direct economic cost. While recent cost data on PrUs in the SCI population is difficult to obtain, it has been estimated that the cost of care for PrUs is approximately \$1.2 to \$1.3 billion annually with prevention costs about one tenth of this (63,71,72). The costs to heal ulcers vary by their severity, with less serious PrUs ranging up to \$30,000 and the cost to heal a complex full-thickness PrU estimated at \$70,000 (1). These costs are higher when taking into account increased attendant and skilled care and long-term hospitalization postsurgical intervention. PrUs also have indirect costs including the loss of income, productivity, progress toward rehabilitation and vocational goals, independence, self-esteem, and sense of self-worth (73).

LOCATION AND SEVERITY OF PRESSURE ULCERS

PrUs usually develop over bony prominences. Model Systems data from SCI patient's initial hospitalization and rehabilitation show that the most common sites of ulcers are the sacrum (37.4%), followed by the heels (15.9%), and ischium (9.2%). Severe ulcers (stages III and IV) occurred most often at the same sites: sacrum (50.9%), heels (12.5%), and ischium (6.3%) (55). After discharge, there is a change in the sites of the development of PrUs with the most common sites after 1 year the sacrum (20.5%), ischium (18.3%), heels (16.6%), and trochanters (12.4%) with the most severe ulcers at the sacrum (25.0%), trochanters (23.4%), and ischium (22.7%) (55). This increase in the percentages of ulcers at the ischium is associated with the patient's progression from lying supine to spending more time in the sitting position in the wheelchair. At year 2 postinjury, the most common sites of PrUs are the ischium (24.3%), sacrum (20.3%), and trochanters (12.5%) with the highest number of severe ulcers found at the ischium (30.9%), trochanter (26.5%), and sacrum (17.6%). Neurologically complete patients are more likely to have PrUs at multiple sites (35,55).

RISK ASSESSMENT SCALES

Risk assessment scales assign numerical equivalents to risk factors for PrU development and stratify that person's risk based on an overall numerical score. A review of these scales in the SCI population was conducted by Mortenson and Miller (74). Two scales have been developed specifically for the SCI population: the SCIPUS and SCIPUS-A (40). These scales, however, require further testing as they reportedly lack reliability data and were developed and tested using the same retrospective data, limiting their validity (74). The Braden Scale (75) was recommended by Mortenson and Miller, and is composed of six subscales: activity, mobility, sensory perception, nutritional status, skin moisture, and friction and shear (Table 14.2). The subscales (rated from highest risk (1) to lowest risk (4) with total scores ranging from 6 to 23) measure functional capabilities of the patient that contribute to either higher intensity and duration of pressure or lower tissue tolerance for pressure. A lower Braden Scale score indicates lower levels of functioning and, therefore, higher levers of risk for PrU development. Patients with a total score of 15 to 18 are considered to be at mild risk of developing PrUs; 13 to 14 = moderate risk; 10 to 12 = high risk, and 6 to 9 = very high risk. If the Braden score is 18 or lower, recommendations for preventive interventions for each category should be initiated.

TABLE 14.2

BRADEN RISK ASSESSMENT SCALE

Subscale					Patient score
Sensory perception	1. Completely limited	2. Very limited	3. Slightly limited	4.No impairment	
Moisture	1. Constantly moist	2. Very moist	3. Occasionally moist	4. Rarely moist	
Activity	1.Bedfast	2. Chairfast	3. Walks occasionally	4. Walks frequently	
Mobility	1. Completely immobile	2. Very limited	3. Slightly limited	4. No limitation	
Nutrition	1. Very poor	2. Probably inadequate	3. Adequate	4. Excellent	
Friction and shear	1. Requires moderate to maximum assistance in moving	2. Moves freely or requires minimum assistance	3. Moves independently		

PRESSURE ULCER PREVENTION

A comprehensive educational program for SCI patients and their family/caregivers should begin from the onset of the SCI, continued through the initial rehabilitation and updated throughout the continuum of care. Information should be presented at an appropriate level for the target audience that includes emphasizing the ramifications of PrU development. The educational program should include information on etiology, risk factors, proper positioning, equipment (i.e., cushions), complications, principles of wound prevention, skin care, wound treatment, and when to seek medical attention. This education should be reinforced especially for the individual who has developed an ulcer. Studies have shown that compliance is greater and the treatment more successful when the patient actively participates in the learning process (76,77). There is level II evidence that providing PrU prevention education is effective in helping persons with SCI gain and retain this knowledge. However, no evidence exists regarding whether this enhanced education results in a reduction in PrU formation (78).

Prevention recommendations (Table 14.3) include examining the skin at least daily, with particular attention to the bony prominences, to allow for early detection of a PrU; shifting body weight in bed and wheelchair on a regular basis independently or with assistance; keeping moisture accumulation to a minimum and cleaning and drying skin promptly after soiling; having an individually prescribed wheelchair, pressure redistribution cushion, and power tilt mechanism if manual pressure relief is not possible; ensuring all equipment is maintained and functioning properly; nutritionally complete diet and maintaining appropriate body weight; and decreasing or stopping smoking and limiting alcohol intake (1,51,78).

Patients and their family/caregivers should be instructed to inspect their skin at least twice daily, with particular attention to the bony prominences, for early signs of skin breakdown. Equipment such as a long-handled flexible mirror may assist in the skin inspection. Health care professionals must assist persons with SCI to determine which preventive strategies are realistic for them to implement based on their life circumstances, and help them identify ways to integrate these preventive strategies into daily schedules.

Specialized seating clinics incorporated into both inpatient and outpatient rehabilitation programs with the use of verbal and video feedback and recommending appropriate seating systems guided by technology-based evaluations, have been shown to reduce the incidence of PrUs and readmission rates (79). Level II evidence reported by Regan et al. (78) shows that early attendance and specialized seating assessment clinics increase the skin management abilities of a person after SCI as an adjunct to a comprehensive skin management program.

Pressure mapping, a computerized pressure-sensitive mat that quantifies interface pressure (pressure between the skin and the sitting surface) under a seating surface, is often used to determine the risk of PrU development, to analyze and understand different sitting postures, to educate about weight shifting techniques, and to compare different surfaces. Unfortunately, no clear cutoff point for interface pressure for the development of PrUs has been established. A systematic review was performed to see whether interface pressures can be used to predict the development of PrUs or to determine the prognosis of an ulcer once developed (80). This review concluded that there is a relation between the magnitude of the pressure and the time to development or healing of the PrU. This is qualitative evidence (i.e., higher pressures are related to higher incidence of PrUs) as no definitive clinical thresholds exist.

TABLE 14.3

PREVENTION PRINCIPLES

1. Daily visual and tactile skin inspections.
2. Assess PrU risk factors.
3. Assess the nutritional status and supplement as needed.
4. Turning and repositioning in bed with appropriate mattress.
5. Provide an individually prescribed wheelchair with appropriate pressure-reducing seating system.
6. Reinforce weight shifting for pressure relief.
7. Provide education to patients, their families, etc., on effective strategies for the prevention and management of PrUs.

Positioning and Equipment

Proper patient positioning and pressure relief should begin immediately after SCI, as soon as the emergency medical condition and spinal stabilization status allow (1,81,82). Since PrUs occur over bony prominences, depending on the patient's position, different bony prominences are at risk. When sitting, the ischial tuberosities (ITs) bear the weight of the upper body and are therefore at greatest risk. In side lying, the greater trochanters become at risk; in the supine position, the sacrum, heels, and occiput (especially in infants) are at risk for PrU development. When in bed, maintaining the bed at a 30-degree elevation and at 30 degrees for side lying can decrease pressure over bony prominences. The prone position has a large surface area of low pressure and a smaller surface area of high pressure, although many patients cannot tolerate this position.

Pillows can be used to assist in maintaining the desired position, provide additional padding to bony prominences (83), or to suspend or provide pressure reduction over bony prominences, being placed proximally and distally, a technique known as bridging. Most persons can be treated with proper bed positioning and turns every 2 hours. Turning techniques should avoid shearing the soft tissues and the patient should be alternated from side to side and placed prone if medically indicated and tolerated. Although it is common for an SCI patient to extend the 2-hour turn schedule once discharged to home, with no increase in PrUs probably secondary to improved tissue tolerance or perfusion, further research is needed to define which patients can and at what point they can increase their turning intervals.

Numerous mattress replacements, mattress overlays, and integrated bed systems have been developed to help prevent PrUs. Although there is a large body of literature available on support surfaces, there is insufficient evidence to recommend one specific support surface over another for cost effectiveness and appropriate patient characteristics of a specific mattress (84). Surfaces are classified as reactive or active. ***A reactive support surface,*** previously referred to as a static surface, is a nonpowered or powered support surface with the capability to change its load distribution properties only in response to applied load. Examples of these include all types of foam

TABLE 14.4

EXAMPLES OF REACTIVE SUPPORT SURFACES

Foam	Air	Gel/Water
Eggcrate	Roho (Roho)	Rik Fluid Overlay (KCI)
Geo-Matt (Span America)	Sof-Care (Gaymar Industries)	
Comfortline (Hill-Rom)	First Step (Kinetic Concepts)	

(viscoelastic, elastic, closed and open cell), gel, water, and air. Static support surfaces redistribute pressure only if the patient is able to reposition oneself. These can be used for an individual without an ulcer or for an individual with a PrU who can position oneself without weight bearing on the ulcer. In those at high risk of PrU development and unable to reposition themselves, an integrated alternating pressure system is indicated. Standard hospital mattresses are usually made of foam and not indicated for patients at high risk for PrU development. Examples of static support surfaces are in Table 14.4.

An active support surface or dynamic support surface should be used if the individual is unable to reposition himself, if there is no evidence of ulcer healing, or if a new ulcer develops. An active or dynamic support surface is a powered support surface with the capability to change its load distribution properties with or without applied load. These include a pulsating low-air-loss bed, overlay, or replacement mattress, and alternating pressure mattress or integrated bed system, and an air-fluidized bed. Examples of dynamic support surfaces are seen in Table 14.5.

Low-air-loss, alternating pressure, and air-fluidized beds (AFB) should be used if there are multiple PrUs or with large stage III or IV PrUs or after myocutaneous flap surgery. In comparison to air-fluidized beds, in general, low-air-loss beds, alternative pressure integrated bed system, and overlays are lighter and patient transfers are more easily managed. Mattress overlays are less often prescribed than previously because of the increased risk of patients falling and the added height to the sleeping surface. Table 14.6 lists some of the characteristics of different support surfaces.

AFB have been shown to increase the rate of healing PrUs over other mattress types and provides cost-effective PrU treatment for stage III and IV wounds (85–92). The specific benefits include decrease pressure and shearing forces, allows for easier care from others (i.e., turning in the bed), decreases maceration, and maintains a clean dry surface for patients with heavy wound exudates, and the ceramic-fluidized beads have a bactericidal effect due to the sequestration and desiccation of microorganisms (1,92–94). A contraindication to usage is an unstable spine. Concerns with AFB include dehydration in approximately 3% of patients (92,95), and the need for more aggressive pulmonary toilet in patients with congestion (96) (although the use of the Clinitron Rite-Hite may obviate this need since it only has the fluidization in the lower part of the body), confusion or disorientation, increased room temperature, and more difficulty for patient transfers in and out of the bed (92). An advantage is that patients can lie on an AFB immediately after surgical flap procedures.

The turning schedule when on an ATB may be lengthened from the every 2-hour schedule to an every 4-hour schedule. Even though turning is not required as frequently with ATB for pressure redistribution, the patient may be repositioned to retain lung expansion, pulmonary clearance, and joint mobility (92,97).

WEIGHT SHIFTING

Repositioning is an important component in the management of PrUs. While sitting, weight shifting will allow for reoxygenation. Weight shifts can be performed by the patient with or without assistance. To perform an anterior weight shift, the patient bends forward at the waist so that their head is between their thighs and knees. To perform a lateral weight shift, the patient will remove the armrest on one side and lean to that side with their hand supporting their body weight on a stable surface and then the procedure is repeated on the other side. Finally, to perform a press-up weight shift, the most difficult type, the patient will place their hands on the armrests and extend their elbows so that their buttocks are suspended over the wheelchair cushion. If the patient is unable to perform their own weight shift, the patient's caregiver tilts the chair posteriorly so that the patient's weight is no longer on their ITs. All these weight shifts maneuvers will relieve the pressure from the buttocks and ITs and redistribute it to other areas to allow reperfusion of the ischial areas.

Although repositioning is universally advocated, confusion exists regarding the frequency and exact method of repositioning required. For repositioning in bed, the Agency for Health Care Policy and Research (AHCPR) (15) advocates 2-hourly

TABLE 14.5

EXAMPLES OF ACTIVE SUPPORT SURFACES

Low-air-loss overlays	Low-air-loss beds	Alternating pressure mattress or integrated bed system	Air fluidized beds
Micro Air (Invacare)	Flexicair (Support Systems International)	Nimbus 3 (Arjo Huntleigh)	Clinitron (Support Systems International)
Clini-Care (Gaymar)	Kinair (Kinetic Concepts)	Excell 8000	Skyton (Skytron)
First Step Select (KCI)	Mediscus (Mediscus Group)		FluidAir (Kinetic Concepts)
	Air II Pulsating Mattress (Stryker)		

TABLE 14.6

SUPPORT SURFACE CHARACTERISTICS

Performance characteristics	Air fluidized	Low air loss	Alternating air	Static flotation	Foam	Standard mattress
Increased support area	Yes	Yes	Yes	Yes	Yes	No
Low moisture retention	Yes	Yes	No	No	No	No
Reduced heat accumulation	Yes	Yes	No	No	No	No
Shear reduction	Yes	Yes	Yes	Yes	No	No
Pressure reduction	Yes	Yes	Yes	Yes	Yes	No
Dynamic	Yes	Yes	Yes	No	No	No
Cost per day	High	High	Moderate	Low	Low	Low

repositioning, whereas other guidelines do not have specific timelines (98,99). A Cochrane review in 2010 was unable to identify any randomized controlled trial (RCT) evidence that addresses this question to provide specific guidance for practice of repositioning and healing of PrUs (100). It is clear, however, that weight bearing directly on an existing PrU will cause pressure and vascular obstruction that will interfere with capillary blood flow to the ulcer and deprive the area of oxygen and nutrients.

While previously recommended that weight shifts in the wheelchair be performed every 15 to 30 minutes for 30 seconds (101,102), Coggrave and Rose, in a retrospective review, assessed the duration of various pressure relief positions required for loaded transcutaneous oxygen tension ($tCPO_2$) to recover to unloaded levels (103). They reported that it took approximately 2 minutes of pressure relief to raise tissue oxygen to unloaded levels for most subjects. This length of pressure relief was more easily sustained by the subjects leaning forward, side to side, or having the wheelchair tipped back at greater than 65 degrees compared to a push-up pressure relief lift. Similarly, Makhsous et al. (104) demonstrated full recovery of $tcPO_2$ with a dynamic protocol in the off loading configuration and it took greater than 2 minutes to achieve this result. Those individuals with paraplegia using a wheelchair push-up were only able to sustain the lift for 49 seconds leading to incomplete recovery of tissue perfusion. Therefore, it is important to perform reliefs for a greater time period than previously recommended and to recognize that push-up weight shifts may not offer adequate weight relief for the long term.

Wheelchairs can also provide weight shifts through mechanical means and a power weight shifting system should be prescribed for individuals who are unable to independently perform an effective weight shift, especially if they do not have a caregiver with them at all times. Hobson showed that for individuals with SCI, changes in posture can reduce maximum pressures that occur while seated. Recline of the backrest to 120 degrees, full body tilt to 20 degrees, forward flexion to 50 degrees, and lateral bending to 15 degrees all resulted in decreases in maximum pressures (105). The mechanical weight shift redistributes the pressure off of the buttocks and onto the back and a minimum of 45 degrees of backward tilt is required for adequate pressure distribution (105). Tilt-in-space mechanisms can be selected over reclining methods to avoid shear and if there is significant spasticity of spinal origin, which may be triggered with changes in body angles (106).

Proper positioning and alignment in the wheelchair can help prevent PrUs on the buttocks. Significant reduction in the force on the buttocks while sitting can be obtained using armrests, which can support up to 10% of the body's weight (107). The sling back wheelchair in the absence of patient trunk support promotes pelvic obliquity and kyphotic posture with an increased risk of PrUs on the buttocks and sacrum (108). A wheelchair back support system can be prescribed to avoid these complications and keep the normal spinal curves intact, although adding lumbar support to the wheelchairs of individuals with chronic SCI is unlikely to have a role in PrU prevention after SCI (78,109). Wheelchair footplate adjustment should be tailored to the patient to provide for a more neutral sitting position of the pelvis, as any imbalance of the normal sitting position places the patient at greater risk for PrU development (110).

Wheelchair cushions compliment bed support surfaces in the prevention of PrUs. Clinically useful computerized systems have been developed to evaluate the pressure exerted on various cushions, although they are limited in their ability to measure shear (111,112). Materials available in wheelchair cushions, as for bed support surfaces, include foam, air, and gel in static cushions as well as low-air-loss cushions. As with bed supports, the use of donut-shaped ring cushions should be avoided, as the ring will prevent perfusion of the central area (113). Examples of the different types of cushions are listed in Table 14.7.

No one cushion is suitable for all individuals with SCI. Cushion selection should be based on a combination of pressure mapping results, clinical knowledge of the prescriber, individual characteristics, and preferences. More research is needed to see if decreasing ischial pressures or decreasing risk factors such as skin temperature via the use of specialty cushions will help prevent PrUs after SCI.

Seat cushions can be made from various materials and they may be incorporated into upright, power tilt, or reclined wheelchairs. Cushions may also be static or dynamic (typically

TABLE 14.7

EXAMPLES OF WHEELCHAIR CUSHIONS

Foam	Gel	Air	Alternating air
Stimulite (Sepracor)	The Cloud (Otto Bock)	Roho (Roho)	Altern8 (Pegasus)
Combi (Jay Medical)	Jay (Jay Medical)	Nexus (Roho)	ErgoDynamic (ErgoAir)
Varilite (Cascade Designs)			

accomplished with air bladders). Dynamic cushions will have alternating sections of the cushion inflated at different times, offering periods of weight relief over the ITs. In a study conducted by Burns and Betz (114), three wheelchair cushions were tested including a dynamic cushion. The dynamic cushion in an upright wheelchair demonstrated greater pressure relief at the IT during the low-pressure portion of the cycle than gel and dry flotation cushions with a 45-degree tilted wheelchair. However, for the dynamic cushion, during the high-pressure portion of the cycle, the pressures over the IT were higher than with either of the other two cushions (114). In earlier studies of various cushions, while there was variability in individual pressures, air-filled cushions had the best pressure readings and were most often prescribed, especially in patients with tetraplegia (115,116). Further study is needed in this area.

Age-associated changes in the SCI patient's skin and mobility mean that the support surface, wheelchair, and wheelchair cushion initially prescribed may not be the most appropriate across the life span. It is therefore recommended that routine and regular assessment of each patient occurs to determine if a change in equipment or additional equipment is needed prior to development of a PrU.

Other Preventive Tools

Researchers have studied the role of electrical stimulation (ES) using implanted as well as surface electrodes on the gluteal muscles in reducing ischial pressures and redistributing seating interface pressures both of which could assist with PrU prevention (117,118). More research is needed to study the effect of long-term ES on reducing ischial pressures and whether this can be used in a clinical setting to prevent PrUs after SCI (78).

Lastly, while telerehabilitation offers many advantages, there is level IV evidence that telerehabilitation does not make a significant difference in the prevention and treatment of PrUs after SCI (78,119).

Nutrition

Individuals who develop PrUs often have significantly lower calorie and protein intake than those who do not develop them (120). Recommendations for prevention or treatment of a PrU include eating a well-balanced, nutritionally complete diet with appropriate calories, proteins, micronutrients (vitamins and minerals), and fluids. The nutrition plan should be individualized based upon the assessed needs (1,50,121).

Nutritional supplements studied for wound healing include vitamins and minerals such as vitamins C and E, zinc, and arginine. Vitamin C is an antioxidant and necessary for the hydroxylation of proline and lysine during collagen formation, and therefore may help with wound healing. However, it is unclear if supplementation of vitamin C is helpful, as it has been reported to not accelerate healing of PrUs (122) nor does intake of vitamin C predict PrU development (102). Other studies, however, have shown some improvement with vitamin C supplementation (123) and as such the value of supplementation of vitamin C for PrU healing is uncertain (84).Vitamin E is also an antioxidant and although reported to improve the healing of PrUs, there is limited scientific evidence of this (124). Zinc is involved in the structural integrity of collagen and, like vitamin E, there are anecdotal reports of improved healing with supplementation, however scientific evidence is limited (125).

A review of the efficacy of vitamin supplementation for prevention and treatment of PrU that was recently performed (126) found that evidence for prevention of PrU by oral nutritional supplementation is low. Only one RCT was found that assessed PrU healing and reported that patients with higher intake of vitamin C, zinc, and arginine in high doses may enhance wound healing (127). A more recent observational study also found that arginine supplementation benefited persons with SCI in wound healing (128). For the purposes of assessing nutritional status, several blood tests are available and have been associated with the presence or development of PrUs. Prealbumin is the most sensitive indicator for monitoring nutritional status because of its short half-life (2 to 3 days) and has been found to be significantly lower in patients with PrUs compared to those without (129). In addition, decreases in total protein (less than 6.4 g/dL) and albumin (less than 3.5 g/dL) have similarly been found to be associated with PrU development (111,130,131). Factors associated with hypoalbuminemia include losses of protein and albumin in PrU exudate and the presence of a chronic inflammatory state (129,131,132).

The individual's weight should be monitored, as an undesirable weight trend has been identified as an early indicator of risk (121). Equations, such as the Harris-Benedict Equation, have been used to estimate the SCI patients' recommended caloric need, both with and without PrUs (133). In addition, the AHCPR Guidelines recommend that an individual without a PrU should intake 1.0 to 1.25 g/kg of body weight per day of protein and with a PrU this should increase to 1.25 to 1.5 g/kg/d (102). This should be individualized and reassessed as the patient's condition changes. Further, renal function is critical to assess in order to ensure that higher levels of protein are appropriate and can be tolerated.

Indirect calorimetry is the best method of determining the energy expenditures in SCI individuals who have PrU (134,135). Increases or decreases in weight may alter contributing factors to PrU development. For example, if an individual gains weight, they may become more susceptible to developing an ulcer from shear, especially if their own strength or that of their caregivers is insufficient to transfer without sliding along the surface. Additionally, weight gain may lead to a piece of equipment no longer fitting properly, thereby increasing pressure on bony surfaces.

With injury or chronic debilitation, there are decreased levels of the normal anabolic hormones, human growth, and testosterone (136,137). Because of this, several investigators have used the anabolic agent oxandrolone, combined with good nutrition, to restore weight and accomplish a significant increase in the healing rate of wounds (137–139). Spungen in a case series of nine subjects with stage III and IV PrUs demonstrated healing in eight of nine subjects 3 to 12 months after daily administration of 20 mg of oxandrolone (139). There is, however, limited level IV evidence to support the use of anabolic steroid agents (oxandrolone) to promote to the healing of stage III and IV PrUs (78) and further study is needed.

PRESSURE ULCER TREATMENT

PrUs are most easily treated when diagnosed early and the interventions promptly initiated. The general principles of PrU treatment are to relieve pressure, eliminate reversible underlying predisposing conditions, avoid friction, shear, tissue maceration, manage moisture, keep the wound bed moist, and debride devitalized tissue. Treatment of the SCI patient who has developed a PrU involves local wound care, as well as an evaluation of causative factors, and implementation of interventions, including additional equipment, to minimize the risk of both chronic wounds and repeated PrUs (see Table 14.8).

Assessment

A comprehensive history and physical examination should be performed on every patient with a PrU. The PrU should be assessed in the context of the patient's overall physical and psychosocial health. Identification of comorbid factors may influence the plan of treatment, healing of the ulcer, and avoidance of additional and future PrUs. In addition, every patient should be assessed for ulcer-related pain including during turning, dressing changes, and debridement. Up to 63% of patients report pain related to either the ulcer or its treatment (140) and these studies suggest that PrU pain changes over time (141).

TABLE 14.8

TREATMENT PRINCIPLES

1. Assess and document wound (size, stage, wound bed appearance, wound edges, exudates, necrosis, odor, signs of infection, surrounding skin, undermining, sinus formation, tunneling, and granulation tissue epitheliazation).
2. Observe and document wound healing progress.
3. Avoid antiseptics (povidone-iodine, H2O2, etc) because of cytotoxicity.
4. Keep periwound skin dry, control exudates, and eliminate dead space.
5. Use dressings that keep ulcer bed moist to allow for optimal cell migration, proliferation, and revascularization.
6. Clean wound at every dressing change using minimal mechanical force.
7. Create optimum wound environment by using modern dressings (hydrocolloids, hydrogels, foams, alginates, soft silicone) rather than gauze.
8. Consider adjunctive therapies (ES, NPWT, etc.) to enhance healing.
9. Consider 2-wk trial of topical antibiotics for clean, non-healing PrUs (i.e., silver sulfadiazine, iodosorb).
10. Manage infection with wound cleansing, systemic antibiotics, and debridement.
11. Ensure adequate nutritional intake.
12. Manage tissue loads through positioning techniques and appropriate support surfaces. Limit time in chair if PrU is on sitting surface.
13. Remove necrotic tissue.

Adapted from Jones KR, Fennie K, Lenihan A. Evidence-based management of chronic wounds. *Adv Skin Wound Care* 2007;20(11):591–600.

To plan treatment of a PrU and to assess the effects of the treatment, the PrU should be monitored at every dressing change and the treatment reassessed at least weekly (142,143). Although staging of the wound is frequently used alone as an assessment, other assessment scales have been developed for assessment including the Pressure Ulcer Scale for Healing (PUSH Tool) (144), the Pressure Sore Status Tool (PSST) (145), the Sessing Scale (146), and the Wound Healing Scale (147). The PUSH Tool is a valid and reliable instrument to track PrUs over time. There is no consensus, however, on how to use these tools for making treatment decisions (148).

Assessment of the PrU should include in addition to the staging, the location, depth, and size; the presence of sinus tracts, undermining, or tunneling; exudate, necrotic tissue; and the presence of granulation tissue and epithelialization. All of these wound variables are important to determine the goal and plan of care. The condition of the skin surrounding the PrU should also be assessed. A photographic record can be a useful aid in documenting progress of a PrU.

Managing Tissue Load

Care must be taken to eliminate direct pressure on the wound, avoiding a delay in healing. Use of a specialized support surface will provide an environment in which existing ulcers improve and may help prevent new ulcers from developing. The decision often needs to be made, for example, if the wound is on the IT, whether limited sitting to complete bed rest is required. While the patient is restricted in bed, a written repositioning schedule should be established to protect uninvolved areas, keeping in mind repositioning so as to avoid higher intensity or longer duration of pressure.

Debridement and Cleansing

Optimal wound healing can only occur in a clean wound environment. Cleaning the wound of inflammatory stimuli such as devitalized tissue and reactive chemicals involves debridement and cleansing. In addition, effective wound cleansing and debridement can reduce the bioburden and minimize colonization in the ulcers, while limiting their cytotoxic effects on white blood cells and fibroblasts, all critical cells in wound repair. For the majority of wounds, isotonic saline is adequate. Water is also an alternative provided it is free of any contaminants. In a Cochrane review, Fernandez et al. (149) found in 11 trials that where tap water is of high quality, it is as effective as other methods such as sterile water or saline for cleaning wounds. Commercial cleaning agents have surfactants that break the bonds that attach wound contaminants; therefore, it is important to weigh the capacity of cleaning agents against their toxicity to wound cells. In 1993, Foresman et al. studied the relative toxicity of nine wound cleansers and seven skin cleansers to determine their relative safety and effect on cell viability and phagocytic function. They defined the toxicity index of any cleansing solution as the amount of dilution required for both viability and phagocytic efficiency to be similar to cells exposed to a balanced salt solution. The toxicity index was the denominator of that dilution. For example, if the nontoxic dilution was 1/1,000, the toxicity index would be 1,000. Generally, the toxic levels of wound cleansers range from 10 to 1,000, while skin cleansers range from 1,000 to 100,000, suggesting that skin cleansers are toxic to polymorphonuclear cells and therefore should never be used for wounds. Wound cleansers with a toxicity index of greater than 10 were found to inhibit cell viability and function (150). For example, in a study by Rabenberg et al. (151), betadine in saline at a 1:10 dilution in the commercially purchased solution was found to be effective in killing both gram-positive and gram-negative bacteria but were not harmful to human fibroblast cells.

Wounds should be cleansed at each dressing change using a technique and solution that minimizes trauma to healthy wound tissue. Cleansing uses specific type of fluid, usually saline based to remove loosely adherent foreign material so as to facilitate wound healing (152). For dirty wounds, stronger cleansing solution may be required and clinicians can use commercial cleansing agents containing surfactants. As the wound becomes cleaner, because surfactants are harmful to wound cells, the strength of the cleansing solution should be decreased (152). While there is evidence to use cleansers for wounds, there is little evidence to guide practitioners to exact choice of product or regimen (153).

Cleansers should be applied gently so as to minimize trauma to healthy tissue. Irrigation streams must keep the impact force below 15 psi. Wound irrigation pressures of 10 to 15 psi are superior to those of 1 or 5 psi and direct application should only be with the smoothest and softest device available (146). As seen in Table 14.9 below, irrigation with a 35-mL syringe and a 19-guage needle or angiocatheter meets these requirements.

Chronic wounds may persist because of chronic inflammation secondary to devitalized tissue, wound exudate, and bacteria. Debridement can be accomplished in a variety of ways, the most common methods include mechanical, autolytic, chemical (enzymatic), biologic, conservative sharp, or surgical.

Conservative sharp debridement is a selective debridement method using sterile instruments such as a forcep and a scalpel with No. 10 and No. 15 blades, curette, or scissors. It is the quickest way to remove loosely adherent devitalized tissue. In a multicenter study, Steed et al. (154) reported a lower rate of healing in those centers that performed less frequent debridement, independent of treatment. These findings suggest a correlation between aggressive wound debridement and improved wound healing.

TABLE 14.9

IRRIGATION PRESSURES BY VARIOUS DEVICES

Device	Irrigation impact pressure (psi)
Bulb syringe	2.0
Piston irrigation syringe (60 mL) with catheter tip	4.2
Saline squeeze bottle (250 mL) with irrigation cap	4.5
Water-Pik at lowest setting (No. 1)	6.0
35-mL syringe with 19-gauge needle or angiocatheter	8.0
Water-Pik at middle setting (No. 3)	42
Water-Pik at highest setting (No. 5).	>50

Mechanical debridement consists of applying saline-moistened gauze to the wound bed and allowing it to dry on the wound, thereby trapping debris. Once dry, usually about 4 to 6 hours after application, the dressing is pulled off along with the trapped debris, thereby cleaning the wound bed. Not only is this method painful for persons with sensation, this method is nonselective and can remove healthy tissue, therefore, alternative methods are recommended. Although a variety of gauzes are available, the most effective gauzes for mechanical debridement are coarse and have large pores (155). Other mechanical debridement methods include hydrotherapy or high-pressure irrigation and pulsatile high-pressure lavage. High-pressure irrigation uses irrigation of the necrotic wound with fluid delivered at 8 to 12 psi, such as with a 35-mL syringe and a 19-guage angiocatheter. This force is believed to remove debris without damaging healthy tissue. Pulsatile high-pressure lavage uses a machine that provides intermittent high-pressure irrigation combined with suction to remove the irrigant and wound debris. It loosens necrotic tissue and facilitates removal by other methods of debridement. This may be used as an alternative to whirlpool treatment.

Autolytic debridement is the process of keeping devitalized tissue hydrated and allowing reactive enzymes within the wound to digest the denatured tissues. This can be accomplished by applying a moisture-retentive dressing, such as a hydrocolloid, or the use of hydrogels to moisturize the devitalized tissue. The dressing should be left undisturbed for a reasonable length of time. When autolytic debridement is used, the wound should be frequently cleansed to wash out partially degraded tissue fragments. Overall, autolytic debridement is selective, leaving viable tissue intact, and less traumatic to the surrounding tissue and healthy wound tissue than mechanical debridement (152).

Enzymatic debridement is another selective method of debridement. This method works by directly digesting the components of slough such as fibrin, bacteria, leukocytes, cell debris, exudate, or by dissolving the collagen anchor that secures the devitalized tissue to the underlying wound bed. Debridement is accomplished by using commercially prepared enzymes. The only product available is Collagenase (Santyl).

Biologic debridement involves the use of sterilized eggs of *Lucilia sericata* (the greenbottle fly), commonly known as *maggot therapy*. The sterile larvae, contained within special dressings that prevent them from leaving the wound, are applied to the wound at a dose of 5 to 10 larvae per square centimeter of wound surface and are left within their dressing for 48 to 72 hours. At that point, if they are satiated and have completed their work, they can be removed. MT is believed to work through three processes: debridement of necrotic tissue (secreting digestive enzymes that dissolve necrotic tissue), disinfection of the wound, and promotion of tissue growth (156). Maggot therapy may be useful as an added treatment when stage III and IV PrUs are not healing after SCI (78,156). Because of the emergence of resistant organisms, there is renewed interest in some wound care centers (157).

ANTIBIOTICS AND PRESSURE ULCERS

While most PrUs are colonized by bacteria, antibiotic treatment is not warranted unless an infection is present. Bacteria present in the ulcer bed do not necessarily predict a failure to heal. The AHCPR and Quality Pressure Guidelines recommend a 2-week trial of topical antibiotics, such as neomycin, mupirocin, bacitracin, or polymyxin B, but used for clinically uninfected PrUs that remain unhealed or produce exudates following 2 to 4 weeks of proper care (158). Topical metronidazole has also been used for reducing odor and decreasing the anaerobic bacterial count (159).

Topical silver preparations are associated with little or no resistance due to its unique mechanism of action. Silver's positive ionic charge allows it to bind to bacterial cells at multiple sites, damaging those cells and preventing further replication. Silver decreases inflammation and bacterial exotoxin release. Silver is also a nonselective broad-spectrum topical agent that covers gram-positive and gram-negative microorganisms (160).

Various silver impregnated wound dressings are available for the management of colonized and locally infected wounds, and include gel, cream, or foam. The dressings differ in structure and physical properties in the form and amount of silver contained in the dressing and the mechanism by which the silver is delivered (161). Overall, silver dressings are mostly well tolerated. Some limitations to its use include poor penetration into deeper wounds and its rapid inactivation in the wound bed, which limits its efficacy in deeper wound infections and leads to necessity for multiple applications. It may also stain tissue a blue-gray hue due to deposition (160). Systemic toxicity may occur if large portions of the body are covered or for smaller wounds with treatment or greater than 30 days (162). Silver impregnated dressings are contraindicated in neonates, pregnancy, in patients with significant renal or hepatic impairment, and in those with sensitivity to sulphonamides or large open wounds (163).

Unfortunately, there are few well-designed studies making conclusions difficult on when to use silver dressings. If using a silver dressing, the wound should be reassessed regularly and discontinued if the wound does not respond, worsens or improves to the point that a different dressing can be used. It is important to remember that the benefit of topical antibiotics is limited to superficial infections (160). Systemic antibiotics are generally only warranted when there is bacteremia, sepsis, advancing cellulitis, or osteomyelitis.

Evidence of infection in a PrU includes the clinical signs of erythema, fever, increased white blood cell count, induration, purulence, and a foul odor. Swab cultures are not useful in determining the presence of infection of PrUs and only reflect the bacteria on the surface of the PrU (164). Tissue biopsy can determine if there are bacteria within the tissue and if the bacterial count is greater than 10^5, wound healing may be impaired (165). Advancing cellulitis is indicative of invasive tissue infection and must be treated with appropriate antibiotics. Approximately 25% of nonhealing PrUs have underlying osteomyelitis (165). Because the clinical diagnosis of osteomyelitis is unreliable, bone biopsy remains the definitive method to diagnoses osteomyelitis and identify the organism (166,167). Bone scans have a high false-positive rate due to surround inflammation inherent in open wounds (166). Once the diagnosis is made, debridement and long-term antibiotic therapy are essential. Untreated osteomyelitis can result in delayed healing, more extensive tissue damage, a longer length of hospitalization, and higher mortality rates.

Dressings and Adjunctive Therapies

PrUs require dressings to maintain physiological integrity and to protect the wound. The ideal dressing should maintain a moist wound environment, facilitate autolytic debridement, be comfortable, and be able to fill tunnels and undermining if needed. In addition, dressings should come in numerous shapes and sizes, be absorbent, provide insulation and bacterial barrier, and reduce or eliminate pain at the wound site and not cause pain on removal.

Although wounds heal better in a moist environment, excessive exudate can macerate surround tissue, cause hypergranulation, and prolong healing time. The choice of wound dressing requires careful consideration of all factors. These include number of days the dressing can remain in place; ease of dressing application and removal; frequency of wound changes; cost, size, location, and character of the wound bed; and evaluation of the goals and principles of the wound care. Various dressing types used in the SCI population have been investigated (see Table 14.10).

Hydrocolloid

Hydrocolloid dressings are indicated for partial- and full-thickness wounds with minimal to moderate exudates. The main function of a hydrocolloid is the absorption of exudates as well as donation of moisture to the wound bed. Hydrocolloids create a moist wound environment and act by autolytic debridement. It acts as an impermeable barrier from surrounding contaminants. They are cost effective because the patients can wear the dressing for 3 to 5 days and they are available in a sheet form as well as a paste or granules that are used to build deeper wounds such as stage II and III PrUs (1,168).

Hydrogel

These are available in three-dimensional sheets, amorphous gel delivered from a tube, or impregnated into strip packing material. These are indicated for necrotic or infected partial- and full-thickness wounds that are dry to minimally exudative and work by donating fluid to the wound bed, thus creating the ideal healing environment by retaining moisture and rehydrating tissue; promoting rapid autolysis. Hydrogel dressings promote healing, provide a protection against wound contamination, are acceptable to patients, decrease pain, and have been found to be cost effective (78,169).

Impregnated Gauze

This packing material is made of woven sponges that are impregnated with chemical compounds and agents (e.g., hypertonic or normal saline, petrolatum, zinc, iodoform). This is indicated for partial- or full-thickness infected or noninfected wounds, and for wounds with cavities or tracts. This dressing delivers antimicrobial medications, nutrients, and moisture. This is also used to loosely fill a wound cavity and fill a tract for easy retrieval.

Alginates

Alginates are derived from seaweed in rope or pad form, nonwoven pad, or fibers composed of alginate salts. Alginates are effective and easy to use for full-thickness wound cavities, undermined areas or tunnels with moderate to heavy exudate, contaminated and infected wounds, including malodorous wounds with or without slough. As the sodium in the wound exudate comes in contact with the alginate, it starts to gel.

TABLE 14.10

DRESSINGS[a]

Transparent films	Hydrocolloids	Hydrogels	Foams	Alginates	Gauze dressings
Tegaderm (3M Healthcare)	Duoderm (ConvaTech)	Aquasorb (DeRoyal Wound Care)	Lyofoam (Ultra)	Sorbsan (Bertek Pharm.)	Kendall Curity (Tyco Healthcare)
Opsite (Smith and Nephew)	Comfeel (Coloplast)	Carrasyn (Carrington)	Allevyn (Smith and Nephew)	Algisite (Smith and Nephew)	Kendall Telfa (Kendall Health-care)
DermaFilm (CWI Medical)	Tegasorb (3M)	Curasol (Healthpoint)	Polymem (Ferris Manufacturing)	Seasorb (Coloplast)	
Polyskin II (Kendall)	Restore (Hollister Wound Care) NuDerm (Obagi)		Biatain (Coloplast) Contreet (Coloplast) Xtrasorb (Derma Sciences) Mepilex (Molnlycke Health Care)	Acticoat (Smith & Nephew) Melgisorb (Molnlycke Health Care)	
Retains moisture; promotes autolysis; suitable for stage I and II ulcers. Used for noninfected wounds. Adhesive (so does not require a secondary dressing) and semipermeable (not to bacteria). May be used with hydrogel or hydrocolloid dressings.	Available in various forms. Promotes autolysis. May be used as primary or secondary dressing for stage I and II ulcers with minimum to moderate exudates. Impermeable to bacteria and other contaminants.	Water or glycerin based. Promotes autolysis and a moist healing environment. Good for stages II–IV with minimum exudate. Can be used for packing.	For partial- to full-thickness wounds with minimum to moderate exudate. May be a primary or secondary dressing for stages II–IV. Provides moist environment and thermal insulation.	Highly absorbent. Absorbs up to 20× its weight. Forms a gel within the wound, conforming to the shape of the wound. Facilitates autolysis. For partial- to full-thickness wounds with moderate to heavy exudate. Good for packing tunnels, cavities, or sinus tracks. Requires secondary dressing.	Good for packing dead space. Generally requires a secondary dressing. Need frequent dressing changes.

[a]Representative samples only and not an exhaustive list of all products on the market.
Other dressings include nonadherent dressings (i.e., Adaptic, Telfa, Vaseline Guaze) and impregnated gauzes (i.e., Xeroform, Mesalt).

This dressing conforms to the wound, is moisture retentive, and insulates the wound effectively.

Contact Layers

These are nonadherent, woven polyamide net placed in contact with the wound bed and allow exudate to pass through from the wound to a secondary dressing. These are used for large or deep wounds to protect the wound bed, often when blood vessels or organs are exposed. They are indicated for full-thickness granular wounds with minimal to heavy exudates. It is especially common to use on donor sites, split-thickness skin grafts, and in combination with negative pressure wound therapy (NPWT).

Foam

Foam is semipermeable, hydrophilic and an impermeable barrier, which is indicated for absorption of partial- and full-thickness wounds with minimal to heavy exudate. These are often used as a secondary dressing in combination with other dressing materials, such as alginates, hydrogels, and powders. It is conformable to the shape around angular body contours. Frequency of change is determined by the amount of exudate absorbed by the dressing.

Transparent Film

This is made up of a thin, transparent polyurethane adhesive film that is impermeable and ideal for partial-thickness minimally draining or closed wounds. Used as a primary dressing, it promotes autolysis, but this is now more commonly used as a secondary dressing.

Hydrofiber

This dressing is made from sodium carboxymethylcellulose, which interacts with wound fluid or exudate to form a gel. These dressings may also contain controlled-released ionic silver. This dressing is effective in maintaining a moist wound environment. This requires a secondary dressing.

Collagen

Derived from bovine, porcine, or avian sources, this is used to stimulate wound healing for partial- and full-thickness wounds, contaminated and infected, with minimal to moderate exudate. They are highly absorptive hydrophilic moist wound dressing. Although collagen is available in pouches, vials, or gels loaded into syringes, pads, powders, and freeze-dried sheets, it is best to use powders, particles, and pads for highly exudating wounds. For moderately exudating wounds, sheets should be used, and if the wound is dry, gels should be used. These dressings require a secondary dressing for securement.

Electrical Stimulation (ES)

Adjunctive therapies have long been described in the PrU literature and the AHCPR critically evaluated the strength of the literature on adjunctive therapies. Based on the clinical evidence available, only ES-merited recommendation is to be considered for stage II, III, and IV PrUs that are unresponsive to conventional therapy.

There remains a lack of clear understanding about how ES works to promote healing. Some of the effects of ES on wound healing include decreased healing time, increased collagen synthesis, increased wound tensile strength, increased rate of wound epithelialization, and enhanced bacteriocidal effects (170). ES has also been shown to improve tissue perfusion and reduce edema formation indirectly stimulating healing by improving oxygen delivery to tissue. The literature shows high variability about which type of electric current and application protocols are effective for specific patient or ulcer type. However, many of the studies have demonstrated that when used in conjunction with standard wound management, ES can accelerate the healing rate of PrUs in patients with SCI (78,171–174).

Other Modalities

Hydrotherapy should be considered for PrUs containing large amounts of exudate and necrotic tissue, where it can assist in debridement. However, once the wound is clean and has healthy granulation tissue, the agitating water may cause damage to the delicate new tissue and should be discontinued. The therapeutic efficacy of hyperbaric oxygen, infrared, ultraviolet, and low-energy laser irradiation, and ultrasonography have not been sufficiently established for recommendation in the treatment of PrUs. The consortium guidelines did not identify enough supporting evidence to recommend lasers as a treatment. Regan reported that there is level I evidence from two RCTs to suggest that laser treatment has no added benefit in PrU healing after SCI over standard wound care alone (78,175,176).

The consortium guidelines found minimal data specific to the use of ultrasound or ultraviolet-C radiation to treat PrUs in SCI (1). Electromagnetic energy acts during the proliferative stage of wound healing to increase production of granulation tissue formation. Other beneficial effects include increased blood and oxygen availability to tissues and decreased tissue edema (78). One RCT supported the efficacy of pulsed electromagnetic energy (PEE) to accelerate the healing of stage II and III PrUs after SCI (177). PEE may improve wound healing in stage II and III PrUs after SCI. A Cochrane review found that there was no strong evidence at this time to recommend PEE in PrU healing in individuals after SCI (178). Further research is recommended (78,178).

PLATELET-DERIVED GROWTH FACTORS

Platelet-derived growth factors (PDGFs) are applied directly to the wound surface to promote growth of skin, soft tissue, and blood vessels. Recombinant DNA technology has been used to produce a recombinant human platelet-derived growth factor (rPDGF, rPDGF-BB, or rhPDGF-BB). Becaplermin (tradename Regranex Gel) is not an autologous product, but is a commercially prepared biotechnology product with recombinant PDGF as the active ingredient. The growth factor is produced in the laboratory by inserting a gene into yeast. Autologel and SafeBlood are autologous preparations in which blood is drawn from the patient and centrifuged to create platelet-rich plasma that is applied to the wound.

Results of studies evaluating recombinant PDGF or becaplermin (Regranex) demonstrated that becaplermin, in conjunction with good wound care, is efficacious in accelerating wound closure of chronic diabetic ulcers (179,180). Significant increases in the incidence of complete wound closure and decreases in the time to achieve complete wound healing were observed in patients receiving the study medication compared with those receiving placebo (181). However, this product carries a boxed warning indicating that patients who use in excess of three tubes may experience increased mortality due to malignancy. Therefore, while growth factors appear to be useful adjuvant therapy, more information on safety with long-term use is necessary (182).

AUTOLOGOUS PLATELET-DERIVED GROWTH FACTORS

A prospective, randomized, controlled, blinded, multicenter study initially included 72 patients with diabetic foot ulcers who were treated with autologous platelet-rich plasma gel or control (saline gel). In this study, significantly more wounds healed in patients treated with platelet-rich plasma gel (13 out of 16 or 81.3%) than patients treated with control gel (8 out of 19 or 42.1%) (183). Likewise, Mazzucco et al. (184) evaluated patients with dehiscent sternal wounds and patients with necrotic skin ulcers who were treated with autologous platelet gel and retrospectively compared with patients having similar lesions but undergoing traditional treatment. In patients with dehiscent sternal wounds, the healing rate and hospital stay were significantly reduced. Patients with necrotic skin ulcers required a shorter time to have surgery (184). Margolis et al. conducted a retrospective cohort study of 26,599 patients from the Curative Health Services database who were treated with platelet releasate or standard wound therapy. The authors determined that more diabetic neuropathic foot ulcers treated with platelet releasate healed by 32 weeks than ulcers treated with standard wound therapy (50% versus 41%, respectively) (185). No studies have been found in SCI.

Cellular Therapy, Tissue-Engineered Skin Substitutes

The principles underlying the use of skin substitutes apply to extensive wounds that cannot heal spontaneously because of their depth and a large percentage of total body surface. They also apply to smaller wounds that cannot heal. It is indicated for wounds that would heal of their own accord but there is a need for faster and/or better quality of healing.

Skin substitutes are either native biological substitutes with or without living cells or biomedically engineered. Native biological substitutes are made up of fresh, cryopreserved, or glycerolized cadaveric skin, porcine disinfected skin, cryopreserved amniotic membrane, porcine small intestine submucosa, or porcine dermal collagen. Tissue-engineered products are epidermal, dermal, or bilayer substitutes and are used during the various phases of wound healing. Some are used for temporary coverage because they do not provide autologous keratinocytes for epithelialization. They must be covered by an epidermal substitute that will restore the epidermal barrier function. Those designed to provide permanent coverage must have keratinocytes to promote proliferation and to sustain epithelialization and restore the epidermal barrier (186,187).

Negative Pressure Wound Therapy (Subatmospheric Pressure Therapy)

NPWT distributes negative pressure (subatmospheric pressure) across a wound surface via a special dressing and can be applied continuously or intermittently. The intent of NPWT is to promote wound healing and it has been used to treat a variety of acute and chronic wounds including PrUs (188,189). An airtight system is created using special foam, sterile tubing and canister, and an adhesive film drape (190). Vacuum (subatmospheric pressure—125 mm Hg below ambient) is applied via a suction bottle or pump (191). The negative pressure in the wound bed increases blood flow, reduces local tissue edema, decreases bacterial colonization, and increases granulation tissue formation and mechanical wound closure (188–190). NPWT when applied to a PrU may improve healing in SCI. It has been shown to be cost effective in the home care of chronic wounds. More research is needed, however.

Normothermia

Normothermia employs the use of a radiant heat dressing to hasten wound healing. Normothermia has been shown in one small study involving patients with SCI with stage III and IV PrUs to decrease the mean wound surface area by 61% over a 4-week period (192). As with negative pressure therapy, use of a normothermic dressing may improve healing of PrUs after SCI but more research is needed.

Surgical Management

In general, stage I and II PrUs are usually treated with local care nonsurgically. Stage III and IV PrUs, because of their high rate of recurrence as well as the long duration necessary for wound closure, often require surgical intervention. In general, the goals of surgical wound closure can include reduction in the time to healing, lower costs, improve patient hygiene and appearance, decrease in amount of care needed, and prevention of secondary complications including renal amyloidosis and Marjolin ulcer (193). Proper selection of the surgical candidate is important because of the cost and postoperative recovery time, both of which can be extensive. In addition, if musculocutaneous flaps are performed, there are only a limited number that can be performed, which may be of consequence if the individual has repeated PrUs or additional risk factors are added with aging.

Operative procedures to repair PrUs include direct closure, skin grafting, skin flaps, musculocutaneous flaps, fasciocutaneous flaps, and free flaps. Free flaps, skin flaps, and skin grafts are rarely used for PrUs in SCI, as they are poorly able to tolerate any future pressure or shear. Direct closure is rarely of benefit unless the source of the pressure has been eradicated and the wound is small. Musculocutaneous and fasciocutaneous flaps have become the coverage of choice for SCI patients who require surgical closure of the ulcer. Because of their blood supply, these flaps are better able to withstand pressure and shear and can be particularly useful in osteomyelitis, by bringing highly vascularized muscle tissue into the area of infection. The decision to use a particular flap or type depends on the surgeons' expertise and the size and position of the ulcer. Surgical interventions for PrUs have been found to offer more rapid healing, improvement in quality of life, and an increase in participation in rehabilitation with long-term results (194,195).

Factors that impair postoperative healing include smoking, spasticity, nutritional concerns, and bacterial colonization. Smoking is one of the strongest inhibitors of wound healing as a result of carbon monoxide and nicotine, both of which are potent vasoconstrictors. In addition to compromises in arterial blood flow and oxygen delivery, smoking increases blood viscosity and increases oxidase release by neutrophils, all of which impair wound healing. Nicotine patches should not be used as they provide the same effects as cigarettes. Spasticity can also impair postoperative healing through repeated contraction of muscles causing joint movement during the period of postoperative immobilization. In addition, significant contractures may impair pressure-relief efforts. Adequate nutrition must be maintained during the postoperative period to allow for wound healing, although serum albumin and total protein levels have not been found to correlate with postoperative wound outcome (48). Exposure to bacterial contamination, particularly of urine and feces, increases colonization of wounds and is associated with slower rates of healing. Constipating medications may on occasion be administered and a low-fiber diet may be used to avoid fecal contamination of the surgical site, although bowel programs still need to be performed given the length of immobilization postoperatively. If there is a great deal of stool incontinence interfering with the wound, or suspected to interfere with postoperative healing of PrUs over the sacrum and ITs, a temporary diverting colostomy may be considered; however, it should be noted that most PrUs heal postoperatively without such procedures (196,197).

At the sacral area, the gluteus maximus muscle may be used entirely or in portions. At the ischium, a posterior thigh fasciocutaneous flap, inferior gluteus maximus myocutaneous flap, hamstring V-Y advancement flap, and tensor fascia lata fasciocutaneous flap can all be used to cover defects in this region. Prophylactic unilateral or bilateral ischiectomy is not recommended. Unilateral ischiectomy, because weight is diverted to the contralateral ischium, is associated with occurrence of a contralateral ischial ulcer (198). Bilateral ischiectomy will transfer weight bearing to the anterior pelvis and perineum, causing perineal ulcer and urethral fistulae (199,200). At the greater trochanter, the tensor fascia lata fasciocutaneous flap is considered the flap of choice in this area, although alternatives include use of the vastus lateralis, inferior gluteus maximus, and rectus femoris muscles. Girdlestone arthroplasty for ulcers that communicate with the hip joint may be necessary, although patients may experience a pistoning of the distal femur after this procedure, which may be detrimental to the flap (201).

Postoperatively, strict bed rest is prescribed with immobilization and pressure relief. It is important to keep pressure off the surgical site as much as possible. Usually, a low- air-loss mattress or an air-fluidized bed is prescribed. For repairs of the sacrum or IT, the head of the bed should not be elevated greater than 15 degrees since this position increases the risk of shear on the repaired ulcer site (1). Bed rest should be maintained postoperatively to allow sufficient time for the surgical site to heal before mobilization. There is no consensus in the literature on the necessary length of immobilization postflap and is variable depending upon the size of the flap as well as on the individual surgeons protocol; and ranges from 2 to 6 weeks (202,203).

Once healing occurs, passive range of motion of the hips in preparation for sitting can be initiated. Once the hip ROM is at 90 degrees without stress on the surgical site, sitting is initiated, starting with short intervals; that is, 15 minutes, and then with return to bed for evaluation of the surgical site. A progressive sitting program ensues, with an increase in sitting by 15 minutes once to twice per day. Usually over a course of 2 to 3 weeks, the patient can progress to sitting up to 5 h/d, with return to complete mobilization from surgery of approximately 8½ weeks (1). Institutional protocols vary, with some faster and others with slower remobilization timing.

PrU recurrence is relatively common. Overall, an 11% to 61% recurrence rate has been reported following a PrU and surgical repair of PrUs (57,204–212). A recent study by Bates-Jensen et al. (206) reported that most PrUs recurred in the same location, most commonly at the ITs (63%). Yamamoto et al. (208) also found higher recurrence rates for the IT site (49%) compared to the sacrum (21%). These findings are intuitive in this population because the ischial sites are subjected to the greatest pressure when in the seated position and persons with SCI spend significant amount of time in the wheelchair. Smoking, diabetes mellitus, and cardiovascular disease were associated with the highest rates of recurrence in these studies (205).

OSTEOMYELITIS

Unilateral osteomyelitis often leads to nonhealing ulcers. Approximately 25% of all nonhealing ulcers are infected (213) and this should be ruled out if there is reasonable suspicion. Bone biopsy is the most sensitive test, although surgeons are often reluctant to perform this unless there are other compelling indications for surgery. In the outpatient setting, osteomyelitis is most easily diagnosed by imaging studies. Conventional bone scan is more sensitive for osteomyelitis than plain films. Although specificity is approximately 50% because of difficulty in differentiating soft tissue infection from bone infection, indium leukocyte scans improve the sensitivity and specificity. MRI reveals anatomic detail and is sensitive to the presence of marrow edema on the T2-weighted image (214). Treatment of osteomyelitis includes appropriate antibiotics for 6 to 12 weeks.

ADDITIONAL PRESSURE ULCER COMPLICATIONS

PrUs have been associated with many complications including endocarditis (213), heterotopic bone formation, maggot infestation, perineal urethral fistula, septic arthritis, sinus tract or abscess, squamous cell carcinoma in the ulcer, and, specifically in SCI, contractures (199,215–222). Long-standing ulcers (20 years or more) can, although rarely (less than 0.5%), develop Marjolin ulcers, a type of squamous cell carcinoma. Biopsy can identify the carcinoma that is suspected clinically with pain, increasing discharge, verrucous hyperplasia, and bleeding (223).

Pain and Pressure Ulcers

Pain is often present in persons with PrUs (224,225) although unclear as to the prevalence in the SCI population. Potential treatments include opioid gel treatment treatments (226,227) although this is not as of yet available in the United States, benzydamine cream (228), lidocaine/prilocaine for local treatment (229), or systemic medication as needed.

CONCLUSION

Despite advances in education, equipment, and technology, and our understanding of their pathophysiology, PrUs remain a significant psychological, financial, and functional barrier to many patients after their SCI. Structured prevention education helps individuals after SCI gain and retain knowledge of PrU prevention practices and the use of specialized equipment assists in PrU prevention. Once ulcers occur, they have wide-ranging effects upon the individual socially, psychologically, vocationally, and medically and it is imperative that maximize wound healing occur as well as interventions necessary to prevent wound recurrence. Further research is needed in all areas of pressure sore prevention and management so as to minimize its impact on the individual following their SCI.

References

1. Consortium for Spinal Cord Medicine. Pressure ulcer prevention and treatment following spinal cord injury: a clinical practice guideline for health care professionals. *J Spinal Cord Med.* 2001;24(Suppl1):S.40–S101
2. Richards JS, Waites K, Chen YY, et al. The epidemiology of secondary conditions following spinal cord injury. *Top Spinal Cord Inj Rehabil* 2004;10:15–29.
3. National Pressure Ulcer Advisory Panel (NPUAP). Pressure ulcers prevalence, cost and risk assessment: Consensus development conference statement. *Decubitus* 1989;2:24–28.
4. National Pressure Ulcer Advisory Panel. Pressure Ulcer Stages Revised by NPUAP. NPUAP 2007. http://www.npuap/pr2.htm. Published February 2007.
5. Lamid S, El Ghatit AZ. Smoking, spasticity and pressure sores in spinal cord injured patients. *Am J Phys Med* 1983;62:300–306.
6. Crenshaw RP, Vistnes LM. A decade of pressure sore research: 1977–1987. *J Rehabil Res Dev* 1989;26:63–74.
7. Bogie KM, Nuseibeh I, Bader DL. Early progressive changes in tissue viability in the seated spinal cord injured subject. *Paraplegia* 1995;33:141–147.
8. Landis EM. Micro-injection studies of capillary blood pressure in human skin. *Heart* 1930;15:209–228.
9. Garber SL, Krouskop TA. Body build and its relationship to pressure distribution in the seated wheelchair patient. *Arch Phys Med Rehabil* 1982;63:17–20.
10. Seiler WO, Allen S, Stahelin HB. Influence of the 30 degrees laterally included position and the "supersoft" 3-piece mattress on skin oxygen tension on areas of maximum pressure—implications for pressure sore prevention. *Gerontology* 1986;32:158–166.
11. Daniel RK, Wheatley D, Priest D. Pressure sores and paraplegics: an experimental model. *Ann Plast Surg* 1985;15:41–49.
12. Kosiak M, Kubicek WG, Olso M, et al. Evaluation of pressure as a risk factor in the production of ischial ulcers. *Arch Phys Med Rehabil* 1958;39:623–629.
13. Kosiak M. Etiology and pathology of ischemic ulcers. *Arch Phys Med Rehabil* 1959;40:62–69.
14. Agency for Health Care Policy and Research. *Pressure ulcers in adults: prediction and prevention.* Clin Pract Guideline number 3. Rockville, MD: Public Health Services. US Department of Human and Health Services, 1992.
15. Stass WE Jr, Cioschi HM. Pressure sores: a multifaceted approach to prevention and treatment. *West J Med* 1991;154:539–544.
16. Daniel RK, Hall EJ, MacLeod MK. Pressure sores: a reappraisal. *Ann Plat Surg* 1979;3:53–63.
17. Husain T. An experimental study of some pressure effects on tissues in reference to the bedsore problems. *J Pathol Bacteriol* 1953;66:347–358.
18. Daniel RK, Priest DL, Wheatley DC. Etiologic factors in pressure sores: an experimental model. *Arch Phys Med Rehabil* 1981;62:492–498.
19. Nola GT, Vistnes LM. Differential response of skin and muscle in the experimental production of pressure sores. *Plast Reconstr Surg* 1980;66:728–733.
20. Reichel S. Shearing force as a factor in decubitus ulcers in paraplegics. *JAMA* 1958;166:762–763.
21. Dinsdale S. Decubitus ulcers: role of pressure and friction in causation. *Arch Phys Med Rehabil* 1974;55:147–152.
22. Bryant R. Skin pathology and types of damage. In: Bryant R, ed. *Acute and chronic wounds; nursing management.* St Louis, MO: Mosby, 2000.
23. Bergstrom N, Braden B, Kemp M, et al. Multi-site study of incidence of pressure ulcers and the relationship between risk level, demographic characteristics, diagnoses, and prescription of preventative interventions. *J Am Geriatr Soc* 1996;44:22–30.
24. Rochon PA. Beaudet MP. McGlinchey-Berroth R, et al. Risk assessment for pressure ulcers: an adaptation of the National Pressure Ulcer Advisory Panel risk factors to spinal cord injured patients. *J Am Paraplegia Soc* 1993;16:169–177.
25. Rodriguez GP, Claus-Walker J. Biomechanical changes in skin composition in spinal cord injury: a possible contribution to decubitus ulcers. *Paraplegia* 1988;26:302–309.
26. Rodriguez GP, Claus-Walker J, Kent MC, et al. Collagen metabolite excretion as a predictor of bone and skin related complications in spinal cord injury. *Arch Phys Med Rehabil* 1989;70:442–444.
27. Teasell RW, Arnold JM, Krassioukov A, et al. Cardiovascular consequences of loss of supraspinal control of the sympathetic nervous system after spinal cord injury. *Arch Phys Med Rehabil* 2000;81:506–516.
28. Rodriguez GP, Claus-Walker J, Kent MC, et al. Adrenergic receptors in insensitive skin of spinal cord injury patients. *Arch Phys Med Rehabil* 1986;67:177–180.
29. Hagisawa, Ferguson-Pell SM, Cardi M. Assessment of skin blood content and oxygenation in spinal cord injured subjects during reactive hyperemia. *J Rehabil Res* 1994;31:1–14.
30. Thornfinn J, Sjorberg F, Lidman D. Sitting pressure and perfusion on buttock skin in paraplegia and tetraplegia patients and in health subjects in comparative study. *Scand J Plast Reconstr Surg Hand Surg* 2002;36:279–283.
31. Fuhrer MJ, Garber SL, Rintala DH, et al. Pressure ulcers in community resident persons with spinal cord injury: prevalence and risk factors. *Arch Phys Med Rehabil* 1993;74:1172–1177.
32. Garber SL, Rintala DH, Hart KA, et al. Pressure ulcer risk in spinal cord injury: predictors of ulcer status over 3 years. *Arch Phys Med Rehabil* 2000;81:465–471.
33. Krause JS. Skin sores after spinal cord injury: relationship to life adjustment. *Spinal Cord* 1998;36:51–56.
34. Gelis A, Dupeyron A, Legros P, et al. Pressure ulcer risk factors in persons with spina cord injury (part II): the chronic stage. *Spinal Cord* 2009;47:651–661.
35. McKinley WO, Jackson AB, Cardenas DD, et al. Long-term medical complications after traumatic spinal cord injury: a regional model systems analysis. *Arch Phys Med Rehabil* 1999;80:1402–1410.
36. Lehman CA. Risk factors for pressure ulcers in the spinal cord injured in the community. *Sci Nurs* 1995;12: 110–114.
37. Vidal J, Sarrias M. An analysis of the diverse factors concerned with the development of pressure ulcers in spinal cord injured patients. *Paraplegia* 1991;29:261–267.

38. Young ME, Rintala DH, Rossi CD, et al. Alcohol and marijuana use in a community-based sample of persons with spinal cord injury. *Arch Phys Med Rehabil* 1995;76:525–532.
39. Chen Y, DeVivo MJ, Jackson AB. Pressure ulcer prevalence in people with spinal cord injury: age-period-duration effects. *Arch Phys Med Rehabil* 2005;86:1208–1213.
40. Salzberg CA, Byrne DW, Cayten CG, et al. Predicting and preventing pressure ulcers in adults with paralysis. *Adv Wound Care* 1998;11:237–246.
41. Fuhrer MJ, Rintala DH, Hart KA, et al. Depressive symptomatology in persons with spinal cord injury who reside in the community. *Arch Phys Med Rehabil* 1993;74:255–260.
42. Rintala DH, Young ME, Hart KA, et al. Social support and the well-being of persons with spinal cord injury living in the community. *Rehabil Psychol* 1992;37:155–163.
43. Richardson RR, Meyer PR. Prevalence and incidence of pressure sores in acute spinal cord injuries. *Paraplegia* 1981;19:235–247.
44. Saladin LK, Krause JS. Pressure ulcer prevalence and barriers to treatment after spinal cord injury: comparisons of four groups based on race-ethnicity. *Neuro Rehabil* 2009;24(1):57–66.
45. Guihan M, Garber SL, Bombardier CH, et al. Predictors of pressure ulcer recurrence in veterans with spinal cord injury. *J Spinal Cord Med* 2008;31(5):551–559.
46. Redelings MD, Lee NE, Sorvillo F. Pressure ulcers: more lethal than we thought? *Adv Skin Wound Care* 2005;18(7):367–372.
47. Saunders LL, Krause JS, Peters BA, et al. The relationship of pressure ulcers, race, and socioeconomic conditions after spinal cord injury. *J Spinal Cord Med* 2010;33(4):387–395.
48. Goodman CM, Cohen V, Armenta A, et al. Evaluation of results and treatment variables for pressure ulcers in 48 veteran spinal cord-injured patients. *Ann Plastic Surg* 1999;42:665–672.
49. Sheerin F, Gillick A, Doyle B. Pressure ulcers in spinal cord injury: incidence among admissions to the Irish National Specialist Unit. *J Wound Care* 2005;14:112–115.
50. Curry K, Casaty L. The relationship between extended periods of immobility and decubitus ulcer formation in the acute spinal cord injured individual. *J Neurosci Nurs* 1992;24:185–189.
51. Caliri MHL. Spinal cord injury and pressure ulcers. *Nurs Clin N Am* 2005;40:337–347.
52. Mawson AR, Biundo JJ, Neville P, et al. Risk factors for early occurring pressure ulcers following spinal cord injury. *Am J Phys Med Rehabil* 1988;67(3):123–127.
53. Chen D, Apple DF Jr, Hudson LM, et al. Medical complications during acute rehabilitation following spinal cord injury—current experience of the Model Systems. *Arch Phys Med Rehabil* 1999;80:1397–1401.
54. Ploumis A, Kolli S, Patrick M, et al. Length of stay and medical stability for spinal cord-injured patients on admission to an inpatient rehabilitation hospital: a comparison between a model SCI trauma center and non-SCI trauma center. *Spinal Cord* 2011;49:411–415.
55. Yarkony GM, Heinemann AW. Pressure ulcers. In: Stover SL, DeLisa JA, Whiteneck GG, eds. *Spinal cord injury: clinical outcomes from the model systems.* Gaithersburg, MD: Aspen Publishing, 1995.
56. Krause JS, Broderick L. Patterns of recurrent pressure ulcers after spinal cord injury: identification of risk and protective factors 5 or more years after onset. *Arch Phys Med Rehabil* 2004;85(8):1257–1264.
57. Niazi ZB, Salzberg CA, Byrne DW, et al. Recurrence of initial pressure ulcer in persons with spinal cord injuries. *Adv Wound Care* 1997;10:38–42.
58. Guihan M, Garber SL, Bombardier CH, et al. Lessons Learned in Conducting a Trial to Prevent Pressure Ulcers in Veterans with Spinal Cord Injury. *Arch Phys Med Rehabil.* 2007 Jul;88(7):858–61.
59. Vogel LC, Krajci KA, Anderson CJ. Adults with pediatric-onset spinal cord injuries: part 3: impact of medical complications. *J Spinal Cord Med* 2002;25(4):297–305.
60. Young JS, Burns PE. Pressure sores and the spinal cord injured: part II. *SCI Digest* 1981;3:11–26.
61. Whiteneck GG, Carter RE, Charlifue SW, et al. A collaborative study of high quadriplegia. Final report to the National Institute of Handicapped Research. Englewood, CO: Rocky Mountain regional Spinal Injury System, 1985.
62. Cardenas DD, Hoffman JM, Kirshblum S, et al. Etiology and incidence of rehospitalization after traumatic spinal cord injury: a multicenter analysis. *Arch Phys Med Rehabil* 2004;85(11):1757–1763.
63. Byrne DW, Salzberg CA. Major risk factors for pressure ulcers in spinal cord disabled: a literature review. *Spinal Cord* 1996;34(5):255–263.
64. Delisa JA, Mikulit MA. Pressure ulcers: what do we do if preventive management fails. *Pressure Ulcers* 1985;77:209–212.
65. Thomas AC, Wysocki AB. The healing wound: a comparison of three useful clinical methods of measurement. *Decubitus* 1990;3:18–25.
66. Kundin JI. Designing and developing a new measuring instrument. *Perioper Nurs* 1975;1:40–45.
67. Mayrovitz HN, Soontupe LB. Wound areas by computerized planimetry of digital images: Accuracy and reliability. *Adv Skin Wound Care* 2008;22(5):222–229.
68. Ahn C, Salcido R. Advances in wound photography and assessment methods. *Adv Skin Wound Care* 2008;21(2);85–93.
69. Lucas C, Classen J, Harrison D, et al. Pressure ulcer surface area measurement using instant full-scale photography and transparency tracings. *Adv Skin Wound Care* 2002;15(1):17–23.
70. Dyson M, Moodley S, Verjee L, et al. Wound healing assessment using 20 MHz ultrasound and photography. *Skin Res Technol* 2004;9(2):116–121.
71. Jones ML, Mathewson CS, Adkins VK, et al. Use of behavioral contingencies to promote prevention of recurrent pressure ulcers. *Arch Phys Med Rehabil* 2003;84:796–802.
72. Bogie KM, Reger SI, Levine ST, et al. Electrical stimulation for pressure prevention and wound healing. *Assist Technol* 2000;12:50–66.
73. LaMantia JG, Hirschwald JF, Goodman CL, et al. Pressure sore readmission program: a method to reduce

chronic readmissions for pressure sore problems. *Rehabil Nurs* 1987;12:22–25.

74. Mortenson WB, Miller WC. A review of scales for assessing the risk of developing a pressure ulcer in individuals with SCI. *Spinal Cord* 2008;46:168–175.
75. Bergstrom N, Braden BJ, Laguzza A, et al. The Braden Scale for predicting pressure sore risk. *Nurs Res* 1987;36:205–210.
76. Braun J, Silvetti A, Zakellis G. What really works for pressure scores. *Patient Care* 1992;26:63–76.
77. Yarkony GM. Pressure ulcers: a review. *Arch Phys Med Rehabil* 1994;75:908–917.
78. Regan MA, Teasell RW, Wolfe DL, et al. A systemic review of therapeutic interventions for pressure ulcers after spinal cord injury. *Arch Phys Med Rehabil* 2009;19:213–231.
79. Dover H, Pickard W, Swain I, et al. The effectiveness of a pressure clinic in preventing pressure sores. *Paraplegia* 1992;30:267–272.
80. Reenalda J, Jannink M, Nederhand M, et al. Clinical use of interface pressure to predict pressure ulcer development: a systematic review. *Assist Technol* 2009;21(2):76–85.
81. Parnham A. Interface pressure measurements during ambulance journeys. *J Wound Care* 1999;8:279–282.
82. Linares HA, Mawson AR, Suarez E, et al. Association between pressure sores and immobilization in the immediate post-injury period. *Orthopedics* 1987;10:571–573.
83. Land L. A review of pressure damage preventing strategies. *J Adv Nurs* 1995;22:329–337.
84. Reddy M, Gill SS, Kalkar SR, et al. Treatment of pressure ulcers: a systematic review. *JAMA* 2008;300(22):2647–2662.
85. Allman RM, Walker JM, Hart MK, et al. Air-fluidized beds or conventional therapy for pressure sores. A randomized trial. *Ann Intern Med* 1987;107(5):641–648.
86. Strauss MJ, Gong J, Gary BD, et al. The cost of home air-fluidized therapy for pressure sores. A randomized controlled trial. *J Fam Pract* 1991;33(1):52–59.
87. Greer DM, Morris J, Walsh NE, et al. Cost-effectiveness and efficacy of air-fluidized therapy in the treatment of pressure ulcers. *J Enterostomal Ther* 1988;15(6):247–251.
88. Ochs RF, Horn SD, van Rijswijk L, et al. Comparison of air-fluidized therapy with other support surfaces used to treat pressure ulcers in nursing home residents. *Ostomy Wound Manage* 2005;51(2):38–68.
89. Barnes S, Rutland BS. Air-fluidized therapy as a cost-effective treatment for a "worst case" pressure necrosis. *J Enterostomal Ther* 1986;13(1):27–29.
90. Cuddigan J, Ayello E. Treating severe pressure ulcers in the home setting: faster healing and lower cost with air fluidized therapy (AFT). Supplement to the Remington Report. May–June 2004.
91. Munro BH, Brown L, Heitman BB. Pressure ulcers: one bed or another? *Geriatr Nurs* 1989;10(4):190–192.
92. VanGilder C, Lachenbruch CA. Air-fluidized therapy: physical properties and clinical uses. *Ann Plast Surg* 2010;65(3):364–370.
93. Sharbaugh RJ, Hargest TS, Wright FA. Further studies on the bactericidal effect of the air-fluidized bed. *Am Surg* 1973;39:253–256.
94. Sharbaugh RJ, Hargest TS. Bactericidal effect of the air-fluidized bed. *Am Surg* 1971;37:583–586.
95. Newsome MW, Johns LA, Pruitt BA Jr. Use of an air-fluidized bed in the care of patients with extensive burns. *Am J Surg* 1972;124(1):52–56.
96. Nicholson GP, Scales JT, Clark RP, et al. A method for determining the heat transfer and water vapour permeability of patient support systems. *Med Eng Phys* 1999;21(10):701–712.
97. Sanchez DG, Bussey B, Petorak M. How air-fluidized beds revolutionize skin care. *RN* 1983;46(6):46–48.
98. European Pressure Ulcer Advisory Panel. Policy statement on the prevention of pressure ulcers. *Br J Nurs* 1998;7(1):888–890.
99. National Institute for Health and Clinical Excellence. The management of pressure ulcers in primary and secondary care. Clinical Guideline Number 29. London, UK, http://www.nice.org.uk/nicemedia/pdf/CG029fullguideline.pdf Published September 22, 2005:1–245.
100. Moore ZE, Cowman S. Repositioning for treating pressure ulcers. *Cochrane Database Syst Rev* 2009;(2):CD006898.
101. Nixon V. Pressure relief. In: *Spinal cord injury: a guide to functional outcomes in physical therapy management.* 1st ed. Rockville, MD: Aspen Publishers, 1985:67–75.
102. Bergstrom N, Bennett MA, Carlson CE. Clinical Practice Guideline Number 3. Pressure ulcers in adults: prediction and prevention. Rockville, MD: US Department of Health and Human Services. Agency for Health Care Policy and Research, 1992. AHCPR Publication No 92-0047.
103. Coggrave MJ, Rose LS. A specialist seating assessment clinic: changing pressure relief practice. *Spinal Cord* 2003;41(12):692–695.
104. Makhsous M, Priebe M, Bankard J, et al. Measuring tissue perfusion during pressure relief maneuvers: insights into preventing pressure ulcers. *J Spinal Cord Med* 2007;30(5):497–507.
105. Hobson DA. Comparative effects of posture on pressure and shear at the body-seat interface. *J Rehabil Res Dev* 1992;15:21–31.
106. Goossens RH, Snijders CJ, Holscher TG, et al. Shear stress measured on beds and wheelchairs. *Scand J Rehabil Med* 1997;29:131–136.
107. Gilsdorf P, Patterson R, Fisher S. Thirty-minute continuous sitting force measurement with different support surfaces in the spinal cord injured and able-bodied. *J Rehabil Res Dev* 1991;28:33–38.
108. Yarkony GM, Chen D. Rehabilitation of patients with spinal cord injuries. In: *Physical medicine rehabilitation.* 1st ed. Philadelphia, PA: WB Saunders, 1996:1149–1179.
109. Shields RK, Cook TM. Lumbar support thickness: effect on seated buttock pressure in individuals with and without spinal cord injury. *Phys Ther* 1992;72:218–226.
110. Koo TK, Mak AF, Lee YL. Posture effect on eating interface biomechanics: Comparison between two seating systems. *Arch Phys Med Rehabil* 1996;77:40–47.
111. Salcido R, Hart D, Smith AM. The prevention and management of pressure ulcers. In: Braddom R, Buschbacher RM, Dumitru D, Johnson EW, Matthews

D, Sinaki M, eds. *Physical Medicine Rehabilitation.* 1st ed. Philadelphia, PA: WB Saunders; 1996:630-648
112. Barr CA. Evaluation of cushions using dynamic pressure measurement. *Prosthet Orthot Int.* 1991;15:232–240.
113. Crewe RA. Problems of rubbering nursing cushions and a clinical survey of alternative cushions for ill patients. *Case SCI Pract* 1987;5:9–11.
114. Burns SP, Betz KL. Seating pressures with conventional and dynamic wheelchair cushions in tetraplegia. *Arch Phys Med Rehabil* 1999;80:566–571.
115. Seymour RJ, Lacefield WE. Wheelchair cushion effect on pressure and skin temperature. *Arch Phys Med Rehabil* 1985;66:103–108.
116. Garber SL. Wheelchair cushions for spinal cord injured individuals. *Am J Occup Ther* 1985;39:722–725.
117. Bogie KM, Wang X, Triolo RJ. Long-term prevention of pressure ulcers in high-risk patients: a single case study of the use of gluteal neuromuscular electric stimulation. *Arch Phys Med Rehabil* 2006;87:585–591.
118. van Londen A, Herwegh M, van der Zee CH, et al. The effect of surface electric stimulation of the gluteal muscles on the interface pressure in seated people with spinal cord injury. *Arch Phys Med Rehabil* 2008;89(9):1724–1732.
119. Vesmarovich S, Walker T, Hauber RP, et al. Innovations in practice; use of telerehabilitation to manage pressure ulcers in persons with spinal cord injuries. *Adv Wound Care* 1999;12:264–269.
120. Tourtual DM, Riesenberg LA, Korutz CJ, et al. Predictors of hospital acquired heel pressure ulcers. *Ostomy Wound Manage* 1997;43:24–28, 30.
121. Keast DH, Parslow N, Houghton PE, et al. Best practice recommendations for the prevention and treatment of pressure ulcers: update 2006. *Adv Skin Wound Care.* 2007 Aug;20(8):447–60
122. terRiet G, Kessels A, Knipschild P. Randomized clinical trial of ascorbic acid in the treatment of pressure ulcers. *J Clin Epidemiol* 1995;48:1453–1460.
123. Taylor TV, Rimmer S, Day B, et al. Ascorbic acid supplementation in the treatment of pressure-sores. *Lancet* 1974;2(7880):544–546.
124. Houwing R, Overgoor M, Kon M, et al. Pressure-induced skin lesions in pigs: reperfusion injury and the effects of vitamin E. *J Wound Care* 2000;9:36–40.
125. Kohn S, Kohn D, Schiller D. Effect of zinc supplementation on epidermal Langerhans' cells of elderly patients with decubital ulcers. *J Derm* 2000;27:258–263.
126. Ellinger S, Stehle P. Efficacy of vitamin supplementation in situations with wound healing disorders: results from clinical intervention studies. *Curr Opin Clin Nutr Metab Care* 2009;12(6):588–595.
127. Desneves KJ, Todorovic BE, Cassar A, et al. Treatment with supplementary arginine, vitamin C and zinc in patients with pressure ulcers: a randomized controlled trial. *Clin Nutr* 2005;24(6):979–987.
128. Brewer S, Desneves K, Pearce L, et al. Effect of an arginine-containing nutritional supplement on pressure ulcer healing in community spinal patients. *J Wound Care* 2010;19(7):311–316.
129. Bonnefoy M, Coulon L, Bienvenu J, et al. Implication of cytokines in the aggravation of malnutrition and hypercatabolism in elderly patients with severe pressure sores. *Age Ageing* 1995;24:37–42.
130. Blaylock B. A study of risk factors in patients placed on specialty beds. *J Wound Ostomy Continence Nurs* 1995;22:263–266.
131. Allman RM, Goode PS, Patrick MM, et al. Pressure ulcer risk factors among hospitalized patients with activity limitation. *JAMA* 1995;273:865–870.
132. Segal JL, Gonzales E, Yousefi S, et al. Circulating levels of IL-2R, ICAM-1, and IL-6 in spinal cord injuries. *Arch Phys Med Rehabil* 1997;78:44–47.
133. Chin D, Kearns P. Nutrition in the spinal-injured patient. *Nutr Clin Pract* 1997;6:213–222.
134. Alexander LR, Spungen AM, Liu MH, et al. Resting metabolic rate in subjects with paraplegia: the effect of pressure sores. *Arch Phys Med Rehabil* 1995;76:819–822.
135. Liu MH, Spungen AM, Fink L, et al. Increased energy needs in patients with quadriplegia and pressure ulcers. *Adv Wound Care* 1996;9:41–45.
136. Jeevendra M, Ramos L, Shamos R, et al. Decreased growth hormone levels in the catabolic phase of severe injury. *Surgery* 1992;111:495–502.
137. Demling R, DeSanti L. Oxandrolone, an anabolic steroid significantly increases weight gain in the recovery phase after major burns. *J Trauma* 1997;43:47–51.
138. Demling R, DeSanti L. Closure of the "non-healing wound" corresponds with correction of weight loss using the anabolic agent oxandrolone. *Ostomy/Wound Manage* 1998;44:58–68.
139. Spungen AM, Koehler KM, Modeste-Duncan R, et al. Nine clinical cases of nonhealing pressure ulcers in patients with spinal cord injury treated with an anabolic agent: a therapeutic trial. *Adv Skin Wound Care* 2001;14:139–144.
140. van Rijswijk L. Full-thickness pressure ulcers: patient and wound healing characteristics. *Decubitus* 1993;6:16–21.
141. Dallam L, Smyth C, Jackson BS, et al. Pressure ulcer pain: assessment and quantification. *J Wound Ostomy Continence Nurs* 1995;22:211–215.
142. van Rijswijk L, Braden BJ. Pressure ulcer patient and wound assessment: an AHCPR clinical practice guideline update. *Ostomy Wound Manage* 1999;45(1A suppl):56S–67S.
143. Jones KR, Fennie K, Lenihan A. Evidence-based management of chronic wounds. *Adv Skin Wound Care* 2007;20(11):591–600.
144. Thomas DR, Rodeheaver GT, Bartolucci AA, et al. Pressure ulcer scale for healing: derivation and validation of the PUSH tool. The PUSH Task Force. *Adv Wound Care* 1997;10:96–101.
145. Bates-Jensen B. New pressure ulcer status tool. *Decubitus* 1990;3:14–15.
146. Ferrell BA. The Sessing Scale for measurement of pressure ulcer healing. *Adv Wound Care* 1997;10(5):78–80.
147. Krasner D. Wound Healing Scale, version 1.0: a proposal. *Adv Wound Care* 1997;10:82–85.
148. Mullins M, Thomason SS, Legro M. Monitoring pressure ulcer healing in persons with disabilities. *Rehabil Nurs* 2005;30(3):92–99.

149. Fernandez R, Griffiths R. Water for wound cleansing. *Cochrane Database Syst Rev* 2008;(1. Art. No.):CD003861. DOI: 10.1002/14651858.CD003861.pub2.
150. Foresman PA, Payne DS, Becker D, et al. A relative toxicity index for wound cleansers. *Wounds* 1993;5(5):226–231.
151. Rabenberg VG, Ingersoll CD, Sandrey MA, et al. The bactericidal and cytotoxic effects of antimicrobial wound cleansers. *J Athl Train* 2002;37(1):51–54.
152. Rodeheaver GT. Pressure ulcer debridement and cleansing: a review of current literature. *Ostomy/Wound Manage* 1999;45(suppl 1A):80S–85S.
153. Moore Z, Cowman S. A systematic review of wound cleansing for pressure ulcers. *J Clin Nurs* 2008;17(15):1963–1972.
154. Steed DL, Donohoe D, Webster MW, et al. Effect of extensive debridement and treatment on the healing of diabetic foot ulcers. Diabetic Ulcer Study Group. *J Am Coll Surg* 1996;183:61–64.
155. Mulder GD. Evaluation of three nonwoven sponges in the debridement of chronic wounds. *Ostomy/Wound Manage* 1995;41:62–67.
156. Sherman RA, Wyle F, Vulpe M. Maggot therapy for treating pressure ulcers in spinal cord injury patients. *J Spinal Cord Med* 1995;18:71–74.
157. Sherman RA. Maggot therapy takes us back to the future of wound care: new and improved maggot therapy for the 21st century. *J Diabetes Sci Technol* 2009;3(2):336–344.
158. Bergstrom N, Bennett MA, Carlson CE, et al. *Treatment of pressure ulcers.* Clinical Practice Guideline, No. 15. Rockville, MD: US Department of Health and Human Services. Public Health Service, Agency for Healthcare Policy and Research. AHCPR Publication #95-0652 December of 1994.
159. Cannon BC, Cannon JP. Management in pressure ulcers. *Am J Health Syst Pharm* 2004;61:1895–1905.
160. Tomaselli N. The role of topical silver preparations in wound healing. *J Wound Ostomy Continence Nurs* 2006;33:367–380.
161. Barnea Y, Weiss J, Gur E. A review of the applications of the hydrofiber dressing with silver (aquacel ag) in wound care. *Ther Clin Risk Manag* 2010;6:21–27.
162. Cutting K, White R, Edmonds M. The safety and efficacy of dressings with silver - addressing clinical concerns. *Int Wound J* 2007;4(2):177–184.
163. Silver dressings—do they work? *Drug Ther Bull* 2010;48(4):38–42.
164. Rousseau P. Pressure ulcers in an aging society. *Wounds* 1989;1:135–141.
165. Sapico FL, Ginunas VJ, Thornhill-Joynes M, et al. Quantitative microbiology of pressure sores in different stages of healing. *Diagn Microbiol Infect Dis* 1986;5:31–38.
166. Lewis VL Jr, Bailey MH, Pulawski G, et al. The diagnosis of osteomyelitis in patients with pressure sores. *Plast Reconstr Surg* 1988;81:229–232.
167. Sugarman B. Pressure sores and underlying bone infection. *Arch Intern Med* 1987;147:553–555.
168. Heyneman A, Beele H, Vanderwee K, et al. A systematic review of the use of hydrocolloids and the treatment of pressure ulcers. *J Clin Nurs* 2008;17:1164–1173.
169. Whittle H, Fletcher C, Hoskin A, et al. Nursing management of pressure ulcers using a hydrogel dressing protocol: four case studies. *Rehabil Nurs* 1996;21:239–242.
170. Kloth LC, Fedar JA. Acceleration of wound healing with high voltage, monophasic, pulsed current. *Phys Ther* 1988;68:503–508.
171. Baker LL, Rubayi S, Villar F, et al. Effect of electrical stimulation waveform on healing of ulcers in human beings with spinal cord injury. *Wound Repair Regen* 1996; 4:21–28.
172. Griffin JW, Tooms RE, Mendius RA, et al. Efficacy of high voltage pulsed current for healing of pressure ulcers in patients with spinal cord injury. *Phys Ther* 1991;71:433–444.
173. Houghton PE, Campbell KE, Fraser CH, et al. Electrical stimulation therapy increases rate of healing of pressure ulcers in community-dwelling people with spinal cord injury. *Arch Phys Med Rehabil* 2010;91(5):669–678.
174. Adegoke BO, Badmos KA. Acceleration of pressure ulcer healing in spinal cord injured patients using interrupted direct current. *Afr J Med Med Sci* 2001;30(3):195–197.
175. Taly AB, Sivaraman, Nair KP, et al. Efficacy of multiwavelength light therapy in the treatment of pressure ulcers in subjects with disorders of the spinal cord: a randomized double blind control trial. *Arch Phys Med Rehabil* 2004;85:1657–1661.
176. Nussbaum EL, Biemann I, Mustard B. Comparison of ultrasound/ultraviolet-C and laser for treatment of pressure ulcers in patients with spinal cord injury. *Phys Ther* 1994;74:812–823.
177. Salzberg CA, Cooper-Vastola SA, Perez F, et al. The effects of non-thermal pulsed electromagnetic energy on wound healing of pressure ulcers in spinal cord injured patients: a randomized, double blind study. *Ostomy Wound Manage* 1995;41:42–44, 46, 48.
178. Aziz Z, Flemming K, Cullum NA, et al. Electromagnetic therapy for treating pressure ulcers. *Cochrane Database Syst Rev*. 2010;11:CD002930.
179. Embil JM, Papp K, Sibbald G, et al. Recombinant human platelet-derived growth factor-BB (becaplermin) for healing chronic lower extremity diabetic ulcers: an open-label clinical evaluation of efficacy. *Wound Repair Regen* 2000;8(3):162–168.
180. Bao P, Kodra A, Tomic-Canic M, et al. The role of vascular endothelial growth factor in wound healing. *J Surg Res* 2009;153(2):347–358.
181. Franz MG, Robson MC, Steed DL, et al. Wound healing society. Guidelines to aid healing of acute wounds by decreasing impediments of healing. *Wound Repair Regen* 2008;16(6):723–748.
182. Mao CL, Rivet AJ, Sidora T, et al. Update on pressure ulcer management and deep tissue injury. *Ann Pharmacother* 2010;44(2):325–332.
183. Driver VR, Hanft J, Fylling CP, et al. Autologel Diabetic Foot Ulcer Study Group. A prospective, randomized, controlled trial of autologous platelet-rich plasma gel for the treatment of diabetic foot ulcers. *Ostomy Wound Manage* 2006;52(6):68–70, 72, 74.
184. Mazzucco L, Medici D, Serra M, et al. The use of autologous platelet gel to treat difficult-to-heal wounds: a pilot study. *Transfusion* 2004;44:1013–1018.

185. Margolis DJ, Kantor J, Santanna J, et al. Effectiveness of platelet releasate for the treatment of diabetic neuropathic foot ulcers. *Diabetes Care* 2001;24(3):483–488.
186. Auger FA, Lacroix D, Germain L. Skin substitutes and wound healing. *Skin Pharmacol Physiol* 2009;22:94–102.
187. Metcalfe AD, Ferguson MWJ. Tissue-engineering of replacement skin: the crossroads of biomaterials, wound healing, embryonic development, stem cells and regeneration. *J R Soc Interface* 2007;4:413–437.
188. Smith APS, Kieswetter K, Goodwin AL, et al. Negative pressure wound therapy. In: Krasner DL, Rodeheaver GT, Sibbald RG, eds. *Chronic wound care: a clinical source book for healthcare professionals.* Malvern, PA: HMP Communications, 2007:271–286.
189. Argenta LC, Morykwas MJ. Vacuum-assisted closure: a new method for wound control and treatment: clinical experience. *Ann Plast Surg* 1997;38:563–576.
190. Houghton PE, Campbell KE. Therapeutic modalities in the treatment of chronic recalcitrant wounds. In: Krasner DL, Rodeheaver GT, Sibbald RG, eds. *Chronic wound care: a clinical source book for healthcare professionals.* Malvern, PA: HMP Communications, 2007:403–415.
191. Mullner T, Mrkonjic L, Kwasny O, et al. The use of negative pressure to promote the healing of tissue defects: a clinical trial using the vacuum sealing technique. *Br J Plast Surg* 1997;50:194–199.
192. Peirce B, Gray M. Radiant heat dressings for chronic wounds. *J Wound Ostomy Continence Nurs* 2001;28(6):263–266.
193. Daniel RK, Faibusoff B. Muscle coverage of pressure points: the role of myocutaneous flaps. *Ann Plast Surg* 1982;8:446–452.
194. Zogovska E, Novevski L, Agai LI, et al. Our experience in treating pressure ulcers by using local cutaneous flaps. *Prilozi* 2008;29(1):199–210.
195. Singh R, Singh R, Rohilla RK, et al. Surgery for pressure ulcers improves general health and quality of life in patient's with spinal cord injury. *J Spinal Cord Med* 2010;33(4):396–400.
196. de la Fuente SG, Levin LS, Reynolds JD, et al. Elective stoma construction improves outcomes in medically intractable pressure ulcers. *Dis Colon Rectum* 2003;46(11):1525–1530.
197. Deshmukh GR, Barkel DC, Sevo D, et al. Use or misuse of colostomy to heal pressure ulcers. *Dis Colon Rectum* 1996;39(7):737–738.
198. Arregui J, Canon B, Murray JE. Long-term evaluation of ischiectomy in the treatment of pressure ulcers. *Plast Reconstr Surg* 1965;36:583–590.
199. Hackler RH, Zampieri TA. Urethral complications following ischiectomy in spinal cord injury patients: a urethral pressure study. *J Urol* 1987;137:253–255.
200. Karaca AR, Binns JH, Blumenthal FS. Complications of total ischiectomy for the treatment of ischial pressure sores. *Plast Reconstr Surg* 1978;62:96–99.
201. Evans GR, Lewis VL Jr, Manson PN, et al. Hip joint communication with pressure sore: the refractory wound and the role of Girdlestone arthroplasty. *Plas Reconstr Surg* 1993;91:288–294.
202. Stal S, Serure A, Donovan W, et al. The perioperative management of the patient with pressure sores. *Ann Plast Surg* 1983;11:347–356.
203. Dolezal R, Cohen M, Schultz RC. The use of Clinitron therapy unit in the immediate postoperative care of pressure ulcers. *Ann Plast Surg* 1985;14(1):33–36.
204. Tavakoli K, Rutkowski S, Cope C, et al. Vandervord J. Recurrence rates of ischial sores in para- and tetraplegics treated with hamstring flaps: an 8-year study. *Br J Plast Surg* 1999;52:476–479.
205. Disa JJ, Carlton JM, Goldberg NH. Efficacy of operative cure in pressure sore patients. *Plast Recons Surg* 1992;89:272–278.
206. Bates-Jensen B, Guihan M, Garber SL, et al. Characteristics of recurrent pressure ulcers in veterans with spinal cord injury. *J Spinal Cord Med* 2009:32(1)34–42.
207. Kieerney PC, Engrav LH, Isik FF, et al. Results of 268 pressure sores in 158 patients managed jointly by plastic surgery and rehabilitation medicine. *Plast Reconstr Surg* 1998;102(3):765–767.
208. Yamamoto Y, Tsutusmida A, Murazumi M, et al. Long-term outcome of pressure sores treated with flap coverage. *Plast Reconstr Surg* 1997;100(5):1212–1217.
209. Krause JS, Vines CL, Farley TL, et al. Exploratory study of pressure ulcers after spinal cord injury: relationship to protective behavior and its risk factors. *Arch Phys Med Rehabil* 2001;82(1):107–113.
210. Holmes SA, Rintala D, Garber SL, et al. Prevention of recurrent pressure ulcers after myocutaneous flap. *J Spinal Cord Med* 2002;25(suppl 1):S23.
211. Sorensen JL, Jorgensen B, Gottrup F. Surgical treatment of pressure ulcers. Am *J Surg* 2004;188(suppl):42S–51S.
212. Aggarwal A, Sangwan SS, Siwach RC, et al. Gluteus maximus island flap for the repair of sacral pressure ulcers. *Spinal Cord* 1996;34(6):346–350.
213. Goldman P. Pressure ulcers. In: Forcia MA, Lavizzo-Mourey R, Schwab EP, eds. *Geriatric secrets.* 2nd ed. Philadelphia, PA: Hanley & Belfus, 2000:272–276.
214. Enderle MD, Coerper S, Schweizer HP, et al. Correlation of imaging techniques to histopathology in patients with diabetic foot syndrome and clinical suspicion of chronic osteomyelitis. The role of high-resolution ultrasound. *Diabetes Care* 1999;22(2):294–299.
215. Schwartz IS, Pervez N. Bacterial endocarditis associated with permanent transvenous cardiac pacemaker. *JAMA* 1971;218:736–737.
216. Roche S, Cross S, Burgess I, et al. Cutaneous myiasis in an elderly debilitated patient. *Postgrad Med J* 1990;66:776–777.
217. Klein NE, Moore T, Capen D, et al. Sepsis of the hip in paraplegic patients. *J Bone Joint Surg* 1988;70:839–843.
218. Putnam T, Calenoff L, Betts HB, et al. Sinography in management of decubitus ulcers. *Arch Phys Med Rehabil* 1978;59:243–245.
219. Berkwits L, Yarkony GM, Lewis V. Marjolin's ulcer complicating a pressure ulcer: case report and literature review. *Arch Phys Med Rehabil* 1986;67:831–833.
220. Johnson CA. Hearing loss following the application of topical neomycin. *J Burn Care Rehabil* 1988;9:162–164.
221. Shetty KR, Duthie EH Jr. Thyrotoxicosis induced by topical iodine application. *Arch Intern Med* 1990;150:2400–2401.

222. Dalyan M, Sherman A, Cardenas DD. Factors associated with contractures in acute spinal cord injury. *Spinal Cord* 1998;36:405–408.
223. Dumurgier C. Pujol G. Chevalley J. et al. Stchepinsky P. Pressure sore carcinoma: a late but fulminant complication of pressure sores in spinal cord injury patients: case reports. *Paraplegia* 1991;29:390–395.
224. Pieper B, Langemo D, Cuddigan J. Pressure ulcer pain: a systematic literature review and national pressure ulcer advisory panel white paper. *Ostomy Wound Manage* 2009;55(2):16–31.
225. Langemo DK, Melland H, Hanson D, et al. The lived experience of having a pressure ulcer: a qualitative analysis. *Adv Skin Wound Care* 2000;13(5):225–235.
226. Zeppetella G, Paul J, Ribeiro MD. Analgesic efficacy of morphine applied topically to painful ulcers. *J Pain Symptom Manage* 2003;25(6):555–558.
227. Flock P. Pilot study to determine the effectiveness of diamorphine gel to control pressure ulcer pain. *J Pain Symptom Manage* 2003;25(6):547–554.
228. Prentice WM, Roth LJ, Kelly P. Topical benzydamine cream and the relief of pressure pain. *Palliat Med* 2004;18(6):520–524.
229. Rosenthal D, Murphy F, Gottschalk R, et al. Using a topical anaesthetic cream to reduce pain during sharp debridement of chronic leg ulcers. *J Wound Care* 2001;10(1):503–505.

CHAPTER 15 ■ SPASTICITY

AMANDA L. HARRINGTON AND WILLIAM L. BOCKENEK

INCIDENCE AND PREVELANCE

Spasticity is a common problem after spinal cord injury (SCI). It is estimated to affect 40% to 78% of persons after injury (1–4). The epidemiology of spasticity is complex. Although it has been suggested that there is no difference in spasticity based on gender (1), Levi reported that males had more problems with spasticity than females (5). Persons with cervical lesions report more spasticity than those with thoracic injuries, and persons with lumbar or sacral lesions are least likely to have spasticity (1–3,5). Lower limb spasticity is more problematic than upper limb spasticity, even in those with cervical injuries (3). Although persons with complete SCI report more spasticity than those with incomplete lesions, spasticity tends to be more problematic in persons with incomplete injuries (2,3,5,6). During the period of spinal shock following initial injury, there is a notable absence of spasticity. Over time, spasticity may develop and intensify. Thus, spasticity that may not have required treatment during initial rehabilitation more commonly requires treatment during follow-up (1). In general, the development of spasticity does not appear to be related to age at injury or to duration of injury (3,5).

NORMAL REFLEX PHYSIOLOGY

The human musculoskeletal system contains muscle stretch receptors that function to carry information about muscle length, tension, and velocity of stretch to the central nervous system (CNS). Reflexes exist to provide sensory information to the spinal cord to allow for quick corrections to motor activity (7). Muscles are predominantly composed of extrafusal fibers, which are innervated by alpha motor neurons from the spinal cord. Golgi tendon organs are specialized receptors for muscle tension and are located in series with extrafusal fibers. Golgi tendon organs can be activated by lengthening of the muscle during stretch or by shortening of the muscle during contraction. Specialized receptors for muscle length, known as muscle spindles, are composed of intrafusal fibers, run in parallel with extrafusal fibers, and are innervated by gamma motor neurons. Muscle spindles are activated by stretch and lengthening but are unloaded with active contraction or muscle shortening. Thus, passive stretching of a muscle causes afferents from both Golgi tendon organs and muscle spindles to fire, but active muscle contraction silences input from muscle spindles, while causing Golgi tendon organs to fire at a faster rate.

The muscle stretch reflex has both phasic and tonic components. The phasic component, manifested by tendon jerk reflexes, is short acting, monosynaptic, and is triggered by movement of the limb or a change in muscle length. The tonic component is manifested by postural reflexes, is long acting, polysynaptic, and is determined by muscle stretch.

A complex interneuron system of inhibition and facilitation helps to stabilize reflex firing. Glutamate acts as the predominant excitatory neurotransmitter, whereas gamma-aminobutyric acid (GABA) and glycine act as inhibitory neurotransmitters. Afferent fibers from myelinated nerves are subdivided based on size and conduction velocity. Group Iav and group II fibers provide input from muscle spindles as primary and secondary afferents, whereas group Ib fibers provide sensory information from Golgi tendon organs (7). Ia fibers have excitatory monosynaptic connections to the alpha motor neurons from which they originate and to the alpha motor neurons of synergistic muscles. In addition, they have excitatory connections to inhibitory interneurons of antagonist muscles. Thus, via reciprocal inhibition, the stretching of a muscle group will lead to inhibition of antagonist muscles (8). Inhibitory interneurons can also reduce Ia firing at alpha motor neurons from which they originate through presynaptic Ia inhibition (7). This helps to maintain a static inhibitory influence on the reflex arc. A specialized inhibitory interneuron, called the Renshaw cell, functions to limit Ia reflex responses through a mechanism known as recurrent inhibition (8). Inhibitory signals from Renshaw cells suppress alpha motor neurons and gamma motor neurons (7). Another inhibitory pathway involves Ib fibers from Golgi tendon organs, which synapse via interneurons to produce a nonreciprocal inhibition of alpha motor neurons (8) (see Fig. 15.1).

PATHOPHYSIOLOGY OF SPASTICITY

Definition

Spasticity has been defined as a "velocity-dependent increase in tonic stretch reflexes (muscle tone) with exaggerated tendon jerks, resulting from hyperexcitability of the stretch reflex, as one component of the upper motor neuron syndrome" (9). This increased resistance to passive stretch manifests as increased tone and represents the static component of the reflex arc (10). In disorders of spasticity, the phasic component of the reflex arc is manifested by hyperactive tendon jerks (10).

Mechanisms

Spasticity occurs as a component of the upper motor neuron (UMN) syndrome, which in SCI occurs after a lesion to the corticospinal tract and surrounding structures (11). The

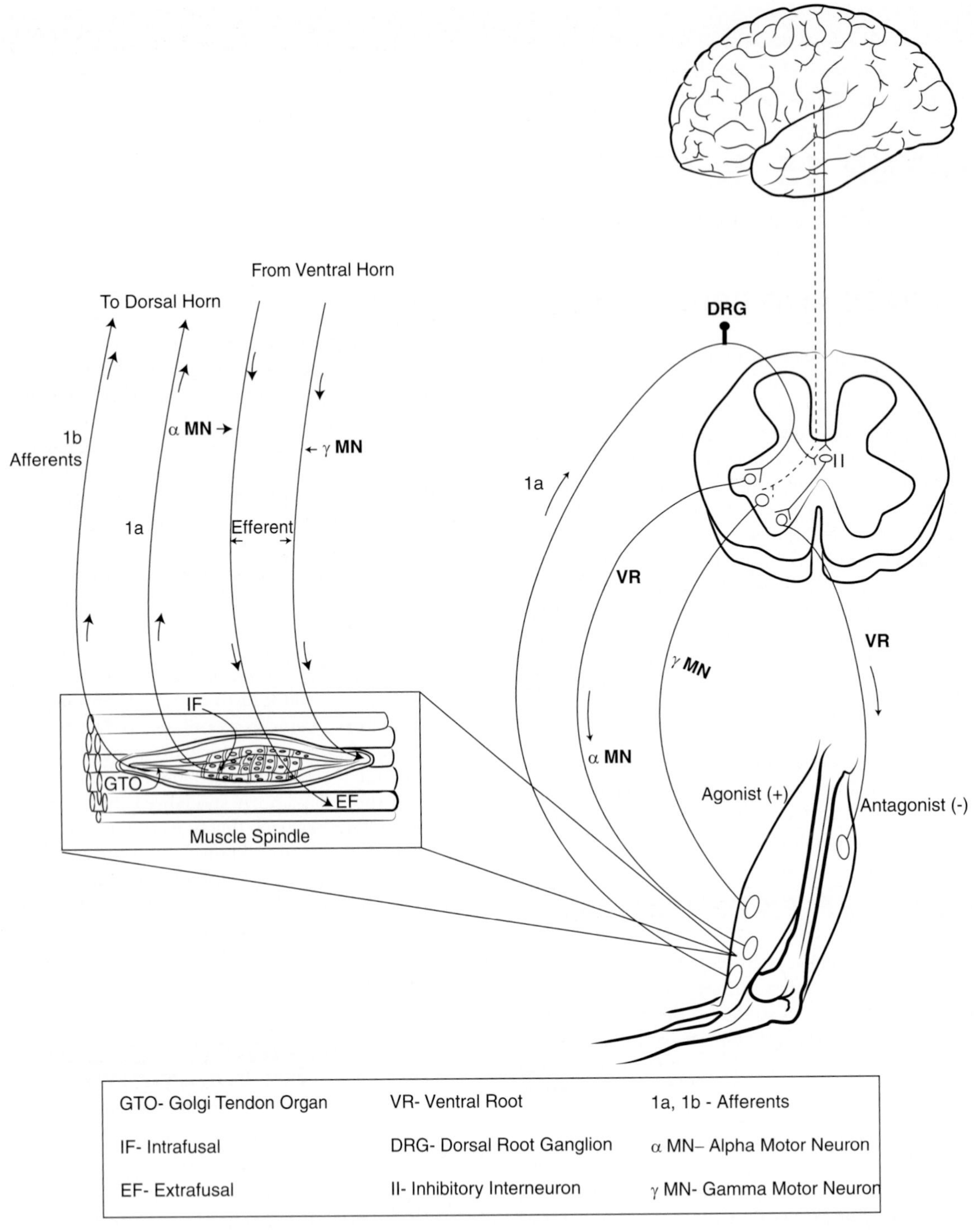

FIGURE 15.1 Components of normal reflex physiology including supraspinal influences, antagonist and agonist muscle reciprocal inhibition, the complex interneuron system, and the muscle spindle. The precise mechanism of spasticity is unknown, however, disruption of the net inhibitory effect of the normal central nervous system on the reflex arc is thought to be the likely etiology. Supraspinal dotted line=inhibitory influences, Supraspinal solid line =facilitatory influences.

UMN syndrome has both positive and negative components. Negative symptoms include weakness, fatigability, and loss of coordination and dexterity. Spasticity is a positive symptom of the UMN syndrome. Other positive clinical manifestations include involuntary spasms, clonus, abnormal primitive reflexes, and autonomic hyperreflexia (8).

Spinal reflexes remain intact after SCI. Spasticity is thought to be caused by an exaggeration of normal reflexes. The exact mechanisms that lead to spasticity are complex and are thought to be multifactorial, although leading theories involve a loss of reflex inhibition (8). Although many theories exist to explain the precise etiology of spasticity, true mechanisms are not known.

In the normal CNS, there is a net inhibitory effect on reflexes, as explained by the complex interneuron system. After injury, the regular suppression of reflexes is lost and the spinal cord becomes hyperexcitable (10). The most common theories of how this hyperexcitable state develops involve changes to inhibitory pathways of spinal reflexes. One possible mechanism for spasticity involves impaired reciprocal inhibition by Ia interneurons. When reciprocal inhibition is decreased, then antagonist muscles will not be suppressed when agonists are activated (7). Resulting inappropriate co-contraction of agonist and antagonist muscles can contribute to increased tone (11). Presynaptic group Ia inhibition of the spinal cord may also be depressed after SCI, leading to heightened firing of alpha motor neurons, when they no longer receive baseline inhibition (7). Normal Ib nonreciprocal inhibition from Golgi tendon organs may also be suppressed after SCI, thus the net inhibitory effect is gone, and reflexes are more prominent (7,8). Other possible mechanisms, which have been described, but are not thought to be accurate, include (a) hyperactivity of muscle spindle systems, (b) hyperexcitability of alpha motor neurons due to changes in neurotransmitter receptors or membrane properties, (c) decreased recurrent inhibition via Renshaw cells, and (d) changes in muscle fiber properties (7,8).

ASSESSMENT

There are many different methods of assessing spasticity. Numerous scales and instruments have been described using clinical, mechanical, or electrophysiological principles. Because there is no set gold standard for spasticity assessment, often a combination of tools is utilized in the clinical setting. In practice, assessment of the extent to which spasticity interferes with functional activities, such as mobility or activities of daily living, or the extent to which spasticity causes pain or discomfort, is often the most important measure of spasticity and the reason that medical and/or surgical treatment is offered.

Clinical Assessment

The first objective scale used to assess spasticity was described by Ashworth in 1964 in a study of persons with multiple sclerosis (12). This original Ashworth scale assessed resistance to passive movement through the full range of movement by grading tone on an ordinal scale (Table 15.1). Later, in attempt to create a more sensitive test in persons with only a small amount of tone, a Modified Ashworth Scale was proposed (13) (Table 15.1). There have been multiple studies evaluating the interrater reliability and utility of both scales. While some studies have found the interrater reliability of both the Ashworth and the Modified Ashworth scales to be high (13,14), more recent studies suggest interrater reliability is low (15). The scales may be of limited use in persons with SCI (16), particularly when describing spasticity in lower limbs (17). Another tool often utilized in research studies and clinical practice is the Penn Spasm Frequency Scale (18). Penn utilized frequency of spasms when measuring spasticity of spinal origin. Spasms are ranked on an ordinal scale based on how many spasms occur in a 1-hour period (Table 15.2). Of note, little correlation was noted between the Ashworth Scale and the Penn Spasm Frequency Scale in one study of persons with SCI (19). The modified Penn Spasm Frequency Scale utilized by Preibe et al. is a self-reported scale that separates spasm frequency from spasm severity, which is graded on a 3-point scale (Table 15.2).

TABLE 15.1

ASHWORTH AND MODIFIED ASHWORTH SCALES

Ashworth scale	
0	No increase in tone
1	Slight increase in tone; catch with limb movement
2	Marked increase in tone, but limb easily moved
3	Considerable increase in tone; passive movement difficult
4	Limb rigid or contracted
Modified Ashworth scale	
0	No increase in tone
1	Slight increase in tone with a catch, or minimal resistance at the end of the ROM
1+	Slight increase in tone with a catch, followed by minimal resistance throughout the remainder (less than half) of the ROM
2	Marked increase in tone through most of the ROM, but limb easily moved
3	Considerable increase in tone; passive movement difficult
4	Limb rigid or contracted

ROM, range of motion.
Adapted from Ashworth B. Preliminary trial of carisoprodol in multiple sclerosis. *Practitioner* 1964;192:540–542; and Bohannon RW, Smith MB. Interrater reliability of a Modified Ashworth Scale of muscle spasticity. *Phys Ther* 1987;67(2):206–207.

Assessments using other components of a neurologic exam have also been described. Loubser (20) described a neurologic reflex scale to grade spasticity and clonus in persons with SCI. However, differences in spasticity, which were found using the Ashworth scale, were not present using this reflex scale in the same patient population. Van Gijn (21) utilized the plantar reflex to assess flexion response in persons with

TABLE 15.2

PENN SPASM FREQUENCY SCORE (PSFS) AND MODIFIED PSFS

PSFS	
Spasm score	**Frequency of spasms**
0	No spasms
1	Mild spasms (brought on by stimulus)
2	Infrequent spasms (occurring <1 time/h)
3	Spasms occurring >1 time/h
4	Spasms occurring >10 times/h
Modified PSFS addition	
Severity score	**Severity**
1	Mild
2	Moderate
3	Severe

Adapted from Penn RD, Savoy SM, Corcos D, et al. Intrathecal baclofen for severe spinal spasticity. *N Engl J Med* 1989;320:1517–1521. and Priebe MM, Sherwood AM, Thornby JI, et al. Clinical assessment of spasticity in spinal cord injury: a multidimensional problem. *Arch Phys Med Rehabil* 1996;77:713–716.

UMN syndromes; however, only eight persons with SCI were included in the study and no further validity testing has been done. The Tardieu Scale, like the Ashworth and Modified Ashworth, measures passive resistance to stretch but incorporates movement at both fast and slow speeds to utilize velocity of stretch as a component of the measurement (22). The Tardieu Scale describes presence of a catch and severity of clonus at three different speeds, with associated measures of range of motion (22,23). The scale has been modified extensively and is not often used in SCI, and studies on validity and reliability have been inconclusive (22). The Oswestry Scale of Grading, described by Goff (24), incorporates quality of movement into an ordinal scale to measure spasticity; however, no interrater reliability studies have been preformed. Although mention of the assessment scales described in this paragraph is important from a historical standpoint, none of these scales are routinely utilized in spasticity assessment in SCI.

In recent years, newer tools to assess spasticity in SCI have been developed (Table 15.3). The Spinal Cord Assessment Tool for Spastic reflexes (SCATS) was developed to better define clonus, flexor spasms, and extensor spasms (25). The SCATS has been validated using kinematic and EMG measurements and is thought to provide additional information to clinicians when attempting to describe spastic hypertonia (25). The Spinal Cord Injury Spasticity Evaluation Tool (SCI-SET) is a new self-report measure to determine impact of spasticity on daily life (26). The SCI-SET was developed to assess both problematic and beneficial components of spasticity related to daily function. The SCI-SET is a 35-question tool that evaluates spasticity on a scale of −3 to +3 over the preceding 7 days. It has been found to be both valid and reliable (26). Another new self-reported assessment tool is the Patient Reported Impact of Spasticity Measure (PRISM) (27). The PRISM tool evaluates patient-perceived positive (or negative) physical, functional, psychological, and social aspects of spasticity. Utilizing self-report as a component of spasticity assessment is an important tool in the clinical setting, as clinical scales have been found to correlate poorly with each other, and often do not correlate with patient-perceived levels of spasticity (3,19,28). A recent review of spasticity outcome measures after SCI suggests that individual spasticity assessment scales measure different components of spasticity and thus might best be utilized in combination (29).

TABLE 15.3

SCATS, SCI-SET, AND PRISM SPASTICITY SCALES

Spinal cord assessment tool for spastic reflexes (SCATS)	
Clonus of ankle plantar flexors with rapid passive dorsiflexion of foot	
0	No reaction
1	Mild: clonus < 3 s
2	Moderate: clonus lasts between 3 and 10 s
3	Severe: clonus > 10 s
Flexor spasms in response to pinprick on foot plantar surface with leg and hip in full extension	
0	No reaction
1	Mild: extension of great toe or <10 degrees of hip/knee flexion
2	Moderate: 10 to 30 degrees of hip/knee flexion
3	Severe: >30 degrees of hip/knee flexion
Extensor spasms of quadriceps muscle after extension of leg from a position of hip/knee flexion	
0	No reaction
1	Mild: spasms last <3 s
2	Moderate: spasms last between 3 and 10 s
3	Severe: spasms last >10 s
Spinal cord injury spasticity evaluation tool (sci-set)	
Evaluation of spasticity effects on components of daily life over a 7-d period	
−3	Extremely problematic
−2	Moderately problematic
−1	Somewhat problematic
0	No effect
+1	Somewhat helpful
+2	Moderately helpful
+3	Extremely helpfult
Patient reported impact of spasticity measure (prism)	
Evaluation of spasticity effects on life experiences over a 7-d period	
0	Never true for me
1	Rarely true for me
2	Sometimes true for me
3	Often true for me
4	Very often true for me

Modified from Benz EN, Hornby TG, Bode RK, et al. A physiologically based clinical measure for spastic reflexes in spinal cord injury. *Arch Phys Med Rehabil* 2005;86:52–59; Adams MM, Martin Ginis KA, Hicks AL, The spinal cord injury spasticity evaluation tool: development and evaluation. *Arch Phys Med Rehabil* 2007;88:1185–1192; and Cook KF, Teal CR, Engebretson JC, et al. Development and validation of Patient Reported Impact of Spasticity Measure (PRISM). *J Rehabil Res Dev* 2007;44:363–372.

Mechanical Assessment

Mechanical assessment tools are designed to objectively test the resistance to passive movement of a joint and may be helpful in describing the tonic components of spasticity. Wartenberg (30) first described a technique by which pendulum-like movements of the legs were used as a diagnostic test of lower limb spasticity. When a patient is seated on the edge of a table with his or her legs hanging freely, the examiner lifts both legs to the same horizontal level and releases them. Swinging time and swing quality are then assessed. Bajd and Vodovnik (31) improved on this assessment, by adding knee angle recordings with an electrogoniometer and measuring knee joint velocity with a tachometer. Use of an isokinetic or handheld dynamometer to quantify spasticity can be accomplished by measuring the resistive torque of the knee or ankle at variable constant angular velocities (32,33). An additional mechanical assessment of spasticity measures the oscillation of the ankle joint on a horizontal axis (34). In this setup, a Spasticity Measurement Device (SMD) creates sinusoidal motion of the ankle and allows for viscous and elastic stiffness measurements to be calculated. Although these mechanical assessments may be valuable in providing a quantitative measure of resistance to movement, their use is more beneficial in the research climate (35). Use of mechanical assessment techniques in clinical practice is limited by both time and equipment. Simple and reliable qualitative measurements have yet to be developed for use in the clinical setting.

Electrophysiologic Assessment

In the lower limbs, experimental measurement of spasticity can quantify reflex activity using EMG in association with knee position and torque measurements (36). As a spastic limb is moved into extension, the joint angle, torque, and EMG may be recorded with both slow and rapid stretches. In a spastic limb, the rapid stretch induces an earlier and larger EMG response when compared to the slow manual stretch (36). More recent techniques allow the entire range of motion of the knee to be assessed at variable speeds (37). The Brain Motor Control Assessment (BMCA) has been evaluated using surface EMG recording and was argued to be superior to the Ashworth scale in objective quantification of spasticity after SCI (38).

In addition to manual limb movement, EMG responses may also be evoked by tendon tap, flexion withdrawal reflex, or electrical stimulation (35,39). Utilization of the H-reflex amplitude and H/M ratio may be used to follow response to medications. In the presence of spasticity, the H-reflex amplitude, as well as H/M ratio, is generally increased compared to normal limits (39). Although less useful than the H reflex, changes to the F-wave amplitude have been measured before and after antispasticity medication administration (39). Similar to mechanical assessment techniques, EMG quantification of spasticity has little value in clinical practice (35). However, the use of electrophysiological techniques as adjunct to clinical assessment may be most helpful when measuring response to spasticity medications (39).

MANAGEMENT

Indications for Treatment

Identification of spasticity after SCI does not necessarily indicate the need for treatment. Although spasticity is common after injury, many persons with SCI are able to tolerate spasticity without treatment. In some cases, spasticity may be beneficial to persons with SCI, with 23% to 40% of individuals reporting spasticity having a positive impact on their lives (3,27). Many persons with SCI may utilize tone from spasticity to assist with positioning, standing, ambulation, or activities of daily living. Some people may utilize spasticity to aid in transfers or pressure relief (6). Other positive benefits of spasticity include preservation of muscles that would otherwise be prone to atrophy and utilization of worsening spasticity as an indicator of new medical problems, such as urinary tract stone, infection, or pressure ulcer (40,41). Although there are times when spasticity may have positive effects on individuals with SCI, negative effects may be more common. Treatment of spasticity is indicated when spasticity causes pain, skin breakdown, or contractures, or when it interferes with sleep, positioning, hygiene, or function. Treatment plans are individualized and may include nonpharmacologic or pharmacologic management.

NONPHARMACOLOGIC MANAGEMENT

Reduction of Nociception

Spasticity may be exacerbated by noxious stimuli; therefore, an important component of spasticity management is the amelioration of nociception. Although noxious stimuli alone are not likely to create severe spasticity, it should be considered in the workup of increased or worsening spasticity. Before changing treatment plans, care should be taken to evaluate for nociceptive input, which may be contributing to increased spasticity. Common causes of nociception include bladder and bowel dysfunction, including urinary tract infections, bladder calculi, blocked urinary catheters, hemorrhoids, and bowel impaction. Other causes of pain or nociception, which may exacerbate spasticity, include ingrown toenails, fractures, pressure ulcers, deep vein thrombosis, heterotopic ossification, or abdominal processes such as menstrual cramping, appendicitis, or cholecystitis. Medication interactions and neurologic complications such as syringomyelia should also be considered and ruled out prior to changing treatment plans. The addition of new medications, such as selective serotonin reuptake inhibitors, may worsen spasticity; therefore, monitoring for increased spasticity as a side effect is recommended (42).

Stretching and Positioning

Stretching is often considered the mainstay of treatment for spasticity, and is important in contracture prevention. Particular attention is often paid to muscles at risk for contractures, including shoulder adductors and internal rotators, elbow and finger flexors, hip and knee flexors, and ankle plantar flexors. Stretching, either by manual or by mechanical means, provides tension to soft tissue structures surrounding a joint. Techniques may vary by duration, velocity, and intensity of stretch (43). The number of repetitions per session and frequency of stretching sessions are also variable. Many studies that investigate stretching as a treatment for spasticity utilize different methods, techniques, and outcome measures, and a recent review of the literature found the evidence to support stretching to be inconclusive (44). Although no standards or guidelines exist for stretching programs, once or twice daily stretching of spastic muscles is considered a normal component of spasticity management (45). Stretching is often combined with passive range of motion therapies in acute rehabilitation or in home exercise programs (43).

Spasticity may also be affected by body position. The use of tilt table or standing frame to allow vertical positioning while loading the joints may reduce spasticity by providing prolonged stretch (46–48). Proper positioning of the limbs and trunk when seated or lying down is also thought to reduce spasticity (48). Suggested wheelchair positioning includes firm seat and back, knees and ankles at 90-degree angles, and minimal dump of seat (i.e., keeping anterior to posterior seat angle relatively level) (45).

Orthotic Management

Use of splints and orthotics may be beneficial is providing prolonged stretch to spastic muscles. Static splints and orthotics are light, removable, and easy to use. The ease of static splints allows for monitoring of skin, changes in range of motion, and an acceptable wearing schedule for patients (43). Recently, the use of bilateral tone-reducing ankle-foot orthotics was found to increase step length and gait velocity in an individual with incomplete SCI (49).

Dynamic splints can adjust to improved range of motion during wear by increasing stretch, while concurrently allowing for functional activities to be performed (23,43,48). Casting of a stretched joint allows for more chronic stretch and has been suggested to be more effective at reducing tone and preventing contracture than orthotic splinting (50). Serial casting may be beneficial by facilitating stretch as range of motion improves (48).

Cryotherapy and Heat Modalities

Both cold and heat have been used in treatment of spasticity and may be of particular benefit in focal areas of spasticity. Cold is typically applied as ice packs or ice massage for 10- to 20-minute intervals but can also be delivered as a cold bath (48). The application of cold is thought to decrease exaggerated stretch reflex activity by directly effecting muscle spindle excitability (51). Studies of cryotherapy, showing a reduction in spasticity, have not shown universal response; thus, clinical results may be variable among patients treated with cold modalities (52,53). Effects of heat are also thought to be variable, with reductions in spasticity thought to be related to increased extensibility of connective tissue (54). Deep heat may be applied using ultrasound, and superficial heat may be applied with hot packs, fluidotherapy, paraffin, or whirlpool (48). Effects of cryotherapy or heat therapy rarely last more than 30 to 60 minutes (53), thus may have limited use in chronic, severe spasticity. Modalities are thought to be most beneficial when used in combination with other treatments, including a daily stretching program (55). Clinicians must use precaution when utilizing heat or cold modalities in SCI patients with insensate skin as they are at risk for burn and skin damage.

Electrical Stimulation

Many studies have investigated the uses of various forms of electrical stimulation on spasticity, and results are variable. Surface electrical stimulation using laboratory techniques or via transcutaneous electrical nerve stimulation (TENS) at high frequency has been suggested to help reduce spasticity with short-term benefits (56–59). However, long-term surface electrical stimulation has been suggested to increase spasticity after SCI, particularly in those with incomplete lesions (60). Implantable functional electrical stimulation (FES) systems utilized for walking programs or standing have been suggested to reduce overall stiffness and tone, as well decrease perception of spasm frequency and severity (61–63). Although spasticity has been reported to decrease for a short period of time following FES (64), reduction of spasticity was not found after long-term FES cycling (65). Spinal cord electrical stimulation, although typically used for pain management, has also been investigated for use in spasticity management with variable results (66,67).

Rectal probe electrical stimulation used for fertility purposes has been found to reduce spasticity after SCI for up to 24 hours after electroejaculation (68,69). Because it is not feasible to utilize rectal probe stimulation in a daily home program, penile vibratory stimulation has been studied as an alternative technique. Reduction in spasticity after vibration was found to last 3 to 6 hours after stimulation with variable results on frequency and severity of spasms (70,71).

Other Nonpharmacologic Treatments

Typical physical or occupational therapy sessions may utilize stretching, positioning, or modalities as described previously. Few studies look at alternative therapeutic interventions to reduce spasticity after SCI. Persons with SCI who underwent hydrotherapy for 20 minutes, three times a week at 71°F were found to have significantly less spasticity than controls, suggesting that hydrotherapy may be a beneficial adjuvant treatment (72). Conversely, the use of passive cycling as a component to therapy was not found to significantly reduce spasticity (73). An alternative form of therapy is hippotherapy, which utilizes the movements of horses to provide sensory input to the rider via their positioning and trunk movements (74). Hippotherapy has been found to reduce spasticity in the lower limbs in persons with SCI in addition to providing short-term positive effects on mental well-being (74,75).

Acupuncture and massage have both been suggested as treatments for spasticity (48); however, most acupuncture studies have been done in persons with stroke, and have had variable results (76–78). Repetitive magnetic stimulation has been evaluated in persons with SCI, multiple sclerosis, and stroke. Repetitive magnetic stimulation at the lumbar nerve roots was shown to decrease lower limb spasticity after SCI without any adverse effects (79), and transcranial repetitive magnetic stimulation was found to reduce spasticity in persons with both multiple

TABLE 15.4

MECHANISM OF ACTION AND TYPICAL DOSING OF COMMONLY USED ORAL ANTISPASTICITY MEDICATIONS

Medication	Mechanism of action	Dosing	Half-life
Baclofen	GABA-B agonist at mono- and polysynaptic spinal reflexes	5–20 mg q6–8 h	2–5.5 h
Diazepam	GABA-A receptor agonist	2–10 mg q6–8 h	30–60 h
Clonidine	Alpha-2 agonist	0.1–0.3 mg q12 h	12–16 h
Tizanidine	Centrally acting alpha-2 agonist	4–8 mg q6–8 h	2.5 h
Dantrolene	Blocks calcium release from the sarcoplasmic reticulum to prevent muscle contraction	25–100 mg q8–12 h	4–8 h

GABA, gamma-aminobutyric acid; Q, every; mg, milligrams.
Thomson Reuters Healthcare Community. PDR.net. Available at: http://www.pdr.net. Accessed November 26,2008; Thomson Healthcare. Micromedex Healthcare Series. Available at: http://www.thomsonhc.com. Accessed February 2, 2009.

sclerosis and stroke (80,81). Although not yet studied for treatment of SCI spasticity, whole-body vibration was shown to reduce knee extensor spasticity in cerebral palsy (82).

PHARMACOLOGIC MANAGEMENT

Oral Medications

Oral medications are commonly used for treatment of spasticity. Unfortunately, there is not one medication that works universally in all patients. All medications have side effects, and most antispasticity medications cause sedation and fatigue. Due to side effect profile and variable efficacy, oral medications must be trialed on an individual basis. Often changes in medication or dose are necessary to achieve desired effects. The use of multiple medications is often necessary. Commonly used medications are detailed below and summarized in Table 15.4. Common side effects and suggested areas of monitoring are outlined in Table 15.5.

Because the loss of baseline inhibition is thought to be one of the main mechanisms of spasticity, medications that upregulate inhibitory neurotransmitters or activate their receptors are thought to decrease effects of spasticity. Many oral medications act by potentiating the effects of the inhibitory neurotransmitter GABA or by acting as GABA receptor agonists.

Baclofen (LIORESAL) is one of the most commonly used antispasticity medications and is often the first agent used in treatment of spasticity of spinal origin. Baclofen is a GABA analog that can inhibit monosynaptic and polysynaptic reflexes at the spinal level as a GABA-B receptor agonist (83). Baclofen is FDA approved for treatment of spasticity (84). Suggested starting dose is 5 mg three times daily, with titration up to 20 mg four times daily (total dose 80 mg/day) (83). Many practitioners will titrate up even higher than recommended maximum daily dose, with doses as high as 240 mg daily having been described with minimal side effects (85). Dose must gradually be titrated down when coming off the medication, as withdrawal can be a problem. Symptoms of withdrawal include worsening spasticity, fever, mental status changes, and multisystem organ failure (84). The most common side effects of baclofen administration are related to sedation, fatigue, and drowsiness, although dizziness, nausea, constipation, weakness, and confusion may also result (83). Headache, hypotension, and urinary frequency have also been reported. Baclofen may lower the seizure threshold, so monitoring is necessary

TABLE 15.5

COMMON SIDE EFFECTS AND SUGGESTED MONITORING OF ANTISPASTICITY MEDICATIONS

Medication	Side effects	Suggested monitoring
Baclofen	Sedation, nausea, constipation, dizziness, weakness, confusion, decreased seizure threshold	Renal function, CNS depression
Diazepam	Drowsiness, weakness, fatigue, confusion, neutropenia, ataxia, respiratory depression	Liver enzymes, CNS depression, CBC with long-term use
Clonidine	Drowsiness, dry mouth, dizziness, constipation, sedation	Renal function at baseline, rebound hypertension
Tizanidine	Dry mouth, somnolence, dizziness, urinary frequency, rhinitis, constipation, blurred vision	Periodic liver enzymes, renal function at baseline
Dantrolene	Elevated liver enzymes, fatigue, dizziness, somnolence, weakness, GI disturbance	Periodic liver enzymes

CNS, central nervous system; CBC, complete blood count; GI, gastrointestinal.
Thomson Reuters Healthcare Community. PDR.net. Available at: http://www.pdr.net. Accessed November 26,2008; Thomson Healthcare. Micromedex Healthcare Series. Available at: http://www.thomsonhc.com. Accessed February 2, 2009.

in persons with known history of seizures. Because baclofen is predominantly excreted in the urine, monitoring is recommended in persons with impaired renal function, and its use should be avoided in patients with acute or chronic renal failure (83). Studies in persons with SCI and multiple sclerosis have shown that baclofen can reduce the frequency of involuntary spasms, the severity of spasms, nocturnal awakenings due to spasticity, and resistance to passive movement of the legs (86,87). Baclofen has also been shown to reduce Ashworth scores, pendulum test scores, and vibratory inhibition of the H reflex (88).

Long-acting *benzodiazepines* such as diazepam (VALIUM), clonazepam (KLONOPIN), and chlorazepate (TRANXENE) can also be used to treat spasticity. Benzodiazepines are GABA-A receptor agonists and are indicated for skeletal muscle spasms (84). The most commonly used benzodiazepine is diazepam, which has been shown to reduce spasticity after SCI with few side effects if used appropriately (89). Diazepam is typically dosed at 2 to 10 mg two or three times daily. Common side effects include drowsiness, ataxia, hypotension, weakness, somnolence, fatigue, and respiratory depression (83). Because benzodiazepines may cause respiratory depression, they should be used with caution in persons with severe respiratory insufficiency or sleep apnea (84). Benzodiazepines are metabolized in the liver, and caution is advised in persons with liver failure. Because they may cause sedation or drowsiness, benzodiazepines should not be used in combination with other CNS depressants or alcohol (83). Benzodiazepines should be used in caution in persons with a history of drug or alcohol abuse, and they may cause psychiatric side effects, especially in persons with underlying psychiatric disease (83). If discontinuing dose, benzodiazepines should be tapered off gradually, as abrupt withdrawal can cause seizures, hyperthermia, or mental status changes. Although the potential for side effects or addiction exists, the use diazepam for periods exceeding 10 years has been described after SCI (90).

Clonidine (CATAPRES) is an antihypertensive medication that works as an alpha-2 receptor agonist. Starting dose is typically 0.1 mg twice daily and may be titrated up to a total dose of 0.6 mg/day. Common side effects include dizziness, fatigue, sedation, somnolence, dry mouth, constipation, weakness, and headache. Clonidine may also cause orthostatic hypotension, palpitations, nervousness, and gastrointestinal side effects (83,84). As clonidine may cause rebound hypertension, doses must be titrated carefully when weaning (84). Clonidine is metabolized in the liver and is partially secreted from the kidneys, so it is often recommended to check baseline renal function. Persons with SCI have reported a subjective improvement in spasticity after treatment with clonidine (91,92). Clonidine has been shown to reduce Ashworth scores and improve pendulum test scores in persons with SCI (88). In addition, the vibratory inhibition index using H-reflex assessment has been reported to be reduced after treatment with clonidine (88,93). Although oral administration is most commonly seen in SCI, transdermal clonidine has also been utilized, and appears to be effective in reducing spasticity (94,95). In addition to reducing effects of spasticity, clonidine has also been shown to help improve locomotor patterns and increase walking speed in individuals with incomplete SCI (96,97).

Tizanidine (ZANAFLEX) is a centrally acting skeletal muscle relaxant that binds to alpha-2 receptors to increase presynaptic inhibition of motor neurons (83). It is FDA approved for treatment of spasticity (84). Tizanidine may cause sedation, so doses are typically initiated prior to sleep at 2 to 4 mg each evening. In persons who do not have sedating side effects, the dose can be titrated up to 8 mg three to four times daily. Common side effects include dry mouth, somnolence, dizziness, urinary frequency, rhinitis, and constipation (83). Tizanidine may also cause hypotension and bradycardia. Tizanidine is metabolized in the liver and may cause elevated liver enzymes; therefore, liver enzymes should be monitored periodically (84). The use of tizanidine in combination with CYP1A2 inhibitors such as fluvoxamine, ciprofloxacin, and some oral contraceptives is not recommended as the plasma levels of tizanidine may be affected (83). It should also be noted that absorption of the tablet and capsule forms vary if taken with food; thus, side effects may be increased if the tablet is not taken on an empty stomach or if the capsule is opened (98). Studies of tizanidine use in SCI have shown reductions of subjective assessment of spasticity, Ashworth score, pendulum test scores, and frequency of daytime spasms (99,100,101). High-dose tizanidine (16 to 32 mg/day) has been reported to reduce passive resistance to movement and to improve motor function (102).

Dantrolene (DANTRIUM) is an FDA-approved antispasticity medication, which acts at the muscular level. Dantrolene blocks the release of calcium from the sarcoplasmic reticulum, thereby preventing muscle contraction (84). Dose should be started at 25 mg a day and titrated up slowly to a maximum of 400 mg/day in divided doses (83). Dantrolene may cause lightheadedness, gastrointestinal side effects, dizziness, headache, somnolence, fatigue, and visual disturbance (83,84). Dantrolene is metabolized in the liver and excreted through the kidneys. It may cause elevated liver enzymes and liver toxicity; thus, liver enzymes should be monitored periodically (83). Because dantrolene acts at the level of the muscle, it is thought to have less cognitive side effects, and has traditionally been used in spasticity of cerebral origin, such as brain injury or stroke. Muscle weakness may be a side effect of dantrolene; thus, it may not be a good choice in persons with new spinal cord injuries who have potential for motor recovery (103). The concern for weakness in persons with motor deficits may limit its use after SCI. However, in studies of persons with SCI, dantrolene has been found to cause positive clinical response, reduce resistance to passive stretch, reduce tendon jerk response, improve ADL assessment, reduce spasm frequency, reduce nocturnal cramps, and reduce clonus (103–105).

Gabapentin (NEURONTIN) was initially developed as an anticonvulsant. It is not FDA approved for spasticity but is often used in persons who have both spasticity and neuropathic pain. The exact mechanism of action is not known, but gabapentin is thought to be a GABA analog (83). Starting dose is typically 100 or 300 mg three times a day, and is titrated up to a maximum dose of 3,600 mg/day (83). Common side effects include peripheral edema, myalgias, dizziness, headaches, somnolence, tremor, ataxia, fatigue, mood swings, slurred speech, weight gain, and double vision (83,84). Side effects may diminish with smaller doses. Caution must be used in persons with renal impairment as it is excreted in the urine (84). Studies in persons with multiple sclerosis and SCI have shown that gabapentin can reduce patient rating of spasticity and Ashworth scores, reduce pain associated with spasticity, and improve rating of disability (106,107). High-dose gabapentin has also been found to improve spasticity scores when measured with surface EMG (108). Pregabalin (LYRICA) is similar to gabapentin in that it is a GABA derivative that is used for treatment of both seizures and pain (83). Doses range from 150 to 300 mg/daily, given in divided doses, and common side effects include dry mouth, dizziness, somnolence, edema, weight gain, blurred vision, and abnormal thinking (83). One recent retrospective case series of persons with spasticity of varying etiology suggested that pregabalin may reduce symptoms of spasticity in some individuals (109).

Many other medications have been trialed for use as antispasticity agents. Cyproheptadine (PERIACTIN) is a serotonin and histamine antagonist that can reduce spontaneous spasms and clonus in spasticity of spinal origin when given in doses of 6 to 24 mg/day (110,111). The mechanism is thought to be due to the reduction of excitatory input to motor neurons (110). Cyproheptadine has been shown to improve Ashworth scores, improve pendulum test scores, and diminish vibratory inhibition of the H reflex after SCI (88). In addition, cyproheptadine has been shown to enhance locomotor function and increase walking speed in persons with incomplete SCI (111,112). Persons with SCI using cannabis have reported reductions of spasticity (113). Both oral and rectal Δ^9-tetrahydrocannabinol (THC) have been found to be both safe and effective for treatment of spasticity after SCI, with reductions in both Modified Ashworth score and self-ratings of spasticity (114). 4-Aminopyridine (FAMPRIDINE-SR), a potassium channel blocker thought to restore nerve conduction after demyelination, has also been suggested as an agent that may improve spasticity (115,116). In SCI, 4-aminopyridine was found to reduce spasticity in those who had spasticity prior to starting treatment, and in multiple sclerosis, it was found to increase walking speed and improve lower extremity strength (116,117). This medication is pending approval by the FDA at the time of this writing. The amino acid glycine and its precursor L-threonine act as inhibitory neurotransmitters and have been suggested for use as antispasticity agents (118,119). Other medications that have been trialed for spasticity treatment include the antiparkinsonian agent orphenadrine citrate (120), the calcium channel blocker ziconotide (121), phenytoin, and chlorpromazine (122). Muscle relaxants such as cyclobenzaprine (FLEXERIL) have not been shown to reduce spasticity after SCI (123).

Intrathecal Medications and Pumps

When generalized spasticity is the predominant problem, oral agents alone may not be strong enough to reduce tone. In addition, some patients with spasticity cannot tolerate the side effects of high-dose oral treatment. An alternative to oral antispasticity treatment is medication via an intrathecal route. By delivering medication directly into the CNS, generalized spasticity can be treated with fewer systemic side effects. Multiple medications have been studied for intrathecal delivery via pumps. The first medication studied for intrathecal use was morphine (124,125). Morphine can both decrease spasticity and control pain by diminishing sensory input into the CNS via disruption of multisynaptic reflex arches (124). Although drug tolerance may inhibit the ability to treat spasticity long-term with morphine, its use has been suggested in cases of intrathecal baclofen (ITB) tolerance (125,126). Intrathecal use of clonidine has also been studied. Similar to morphine, intrathecal clonidine is more often associated with treatment of pain, than with management of spasticity. Intrathecal clonidine has been shown to reduce spasticity and improve function in a dose-dependent manner (127). As expected, the biggest adverse effect is hypotension, which appears to be dose dependent (127). Lidocaine and fentanyl have also been studied for intrathecal use; however, their use is not routinely seen in clinical practice (128).

The most commonly used intrathecal medication is baclofen. Baclofen has been FDA approved for intrathecal use for the treatment of spasticity, and has been studied extensively in SCI (18,20,129–133). Baclofen is a GABA-B agonist and is thought to inhibit both monosynaptic and polysynaptic reflexes at the spinal level by blocking the release of neurotransmitters (132,134). In the spinal cord, GABA-B receptors can easily be accessed by low concentrations of ITB, allowing the medication to be given at much lower doses than are required orally (36). ITB has been shown to reduce spasticity, reduce pain, improve function, and improve quality of life (129–131,133,135–138). Proper patient selection is key to successful treatment with ITB. Patients who have failed treatment with oral medication or who cannot tolerate side effects of oral medications are appropriate for consideration. Because pump maintenance and refill is crucial, patients with a history of medical noncompliance and poor social support may be excluded. Prior to pump placement, other medical causes for worsening spasticity, such as syringomyelia, renal stones, heterotopic ossification, and infection, should be ruled out. Clear functional goals should be set prior to pump implantation. It is important to emphasize to patients that improved control of spasticity and further improvements in function are the goal of ITB pump placement.

Prior to implantation, all potential candidates undergo a trial via lumbar puncture. The suggested test dose is 50 μg (micrograms) of baclofen. After approximately 1 hour, the initial effect should be apparent, with peak effect apparent at 4 hours. Generally, the test dose effect is lost after 8 hours. Before the test dose, and at 2-hour intervals thereafter, assessment by the Modified Ashworth or Penn Spasm Frequency Scale is completed. Efficacy is typically defined as a decline in mean Ashworth score and/or Penn spasm scale of 2 (18). Although trial results vary by patient, the results of the trial are determined to be either positive or negative, in that there was either a reduction of spasticity or no change. Evaluation of functional goals during test dose administration may also help patients assess how function may be improved with pump placement (130). It is important to remind patients that response to test dose is not indicative of their level of spasticity after implantation, as actual dosing can be titrated to their individual need. If initial test dose produces no results, subsequent trials with 75, 100, or 150 μg doses may be preformed. Failure of a 150-μg trial suggests that implantation is not likely to be successful.

After a positive response to a test dose, pump implantation can be scheduled. Pumps are typically placed subcutaneously or subfascially in the abdomen, inferior and lateral to the umbilicus. The catheter is tunneled subcutaneously to the spine, enters the spinal canal the L4/L5 interspace, and is then threaded cranially to the spinal level of choice, where it resides within the subarachnoid space. Traditional catheter placement is in the intrathecal space between T10 and L2 (20,133).

When medication is infused into the spinal canal, drug concentration within the cerebral spinal fluid is higher caudally compared to more cranial locations (139). Because there is incomplete ascent of the medication in the spinal canal, lower limb spasticity is better controlled than upper limb spasticity (132). Placement of catheter tip more cranially in high cervical level tetraplegics, to approximately the T6 level, is thought to improve control of upper limb spasticity (140). However, if the goal is to preserve upper limb strength and function in tetraplegics with residual upper limb strength, more caudal catheter placement may be reasonable. Regardless of catheter location, upper limb spasticity will not be as well controlled as lower limb spasticity (129,130).

The initial dose of ITB is typically considered to be twice the effective trial dose, given over a 24-hour period (18,131). If a prolonged effect (greater than 8 hours) is seen at the trial, a smaller starting dose may be selected. Following pump implantation, attempts are made to wean patients off oral medications, as intrathecal dose is titrated up. Pumps store data in their internal memory, and dose adjustments are made by a remote programmer. Dose adjustments are often necessary postimplantation until optimal dose has been determined. It typically takes 6 months of dose titration to reach a desirable level of spasticity reduction (130,133). Dose may be increased 5% to 20% per adjustment, as frequently as every 24 hours postimplantation. Proper dose of ITB is determined by patient response to medication. Reduction of pain and improvement of functional goals should help determine correct titration dose. Because some persons with spasticity utilize their tone for functional tasks, it is important to make sure baclofen dose does not reduce spasticity to the point of causing weakness (18,133,136). The average maintenance dose for ITB treatment of SCI spasticity ranges between 50 and 1,500 μg/day, with average doses at 400 to 600 μg/day (141).

Tolerance to baclofen has been reported to occur in up to 15% of cases; however, true tolerance is rare (142). Because ITB dose typically stabilizes after the first 6 to 12 months of treatment, long-term dose titration is uncommon (129,130,132,143). In cases of tolerance, alternative medications via intrathecal route can be trialed, or utilized for a "drug holiday" from baclofen (36,125,126,141). The most common intrathecal drug used during baclofen drug holiday is morphine (125,126,129,131,133). Combining baclofen with other medications such as clonidine or morphine within the same intrathecal pump has also been studied; however, such use is not common (144,145).

Newer pumps allow for flexible dosing, which can vary throughout the week or throughout a day. Variable dosing during the week can be arranged when patients experience changes in spasticity based on activity fluctuations, such as a reduction in spasticity over the weekend. Variable doses can also be given in a 24-hour period, by programming a sustained basal rate throughout the day, with increased dosing at times of worsening spasticity (36). Refill of medication is performed via a simple percutaneous injection of drug into the pump reservoir, and can be performed in the outpatient clinic using a prepared refill kit. Time between refills is dependent on dose. Newer pumps, with a reservoir of 40 mL, hold a greater volume of medication and may only need to be refilled every 6 months. At a minimum, ITB pumps should be emptied and refilled at least every 6 months in order to replace the medication (134). Patients are made aware of alarm dates, so that refills are performed before medication is scheduled to run out. It is important to emphasize the need to keep refill appointments with patients, as ITB withdrawal can be severe.

Adverse effects of ITB are much less common than with oral dosing; however, effects of withdrawal or overdose are more severe. Baclofen delivered via intrathecal route causes fewer cognitive side effects than oral baclofen, and noticeable less sedation (141). Reported side effects include dizziness, nausea, hypotension, headache, weakness, urinary retention, and seizures (141). Although up to 16% of patients report adverse drug effects, discontinuation of therapy in persons with SCI is rare (131,142,146). Overdose is usually caused by mechanical problems and may present as respiratory depression, lethargy, dizziness, nausea, hypotension, and weakness. Rates of overdose have been reported to range from 0% to 14% (142). Decreasing the dose or temporarily stopping the pump will typically reverse symptoms. Supportive care with ventilator support may be necessary in cases of severe overdose (138,141). The use of physostigmine as an antidote has been described, but its routine use in cases of overdose is not common (131,134).

Mechanical problems with the baclofen pump can occur and include catheter microfracture, catheter kinking, catheter displacement, and pump failure by a number of mechanisms (138,141,147). Although rare, granuloma formation at the distal end of the catheter has also been described (148). If the baclofen pump or catheter fails, patients may experience withdrawal. Reported signs of withdrawal include worsening spasticity, itching, tachycardia, hyperthermia, hypotension, and mood changes (149). If withdrawal becomes severe, seizures, rhabdomyolysis, or multisystem organ failure may occur (147,149). Patients should always be given a backup supply of oral baclofen, which can be taken if symptoms that could be related to pump failure occur. Oral diazepam at 5 to 10 mg every 6 to 12 hours and cyproheptadine in doses of 4 to 8 mg every 6 to 8 hours have also been used during acute withdrawal (150). Intrathecal injection of baclofen via lumbar puncture can help ameliorate effects of withdrawal while the problem is being assessed and corrected. Workup for pump failure includes catheter check and pump evaluation for both programming errors and mechanical failure (147). AP and lateral spine x-rays with KUB films are the initial step in diagnosis of pump malfunction. CT scan with contrast injected into the side port of the pump is the next step in trouble shooting (147). The implanting surgeon should be notified if failure is a concern. All pumps now come with alarms. Critical alarms will sound if a pump reservoir is empty, if the pump motor stalls, or if there is an error with pump memory (134). Pump replacement will be necessary once battery life has ended, approximately every 5 to 10 years. Infection near site of pump implantation can occur, but meningitis is rare (141). Infection is typically treated with antibiotics and infected equipment is removed.

NERVE BLOCKS

Although spasticity associated with SCI is often a diffuse process, there are cases when localized areas of spasticity can be particularly problematic. If focal areas of spasticity lead to pain or functional limitations in transfers, positioning, dressing, or hygiene, localized treatment of spasticity may be beneficial (151). Treatment of focal areas of spasticity can best be managed with localized injection of pharmacologic agents. By delivering concentrated amounts of medication to affected muscles, systemic effects as seen with oral and intrathecal agents can be reduced. In order to achieve focal delivery, medication is aimed at peripheral nerves or motor points of affected muscles.

Because they are of short duration, nerve blocks using anesthetic agents such as lidocaine are not helpful in management of focal spasticity. In contrast, neurolysis by phenol or alcohol results in destruction of the axon; thus, the effect of the nerve block may be present from 1 month to 3 years (152–154). Average duration of response after phenol injection is around 3 to 9 months (155). Phenol and alcohol act by denaturation of nerve fiber proteins and destruction of nerve tissue, leading to neuropraxia and axonal degeneration (152,154,156). At the muscular level, atrophy and fiber necrosis are apparent (154). One to 20 mL of aqueous phenol in concentrations between 2% and 7% and ethyl alcohol concentrations between 35% and 100% are used for chemical denervation (153–155,157–159). Higher concentrations are thought to prolong treatment effect (156,157). Injection sites are determined by anatomical localization, with a nerve stimulator used for confirmation and better localization (153,156,157). Sterile technique is preferred. Common injections sites include the musculocutaneous nerve, obturator nerve, and tibial nerves, to reduce spasticity at elbow flexors, hip adductors, and plantar flexors, respectively. Open phenol injections of an exposed nerve can be done surgically (152,156,160). After phenol injection, local anesthetic effect and improved range of motion is seen immediately.

Often, intense stretching programs, splinting, or serial casting are utilized after phenol or alcohol injections to improve range of motion and optimize results (153,161). Return of tone occurs with remyelination and axonal regrowth (161). As with any injection, complications can include injection site pain, bleeding, and infection. Drawing back on the syringe prior to injection reduces risk for intravascular injection, which in the case of phenol block could cause seizures, cardiovascular collapse, or CNS compromise (156). Although neurolysis can improve range of motion and reduce spasticity, there is also a risk for increased weakness (161). Dysesthesias resulting from phenol injection are of concern and are estimated to occur in 0% to 32% of cases (154,161). Phenol affects both motor and sensory nerves, and dysesthesias are more likely to occur in mixed nerves, or those with large sensory components (156–161). Injection into the motor branch of a mixed nerve or directly into the motor point is thought to decrease risk for dysesthesias (152,156). If dysesthesias occur, they can often be eliminated by repeat block at the same site, or treated with anticonvulsants, such as gabapentin (161). Because phenol is a low-cost medication and duration of effect is longlasting, there are many advantages to utilizing it in areas of focal tone. However, complex and sometimes tedious injection technique, risk for dysesthesias, and risk of weakness may limit its use in many clinical situations.

CHEMODENERVATION WITH BOTULINUM TOXIN

Chemical denervation can also be accomplished with the use of botulinum toxin. Although most studies on botulinum toxin for spasticity have been completed in cerebral palsy, stroke, and brain injury populations, use in SCI is widely accepted (151,162–164). Botulinum toxin acts at the presynaptic membrane of the neuromuscular junction to prevent the release of acetylcholine (ACh). After the toxin is internalized, toxin internal bonds are cleaved, and the toxin light chain interrupts ACh vesicle release by blocking the proteins that normally allow ACh vesicles to fuse with the membrane (165,166). There are multiple serotypes of botulinum toxin (A though G), and each has a slightly different mechanism of action by acting at a different docking protein. Whereas botulinum toxin A cleaves synaptosomal-associated protein (SNAP-25), botulinum toxin B cleaves vesicle-associated membrane protein (VAMP)/synaptobrevin (165,166). Only serotypes A and B have been approved for use in the United States. Botulinum toxin type A (BOTOX) has been FDA approved for treatment of cervical dystonia, axillary hyperhidrosis, strabismus, blepharospasm, and cosmesis (PDR). Botulinum toxin type B (MYOBLOC) has been FDA approved for cervical dystonia (PDR). Both are often used off-label for focal treatment of spasticity. As of April 30, 2009, the FDA approved the use of botulinum toxin type A (DYSPORT) for the treatment of cervical dystonia. (167). Several other botulinum toxin preparations are approved for use outside the United States and include another form of botulinum toxin A (XEOMIN) and botulinum toxin type B (NEUROBLOC). New names have recently been established for the currently available botulinum toxin preparations. BOTOX is now known as onabotulinumtoxinA, MYOBLOC is now known as rimabotulinumtoxinB, and DYSPORT is referred to as abobotulinumtoxinA (168).

Vials of botulinum toxin type A come in 100-unit doses and can be reconstituted into different concentrations based on practitioner preference (83). There are only a few studies that investigate the effect of concentration on treatment response. Some suggest that a more dilute concentration may improve response (169), but no studies looking at the effect of dilution in SCI spasticity have been reported (170). Although dilution concentrations ranging from 20 to 200 U/mL have been described, a concentration of 50 U/mL is most commonly seen, with no more than 0.5 to 1 mL injected per site (154,164,170–172). Botulinum toxin type B is supplied as an injectable solution, containing 2,500, 5,000, or 10,000 units per vial (83). Direct dose conversions of differing types of botulinum toxin are not known; however, a ratio of approximately 1:50 for botulinum toxin type A (BOTOX) to type B (MYOBLOC) has been described (173).

Correct localization of the motor endplate is thought to optimize treatment effect. Anatomic localization texts offer techniques to determine muscle location based on surface anatomy. Many clinicians utilize nerve stimulator or electromyography for more precise localization (154,171). Commonly injected muscles and dose range of botulinum toxin type A (BOTOX) are seen in Table 15.6. Initial starting doses from 10 to 100 units in upper limbs and from 50 to 200 units in lower limbs have been described (171). Although higher doses have been shown to yield greater response, no dose-response studies in persons with SCI have been published (151,170,174). The number of injection sites per muscle is variable, often related to muscle size and clinician preference (151,171). Small individual muscles such as those found in the hand may only need one injection per muscle, whereas

TABLE 15.6

DOSE RANGE FOR SPASTICITY TREATMENT USING BOTULINUM TOXIN TYPE A (BOTOX)

Muscle	Dose range (units)
Upper limbs	
Pectoralis	60–150
Teres major	25–100
Biceps	30–200
Brachialis	20–100
Brachioradialis	15–80
Triceps	50–200
Pronator teres	10–90
Flexor carpi ulnaris	20–75
Flexor carpi radialis	10–100
Flexor digitorum superficialis	20–150
Flexor digitorum profundus	25–120
Flexor pollicis longus	5–30
Lumbricals/Interossei	10–50 per hand
Lower limbs	
Quadriceps complex	30–200
Hip adductor complex	50–400
Hamstring complex	40–300
Tibialis anterior	30–150
Extensor hallucis longus	40–100
Extensor digitorum	50–100
Peroneus tertius/longus	50–120
Gastrocnemius/Soleus	40–300
Tibialis posterior	40–200
Flexor hallucis longus/brevis	10–80

Note: Number of injections per site may range from 1 to 6. Adapted from Al-Khodairy AT, Gobelet C, Rossier AB. Has botulinum toxin type A a place in the treatment of spasticity in spinal cord injury patients? *Spinal Cord* 1998;36:854–858; Marciniak C, Rader L, Gagnon C. The use of botulinum toxin for spasticity after spinal cord injury. *Am J Phys Med Rehabil* 2008;87:312–320; Brin MF. Dosing, administration, and a treatment algorithm for use of botulinum toxin A for adult-onset spasticity. *Muscle Nerve* 1997;20(Suppl 6):S208–S220; Francisco GE. Botulinum toxin: dosing and dilution. *Am J Phys Med Rehabil* 2004;83(Suppl):S30–S37; and Dunne JW, Heye N, Dunne SL. Treatment of chronic limb spasticity with botulinum toxin A. *J Neurol Neurosurg Psychiatry* 1995;58:232–235.

large complexes of muscles in the proximal leg may need up to six injection sites per muscle group (171). Maximum dosage per session is recommended to be 400 to 600 U for botulinum toxin type A and 10,000 units for botulinum toxin type B, although higher doses may be used in clinical practice (151,170,171,175). Most clinicians will utilize smaller total doses at initial injection and titrate dose based on initial response (170).

Duration of treatment effect is variable and is often affected by dose. Initial effect is typically seen within 1 to 10 days of injection, with peak effect seen in the first 1 to 6 weeks, and total effect lasting between 3 and 6 months (154,171). Reinjection is often necessary once treatment effects fade and spasticity returns. Stretching and splinting postinjection may help to lengthen time between injections. Some clinicians advocate for electrical stimulation to muscles after injection as it may increase uptake of the toxin (176).

Adverse effects to botulinum toxin injection include injection site pain, bleeding, bruising, rash, or infection, as well as dysphagia, and dry mouth (83). Flu-like symptoms and low-grade fever are rarely reported (164). Dry mouth is thought to occur more frequently with use of botulinum toxin type B (175). A recent announcement by the FDA included that boxed warnings have been added to all botulinum toxin preparations regarding the risk of spread of the medication beyond the area of injection and can cause symptoms similar to clinical botulism. These symptoms can include potentially life-threatening swallowing and breathing difficulties and even death (168). Cost is significant compared to phenol or alcohol, thus limiting use in some patient populations. Antibodies to the toxin can develop, which decreases response to subsequent injections (177). Waiting at least 3 months between injections is thought to decrease the risk of antibody formation (170). If antibody resistance occurs, switching treatment to another form of botulinum toxin is thought to improve response (163).

SURGICAL INTERVENTIONS

At times, spasticity and associated problems of contracture, pain, and loss of function can be resistant to medical treatment. When conservative treatment fails, surgical referral may be the most appropriate option. Although surgical procedures involve risk of anesthesia, wound infection, and other surgical complications, the benefits of treatment often outweigh the risks if greater function can be restored to the patient. Surgical intervention for spasticity management is more common in the pediatric population; however, options should be considered in persons with SCI who have ongoing problems with spasticity.

Neurosurgical procedures, which may be used for treatment of spasticity or pain, range from severely destructive procedures such as cordectomy, cordotomy, and myelotomy to more local treatment such as selective dorsal rhizotomy or dorsal root entry zone procedure (178,179). Myelotomy, cordectomy, and cordotomy involve destruction of the spinal cord and thus can cause muscle atrophy and weakness in persons with incomplete injury (178). Because of their side effect profile and the availability of newer procedures, these destructive procedures are rarely done (180). A selective dorsal rhizotomy procedure involves ablation of sensory roots, while leaving motor roots intact (178). Maintenance of motor roots is particularly important in patients with incomplete injuries who are able to stand. Not only is motor function preserved but muscle atrophy is avoided. The dorsal root entry zone procedure involves ablation of nociceptive fibers of dorsal roots near their entry in the spinal cord, providing similar results to a dorsal rhizotomy (45,180). Although some treatments may reduce both spasticity and pain, many neurosurgical interventions, which are beneficial for pain management, appear to have minimal effects on spasticity. Spinal cord stimulator implantation, for example, has not shown consistent results in treatment of spasticity after SCI (178,179).

Orthopaedic procedures may be preferred in persons with SCI and include tendon lengthening, tendon transfers, tenotomy, neurotomy, neurectomy, myotomy, capsulotomy, or osteotomy (181). Reducing joint contracture can often help to improve positioning and hygiene in persons with severe spasticity. Tendon transfers, particularly in the upper limbs of tetraplegic patients, may also help restore function.

References

1. Maynard FM, Karunas RS, Waring WP. Epidemiology of spasticity following traumatic spinal cord injury. *Arch Phys Med Rehabil* 71;1990:566–569.
2. Noreau L, Proulx P, Gagnon L, et al. Secondary impairments after spinal cord injury: a population-based study. *Am J Phys Med Rehabil* 2000;79(6):526–535.
3. Sköld C, Levi R, Seiger Å. Spasticity after traumatic spinal cord injury: nature, severity and location. *Arch Phys Med Rehabil* 1999;80:1548–1557.
4. Walter JS, Sacks J, Othman R, et al. A database of self-reported secondary medical problems among VA spinal cord injury patients: its role in clinical care and management. *J Rehabil Res Dev* 2002;39(1):53–61.
5. Levi R, Hultling C, Seiger Å. The Stockholm spinal cord injury study: 2. Associations between clinical patient characteristics and post-acute medical problems. *Paraplegia* 1995;33:585–594.
6. Little JW, Micklesen P, Umlauf R, et al. Lower extremity manifestations of spasticity in chronic spinal cord injury. *Am J Phys Med Rehabil* 1989;68(1):32–36.
7. Sehgal N, McGuire JR. Beyond Ashworth: electrophysiologic quantification of spasticity. *Phys Med Rehabil Clin N Am* 1998;9(4):949–979.
8. Young RR. Spasticity: a review. *Neurology* 1994;44(Suppl 9):S12–S20.
9. Lance JW. Symposium synopsis. In: Feldman RG, Young RR, Koela WP, eds. *Spasticity: disordered motor control.* Chicago, IL: Year Book Medical, 1980:487–489.
10. Mayer NH. Clinicophysiologic concepts of spasticity and motor dysfunction in adults with an upper motorneuron lesion. *Muscle Nerve* 1997;20(Suppl 6):S1–S13.
11. Ivanhoe CB, Reistetter TA. Spasticity: the misunderstood part of the upper motor neuron syndrome. *Am J Phys Med Rehabil* 2004;83(Suppl):S3–S9.
12. Ashworth B. Preliminary trial of carisoprodol in multiple sclerosis. *Practitioner* 1964;192:540–542.
13. Bohannon RW, Smith MB. Interrater reliability of a modified Ashworth scale of muscle spasticity. *Phys Ther* 1987;67(2):206–207.
14. Lee K, Carson L, Kinnin E, et al. The Ashworth scale: a reliable and reproductive method of measuring spasticity. *J Neuro Rehab* 1989;3:205–209.
15. Ansari NN, Naghdi S, Moammeri H, et al. Ashworth scales are unreliable for the assessment of muscle spasticity. *Physiother Theory Pract* 2006;22(3):119–125.
16. Haas BM, Bergström E, Jamous A, et al. The inter rater reliability of the original and of the modified Ashworth scale for the assessment of spasticity in patients with spinal cord injury. *Spinal Cord* 1996;34:560–564.
17. Pandyan AD, Johnson GR, Price CIM, et al. A review of the properties and limitations of the Ashworth and modified Ashworth Scales as measures of spasticity. *Clin Rehabil* 1999;13:373–383.
18. Penn RD, Savoy SM, Corcos D, et al. Intrathecal baclofen for severe spinal spasticity. *N Engl J Med* 1989;320: 1517–1521.
19. Priebe MM, Sherwood AM, Thornby JI, et al. Clinical assessment of spasticity in spinal cord injury: a multidimensional problem. *Arch Phys Med Rehabil* 1996;77:713–716.
20. Loubser PG, Narayan RK, Sandin KJ, et al. Continuous infusion of intrathecal baclofen: Long-term effects on spasticity in spinal cord injury. *Paraplegia* 1991;29:48–64.
21. Van Gijn J. The Babinski sign and the pyramidal syndrome. *J Neurol Neurosurg Psychiatry* 1978;41:865–873.
22. Haugh AB, Pandyan AD, Johnson GR. A systematic review of the Tardieu scale for the measurement of spasticity. *Disabil Rehabil* 2006;28(15):899–907.
23. Gracies J-M, Marosszeky JE, Renton R, et al. Short-term effects of dynamic Lycra splints on upper limb in hemiplegic patients. *Arch Phys Med Rehabil* 2000;81: 1547–1555.
24. Goff B. Grading of spasticity, and its effect on voluntary movement. *Physiotherapy* 1976;62(11):358–361.
25. Benz EN, Hornby TG, Bode RK, et al. A physiologically based clinical measure for spastic reflexes in spinal cord injury. *Arch Phys Med Rehabil* 2005;86:52–59.
26. Adams MM, Martin Ginis KA, Hicks AL. The spinal cord injury spasticity evaluation tool: development and evaluation. *Arch Phys Med Rehabil* 2007;88:1185–1192.
27. Cook KF, Teal CR, Engebretson JC, et al. Development and validation of Patient Reported Impact of Spasticity Measure (PRISM). *J Rehabil Res Dev* 2007;44: 363–372.
28. Lechner HE, Frotzler A, Eser P. Relationship between self- and clinically rated spasticity in spinal cord injury. *Arch Phys Med Rehabil* 2006;87:15–19.
29. Hsieh JTC, Wolfe DL, Miller WC, et al. Spasticity outcome measures in spinal cord injury: psychometric properties and clinical utility. *Spinal Cord* 2008;46:86–95.
30. Wartenberg R. Pendulousness of the legs as a diagnostic test. *Neurology* 1951;1:18–24.
31. Bajd T, Vodovnik L. Pendulum testing of spasticity. *J Biomed Eng* 1984;6:9–16.
32. Firoozbakhsh KK, Kunkel CF, Scremin AME, et al. Isokinetic dynamometric technique for spasticity assessment. *Am J Phys Med Rehabil* 1993;72:379–385.
33. Lamontagne A, Malouin F, Richards CL, et al. Evaluation of reflex- and nonreflex-induced muscle resistance to stretch in adults with spinal cord injury using hand-held and isokinetic dynamometry. *Phys Ther* 1998;78(9):964–978.
34. Hinderer SR, Lehmann JF, Price R, et al. Spasticity in spinal cord injured persons: quantitative effects of baclofen and placebo treatment. *Am J Phys Med Rehabil* 1990;69(6):311–317.
35. Biering-Sørensen F, Nielsen JB, Klinge K. Spasticity-assessment: A review. *Spinal Cord* 2006;44:708–722.
36. Penn RD. Intrathecal baclofen for severe spasticity. *Ann NY Acad Sci* 1988;531:157–166.
37. van der Salm A, Veltink PH, Hermens HJ, et al. Development of a new method for objective assessment of spasticity using full range passive movements. *Arch Phys Med Rehabil* 2005;86:1991–1997.
38. Sherwood AM, Graves DE, Priebe MM. Altered motor control and spasticity after spinal cord injury: subjective and objective assessment. *J Rehabil R D* 2000;37(1):41–52.
39. Yablon SA, Stokic DS. Neurophysiologic evaluation of spastic hypertonia: implications for management of the patient with the intrathecal baclofen pump. *Am J Phys Med Rehabil* 2004;83(Suppl):S10–S18.

40. Gorgey AS, Dudley GA. Spasticity may defend skeletal muscle size and composition after incomplete spinal cord injury. *Spinal Cord* 2008;46:96–102.
41. Mahoney JS, Engebretson JC, Cook KF, et al. Spasticity experience domains in persons with spinal cord injury. *Arch Phys Med Rehabil* 2007;88:287–294.
42. Stolp-Smith KA, Wainberg MC. Antidepressant exacerbation of spasticity. *Arch Phys Med Rehabil* 1999;80: 339–342.
43. Gracies J-M. Pathophysiology of impairment in patients with spasticity and use of stretch as a treatment of spastic hypertonia. *Phys Med Rehabil Clin N Am* 2001;12(4):747–768.
44. Bovend'Eerdt TJ, Newman M, Barker K, et al. The effects of stretching in spasticity: a systematic review. *Arch Phys Med Rehabil* 2008;89:1395–1406.
45. Kirshblum S. Treatment alternatives for spinal cord injury related spasticity. *J Spinal Cord Med* 1999;22(3):199–217.
46. Bohannon RW. Tilt table standing for reducing spasticity after spinal cord injury. *Arch Phys Med Rehabil* 1993;74:1121–1122.
47. Kunkel CF, Scremin AME, Eisenberg B, et al. Effect of "standing" on spasticity, contracture, and osteoporosis in paralyzed males. *Arch Phys Med Rehabil* 1993;74:73–78.
48. Watanabe T. The role of therapy in spasticity management. *Am J Phys Med Rehabil* 2004;83(Suppl):S45–S49.
49. Nash B, Roller JM, Parker MG. The effects of tone-reducing orthotics on walking of an individual after incomplete spinal cord injury. *J Neurol Phys Ther* 2008;32:39–47.
50. Hill J. The effects of casting on upper extremity motor disorders after brain injury. *Am J Occup Ther* 1994;48(3):219–224.
51. Miglietta O. Action of cold on spasticity. *Am J Phys Med* 1973;53(4):198–205.
52. Knutsson E. Topical cryotherapy in spasticity. *Scand J Rehab Med* 1970;2:159–163.
53. Price R, Lehmann JF, Boswell-Bessette S, et al. Influence of cryotherapy on spasticity at the human ankle. *Arch Phys Med Rehabil* 1993;74:300–304.
54. Lehmann J, Masock A, Warren C, et al.. Effect of therapeutic temperatures on tendon extensibility. *Arch Phys Med Rehabil* 1970;51:481–487.
55. Lee JM, Warren MP. Ice, relaxation and exercise in reduction of muscle spasticity. *Physiotherapy* 1974;60(10):296–302.
56. Aydin G, Tomruk S, Kele? I, et al. Transcutaneous electrical nerve stimulation versus baclofen in spasticity: clinical and electrophysiologic comparison. *Am J Phys Med Rehabil* 2005;84:584–592.
57. Bjad T, Eng D, Gregoric M, et al. Electrical stimulation in treating spasticity resulting from spinal cord injury. *Arch Phys Med Rehabil* 1985;66:515–517.
58. Ji-sheng H, Xiao-hong C, Yu Y, et al. Transcutaneous electrical nerve stimulation for treatment of spinal spasticity. *Chin Med J* 1994;107(1):6–11.
59. Robinson CJ, Kett NA, Bolam JM. Spasticity in spinal cord injured patients: 1. Short-term effects of surface electrical stimulation. *Arch Phys Med Rehabil* 1988;69:598–604.
60. Robinson CJ, Kett NA, Bolam JM. Spasticity in spinal cord injured patients: 2. Initial measures and long-term effects of surface electrical stimulation. *Arch Phys Med Rehabil* 1988;69:862–868.
61. Granat MH, Ferguson ACB, Andrews BJ, et al. The role of functional electrical stimulation in the rehabilitation of patients with incomplete spinal cord injury-observed benefits during gait studies. *Paraplegia* 1993;31:207–215.
62. Mirbagheri MM, Ladouceur M, Barbeau H, et al. The effects of long-term FES-assisted walking on intrinsic and reflex dynamic stiffness in spastic spinal-cord-injured subjects. *IEEE Trans Neural Syst Rehabil Eng* 2002;10(4):280–288.
63. Agarwal S, Triolo RJ, Kobetic R, et al. Long-term user perceptions of an implanted neuroprosthesis for exercise, standing, and transfers after spinal cord injury. *J Rehabil Res Dev* 2003;40(3):241–252.
64. Krause P, Szecsi J, Straube A. Changes in spastic muscle tone increase in patients with spinal cord injury using functional electrical stimulation and passive leg movements. *Clin Rehabil* 2008;22(7):627–637.
65. Sköld C, Lönn L, Harms-Ringdahl K, et al. Effects of functional electrical stimulation training for six months on body composition and spasticity in motor complete tetraplegic spinal cord- injured individuals. *J Rehabil Med* 2002;34:25–32.
66. Barolat G, Myklebust JB, Wenninger W. Effects of spinal cord stimulation on spasticity and spasms secondary to myelopathy. *Appl Neurophysiol* 1988;51:29–44.
67. Gybels J, Van Roost D. Spinal cord stimulation for spasticity. *Adv Tech Stand Neurosurg* 1987;15:63–96.
68. Halstead LS, Seager SW. The effects of rectal probe electrostimulation on spinal cord injury spasticity. *Paraplegia* 1991;29(1):43–47.
69. Halstead LS, Seager SW, Houston JM, et al. Relief of spasticity in SCI men and women using rectal probe electrostimulation. *Paraplegia* 1993;31:715–721.
70. Læssøe L, Nielsen JB, Biering-Sørensen F, et al. Antispastic effect of penile vibration in men with spinal cord lesion. *Arch Phys Med Rehabil* 2004;85:919–924.
71. Alaca R, Goktepe AS, Yildiz N, et al. Effect of penile vibratory stimulation on spasticity in men with spinal cord injury. *Am J Phys Med Rehabil* 2005;84:875–879.
72. Kesiktas N, Parker N, Erdoan N, et al. The use of hydrotherapy for the management of spasticity. *Neurorehabil Neural Repair* 2004;18(4):268–273.
73. Kakebeeke TH, Lechner HE, Knapp PA. The effect of passive cycling movements on spasticity after spinal cord injury: preliminary results. *Spinal Cord* 2005;43:483–488.
74. Lechner HE, Feldhaus S, Gudmundsen L, et al. The short-term effect of hippotherapy on spasticity in patients with spinal cord injury. *Spinal Cord* 2003;41:502–505.
75. Lechner HE, Kakebeeke TH, Hegemann D, et al. The effect of hippotherapy on spasticity and on mental well-being of persons with spinal cord injury. *Arch Phys Med Rehabil* 2007;88:1241–1248.
76. Fink M, Rollnik JD, Bijak M, et al. Needle acupuncture in chronic poststroke leg spasticity. *Arch Phys Med Rehabil* 2004;85:667–672.

77. Moon S-K, Whang Y-K, Park S-U, et al. Antispastic effect of electroacupuncture and moxibustion in stroke patients. *Am J Chin Med* 2003;31(3):467–474.
78. Mukherjee M, McPeak LK, Redford JB, et al. The effect of electro-acupuncture on spasticity of the wrist joint in chronic stroke survivors. *Arch Phys Med Rehabil* 2007;88:159–166.
79. Krause P, Straube A. Repetitive magnetic and functional electrical stimulation reduce spastic tone increase in patients with spinal cord injury. *Suppl Clin Neurophysiol* 2003;56:220–225.
80. Centonze D, Koch G, Versace V. Repetitive transcranial magnetic stimulation of the motor cortex ameliorates spasticity in multiple sclerosis. *Neurology* 2007;68: 1045–1050.
81. Málly J, Dinya E. Recovery of motor disability and spasticity in post-stroke after repetitive transcranial magnetic stimulation (rTMS). *Brain Res Bull* 2008;76:388–395.
82. Ahlborg L, Andersson C, Julin P. Whole-body vibration training compared with resistance training: effect on spasticity, muscle strength, and motor performance in adults with cerebral palsy. *J Rehabil Med* 2006;38(5):302–308.
83. Thomson Reuters Healthcare Community. PDR.net. Available at: http://www.pdr.net. Accessed November 26,2008.
84. Thomson Healthcare. Micromedex® Healthcare Series. Available at: http://www.thomsonhc.com. Accessed February 2, 2009.
85. Aisen ML, Dietz MA, Rossi P, et al. Clinical and pharmacokinetic aspects of high dose oral baclofen therapy. *J Am Paraplegia Soc* 1992;15(4):211–216.
86. Duncan GW, Shahani BT, Young RR. An evaluation of baclofen treatment for certain symptoms in patients with spinal cord lesions. *Neurology* 1976;26:441–446.
87. Shahani BT, Young RR. Management of flexor spasms with Lioresal. *Arch Phys Med Rehabil* 1974;55:465–467.
88. Nance PW. A comparison of clonidine, cyproheptadine and baclofen in spastic spinal cord injured patients. *J Am Paraplegia Soc* 1994;17:150–156.
89. Corbett M, Frankel HL, Michaelis L. A double-blind, cross-over trial of valium in the treatment of spasticity. *Paraplegia* 1972;10:19–22.
90. Broderick CP, Radnitz CL, Bauman WA. Diazepam usage in veterans with spinal cord injury. *J Spinal Cord Med* 1997;20:406–409.
91. Donovan WH, Carter RE, Rossi CD. Clonidine effect on spasticity: a clinical trial. *Arch Phys Med Rehabil* 1988;69:193–194.
92. Maynard FM. Early clinical experience with clonidine in spinal spasticity. *Paraplegia* 1986;24:175–182.
93. Nance PW, Shears AH, Nance DM. Reflex changes induced by clonidine in spinal cord injured patients. *Paraplegia* 1989;27:296–301.
94. Yablon SA, Sipski ML. Effect of transdermal clonidine on spinal spasticity. A case series. *Am J Phys Med Rehabil* 1993;72:154–157.
95. Weingarden SI, Belen JG. Clonidine transdermal system for treatment of spasticity in spinal cord injury. *Arch Phys Med Rehabil* 1992;73:876–877.
96. Stewart JE, Barbeau H, Gauthier S. Modulation of locomotor patterns and spasticity with clonidine in spinal cord injured patients. *Can J Neurol Sci* 1991;18:321–332.
97. Norman KE, Pépin A, Barbeau H. Effects of drugs on walking after spinal cord injury. *Spinal Cord* 1998;36:699–715.
98. Shah J, Wesnes KA, Kovelesky RA, et al. Effects of food on the single-dose pharmacokinetics/pharmacodynamics of tizanidine capsules and tablets in healthy volunteers. *Clin Ther* 2006;28:1308–1317.
99. Mathias CJ, Luckitt J, Desai P, et al. Pharmacodynamics and pharmacokinetics of the oral antispastic agent tizanidine in patients with spinal cord injury. J Rehabil Res Dev 1989;26(4):9–16.
100. Nance PW, Bugaresti J, Shellenberger K, et al. Efficacy and safety of tizanidine in the treatment of spasticity in patients with spinal cord injury. *Neurology* 1994;44(Suppl 9):S44–S52.
101. Newman PM, Nogues M, Newman PK, et al. Tizanidine in the treatment of spasticity. *Eur J Clin Pharmacol* 1982;23:31–35.
102. Knutsson E, Mårtensson A, Gransberg L. Antiparetic and antispastic effects induced by tizanidine in patients with spastic paresis. *J Neurol Sci* 1982;53:187–204.
103. Weiser R, Terenty T, Hudgson P, et al. Dantrolene sodium in the treatment of spasticity in chronic spinal cord disease. *Practitioner* 1978;221(1321):123–127.
104. Glass A, Hannah A. A comparison of dantrolene sodium and diazepam in the treatment of spasticity. *Paraplegia* 1974;12:170–174.
105. Monster AW. Spasticity and the effect of dantrolene sodium. *Arch Phys Med Rehabil* 1974;55:373–383.
106. Gruenthal M, Mueller M, Olson WL, et al. Gabapentin for the treatment of spasticity in patients with spinal cord injury. *Spinal Cord* 1997;35:686–689.
107. Mueller ME, Gruenthal M, Olson WL, et al. Gabapentin for relief of upper motor neuron symptoms in multiple sclerosis. *Arch Phys Med Rehabil* 1997;78:521–524.
108. Priebe MM, Sherwood AM, Graves DE. Effectiveness of gabapentin in controlling spasticity: a quantitative study. *Spinal Cord* 1997;35:171–175.
109. Bradley LJ, Kirker GB. Pregabalin in the treatment of spasticity: a retrospective case series. *Disabil Rehabil* 2008;30(16):1230–1232.
110. Barbeau H, Richards CL, Bédard PJ. Action of cyptoheptadine in spastic paraparetic patients. *J Neurol Neurosurg Psychiatry* 1982;45:923–926.
111. Wainberg M, Barbeau H, Gauthier S. The effects if cyproheptadine on locomotion and on spasticity in patients with spinal cord injuries. *J Neurol Neurosurg Psychiatry* 1990;53:754–763.
112. Wainberg M, Barbeau H, Gauthier S. Quantitative assessment of the effect of cyproheptadine on spastic paretic gait: a preliminary study. *J Neurol* 1986;233:311–314.
113. Malec J, Harvey RF, Cayner JJ. Cannabis effect on spasticity in spinal cord injury. *Arch Phys Med Rehabil* 1982;63:116–118.
114. Hagenbach U, Luz S, Ghafoor N, et al. The treatment of spasticity with Δ^9-tetrahydrocannabinol in persons with spinal cord injury. *Spinal Cord* 2007;45:551–562.

115. Potter PJ, Haynes KC, Segal JL, et al. Randomized double-blind crossover trial of fampridine-SR (sustained release 4-aminopyridine) in patients with incomplete spinal cord injury. *J Neurotrauma* 1998;15(10): 837–849.
116. Cardenas DD, Ditunno J, Graziani V, et al. Phase 2 trial of sustained-release fampridine in chronic spinal cord injury. *Spinal Cord* 2007;45:158–168.
117. Korenke AR, Rivey MP, Allington DR. Sustained-release fampridine for symptomatic treatment of multiple sclerosis. *Ann Pharmacother* 2008;42:1458–1465.
118. Stern P, Bokonjić R. Glycine therapy in 7 cases of spasticity. *Pharmacology* 1974;12:117–119.
119. Lee A, Patterson V. A double-blind study of L-threonine in patients with spinal spasticity. *Acta Neurol Scand* 1993;88:334–338.
120. Casale R, Glynn CJ, Buonocore M. Reduction of spastic hypertonia in patients with spinal cord injury: a double-blind comparison of intravenous orphenadrine citrate and placebo. *Arch Phys Med Rehabil* 1995;76:660–665.
121. Ridgeway B, Wallace M, Gerayli A. Ziconotide for the treatment of severe spasticity after spinal cord injury. *Pain* 2000;85:287–289.
122. Cohan SL, Raines A, Panagakos J, et al. Phenytoin and chlorpromazine in the treatment of spasticity. *Arch Neurol* 1980;37:360–364.
123. Ashby P, Burke D, Rao S, et al. Assessment of cyclobenzaprine in the treatment of spasticity. *J Neurol Neurosurg Psychiatry* 1972;35:599–605.
124. Erickson DL, Blacklock JB, Michaelson M, et al. Control of spasticity by implantable continuous flow morphine pump. *Neurosurgey* 1985;16:215–217.
125. Erickson DL, Lo J, Michaelson M. Control of intractable spasticity with intrathecal morphine sulfate. *Neurosurgey* 1989;24:236–238.
126. Soni BM, Mani RM, Oo T, et al. Treatment of spasticity in a spinal cord-injured patient with intrathecalmorphineduetointrathecalbaclofentolerance–a case report and review of literature. *Spinal Cord* 2003;41:586–589.
127. Rémy-Néris O, Denys P, Bussel B. Intrathecal clonidine for controlling spastic hypertonia. *Phys Med Rehabil Clin N Am* 2001;12(4):939–951.
128. Chabal C, Jacobson L, Schwid HA. An objective comparison of intrathecal lidocaine versus fentanyl for the treatment of lower extremity spasticity. *Anesthesiology* 1991;74:643–646.
129. Abel NA, Smith RA. Intrathecal baclofen for treatment of intractable spinal spasticity. *Arch Phys Med Rehabil* 1994;75:54–58.
130. Azouvi P, Mane M, Thiebaut J, et al. Intrathecal baclofen administration for control of severe spinal spasticity: functional improvement and long-term follow-up. *Arch Phys Med Rehabil* 1996;77:35–39.
131. Coffey RJ, Cahill D, Steers W, et al. Intrathecal baclofen for intractable spasticity of spinal origin: results of a long-term multicenter study. *J Neurosurg* 1993;78:226–232.
132. Meythaler JM, Steers WD, Tuel SM, et al. Continuous intrathecal baclofen in spinal cord spasticity. *Am J Phys Med Rehabil* 1992;71:321–327.
133. Orida JI, Fisher E, Adamski E, et al. Chronic intrathecal delivery of baclofen by a programmable pump for the treatment of severe spasticity. *J Neurosurg* 1996;85:452–457.
134. Medtronic, Inc. Lioresal® Intrathecal (baclofen injection). Avaliable at: http://www.medtronic.com/physician/itb/index.html. Accessed November 26, 2008.
135. Boviatsis EJ, Kouyialis AT, Korfias S, et al. Functional outcome of intrathecal baclofen administration for severe spasticity. *Clin Neurol Neurosurg* 2005;107(4):289–295.
136. Guillaume D, Van Havenbergh A, Vloeberghs M, et al. A clinical study of intrathecal baclofen using a programmable pump for intractable spasticity. *Arch Phys Med Rehabil* 2005;86(11):2165–2171.
137. Middel B, Kuipers-Upmeijer H, Bouma J, et al. Effect of intrathecal baclofen by an implanted programmable pump on health related quality of life in patients with severe spasticity. *J Neurol Neurosurg Psychiatry* 1997;63:204–209.
138. Teddy P, Jamous A, Gardner B, et al. Complications of intrathecal baclofen delivery. *Br J Neurosurg* 1992;6:115–118.
139. Kroin JS, Ali A, York M, et al. The distribution of medication along the spinal canal after chronic intrathecal administration. *Neurosurgery* 1933;33:226–230.
140. Burns AS, Meythaler JM. Intrathecal baclofen in tetraplegia of spinal origin: efficacy for upper extremity hypertonia. *Spinal Cord* 2001;39(8):413–419.
141. Penn RD. Intrathecal baclofen for spasticity of spinal origin: seven years of experience. *J Neurosurg* 1992;77:236–240.
142. Dario A, Scamoni C, Picano M, et al. Pharmacological complications of the chronic baclofen infusion in the severe spinal spasticity: personal experience and review of the literature. *J Neurosurg Sci* 2004;48(4):177–181.
143. Akman MN, Loubser PG, Donovan WH, et al. Intrathecal baclofen: does tolerance occur? *Paraplegia* 1993;31(8):516–520.
144. Middleton JW, Siddall PJ, Walker S, et al. Intrathecal clonidine and baclofen in the management of spasticity and neuropathic pain following spinal cord injury: a case study. *Arch Phys Med Rehabil* 1996;77:824–826.
145. Sadiq SA, Poopatana CA. Intrathecal baclofen and morphine in multiple sclerosis patients with severe pain and spasticity. *J Neurol* 2007;254(10):1464–1465.
146. Lewis KS, Mueller WM. Intrathecal baclofen for severe spasticity secondary to spinal cord injury. *Ann Pharmacother* 1993;27:767–774.
147. Pasquier Y, Cahana A, Schnider A. Subdural catheter migration may lead to baclofen pump dysfunction. *Spinal Cord* 2003;41:700–702.
148. Murphy PM, Skouvaklis DE, Amadeo RJJ. Intrathecal catheter granuloma associated with isolated baclofen infusion. *Anesth Analg* 2006;102:848–852.
149. Green LB, Nelson VS. Death after acute withdrawal of intrathecal baclofen: case report and literature review. *Arch Phys Med Rehabil* 1999;80:1600–1604.
150. Meythaler JM, Roper JF, Brunner RC. Cyproheptadine for intrathecal baclofen withdrawal. *Arch Phys Med Rehabil* 2003;84(5):638–642.
151. Marciniak C, Rader L, Gagnon C. The use of botulinum toxin for spasticity after spinal cord injury. *Am J Phys Med Rehabil* 2008;87:312–320.
152. Botte MJ, Abrams RA, Bodine-Fowler SC. Treatment of acquired muscle spasticity using phenol peripheral nerve blocks. *Orthopedics* 1995;18:151–159.

153. Chua KSG, Kong K-H. Alcohol neurolysis of the sciatic nerve in the treatment of hemiplegic knee flexor spasticity: Clinical outcomes. *Arch Phys Med Rehabil* 2000;81:1432–1435.
154. Tilton AH. Injectable neuromuscular blockade in the treatment of spasticity and movement disorders. *J Child Neurol* 2003;18:S50–S66.
155. Elovic E. Principles of pharmaceutical management of spastic hypertonia. *Phys Med Rehabil Clin N Am* 2001;12(4):793–816.
156. Zafonte RD, Munin MC. Phenol and alcohol blocks for the treatment of spasticity. *Phys Med Rehabil Clin N Am* 2001;12(4):817–832.
157. Chua KSG, Kong K-H. Clinical and functional outcome after alcohol neurolysis of the tibial nerve for ankle-foot spasticity. *Brain Inj* 2001;15(8):733–739.
158. Khalili AA, Harmel MH, Forster S, et al. Management of spasticity by selective peripheral nerve block with dilute phenol solutions in clinical rehabilitation. *Arch Phys Med Rehabil* 1964;45:513–519.
159. Kong K-H, Chua KSG. Outcome of obturator nerve block with alcohol for the treatment of hip adductor spasticity. *Int J Rehab Res* 1999;22:327–329.
160. Garland DE, Lucie RS, Waters RL. Current use of open phenol nerve block for adult acquired spasticity. *Clin Orthop Relat Res* 1982;165:217–222.
161. Glenn MB, Elovic E. Chemical denervation for the treatment of hypertonia and related motor disorders: Phenol and botulinum toxin. *J Head Trauma Rehabil* 1997;12(6):40–62.
162. Al-Khodairy AT, Gobelet C, Rossier AB. Has botulinum toxin type A a place in the treatment of spasticity in spinal cord injury patients? *Spinal Cord* 1998;36:854–858.
163. Fried GW, Fried, KM. Spinal cord injury and use of botulinum toxin in reducing spasticity. *Phys Med Rehabil Clin N Am* 2003;14:901–910.
164. Opara J, Hordyñska E, Swoboda A. Effectiveness of botulinum toxin A in the treatment of spasticity of the lower extremities in adults—preliminary report. *Ortop Traumatol Rehabil* 2007;9(3):277–285.
165. Humeau Y, Doussau F, Grant NJ, et al. How botulinum and tetanus neurotoxins block neurotransmitter release. *Biochimie* 2000;82:427–446.
166. Simpson LL. Identification of the major steps in botulinum toxin action. *Annu Rev Pharmacol Toxicol* 2004;44:167–193.
167. FDA Approves DYSPORT® for Therapeutic and Aesthetic Uses. www.dysport.com/in the news. Accessed August 12, 2009.
168. FDA Gives Update on Botulinum Toxin Safety Warnings; Established Names of Drugs Changed. www.fda.gov/newsevents/newsroom/pressannouncements/ucm175013.htm. Accessed August 12, 2009.
169. Gracies JM, Lugassy M, Weisz DJ, et al. Botulinum toxin dilution and endplate targeting in spasticity: a double-blind controlled study. *Arch Phys Med Rehabil* 2009;90(1):9–16.
170. Francisco GE. Botulinum toxin: dosing and dilution. *Am J Phys Med Rehabil* 2004;83(Suppl):S30–S37.
171. Brin MF. Dosing, administration, and a treatment algorithm for use of botulinum toxin A for adult-onset spasticity. *Muscle Nerve* 1997;20(Suppl 6):S208–S220.
172. Dunne JW, Heye N, Dunne SL. Treatment of chronic limb spasticity with botulinum toxin A. *J Neurol Neurosurg Psychiatry* 1995;58:232–235.
173. Blitzer A. Botulinum toxin A and B: a comparative dosing study for spasmodic dysphonia. *Otolaryngol Head Neck Surg* 2005;133(6):836–838.
174. Childers MK, Brashear A, Jozefczyk P. Dose-dependent response to intramuscular botulinum toxin type A for upper-limb spasticity in patients after a stroke. *Arch Phys Med Rehabil* 2004;85(7):1063–1069.
175. Brashear A, McAfee AL, Kuhn ER, et al. Treatment with botulinum toxin type B for upper-limb spasticity. *Arch Phys Med Rehabil* 2003;84:103–107.
176. Hesse S, Reiter F, Konrad M, et al. Botulinum toxin type A and short-term electrical stimulation in the treatment of upper limb flexor spasticity after stroke: a randomized, double-blind, placebo-controlled trial. *Clin Rehabil* 1998;12:381–388.
177. Greene P, Fahn S, Diamond B. Development of resistance to botulinum toxin type A in patients with torticollis. *Mov Disord* 1994;9(2):213–217.
178. Barolat G. Surgical management of spasticity and spasms in spinal cord injury: an overview. *J Am Paraplegia Soc* 1998;11(1):9–13.
179. Smyth MD, Peacock WJ. The surgical treatment of spasticity. *Muscle Nerve* 2000;23:153–163.
180. Salame K, Ouaknine GER, Rochkind S, et al. Surgical treatment of spasticity by selective posterior rhizotomy: 30 years experience. *Isr Med Assoc J* 2003;5:543–546.
181. Eltorai I, Montroy R. Muscle release in the management of spasticity after spinal cord injury. *Paraplegia* 1990;28:433–440.

CHAPTER 16 ■ NEUROMUSCULOSKELETAL COMPLICATIONS OF SPINAL CORD INJURY

WILLIAM M. SCELZA AND TREVOR A. DYSON-HUDSON

INTRODUCTION

Chronic spinal cord injury (SCI) can lead to numerous complications over the course of an individual's lifetime. Injury to the musculoskeletal system can contribute to pain syndromes that can lead to musculoskeletal complications and neurological decline. This chapter outlines the pathophysiology, clinical presentation, diagnosis, and management of neuromusculoskeletal complications, overuse injuries, and peripheral nerve entrapments after SCI.

NEUROMUSCULOSKELETAL COMPLICATIONS

Fractures

The incidence of fractures in persons with chronic SCI has been reported to be 2% to 6% with the SCI Model Systems database reporting an incidence of 2.5% (1). Studies estimate up to 70% of persons with SCI will sustain a long bone fracture (2,3). Many fractures may go undiagnosed because of impaired sensation and therefore patients may not seek medical attention. Fractures in the SCI population require special consideration in the approach to their management.

After SCI, there is a rapid and dramatic loss of trabecular bone below the level of injury (see Chapter 12), which is the main reason why persons with SCI are at high risk for fractures. Individuals with SCI will lose significant bone mineral density (BMD) within the first year after injury. This is most significant around the knee region and is more severe in women and as such fractures are more common in this region and in women. Fracture patterns have shown to be more prominent in those with complete versus incomplete injuries and in those with paraplegia versus tetraplegia; this may be explained by a greater ability to participate in physical activities, transfers, and sustain falls (4,5). Defining the fracture threshold has been difficult, but evidence suggests those who develop fractures have reduced bone mass versus those who do not develop fractures (6). A BMD fracture threshold of 50% appears to exist for the knee, and this most likely is the fracture threshold for most regions in the body (5,7). As such, preventative measures should be taken with all individuals, and counseling for safe practices should be initiated during the acute rehabilitation phase.

The knee is the most common fracture site in chronic SCI (7). Supracondylar femur fractures are the most common, followed by the tibia (proximal then distal), femoral shaft and neck, and humerus, respectively, with the latter being more common in those with tetraplegia (4,8,9). Falls account for a majority of the fractures but even minimal stresses from range of motion (ROM) or transfers may cause fracture and many times the cause will remain undetermined. Symptoms include typical presence of erythema, swelling, and joint deformity may be present. In those who are sensate, pain may be present but index of suspicion should be high even in the absence of pain given the impaired sensation in the SCI population. Fracture should be considered in the presence of undiagnosed fever, spasticity, malaise, or autonomic dysreflexia. Deep venous thrombosis (DVT) may also coexist and diagnosis should be considered (10). Plain x-ray will diagnose most fractures and may reveal old or chronic undiagnosed fractures as well.

For persons who are ambulatory, management is similar to the non-SCI population. The main approach to treatment of fractures in those who do not have functional use of their lower extremities is to minimize complications, allow satisfactory healing, and preserve function and alignment (11–13). In nonambulatory patients, some degree of shortening and angulation is acceptable. Most fractures are treated nonoperatively with soft-padded splints. A well-padded knee immobilizer is useful for femoral supracondylar, femoral shaft, and proximal tibial fractures; a well-padded ankle immobilizer can be used for distal tibial fractures. A soft splint can be made of a blanket wrapped around the fracture site and fixed with adhesive tape, but this is more difficult to keep clean and to remove/reapply (14).

Methods commonly utilized for non-SCI fracture management (surgery, circumferential casting, external fixation) are usually not indicated in the SCI population because of potential complications. Circumferential plaster casts or traction can cause skin breakdown because of sensory impairment (11,15,16). If used, they should be well padded and bivalved for skin inspection at least twice daily. Any skin breakdown, which develops, even if superficial, must be treated aggressively; the source of the breakdown must be identified and eliminated (11–13). Surgical intervention for femoral shaft and distal femoral fractures is associated with a high complication rate because of bone quality, risk of osteomyelitis, and recurrent bacteremia (12,14,15,17,18). Most fractures will heal using the conservative approach. The patient does not need to remain in bed and should be mobile in the wheelchair within a few days. Having the legs flexed at the hip and knee in a wheelchair with the feet flat on the footrests maintains functional positioning for healing, unless the fracture is close to the knee such that knee extension is required. In this case, an elevating legrest will be required for the wheelchair. Callus formation is usually evident in 3 to 4 weeks (13,14,17). Immobilization can usually be discontinued in 6 to 8 weeks and ROM initiated, though weight bearing (tilt table, standing, and stand-pivot transfers) should be delayed for a longer period. Nonunion of fractures occurs at a reported rate of 2% to 10% (13–15,17–20); however, this is not clinically significant in those who do not weight bear through their lower limbs.

Surgical intervention may be indicated when conservative methods will not control rotational deformity. Surgery may also be required for proximal femur fractures in the setting of severe spasticity, impaired vascular supply, impractical splinting options, or if shortening/angulation will result in impaired function or cosmesis (9,11,13,14,16,21). For these fractures, internal fixation may allow the fastest mobilization and allow for more anatomic alignment. Femoral neck and subtrochanteric fractures are probably the most difficult to manage and internal fixation may be considered if a minimal device such as an intramedullary rod can be used (13). Interlocking intramedullary rods are preferred with proximal femoral shaft fractures that cannot be immobilized successfully. Patients with femoral neck fractures can maintain prefracture mobility and may be mobilized without LE immobilization, since splinting this area may be too difficult. External fixation devices should be avoided if at all possible secondary to complications with pin movement in the osteoporotic bone, patient positioning, and risk of skin breakdown (16,22). Postoperative positioning should allow for foot flat positioning on the footrest and adductor pillows between the legs if hip precautions are indicated.

The etiology of the fracture and the functional impact of the fracture should be considered. Hospitalization is not always required and should be reserved for those who have severe swelling, who require surgery, or who require patient/family training to return home. Vascular studies should be performed if venous thrombosis or arterial injury is suspected. DVT prophylaxis should be considered in all SCI patients with lower limb fractures, for 7 to 14 days (10), though the optimal duration has not been established. The patient may require rehabilitation for functional training; they may need additional assistance in the home and may need an alternate wheelchair, elevating legrests, and wheelchair cushion.

Charcot Arthropathy

Jean Martin Charcot (23) originally described the tabetic neuroarthropathy in 1868 in the era of neurosyphillis. Over the years, several other conditions such as diabetic peripheral neuropathy, tertiary syphilis, and myelomeningocele have led to the development of joint destruction in the light of absent protective sensation and proprioception. This has also been described after traumatic SCI with regard to the spine, possibly leading to neuropathic spinal arthropathy or Charcot spine (24).

After traumatic SCI, disruption to the bony elements and supporting ligamentous structures will often require operative stabilization of the spine (24–26). Postsurgery, the fused segments will not retain their normal flexion, extension, or rotational mobility. This immobility can lead to repetitive flexion and extension stresses above and below the fused spinal segments. Although not commonly used during this era, extensive multilevel laminectomies may contribute to adjacent segmental instability that may exert similar forces over these regions placing them at risk for degenerative changes (27–29).

Repetitive trauma secondary to the elevated stresses is believed to lead to erosive bony destruction and inflammation. Impaired proprioception and sensation takes away protective mechanisms that could alert the individual to the destructive processes that are continuing (30). Weakness of spinal stabilizing musculature may contribute to the extremes of motion and lack of postural support can perpetuate this situation. Repetitive stress may also be placed on the spine with poor seating position, transfers, recreational activities, and other daily necessities that injured patients will need to accomplish over their lifetime.

As a result of this repetitive motion, a cascade of degeneration can develop. These processes can occur simultaneously such as cartilaginous destruction, erosive bony degradation of subchondral bone, fracture of subchondral bone, and the development of a spinal pseudoarthrosis. Ultimately, vertebral collapse and frank spinal instability may ensue. It has also been reported that such severe repetitive stresses have led to the development of a ball and socket joint pseudoarthrosis and the complete disruption and transection of the spinal cord.

Signs and symptoms of a neuropathic spinal arthropathy may present at any time and have been reported as far as several decades from the original injury (26,31). Patients most commonly complain of low back pain (4,7). This can be the presentation even in a relatively insensate area, although it is unclear of the etiology of such pain. Other symptoms may include a descending or ascending neurological deficit such as new muscle weakness or sensory deficit if frank spinal instability leads to spinal cord compression. A descending neurological deficit should be sought as a majority of the cases tend to occur approximately two to three segments below fusion levels in the thoracolumbar region. A patient with a low thoracic injury who develops neuropathic spinal arthropathy in segments below the injury can lead to disruption of the lumbosacral nerve roots. This can lead to the loss of reflexive bladder control, loss of reflexogenic erectile control, muscle flaccidity, and the loss of spasticity. Almost all patients will describe audible spinal crepitus and its presence should give the clinician a high clinical suspicion of a neuropathic spinal arthropathy. Individuals with SCI may also present with changes in their sitting balance and the development of new pressure ulcers from altered seating positioning (26,29,32).

There is often a delay in formal diagnosis and treatment from the first presentation of symptoms (26,31). Neurological exam can be an effective tool in conjunction with the history to raise suspicion of worsening neurological deficits, both ascending and descending. Serial and periodic examinations can help identify any significant changes. The evaluation of lower extremity muscle tone and spasticity are helpful to suggest descending injury patterns. Any changes in urodynamic examinations including the loss of reflexive bladder contractions or loss of detrusor sphincter dyssynergia may heighten the clinical suspicion of a cauda equina injury.

Radiological imaging is essential to assess for a neuropathic spinal arthropathy. Plain films of the spine can often show early changes of erosion of the facets as some of the first signs

(27,30). Flexion/extension views may be the most helpful to identify instability in spinal segments that may not be readily identifiable in plain films or static computerized tomography (CT) scan. CT scanning will provide greater detail in specific bony structures and assess central or foraminal canal stenosis encroaching on the neural structures and can be used in conjunction with myelography. Posterior elements are also imaged in greater detail and may show fracture or pseudoarthrosis that may not be visible on plain films. This may be especially useful in those who may be having new neurological deficits or those unable to undergo magnetic resonance imaging (MRI) due to artifact from metallic hardware or other contraindications.

MRI can provide valuable information in the soft tissue structures as there may be some degree of ligamentous injury not visualized with conventional radiographs or CT scanning. Furthermore, MRI is the study of choice to evaluate for infection, tumor, syringomyelia, or other soft tissue or ligamentous injury. It is important to evaluate any new destructive lesion of the spine for infectious etiology. Osteomyelitis, diskitis, septic pseudoarthrosis as well as metastatic lesions or other primary malignant tumors must be considered in the differential diagnosis (25).

Once identified, the treatment of a neuropathic spinal arthropathy is best accomplished with surgical intervention. This may include a staged posterior instrumented fusion followed by an anterior debridement and bone grafting. Conservative management could include prolonged immobilization with bracing, but this could ultimately lead to complications from immobility including pressure ulcers and worsening neurological deficit. The underlying instability also may never be definitively addressed leaving the likelihood that surgical fixation will need to be completed (25,27). Surgical intervention should not be taken lightly, however. Some have suggested that after surgical correction the individual is at further risk of redeveloping similar degenerative changes below the surgical revision of the spinal segments and thus these patients should be monitored with serial imaging (30). The focus should also emphasize protective measures that will improve sitting posture as well as transfer techniques to avoid stressing the spine as much as possible (25).

Scoliosis

Scoliosis is defined as an abnormal curvature of the spine. Although it is most prominent in individuals injured as children, adults with traumatic SCI may also be affected (33,34). Those who sustain a lateral compression or burst fractures may develop kyphotic and/or coronal curvature. New compression fractures below the level of injury may occur and may be asymptomatic in terms of pain but could potentially lead to the development of scoliotic curves (27). Individuals with extensive laminectomies may also contribute to spinal curvature over time. In those injured prior to the skeletal maturity, it is estimated that 98% will develop a scoliosis, two thirds of which will require surgical stabilization (34). For children who were injured after puberty, the incidence decreased to 20% with much fewer requiring surgery. These issues are addressed more extensively in Chapter 29. Observation is typically utilized in those with curvature under 20 degrees. Immobilization with bracing can also be used to help slow or stop the progression of the curvature. Should the curvature continue or restrictive pulmonary deficits ensue, surgery may be considered (35).

Neurological Decline

Neurological decline, including new onset weakness or sensory loss, may be present in up to 20% of patients with SCI (36,37). The timeframe in which these changes occur can be as early as a few weeks post injury, or present itself decades after an injury. Patterns of functional decline may present as acute frank weakness to gradual and subtle changes in sensory function. Furthermore, there may be complaints of functional declines and pain below the level of injury that could be attributed to overuse syndromes and musculoskeletal dysfunction that is common in the SCI population.

As such, routine testing of sensory and motor function should be undertaken and documented on a regular basis for individuals with SCI. The exam as described in the International Standards (38) may help to detect gross and distinct changes over time. More challenging are patients with complaints of neurological decline, which may be more vague and subtle in their presentation. In these cases, serial examinations may not be enough and radiological and electrodiagnostic studies are needed (39).

Patients who develop a worsening neurological deficit postinjury should undergo an evaluation for new spinal cord and/or nerve root compression. In any situation where there is an acute presentation of neurological decline or severe and debilitating pain, the clinician must consider an urgent situation as prompt intervention may be required to prevent further worsening of the injury. Significant functional deterioration in patients may also be a clue to an abrupt neurological decline. New or worsening axial spinal pain may also be a presenting symptom that may signify degenerative or bony etiologies. New radiation of pain in radicular patterns or complaints of neuropathic or dysesthetic pain may signify nerve root impingement or peripheral nerve etiologies. Fever or malaise may also signify an infectious process such as diskitis, osteomyelitis, or epidural abscess. The potential for a systemic metabolic or disease process must also be considered in the differential of a neurological decline as well.

Syringomyelia

Syringomyelia is the most common cause of neurological decline in those with SCI (36). Syringomyelia is defined as a fluid-filled cyst within the gray matter of the spinal cord, and has been described by many other terms including a syrinx, hydromyelia, hydrosyringomyelia, and ascending cystic degeneration. The most common cause of syringomyelia after SCI is referred to as posttraumatic syringomyelia (PTS).

PTS is a gray matter cystic structure that develops at the site of injury to the spinal cord. Small intramedullary cysts at the primary site of trauma to the spinal cord are quite common and it is estimated that 39% to 59% of all patients with traumatic SCI will have such posttraumatic cystic structures (40–43). These small posttraumatic cysts do not enlarge in either the rostral or caudal planes and do not cause any neurological decline. They are often identified incidentally on imagining studies such as MRI and remain stable over the course of a patient's lifetime.

Enlarging PTS may be present in 12% to 20% of MRI imaging studies and some postmortem autopsy studies suggest an incidence of syringomyelia in up to 22% of subjects although the precise incidence is not known (40,44–47). The most concerning sequelae of these enlarging cystic cavities is a decline in neurological functioning over time. It is estimated that anywhere from 3% to 8% of individuals with SCI will develop neurological decline (48,49). Expanding PTS can develop relatively soon in the first few months post injury or may present itself after decades. PTS should always be considered in any SCI patient presenting with new neurological complaints (14,50).

While the precise mechanisms and pathophysiology that contributes to PTS remain unknown, there are many theories that contribute to their development. Postinjury, there is usually hemorrhage formation that progresses to liquefaction necrosis. There are also numerous cytotoxic chemicals and inflammatory cascades that evolve post injury that contributes to the secondary injury to the spinal cord (42,51,52). There are also almost certain breaches in the blood-brain barrier that also exist, all of which could contribute to the development of the initial intramedullary cyst formation and myelomalacia or thinning and scarring of the spinal cord.

Inflammatory reactions as a result of the injury may cause arachnoid scarring and adhesions of the injured cord directly to the dural tissue causing impairments of flow of cerebral spinal fluid in the subarachnoid space and cause tension of the spinal cord. Ischemia may ensue from traction of the blood vessels supplying the spinal cord or from the expansion of the intramedullary cysts. Traction may also cause direct injury to the intramedullary spinal cord and allow cerebral spinal fluid to permeate into newly formed cysts (53).

Expansion of these cavities can occur in rostral and/or caudal directions and this is likely directed by the pathways of least resistance. The expansion of the syrinx cavity may also be due to increased pressures within the subarachnoid space. Any increase in intra-abdominal or intrathoracic pressure as may occur with Valsalva maneuvers, bearing down, weight lifting, assisted cough (quad cough), transfers, or with bowel and bladder programs that may occur repeatedly over the lifetime of an individual have been postulated to contribute to a sloshing phenomenon (54–57). The sloshing phenomenon has been postulated to contribute to the formation and enlargement of syrinx cavities by the repetitive and constant small increases in pressure within the syrinx cavity. The constant "slosh and suck" forces contribute to the expansion of the weakened spaces within the intramedullary space allowing growth and expansion of the syrinx cavity (58,59). Several small cavities may also be allowed, with ongoing repetitive stress to form larger, confluent, and more organized syrinx cavities. The impact of these repetitive increases of pressure within the subarachnoid space has not precisely been defined. Prevention of worsening of this phenomenon by avoiding of Valsalva-type maneuvers has been suggested in those who may have syrinx cavities. It must be considered that this may significantly impact an individual's ability to participate in everyday self-care and mobility activities that are necessary for independence, recreational, vocational aspirations of an individual. As such, activity restrictions, while they may be recommended for an individual with an expansive PTS, may significantly impact an individual's independence and quality of life and in some instances be totally unavoidable. Reviewing techniques, strategies, and prescribing assistive devices, especially for transfers, are beneficial to minimize as much as possible the repetitive increases in pressure within the syrinx cavity and expansion of the cavity.

Of note, syringomyelia is also associated with Chiari malformations. These congenital defects are characterized by cerebellar tonsil displacement into the foramen magnum and interruption of cerebral spinal fluid. The syrinx cavity from Chiari malformations usually does communicate directly with the fourth ventricle and is confluent with the central spinal canal, whereas a posttraumatic syrinx is usually restricted to the gray matter of the spinal cord. Thus, PTS is often referred to as a noncommunicating syringomyelia versus communicating syringomyelia with Chiari malformations. Chiari I malformations usually present in childhood of adolescence, whereas Chiari II malformations typically present themselves in infancy (60).

The most common clinical presentation in those with expansive PTS is pain (46). The pain will often be unilateral and neuropathic in description, that is, burning, numbness, and tingling sensation that may or may not radiate. The pain is often located at the site of the original injury or radiate to the neck or upper limbs in cervical injuries. This may make it difficult to distinguish from other peripheral nerve entrapments or radiculopathy, which are also quite common in those with chronic SCI. The symptoms are often vague and nonspecific. The development of a neuropathic arthropathy of the spine or other peripheral joint may also be the initial clinical presentation. Clinical features that may point to the development of a PTS include initial unilateral presentation with progression to bilateral symptomatology. The worsening of symptoms with coughing or Valsalva techniques may also be present. Ascending sensory levels, often asymmetric is the next most common symptom of a syrinx. The sensory loss is often dissociated, with loss of pain and temperature sensation often with the preservation of light touch sensation (44,48,61–63).

The development of new weakness in PTS will not commonly be the presenting symptom but certainly the most concerning as this would potentially have the largest impact on function. Even more concerning would be if the ascending syringomyelia would impact and affect the respiratory control of the diaphragm and brain stem, potentially leading to ventilator dependence, dysphagia, and other bulbar symptoms.

Other common signs and symptoms associated with PTS may be more nonspecific. These include increasing spasticity and the development of a lower motor neuron pattern of neurogenic bowel/bladder function. Autonomic dysfunction may also be a common presentation or symptom. The development of a Horner syndrome, increased sweating, development of orthostatic hypotension or autonomic dysreflexia may be present (44,48,61–63). One must always consider the signs and symptoms from a descending syrinx that present as a decrease in spasticity and may impact autonomic and bowel/bladder function below the injury.

The location of an SCI may also be crucial in the development and presentation of symptoms. For example, in those with a thoracic injury, an ascending sensory level may have very little impact on function and may often go unnoticed. At the same time, ongoing ascending injury may lead to a profound change in a person's clinical abilities that could drastically alter a patient's sitting balance, pain, and weakness in upper extremity muscles that was not present previously.

Individuals with an incomplete injury may also be affected by an expansive syrinx that may interrupt ascending and descending sensory and motor tracts, respectively. Previously ambulatory patients may therefore present with worsening ataxia, falls, or worsening spasticity patterns.

MRI is the most useful tool in the diagnosis of PTS (43,44,63,64) (Fig. 16.1). The use of gadolinium contrast is suggested as it may improve the ability to distinguish from an infectious, vascular, or neoplastic process and can also be useful in identifying the cause of neurological decline as a myelopathy from spinal stenosis, disc herniation, or other pathologic process may be easily identifiable. The limitations of MRI scanning are mostly related to underlying hardware and spinal stabilization instrumentation that may contribute to artifact that limits visualization of the spinal cord. In such cases, CT myelography would be the test of choice (63,65).

MRI scanning also may provide ability to compare serial examinations and evaluate a syrinx for progression. A syrinx may increase in size over time with either a very subtle or no change in clinical symptoms. Often times, the size of the syrinx does not correlate clinically with the extent of neurologic symptoms. However, the largest and most dilated cases of syringomyelia tend to cause the greatest neurological deficits. A syrinx cavity that rapidly progresses and has an early presentation after an injury may tend to be the most clinically destructive and warrant close monitoring and early intervention. A syrinx may be somewhat dynamic in nature and resolve spontaneously.

Electrodiagnostic studies may be important diagnostic tool in the evaluation of PTS. These studies may help distinguish between the development of a brachial plexus lesion, peripheral nerve injury, or peripheral neuropathy. In chronic SCI, injury to the spinal cord, nerve roots, or peripheral nerves may leave one with some persistent electrodiagnostic abnormalities. There may also be a combination of upper and lower motor neuron findings and thus a focused electrodiagnostic examination will be the most useful based upon the patient's clinical appearance and examination and should be used in conjunction with the appropriate neuroimaging. Early abnormalities on electrodiagnostic studies could include prolonged F waves and prolonged descending motor conduction on motor-evoked potential testing. Later findings that would be suggestive of syringomyelia include progressive denervation potentials, a reduced compound motor unit action potential, enlarged motor units to signify compensatory motor unit sprouting in the presence of denervation, and reduced maximal firing rate of motor units (36,39). The clinical sensory and motor examinations may also not be sufficient to detect early and subtle changes enhancing the benefits of electrodiagnostic studies.

Treatment of PTS consists of both conservative and surgical treatments. Conservative treatments primarily consist of observation and serial physical examinations of sensory and motor function, serial imaging, and electrodiagnostic studies. As indicated above, activity restrictions with the avoidance of increased intra-abdominal pressure to keep venous pressures down may be helpful but not precisely defined. Keeping the head elevated above 20 degrees overnight has also been suggested. The use of treatments aiming to alter the pathophysiology of the formation of the syrinx is thought to be more efficacious than methods to drain the cavity (63). Diuretics have been used to decrease the production and accumulation of cerebral spinal fluid. The presence of motor loss alone is

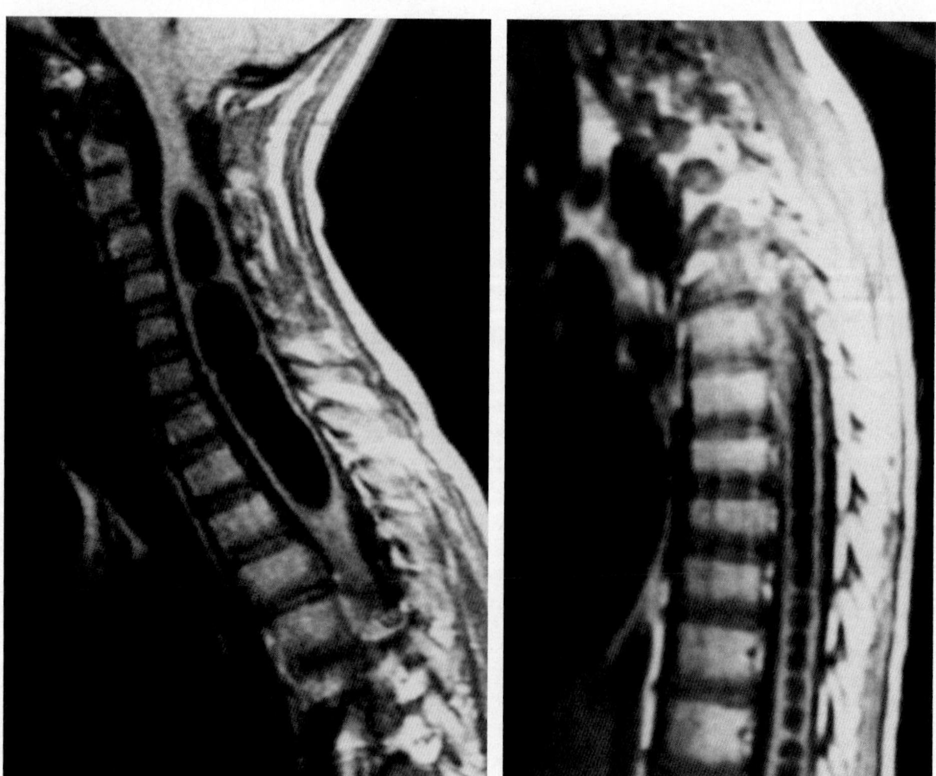

FIGURE 16.1 MRI of spine revealing a syrinx.

not an indication for surgery. Symptomatic management of the symptoms (i.e., aggressive pain relief) during the monitoring phase will also be helpful.

Surgical treatment is indicated if there is notable persistent motor weakness occurring or severe or persistent or worsening (intractable) pain despite the conservative measures. It is recommended that if a rapidly developing course of symptoms occurs that early surgery should be considered to prevent or halt worsening neurological deficits. Surgical treatments include a variety of approaches. Percutaneous drainage with CT guidance has been used with some benefit although reaccumulation can occur within weeks (66). Shunting procedures to the peritoneal, pleural, or subarachnoid spaces are also used with some reporting improvement in motor strength and pain although there is an incidence of up to 50% of shunt malfunction and often reoccurrence of neurological symptoms by 5 years (49,64,67). Shunt procedures can also lead to arachnoiditis, scarring, and cord tethering. Other surgical interventions include the lysis of adhesions contributing to traction of the spinal cord cerebral spinal fluid flow coupled with duraplasty (63,67,68). Cordectomy is limited to only those who have complete injuries.

Goals of surgical treatment are to limit further progression of neurological symptoms and hopefully improve any neurological deficit already incurred. Despite surgical treatment, however, many develop a return of neurological symptoms. Postoperative imaging and neurological examination is indicated to assess for progression or return of syringomyelia. The complete resolution of a syrinx is not necessary for improvement of symptoms, however.

Myelopathy and Radiculopathy

Spinal cord and nerve root compression causing myelopathy and/or radiculopathy are other common causes of neurological decline after SCI. Many individuals may have an underlying congenital spinal stenosis, which may have played a contributing role during the original injury. This may manifest itself in worsening spinal stenosis and myelopathy.

Individuals who have had previous spinal surgery and fusion may also be at risk for adjacent (both rostral and caudal) degenerative changes (69–71). The intravertebral disc appears to be at greatest risk of herniation due to the extensive stresses placed upon this region form the immobile segments above and below (70,72,73). Degenerative changes over the posterior elements and facets joints may also contribute to a degenerative stenosis causing myelopathy (74,75). There may also be components of segmental instability contributing to the development of symptomatic myelopathy. It does appear that risk factors include the use of instrumentation during fusion procedures, which may often be required to provide stability to the highly unstable spine, causes rigidity of the instrumented segments. The length of the fusion causes an increased lever arm that can increase stresses over the free segments adjacent fusion segments as well (69,76). Some studies have also suggested that previous laminectomies and short fusion segments around the thoracolumbar junction may contribute to spinal instability in these regions (77). Residual kyphotic deformity after spinal trauma may also lead to increased pain and neurological change and thus may require anterior and posterior stabilization procedures (27,78).

Nonunion of previous surgical stabilization procedures may also predispose posttraumatic spinal injuries to further neurological decline after surgery. Predisposing factors include poor surgical technique, infection, trauma, osteoporosis, or other metabolic bone disease (79,80). In addition, the use of nonsteroidal anti-inflammatory drugs (NSAIDs) after spinal fusion has also been shown to increase the risk of developing a nonunion and pseudoarthrosis of fusion segments. The use of NSAIDs, particularly in the early postoperative phase, has been demonstrated to have an inhibitory effect of the healing of bone and are likely most detrimental during the inflammatory phase of bone healing. Thus, if individuals requiring NSAIDs for pain control or those who may be on long-term NSAIDs for other chronic conditions, consultation with the spine surgeon would be recommended prior to the resumption of these medications.

The development of a symptomatic nonunion of fusion is three to five times greater in those who are smokers (81–83). The deleterious effects of smoking are most likely multifactorial and are based primarily on the impairments in vascular supply, oxygenation, and the effects of osteoprogenitor cells necessary for the maturation of the fusion (83–85). The effects of smoking are most profound in the early postoperative period after a spinal fusion when blood supply to the fusion is crucial to its maturation, especially when allograft bone is utilized, and do not appear to be influenced by age, sex, or other mitigating factors. Long-term smokers will also have bone that is less robust and will be susceptible to osteoporosis and other metabolic derangements of bone metabolism (83,86).

Excessive motion can also be a contributing factor and patient noncompliance with postoperative bracing can certainly be a component. While nonunion may be asymptomatic in some patients, increase in pain or changing neurological symptoms may be inevitable over time. Any individual with worsening pain or neurological symptoms must be followed with serial neurological exams and neuroimaging. Signs of residual stenosis or signs of instability should warrant consultation with spinal surgeon to determine course of action. Options include immobilization, conservative and symptomatic relief with analgesics, or further spinal stabilization.

Tethered Cord Syndrome

Inflammation and swelling after an SCI can lead to arachnoiditis and potentially cause scarring of the spinal cord to the meningeal lining. This can also be most prevalent in injuries to the lumbosacral spine where arachnoiditis occurs in the cauda equina and tethering of the nerve roots. This may or may not cause symptoms but common presentations include pain, sensory deficits, weakness, or new bowel/bladder symptomatology (87,88). While this may be most problematic in children with SCI where the patient will continue to grow and ongoing tension to the spinal cord may ensue, tethering may also present itself when traction is placed on the spinal cord with repeated flexion/extension of the cervical spine. Ultimately, traction from tethering may cause tension and ischemia to the spinal cord and contribute to the formation of PTS, which is discussed in the previous section. Treatment may include bracing of the cervical spine to prevent repetitive flexion and extension. If symptoms remain severe or progressive, surgical management to relieve to tethered portions of the spinal cord may be indicated. The use of a dural graft to expand the dural space may be used but there always remains a high risk of repeated inflammation and tethering at the surgical sight; thus, surgical intervention requires careful patient selection (87,88).

Aging with SCI

In addition to the previously mentioned causes of neurological decline specific to SCI, individuals with SCI are susceptible to other neurodegenerative disorders, metabolic disorders, or nutritional disorders seen in the general population. For these potential etiologies, clinical suspicion may warrant workup for the suspected disorders. Aging with an SCI may also be a potential cause of the patient's functional changes as well. Over time loss of muscle mass, strength, and abnormalities in sensation, reaction time, and coordination have been described. Age-related loss of anterior horn cells or myelination of neural tracts does occur and one can only extrapolate these effects will be magnified in an individual with an SCI. In these cases, it may be indicated to address the condition of aging with these individuals. Proper nutritional support and discussion of psychological and social barriers may help address the underlying problems. Prescribing therapy may help address functional problems that can be addressed with evaluation of technique and teaching of caregivers on how to assist with patient mobility. The evaluation of assistive devices may also address these problems in the chronic SCI population.

MUSCULOSKELETAL PAIN AND OVERUSE INJURIES

Musculoskeletal pain and peripheral nerve entrapment syndromes*† are a common complication after SCI. Upper limb pain syndromes are most common and are associated with acute strain and/or overuse due to an increased reliance on the upper limbs for mobility and other activities of daily living (ADL) (89–94). Overuse-related musculoskeletal pain syndromes may also occur in the lower limbs in persons with incomplete or lower levels of injury who are able to ambulate. Impaired sensation and/or muscle paralysis can make lower limb joints unstable, increasing the risk of injury to these structures. Intensive training through activities such as body weight–supported treadmill training can further expose lower limb structures to overuse and also warrant close monitoring. Upper and lower limb pain syndromes may also arise from lack of upper limb use or poor positioning as seen in persons with SCI who were recently injured, restricted to bed due to underlying illness, or with cervical-level injuries and impaired limb movement or altered sensation.

*Spinal Cord Injury Pain Task Force of the International Association of the Study of Pain (IASP) taxonomy: nociceptive [tier I], musculoskeletal [tier II], secondary overuse syndromes [tier III]; and neuropathic [Tier I], above-level [tier II], compressive mononeuropathies [tier III], respectively (258).

†Bryce-Ragnarsson SCI Pain Taxonomy (BR-SCI-PT): above-level, nociceptive, mechanical/muscuoskeletal; and above-level, neuropathic, compressive neuropathy, respectively (259)."

Upper Limb Pain Syndromes

Upper limb weight-bearing activities like wheelchair propulsion, transfers, and raised ischial pressure reliefs, as well as repeated reaching from the seated position of a wheelchair, place a great deal of stress on the structures of the upper limb, putting them at risk for overuse injuries and pain. Upper limb pain syndromes can disturb the progress of rehabilitation, as well as interfere with ADL, functional independence, and quality of life (92,95–97). In one study, 30% of all persons with chronic SCI (59% of those with tetraplegia; 41% of those with paraplegia) reported significant upper limb pain requiring analgesic medication, limiting function, or causing pain with two or more ADL (92). Upper limb pain may lead to functional decline and increase the risk for other medical conditions such as obesity, fatigue, depression, pressure ulcers, contractures, and spasticity (98,99). This may also adversely affect vocational activities, with unemployment higher and full-time employment lower in persons with upper limb pain than those without (100). Perhaps most importantantly, permanent damage to the upper limbs may be functionally and economically equivalent to an SCI of a much higher level (92).

Shoulder Overuse Syndromes

Disorders of the shoulder are among the most frequent causes of musculoskeletal pain and disability in persons with SCI, with a prevalence of 30% to 73% (89–92,94,100–109). Overall, all-cause shoulder pain is more common in persons with tetraplegia and in those with neurologically complete injuries (92,101,103,110), especially during the first year after SCI (92,102,111). However, overuse-related shoulder pain is more common in those with paraplegia and is seen in later years after injury. Other risk factors for shoulder pain include female gender (91,112,113), higher body mass index (108), and older age (112). Duration of injury may also be a risk factor (89,104,106,107); however, this is not a consistent finding (100,102,103). The combined affects of aging and duration of injury may be more severe in persons with pediatric-onset SCI given their relatively long life span (105); however, the impact of physical and physiological immaturity at time of injury on shoulder pain risk is uncertain.

Musculotendinous overuse syndromes are the most common cause of shoulder pain in persons with SCI (101). Musculotendinous pain can be separated into 2 broad categories: (a) pain in relation to the rotator cuff tendons and surrounding structures (e.g., bursa, biceps tendon) and (b) pain in the regional muscles of the shoulder and the shoulder girdle (e.g., rotator cuff and scapular stabilizers) (114). Pain in relation to the rotator cuff is most common and is likely a consequence of overuse combined with subacromial impingement rather than acute trauma (115). Common diagnoses include rotator cuff tendinitis, supraspinatus tendinitis, bicipital tendinitis, subacromial bursitis, and impingement syndrome (90,92,116). Since these diagnostic terms refer to the same clinical syndrome and it is often difficult to reliably establish which structure in the shoulder is causing the pain, some advocate using the terms *subacromial pain syndrome* or *rotator cuff disease (syndrome)* (114,117–119).

Pain in the regional muscles of the shoulder and the shoulder girdle may be caused by acute muscle strains or chronic muscle pain. *Acute muscle strains* present as a sudden onset of localized pain during strenuous activities. They are usually caused by a rapid change from an eccentric to concentric contraction, by awkward positioning during transfers, or by sudden bouts of increased activity as seen during rehabilitation after SCI or in persons living in the community. On physical exam, there is tenderness over the strained muscle. Pain-inhibited weakness of the muscle may also be present. Bruising may be present over the affected area if the muscle is torn. Treatment of acute muscle strains consists of rest and ice. Gentle concentric strengthening at submaximal levels may begin 3 days after the injury, followed by gentle stretching a few days later. The eccentric component of strengthening can be added as symptoms improve (120). *Chronic muscle pain*, on the other hand, results from overuse and is often more resistant to treatment (101,121).

Myofascial pain syndromes may also be present and these refer to a specific condition characterized by the presence of trigger points (122). In addition, acromioclavicular and glenohumeral joint osteoarthritis, osteolysis of the distal clavicle, and osteonecrosis of the humeral head are all conditions that have been associated with shoulder overuse in persons with SCI (90,108,112,123,124).

A thorough pain history and physical exam of the neck and upper limbs is critical to develop an accurate diagnosis. Important questions include the quality and characteristics of the pain (e.g., onset, duration, quality, intensity, radiation, and aggravating/alleviating factors). Important information includes the patient's motor and neurological level of injury; handedness; and type and set-up of wheelchair. The history should not focus solely on the shoulder pain, but should include a thorough review of systems to rule out other causes of shoulder pain. Nausea, loss of appetite, fever, chills, or increasing autonomic dysreflexia may be a sign of abdominal or pelvic pathology; new onset weakness, sensory loss, or radiating pain may be a sign of PTS or cervical radiculopathy. Pain in persons with SCI may be complex in that multiple types of pain with different characteristics may exist simultaneously in different regions of the body (125).

Common outcome measures used to assess shoulder pain in persons with SCI include measures of shoulder pain intensity over the past week (average, highest, lowest) using an 11-point numerical rating scale (NRS; 0–10, anchored at the ends by 0 = "no pain" and 10 = "pain as bad as you can imagine") and the Wheelchair Users Shoulder Pain Index (WUSPI) (Fig. 16.2). The WUSPI is a 15-item functional measure of shoulder pain intensity in wheelchair users during various ADLs (126), which is a valid and reliable disease-specific measure of pain intensity, and has been shown to be sensitive to treatments that impact shoulder pain intensity (126–130). Measures of physical functioning such as the pain interference item from the Short Form-36, the 7-item Brief Pain Inventory, and the Multidimensional Pain Inventory may provide useful insight into whether shoulder pain interferes with daily activities (131). The International Spinal Cord Injury Pain Data Set (ISCIPDS) may also be helpful as it contains core questions concerning SCI-related pain and can measure multiple types of pain in the same individual (125).

The physical examination should include ROM, flexibility, strength, and sensory testing of the neck and upper limb structures. Palpation of the supraspinatus tendon at its insertion on the greater tuberosity, the biceps tendon in the bicipital groove, and palpation of acromioclavicular joint, as well as special provocative tests are all commonly used during the physical examination to reproduce symptoms of pain. Common provocative tests for rotator cuff disease include tests for subacromial impingement, such as Neer impingement sign (132), Hawkins-Kennedy impingement sign (133), Yocum test (134), and the painful arc (135), as well as tests of rotator cuff muscle integrity, such as the supraspinatus (Jobe's or "empty can") test (136), Napolean test (137), bear-hug test (138), and the forced internal and external rotation tests (139,140). Other provocative tests such as the Speed's test (141), Yergason's test (141), active-compression (O'Brien's) test (142), and cross-body adduction (Scarf) test (141) are used to identify other shoulder complex abnormalities, such as biceps tendon, superior labral, or acromioclavicular joint abnormalities.

Functional testing should include assessment of the patient's posture, pressure relief techniques, transfer capability and techniques to all surfaces, wheelchair set-up and propulsion, as well as a review of work, home, community, and driving environments.

As previously mentioned, shoulder pain may be referred from structures outside the shoulder region as well. In one study (92), referred pain from the cervical spine accounted for 33% and 13% of the shoulder pain diagnoses in persons with tetraplegia and paraplegia, respectively. Importantly, other types of nociceptive musculoskeletal pain (e.g. degenerative changes and mechanical instability at the cervical spine, spasticity, heterotopic ossification), as well as above-level neuropathic pain (e.g. complex regional pain syndrome Type II) and at-level neuropathic pain (e.g., syringomyelia, nerve root entrapment, transitional zone pain) may all cause shoulder pain in persons with SCI (92,95,106,111,143–147). Nociceptive visceral pain may also refer to the shoulder, so it is especially important to keep in mind that shoulder pain may be an early presenting symptom of the acute abdomen (e.g., appendicitis, cholecystitis, perforated peptic ulcer) or other abdominal or pelvic pathology (e.g., renal calculus) in persons with SCI, especially in those with injuries above the seventh thoracic (T7) level (148–153). It is very important to be aware of any "red flags" or signs of serious illness (e.g., fever, chills, and worsening autonomic dysreflexia) that would warrant further investigation.

Treatment should focus on decreasing the acute pain, addressing any secondary disabilities that may be caused by pain, and prevention (144). Treatment of overuse syndromes in persons with SCI can be broken down into (a) control of pain and inflammation; (b) rest and activity modification; (c) rehabilitation (e.g., restoration of shoulder complex flexibility, muscle strength and balance, and endurance); (d) evaluation of posture and wheelchair set-up; (e) review of ADL; and (f) education. Many of these treatments will also be appropriate for the treatment of other upper limb pain overuse syndrome involving the elbow, wrist, and hand and carpal tunnel syndrome (CTS) that will be discussed later in the chapter. Guidelines on the management and prevention of upper limb overuse injuries in persons with SCI have been published (Table 16.1) and provide additional information on many of the treatments discussed below (94).

Acute pain may be relieved with pharmacological interventions (e.g., NSAIDs, acetaminophen, muscle relaxants), local anesthetic and corticosteroid injections, and modalities, including ice, superficial heat, transcutaneous electrical nerve stimulation (TENS), and ultrasound (144). The use of anti-inflammatory agents like NSAIDs for chronic tendon

WHEELCHAIR USERS SHOULDER PAIN INDEX

Place an "**X**" on the scale to estimate your level of pain with the following activities. Check box at right if the activity was not performed **in the past week.**

Based on your experiences in the past week, how much shoulder pain do you experience when:

				not performed
1. transferring from a bed to a wheelchair?	No Pain [ ]	________	Worst Pain Ever Experienced	[ ]
2. transferring from a wheelchair to a car?	No Pain [ ]	________	Worst Pain Ever Experienced	[ ]
3. transferring from a wheelchair to the tub or shower?	No Pain [ ]	________	Worst Pain Ever Experienced	[ ]
4. loading your wheelchair into a car?	No Pain [ ]	________	Worst Pain Ever Experienced	[ ]
5. pushing your chair for 10 minutes or more?	No Pain [ ]	________	Worst Pain Ever Experienced	[ ]
6. pushing up ramps or inclines outdoors?	No Pain [ ]	________	Worst Pain Ever Experienced	[ ]
7. lifting objects down from an overhead shelf?	No Pain [ ]	________	Worst Pain Ever Experienced	[ ]
8. putting on pants?	No Pain [ ]	________	Worst Pain Ever Experienced	[ ]
9. putting on a t-shirt or pullover?	No Pain [ ]	________	Worst Pain Ever Experienced	[ ]
10. putting on a button down shirt?	No Pain [ ]	________	Worst Pain Ever Experienced	[ ]
11. washing your back?	No Pain [ ]	________	Worst Pain Ever Experienced	[ ]
12. usual daily activities at work or school?	No Pain [ ]	________	Worst Pain Ever Experienced	[ ]
13. driving?	No Pain [ ]	________	Worst Pain Ever Experienced	[ ]
14. performing household chores?	No Pain [ ]	________	Worst Pain Ever Experienced	[ ]
15. sleeping?	No Pain [ ]	________	Worst Pain Ever Experienced	[ ]

FIGURE 16.2 The Wheelchair User's Shoulder Pain Index (WUSP) is a 15-item functional measure of shoulder pain intensity in wheelchair users during various ADL. (From Curtis KA, Roach Ke, Applegate EB, et al. Reliability and validity of the Wheelchair User's Shoulder Pain Index (WUSPI). *Paraplegia.* 1995;33:595–601.)

TABLE 16.1

SUMMARY OF CONSORTIUM FOR SPINAL CORD MEDICINE RECOMMENDATIONS ON THE PRESERVATION OF UPPER LIMB FUNCTION FOLLOWING SCI

Initial Assessment of Acute SCI

1. Educate healthcare providers and persons with SCI about the risk of upper limb pain and injury, the means of prevention, treatment options, and the need to maintain fitness.
2. Routinely assess the patient's function, ergonomics, equipment, and level of pain as part of a periodic health review. This review should include evaluation of
   - Transfer and wheelchair propulsion techniques.
   - Equipment (wheelchair and transfer device).
   - Current health status.

Ergonomics

3. Minimize the frequency of repetitive upper limb tasks.
4. Minimize the force required to complete upper limb tasks.
5. Minimize extreme or potentially injurious positions at all joints.
   - Avoid extreme positions of the wrist.
   - Avoid positioning the hand above the shoulder.
   - Avoid potentially injurious or extreme positions at the shoulder, including extreme internal rotation and abduction.

Equipment Selection, Training, and Environmental Adaptations

6. With high-risk patients, evaluate and discuss the pros and cons of changing to a power wheelchair system as a way to prevent repetitive injuries.
7. Provide manual wheelchair users with SCI a high strength, fully customizable manual wheelchair made of the lightest possible material.
8. Adjust the rear axle as far forward as possible without compromising the stability of the user.
9. Position the rear axle so that when the hand is placed at the top dead-center position on the push rim, the angle between the upper arm and the forearm is between 100 and 120.
10. Educate the patient to
    - Use long, smooth strokes that limit high impacts on the pushrim.
    - Allow the hand to drift down naturally, keeping it below the pushrim when not in actual contact with that part of the wheelchair.
11. Promote an appropriate seated posture and stabilization relative to balance and stability needs.
12. For individuals with upper limb paralysis and/or pain, appropriately position the upper limb in bed and in a mobility device. The following principles should be followed:
    - Avoid direct pressure on the shoulder.
    - Provide support to the upper limb at all points.
    - When the individual is supine, position the upper limb in abduction and external rotation on a regular basis.
    - Avoid pulling on the arm when positioning individuals.
    - Remember that preventing pain is a primary goal of positioning.
13. Provide seat elevation or possibly a standing position to individuals with SCI who use power wheelchairs and have arm function.
14. Complete a thorough assessment of the patient's environment, obtain the appropriate equipment, and complete modifications to the home, ideally to American with Disabilities Act (ADA) standards.
15. Instruct individuals with SCI who complete independent transfers to
    - Perform level transfers when possible.
    - Avoid positions of the impingement when possible.
    - Avoid placing either hand on a flat surface when a hand grip is possible during transfers.
    - Vary the technique used and the arm that leads.
16. Consider the use of transfer-assist device for all individuals with SCI. Strongly encourage individuals with arm pain and/or upper limb weakness to use a transfer-assist device.

Exercise

17. Incorporate flexibility exercises into an overall fitness program sufficient to maintain normal glenohumeral motion and pectoral muscle mobility.
18. Incorporate resistance training as an integral part of an adult fitness program. The training should be individualized and progressive, should be of sufficient intensity to enhance strength and muscular endurance, and should provide stimulus to exercise all the major muscle groups to pain-free fatigue.

Management of Acute and Subacute Upper Limb Injuries and Pain

19. In general, manage musculoskeletal upper limb injuries in the SCI population in a similar fashion as in the unimpaired population.
20. Plan and provide intervention for acute pain as early as possible in order to prevent the development of chronic pain.
21. Consider a medical and rehabilitative approach to initial treatment in most instances of nontraumatic upper limb injury among individuals with SCI.
22. Because relative rest of an injured or postsurgical upper limb in SCI is difficult to achieve, strongly consider the following measures:
    - Use of resting night splints in CTS.
    - Home modifications or additional assistance.
    - Admission to a medical facility if pain cannot be relieved or if complete rest is indicated.
23. Place special emphasis on maintaining optimal ROM during rehabilitation from upper limb injury.
24. Consider alternative technique for activities when upper limb pain or injury is present.
25. Emphasize that the patient's return to normal activity after injury or surgery must occur gradually.
26. Closely monitor results of the treatment, and if the pain is not relieved, continued workups and treatment are appropriate.

(continued)

TABLE 16.1

SUMMARY OF CONSORTIUM FOR SPINAL CORD MEDICINE RECOMMENDATIONS ON THE PRESERVATION OF UPPER LIMB FUNCTION FOLLOWING SCI *(continued)*

27. Consider surgery if the patient has chronic neuromusculoskeletal pain and has failed to regain functional capacity with medical and rehabilitative treatment and the likelihood of a successful surgical and functional outcome outweighs the likelihood of an unsuccessful procedure.
28. Operate on upper limb fractures if indicated and when medically feasible.
29. Be aware of and plan for the recovery time needed after surgical procedures.
30. Assess the patient's use of complementary and alternative medicine techniques and beware of possible negative interactions.

Treatment of Chronic Musculoskeletal Pain to Maintain Function

31. Because chronic pain related to musculoskeletal disorders is a complex, multidimensional clinical problem, consider the use of an interdisciplinary approach to assessment and treatment planning. Begin treatment with a careful assessment of the following:
    - Etiology.
    - Pain intensity.
    - Functional capacities.
    - Psychosocial distress associated with the condition.
32. Treat chronic pain and associated symptomatology in an interdisciplinary fashion and incorporate multiple modalities based on the constellation of symptoms revealed by the comprehensive assessment.
33. Monitor outcomes regularly to maximize the likelihood of providing effective treatment.
34. Encourage manual wheelchair users with chronic upper limb pain to seriously consider use of a power wheelchair.
35. Monitor psychosocial adjustment to secondary upper limb injuries and provide treatment if necessary.

From Consortium for Spinal Cord Medicine. Preservation of upper limb function following spinal cord injury: A clinical practice guideline for health-care professionals. *J Spinal Cord Med* 2005;28:433–470.

injuries is the topic of debate since overuse injuries appear to be a degenerative tendinosis rather than an inflammatory tendinitis (154,155). Analgesic properties associated with NSAIDs may account for their effectiveness in many individuals; however, concerns about deleterious side effects and inhibitory effects on collagen repair have led some to question the use of these agents in chronic tendon injuries (156–158). Injection with a local anesthetic and steroids into the subacromial bursa or other appropriate space has been noted by some to be extremely helpful. Like NSAIDs, however, the use of corticosteroids, a potent anti-inflammatory agent, for chronic tendon injuries is the subject of debate (159–161). They may compromise healing potential, weaken tissue, and predispose an individual to further injury (159). As a result, it is recommended steroid injections be given no more than once every 6 weeks, with a maximum of three times per year (162). Furthermore, it is recommended that people who receive local steroid injections avoid vigorous muscle activity of that joint for at least 2 weeks (163); this may not be possible in persons who rely extensively on their upper limbs for mobility.

Physical modalities like heat (especially when combined with stretching) and ultrasound can have analgesic effects and are thought to help reverse tendinosis by stimulating fibrosis and collagen repair (155,164,165). Cold or cryotherapy is typically used for the treatment of acute tendon injuries; however, it may also serve a role during rehabilitation of chronic tendon injuries and tendinosis. Special care, however, should be taken when using heat or cold on insensate areas of skin in individuals with SCI in order to avoid burns. Acupuncture has also been found to be effective for chronic shoulder pain in persons with SCI and is not associated with the adverse effects associated with pharmacological agents (128,129). A systematic review reported that there may be short-term benefit associated with acupuncture with respect to shoulder pain and function; however, little could be concluded due to the small number of clinical and methodologically diverse trials (166). Manual therapy and magnetic therapy have also been reported to be effective for rotator cuff disease and myofascial pain (121,128).

Unlike able-bodied persons, it is difficult for persons with SCI to rest their upper limbs due to their dependency on these structures for mobility and ADL. In this population, a period of relative rest or *activity modification* may be the only realistic option. This may be achieved by altering the way ADL are performed and by using a variety of adaptive equipment. Altering transfer and pressure relief techniques by transferring to a surface at the same height and alternating transfer directions, respectively, may be helpful (94,167). Using a sliding board to assist with transfers or leaning farther forward with the chest toward the thighs during transfers will shift some of the body weight off of the buttocks and may be less stressful on the shoulders. Raised ischial pressure reliefs may also contribute to or aggravate upper limb pain in persons with SCI (90,100,168). Switching to a power wheelchair, either temporary or long-term, may be an effective conservative treatment for shoulder pain, although this may require additional home or vehicular modifications and may be met with resistance by active manual chair users (102,169). Power-assist wheels that replace the standard wheels of the user's manual wheelchair (Quickie XTender, e-motion M15, Alber Invacare) or manual assist wheelchairs (Tailwind, NEXT Mobility) are another option, offering an alternative between manual wheelchair mobility and electric-powered wheelchair driving (170). Use of these wheels reduces stroke frequency, energy demands, and perceived exertion compared with manual wheelchair propulsion, while increasing distance propelled and improving functional capabilities during certain ADL such as propelling up ramps, over uneven surfaces, and over thick carpets (170–173).

Once pain has subsided, functional rehabilitation should be initiated to restore shoulder complex flexibility, muscle strength and balance, and endurance. Inflexibility of the anterior shoulder muscles is associated with shoulder pain in persons with SCI (126,174,175). Therefore, one of the goals of rehabilitation is to restore full, painless ROM. Pendulum exercises can be used to initiate gentle stretching and can be followed by the "open book" stretch to stretch tight coracoid-based muscles (Fig. 16.3). Passive forward flexion, abduction, extension, internal rotation, and external rotation exercises using a doorway or while lying prone on a bed or therapy mat can also be performed. During stretching, patients should avoid impingement positioning (greater than 70 degrees elevation) until pain begins to improve. Moist heat or ultrasound applied to the shoulder may assist in warming up the muscles prior to stretching and ice may help diminish any inflammation after stretching.

Shoulder strengthening exercises in persons with SCI should consist of a balanced program with strengthening of the posterior musculature and should emphasize four main areas: (a) the scapular stabilizers (trapezius and serratus anterior); (b) the rotator cuff muscles (supraspinatus, infraspinatus, teres minor, and subscapularis); (c) the shoulder adductors; and finally, (d) the primary humeral head movers (deltoid, pectoralis major, and latissimus dorsi) (119,176,177).

Successful strengthening of the rotator cuff muscles requires adequate scapular stabilization; therefore, scapular rehabilitation exercises should precede rotator cuff strengthening

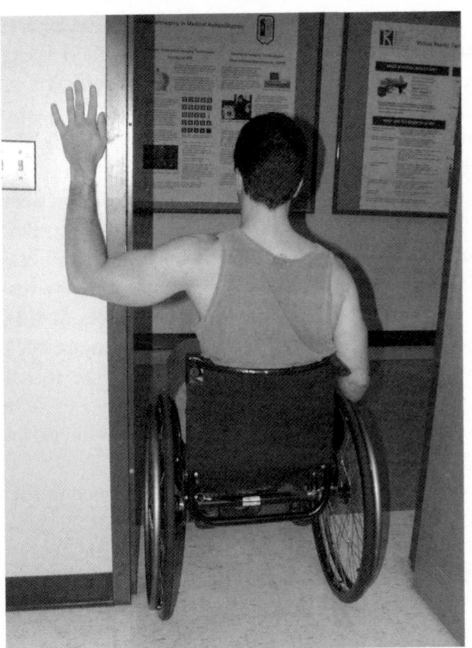

B

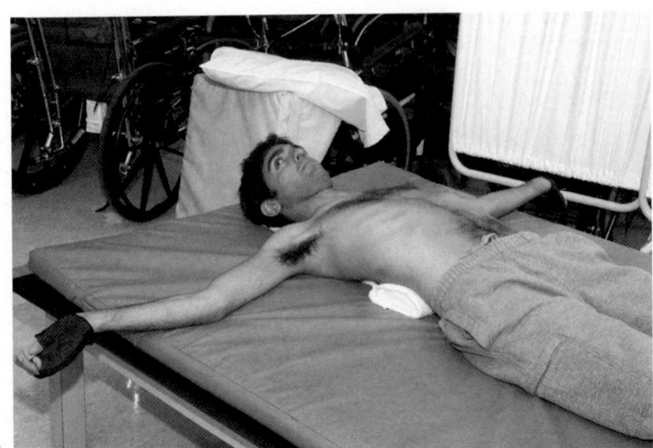

A

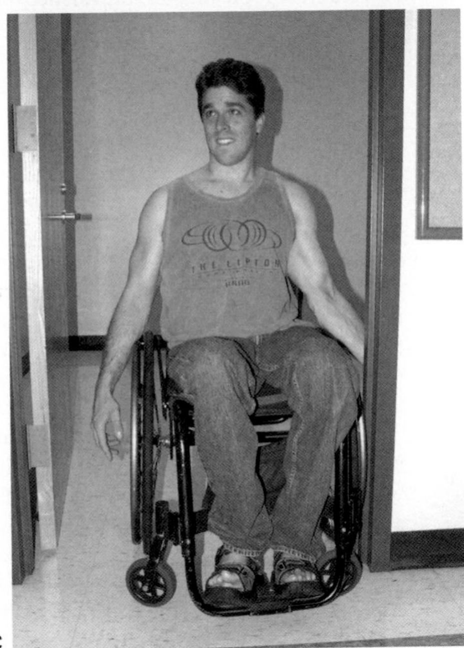

C

FIGURE 16.3 Shoulder stretching exercises include "open book" stretch (**A**) and unilateral corner stretch for pectoralis minor (**B**) and short head of the biceps (**C**).

exercises (119,176). The goal is to restore control of the scapula so that it maintains a position of posterior tilt and external rotation (i.e., retraction). Inferior glide, low row, lawnmower, and robbery exercises are all effective in activating the upper trapezius, lower trapezius, and serratus anterior muscles and do not place the humerus in potential impingement positions of active forward elevation or shoulder abduction (178). These exercises are effective in activating key scapular muscles in task-specific patterns at moderate levels of intensity and can be adopted for use in persons in wheelchairs (Fig. 16.4). Depending on the degree of disability and pain, exercises can begin with simple isometric exercises and then progress to more strenuous open-chain activities using Theraband or weights. Push-up plus exercises are also effective in strengthening the serratus anterior (179) and can be adapted for use in persons with SCI (Fig. 16.5). "Scapular clock exercises" are closed-chain activities in which the individual performs scapular elevation, depression, retraction, and protraction exercises while the arm is abducted 90 degrees and the hand is stabilized against a wall (Fig. 16.6). These activities reproduce the normal physiologic patterns of co-contractions of the scapular stabilizing muscles and the rotator cuff muscles (176). Backwards wheeling also provides another method of strengthening the scapular retractors, although it may not be as effective as the other in activating scapular retractors (180). Overhead exercises like pull-downs should initially be avoided in persons with shoulder pain, unless they can be performed with the arms in neutral rotation and in less than 90 degrees flexion to avoid impingement positioning. Activity-specific exercises like the rickshaw and dips simulate everyday ADL like transfers and press-up weight shifts; however, these exercises should be avoided until adequate strengthening of the humeral head depressors has been achieved.

Rotator cuff muscle strengthening can begin once the scapula is stabilized. Rotator cuff rehabilitation must be graded in intensity of activation and position of activation so as not to place undue strain on the cuff and to avoid injury. Exercises that involve minimal deltoid activity are often desired in order to minimize the amount of superior humeral head migration, thus reducing the chance of subacromial impingement (181,182). Exercises performed in the scapular plane or at 0 degrees abduction show less middle and posterior deltoid activity than those at 90 degrees. The "full can" exercise (i.e., elevation in the scapular plane with glenohumeral external rotation) is the safest and most effective exercise to strengthen the supraspinatus muscle (Fig. 16.7A) (182–184). External rotation with towel roll and external rotation in the scapular plane at 45 degrees of abduction and 30 degrees of horizontal adduction are both effective exercises to strengthen the infraspinatus and teres minor muscles (Fig. 16.7B,C) (185). Internal rotation exercises at 0 degrees can be used to strengthen the subscapularis muscle; however, this action is assisted by several larger muscles, including the pectoralis major, latissimus dorsi, and teres major (Fig. 16.7D,E) (186). The subscapularis muscle is also strengthened during push-up plus exercises described previously (186).

The shoulder adductors (e.g., sternal pectoralis major and latissimus dorsi) are used to elevate the trunk during transfers and raised weight shifts in persons with SCI as long as the hand and humerus are stabilized (168,187). By originating on the thorax and inserting on the proximal humerus, these muscles transfer body weight directly to the supporting arm without loading the glenohumeral joint, thus protecting the rotator cuff against potential impingement. Strengthening of these muscles is, therefore, a critical component of functional rehabilitation in persons with SCI. Resisted adduction exercises can be used for strengthening of sternal pectoralis major and latissimus dorsi muscles instead of exercise regimens that rely on axial loading (127,187).

Since wheelchair propulsion and other ADL place significant demands on the muscles of the shoulder, functional rehabilitation in individuals with SCI should include endurance training exercises as well. Both tetraplegics and paraplegics can improve their cardiovascular fitness and physical work capacity through aerobic exercise training (e.g., arm cycle, wheelchair ergometry), which are moderate intensity, performed 20 to 60 minutes a day, at least three times a week, for a minimum of 6 to 8 weeks (188). Fitness programs such as circuit resistance training (189–191) that incorporate periods of low-intensity high-paced movements interposed within activities performed at a series of resistance training exercises for the shoulder complex may be even better for persons with SCI than arm crank ergometry alone (192).

Postural control is one of the most important factors in preventing and treating shoulder pain (193). Due to impaired abdominal-thoracic musculature, individuals with lower cervical-level (C5-8) and high thoracic-level (T1-7) injuries often assume a "C"-shaped kyphotic trunk position for stability (169,194). This position, which results in excessive scapular protraction, can lead to overstretching and weakening of the scapular retractors (middle trapezius and rhomboids) (127,175). Thoracic kyphosis or excessive scapular protraction can lead to (a) narrowing of the supraspinatus outlet and subacromial space, increasing the risk for impingement and rotator cuff disease (174,176,195,196); (b) disturbances of the normal length-tension relationship of the rotator cuff muscles that can reduce their ability to control the upward migration of the humeral head (176,180); and (c) excessive strain on the anterior band of the inferior glenohumeral ligament that can compromise its ability to provide anterior shoulder stability (197,198). Thoracic kyphosis and scapular protraction may contribute to the higher prevalence of rotator cuff disease seen in persons with higher level SCI (199). Treatment should include postural correction. A low backrest (meeting the lowest ribs) will allow for scapular movement during wheelchair propulsion (200). However, a high backrest may be necessary to provide adequate trunk stabilization; therefore, it is important to place the trunk support as high as the patient needs to feel stable and comfortable (94). A smaller seat-to-back angle or "dump" (i.e., a positive seat plane [front seat to floor > rear seat to floor by approximately 4 inches over 16-inch depth] and a perpendicular backrest [acute inside angle to seat]) can improve pelvic stabilization but can make transfers more difficult so additional transfer training may be needed in order to master transferring independently out of this configuration (94,200).

Manual wheelchair propulsion is a major factor contributing to shoulder pain and is associated with a vertically oriented force that increases during fast and inclined propulsion, as well as with fatigue (201,202). Repetitive internal rotation of the humerus can further increase the potential for impingement (177,203). Clinical practice guidelines (94) recommend that persons with SCI be provided with the lightest possible wheelchair. For manual wheelchairs, proper set-up is paramount to

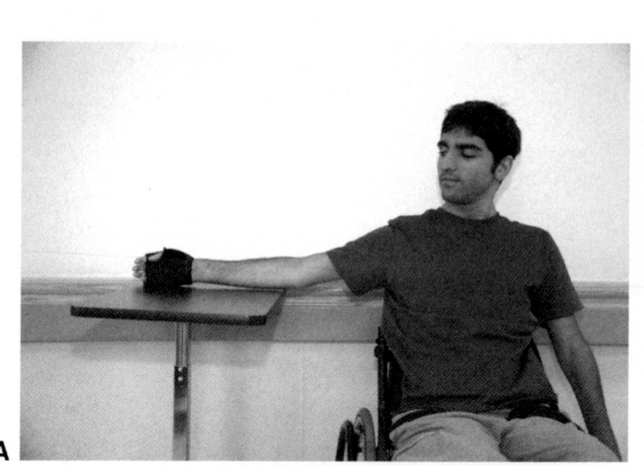
A

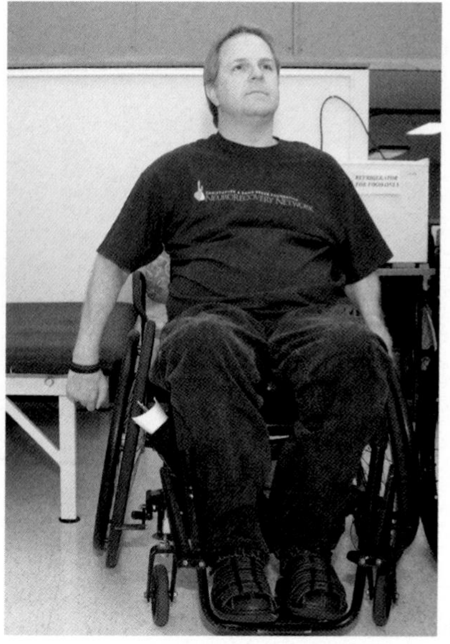
B

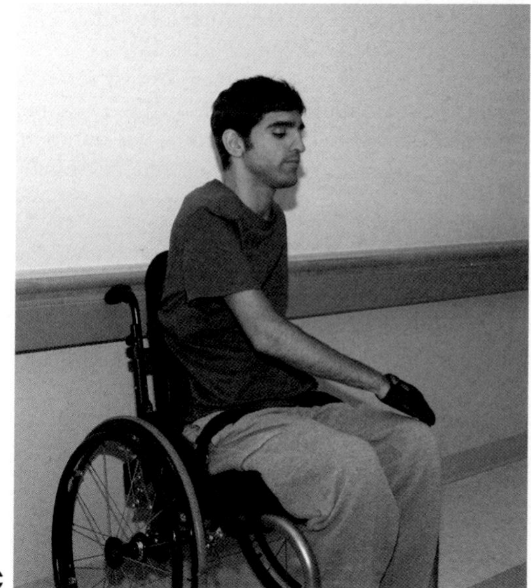
C

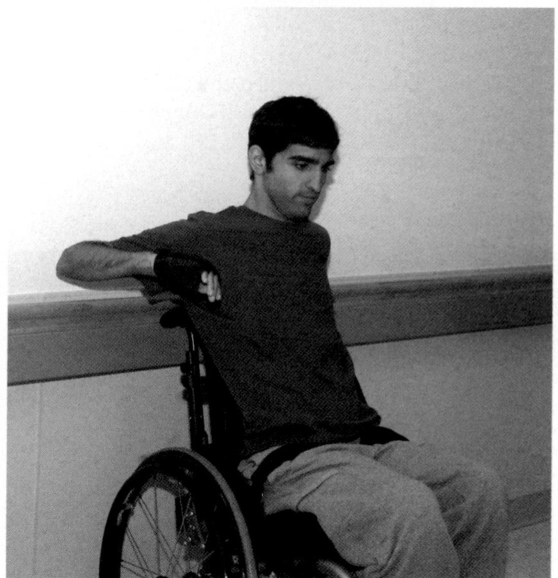
D

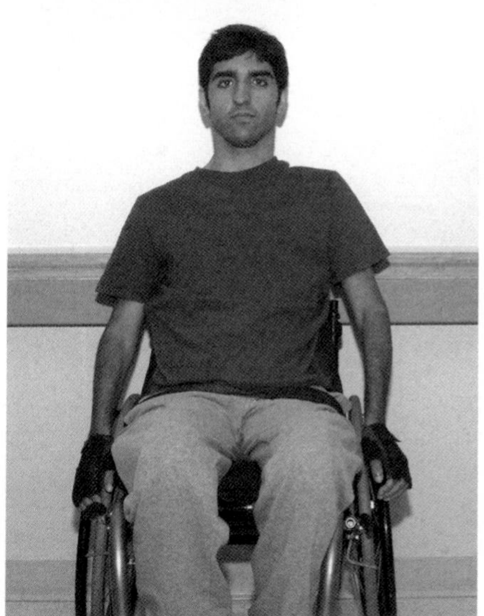
E

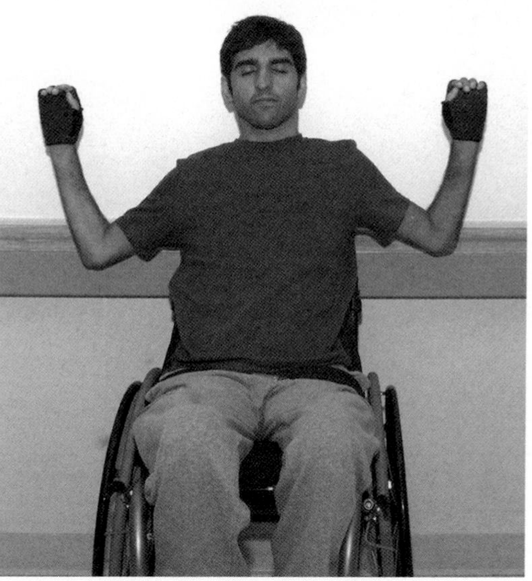
F

FIGURE 16.4 Inferior glide (**A**), low row (**B**), lawnmower (**C,D**), and robbery (**E,F**) exercises are all effective in activating the upper trapezius, lower trapezius, and serratus anterior muscles and do not place the humerus in potential impingement positions of active forward elevation or shoulder abduction.

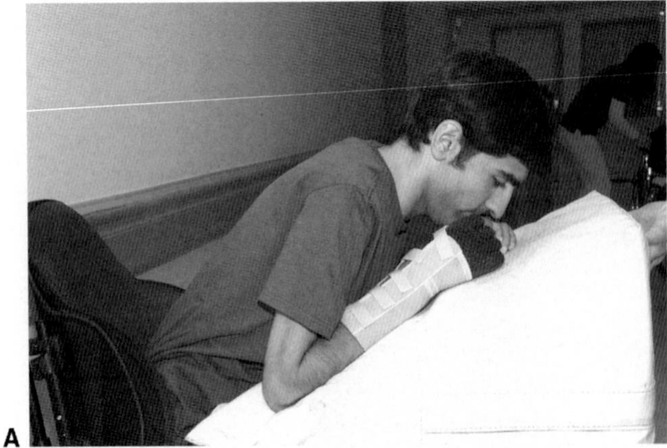

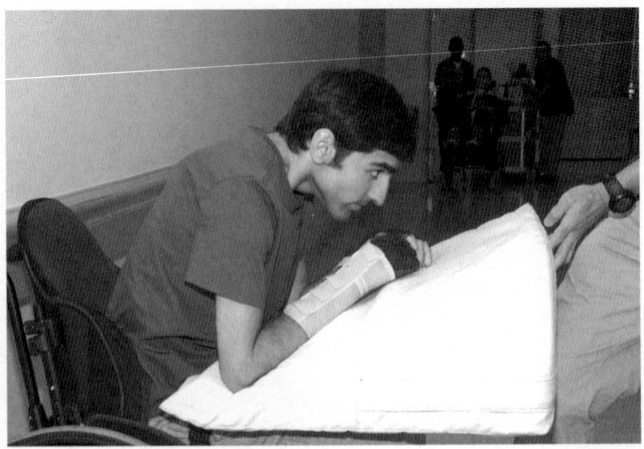

FIGURE 16.5 Push-up plus exercises are also effective in strengthening the serratus anterior and can be adapted for use in persons with SCI. (A) Start and (B) Finish.

ensure fluid motion. Beneficial adjustments include moving the rear axle as far forward as possible without compromising the stability of the user so as to decrease rolling resistance and increase propulsion efficiency (94,204–206) and placing the vertical position of the rear axle so that when the hand is placed at the top dead-center position on the pushrim, the angle between the upper arm and forearm is between 100 and 120 degrees (94,206,207).

Finally, patient education should form the cornerstone of any shoulder injury prevention and rehabilitation program. Early identification of overuse problems may allow intervention before the condition becomes chronic (Table 16.1).

Surgery is often considered a treatment of last resort and is generally reserved for failure of a high-quality program of conservative management. Recommendations for duration of conservative management vary depending on the situation;

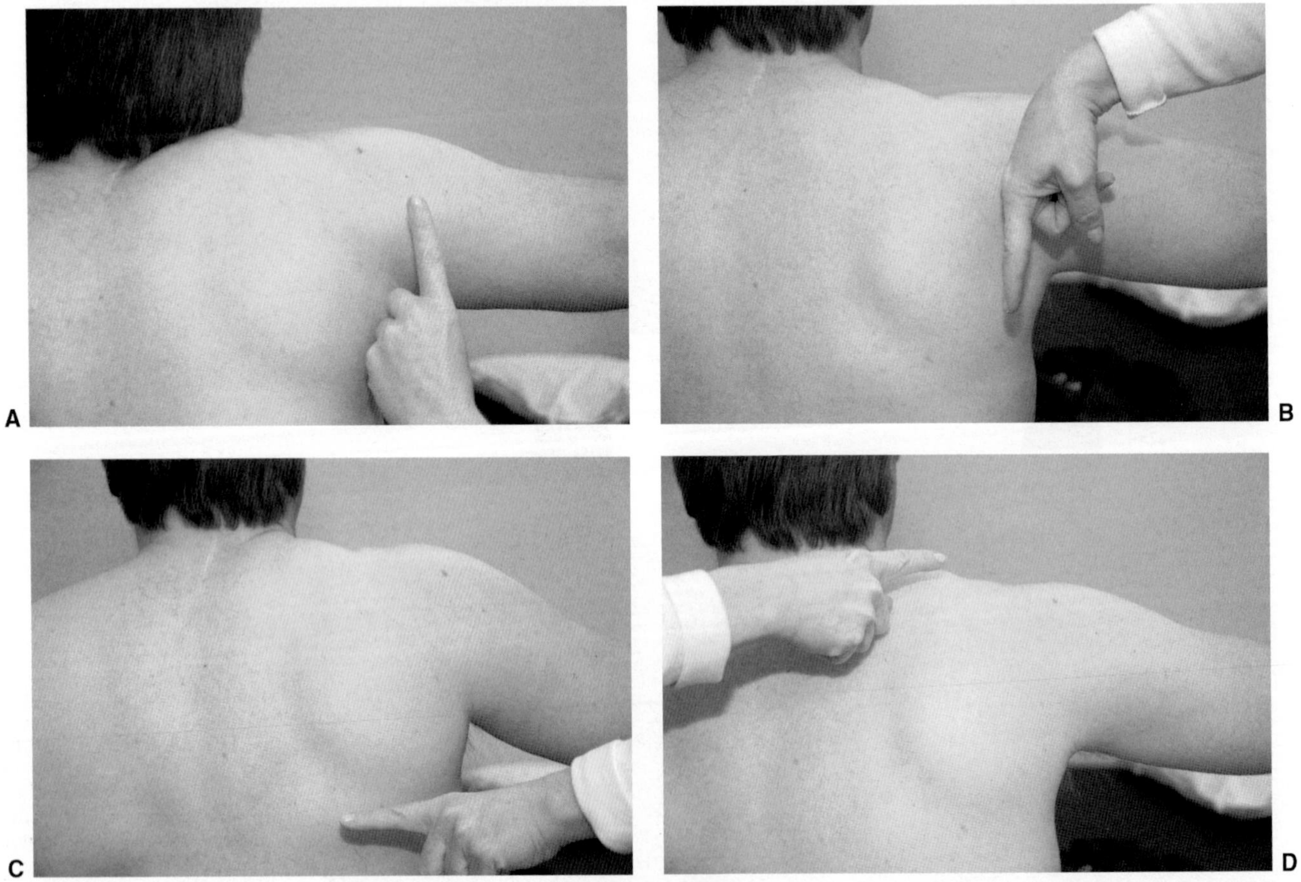

FIGURE 16.6 "Scapular clock" exercises. The hand is stabilized and the scapula is moved in a closed-chain fashion to the points of the clock to simulate elevation to 12:00 (A), depression to 6:00 (B), retraction to 3:00 (C), and protraction to 9:00 (D).

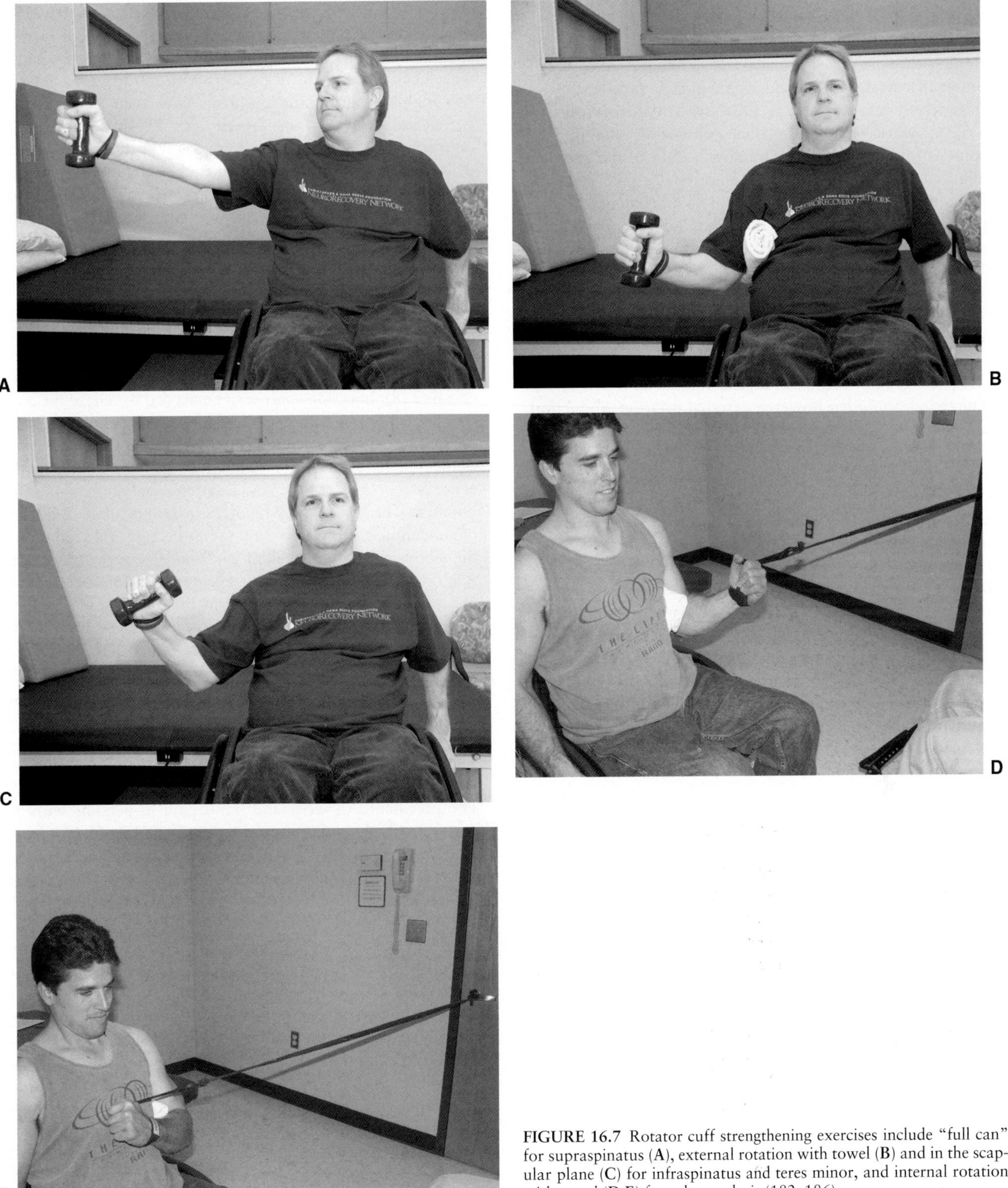

FIGURE 16.7 Rotator cuff strengthening exercises include "full can" for supraspinatus (A), external rotation with towel (B) and in the scapular plane (C) for infraspinatus and teres minor, and internal rotation with towel (D,E) for subscapularis (182–186).

however, a minimum 6-month trial is usually recommended in the able-bodied population (208). Results of studies on rotator cuff surgery outcomes in persons with SCI are limited and conflicting (209–211). However, persons with SCI, especially manual wheelchair users, may be at increased risk of poor outcomes from surgery if manual wheelchair use continues or if other repetitive upper limb tasks are not changed (94). Finally, one must seriously consider the immobilization time frame after surgery and how that may impact an individual's everyday living situation and needs.

Frozen Shoulder

Although thought of as primarily a secondary overuse syndrome, musculoskeletal shoulder pain in SCI may also be seen in less-active persons such as those with high cervical-level injuries or those restricted to their bed during rehabilitation or times of illness (143,212). Immobilization of the shoulder girdle muscles due to upper limb paralysis or pain can limit active joint movement and lead to muscle shortening, shoulder capsule tightness, and frozen shoulder (adhesive capsulitis). Frozen shoulder is characterized by painful and limited active and passive glenohumeral ROM resulting from contracture and loss of compliance of the glenohumeral joint capsule (213). Glenohumeral stiffness may be associated with increased scapulothoracic motion; therefore, it is important to stabilize the scapula in order to determine true glenohumeral motion. There is no general consensus on the amount of ROM loss to define frozen shoulder; however, external rotation, abduction, and internal rotation are the most affected (213,214).

The primary mode of treatment for frozen shoulder is prevention (214). Avoiding prolonged immobilization of the shoulder in newly injured persons or when shoulder pain develops is important. The overall goal of treatment is to relieve pain and restore motion and function in those with SCI who have preserved upper limb movement. Analgesic medications like NSAIDs may be used to alleviate pain. Corticosteroid and analgesic injections may also alleviate pain and inflammation in the early stages and along with stretching may increase ROM. Manipulation under anesthesia and arthroscopic capsular release may be performed in able-bodied persons who have not responded to at least 4 to 6 months of conservative treatment; however, their use in persons with SCI has not been described and is probably not necessary unless associated with severe functional limitations.

Elbow Pain

Upper limb overuse can also lead to elbow pain in persons with SCI, with a reported prevalence of 32% (215). The most common musculoskeletal conditions of the elbow seen in persons with SCI are lateral and medial epicondylitis due to inflammation and chronic degeneration of the extensor and flexor tendons where they attach to the lateral and medial epicondyles of the elbow, respectively, and olecranon bursitis, although the exact prevalence of each condition is not known (216).

Lateral epicondylitis (extensor tendinosis) typically presents with pain over the extensor carpi radialis brevis (ECRB) and weakness of the wrist extensors. In persons with SCI, lateral epicondylitis can arise from excessive pushrim grip forces and poor propulsion technique (217). The pain is often described as a burning pain and may be noted to radiate down the forearm. Physical examination should reveal tenderness over the origin of the ECRB or extensor digitorum communis (EDC), 1 to 2 cm distal to the lateral epicondyle. If the point of maximum tenderness is distal to the level of the radial head, then posterior interosseous nerve entrapment (radial tunnel syndrome; described later) should be suspected. Provocative tests are aimed at reproducing symptoms by loading the injured musculotendinous units.

Medial epicondylitis (flexor tendinosis) typically presents with pain over the flexor-pronator mass. This tends to develop because of excessive flexor-pronator muscle group activity or repeated wrist hyperextension and upper limb axial loading, such as may occur during adduction of the pushrim during wheelchair propulsion in persons with tetraplegia since they are unable to grasp the pushrims with their hands, during wheelchair transfers, or crutch use. Physical examination reveals point tenderness 1 to 2 cm distal to the medial epicondyle, on the lateral side of the flexor-pronator muscle mass. Provocative tests are aimed at reproducing symptoms during resisted flexion and pronation. In contradistinction to lateral epicondylitis, medial epicondylitis causes greater pain with the elbow flexed.

Treatment of lateral and medial epicondylitis includes local ice, heat, and electrical stimulation to promote healing during the acute phase. Avoidance of ADL that increase pain may aid in decreasing the pain associated with the injury. Maintenance of flexibility and wearing a counterforce brace may also be beneficial (218). Injections may also be needed to relieve the pain.

Olecranon bursitis is an inflammatory condition of the bursa overlying the olecranon process at the proximal aspect of the ulna (218). Bursal inflammation may be caused by either acute or repetitive trauma and less commonly infection (septic bursitis). The history may be of an insidious onset of swelling or sudden if secondary to trauma or infection. Examination of the elbow will reveal swelling and tenderness over the bursa. Aspiration is recommended if an infection or other underlying condition (e.g., rheumatoid arthritis, gout) is suspected. Treatment of olecranon bursitis is nonoperative and involves rest, ice, compression, and elevation, which may be difficult for persons with SCI who are dependent on their upper limbs. Treatment of septic bursitis involves intravenous antibiotics.

Wrist and Hand Pain

The prevalence of wrist and hand pain in persons with SCI may be as high as 48% to 64% (92,102,215). *DeQuervain's tenosynovitis* involving the first dorsal compartment of the wrist (containing the abductor pollicis longus and extensor pollicis brevis) may be seen in repetitive wrist motions associated with gripping of the wheelchair pushrim (217). A positive Finkelstein test is highly suggestive of this condition. Pain can also be seen in *scapholunate dissociation instability* arising from a fall on an outstretched hand with impact to the thenar eminence and the wrist positioned in ulnar deviation with intercarpal supination (217). Diagnosis is often delayed until several months after the injury. The differential diagnosis includes *scaphoid fracture*, which may lead to considerable secondary disability in the wheelchair user. Persons with SCI may also be at risk for *carpal instability* due to excessive wrist trauma, with a prevalence of 6% and 18% in those with SCI for more than 20 years (217,219). Persons with carpal instability report daily pain in the wrist or hand on extreme wrist flexion or wrist extension. Physical examination usually reveals substantially limited wrist flexion with preserved wrist extension, point tenderness over the wrist, instability of the scaphoid, and mid-carpal instability. Treatment principles include those previously discussed above, including treatment of pain, avoiding immobilization if possible, re-establishing normal ROM and strength, optimizing posture and set-up, minimizing mechanical loads, correcting poor techniques, and optimizing equipment (216). Treatment for chronic carpal instability is surgical reconstruction with mid-carpal arthrodesis and immobilization that may be met with resistance in upper limb–dependent persons with SCI who rely on their upper limbs for ADL (219).

Kienböck disease is a rare cause of dorsal wrist pain in persons with SCI and is caused by loss of blood supply to the lunate due to trauma (96). Patients present with dorsal wrist pain. Examination may reveal tenderness directly over the lunate bone. Diagnosis may be made by standard x-ray, although the lunate bone may appear normal during early stages. Treatment at early stages includes analgesics, NSAIDs, a protective wrist splint at neutral position at night, and, if possible, temporary cessation of wheelchair propulsion and transfers (96). For more advanced stages, surgery is usually considered to try to reduce the load on the lunate bone.

Lower Limb Overuse Syndromes

Persons with incomplete or lower level injuries who are able to ambulate (even short distances) may be at risk for overuse-related lower limb injuries. Increased susceptibility to fracture due to bone demineralization below the level of injury is a well-known complication associated with SCI; however, little is known about the risks of weight-bearing activities on the joints and muscles of the lower limb. In the absence of normal sensation and joint protecting reflexes, the normal range of lower limb joints is exceeded and articular and periarticular tissues are subjected to mechanical trauma, which may lead to severe joint degeneration and neuropathic arthropathy (a Charcot joint) (220,221). The neuropathic joint presents as a spectrum of radiographic changes, from excessive bone formation to extensive bone resorption (221). We are unaware of anything published to date that suggests that electrical stimulation or treadmill training leads to bone or joint deterioration in persons with SCI (222–224). Although risks for knee injury exist, there is not enough information to justify withholding lower limb training or justify specific treatment (224). Thus, periodic physical exam of the joints with appropriate workup of clinically significant findings, especially in those individuals involved in intense and prolonged exercise/treadmill activities, may be necessary in screening for potential problems (223).

Peripheral Nerve Entrapment Syndromes

Peripheral nerve compression syndromes are common in persons with SCI, especially those with paraplegia (92). Wheelchair propulsion, transfers, raised ischial pressure reliefs, and crutch walking increase the risk of peripheral nerve compression and injury. Cervical cord injury may also lead to "double-crush" syndrome in which cord or root impingement proximally disturbs axonal transport and impairs the capacity of the nerve segment distally to resist focal compressive injury, increasing risk that an otherwise subclinical entrapment neuropathy may become symptomatic (225,226).

Median nerve entrapment at the wrist (Carpal Tunnel Syndrome) and ulnar nerve entrapment at the elbow (cubital tunnel syndrome) are the most common peripheral nerve compression injuries in persons with SCI; however, more proximal nerve entrapments can occur. Compression of the median nerve may also occur at the elbow and can present in one of two forms: pronator syndrome and anterior interosseous nerve syndrome (AINS). Diagnosis, especially in persons with low cervical or high thoracic SCI, poses a unique challenge to clinicians as the sensory and/or motor symptoms associated with these conditions often overlap with each other (e.g., syringomyelia, cervical radiculopathy, brachial plexus injuries, and thoracic outlet syndrome).

Carpal Tunnel Syndrome

Carpal Tunnel Syndrome (CTS) is the most common overuse neuropathy observed in persons with SCI, with a reported prevalence between 40% and 66% based on clinical criteria (92,106,227–231) that may be even higher based on electrodiagnostic criteria (231–233). The prevalence of CTS increases with time from injury, reaching 86% in those injured 20 years or more (92,106,227). CTS is most commonly reported in persons with paraplegia (92).

In persons with SCI, CTS is believed to be caused by a combination of ischemia resulting from repetitive increases in canal tunnel pressures during wrist extension activities such as transfers, weight shifts, and wheelchair propulsion and repetitive trauma to the volar aspect of the extended wrist ("repetitive contact neuropathy") during wheelchair propulsion (92,228,234). Pressure elevation in the carpal tunnel may be even further accentuated by finger flexion when gripping the pushrim and by the combined effects of both wrist extension and externally applied pressure to the distal carpal tunnel during wheelchair propulsion (234). Repeated stress loading of the wrist may alter the configuration and volume characteristics of the carpal canal (234).

Symptoms of CTS include dull, aching discomfort in the hand, forearm, or upper arm; paresthesias of the hand; weakness or clumsiness of the hand; provocation of symptoms during sleep ("night pain"); provocation of symptoms during repetitive hand or wrist activities; and lessening of symptoms by changing hand posture or shaking the wrist (235). On examination, inspection may reveal thenar atrophy in advanced cases. Sensory testing may reveal impaired two-point discrimination (less than 5 mm) in the median nerve distribution; however, this might not be apparent until later in the natural history of the condition. The Semmes-Weinstein monofilament test and the 256-cycle/second vibratory (tuning fork) test have both been found to be more sensitive indications of nerve compression than two-point discrimination (236). Strength testing of the thumb may identify weakness to abduction. Symptoms may be elicited by tapping or direct pressure over the median nerve at the wrist (Tinel's sign or carpal compression test, respectively) or with forced flexion (Phalen's sign) or extension (reverse Phalen's). These tests are highly suggestive for CTS if they are positive; however, they do not rule out the problem if they are negative (235). Electrodiagnostic tests may be more conclusive in diagnosing CTS and can help define the severity (237). Findings include prolongation of median nerve distal motor latency and slowing of sensory conduction across the wrist. Distal sensory latency may be a more sensitive indicator than distal motor latency, and prolongation of the duration of sensory nerve action potential may be seen even before the sensory distal latency is prolonged (238). Although electrodiagnostic findings by themselves and in the absence of clinical symptoms are not diagnostic for CTS (239), some have advocated early testing of median (and ulnar) nerve function within the first 5 years after SCI, even in asymptomatic individuals, with periodic reevaluations as the situation dictates (227).

Treatment for CTS in persons with SCI is initially conservative and includes, if possible, avoidance of activities that cause pain, use of padded gloves when pushing a wheelchair, use of a resting night splint, analgesic medications, NSAIDs, and the judicious use of steroid injections into the carpal canal (232). As with the other upper limb overuse syndromes described previously, functional training to correct poor techniques and optimization of equipment and environment are necessary. The use of ergonomic pushrims may also reduce hand and wrist pain (240,241). Hand and wrist protection in the form of a splint or glove per splint combination can reduce hyperextension of the wrist without interfering with wheelchair propulsion (242). If relief is not obtained, surgical release may be required; however, the postoperative recovery time must be weighed against the long-term benefits of the procedure.

Pronator Syndrome and Anterior Interosseous Nerve Syndrome

Pronator syndrome is a compression neuropathy caused by median nerve entrapment in the proximal forearm. It may present with symptoms of numbness or paresthesia involving the thumb, index, middle, and radial half of the ring fingers that can easily be confused with CTS, which is much more common and presents with similar sensory symptoms (243). Grip-intensive activities and repetitive and forceful pronation and supination have been indicated as possible causes of pronator syndrome (244).

Findings on physical exam include tenderness or firmness of the pronator teres muscle, a positive Tinel's sign on percussion of the proximal muscle mass, and marked increase in paresthesias in the affected digits after mild compression of the proximal muscle mass of the pronator teres for 30 seconds or less ("pronator compression test") (243,245). There may be weakness in the proximal median nerve innervated muscles (flexor pollicis longus and flexor digitorum profundus), in addition to the abductor pollicis brevis muscle (246). Unlike CTS, there should be an absence of any night pain in pronator syndrome and the Phalen's sign and the reverse Phalen's sign should be negative. Another finding that distinguishes pronator syndrome from CTS is decreased sensation in the palm over the thenar eminence since this area is innervated by the palmar cutaneous nerve, which branches from the median nerve proximal to the carpal tunnel.

Electrodiagnostic studies in pronator syndrome are frequently normal. They are useful in ruling out a concurrent case of CTS ("double-crush" syndrome) or other conditions (244,247).

Anterior interosseous nerve syndrome (AINS) is also caused by median nerve entrapment in the proximal forearm. The anterior interosseous nerve can be compressed at the fibrous arch of the flexor digitorum superficialis and the pronator teres. AINS presents purely as a motor palsy. Patients often complain of weakness of pinch that can affect activities such as writing and picking up small objects. There may be a history of spontaneous forearm pain that only lasted a few hours followed by progressive weakness of the hand. Repetitive elbow flexion and forearm pronation have been proposed as dynamic causes of compression of the anterior interosseous nerve in the proximal forearm (248). Physical exam findings include inability to flex the terminal phalanges of the thumb and forefinger. This can be tested by asking the patient to make the "OK sign" by firmly opposing the tip of the thumb and index finger. A person with anterior interosseous nerve palsy will compensate with a key or lateral pinch with extension of the distal interphalangeal joint of the index finger and hyperextension of the interphalangeal joint of the thumb. There will also be weakness of the pronator quadratus muscle, but this must be tested with the elbow fully flexed to minimize the action of the pronator teres (238). Electromyography will reveal abnormalities in the flexor pollicis longus, the radial portion of the flexor digitorum profundus, and the pronator quadratus. The flexor pollicis may occasionally receive a branch directly from the main trunk of the median nerve and may appear normal; however, the pronator quadratus is always supplied by the anterior interosseous nerve and should be abnormal (238).

Treatment of pronator syndrome or AINS includes, if possible, the avoidance of activities that involves repetitive flexion, forearm pronation, or forceful gripping. Changing wheelchair propulsion technique to avoid excessive pronation may be helpful (249). Oral NSAIDs may be helpful (248). Operative decompression may be indicated in those who do not respond to conservative management. As with other surgical procedures in this population, the postoperative recovery time must be weighed against the long-term benefits of the procedure.

Ulnar Nerve Compression Syndromes

Ulnar neuropathy is the second most common upper limb neuropathy observed in persons with SCI, with prevalence between 19% and 45% (227,229–231,250). Ulnar nerve compression in persons with SCI can occur at the elbow (cubital tunnel syndrome) (217,227,230,250–252) or at the wrist (ulnar tunnel syndrome, "Guyon's canal") (217,229–231,251,252). These can be caused by repetitive elbow flexion and contraction of the flexor carpi ulnaris muscle as occurs during wheelchair propulsion, direct pressure on the forearm as occurs in persons who rest their elbows on the armrest of their wheelchair or their vehicle while driving, or prolonged elbow flexion as occurs in patients who are confined to bed for extended periods of time (231,250,251,253).

Cubital Tunnel Syndrome usually presents as numbness in the little and ring finger and can vary in severity depending on the degree and duration of nerve compression. Motor symptoms usually occur later than sensory symptoms and, therefore, may be subtle with the patient complaining of clumsiness or early fatigue in the hand. Weakness more commonly affects the intrinsic muscles of the hand than the extrinsic muscles in the forearm as the motor fascicles to intrinsic muscles, as well as the sensory fascicles, are situated superficial in the ulnar nerve at the elbow relative to the motor fascicles to the extrinsic muscles, and are more vulnerable to compression (253). Physical examination findings include decreased sensation on both sides of the little finger and the medial half of the ring finger. A sensory deficit over the dorsoulnar aspect of the hand and dorsum of the little finger aids in differentiating an ulnar neuropathy at the elbow from one at the wrist. Dorsal sensibility remains intact in ulnar nerve compression at the wrist (ulnar tunnel syndrome) because that area is innervated by the dorsal cutaneous branch of the ulnar nerve that comes off proximal to Guyon's canal (253). Other physical examination findings include a positive Tinel's sign over the cubital tunnel or medial side of the humerus, clawing of the ring and little finger ("ulnar claw"), a positive Froment's sign (flexion of the interphalangeal joint of the thumb while pulling on a paper), or a positive Wartenberg sign (little finger abduction). More severe cases may involve increased two-point discrimination (less than 5 mm) over the little finger digit (139). The elbow flexion test, which involves maintaining the elbow in full flexion with the wrist in full extension for 1 minute, may be useful in reproducing symptoms (253). Electrodiagnostic studies demonstrating a significant loss of conduction velocity across the elbow can help to localize the lesion, but may be misleading as false negatives are not uncommon (253,254).

Treatment includes educating the patient to avoid putting pressure on the medial aspects of their elbows and to avoid keeping their elbows flexed for prolonged periods of time. Ice and NSAIDs may also be used, but immobilization is usually more effective. Local steroid injections around the nerve should be avoided. If conservative treatment is not successful or weakness develops, then surgery may be indicated (253).

Ulnar Tunnel Syndrome occurs when the ulnar nerve is compressed at the wrist during its path through the ulnar tunnel ("Guyon's canal"). It may be caused by repetitive trauma or forces to the hypothenar area of the palm of the hand that can occur during wheelchair propulsion or crutch walking or from a fracture of the hamate or pisiform (217,251,255). Clinical symptoms overlap with those of ulnar nerve injury at the elbow, but can be purely sensory, purely motor, or both depending on the site of compression (253,255). Sensory findings include numbness and/or paresthesias of the little finger and the medial half of the ring finger that is confined to the volar surface of the digits as the dorsal surface is innervated by the dorsal cutaneous branch of the ulnar nerve that comes off the main branch proximal to Guyon's canal. There may be a positive Tinel's sign over Guyon's canal. Motor findings include weakness of the interossei muscles, which may result in a clawing of the ring and little finger ("ulnar claw"), and the adductor pollicis muscle, which compromises pinch. There may be a positive Froment's sign (flexion of the interphalangeal joint of the thumb while pulling on a paper) or a positive Wartenberg sign (little finger abduction) due to unopposed extensor digiti minimi action (139,253,254). Treatment involves changing activities to avoid pressure on the palm in the hypothenar and hook of the hamate areas of the palm. NSAIDs may be prescribed and rest and avoidance of activities may be required. Failure of conservative therapy is an indication for surgical decompression of the nerve at Guyon's canal.

Radial Nerve Compression Syndromes

Although less common than median nerve or ulnar nerve compression syndromes, radial nerve compression syndromes may also be seen in persons with SCI (96,217,228,256). The radial nerve is susceptible to compressive neuropathy at three levels, above the elbow, at the elbow, and at the wrist. High radial nerve compression above the elbow may result from crutch use and the well-known "Saturday night palsy"; however, it is probably very rare in persons with SCI.

Compression of the radial nerve at the elbow can present in one of two forms: *radial tunnel syndrome* or *posterior interosseous nerve syndrome* (PINS). Patients with radial tunnel syndrome complain of lateral elbow pain that can easily be confused with lateral epicondylitis. There may be weakness secondary to pain; however, motor involvement is rare. Patients with PINS, on the other hand, present with a motor palsy (248). Both radial tunnel syndrome and PINS have the same sites of compression: fibrous bands at the radiocapitellar joint; the radial recurrent vessels (vascular leash of Henry); the tendinous origin of the ECRB; the arcade of Frohse (tendinous proximal border of the supinator); or the distal edge of the supinator (248,254,257).

Patients with radial tunnel syndrome will often complain of pain in the proximal dorsal forearm. Symptoms may occur at night and may be aggravated by repetitive pronation-supination, elbow flexion, and maximum wrist flexion-extension. Radial tunnel syndrome should always be considered in cases of resistant lateral epicondylitis (248). Physical exam findings include tenderness over the mobile wad (i.e., extensor muscle mass; ECRB, extensor carpi radialis longus [ECRL], and brachioradialis), about 4 cm distal to the lateral humeral epicondyle, rather than over the lateral epicondyle. Provocative tests include pain with resisted supination with the elbow extended, made worse with wrist flexion, and pain with resisted middle finger extension with the elbow in extension ("middle finger extension test") (254). The sensory exam is unremarkable and there are no motor strength deficits. Electrodiagnostic testing is not especially helpful in this condition (257).

PINS may result from compression secondary to overuse of the extensor musculature or repetitive pronation-supination (254). Patients may present with transient episodes of forearm pain followed by progressive weakness of the digital extensors as well as the extensor carpi ulnaris; however, the muscles of the mobile wad are usually spared. There may be tenderness over the lateral epicondyle or more distally over the arcade of Froshe. Provocative maneuvers include pain with resisted forearm supination from a pronated position along with wrist flexion, as well as pain with resisted extension of the middle finger. A key diagnostic sign of PINS is if the wrist dorsiflexes radially, there is an indication of an intact ECRL but an impaired extensor carpi ulnaris (217). In differentiating between a radial and an ulnar nerve injury, the partial radial nerve injury results in "pseudo claw hand" with inability to extend the fourth and fifth digits, but the metacarpophalangeal joints do not hyperextend as in a true ulnar nerve injury (217).

Treatment of radial tunnel syndrome and PINS includes avoidance of activities, NSAIDs, and splinting of the elbow in 90 degrees of flexion and supination. In radial tunnel syndrome, treatment of lateral epicondylitis should also be instituted because it is often present concomitantly. Use of a Count' R-Force brace commonly used in lateral epicondylitis may exacerbate the symptoms of radial tunnel syndrome. Most cases of radial tunnel syndrome respond well to conservative treatment; however, posterior interosseous nerve release and decompression may be considered if conservative management fails (257). For patients with PINS, surgery should be considered in cases of progressive weakness, late presentation with severe weakness and atrophy, or absence of improvement after four to twelve weeks of conservative treatment (248).

Radial nerve compression may also occur at the wrist in persons with SCI. Persons with C6 tetraplegia may especially be at risk for *distal posterior interosseous nerve syndrome* since they only have wrist extensor muscle activity for joint stability due to paralysis of the wrist flexor muscles (96). Symptoms of distal PINS include pain with repetitive wrist extension. Examination may reveal point tenderness over the fourth extensor compartment and reproduced pain on extreme wrist extension. Diagnosis can be confirmed by relief of symptoms with lidocaine injection to the distal posterior interosseous nerve region, 2 cm proximal to the wrist joint. Rest from transfers and wheelchair propulsion, a protective wrist splint at neutral position at night, and/or anesthetic injections have been reported to be effective for dorsal wrist joint pain (96).

Wartenberg syndrome involves compression of the sensory branch of the radial nerve as it passes under the brachioradialis muscle (139,255). Wartenberg syndrome in persons with SCI may be caused by repetitive wrist extension and wrist joint loading during wheelchair propulsion (96). Symptoms include nocturnal pain along the dorsum of the wrist, thumb, and web space (139). Examination may reveal a Tinel's sign, reproducing symptoms over the nerve as it exits under the brachioradialis muscle (255). Symptoms may be provoked by wrist extension and ulnar deviation. Treatment includes rest, ice, analgesics, and use of a palmar cock-up wrist splint (96,255). Decompression of the fascia between the brachioradialis and the extensor carpi radialis tendons and neurolysis of the nerve followed by use of a soft dressing and early motion has been reported to be effective in non-SCI population who do not respond to conservative therapy (255).

References

1. McKinley WO, Jackson AB, Cardenas DD, et al. Long-term medical complications after traumatic spinal cord injury: a regional model systems analysis. *Arch Phys Med Rehabil* 1999;80:1402–1410.
2. Eser P, Frotzler A, Zehnder Y, et al. Assessment of anthropometric, systemic, and lifestyle factors influencing bone status in the legs of spinal cord injured individuals. *Osteoporos Int* 2005;16:26–34.
3. Frey-Rindova P, de Bruin ED, Stussi E, et al. Bone mineral density in upper and lower extremities during 12 months after spinal cord injury measured by peripheral quantitative computed tomography. *Spinal Cord* 2000;38:26–32.
4. Garland DE. Pathologic fractures and bone mineral density at the knee. *J Spinal Cord Med* 1999;22:335.
5. Garland DE, Adkins RH, Kushwaha V, et al. Risk factors for osteoporosis at the knee in the spinal cord injury population. *J Spinal Cord Med* 2004;27:202–206.
6. Lazo MG, Shirazi P, Sam M, et al. Osteoporosis and risk of fracture in men with spinal cord injury. *Spinal Cord* 2001;39:208–214.
7. Garland DE, Adkins RH, Stewart CA. Fracture threshold and risk factors for osteoporosis and pathological fractures in individuals with spinal cord injury. *Top Spinal Cord Inj Rehabil* 2005;11(1):61–69.
8. Frisbie JH. Fractures after myelopathy: the risk quantified. *J Spinal Cord Med* 1997;20:66–69.
9. Rogers T, Shokes LK, Woodsworth PH. Pathologic extremity fracture care in spinal cord injury. *Top Spinal Cord Inj Rehabil* 2005;11(1):70–78.
10. Bick RL, Haas SK. International consensus recommendations. Summary statement and additional suggested guidelines. European Consensus Conference, November 1991; American College of Chest Physicians consensus statement of 1995. International Consensus Statement, 1997. *Med Clin North Am* 1998;82:613–633.
11. McMaster WC, Stauffer ES. The management of long bone fracture in the spinal cord injured patient. *Clin Orthop Relat Res* 1975:44–52.
12. Ragnarsson KT, Sell GH. Lower extremity fractures after spinal cord injury: a retrospective study. *Arch Phys Med Rehabil* 1981;62:418–423.
13. Freehafer AA. Limb fractures in patients with spinal cord injury. *Arch Phys Med Rehabil* 1995;76:823–827.
14. Freehafer AA, Mast WA. Lower extremity fractures in patients with spinal-cord injury. *J Bone Joint Surg Am* 1965;47:683–694.
15. Eichenholtz SN. Management of long bone fractures in paraplegic patients. *J Bone Joint Surg Am* 1963;45(2):299–310.
16. Baird RA, Kreitenberg A, Eltorai I. External fixation of femoral shaft fractures in spinal cord injury patients. *Paraplegia* 1986;24:183–190.
17. Comarr AE, Hutchinson RH, Bors E. Extremity fractures of patients with spinal cord injuries. *Am J Surg* 1962;103:732–739.
18. Freehafer AA, Hazel CM, Becker CL. Lower extremity fractures in patients with spinal cord injury. *Paraplegia* 1981;19:367–372.
19. Michaelis LS. *Orthopedic Surgery of the Limbs in Paraplegia*. Berlin, Germany: Springer-Verlag, 1964.
20. Nottage WM. A review of long-bone fractures in patients with spinal cord injuries. *Clin Orthop Relat Res* 1981: 65–70.
21. Martinez A, Cuenca J, Herrera A, et al. Late lower extremity fractures in patients with paraplegia. *Injury* 2002;33:583–586.
22. Levine AM, Krebs M, Santos-Mendoza N. External fixation in quadriplegia. *Clin Orthop Relat Res* 1984:169–172.
23. Charcot JM. Sur quelques arthropathies qui paraissant dependre dune lesion due cerveau ou de la moelle epiniere. *Arch Physiol Norm Pathol* 1868;1:161.
24. Slabaugh PB, Smith TK. Neuropathic spine after spinal cord injury. A case report. *J Bone Joint Surg Am* 1978;60:1005–1006.
25. Suda Y, Shioda M, Kohno H, et al. Surgical treatment of Charcot spine. *J Spinal Disord Tech* 2007;20:85–88.
26. Standaert C, Cardenas DD, Anderson P. Charcot spine as a late complication of traumatic spinal cord injury. *Arch Phys Med Rehabil* 1997;78:221–225.
27. Vaccaro AR, Silber JS. Post-traumatic spinal deformity. *Spine* 2001;26:S111–S118.
28. Bolesta M, Bohlman HH. Late sequealae of thoracolumbar fractures and fracture-dislocations: Surgical treatment. In: Frymoyer JW, ed. *The Adult Spine: Principles and Practice*. 2nd ed. Philadelphia, PA: Lippincott-Raven, 1997:1513–1533.
29. Sobel JW, Bohlman HH, Freehafer AA. Charcot's arthropathy of the spine following spinal cord injury. A report of five cases. *J Bone Joint Surg Am* 1985;67:771–776.
30. Brown CW, Jones B, Donaldson DH, et al. Neuropathic (Charcot) arthropathy of the spine after traumatic spinal paraplegia. *Spine* 1992;17:S103–S108.
31. McBride GG, Greenberg D. Treatment of Charcot spinal arthropathy following traumatic paraplegia. *J Spinal Disord* 1991;4:212–220.
32. Glennon TP, Madewell JE, Donovan WH, et al. Neuropathic spinal arthropathy after spinal cord injury. A report of three cases. *Spine* 1992;17:964–971.
33. Bergstrom EM, Short DJ, Frankel HL, et al. The effect of childhood spinal cord injury on skeletal development: a retrospective study. *Spinal Cord* 1999;37:838–846.
34. Dearolf WW III, Betz RR, et al. Scoliosis in pediatric spinal cord-injured patients. *J Pediatr Orthop* 1990;10: 214–218.

35. Betz RR. Unique management needs of pediatric spinal cord injury patients: orthopedic problems in the child with spinal cord injury. *J Spinal Cord Med* 1997;20:14–16.
36. Bursell JP, Little JW, Stiens SA. Electrodiagnosis in spinal cord injured persons with new weakness or sensory loss: central and peripheral etiologies. *Arch Phys Med Rehabil* 1999;80:904–909.
37. Bosch A, Stauffer ES, Nickel VL. Incomplete traumatic quadriplegia. A ten-year review. *JAMA* 1971;216:473–478.
38. Marino RJ, Barros T, Biering-Sorensen F, et al. International standards for neurological classification of spinal cord injury. *J Spinal Cord Med* 2003;26(Suppl 1): S50–S56.
39. Little JW, Stiens SA. Electrodiagnosis in spinal cord injury. *Phys Med Rehabil Clin N Am* 1994;5:571–593.
40. Sett P, Crockard HA. The value of magnetic resonance imaging (MRI) in the follow-up management of spinal injury. *Paraplegia* 1991;29:396–410.
41. Backe HA, Betz RR, Mesgarzadeh M, et al. Post-traumatic spinal cord cysts evaluated by magnetic resonance imaging. *Paraplegia* 1991;29:607–612.
42. Silberstein M, Hennessy O. Cystic cord lesions and neurological deterioration in spinal cord injury: operative considerations based on magnetic resonance imaging. *Paraplegia* 1992;30:661–668.
43. Perrouin-Verbe B, Lenne-Aurier K, Robert R, et al. Post-traumatic syringomyelia and post-traumatic spinal canal stenosis: a direct relationship: review of 75 patients with a spinal cord injury. *Spinal Cord* 1998;36:137–143.
44. Carroll AM, Brackenridge P. Post-traumatic syringomyelia: a review of the cases presenting in a regional spinal injuries unit in the north east of England over a 5-year period. *Spine* 2005;30:1206–1210.
45. Squier MV, Lehr RP. Post-traumatic syringomyelia. *J Neurol Neurosurg Psychiatry* 1994;57:1095–1098.
46. Frisbie JH, Aguilera EJ. Chronic pain after spinal cord injury: an expedient diagnostic approach. *Paraplegia* 1990;28:460–465.
47. Wozniewicz B, Filipowicz K, Swiderska SK, et al. Pathophysiological mechanism of traumatic cavitation of the spinal cord. *Paraplegia* 1983;21:312–317.
48. Edgar R, Quail P. Progressive post-traumatic cystic and non-cystic myelopathy. *Br J Neurosurg* 1994;8:7–22.
49. Umbach I, Heilporn A. Review article: post-spinal cord injury syringomyelia. *Paraplegia* 1991;29:219–221.
50. Yarkony GM, Sheffler LR, Smith J, et al. Early onset posttraumatic cystic myelopathy complicating spinal cord injury. *Arch Phys Med Rehabil* 1994;75:102–105.
51. Biyani A, el Masry WS. Post-traumatic syringomyelia: a review of the literature. *Paraplegia* 1994;32:723–731.
52. Williams B. Pathogenesis of post-traumatic syringomyelia. *Br J Neurosurg* 1992;6:517–520.
53. Cho KH, Iwasaki Y, Imamura H, et al. Experimental model of posttraumatic syringomyelia: the role of adhesive arachnoiditis in syrinx formation. *J Neurosurg* 1994;80:133–139.
54. Williams B, Terry AF, Jones F, et al. Syringomyelia as a sequel to traumatic paraplegia. *Paraplegia* 1981;19: 67–80.
55. Vernon JD, Silver JR, Symon L. Post-traumatic syringomyelia: the results of surgery. *Paraplegia* 1983;21:37–46.
56. Balmaseda MT Jr, Wunder JA, Gordon C, et al. Posttraumatic syringomyelia associated with heavy weightlifting exercises: case report. *Arch Phys Med Rehabil* 1988;69:970–972.
57. Tator CH, Briceno C. Treatment of syringomyelia with a syringosubarachnoid shunt. *Can J Neurol Sci* 1988;15:48–57.
58. Jensen F, Reske-Nielsen E. Post-traumatic syringomyelia. Review of the literature and two new autopsy cases. *Scand J Rehabil Med* 1977;9:35–43.
59. Kruse A, Rasmussen G, Borgesen SE. CSF-dynamics in syringomyelia: intracranial pressure and resistance to outflow. *Br J Neurosurg*. 1987;1:477–484.
60. Hurlbert RJ, Fehlings MG. The Chiari malformations. In: Engler GI, Cole J, Merton WL, eds. *Spinal Cord Diseases: Diagnosis and Treatment*. New York: Mercel Decker, Inc., 1998:65–100.
61. Lyons BM, Brown DJ, Calvert JM, et al. The diagnosis and management of post traumatic syringomyelia. *Paraplegia* 1987;25:340–350.
62. Rossier AB, Foo D, Shillito J, et al. Posttraumatic cervical syringomyelia. Incidence, clinical presentation, electrophysiological studies, syrinx protein and results of conservative and operative treatment. *Brain* 1985;108 (Pt 2):439–461.
63. Lee TT, Alameda GJ, Camilo E, et al. Surgical treatment of post-traumatic myelopathy associated with syringomyelia. *Spine* 2001;26:S119–S127.
64. Asano M, Fujiwara K, Yonenobu K, et al. Post-traumatic syringomyelia. *Spine* 1996;21:1446–1453.
65. Quencer RM, Green BA, Eismont FJ. Posttraumatic spinal cord cysts: clinical features and characterization with metrizamide computed tomography. *Radiology* 1983;146:415–423.
66. Sgouros S, Williams B. Management and outcome of posttraumatic syringomyelia. *J Neurosurg* 1996;85:197–205.
67. Schaller B, Mindermann T, Gratzl O. Treatment of syringomyelia after posttraumatic paraparesis or tetraparesis. *J Spinal Disord* 1999;12:485–488.
68. Batzdorf U, Klekamp J, Johnson JP. A critical appraisal of syrinx cavity shunting procedures. *J Neurosurg* 1998;89:382–388.
69. Park P, Garton HJ, Gala VC, et al. Adjacent segment disease after lumbar or lumbosacral fusion: review of the literature. *Spine* 2004;29:1938–1944.
70. Chen WJ, Lai PL, Niu CC, et al. Surgical treatment of adjacent instability after lumbar spine fusion. *Spine* 2001;26:E519–E524.
71. Phillips FM, Carlson GD, Bohlman HH, et al. Results of surgery for spinal stenosis adjacent to previous lumbar fusion. *J Spinal Disord* 2000;13:432–437.
72. Chow DH, Luk KD, Evans JH, et al. Effects of short anterior lumbar interbody fusion on biomechanics of neighboring unfused segments. *Spine* 1996;21:549–555.
73. Weinhoffer SL, Guyer RD, Herbert M, et al. Intradiscal pressure measurements above an instrumented fusion. A cadaveric study. *Spine* 1995;20:526–531.
74. Wiltse LL, Radecki SE, Biel HM, et al. Comparative study of the incidence and severity of degenerative change in the transition zones after instrumented versus noninstrumented fusions of the lumbar spine. *J Spinal Disord* 1999;12:27–33.

75. Aota Y, Kumano K, Hirabayashi S. Postfusion instability at the adjacent segments after rigid pedicle screw fixation for degenerative lumbar spinal disorders. *J Spinal Disord* 1995;8:464–473.
76. Selby DK, Henderson RJ, Blumenthal S, et al. Anterior lumbar fusion. In: White AH, Rothman RH, Ray CD, eds. *Lumbar spine surgery: techniques and complications.* St. Louis, MO: CV Mosby, 1987:222–236.
77. Keene JS, Lash EG, Kling TF Jr. Undetected posttraumatic instability of "stable" thoracolumbar fractures. *J Orthop Trauma* 1988;2:202–211.
78. Abel R, Gerner HJ, Smit C, et al. Residual deformity of the spinal canal in patients with traumatic paraplegia and secondary changes of the spinal cord. *Spinal Cord* 1999;37:14–19.
79. Lee C, Dorcil J, Radomisli TE. Nonunion of the spine: a review. *Clin Orthop Relat Res* 2004:71–75.
80. Rothman RH, Booth R. Failures of spinal fusion. *Orthop Clin North Am* 1975;6:299–304.
81. Wetzel FT, Hoffman MA, Arcieri RR. Freeze-dried fibular allograft in anterior spinal surgery: cervical and lumbar applications. *Yale J Biol Med* 1993;66:263–275.
82. Brown CW, Orme TJ, Richardson HD. The rate of pseudarthrosis (surgical nonunion) in patients who are smokers and patients who are nonsmokers: a comparison study. *Spine* 1986;11:942–943.
83. Hadley MN, Reddy SV. Smoking and the human vertebral column: a review of the impact of cigarette use on vertebral bone metabolism and spinal fusion. *Neurosurgery* 1997;41:116–124.
84. Burchardt H. The biology of bone graft repair. *Clin Orthop Relat Res* 1983:28–42.
85. Prolo DJ, Rodrigo JJ. Contemporary bone graft physiology and surgery. *Clin Orthop Relat Res* 1985;322–342.
86. Hopper JL, Seeman E. The bone density of female twins discordant for tobacco use. *N Engl J Med* 1994;330:387–392.
87. Haro H, Komori H, Okawa A, et al. Long-term outcomes of surgical treatment for tethered cord syndrome. *J Spinal Disord Tech* 2004;17:16–20.
88. Falci SP, Lammertse DP, Best L, et al. Surgical treatment of posttraumatic cystic and tethered spinal cords. *J Spinal Cord Med* 1999;22:173–181.
89. Nichols PJ, Norman PA, Ennis JR. Wheelchair user's shoulder? Shoulder pain in patients with spinal cord lesions. *Scand J Rehabil Med* 1979;11:29–32.
90. Bayley JC, Cochran TP, Sledge CB. The weight-bearing shoulder. The impingement syndrome in paraplegics. *J Bone Joint Surg Am* 1987;69:676–678.
91. Pentland WE, Twomey LT. The weight-bearing upper extremity in women with long term paraplegia. *Paraplegia* 1991;29:521–530.
92. Sie IH, Waters RL, Adkins RH, et al. Upper extremity pain in the postrehabilitation spinal cord injured patient. *Arch Phys Med Rehabil* 1992;73:44–48.
93. Pentland WE, Twomey LT. Upper limb function in persons with long term paraplegia and implications for independence: Part II. *Paraplegia* 1994;32:219–224.
94. Consortium for Spinal Cord Medicine. Preservation of upper limb function following spinal cord injury: A clinical practice guideline for health-care professionals. *J Spinal Cord Med* 2005;28:433–470.
95. Ohry A, Brooks ME, Steinbach TV, et al. Shoulder complications as a cause of delay in rehabilitation of spinal cord injured patients. (Case reports and review of the literature). *Paraplegia* 1978;16:310–316.
96. Hara Y. Dorsal wrist joint pain in tetraplegic patients during and after rehabilitation. *J Rehabil Med* 2003;35: 57–61.
97. Alm M, Saraste H, Norrbrink C. Shoulder pain in persons with thoracic spinal cord injury: prevalence and characteristics. *J Rehabil Med* 2008;40:277–283.
98. Gerhart KA, Bergstrom E, Charlifue SW, et al. Long-term spinal cord injury: functional changes over time. *Arch Phys Med Rehabil* 1993;74:1030–1034.
99. Curtis KA, Roach KE, Applegate EB, et al. Development of the Wheelchair User's Shoulder Pain Index (WUSPI). *Paraplegia* 1995;33:290–293.
100. Dalyan M, Cardenas DD, Gerard B. Upper extremity pain after spinal cord injury. *Spinal Cord* 1999;37:191–195.
101. Dyson-Hudson TA, Kirshblum SC. Shoulder pain in chronic spinal cord injury, Part I: Epidemiology, etiology, and pathomechanics. *J Spinal Cord Med* 2004;27:4–17.
102. Subbarao JV, Klopfstein J, Turpin R. Prevalence and impact of wrist and shoulder pain in patients with spinal cord injury. *J Spinal Cord Med* 1995;18:9–13.
103. Curtis KA, Drysdale GA, Lanza RD, et al. Shoulder pain in wheelchair users with tetraplegia and paraplegia. *Arch Phys Med Rehabil* 1999;80:453–457.
104. Ballinger DA, Rintala DH, Hart KA. The relation of shoulder pain and range-of-motion problems to functional limitations, disability, and perceived health of men with spinal cord injury: a multifaceted longitudinal study. *Arch Phys Med Rehabil* 2000;81: 1575–1581.
105. Vogel LC, Krajci KA, Anderson CJ. Adults with pediatric-onset spinal cord injury: part 2: musculoskeletal and neurological complications. *J Spinal Cord Med* 2002;25:117–123.
106. Gellman H, Sie I, Waters RL. Late complications of the weight-bearing upper extremity in the paraplegic patient. *Clin Orthop* 1988;233:132–135.
107. Pentland WE, Twomey LT. Upper limb function in persons with long term paraplegia and implications for independence: Part I. *Paraplegia* 1994;32:211–218.
108. Boninger ML, Towers JD, Cooper RA, et al. Shoulder imaging abnormalities in individuals with paraplegia. *J Rehabil Res Dev* 2001;38:401–408.
109. Jensen MP, Hoffman AJ, Cardenas DD. Chronic pain in individuals with spinal cord injury: a survey and longitudinal study. *Spinal Cord* 2005;43:704–712.
110. Noreau L, Proulx P, Gagnon L, et al. Secondary impairments after spinal cord injury: a population-based study. *Am J Phys Med Rehabil* 2000;79:526–535.
111. Silfverskiold J, Waters RL. Shoulder pain and functional disability in spinal cord injury patients. *Clin Orthop* 1991;272:141–145.
112. Lal S. Premature degenerative shoulder changes in spinal cord injury patients. *Spinal Cord* 1998;36: 186–189.
113. Schultz MM, Lee TQ, Nance PW. Musculoskeletal and neuromuscular implications of gender in spinal cord injury. *Top Spinal Cord Inj Rehabil* 2001;7:72–86.

114. Norregaard J, Jacobsen S, Kristensen JH. A narrative review on classification of pain conditions of the upper extremities. *Scand J Rehabil Med* 1999;31:153–164.
115. Soslowsky LJ, Thomopoulos S, Esmail A, et al. Rotator cuff tendinosis in an animal model: role of extrinsic and overuse factors. *Ann Biomed Eng* 2002;30:1057–1063.
116. Escobedo EM, Hunter JC, Hollister MC, et al. MR imaging of rotator cuff tears in individuals with paraplegia. *AJR Am J Roentgenol* 1997;168:919–923.
117. Wolf WB III. Shoulder tendinoses. *Clin Sports Med* 1992;11:871–890.
118. McFarland EG, Selhi HS, Keyurapan E. Clinical evaluation of impingement: what to do and what works. *J Bone Joint Surg Am* 2006;88:432–441.
119. Morrison DS, Greenbaum BS, Einhorn A. Shoulder impingement. *Orthop Clin North Am* 2000;31:285–293.
120. Barr KP. Review of upper and lower extremity musculoskeletal pain problems. *Phys Med Rehabil Clin N Am* 2007;18:747–760, vi–vii.
121. Panagos A, Jensen M, Cardenas DD. Treatment of myofascial shoulder pain in the spinal cord injured population using static magnetic fields: a case series. *J Spinal Cord Med* 2004;27:138–142.
122. Simons DG, Travell JG, Simons LS, et al. Travell & Simons' Myofascial Pain and Dysfunction: *The Trigger Point Manual*. 2nd ed. Baltimore, MD: Lippincott Williams & Wilkins, 1999.
123. Roach NA, Schweitzer ME. Does osteolysis of the distal clavicle occur following spinal cord injury? *Skeletal Radiol* 1997;26:16–19.
124. Barber DB, Gall NG. Osteonecrosis: an overuse injury of the shoulder in paraplegia: case report. *Paraplegia* 1991;29:423–426.
125. Widerström-Noga E, Biering-Sørensen F, Bryce T, et al. The International Spinal Cord Injury Pain Basic Data Set. *Spinal Cord* 2008.
126. Curtis KA, Roach KE, Applegate EB, et al. Reliability and validity of the Wheelchair User's Shoulder Pain Index (WUSPI). *Paraplegia* 1995;33:595–601.
127. Curtis KA, Tyner TM, Zachary L, et al. Effect of a standard exercise protocol on shoulder pain in long-term wheelchair users. *Spinal Cord* 1999;37:421–429.
128. Dyson-Hudson TA, Shiflett SC, Kirshblum SC, et al. Acupuncture and Trager psychophysical integration in the treatment of wheelchair user's shoulder pain in individuals with spinal cord injury. *Arch Phys Med Rehabil* 2001;82:1038–1046.
129. Dyson-Hudson TA, Kadar P, LaFountaine M, et al. Acupuncture for chronic shoulder pain in persons with spinal cord injury: a small-scale clinical trial. *Arch Phys Med Rehabil* 2007;88:1276–1283.
130. Felix ER, Cruz-Almeida Y, Widerstrom-Noga EG. Chronic pain after spinal cord injury: What characteristics make some pains more disturbing than others? *J Rehabil Res Dev* 2007;44:703–716.
131. Bryce TN, Budh CN, Cardenas DD, et al. Pain after spinal cord injury: an evidence-based review for clinical practice and research. Report of the National Institute on Disability and Rehabilitation Research Spinal Cord Injury Measures meeting. *J Spinal Cord Med* 2007;30:421–440.
132. Neer CS II. Anterior acromioplasty for the chronic impingement syndrome in the shoulder: a preliminary report. *J Bone Joint Surg Am* 1972;54:41–50.
133. Hawkins RJ, Kennedy JC. Impingement syndrome in athletes. *Am J Sports Med* 1980;8:151–158.
134. Yocum LA. Assessing the shoulder. History, physical examination, differential diagnosis, and special tests used. *Clin Sports Med* 1983;2:281–289.
135. Kessel L, Watson M. The painful arc syndrome. Clinical classification as a guide to management. *J Bone Joint Surg Br* 1977;59:166–172.
136. Jobe FW, Jobe CM. Painful athletic injuries of the shoulder. *Clin Orthop Relat Res* 1983;117–124.
137. Burkhart SS, Tehrany AM. Arthroscopic subscapularis tendon repair: Technique and preliminary results. *Arthroscopy* 2002;18:454–463.
138. Barth JR, Burkhart SS, De Beer JF. The bear-hug test: a new and sensitive test for diagnosing a subscapularis tear. *Arthroscopy* 2006;22:1076–1084.
139. Magee DJ. *Orthopedic physical assessment*. 3rd ed. Philadelphia, PA: W.B. Saunders Co., 1997.
140. Kelly BT, Kadrmas WR, Speer KP. The manual muscle examination for rotator cuff strength. An electromyographic investigation. *Am J Sports Med* 1996;24:581–588.
141. Ellenbecker TS. *Clinical examination of the shoulder*. St. Louis, MO: Elsevier Saunders, 2004.
142. O'Brien SJ, Pagnani MJ, Fealy S, et al. The active compression test: a new and effective test for diagnosing labral tears and acromioclavicular joint abnormality. *Am J Sports Med* 1998;26:610–613.
143. Waring WP, Maynard FM. Shoulder pain in acute traumatic quadriplegia. *Paraplegia* 1991;29:37–42.
144. Kirshblum S, Druin E, Planten K. Musculoskeletal conditions in chronic spinal cord injury. *Top Spinal Cord Inj Rehabil* 1997;2:23–35.
145. Tully JG Jr, Latteri A. Paraplegia, syringomyelia tarda and neuropathic arthrosis of the shoulder: a triad. *Clin Orthop* 1978;134:244–248.
146. Rhoades CE, Neff JR, Rengachary SS, et al. Diagnosis of post-traumatic syringohydromyelia presenting as neuropathic joints. Report of two cases and review of the literature. *Clin Orthop* 1983;180:182–187.
147. Aisen PS, Aisen ML. Shoulder-hand syndrome in cervical spinal cord injury. *Paraplegia* 1994;32:588–592.
148. Walsh JJ, Nuseibeh I, el-Masri W. Proceedings: Perforated peptic ulcer in paraplegia. *Paraplegia* 1974;11:310–313.
149. Frankel HL. Proceedings: accidental perforation of the rectum. *Paraplegia* 1974;11:314–316.
150. Charney KJ, Juler GL, Comarr AE. General surgery problems in patients with spinal cord injuries. *Arch Surg* 1975;110:1083–1088.
151. Juler GL, Eltorai IM. The acute abdomen in spinal cord injury patients. *Paraplegia* 1985;23:118–123.
152. Neumayer LA, Bull DA, Mohr JD, et al. The acutely affected abdomen in paraplegic spinal cord injury patients. *Ann Surg* 1990;212:561–566.
153. Bar-On Z, Ohry A. The acute abdomen in spinal cord injury individuals. *Paraplegia* 1995;33:704–706.
154. Nirschl RP. Rotator cuff tendinitis: basic concepts of pathoetiology. *Instr Course Lect* 1989;38:439–445.

155. Khan KM, Cook JL, Bonar F, et al. Histopathology of common tendinopathies. Update and implications for clinical management. *Sports Med* 1999;27:393–408.
156. Weiler JM. Medical modifiers of sports injury. The use of nonsteroidal anti- inflammatory drugs (NSAIDs) in sports soft-tissue injury. *Clin Sports Med* 1992;11:625–644.
157. Amadio P Jr, Cummings DM, Amadio PB. NSAIDs revisited: selection, monitoring, and safe use. *Postgrad Med* 1997;101:257–260, 263–267, 270–271.
158. Kaplan RJ. Current status of nonsteroidal anti-inflammatory drugs in physiatry: balancing risks and benefits in pain management. *Am J Phys Med Rehabil* 2005;84:885–894.
159. Kennedy JC, Willis RB. The effects of local steroid injections on tendons: a biomechanical and microscopic correlative study. *Am J Sports Med* 1976;4:11–21.
160. Tillander B, Franzen LE, Karlsson MH, et al. Effect of steroid injections on the rotator cuff: an experimental study in rats. *J Shoulder Elbow Surg* 1999;8:271–274.
161. Speed CA. Fortnightly review: Corticosteroid injections in tendon lesions. *BMJ* 2001;323:382–386.
162. van der Heijden GJ, van der Windt DA, Kleijnen J, et al. Steroid injections for shoulder disorders: a systematic review of randomized clinical trials. *Br J Gen Pract* 1996;46:309–316.
163. Park HB, Lin SK, Yokota A, et al. Return to play for rotator cuff injuries and superior labrum anterior posterior (SLAP) lesions. *Clin Sports Med* 2004;23: 321–334, vii.
164. Rivenburgh DW. Physical modalities in the treatment of tendon injuries. *Clin Sports Med* 1992;11:645–659.
165. Lehmann JF, Masock AJ, Warren CG, et al. Effect of therapeutic temperatures on tendon extensibility. *Arch Phys Med Rehabil* 1970;51:481–487.
166. Green S, Buchbinder R, Hetrick S. Acupuncture for shoulder pain. *Cochrane Database Syst Rev* 2005;CD005319.
167. Wang YT, Kim CK, Ford HT III, et al. Reaction force and EMG analyses of wheelchair transfers. *Percept Mot Skills* 1994;79:763–766.
168. Reyes ML, Gronley JK, Newsam CJ, et al. Electromyographic analysis of shoulder muscles of men with low-level paraplegia during a weight relief raise. *Arch Phys Med Rehabil* 1995;76:433–439.
169. Minkel JL. Seating and mobility considerations for people with spinal cord injury. *Phys Ther* 2000;80: 701–709.
170. Algood SD, Cooper RA, Fitzgerald SG, et al. Effect of a pushrim-activated power-assist wheelchair on the functional capabilities of persons with tetraplegia. *Arch Phys Med Rehabil* 2005;86:380–386.
171. Algood SD, Cooper RA, Fitzgerald SG, et al. Impact of a pushrim-activated power-assisted wheelchair on the metabolic demands, stroke frequency, and range of motion among subjects with tetraplegia *Arch Phys Med Rehabil* 2004;85:1865–1871.
172. Cooper RA, Fitzgerald SG, Boninger ML, et al. Evaluation of a pushrim-activated, power-assisted wheelchair. *Arch Phys Med Rehabil* 2001;82:702–708.
173. Nash MS, Koppens D, van Haaren M, et al. Power-assisted wheels ease energy costs and perceptual responses to wheelchair propulsion in persons with shoulder pain and spinal cord injury. *Arch Phys Med Rehabil* 2008;89:2080–2085.
174. Burnham RS, May L, Nelson E, et al. Shoulder pain in wheelchair athletes. The role of muscle imbalance. *Am J Sports Med* 1993;21:238–242.
175. Burnham RS, Curtis KA, Reid DC. Shoulder problems in the wheelchair athlete. In: Petrone FA, ed. *Athletic injuries of the shoulder*. New York: McGraw-Hill, Inc., 1995:375–381.
176. Kibler WB. The role of the scapula in athletic shoulder function. *Am J Sports Med* 1998;26:325–337.
177. Mulroy SJ, Gronley JK, Newsam CJ, et al. Electromyographic activity of shoulder muscles during wheelchair propulsion by paraplegic persons. *Arch Phys Med Rehabil* 1996;77:187–193.
178. Kibler WB, Sciascia AD, Uhl TL, et al. Electromyographic analysis of specific exercises for scapular control in early phases of shoulder rehabilitation. *Am J Sports Med* 2008;36:1789–1798.
179. Decker MJ, Hintermeister RA, Faber KJ, et al. Serratus anterior muscle activity during selected rehabilitation exercises. *Am J Sports Med* 1999;27:784–791.
180. Olenik LM, Laskin JJ, Burnham R, et al. Efficacy of rowing, backward wheeling and isolated scapular retractor exercise as remedial strength activities for wheelchair users: application of electromyography. *Paraplegia* 1995;33:148–152.
181. Malanga GA, Jenp YN, Growney ES, et al. EMG analysis of shoulder positioning in testing and strengthening the supraspinatus. *Med Sci Sports Exerc* 1996;28: 661–664.
182. Reinold MM, Macrina LC, Wilk KE, et al. Electromyographic analysis of the supraspinatus and deltoid muscles during 3 common rehabilitation exercises. *J Athl Train* 2007;42:464–469.
183. Itoi E, Kido T, Sano A, et al. Which is more useful, the "full can test" or the "empty can test," in detecting the torn supraspinatus tendon? *Am J Sports Med* 1999;27:65–68.
184. Reinold MM, Escamilla RF, Wilk KE. Current concepts in the scientific and clinical rationale behind exercises for glenohumeral and scapulothoracic musculature. *J Orthop Sports Phys Ther* 2009;39:105–117.
185. Reinold MM, Wilk KE, Fleisig GS, et al. Electromyographic analysis of the rotator cuff and deltoid musculature during common shoulder external rotation exercises. *J Orthop Sports Phys Ther* 2004;34:385–394.
186. Decker MJ, Tokish JM, Ellis HB, et al. Subscapularis muscle activity during selected rehabilitation exercises. *Am J Sports Med* 2003;31:126–134.
187. Perry J, Gronley JK, Newsam CJ, et al. Electromyographic analysis of the shoulder muscles during depression transfers in subjects with low-level paraplegia. *Arch Phys Med Rehabil* 1996;77:350–355.
188. Warburton DER, Sproule S, Krassioukov A, et al. Cardiovascular health and exercise following spinal cord injury. In: Teasell RW, Miller WC, Wolfe DL, et al., eds. *Spinal cord injury rehabilitation evidence*. Vancouver, 2006:7.1–7.28.
189. Jacobs PL, Nash MS, Rusinowski JW. Circuit training provides cardiorespiratory and strength benefits

in persons with paraplegia. *Med Sci Sports Exerc* 2001;33:711–717.

190. Nash MS, Jacobs PL, Woods JM, et al. A comparison of 2 circuit exercise training techniques for eliciting matched metabolic responses in persons with paraplegia. *Arch Phys Med Rehabil* 2002;83:201–209.
191. Nash MS, van de Ven I, van Elk N, et al. Effects of circuit resistance training on fitness attributes and upper-extremity pain in middle-aged men with paraplegia. *Arch Phys Med Rehabil* 2007;88:70–75.
192. Dyson-Hudson TA, Sisto SA, Bond Q, et al. Arm crank ergometry and shoulder pain in persons with spinal cord injury. *Arch Phys Med Rehabil* 2007;88:1727–1729.
193. Hastings J, Goldstein B. Paraplegia and the shoulder. *Phys Med Rehabil Clin N Am* 2004;15:vii, 699–718.
194. Hobson DA, Tooms RE. Seated lumbar/pelvic alignment. A comparison between spinal cord- injured and noninjured groups. *Spine* 1992;17:293–298.
195. Solem-Bertoft E, Thuomas KA, Westerberg CE. The influence of scapular retraction and protraction on the width of the subacromial space. An MRI study. *Clin Orthop* 1993;296:99–103.
196. Fu FH, Harner CD, Klein AH. Shoulder impingement syndrome. A critical review. *Clin Orthop* 1991;269: 162–173.
197. Weiser WM, Lee TQ, McMaster WC, et al. Effects of simulated scapular protraction on anterior glenohumeral stability. *Am J Sports Med* 1999;27:801–805.
198. Lee TQ, McMahon PJ. Shoulder biomechanics and muscle plasticity: implications in spinal cord injury. *Clin Orthop* 2002;403(suppl):S26–S36.
199. Sinnott KA, Milburn P, McNaughton H. Factors associated with thoracic spinal cord injury, lesion level and rotator cuff disorders. *Spinal Cord* 2000;38:748–753.
200. Hastings JD, Fanucchi ER, Burns SP. Wheelchair configuration and postural alignment in persons with spinal cord injury. *Arch Phys Med Rehabil* 2003;84: 528–534.
201. Kulig K, Rao SS, Mulroy SJ, et al. Shoulder joint kinetics during the push phase of wheelchair propulsion. *Clin Orthop* 1998;354:132–143.
202. Rodgers MM, Gayle GW, Figoni SF, et al. Biomechanics of wheelchair propulsion during fatigue. *Arch Phys Med Rehabil* 1994;75:85–93.
203. Newsam CJ, Rao SS, Mulroy SJ, et al. Three dimensional upper extremity motion during manual wheelchair propulsion in men with different levels of spinal cord injury. *Gait Posture* 1999;10:223–232.
204. Majaess GG, Kirby RL, Ackroyd-Stolarz SA, Charlebois PB. Influence of seat position on the static and dynamic forward and rear stability of occupied wheelchairs. *Arch Phys Med Rehabil* 1993;74:977–982.
205. Brubaker CE. Wheelchair prescription: an analysis of factors that affect mobility and performance. *J Rehabil Res Dev* 1986;23:19–26.
206. Boninger ML, Baldwin M, Cooper RA, et al. Manual wheelchair pushrim biomechanics and axle position. *Arch Phys Med Rehabil* 2000;81:608–613.
207. van der Woude LH, Veeger DJ, Rozendal RH, et al. Seat height in handrim wheelchair propulsion. *J Rehabil Res Dev* 1989;26:31–50.
208. Bigliani LU, Levine WN. Subacromial impingement syndrome. *J Bone Joint Surg Am* 1997;79:1854–1868.
209. Robinson MD, Hussey RW, Ha CY. Surgical decompression of impingement in the weightbearing shoulder. *Arch Phys Med Rehabil* 1993;74:324–327.
210. Goldstein B, Young J, Escobedo EM. Rotator cuff repairs in individuals with paraplegia. *Am J Phys Med Rehabil* 1997;76:316–322.
211. Popowitz RL, Zvijac JE, Uribe JW, et al. Rotator cuff repair in spinal cord injury patients. *J Shoulder Elbow Surg* 2003;12:327–332.
212. Turner JA, Cardenas DD, Warms CA, et al. Chronic pain associated with spinal cord injuries: a community survey. *Arch Phys Med Rehabil* 2001;82:501–509.
213. Kelley MJ, McClure PW, Leggin BG. Frozen shoulder: evidence and a proposed model guiding rehabilitation. *J Orthop Sports Phys Ther* 2009;39:135–148.
214. Harrast MA, Rao AG. The stiff shoulder. *Phys Med Rehabil Clin N Am* 2004;15:v, 557–573.
215. Blankstein A, Shmueli R, Weingarten I, et al. Hand problems due to prolonged use of crutches and wheelchairs. *Orthop Rev* 1985;14:29–34.
216. Goldstein B. Musculoskeletal conditions after spinal cord injury. *Phys Med Rehabil Clin N Am* 2000;11:91–108, viii–ix.
217. Groah SL, Lanig IS. Neuromusculoskeletal syndromes in wheelchair athletes. *Semin Neurol* 2000;20:201–208.
218. Budoff JE, Nirschl RP. Tendinopathaties of the elbow. In: Garrett WE Jr, Speer KP, Kirkendall DT, eds. *Principles and Practice of Orthopaedic Sports Medicine.* Philadelphia, PA: Lippincott Williams & Wilkins, 2000:289–327.
219. Schroer W, Lacey S, Frost FS, et al. Carpal instability in the weight-bearing upper extremity. *J Bone Joint Surg Am* 1996;78:1838–1843.
220. O'Connor BL, Palmoski MJ, Brandt KD. Neurogenic acceleration of degenerative joint lesions. *J Bone Joint Surg Am* 1985;67:562–572.
221. Brower AC. The acute neuropathic joint. *Arthritis Rheum* 1988;31:1571–1573.
222. Nash MS, Tehranzadeh J, Green BA, et al. Magnetic resonance imaging of osteonecrosis and osteoarthrosis in exercising quadriplegics and paraplegics. *Am J Phys Med Rehabil* 1994;73:184–192.
223. Rizzo M, Betz RR, Mulcahey MJ, et al. Magnetic resonance imaging data in the evaluation of effects of functional electrical stimulation on knee joints of adolescents with spinal cord injury. *J Spinal Cord Med* 1998;21:124–130.
224. Ferro FP, Gonzalez HJ, Ferreira DM, et al. Electrical stimulation and treadmill gait in tetraplegic patients: assessment of its effects on the knee with magnetic resonance imaging. *Spinal Cord* 2008;46:124–128.
225. Upton AR, McComas AJ. The double crush in nerve entrapment syndromes. *Lancet* 1973;2:359–362.
226. Wilbourn AJ, Gilliatt RW. Double-crush syndrome: a critical analysis. *Neurology* 1997;49:21–29.
227. Aljure J, Eltorai I, Bradley WE, et al. Carpal tunnel syndrome in paraplegic patients. *Paraplegia* 1985;23: 182–186.
228. Gellman H, Chandler DR, Petrasek J, et al. Carpal tunnel syndrome in paraplegic patients. *J Bone Joint Surg Am* 1988;70:517–519.

229. Tun CG, Upton J. The paraplegic hand: electrodiagnostic studies and clinical findings. *J Hand Surg [Am]* 1988;13:716–719.
230. Davidoff G, Werner R, Waring W. Compressive mononeuropathies of the upper extremity in chronic paraplegia. *Paraplegia* 1991;29:17–24.
231. Burnham RS, Steadward RD. Upper extremity peripheral nerve entrapments among wheelchair athletes: prevalence, location, and risk factors. *Arch Phys Med Rehabil* 1994;75:519–524.
232. Jackson DL, Hynninen BC, Caborn DN, et al. Electrodiagnostic study of carpal tunnel syndrome in wheelchair basketball players. *Clin J Sport Med* 1996;6:27–31.
233. Liang HW, Wang YH, Pan SL, et al. Asymptomatic median mononeuropathy among men with chronic paraplegia. *Arch Phys Med Rehabil* 2007;88:1193–1197.
234. Goodman CM, Steadman AK, Meade RA, et al. Comparison of carpal canal pressure in paraplegic and nonparaplegic subjects: clinical implications. *Plast Reconstr Surg* 2001;107:1464–1471; discussion 1472.
235. Practice parameter for carpal tunnel syndrome (summary statement). Report of the Quality Standards Subcommittee of the American Academy of Neurology. *Neurology* 1993;43:2406–2409.
236. Gelberman RH, Hergenroeder PT, Hargens AR, et al. The carpal tunnel syndrome. A study of carpal canal pressures. *J Bone Joint Surg Am* 1981;63:380–383.
237. Practice parameter for electrodiagnostic studies in carpal tunnel syndrome (summary statement). American Academy of Neurology, American Association of Electrodiagnostic Medicine, and American Academy of Physical Medicine and Rehabilitation. *Neurology* 1993;43:2404–2405.
238. Wertsch JJ, Melvin J. Median nerve anatomy and entrapment syndromes: a review. *Arch Phys Med Rehabil* 1982;63:623–627.
239. Redmond MD, Rivner MH. False positive electrodiagnostic tests in carpal tunnel syndrome. *Muscle Nerve* 1988;11:511–518.
240. Koontz AM, Yang Y, Boninger DS, et al. Investigation of the performance of an ergonomic handrim as a pain-relieving intervention for manual wheelchair users. *Assist Technol* 2006;18:123–143; quiz 145.
241. Richter WM, Rodriguez R, Woods KR, et al. Reduced finger and wrist flexor activity during propulsion with a new flexible handrim. *Arch Phys Med Rehabil* 2006;87:1643–1647.
242. Malone LA, Gervais PL, Burnham RS, et al. An assessment of wrist splint and glove use on wheeling kinematics. *Clin Biomech (Bristol, Avon)* 1998;13:234–236.
243. Johnson RK, Spinner M, Shrewsbury MM. Median nerve entrapment syndrome in the proximal forearm. *J Hand Surg [Am]* 1979;4:48–51.
244. Rehak DC. Pronator syndrome. *Clin Sports Med* 2001;20:531–540.
245. Gainor BJ. The pronator compression test revisited. A forgotten physical sign. *Orthop Rev* 1990;19:888–892.
246. Morris HH, Peters BH. Pronator syndrome: clinical and electrophysiological features in seven cases. *J Neurol Neurosurg Psychiatry* 1976;39:461–464.
247. Werner CO, Rosen I, Thorngren KG. Clinical and neurophysiologic characteristics of the pronator syndrome. *Clin Orthop Relat Res* 1985;231–236.
248. Tsai P, Steinberg DR. Median and radial nerve compression about the elbow. *J Bone Joint Surg Am* 2008;90:420–428.
249. D'Agostino RB SR, Vasan RS, Pencina MJ, et al. General cardiovascular risk profile for use in primary care: the Framingham Heart Study. *Circulation* 2008;117:743–753.
250. Stefaniwsky L, Bilowit DS, Prasad SS. Reduced motor conduction velocity of the ulnar nerve in spinal cord injured patients. *Paraplegia* 1980;18:21–24.
251. Dozono K, Hachisuka K, Hatada K, et al. Peripheral neuropathies in the upper extremities of paraplegic wheelchair marathon racers. *Paraplegia* 1995;33:208–211.
252. Boninger ML, Robertson RN, Wolff M, et al. Upper limb nerve entrapments in elite wheelchair racers. *Am J Phys Med Rehabil* 1996;75:170–176.
253. Posner MA. Compressive neuropathies of the ulnar nerve at the elbow and wrist. *Instr Course Lect* 2000;49: 305–317.
254. Plancher KD, Peterson RK, Steichen JB. Compressive neuropathies and tendinopathies in the athletic elbow and wrist. *Clin Sports Med* 1996;15:331–371.
255. Nunley JA, Goetz T. Injuries to the soft tissues of the wrist. In: Garrett WE Jr, Speer KP, Kirkendall DT, eds. *Principles and Practice of Orthopaedic Sports Medicine* Philadelphia, PA: Lippincott Williams & Wilkins, 2000:273–288.
256. Nemchausky BA, Ubilluz RM. Upper extremity neuropathies in patients with spinal cord injuries. *J Spinal Cord Med* 1995;18:95–97.
257. Lintner S. Nerve injuries in the upper extremity. In: Garrett WE Jr, Speer KP, Kirkendall DT, eds. *Principles and practice of orthopaedic sports medicine*. Philadelphia, PA: Lippincott Williams & Wilkins, 2000:543–550.
258. Siddall PJ, Yezierski RP, Loeser JD. Pain following spinal cord injury: clinical features, prevalence, and taxonomy. *IASP Newslett* 2000;3:3–7.
259. Bryce TN, Ragnarsson KT. Pain after spinal cord injury. *Phys Med Rehabil Clin N Am* 2000;11:157–168.

CHAPTER 17 ■ REHABILITATION OF SPINAL CORD INJURY

STEVEN KIRSHBLUM, JESSICA BLOOMGARDEN, ISA McCLURE, CINDY NEAD, GAIL FORREST, AND JANE MITCHELL

> The neurologic impairment is not nearly as important as the quality of rehabilitation, the social support system and possibly the personality and mind set of persons with SCI themselves that determine coping and ultimately satisfaction with life after injury.
>
> Sam Stover

INTRODUCTION

Before the second half of the 20th century, persons who sustained a traumatic spinal cord injury (SCI) were given little hope for survival. Since that time, there has been great progress in the medical care and rehabilitation of those who sustain an SCI, improving functional capability and community reintegration. "Rehabilitation," including meeting SCI-specific medical and rehabilitative needs, is extremely important to help the injured individuals reach their physical, social, emotional, recreational, vocational, and functional potential. While the search for cure has brought a greater understanding of SCI, rehabilitation is the only treatment currently available to enhance function after injury. Because of this, rehabilitation in the acute, subacute, and chronic phases after injury is of utmost importance.

REHABILITATION IN ACUTE CARE

Rehabilitation should begin as soon as possible after injury. Once lifesaving measures have been initiated in the acute care hospital, early intervention by rehabilitation specialists can prevent complications, such as atelectasis, thromboembolic disorders, pressure ulcers, and contractures (1).The majority of complications in traumatic SCI occur early after injury (2), and studies have shown a decrease in these complications in patients who were treated in specialized SCI units (3–7). Early intervention by rehabilitation specialists may shorten lengths of stay during the acute hospitalization phase by preventing secondary complications, initiating education about the rehabilitation process, and encouraging participation in discharge planning discussions, thus facilitating discharge to the next level of care (1,5,6,8,9). This decreases the total rehabilitation time and cost of care, as well as the degree of human suffering (10).

The medical aspects of the SCI specialist's acute recommendations are covered in Chapters 6 and 8, as well as in the Consortium Guidelines (1). The most important rehabilitation interventions in the acute care setting include bowel, bladder, and pulmonary management; thromboembolic and gastrointestinal prophylaxis; and proper positioning in bed with turning at least every 2 hours to prevent skin breakdown. Once the spine is stabilized, active, active assistive, and passive range of motion (ROM) should be performed by staff or family at least daily to help prevent contractures. Shoulder, elbow, hip flexor, and heel cord contractures are most frequently observed on presentation to the acute rehabilitation unit and can potentially serve as a source of pain and functional limitation; therefore, these joints are the most important to range. Resting splints for paralyzed upper extremities (UEs) can help prevent contractures and increase comfort. Functional UE splints may also be useful for feeding and other self-care skills in the early period. Muscles that are innervated should be exercised to prevent disuse atrophy and weakness. Sitting tolerance can be initiated at the bedside with weight relief (shifts) every 20 to 30 minutes. If the patient is medically stable, mat training can begin in the therapy setting. Speech and language pathologists can perform bedside screening for dysphagia. For persons with acute high-level tetraplegia with a tracheostomy, early introduction of communication aids (letter boards, speaking valve, etc.) is important. Once the patient is medically stable and after spinal stabilization, the patient should be transferred to a specialized spinal cord rehabilitation unit.

REHABILITATION TEAM

The interdisciplinary approach of the rehabilitation team is important for the optimal care of the individual with SCI. Members of the team include the rehabilitation nurse and aides; physical, occupational, speech, recreational, and vocational therapists; psychologist; and the social worker/case manager. Additional team members include the orthotist, driving instructor, SCI educator, peer mentor, nutritionist, and rehabilitation engineer. Everyone should keep in mind that the patient and family are also full members of the team. The physician specializing in the care of the SCI person (most commonly a physiatrist, preferably with subspecialty board certification in SCI Medicine) is the team leader. Responsibilities of the physician include preventing and treating SCI-specific medical issues, formulating the therapeutic goals and prescriptions, solving team member conflicts, and discussing prognosis with the patient and family.

The team members should not work in isolation, but rather as a cohesive unit toward the common goal of maximizing the patient's potential. The collective wisdom of the interdisciplinary team will provide the person with SCI the best possible opportunity of achieving functional outcomes (10). The role of each team member is valuable, and although there is occasional overlap between disciplines, this serves as reinforcement for the patient rather than as a duplication of services. All team members provide education, assist in adjustment issues for the patient and family, and help with preparation for discharge and reintegration into the community. The more educated the patients and their family, the better the outcome with respect to health function and quality of life.

The rehabilitation nurse performs typical nursing tasks and has the added responsibility of serving as an educator, motivator, listener, and assistant coordinator of discharge planning. The rehabilitation nurse helps the patient and family recognize medical issues and prevent complications. This includes training in bowel and bladder care, monitoring of skin and nutritional needs, and reinforcing ROM and transfer techniques. Nurses are the front line in encouraging the patient to be an active participant in the rehabilitation process. For discharge, the rehabilitation nurse assists in listing the patient's supplies and equipment needs.

Physical and occupational therapists should work together to help the patient achieve his or her optimal level of self-care and mobility. An integrated program encompassing ROM, strengthening, functional training, patient and family education, and equipment training is just a part of the therapist responsibilities. Other important aspects of care include an assistive technology evaluation and training (including environmental control units [ECUs]), a home evaluation and recommendations for modifications, and specialty equipment recommendations, that is, wheelchair, cushion, orthotics, assistive devices, bed, and mattress. The therapist also serves as a motivator, listening to the patient's frustrations and attempting to channel those emotions into the rehabilitation process. The most commonly used techniques in therapy are discussed later in this chapter.

The speech pathologist is involved in the care of swallowing, communication, and cognitive deficits. Swallowing deficits are more common in persons with a high-level cervical injury, who have a tracheostomy tube, or who have undergone anterior approach spinal surgery (11). Training for swallowing as well as voice control can be undertaken.

The psychologist assesses the patient's cognitive status, adjustment to disability, and emotional status. Working with other team members as well as the patient and family, the psychologist can help identify problem issues and suggest appropriate interventions to assist in attaining the rehabilitation goals.

Recreational therapy helps the patient focus on leisure activities that are possible both as an inpatient and after discharge from the rehabilitation hospital. The team should encourage participation in previous recreational interests and look for new activities that the patient may enjoy. Often, patients and families are unaware of the scope of activities that are available for the injured person, and education is needed to change the focus from those activities that they can no longer participate in to the many activities that they can. Community outings frequently take place during the inpatient stay (to a shopping mall, movie theatre, etc.) to start reintegrating the patient into community settings.

The social worker or case manger (often trained as a nurse) helps the patient and family with insurance/financial issues in order to maximize benefits. They can also identify and coordinate other community and governmental resources available to assist with the patient's care. Responsibilities include helping to identify potential barriers for community reintegration and facilitating discharge planning to ensure a smooth transition to the discharge destination. Home care equipment delivery and outpatient programs should be scheduled before discharge, and continuity of medical care should be ensured. Family counseling throughout this period is crucial.

Team conferences should be held at least once weekly to allow all team members to address the clinical problems, report progress, and update goals, as well as to secure a proper and safe discharge. Frequently, a home evaluation performed early in the inpatient stay is especially valuable to assess for necessary home modifications and adaptive equipment. In addition, a work place evaluation may be recommended either as part of the inpatient stay or as part of the outpatient program. As the length of stay (LOS) shortens in acute rehabilitation, coordination of the entire team is of even greater importance to allow for a timely and safe discharge.

INPATIENT REHABILITATION

There are many locations where one can receive inpatient rehabilitation, and the choice of facility should be made carefully. Facilities should be evaluated on the level of experience of the staff (including the physicians, therapists, and nurses) and the number of SCI patients served by that facility per year. The Model SCI System included in their most recent criteria a minimum of 30 admissions a year for eligibility (12). Caring for a volume of patients can indicate the degree of expertise of services that may be available, including medical care, therapies, full-time psychology, vocational and SCI educational services, and an active peer support program. The ability for an individual to undergo rehabilitation with others who have similar impairments is extremely helpful. Additional opportunities available at larger centers include the ability to trial equipment (i.e., wheelchairs, cushions, bathroom equipment), availability of high-level assistive technology, and a specialized seating program.

At admission, the SCI physician performs a comprehensive evaluation, establishing the motor, sensory, and neurological level of injury (LOI) and the ASIA Impairment Scale (AIS) classification (see Chapter 6). A problem list (Table 17.1) with long-term and short-term goals should be established by the team based upon their evaluations. Keeping those goals in mind, specific therapy prescriptions for all of the involved team members should be established by the physician (Table 17.2).

Therapy usually begins at a minimum of 3 h/d, although some patients may need to work up to this level of endurance. At first, therapy may take place at the bedside, progressing as tolerated into the therapy gym. Mobilization begins slowly, using a reclining wheelchair to help patients accommodate to the upright position. An abdominal binder and lower extremity (LE) ace wraps/stockings are recommended to prevent orthostasis. In therapy, a tilt table may be utilized. Over the course of days, the patient is usually able to tolerate a more upright position, thus improving endurance for wheelchair mobility and therapy.

FUNCTIONAL GOALS

The most important factor in determining functional outcome is the motor level and the degree of impairment, that is, AIS Classification (i.e complete versus incomplete status). Table 17.3 lists the functional goals expected to be achieved at 1 year for each key LOI in a person with a motor complete injury. Table 17.4 lists equipment usually prescribed by LOI. The ideal outcome may not always be achieved for each patient, as there is a significant

TABLE 17.1

SAMPLE PROBLEM LIST

Problem list	Interventions
Medical	
Respiratory	Monitor vital capacity. Perform incentive spirometry, assisted cough, deep breathing techniques, chest PT, and respiratory treatments.
Gastrointestinal	Stress ulcer prophylaxis
Nutrition	Perform calorie count. Monitor weekly weights.
Neurogenic bowel	Initiate bowel program and adjust as needed. Patient and family training.
Neurogenic bladder	Proper intake and output. Discuss bladder options. Family training.
DVT prophylaxis	Check admission Doppler study. Adequate pharmacological prophylaxis. Monitor LE circumference.
Skin	Proper mattress. Turn Q 2 degrees initially. Heel protectors. Frequent weight shifts in wheelchair. Proper cushion. Teach patient to use mirror to check skin.
Orthostasis	Change positions slowly. Ace wrap or LE stockings and abdominal binder. Use tilt table. Pharmacological intervention if needed.
H.O.	Monitor hip and knee ROM. X-rays and bone scan if suspect.
Spasticity	Stretching/ROM. Modalities. Medications. Injections. Intrathecal baclofen.
AD	Monitor closely.
Hypercalcemia	Monitor for symptoms. Fluids, medications.
Rehabilitation issues	
Mobility	ADL
Adjustment to disability	Cognitive
Communication	Swallowing
SCI education	Vocational
Sexuality	Driving
Recreation	Family training
Discharge planning	Equipment evaluation

AD - autonomic dysreflexia; ADL - activities of daily living; LE - lower extremity; PT - physical therapy; ROM - range of motion.

amount of variability in individual outcomes despite similar LOI. Functional outcomes are dependent upon the age of the individual and coexistent conditions such as body habitus, cognitive impairment (i.e., dual diagnosis of SCI with concomitant brain injury), brachial plexus injury, secondary complications, or preexistent conditions. In addition, complications such as pain, spasticity, contractures, and depression may also interfere with the achievement of expected long-term goals. Persons who are highly motivated and those with good social support may exceed the expected functional outcome for their respective LOI (13).

Persons with motor complete injuries are usually expected to gain one motor level of function from their initial examination (performed 72 hours to 1 week after injury) to the subsequent months (see Chapter 8). If the patient is expected to remain in rehabilitation during that period of time, typical recovery patterns should be kept in mind when determining goals. For individuals with incomplete injuries, recovery occurs most rapidly in the first 2 months after injury and slows after 3 to 6 months, but motor and functional recovery may continue up to 2 years postinjury.

The treatment team is guided by long-term functional goals, but the rehabilitation program should be individualized to meet each person's strengths, weaknesses, and individual circumstances. Short-term goals are progressive steps that should be attained on the way to achieving the long-term goals. Progress toward the functional goals should be monitored at the team conference in order to identify limiting factors and additional needs. Understanding the goals allows the patient to become an active participant in his or her program.

TABLE 17.2

SAMPLE PHYSICAL AND OCCUPATIONAL THERAPY PRESCRIPTION:

Diagnosis: C7 ASIA A Tetraplegia
Goals: (see outlined goals in Table 17.3)
Precautions: Skin, respiratory, sensory, orthostasis, safety, risk for AD, and others as needed for the specific patient (i.e., orthosis, bleeding if on Coumadin).

Physical Therapy
PROM to bilateral LE, with stretching of shoulders, hamstrings and hip extensors.
Mat activities.
Tilt table as tolerated. Start at 15 degrees progress 10 degrees every 15 min within precautions up to 80 degrees.
Sitting balancing (static and dynamic).
Transfer training from all surfaces including mat, bed, wheelchair, and floor.
Wheelchair propulsion training and management.
Teach and encourage weight shifting.
Standing table as tolerated.
Deep breathing exercises.
FES for appropriate candidates.
Family training.
Community skills.
Teach HEP.

Occupational Therapy
Passive, active assisted, active ROM/exercises to bilateral UEs.
Allow for some finger tightness to enhance grasp in C5 and C6 patients.
Bilateral UE strengthening.
Motor coordination skills.
ADL program with adaptive equipment as needed (dressing, grooming, feeding).
Functional transfer training (bathroom, tub, car, etc.).
Splinting and adaptive equipment evaluation.
Desk top skills.
Shower program.
Kitchen and homemaking skills.
Wheelchair training (parts and management).
Home evaluation.
Family training.
Teach HEP.

HEP - home exercise program; FES - functional electrical stimulation; PROM - passive range of motion; UE - upper extremity.

TABLE 17.3

PROJECTED FUNCTIONAL OUTCOMES AT 1 YEAR POSTINJURY BY LEVEL

	C1-4	C5	C6	C7	C8-T1
Feeding	Dependent	Modf ind with adaptive equipment after set up	Modf ind. with adaptive equipment	Independent	Independent
Grooming	Dependent	Min assist with equip. after set up	Modf ind to CG w/ adaptive equipment	Modf ind	Independent
UE dressing	Dependent	Requires assistance	Modf ind	Independent	Independent
LE dressing	Dependent	Dependent	Some assist	Modf ind -CG	Modf ind
Bathing	Dependent	Max to Mod A	Min assist w/ equipment	CG to Modf ind with equipment	Modf ind with equipment
Bed mobility	Dependent	Max to Mod	CG to CS	Modf ind	Independent
Weight shifts	Ind. in power. Dep. in manual w/c	Ind w/ power w/c Mod w/ manual	Independent	Independent	Independent
Transfers	Dependent	Max to mod	CG on level surfaces	Ind. with or without board for level surfaces	Independent
W/C propulsion	Ind. with power Dependent in manual	Modf ind power Modf ind power assist wheels Modf ind manual on level surfaces	Ind—manual with coated rims on level surfaces	Ind—except curbs and uneven terrain	Independent
Driving	Modified passenger van	Modf ind w/ van conversion	Modf ind w/ adaptations	Car with hand controls or adapted van	Car with hand control or adapted van

POTENTIAL OUTCOMES IN COMPLETE PARAPLEGIA

	T2-9	T10-L2	L3-S5
ADL (grooming, feeding, dressing, bathing)	Independent	Independent	Independent
Bowel and bladder	Independent	Independent	Independent
Transfers[a]	Independent	Independent	Independent
Ambulation[a]	Standing in frame, tilt table or standing wheelchair Exercise only	Household ambulation with orthoses Can trial ambulation outdoors	Community ambulation is possible
Braces[a]	Bilateral KAFO with forearm crutches or walker	KAFOs, with forearm crutches	Possibly KAFO or AFOs, with canes/crutches

[a]Account for PMH and functional strength.
Modf, modified; Ind, independent; Dep, dependent; CS, close supervision; CG, contact guard.

The rehabilitation program can then be modified to help the patient meet individual expectations.

Lengths of stay have been decreasing in the United States, both for acute care and for rehabilitation over the last 30 years (8,14). Comparison of model SCI system data reveals that mean adjusted LOS has been reduced by 62.6 days from 1973–1981 to 2002–2006 (14). The percentage of patients discharged home has not been adversely affected, although functional independence at discharge has been reduced as a result. Patients with higher injury levels, more severe injuries, and lower function have longer rehabilitation LOS (8). It is no longer possible to achieve all of the rehabilitation goals in the number of days that are being certified by third-party payers. Discharge planning should be discussed as early as the first team conference, assuring a timely and safe discharge. Excessively short rehabilitation LOS has been linked to negative consequences including increased incidence of secondary complications and rehospitalization (8). Most patients receive outpatient therapy to help them reach the levels of functional independence formerly achieved while still an inpatient (15); however, there are no studies comparing the cost effectiveness of these approaches.

If rehabilitation services are to be relevant and effective in meeting the needs of individuals with SCI, they must be aware of the patient's perspective. In a meta-synthesis of research studying the experience of inpatient rehabilitation from a patient's perspective, a number of conclusions were reached (16). These include the following: (a) the importance of specific staff qualities (i.e., staff who treat patients as unique individuals rather than as rehabilitation clients, who are perceived as caring, interact in a personal rather than a professional manner, and treat patients as partners in the rehab process);

TABLE 17.4

SUGGESTED EQUIPMENT FOR COMPLETE TETRAPLEGIA (EACH PATIENT VARIES)

	C1-3	C4-5	C6-7	C8-T1
Durable medical equipment				
Tilt-in-space shower/commode chair	X	X		
Standard shower/commode			X	X
Padded tub bench			X	X
Padded drop arm commode			X	X
Hospital bed full electric	X	X	X	X
Low air loss mattress	X	X	X	
Low air loss overlay			X	X
Patient lifter (power)	X	X		
Patient lifter (mechanical)		X		
Transfer board	X	X	X	X
Power w/c with tilt/recline	X	X	?	-
Power w/c			X	
Power asst w/c		?	X	X
Manual w/c	X	X	X	X
Assistive devices				
Balance forearm orthosis		X		
Dorsal ADL cuff		X		
Universal cuff		X	X	
U-shaped holder for toothbrush		X		
Plate guard		X	X	
Vertical holder and fork		X		
Quad rocker knife			X	
Dycem		X	X	
Skin inspection mirror		X	X	X
Wash mitt		X		
Dressing stick			X	X
Soft loops			X	X
Rings/adaptations to closures			X	
Universal cuff with catheter clip			X	
Digital stimulator			X	X
Suppository Inserter			X	X
Pants holder			X	X
Typing pegs		X	X	
Wanchik writer		X	X	
Pencil grip				X
Splints				
Resting hand splint	X	X		
Wrist support	X	X		
Long opponent splint		X		
Short opponent splint			X	
Spiral splint		X		
Powered tenodesis splint		X		
Elbow extension		X		
RIC tenodesis splint			X	
Wrist driven tenodesis			X	
Lumbrical (MC block)			X	X

(b) a vision of future life possibilities (i.e., convey a sense of hope, are willing to talk about the patients' priorities, and refer patients to peers); (c) importance of peers (to provide a resource for advice on problem solving, knowledge, experience, and inspiration); (d) relevance of program content (i.e., the importance of staff and program flexibility); (e) institutional context of rehabilitation (i.e., tailoring the program to the patients' needs); (f) importance of reconnecting the past with the future (i.e., focusing on more than just physical activities); and (g) the importance of meeting the needs of the real world (rather than just the rehabilitation setting). This review concludes that the most important dimension of rehabilitation for people with SCI is the caliber and vision of the rehabilitation staff (16).

C1-4 Level

The muscles available with lesions at or above C3 include the cervical paraspinals, sternocleidomastoid, neck accessory muscles, and partial innervation of the diaphragm. Functionally, this allows for neck flexion, extension, and rotation.

At the C4 level, there is further innervation of the diaphragm and paraspinal muscles, with additional inspiratory strength and functional scapular elevation.

Persons with motor levels at or above C3 will usually require long-term ventilator assistance, whereas most with lesions at C4 will be able to wean off the ventilator (see Chapter 9). For persons requiring a ventilator, two ventilators are recommended; one to be the backup (13). Additional respiratory equipment will be needed, including a method for secretion management (i.e., suction, mechanical insufflator/exsufflator), backup batteries, and a generator in case of power failure. The local power company and emergency services should be alerted prior to discharge.

Individuals with these high levels of injury, whether requiring a ventilator or not, are dependent in self-care activities and mobility. They should, however, be independent in instructing others in how to provide their care, including performing weight shifts, ROM, positioning in bed, donning orthoses, transferring (with and without mechanical lifts), monitoring skin for breakdown, and setting up their ECU. They should also be independent in instructing others in how to manage in the event of an emergency (i.e., autonomic dysreflexia [AD]) or equipment failure. Persons at this level require total assistance with their bowel and bladder management. It is often difficult to assure that there is always a trained person available to perform intermittent catheterization (IC); therefore, other bladder options should be discussed.

For mobility, persons at this level should be independent in the use of a power wheelchair using breath control, mouth stick, tongue, or chin control mechanisms (see Chapter 18). If the patient can control a power chair, then both a power (recline and/or tilt wheelchair) and a manual wheelchair should be prescribed. The manual wheelchair is used when accessibility for a power wheelchair is not available or if the patient is unable for some reason to use the power wheelchair. These persons are not able to drive, but would benefit from an adapted van for accessibility. Once properly set up, persons at these levels of injury should be independent in ECU control (see later).

Persons with a C4 NLI who have some elbow flexion and deltoid strength may be able to use a mobile arm support (MAS) or balanced forearm orthosis (BFO) to assist with feeding, grooming, and hygiene (Fig. 17.1). These devices may also enable patients with limited shoulder flexion to increase the strength and endurance of this motion through repetition. Once the deltoid and biceps muscles have strength of 3+/5 with adequate endurance, the MAS is no longer needed. The patient should also have a long straw or a bottle that allows access to drink fluids.

Specialized acute rehabilitation for persons with high LOI is justifiable even if unable to initially tolerate 3 hours a day of therapy, and despite having what some might consider limited functional goals. The SCI specialized care during the first few months after injury are crucial for monitoring, treating, and preventing medical complications that can lead to future morbidity and mortality. The patient and family education, emotional and social support, and exposure to advanced technology that may allow independence in the proper environment (i.e., power mobility, ECU) may be the difference between returning to their family/community versus spending their life in a nursing home.

Families should be trained by the team (i.e., physician, nursing, and therapists) in respiratory management (i.e., "quad coughing"), skin management, ROM activities, transfers both with and without equipment, positioning, and weight shifting. They should also be trained to handle medical issues such as orthostasis, AD, and bowel and bladder programs. Several sessions may be needed to complete the training. It is recommended that the training be documented in the medical record.

C5 Level

The C5 level adds the key muscle group of the biceps (elbow flexors), as well as the deltoids, rhomboids, and partial innervation of the brachialis, brachioradialis, supraspinatus, infraspinatus, and serratus anterior. These muscles allow for shoulder flexion, extension, and abduction; elbow flexion and supination; and weak scapular adduction and abduction. The individual can be partially independent with skills such as feeding and grooming with splints. It is extremely important to prevent elbow flexion and forearm supination contractures caused by unopposed biceps activity. Continued stretching should be performed both acutely and chronically. Shoulder

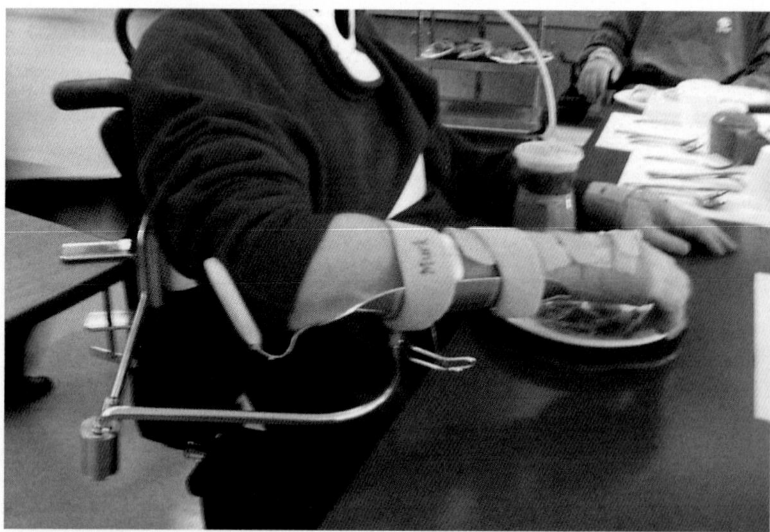

FIGURE 17.1. Balanced Forearm Orthosis. Also note the long handled straw, plate guard, and Dycem.

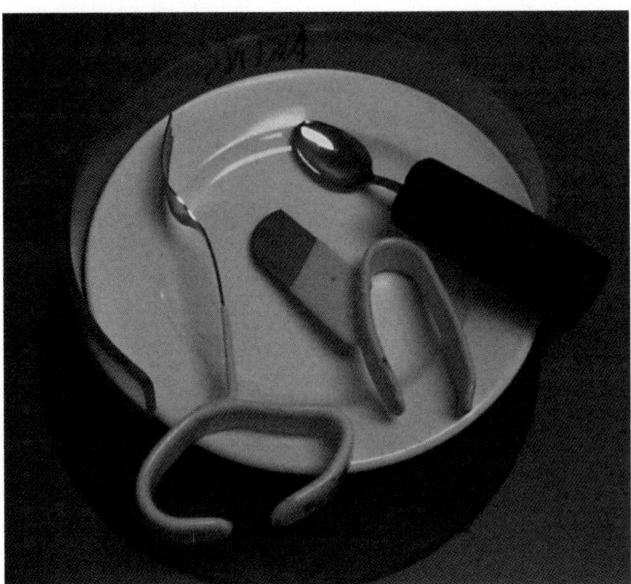

FIGURE 17.2. Adaptive feeding equipment. Dycem, plate guard, adapted utensils.

external rotation should be encouraged. An MAS may be needed initially; however, the person should regain adequate strength to perform activities without its use.

The addition of the elbow flexors should allow for use of a joystick on a power wheelchair and for manual wheelchair propulsion on level surfaces with either rim projections (lugs) or plastic coated handrims with a protective glove. Power wheelchairs, with a power recline and/or tilt mechanism, are usually still required in addition to the manual wheelchair. The lighter the manual wheelchair, the easier to propel. A manual wheelchair with power assist wheels (see Chapter 18) can be very useful for individuals with this LOI. Driving a specially modified van is possible at this level.

A long opponent splint, with a pocket for inserting different utensils (i.e., Universal Cuff), is extremely important to assist with many tasks, including feeding, hygiene, grooming, and writing. Various adaptive devices are represented in Figs. 17.2–17.4. Most functional activities will require the use of assistive devices, and tendon transfers may be considered after neurological recovery is complete (see Chapter 28).

Persons at this level will require almost total assistance for their bowel program. Bladder management method is a decision based upon discussion with the SCI specialist and urologist, urodynamic results, amount of assistance available, and lifestyle circumstances. IC usually cannot be performed independently. If using a leg bag, electronic devices to help empty the bag are available.

C6 Level

The C6 level adds the key muscle group of the extensor carpi radialis (ECR) longus that performs wrist extension. Additional muscles partially innervated include the ECR brevis, supinator, pronator teres, and latissimus dorsi. Movements gained include scapular abduction and radial wrist extension. Active wrist extension can allow for "tenodesis," the opposition of the thumb and index finger as the finger flexor tendons are stretched with wrist extension. One should avoid overly stretching the finger flexors initially after injury in C5 and C6 motor level patients to avoid potentially losing tenodesis. Tenodesis splints can be fabricated but are frequently discarded by patients; however, the use of these splints should be encouraged so that the patient can develop a functional grasp.

Individuals with a C6 level are usually independent after assistance with setup in feeding, grooming, and UE hygiene. Clothing modifications such as Velcro closures on shoes, loops on zippers, and pullover garments are usually advised. Assistance for meal preparation and homemaking tasks is required.

Transfers may be possible using a transfer board and loops for LE management, but usually requires assistance. Although persons with a C6 motor level can propel a manual wheelchair with plastic coated rims, a power wheelchair is often required for long distances, especially if the individual will be returning to the workplace. A manual wheelchair with power assist wheels can be very useful for individuals with this LOI. Driving a modified van is a goal, with a lift for access allowing the patient be fully independent.

The person at this level will require assistance with the bowel program. IC is possible for males after assistance for setup with adaptive devices, but this technique is more difficult for females.

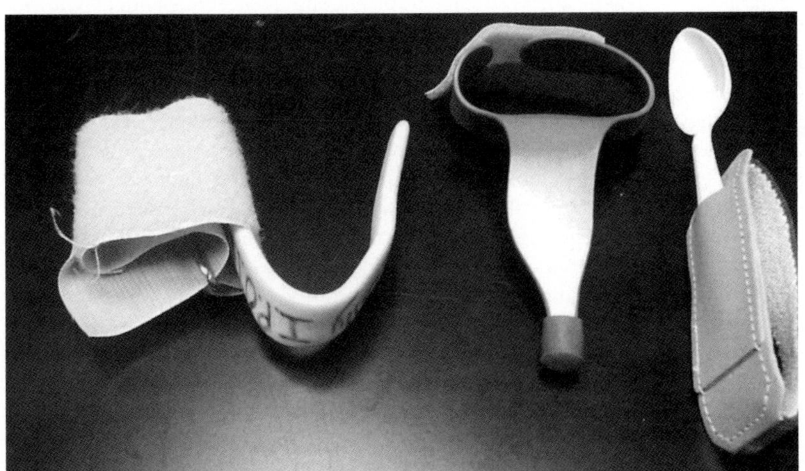

FIGURE 17.3. Adaptive utensils including (from left to right) a quad phone holder, typing peg, and universal cuff with a plastic spoon attached.

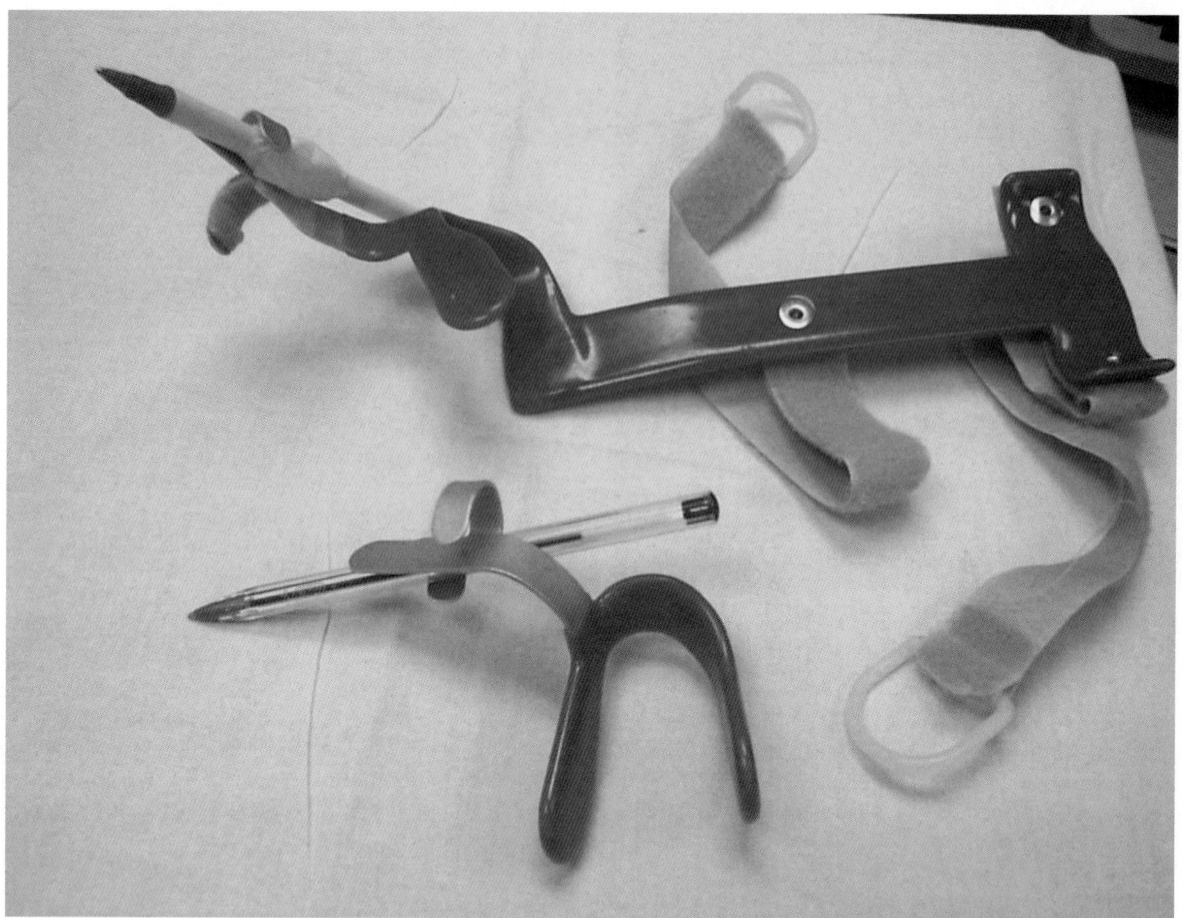

FIGURE 17.4. Adaptive writing utensils.

C7-8 Levels

The C7 level adds the triceps (elbow extensors) as the key muscle group; C8 adds the flexor digitorum profundus (long finger flexors). At C7, in addition to elbow extension, ulnar wrist extension, wrist flexion, and some finger extension are added. At the C8 level, the long finger flexors become functional, allowing for improved hand and finger function. Additional muscles with some innervation at these levels include the flexor carpi radialis, extensor carpi ulnaris, pronator quadratus, flexor digitorum superficialis, abductor pollicis, and lumbricals.

The C7 level is considered the key level for becoming independent in most activities at the wheelchair level. Persons with a C7 motor level are usually independent for weight shifts, transfers between level surfaces, feeding, grooming, and upper body dressing. Uneven surface transfers and lower body dressing may require assistance. These individuals should be independent in light meal preparation; although, they will require some to total assist for complex meal preparation and house cleaning. Persons with this LOI should be independent in manual wheelchair propulsion for indoor and outdoor terrain, but may require some assistance for uneven surfaces. Driving should be independent in a modified van or a car if they can transfer and load/unload their wheelchair independently.

IC in males can be performed, but it is more difficult for females, especially if LE spasticity is present. Bowel care may still require assistance, although independence can be achieved with adaptive devices that aid in suppository insertion and digital stimulation.

Thoracic Levels

It is best to separate persons with a thoracic injury into upper (T1-6) and lower level injuries (T7-12) because of improved trunk control and core stability in the latter group. Persons with all levels of paraplegia should be independent with all ADL and mobility skills at the wheelchair level on even and uneven surfaces. Advanced wheelchair training (described later) should be undertaken. They should be able to drive a car with adaptations, although loading/unloading the wheelchair may still be difficult. They also should be able to prepare meals in an adapted environment and perform light housekeeping, but may still require assistance with heavy housekeeping.

The lower the LOI, the greater the trunk control due to abdominal and paraspinal muscle innervation. Although individuals with high and mid-thoracic level thoracic injuries may be interested in gait training and should undergo this if there are no medical contraindications (i.e., hip flexion contractures, LE fractures), ambulation is usually not a primary inpatient goal. Persons with lower thoracic levels of paraplegia can participate in ambulation training with bilateral LE orthoses as an exercise and for short distance ambulation (see Ambulation section). Persons with these LOI should be independent in their bowel and bladder programs, with any technique they choose.

Lumbar Paraplegia

The lower the LOI, the greater the opportunity for the patient to become independent in ambulation. As muscle strength increases, less bracing is necessary, and ambulation becomes more functional over greater distances.

L1-2 Levels

Muscles gained at these levels include the hip flexors and part of the knee extensors. While the person can walk for short distances, a wheelchair will still be required. Individuals with these levels of injury can drive a car with hand controls.

Individuals with these levels of injury should be independent in their bowel and bladder programs, with any techniques they choose. Bladder care is usually by IC.

L3-4 Levels

The knee extensors are fully innervated and ankle dorsiflexion regains some strength. Ambulation usually requires ankle foot orthoses (AFOs) with assistive devices (i.e., canes or crutches). Bowel and bladder management depends on whether there is upper (UMN) or lower motor neuron (LMN) damage. In either case, the person should be independent. If there is an LMN injury, bowel management is by contraction of abdominal muscles and manual disimpaction. Suppositories will not be effective because of the loss of reflexes. Bladder management is usually performed via IC or Valsalva maneuver if postvoid residuals are within normal limits, and urological workup reveals no contraindication to this method. Absorbent pads can be used. If there is an UMN injury, digital stimulation will usually suffice for bowel management, and bladder management is similar to thoracic level paraplegia.

L5 and Below

These individuals should be independent in all activities unless there are associated problems, that is, severe pain, cardiac conditions, etc.

SPINAL ORTHOTICS IN REHABILITATION

Chapter 19 describes the different orthotics available for individuals with SCI. When an orthosis is used to protect the spine during fracture healing or postoperatively after a surgical fusion, it generally is worn for 10 to 12 weeks. This timeframe may vary by surgeon and technique performed. To insure that a patient's spinal stability is not compromised, there may be limits placed on participation in certain functional activities (i.e., certain types of transfers or weight shifts, prone or high-level position changes, advanced wheelchair skills) while in the orthosis. These precautions should be clearly communicated between the physician and treating therapists.

While spinal orthoses provide a degree of immobilization of the spine, they also restrict the general mobility of the patient and may interfere with the rehabilitation program and achievement of functional goals in a timely manner. In general, cervical and lumbosacral orthoses are less restrictive than the Halo device or a custom-molded TLSO; the more restrictive orthoses place greater limitations on the rehabilitation program. Delaying admission to an acute SCI rehabilitation unit after the orthosis is removed, however, is not usually recommended because the person with SCI can participate in many aspects of the SCI program and make significant gains. Important issues that can still be addressed include prevention of medical complications and dealing with social and psychological reactions to injury. The patients can exercise to strengthen innervated muscles, participate in training of bladder and bowel programs, engage in SCI educational programs and psychological counseling, train with adaptive equipment, and make preparations for discharge to home. Once the restrictive spinal orthosis is removed, achievement of goals in activities of daily living and mobility usually occurs swiftly. Often the rehabilitation stay can be divided: patients can participate for a shorter time period initially and then return when the orthosis is removed to complete the program and achieve their goals. It is recommended to delay wheelchair prescription while a restrictive orthosis, especially a Halo or TLSO, is in place. Once the orthosis is removed, patients can adequately trial wheelchairs before final prescription.

SPECIFIC ACTIVITIES IN THERAPY

This chapter will outline some of the key aspects of the rehabilitation of persons with SCI. The reader is referred elsewhere for details regarding specific techniques (17).

Range of Motion

ROM prevents contractures and maintains functional capabilities. Decreased ROM of a joint can result from structural bony changes as seen in heterotopic ossification or from soft tissue tightness in muscles and supportive tissues around the joint. ROM activities, whether active assisted in those areas with partial functional strength or passive in areas with minimal or no strength, should be performed at least daily.

The LOI will determine the areas requiring passive ROM. In both paraplegia and tetraplegia, the hips, knees, and ankles are of primary importance. The hips often develop flexion tightness and/or contractures secondary to frequent side-lying and sitting in a wheelchair, as well as from spasticity. Hip ROM should involve flexion and extension, abduction and adduction, and internal and external rotation. The goal of knee ROM should be to maintain a 120 degree arc. Ankle ROM occurs in all planes, but prevention of heel cord tightness and contracture is of utmost importance for proper positioning of the feet on the wheelchair footplate. Stretching of the lumbar spine is initiated when tightness or spasticity interferes with function, but is often avoided to provide the patient with increased postural stability and balance in the short and long sitting positions.

Tetraplegia introduces unique challenges not seen in paraplegia. Individuals with high-level tetraplegia (C1-4) lack active shoulder movement and can develop limited ROM with or without spasticity. Natural shoulder movements should be replicated with ROM exercises in flexion and extension, abduction and adduction, and internal and external rotation. The scapula must be stabilized with all UE ROM and brought through the normal kinematics of scapulohumeral rhythm at the elbow, flexion and extension, as well as supination and pronation, should be addressed because both elbow flexion and supination contractures can develop in individuals without active triceps function (C5 and C6 motor level patients). Existing wrist and hand motor function will determine whether a stretching or tightening program will be implemented. Individuals with high-level injuries and no motor function at the wrist or hand can have their wrist and fingers stretched to lie open and flat to accommodate the wheelchair arm tray. For those with active wrist extension and weak or no finger function, the finger flexors should not be fully stretched, but instead, allowed to tighten somewhat ("selective tightening") and naturally curl to improve grip strength and function utilizing a tenodesis action (18). Maintaining relative tightness of the long finger flexors can occur while performing finger ROM if performed properly. Tenodesis occurs as the fingers are passively flexed when the wrist is extended, and extended when the wrist is in flexion.

Mat Activities

Mat activities focus on training balance, strength, and endurance for reaching, sitting and transferring. As one of the first steps in therapy, mat activities are important to bridge the gap between immobility and functional activities. The functional goals of mat activities include training for bed mobility; preparing the individual to sit up in bed or wheelchair; preparing the individual for further complex functional activities, such as dressing and transfers; and preventing complications of a prolonged stay in bed, including deconditioning, pressure sores, atelectasis and pneumonia, orthostasis, and social isolation.

Mat activities begin with simple, passive tasks, and then progress to more active and complex tasks, including bed mobility. ROM and strengthening exercises of muscles, such as the shoulder and scapular stabilizers, that are used for functional activities are performed. As the individual progresses, rolling activities may begin. Once rolling has been achieved, the UEs and shoulders can be strengthened through the use of various prone and supine positions, such as prone-on-elbows, prone-on-hands, and supine-on-elbows. As the individual tolerates sitting up, static and dynamic balance training and pushing up on the mat should be started in preparation for transferring into the wheelchair. In individuals with paraplegia, tall kneeling and the quadruped position can also be included. All of these skills teach strengthening of the trunk and UE muscles, use of the head and neck muscles for balance and positioning, hand-eye coordination, and safety to prevent falls.

Modalities

Modalities such as heat, cold, and ultrasound can be used above the level of sensory loss. In areas that have diminished or no sensation, one must be extremely cautious when using such modalities. The risk of causing a burn is high, and, therefore, alternatives should be sought. The use of fluidotherapy or whirlpool at neutral temperatures is an alternative for the extremities.

Weight Shifts

Weight shifts are performed to prevent the occurrence of pressure ulcers. Patients need to be instructed in proper pressure relief techniques prior to sitting. The method of pressure relief will vary depending on the LOI and functional capability of the patient. Individuals with injuries at C5 and above will usually require a power wheelchair with a tilt or recline mechanism. A full-body tilt seating mechanism is preferred to the reclining type to prevent the shear forces that occur at the body-seat interface (19). Some individuals with C5 injury can perform an anterior weight shift with loops attached to the back of their wheelchair, allowing them to pull themselves back to the upright position. The forward-leaning position is accomplished by leaning forward with the chest toward the thighs at an angle greater than45 degrees from the wheelchair backrest. This position has been shown to be significantly more effective in pressure relief than tipping the wheelchair backwards to 35 or 65 degrees (20). Individuals with C6 tetraplegia lack innervation of triceps muscles and cannot support their body weight in a push-up weight shift. Instead they can perform a lateral or an anterior (forward) weight shift. When performing a lateral weight shift, the person hooks their arm over the back of the chair or through an attached loop to stabilize the trunk and assist in returning to the initial sitting position. Individuals injured at C7 or below have triceps function and are usually capable of performing independent push-up pressure reliefs; although, other forms of weight shifting should still be used to protect the shoulders from overuse injury.

Force sensing array (FSA) pressure mapping is a method used to measure the interface pressure, defined as the perpendicular force per unit area, between the body and support surface. FSA can be used to locate areas of high pressure in the patient's current wheelchair cushion and to teach which pressure relief technique provides the best results. Studies have used FSA pressure mapping to compare various wheelchair cushions with tilting and upright positions (21).

Some authors recommend that patients perform a pressure relief for 1 minute every 30 minutes while in the wheelchair (22). More recently, recommendations are that pressure reliefs need to be almost 2 minutes to fully allow for return of blood flow to the area (23). Regardless of the chosen time frame, it is critical to instill in all patients the importance of regularly scheduled weight shifts and daily skin integrity examinations. The use of a mirror will greatly enhance the ability to monitor the sacral area and ischial tuberosities.

Transfers

Transferring is a complex activity that requires motor planning, strength, and coordination. With incorrect technique, overuse or traumatic injuries may occur, as well as increasing the risk for skin breakdown.

There are many types of transfers, including between different functional surfaces, (i.e., bed to wheelchair; wheelchair to car, commode, or tub), and between level (e.g., bed to chair) and uneven surfaces (e.g., floor to chair) (24). Transfer training involves multiple components, including training the patient and the caregivers (if needed) and educating the patient to be able to give clear instructions to their caregivers.

The presence of spasticity and contractures can influence choice of transfer technique. For instance, in the presence of some spasticity, the individual may be able to weight bear even without antigravity motor strength. This allows transfer methods that require weight bearing through the LEs, for example, stand-pivot transfer, to be considered. Flaccid LEs will not allow standing without extensive bracing, thereby making transfers that require LE weight bearing impractical. Excessive spasms, however, may interfere with the safety of the transfers. Similarly, the presence of contractures in weight-bearing joints may restrict transfer method.

The wheelchair should be in proper position at a 30 to 45 degrees angle from the intended surface and locked before the transfer begins. The footrest and armrest need to be placed out of the way. Safety precautions and the avoidance of impulsive behavior are important to prevent injuries. The transfer technique used should take into account the presence of pressure ulcers at surfaces such as the sacrum and the ischial tuberosity (IT), as well as the greater trochanter. For instance, transfers with a transfer (sliding) board may result in significant shearing force on the IT, and, therefore, should be avoided if a pressure ulcer is present.

Generally speaking, individuals with paraplegia should achieve independence with transfers, whereas those with tetraplegia may have varying levels of transfer independence. In most instances, those with a motor level at or below C7 can perform independent transfers, with or without the use of a transfer board. Some individuals with a C6 LOI may also transfer independently with a transfer board. Individuals with a C5 LOI (and most patients with a C6 motor complete injury) require assistance with or without a transfer board, whereas individuals with an injury at or above the level of C4 will be dependent.

The exact transfer technique used by individuals with SCI varies tremendously. For instance, an individual with a strong upper body who can stand up with the help of an assistive device such as a walker or crutches may be able to perform a stand-pivot transfer independently. Other equipment, such as cushions to raise the seat height or mechanical devices that can help individuals with SCI to stand up, may be very helpful in transfers. The best transfer technique provides a functional solution and is safe and effective for the individual (and caregiver) concerned. This develops over time with training.

Wheelchair Training

Wheelchair training includes basic and advanced activities. Basic skills include wheelchair propulsion on level and uneven surfaces (inclines, carpet, etc.) and transfers from the wheelchair, including into the bathroom and car. The patient and family should be taught how to handle the chair on curbs and inclines, how to fold the wheelchair for placement into a car, and how to trouble shoot maintenance and simple repairs. "*Advanced wheelchair activities*" include negotiating uneven surfaces such as riding on rough terrain, independently negotiating ramps and curbs, performing wheelies, negotiating elevators and escalators, being able to fall safely, and transferring from the floor to the wheelchair. Patients below the T4 level should be independent in advanced wheelchair skills.

Standing

Standing can be achieved after SCI with the use of tilt tables or standing frames. After an acute SCI, standing has been shown to decrease hypercalciuria and may retard or lessen bone loss, although there are conflicting studies (25–29). If started early (within 4 months) and performed for at least 5 d/wk for greater than or equal to 1 hour, less bone loss has recently been reported over a 2-year period (27). Standing alone has not been shown to reverse osteoporosis after it has occurred in chronic SCI (28). Standing may decrease spasticity (30,31) and enhance bowel and bladder programs secondary to the effect of gravity.

An increase in physical self-concept scores and a decrease in depression scores have been reported with standing after SCI (32). Tilt tables can be used early in the rehabilitation process to gradually obtain a vertical position, aiding in the treatment of orthostatic hypotension. Standing should proceed with caution in patients with chronic SCI since bone mineral density is often below fracture threshold (33). There currently is no firm recommendation regarding the level of bone loss at which standing is contraindicated. The clinician should discuss with the patient the risk/benefit ratio of standing and weigh this decision based upon the time from injury, the degree of bone loss, and the perceived goals. The decision to purchase a standing frame after rehabilitation depends upon the motivation of the user to use it on a consistent basis. Standing in the frame for >1 hour at a time is not recommended if a great amount of edema develops.

AMBULATION AND LOWER EXTREMITY ORTHOTICS IN SCI

Ambulation is a primary goal of most individuals with acute SCI. All members of the rehabilitation team, including the patient, should understand the advantages and disadvantages of gait training, the levels of ambulation, and the prognosis for ambulation.

Potential physiologic benefits of walking include decreased progression of osteoporosis, reduced urinary calcinosis, reduced spasticity, improved digestion and bowel function due to the effects of gravity, and prevention of pressure ulcers (27,30,31,34–36). Walking allows access to out-of-reach objects and to areas that are not wheelchair accessible. The psychological benefits, such as allowing the individual to be at eye level with others, also should not be overlooked.

Drawbacks of ambulation, however, do exist. These include increased energy consumption, weight bearing through the UEs, and poor long-term follow-through. When comparing wheelchair propulsion to walking in the same individuals with paraplegia, walking with bilateral knee-ankle-foot orthoses (KAFOs) is slower and requires more energy. On the other hand, speed and energy cost of wheelchair propulsion approximate those for normal walking (37–39). Weight bearing through the UEs may predispose to shoulder, elbow, and wrist injuries. Many individuals who learn to ambulate with bilateral assistive devices will not continue ambulating in the long term (40).

There are four levels of ambulation: community, household, exercise ambulation, and nonambulatory (41). Community ambulators are able to transfer from sit to stand, don and doff orthotics independently, and walk at least 150 ft. Individuals able to walk independently in the home but requiring a wheelchair for longer distances are characterized as household ambulators. Exercise ambulators can stand and take a few steps using LE orthotics, but require use of parallel bars or another person for support. Finally, nonambulatory patients cannot stand or walk and are fully wheelchair dependent.

Hussey and Stauffer studied the sensation and muscle strength required for ambulation (42). Community ambulation requires bilateral hip flexion strength and unilateral knee extension strength of at least 3/5. In terms of orthotic requirements, the maximum bracing required for community ambulation is one long leg brace (i.e., KAFO) and one short leg brace (ankle foot orthosis). Proprioception was also found to be important, with community ambulation requiring intact proprioception in at least the hip and knee joints.

Waters et al. (43) also studied gait performance in SCI, but used the ambulatory motor index (AMI) instead of the standard 0 to 5 motor scoring scale. The AMI is based on motor scores of the bilateral hip flexors, hip abductors, hip extensors, knee extensors, and knee flexors. Each muscle is graded on a 0 to 3 scale, with a maximum total score of 30. The AMI is expressed as a percentage of this maximum possible score. Higher AMI scores were associated with faster gait velocity, increased cadence, decreased oxygen cost per meter of ambulation, and decreased force on UE assistive devices. An AMI of ≥60%, which correlates with a maximum of one long leg brace, was required for community ambulation. Individuals with incomplete tetraplegia required a greater AMI to ambulate than those with paraplegia, due to a decreased ability to use UE assistive devices in the tetraplegic group (43). A later study found good correlation between the AMI and the ASIA LE motor score (44).

Aside from muscle strength, other factors are also important to consider when determining if a patient will be able to ambulate. These factors include the degree of muscle tone present, ROM of the LEs, proprioception, vision, cognitive status, aerobic capacity, and motivation (45). Individuals must also be able to maintain the appropriate posture in standing, termed the "para-stance" position. When standing with bilateral long leg braces, the ankles are in slight dorsiflexion, the knees are fully extended, and the hips are in slight hyperextension. The patient leans posteriorly, with anterior hip joint stability being provided by the iliofemoral ligament and anterior capsule of the hip. In this position, the center of gravity is behind the hip joints and in front of the knee and ankle joints, thus allowing for a stable standing position (46).

Functionality of gait after SCI will depend on multiple factors. These include energy cost, independence, cosmesis, orthotic reliability, and finances. As previously mentioned, walking is slower and requires more energy than wheelchair propulsion. The patient should be independent with orthosis donning and doffing, transfers, walking, sitting, and negotiation of environmental barriers. Cosmetic factors, such as the appearance of the orthosis and resulting gait, will also influence gait utilization. The orthosis and resultant gait must be safe and reliable. Finally, the financial costs will include not just the orthosis itself but the walking aids, fitting and training, and maintenance (47).

Multiple studies have shown that most patients with an injury level at T12 or above will not become community or household ambulators. Those with lesions at L2 or below have the best prognosis for continued community ambulation (27,41,48). Overall, as reported by Waters et al., rate of community ambulation at 1 year has been estimated as follows: complete paraplegia, 5%; incomplete paraplegia, 76%; and incomplete tetraplegia, 46%. The likelihood of community ambulation at 1 year after injury can be predicted using the lower extremity motor score (LEMS) measured at 30 days after injury. For persons with complete paraplegia, the chances of walking at 1 year with a 30-day LEMS of zero is <1%, and with a score of 1 to 9 is 45%. For persons with incomplete paraplegia, the chances of walking at 1 year with a score of zero is 33%, with a score of 1 to 9 is 70%, and with a score of greater than 10 is 100%. For persons with incomplete tetraplegia, the chances of walking at 1 year with a 30-day LEMS of zero is zero, with a score of 1 to 9 is 21%, with a score of 10 to 19 is 63%, and with a score of greater than 20 is 100%. Patients with incomplete tetraplegia require greater LE strength to ambulate than those with incomplete paraplegia because of decreased ability to bear weight on the UEs (49–52). For additional information see Chapter 8.

In predicting walking during the rehabilitation stay (rather than long-term prognosis for walking), Kay et al. (53) reported on persons with traumatic SCI who were admitted to rehabilitation with a mean of 24.0 days post injury and a mean LOS in rehabilitation of 60.4 days. They found that 67.2% of persons with AIS D, 28.3% of those with AIS C, and 0.9% of those with AIS A or B ambulated at discharge. LOI (i.e., tetraplegia versus paraplegia) did not significantly affect walking in AIS grades C or D. The percentage of AIS C ambulators is less than the 67% reported by Burns et al. (54); although, in the latter study, AIS grade was assigned at the time of injury rather than at the time of rehabilitation admission, and data were collected during a time period (1984–1993) when rehabilitation LOS was longer. The rates of AIS C and D ambulation are similar to those found in studies of the nontraumatic population (55). In the study by Kay et al., being 50 years of age or older had a significant negative affect on walking in persons with AIS D, but not AIS C injuries. In other studies, age less than 50 years in AIS C subjects has been shown to have a positive influence on prognosis for ambulation (54,56). The differences may be related to LOS in rehabilitation or to the small sample sizes in each of these studies. Further work in this area is needed.

Even with the above statistics and guidelines in mind, there is still debate over which patients should undergo gait training. We believe that all patients with the potential for ambulation should be given a trial if desired. Each individual should be allowed to discover for himself or herself whether ambulation is feasible. The entire team, including the patient and family, should be clear as to the goals of gait training. For patients with thoracic-level complete injuries, however, gait training should not be initiated until the patient is independent at the wheelchair level, since the majority will utilize the wheelchair as their primary means of mobility.

Ambulation training should take into consideration the types of gait patterns and orthotic devices available, as well as the energy expenditure required. There are two main gait patterns: swing-through and reciprocal. Swing-through gait with crutches is typically used by individuals with complete paraplegia and requires bilateral KAFOs to stabilize the knees.

The arms are used to lift and swing the body forward during the swing phase, while the para-stance position is used for stance phase control. This gait pattern has an average speed of 64% slower than normal ambulation, yet requires an oxygen uptake of 38% more than normal (40,48). Patients lacking the upper body strength or balance required to swing the legs in front of the hands may use a swing-to gait, in which the feet land slightly behind the hands, or drag-to gait, in which the legs do not clear the ground.

A reciprocal (alternating) gait pattern can be used by individuals with hip flexion strength of at least 3/5, or by those able to compensate for absent hip flexion by lifting the hip and performing a posterior pelvic tilt to advance the leg. In patients who can reciprocally ambulate, LEMS is the main determinant of walking ability and is directly related to speed and cadence of ambulation. Oxygen cost of ambulation decreases with an increase in LEMS (44). Even when hip flexion and knee extension strength is sufficient such that KAFOs are not required, reciprocal gait for an individual with SCI still requires an oxygen consumption 15% greater than able-bodied walking (40). Many orthotics, such as the Parawalker, reciprocating gait orthosis (RGO), advanced RGO (ARGO), and Parastep, can facilitate a reciprocal gait pattern and will be discussed below.

ORTHOTICS

Conventional KAFOs, or long leg braces, include a metal double-upright AFO with the addition of knee joints, thigh uprights, and a proximal thigh band. The ankle may have either a posterior pin, allowing for passive dorsiflexion, or both anterior and posterior pins. The knee may be straight-set or offset, with either a ratchet lock or drop lock. Ratchet locks have a catching mechanism that operates in increments as the knee is extended, making this lock advantageous for individuals with knee flexion contractures. Drop locks require full knee extension prior to locking, and fine motor coordination skills are needed to unlock the two drop locks on either side of each brace.

KAFOs may also be made out of thermoplastic, with the advantages of lighter weight, a more cosmetic appearance, and the ability to interchange shoes. Plastic KAFOs, however, cannot be readily modified. Adjustments available at the ankle joint are minimal, and the brace cannot be easily cut down into an AFO if needed. Because of the increased potential for skin breakdown with any changes in fit, a limb with fluctuating edema, increased tone, or decreased sensation may be better served by a KAFO with metal uprights.

Another variation on the KAFO is the Craig-Scott orthosis (CSO) (Fig. 17.5). The CSO is a double-upright KAFO with offset knee joints, bail lock, ankle joint with anterior and posterior pin stops set at 5 to 10 degrees of dorsiflexion, a cushioned heel, and a steel soleplate extending beyond the metatarsal heads. There is a crossbar at the ankle to provide mediolateral stability, an anterior tibial band, and a rigid posterior thigh band. The crossbar at the ankle makes the CSO heavier than a conventional KAFO. The bail lock is a horizontal semicircular lever behind the knee that is attached to the knee joint on each side of the brace. The knee unlocks when the lever is pulled up.

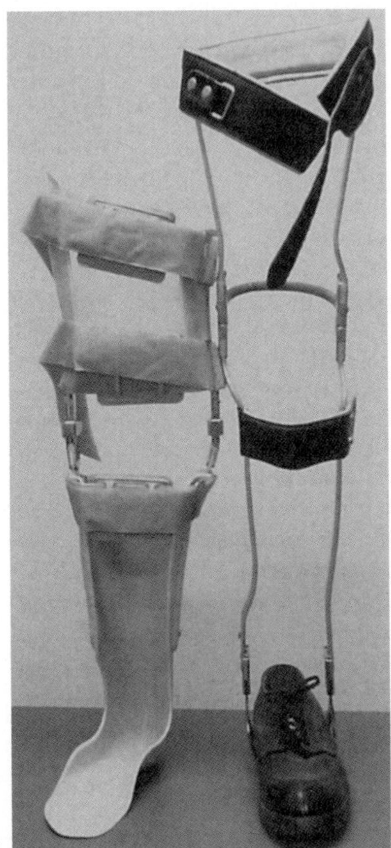

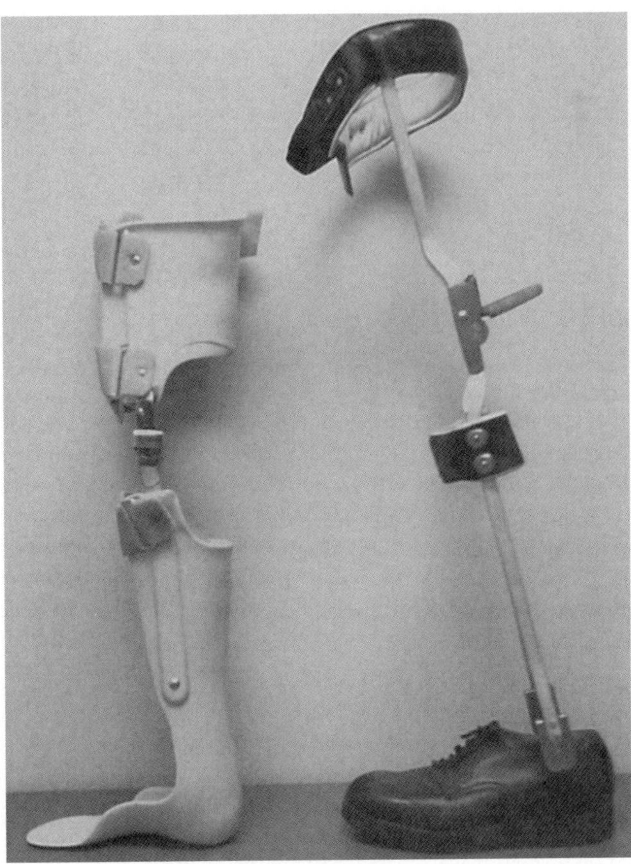

FIGURE 17.5. Knee-ankle-foot orthosis, (**left**) plastic molded, and **right** CSO. **A**: Frontal view. **B**: Lateral view.

The CSO has several advantages when compared with the conventional KAFO. Static standing is more stable with a CSO because the ankle is fixed in dorsiflexion. The bail lock allows the medial and lateral knee joints to be unlocked simultaneously by leaning against a chair. This permits the patient to maintain bilateral UE support on crutches while transferring to a sitting position. The offset knee joint provides an extension moment at the knee, decreasing stress on the locking mechanism and making it easier to unlock. The cushioned heel allows for a softer landing and improved rollover. Gait with a CSO is more energy efficient than with a conventional KAFO, requiring 31% less kcal/min when ambulating with a walker and 25% less kcal/min when ambulating with crutches (57). Disadvantages of the CSO include a greater cost and increased difficulty with standing from the floor due to the fixed ankle. The bail locks may be accidentally unlocked by bumping against objects in the environment, resulting in falls. A four-point gait, in which one leg is moved while the other leg and both crutches are in contact with the floor, is also more difficult with a CSO than a KAFO.

In contrast, advantages of the KAFO include more stability at the knee joint provided by drop locks and additional calf and thigh bands. Standing from the floor and ambulating with a four-point gait are easier than with a CSO. Progression from KAFO to AFO is also easier than with a CSO because the brace can be worn with the knees unlocked. KAFOs are less costly and are easier to cut down into an AFO. Disadvantages include the difficulty associated with donning and doffing the brace and locking and unlocking drop locks, decreased stability in standing, and a less energy efficient gait.

The Swivel Walker enables children with lesions below C6 to ambulate without the use of other walking aids. It consists of a rigid body frame with swiveling foot plates. Ambulation is accomplished by rocking to alternate sides, so that one foot plate is lifted off the ground. The frame then automatically swivels forward under the influence of gravity. Use of the Swivel Walker generally requires assistance to don and doff and to achieve a standing position. Ambulation is slow and restricted to a level surface (47).

The RGO allows for a reciprocal gait pattern with use of a walker or crutches for stabilization. Consisting of bilateral hip KAFO with trunk support, the RGO has Bowden cables linking the orthotic hip joints such that extension of one hip causes the other to flex. In order to take a step, the body is tilted laterally over the stance leg, so that the swing leg is cleared off the floor. Extension of the trunk causes extension of the stance hip. The cables transmit force to the swing hip, which flexes, resulting in a forward step. Gait velocity with the RGO is slow, ranging from 11 to 14 m/min (compared with normal walking speed of 60 to 90 m/min). The energy cost of RGO walking is three to four times greater than normal slow walking (58–60). The abandonment rate of the RGO is high, ranging from 10% to 58% due to discomfort, difficulty donning or doffing the brace, slow speed compared with wheelchair propulsion, or poor fit (61,62).

The RGO may also be used in conjunction with functional electric stimulation (FES). The hybrid orthosis, called the RGO-II, includes a four-channel stimulator with electrodes on the bilateral quadriceps and hamstrings. Pressing one switch that is mounted on a rollator walker will activate the quadriceps and contralateral hamstring, producing the swing phase and contralateral push-off. Pushing both switches simultaneously produces bilateral hip and knee extension, allowing the patient to stand up without assistance. Gait speed with the RGO-II is one fifth of normal (63). Addition of FES to the RGO reduces energy cost by 16% at average walking speeds of 12.5 m/min (64).

In comparison with the RGO, the ARGO has a single control cable that connects to both legs. The technique for taking a forward step is similar to the RGO, but the ARGO is designed to reduce friction and allow the user to transfer from sit to stand or stand to sit more easily. Knee-lock cables connect the hip and knee joints, so that activation of only one lever is required to sit and to stand. When the hip joints are extended, the knee joints automatically lock. Speed of ambulation with the ARGO ranges from 9.6 to 19.8 m/min, again significantly slower than normal walking. Energy cost is approximately eight times higher than normal walking (47,65,66).

The Hip guidance orthosis (HGO), also called the Orlau Parawalker, allows individuals with thoracic paraplegia to ambulate with a reciprocal gait and crutches. It consists of a rigid body brace connected to bilateral KAFOs. The hip joints resist adduction/abduction and have adjustable flexion/extension stops. The knee joints are locked during ambulation and have release mechanisms for sitting. Ambulation is achieved by leaning forward, putting the hips in full extension, and shifting the weight toward the stance side. The swing leg moves forward under the influence of gravity (67). Walking speed with the HGO ranges from 9.8 to 16.9 m/min, and the energy cost is 4.9 times that of normal walking (59,60,68,69).

Like the RGO, the HGO may be used in conjunction with FES. This hybrid orthosis has two channels, with stimulation over the gluteal musculature during stance phase. The stimulation is activated by switches on the crutch handles. Addition of FES reduces energy cost of HGO ambulation by 6% to 8%, with a minimal improvement in speed (70). When comparing the HGO with the RGO, RGO-II, and KAFOs, the combination of RGO with FES (RGO-II) requires the least energy expenditure. The RGO and HGO require a moderate amount of energy, and KAFOs require the greatest expenditure of energy (64,71).

The Parastep is a transcutaneous FES system that allows for reciprocal gait. Electrodes are placed over the bilateral quadriceps muscles to promote knee extension, the bilateral common peroneal nerves to induce a hip flexion reflex, and over bilateral paraspinals or gluteus maximus for trunk stability. The electrodes are connected to a microprocessor unit worn by the patient. The microprocessor is connected to a walker with control switches, allowing for the following commands: stand up, sit down, left step, right step, increase stimulation, and decrease stimulation. Candidates for the Parastep should have a complete thoracic SCI with an intact lumbar and sacral spinal cord. The individual must be able to transfer independently and have intact skin at stimulation sites. Contraindications include a history of long bone stress fractures or osteoporosis, a history of cardiac or respiratory disease, LMN injury, severe scoliosis, morbid obesity, and an implanted cardiac or phrenic nerve pacemaker. Potential benefits of Parastep include an increased muscle mass in the LEs, improved work capacity, decreased spasticity, and improvement in self-concept. Gait velocity with the Parastep ranges from 5 to 14.5 m/min in trained users (72,73).

LOCOMOTOR TRAINING TO REGAIN WALKING FUNCTION

Rehabilitation approaches to facilitate locomotion recovery after SCI have recently been directed away from compensatory strategies (as described above) toward an "activity-based therapy" called locomotor training (LT). LT can best be described as repetitive stepping on a treadmill while using an overhead harness connected to a body weight support system (BWS). Such a BWS treadmill training (BWSTT) system allows for unloading and loading of body weight, improved head, neck and trunk postural alignment, and improved coordination of the lower limbs. This form of rehabilitation therapy was first proposed in the 1980s (74–76), and the efficacy of LT using BWSTT for walking has been extensively researched in animal studies (77–79) and in humans after SCI (76,80–90). Research and commercial development of LT as a rehabilitation therapy has also included development of different BWS systems, robotics, and multimodality approaches to LT.

Evidence from studies on cats demonstrated that after complete transaction, the spinal cord can generate rhythmic movements, resulting in locomotion (91). Initially, the cats were partially supported by a sling around the trunk, and manual assistance was given to provide rhythmic step-like movements of the hind limbs. With continued training, the body support was reduced as locomotion skills improved. After several weeks, the cats could support more of their weight and demonstrated more coordinated stepping movements. The LT provided sensory input into the spinal cord without supraspinal or proprioceptive input, suggesting that movement patterns associated with ambulation can be generated by neurons within the spinal cord. These neurons are known as locomotor or spinal central pattern generators (CPGs) (86,91).

Human studies on LT using BWSTT and manual assistance have reported favorable effects on gait patterns of patients with neurological impairments. Supporting a percentage of body weight while walking on a treadmill symmetrically unloads the LEs and improves timing and structure of leg pattern activity compared to walking with full body weight (80,87–90,92–94). The interaction between LT and BWSTT is important to optimize locomotor movement patterns and ultimately achieve full weight bearing for people with SCI who have incomplete motor function impairment (i.e., AIS C and D) (74,76,81,83,86,90,92,94,95). Loading of the legs (84,96,97), speed of stepping (98), and leg kinematics (99) provide sensory information and facilitate activity-dependent plasticity within the spinal cord to control movement (84,85,96,97). Optimizing these sensory cues with LT using BWSTT can result in improvement of locomotor patterns even within a single stepping session (84,85,96,97,100). Also, after a severe (neurologically complete) SCI, individuals can generate standing and stepping patterns with significant EMG activity recorded during LT when provided with BWS and manual assistance (84,85,96–99,101–103). In addition, there is an improved muscle activation pool (104) and functional response to extended bouts of LT using BWS (100).

TYPES OF LOCOMOTOR TRAINING

There are several different approaches to LT using BWS for individuals after an incomplete or a complete SCI, including (a) suspension systems using an overhead pulley versus pneumatic control, (b) LT with and without FES, (c) robotics for the automation of LT, and (d) a combination of these modalities.

Body Weight Support Suspension Systems

Wernig and Müller (80) used a commercial driven treadmill with variable speed control and a parachute harness suspended from the ceiling by a set of pulleys to train eight persons with incomplete SCI and found significant locomotion gains in the utilization of paralyzed limbs. The system allowed for a variable degree of BWS, and the legs and arms could move freely. Hicks et al. (105) used an LT device called the Woodway Locosystem (Woodway USA, Inc., Foster, CT, USA) treadmill, which allowed for BWS via an overhead system with weight counterbalance. More recently, researchers have used pneumatic BWS (88,106) to counterbalance weight; the harness is connected to an overhead motorized or pneumatic lift (Neuro II, Vigor Equipment Inc., Stevensville, MI 49127) suspended over the treadmill. The advantage of pneumatic systems is the promotion of a loading and unloading walking pattern that is analogous to able-bodied gait.

Within the clinical environment, there are several other different BWS systems, including LiteGait (Tempe, Arizona), Biodex Unweighing system (Biodex Medial Systems, Shirley, New York), and Robomedica (Irvine, CA). These systems differ relative to design and cost. The Biodex system has a single-point or single position suspension to an overhead bar with attachment rings connected to a BWS harness. The LiteGait includes a 4-buckle system with a 2-point attachment. Both LiteGait and Biodex can be used on treadmills or over ground. The Robomedica is a closed loop pneumatic BWS system equipped with a pneumatic lift, an overhead harness and a treadmill. The treadmill and wheelchair ramp are elevated, with seating provided on each side of treadmill for accessibility to the lower limb and foot by a therapist during training. Computer interface is provided for continuous control of BWS. A similar type of system is the Therastride from Innoventor Engineering (St Louis, MO), which includes an integrated pneumatic system with a hardware-software interface to control both treadmill and BWS. An advantage of systems designed to accommodate manual assistance is that the experienced trainer or therapist is able to perceive the level of assistance needed for stepping. The trainer can guide the support needed at the trunk and/or foot during each stepping motion. Disadvantages, however, may involve the physical effort required by three therapists (or technicians) to assist the patient while stepping (107–109) and therapist fatigue, which may limit training.

Functional Electrical Stimulation with LT

A combination approach to LT is described by Field-Fote (107) who used FES with LT and BWS to examine the effect on overground walking speed and treadmill speed for individuals with chronic incomplete SCI. The swing phase of gait was assisted with FES "by using flexion withdrawal response by electrical stimulation to the peroneal nerve of the more impaired limb." During the training sessions, the FES eliminated the use of manual assistance on the treadmill; the amount of treadmill speed and BWS were adjusted to allow subjects to walk as fast as possible while maintaining proper kinematics. For overground walking, individuals were strapped into a harness (for safety) suspended from a ceiling mounted track and trolley assembly; individuals were able to use orthotic devices without the use of BWS or FES when walking overground. The LT-FES combination resulted in a 75% increase in mean overground walking speed (initial mean (and standard deviation) walking speed: 12 (±0.8) m/s to final mean (and standard deviation), 21(±0.15) m/s).

Robotic Training

An alternative to manually assisted LT employs robotics to automate gait retraining (107–109,111). The suggested advantage of a robotic-assisted locomotor setup (108,109) is that it allows for consistent bilateral coordinated stepping consistent with normal kinematics of human gait. Wirz et al. (109) and other authors (111,112) have reported on the effectiveness of LT with a computer-controlled, driven-gait orthosis (DGO) ("Lokomat," Hocoma AG, Zurich, Switzerland) to increase functional mobility in persons with chronic, motor incomplete SCI. With this device, bilateral exoskeleton leg braces are secured to the person at the pelvis and throughout the LE by adjustable cuffs. The ankle is secured in a neutral (90 degree) position by elastic straps around the metatarsal head. The orthosis is adjustable for length of the thigh and lower leg and for position of the leg braces. The individual is supported over a motorized treadmill using a counterweight BWS unloading system, with suspension straps around the breast, waist, and legs. The motorized exoskeleton generates passive guided leg movements consistent with normal gait. Actuators at each joint (knee and hip) are controlled by a position controller. Control of postural stability and setup of the DGO, including user interface and generation of a physiological standardized gait pattern, are described by Colombo et al. (111,112).

Wirz et al. (109) performed a multisite trial using the Lokomat on 20 individuals with incomplete chronic SCI, 16 of whom were able to ambulate overground (greater than 10 m) before the study; although only 4 used ambulation as their only mode of mobility. Overground walking speed and endurance improved for all the ambulators. Only two persons improved according to the WISCI II scale, and all individuals who were nonambulatory at the start were nonambulatory at the end. Hornby et al. (108) described a case series of three subjects (all AIS C, acute and chronic) using the Lokomat to improve functional walking performance. All participants started training using the robotic device and transitioned to LT using manual assistance. This transition occurred when individuals could generate normal stepping kinematics with assistance by one therapist "and assistive devices and braces as required." Two of the three subjects showed an improved WISCI II score.

To date, much of the research in robotic rehabilitation for gait has focused on the Lokomat, but other robotic gait trainers have been developed for the neurologically impaired population (107,113–118). At this time, however, robotic designs are limited by the degrees of freedom to move the joints in the LE. This limitation would potentially effect the repetitive training response of the lower limb; to potentially affect functional performance.

Field-Fote (92) compared walking outcomes for four different LT approaches; 27 subjects with chronic motor incomplete SCI were randomly assigned to one of four groups: BWSTT and manual assistance, BWSTT and FES, overground training using BWS and FES, and robotic training (Lokomat). Across all groups, there was a significant improvement in walking speed, but no significant difference was found between the four treatment approaches. The greatest improvements occurred in those with the slowest walking speeds at baseline. None of the subjects in the study became community ambulators; however, improvements were noted in household ambulation.

LT: Randomized Controlled Trials

Most of the reported research on LT is based on nonrandomized clinical studies in persons with chronic incomplete SCI, where no control or comparison groups were used and a wide range of outcome measures and varying intensities and durations of training were employed (81,86,88,89,103,105,119,120). Only one randomized multicenter controlled trial (RCT) of LT has been performed in persons with acute incomplete SCI (103). This trial compared BWSTT to a control group and found no significant differences in locomotor Functional Independence Measure (FIM) scores or overground walking speed between the two groups 6 months following randomization (107). Results in both groups were better than generally reported in longitudinal studies of recovery of ambulation, with 92% of AIS C and 100% of AIS D subjects ambulating at the end of treatment with a median speed of 1.0 m/s. However, it is important to note some key aspects of this study. First, the control group received up to 1 hour each day of overground mobility training, including standing or stepping. Second, the control group's outcomes were much better than expected, as previous trials found that less than 60% of AIS C patients were ambulating at discharge from inpatient rehabilitation. While inclusion/exclusion criteria may have resulted in a sample of people with better prognosis for recovery, the authors suggested that early intensive weight bearing with repetitive standing and stepping provided task-specific practice that may have contributed to higher functional outcomes than expected.

A recent Cochrane Report incorporated this RCT sample with samples from other clinical trials ($N = 222$) (121) to evaluate efficacy of LT using BWS compared to overground training on ambulation speed and endurance. The four RCTs used different training interventions, different dosing strategies (training sessions per week and total number of training sessions), and different participant demographics (years postinjury, age, etc). There were no significant differences in walking outcomes measures between the different interventions (overground, robotic, or treadmill). Although there are limitations, based on this review there is currently insufficient evidence that any one LT strategy improves walking recovery more than any other for SCI patients. Missing from the literature are (a) an RCT to compare LT to "regular or traditional therapy" and (b) a comprehensive LT predictor model for a "walking outcome measure" using input variables such as treatment dosage, intensity (speed and BWS), and number of treatment sessions, motor score, and progression. Further study is, therefore, needed.

Benefits Beyond the Improvement of Standing and Walking

Beyond using the activity-based therapy of LT for improvement of walking, a number of studies have examined its efficacy on health and physical fitness for individuals after SCI.

Predominantly, the research has concentrated on muscle composition and metabolism, fat mass, bone mass, and cardiovascular factors (100,104,122–128). Although LT may attenuate bone loss (104), for LT to be proven effective in preventing or minimizing bone loss after SCI, research needs to determine the optimum intensity of loading, velocity of treadmill, duration of training at low BWS, and the frequency of training per week.

A number of studies have reported positive results for LT in improving muscle atrophy below the LOI, specifically for improving muscle mass and muscle volume. Stewart et al. (128) trained individuals with chronic incomplete SCI for 6 months (3×/wk) and demonstrated changes in muscle phenotype including hypertrophy and increased oxidative capacity, which subsequently reflected a change in ambulatory capacity. Atrophy, a result of SCI, is a potential source of fatigue due to the large number of motor units required to perform a walking task. LT may counteract this effect by inducing relative muscle hypertrophy. With continued LT and repetitive load-bearing stepping, the hypertrophy would enhance torque around the hip, knee, and ankle joint. Theoretically, improved torque would translate to improvement in walking or standing ability. Along with hypertrophy, the level of muscle activation (shown by EMG activity) would increase a prerequisite for the task of standing or walking. Some authors (127) have suggested that an increase in muscle mass seen with LT may also improve glucose tolerance and increase metabolic rate, leading to less fat deposits and improved skin integrity. This, in turn, may reduce seating pressure and increase peripheral blow flow to reduce pressure ulcers.

Other Activity-Based Therapy

There has been great excitement for activity-based therapies (ABT), in regard to the potential to improve motor activation for functional activities. Specifics include LT (as discussed above), FES (Chapter 25), and task-specific training. All of these interventions are strategies to "stimulate the nervous system" to optimize functional recovery, eliciting abilities initially thought to be lost. Recovery may be via neuroplasticity and reorganization of the nervous system (129). Activity-based programs will also have benefits beyond motor function, including organ system benefits such as cardiac function; health including on bone, muscle, and glucose metabolism; and quality of life.

Much of the work on ABT has been performed with locomotion. Currently, a network of rehabilitation centers whose staffs have been trained in intensive activity-based treatments is working together as part of the NeuroRecovery Network with funding from the Christopher and Dana Reeve Foundation and the Center for Disease Control, to develop and expand access to such therapy to create a comprehensive database to track the success of activity-based therapeutic interventions, identify optimal locomotor training regimens and maintain administrative network that can supply logistical, technical, and personnel-based support for rehabilitation programs. Preliminary results have shown improvements in trunk control, endurance, speed of walking and balance, ability to perform ADL, and decreased dependence on caregivers. In addition, other benefits were seen in cardiovascular, pulmonary, bladder function and bone density, and overall physical well-being and quality of life (130).

Targeting directly the proposed CPG in the lumbar cord, Herman et al. reported on a subject with an incomplete SCI who after LT and implantation of an epidural stimulator (at L2 level) regained the ability to ambulate (131). An additional patient was reported later (132); however, over time increased stimulation was required and there has been no recent follow-up.

There has been question as to whether ABT can enhance neurological (as opposed to functional) recovery, specifically conversion of a neurologically complete to incomplete injury. McDonald et al. reported that after ABT including FES therapy (1 hour 3 times per week), a single subject improved to ASIA C after 5 years, with a 10-fold reduction of rate of infection and use of antibiotics (133). No other reports or prospective trials have been reported to support this and late recovery years after SCI has been reported (134). A prospective trial is needed before neurological change of complete to incomplete injury (as opposed to functional recovery) can be attributed to ABT.

Assistive Technology Devices

Assisted Technology Devices (ATDs) include any product or piece of equipment, whether acquired commercially or customized, that is used to increase, maintain, or improve functional capabilities of an individual with a disability (135). ATDs may be the key to independence for persons with SCI, becoming valuable tools for basic life skills and improving social, recreational, and vocational activities. The person's LOI will determine which ATDs are appropriate. A comprehensive evaluation by an assistive technology specialist and a trial period are important for the correct ATDs to be prescribed. Technology is improving at a rapid speed; therefore, newer modifications of equipment may be available.

Prior to prescribing assistive devices, it is important to identify the patient's capabilities, goals, and environmental barriers. The assessment should incorporate a thorough medical history, current functional status, level of cognition, and mood (i.e., easily frustrated, motivation). This includes testing the patient's strength and ROM, as well as his or her positioning and sitting balance in bed and wheelchair, degree of spasticity, and auditory and visual capability. A trial period should be followed by a prescription and letter of justification to access the funding needed. The proper vendor, especially for high-level devices, is crucial for proper service and delivery.

ATDs can be separated into low versus high level. Low-level technology includes everyday tools such as desktop and feeding items as well as telephone systems; high-level technology includes complex electronic or battery operated devices that require more detailed programming, trialing, and means for funding. Low-level technology items are more affordable and may be commercially available or custom made for the client.

Low-Level Devices

Desktop items are important for vocational and recreational activities, and for socialization. In individuals with a NLI of C1-4, this may include a computer with voice recognition software or a mouth stick with a docking station. For word processing, voice activated systems are available commercially. For those with a lower NLI (C5-7), items such as a Wanchik writer, typing peg, or a universal cuff with a pen/pencil can be prescribed for writing (Figs. 17.3 and 17.4). Adaptive devices for reading in high-level clients may include a battery operated page turner or newer technology (i.e., E-Reader, SONY;

Kindle, Amazon); while for those individuals with lower levels of injury, a typing peg with or without a bookstand is appropriate.

Assistive devices for feeding are extremely important. Items include an MAS or BFO (Fig. 17.1), with a table or wheelchair mount for individuals with C4-5 levels of injury. For persons with a C5-6 motor level, a plate guard or scoop dish, Dycem, long straw, horizontal or vertical fork/spoon, universal cuff, or dorsal splint can be prescribed. (Fig. 17.2)

High-Level ATDs

Electronic aids for daily living (E-ADLs), previously known as ECUs, are devices that either act as remote controls for any electronic equipment or can be modified with electrical power to be controlled through a switch, voice activation, computer interface, or adaptor. The E-ADL is the control center for almost any aspect of the environment, including the patient's radio, television, bed, computer, lights, fan, thermostat controls, etc. An ECU can allow the individual to remain home alone for a short period of time without assistance. Prior to prescribing an E-ADL, one should consider if low-level technology or a commercially available device could meet the goal. Some resources for E-ADLs include www.abledata.com, www.resna.org, www.NATRI.uky.edu, and www.AbilityHub.com/ecu. As technology continues to improve and become commercially available, it may obviate the need for specialized devices. Examples include voice-activated systems for computers, light switches, and so on.

The E-ADL has multiple components, including the control unit, display unit (auditory or visual), switch, and needed cables. The control method may be through infrared, ultrasound, AC house wiring, or radio waves (136). For details regarding the mode of control and switches, the reader is referred elsewhere (137,138).

When addressing high-level ATDs, it is necessary to determine the type of adaptive switch for activation. A person can essentially use any body part to activate a switch as long as he or she can perform the activity consistently with accuracy. Reliable sites can include the head, chin, mouth, shoulder, arm, or hand. Voice activation is also an option. The patient's overall capability (i.e., cognitive status and functional movements) as well as the environment in which the ATD will be utilized should be evaluated to choose the appropriate switch. The Bains Assistive Technology System is an evaluation tool that can determine the proper switch for the individual. It includes four components: the patient, task, device, and environment. The switch's function can be single (on/off activation), dual (i.e., allows scanning and selection options for an ECU or computer), or multiple (i.e., joystick for greater capability). Switch operation can be momentary (remains activated as long as pressure is maintained), latching (stays on/off until switch is activated again), or proportional (degree of activity varies by amount of pressure applied). The switch can be mounted on the patient, their wheelchair, bed, or desk. An ECU can interface with other devices, such as a power wheelchair, and, by connecting a remote ECU package to the serial port in the wheelchair, the client can use a switch already set up for driving as the means to access the ECU. The e-ADL system is only as good as the user's access to it, so it should be placed such that the individual will be comfortable and easily able to activate it. Options for switches available include eye blink or eye tracking, pneumatic, rocker, tongue touch keypad, wobble, pillow, voice activated, scatir, and head array (137).

Phone. Telephone access is an important basic skill to allow for socialization as well in case of medical emergencies. Technological advances in communication have enabled disabled individuals to access telephones independently and privately. Evaluation for telephone access should include the patient's cognitive status, voice quality, endurance, physical ability, environment, and funding sources. Consideration must also be given to the individual's goals and prior experience with cell phone use.

For persons with **C1-4** levels of injury, access to a land line can be via an ECU with telephone functions. The phone features built into the ECU allow for a directory, dial, and hang up, and the system can be controlled by switch or voice. Cell phones with Bluetooth technology mounted either bedside or on the wheelchair can be activated through an appropriate switch or voice activation. Some cell phones are also designed with voice recognition programs to make and receive calls and to access phone features. Another option for the individual who does not have a cell phone is a stand-alone speaker phone with switch or voice activation, making it totally hands free. Keypad functions are possible with use of an adaptive device (i.e., typing peg) or for the able-bodied person. A wireless remote with set distance range allows the individual to be away from the base.

For persons with **C5-7** injuries, low-level ATDs are used. Any telephone or cell phone with or without a wireless headset can be adapted and accessed with an assistive device. Cell phones with Bluetooth technology are extremely useful.

Computers. Persons with SCI can access and utilize a computer in many ways. Individuals with a NLI below C5 can access the computer with their UEs through basic adaptations and assistive devices such as typing pegs. If the patient is unable to use a traditional mouse, a trackball can be tried. For clients with a C1-4 NLI, accessing the computer will require a higher level of assistive technology. This may be via a voice activated or eye-gaze system; some type of operation with their mouth is the next best option.

If the patient is able to use a standard keyboard, there are many software packages available to improve accessibility. StickyKeys is designed for people who cannot hold down two or more keys at a time; it enables the user to press one key at a time instead of pressing them simultaneously (e.g., for use of Shift, Ctrl, or Alt). FilterKeys can be used to ignore brief or repeated keystrokes or to slow the repeat rate. Rate enhancement software will type an entire word after an abbreviation (programmed by the user) is entered. Word prediction software, which generates a list of most frequently used words after a letter is typed, also speeds the rate of typing.

If the patient is unable to access a standard keyboard, there are many alternative options. A keyguard with holes over the keys can be fit over a standard keyboard. Other nonstandard keyboards include onscreen, mini, enlarged, and alternate key arrangement. The onscreen keyboard graphically depicts a keyboard on the computer screen. Letters can be selected using a touch screen and mouth stick, by scanning with a single switch, or by using the mouse or a joystick to point and click. A touch pad can be used, especially if the user can be accurate in pointing with one finger. One can also use a foot mouse for individuals with no functional use of their hands, but with use of their feet (i.e., central cord syndrome). The addition of word prediction software saves keystrokes. The mini keyboard can be used for those with limited ROM who are unable to reach all of the keys on a standard keyboard. An enlarged keyboard is useful for people who have trouble with accuracy. This keyboard also requires very little pressure to activate the keys.

Voice recognition software allows the individual to control any mouse or keyboard functions through use of speech. Adequate voice quality and endurance are essential for accuracy and reliability. To determine if voice recognition is an option for the individual, a tutorial program should be completed prior to purchase. In ventilator-dependent persons, training is required, and their ability to use the software can vary according to level of fatigue, secretions, or noise from the ventilator or environment. Voice recognition software has become less expensive, and better technology is making this method of input a popular choice for all neurological levels of injury. Some voice activated software programs include Dragon Dictate, MacSpeech Dictate:ILIsten, L&H Voice Express, and IBMvia voice. Each program has different features, and knowing the details of each will assist in selection of the correct system.

The head pointer and eye gaze systems are options for high-level patients. In the head pointer system, the user wears a reflective dot on his/her head. A camera mounted on top of the monitor detects the location of the dot and translates it into an onscreen cursor. The user then moves his head very slightly to move the cursor. This system is used with an onscreen keyboard; when the cursor is on a key, the user must "dwell" there for a predetermined period of time to activate the key. Extremely good head and neck control is required. The eye gaze system uses a camera and infrared light to track the user's eye movements, and these movements are translated into an onscreen cursor. Clicks are performed by an eye blink, eye dwelling, or by use of a mechanical switch. Examples of eye gaze products include the Tracker 2000 (Madentec), Mytobii D10 (Window XP base product by Iubi Technologies Inc.), and the Erica standard system (Eye Response Technologies).

Neural Interface Technology

Neural interface technology, also called brain-computer interface (BCI), is a direct communication pathway between the brain and an external device that has the potential to promote neuroplasticity and functional recovery. In a typical BCI, neural signals are recorded and decoded that can be used to control movement of a computer cursor or other external device, such as a robotic arm or a communication aid (i.e., controlling a computer for typing). There is a broad range of devices and systems for neural recording, varying for instance in terms of invasiveness of placing the electrodes (139), and has been described as a potential rehabilitation tool to promote functional recovery for persons with stroke and SCI (140–143).

Exciting possibilities in SCI include the combination of BCI with FES, whereby motor cortical is used to directly control FES devices to control paralyzed limbs, bypassing the injured spinal cord (144,145). CyberKinetics initiated a clinical trial implanting a few patients with the BrainGate system, although this trial has recently been on hold. Further study is forthcoming.

Home Exercise Program

At discharge from acute rehabilitation, all patients should receive an individualized home exercise program (HEP). The HEP should not be new to the patient, but rather should reflect what the patient has been working on in the clinical setting. Key features of the HEP include weight shifting, skin care, and a balanced shoulder strengthening program. All home exercises should be reviewed with the family as well, if they are needed to assist. A database helpful for designing a HEP can be found at www.physiotherapyexercises.com.

Initially upon discharge, home care services may be beneficial. A home care therapist will not only perform a home safety evaluation and assist with training in functional tasks but also assist with and supervise the HEP. Once the client is admitted to an outpatient program, the HEP should be performed on the days that they do not attend therapy. After all outpatient therapy goals have been achieved, the client can then be referred to a local gym or wellness center, with periodic reevaluations by the physician and therapy team.

SPINAL CORD EDUCATION

Formal classes in spinal cord education for patients and families should be held. Topics should include anatomy and classification of SCI; medical issues regarding bowel, bladder, skin, and AD; adjustment to disability issues; sexuality and fertility; and research topics in SCI. As lengths of stay shorten, starting these classes as soon as possible is of great importance. However, formal classes alone are not sufficient. All members of the team should perform spinal cord education. Bedside teaching by the nurses to reinforce proper bowel and bladder techniques and the importance of skin checks with a mirror cannot be over emphasized. Knowledge of the symptoms of AD and going through the steps of management may prove life saving once the patient is discharged. Reviewing proper techniques for ROM, proper placement of splints, and transfer techniques to all surfaces should be incorporated as part of therapy time.

HOME MODIFICATIONS FOR PEOPLE WITH SCI

Evaluating the home for wheelchair accessibility is an important aspect of the rehabilitation process. The patient and family's participation is needed to gather information and begin planning for discharge. A home assessment form will provide the basis for potential home modifications. This form should request measurements of doorways, hallways, and rooms, provide a floor plan, and identify all entries into the home. Photographs are a valuable addition to this process.

The prognosis, age, functional strength, and skill of the SCI individual are factors that will influence the types of home modifications that are recommended. For example, one needs to take into consideration the use of a manual versus power wheelchair and UE strength for opening doors. Goals regarding to return to work or school, the need for a work station, and the social and financial situation (including how much assistance is needed) should also be evaluated before making recommendations. A temporary plan can be made if significant modifications are needed. It is important to keep the home environment as similar as possible to before the accident, and the client's feelings regarding any changes should be discussed.

Modifications to the entrances, bedroom, bathroom, and kitchen will often be needed, and general safety issues should also be addressed (146). Specific recommendations will be discussed below. The rehabilitation team should be familiar with contractors and architects in the local area and have information from previous clients available for the family. In addition, family members may want to see other modified homes before going forward with their own modifications.

Entrances

The entire area from the car to the front door must be evaluated, making sure that the surface is smooth and level. Outdoor walkways must accommodate a slope of 20 inches of length to every 1 inch in height as the maximum grade. Ramps (temporary or permanent) should provide 12 inches (1 ft) length for every 1 inch in rise. The ramp should be a minimum of 3 ft wide, measured inside the railing. A 4 inch curb should be provided on both sides of the ramp to serve as a guardrail. Handrails 32 inches high can be provided on both sides of the ramp for additional safety. Ramps should be of a nonskid, fire-retardant material and divided into 10 to 12 ft sections, with a 5 × 5 ft platform at any point where the ramp changes direction. The base and top portion of the ramp should terminate with a level section of the walkway or driveway or doorway entrance.

A lighted overhead covering can be constructed for protection during the inclement weather. Portable ramps and modular ramps can be considered for those who require transportability for home or travel. Portable ramps should follow the same recommendations as a constructed ramp.

An individual with restricted mobility is especially vulnerable to fire and other hazards. It is therefore recommended to provide two means of entry/exit from any residence to provide the occupant with the ability to vacate the house in the event of an emergency.

Doorways and Hallways

The ramp entrance should be devoid of a storm door. If present it should swing inward, away from the confined space of the porch landing or steps. A 5 × 5 ft exterior landing at the top of the ramp for wheelchair maneuvering during door management should be constructed. The landing should be level with the living space floor.

The exterior doorway width should be at least 32 to 36 inches (depending on the size of the wheelchair, measured door-to-molding, if no turn is involved, with a 5 × 5 ft landing to allow space during door management. Door handles should be the lever type, which are easier to handle for people with limited hand function. Doors should be hung on offset hinges, which allow the door to swing clear of the doorway providing maximum width for access. Pocket doors can replace a standard door when the swing of the door takes up too much floor space or to maximize door width. French style doors can replace sliding glass doors. An automatic door opener accessed by a remote control switch can provide a sense of independence and safety.

A hallway measuring 36 inches minimum will accommodate the wheelchair for a straight entry into the doorway. The hallway space for a manual wheelchair turning into a doorway may need to be up to 5 ft to accommodate a 360 degrees turn.

Bedroom

Unnecessary furniture should be removed from the bedroom, which should only contain the bed, dresser, and possibly a counter space for entertainment/computer activities. The bedroom should accommodate an area of at least 10 × 14 ft, and should allow at least one 5 × 5 ft area clear of furniture for maneuvering the wheelchair. A passageway with a minimum width of 3 ft should be provided on at least one side of the bed, with a passageway of a minimum of 4 ft provided at the end of the bed. A clear floor area, 4 ft in length, should precede dressers and closet space. Light switches should measure 36 inches high. Outlets should follow local town code and be assessable to provide power source to the needed durable medical equipment (DME).

For closet access, if the person with an SCI has adequate arm and hand function, rods should be placed at a height of 3 ft 6 inches to 4 ft. Accessible shelves should be no higher than 4 ft 6 inches and no deeper than 1 ft 4 inches. For a standard closet, bifolding or sliding doors are preferred, with recessed floor mounted door tracks. Four feet of clear floor space in front of the closet doors should allow for wheelchair maneuvering space. For a roll-in closet, the door should have a clearance width of 32 inches. A minimum of a 5 × 5 ft area is needed, clear of shelving and hanging clothing, for wheelchair turning.

Work space may be provided in the bedroom. Equipment, such as stereo systems, computers, etc., is easily accessible from a countertop. Counters should be constructed between 2 ft 6 inches and 2 ft 10 inches in height and a minimum depth of 2 ft. Knee space clearance should have a minimum height of 2 ft 3 inches and a minimum width of 3 ft. Countertop level outlets should be provided.

Bathroom

Depending on the person's LOI, the bathroom is most often the room that needs the greatest modifications. Knowing the DME being prescribed will determine what modifications are necessary. The accessible bathroom should be adjacent to the bedroom if possible and be a minimum of 8 × 10 ft. The swing of the bathroom door should be outward, into the bedroom, and away from the more confined space of the bathroom. An area 5 × 5 ft clear of fixtures, for wheelchair turning radius and maneuvering should be provided.

The sink should be wall mounted without a cabinet beneath, measuring 30 inches wide and 19 inches deep. The sink depth should not exceed 6½ inches. Knee clearance should be provided below the sink that is at least 27 inches high, and varies according to how high the patient sits in their chair. A clear floor space, 4 ft wide and 4 ft in length should be provided in front of the toilet and sink. Sink pipes/drains must be insulated to prevent scrapes and burns. To maximize knee space clearance, it is recommended that pipes be recessed, offset horizontally or located behind the wall. Countertops provided should not have a height that exceeds 34 inches. Counter space and a cabinet for storage of hygiene and toileting supplies are recommended.

A mirror should be hung for viewing from both a seated and standing position. The lower edge mounted no greater than 3 ft 4 inches from the floor, with the top edge mounted no less than 6 ft 2 inches.

A standard height (14 inches rim height) toilet is recommended for use with a standard commode and rehab shower/commode chair. Adequate space of 18 inches from the center of toilet on both sides of the toilet is required to allow the SCI individual or their caregiver access to complete their care.

A roll-in shower is recommended for the patient using a shower commode chair. This is constructed of a tiled, two- or three-sided shower, with no curb or threshold. The floor of the shower should be of nonslip material, a minimum of 5 × 5 ft (longer if a tilt-in-space shower chair is used), and should be slightly pitched for water drainage.

A handheld adjustable height shower hose, ceiling hung curtain, thermostat control, heat light, and exhaust fan are other considerations. A standard tub or shower stall with a curtain and appropriate padded DME is recommended for the SCI individual who is ambulating or have good upper body strength and stability.

Kitchen

Even if the SCI individuals will not be performing basic kitchen skills, they still should be able to access the kitchen for meals and socialization. The SCI individual who has upper body strength and stability may decide to manage in the kitchen by making minimal modifications, by propelling the wheelchair alongside the counter and working off the table, rearranging cabinets and storing frequently used items within reach. For custom modifications, the counters should be 30 to 35 inches above the floor with 24 inches beneath for knee clearance. Providing a pull-out surface for workspace can easily accommodate these specifications. It is recommended that all lower kitchen cabinets have roll-out shelves to facilitate access.

All appliances should be evaluated and recommendations made for access. The stove should contain front or side controls in order to avoid burns while reaching over the burners. Gas is preferred to electric, as it is easier to identify when burners are on. The oven and microwave should be low enough for the person with SCI to be able to reach inside. If the person with SCI has difficulty pressing recessed buttons, a microwave with a dial is preferred. The refrigerator/freezer should be a side-by-side model, keeping the most frequently used items on the lower shelves. "Lazy Susans" can be placed in the refrigerator and cabinets to allow easy access of items.

The faucet should have one-lever controls, preferably mounted on the side of the sink for easy access. The sink height should be 29 to 31 inches with a shallow depth. The cabinets beneath the sink should be removed and the pipes well insulated to prevent burns.

Lifts

It is highly recommended that a lift manufacturer be contacted to determine the appropriate installation for structure stability. An exterior mechanical vertical platform lift may need to be considered when a ramp is not possible due to the size, terrain, and space of the property. Vertical platform lifts have applications for outside and inside the home. Standard features include safety and emergency features, accessible switches, automatic self-lowering folding ramp and lifting weight capacity.

Floor-to-floor access by use of a stair glide can be considered for the SCI individual who has upper body strength and trunk stability. The individual should be independent in transferring to the surface and in maintaining balance while ascending/descending the elevations. The stair glide travels along a track attached to the wall, and some will move around curves. One that folds when not in use will maintain walking space for others. Safety considerations include weight capacity, chair pivots, arm rest and foot plate flip up for safe transfers, a deep padded seating surface and access to the control. A second wheelchair will need to be positioned on the next level, or the wheelchair will need to be carried up by a family member. Interior lifts or elevators can be an option for the SCI individual who has limited to absent upper body strength and trunk stability. The specifications are the same as an exterior lift. Weight capacity and home structure should be evaluated prior to installation. Wheelchair stair lifts are also an option and should follow the same safety standards as an interior lift and stair glide. These platform lifts can be used to access one or more levels inside and outside the home or commercial building. Again, it is imperative that a qualified lift representative evaluate the appropriateness of the stair glide and that a contractor evaluate the structure of the staircase.

General Considerations

When discussing home modifications, occasionally the most accessible room for adaptations may be in a garage or basement area. These areas should have stringent temperature control and insulation. They should be air-conditioned in warm weather and heated in cold weather, with controls that can be operated independently. Often, a zoned system where different areas of the house can be set for different temperatures is best. The patient may need to make one area of the house warmer or cooler than the rest of the house due to the inability to regulate body temperature.

Having a backup generator supplying power to outlets supporting DME, lifts, ventilators, automatic garage and door openers, and appliances for basic needs should be a consideration for the SCI individual who relies heavily on this equipment and also for those who may reside in a rural area. Consultation should take place with knowledgeable contractors and accessibility design professionals prior to any work. Hardwood floors or low-pile carpet makes wheelchair propulsion easier, and rearranging furniture for wheelchair accessibility is important. Smoke and carbon monoxide detectors are recommended. General recommendations for home modifications are listed in Table 17.5. The extensiveness of these modifications depends highly on the person's function, family wishes, and resources. Some resources for home modifications are listed in Table 17.6.

OTHER DURABLE MEDICAL EQUIPMENT

Evaluating and choosing the correct DME for the SCI individual is crucial to achieving functional safety and independence. When working with the patient and family to identify the appropriate piece of equipment, discharge placement and insurance coverage must also be considered.

A shower/commode chair is used in a roll-in shower stall and appropriate for the C1-6 individual. Standard and tilt-in-space styles are considered depending on the individual tolerance to upright position, sitting balance, and episodes of orthostasis or AD. Customizing seating supports can be added to the prescription to provide trunk support and seating stability. A padded tub bench and commode are options for persons with paraplegia with good trunk balance.

TABLE 17.5

GENERAL RECOMMENDATIONS FOR ACCESSIBILITY IN THE HOME

- Consult with a construction company with knowledge in accessibility design.
- Consult with a licensed professional lift vendor when considering interior and exterior lifts.
- The minimum space for turning around is 5 × 5 ft for a manual wheelchair and 6 × 6 ft for a power wheelchair.
- Doorway widths that require a "straight shot" (no turning involved) are 32 inches for a manual chair and 34 inches for a power wheelchair. This space increases to 36 inches if there is a turn involved.
- All thresholds should be no greater than 1 inches to allow the person in the wheelchair to maneuver.
- Install carbon monoxide detectors and smoke alarms throughout the home.
- Low-pile carpeting or hard surface flooring is recommended for wheelchair maneuvering.
- Eliminate throw rugs as they pose a hazard for people who are walking and are difficult for people in wheelchairs to roll over.
- Remove or rearrange furniture that will impede wheelchair access.
- Notify police/fire departments that an individual with a disability resides in the home and provide the bedroom location.
- An intercom system can be useful to allow for communication.
- Backup power should be provided if the person with an SCI is dependent on equipment for life support, such as a ventilator.
- Light switches should be at a height of no more than 36 inches.
- Fireplace/heater cautions: Wheelchairs are generally constructed of some type of metal which may or may not conduct heat; therefore, when a person in a wheelchair is seated near a fireplace or heater, care should be taken to cover the metal parts of the wheelchair that may contact the person's skin to prevent burns.
- Power door openers, controlled by a remote control or wall-mounted push plate, can be installed for people in wheelchairs.

A fully electric hospital bed is recommended for persons with tetraplegia to aid in nursing care, positioning, bed mobility, and self-care. A variety of mattresses and overlays of differing materials, such as air, foam, or gel, are available, both powered and nonpowered. It is recommended that support surfaces be evaluated for adequate pressure relief given the risk for skin breakdown after SCI. A pressure mapping software program with a pressure pad is ideal to complete this evaluation and trial process.

Preparing for Discharge

Preparing the SCI individual and the family begins with the completed home assessment forms, which should prompt trials of appropriate DME, discussion of home modifications, and patient/family training and education. Home modification recommendations should be made according to the patient's prognosis; however, due to shorter acute rehab stays, the SCI individual may be discharged before the modifications are completed. Thus, a temporary setup for the SCI individual's bedroom and bathing area, in addition to home entrances, should be planned with appropriate DME. Special consideration is needed if the injured individual has children at home. A lift or stair glide may be needed to access the children's bedrooms while keeping the patient's living space on the first floor.

TABLE 17.6

RESOURCES AND WEB SITES FOR HOME MODIFICATIONS

www.usrehab.com
www.homemods.org
www.design.ncsu.edu
www.hiri.org
www.makoa.org
www.aema.com
www.hud.gov/news

Discussing Prognosis

Discussing prognosis for significant motor recovery following a neurologically complete SCI (often termed "breaking the bad news") is one of the most difficult tasks for the spinal cord medicine specialist. Learning the skills to facilitate this communication is extremely important to better assist patients in understanding their prognosis as well as to foster hope for their future (147). If bad news is delivered poorly, it can cause confusion, long-lasting distress, and resentment; if done well, it may assist understanding, adjustment, and acceptance.

Prognosticating outcome from a traumatic SCI is of great importance to the patient and family, as well as to the treating rehabilitation team in order to plan realistically for the future following discharge from rehabilitation (148). Some physicians may feel that discussing the poor prognosis for motor recovery with newly injured individuals soon after injury may be a source of depression or anxiety that may in turn affect the person's willingness to participate in their comprehensive rehabilitation. There is no data to support this, and, in other patient populations (e.g., oncology), perceived adequacy of the information patients receive and the success to which the clinician is able to elicit and resolve their concerns may predict risk for developing a depressive and/or an anxiety disorder (149). When it comes to medical issues, withholding bad news in an attempt to protect the patient from the truth is usually an error and reportedly often arises from a desire to protect the holder of the information (150).

Failure to explain the diagnosis and prognosis in a clear manner may interfere with the patient's process of coping and reduce their subjective well-being (151). The manner in which the information is delivered and discussed can have a significant impact on the patient's perspective of illness, compliance with treatment, long-term relationship with the clinician, and both patient and provider satisfaction (152–156).

Certain recommendations have been made regarding the way to discuss the prognosis in this situation (147). An overview of recommendations to facilitate communication is listed in Table 17.7. It should be noted that there may be no ideal

TABLE 17.7

SUGGESTIONS FOR DISCUSSING PROGNOSIS

Preparation
Experienced clinician should lead the conversation.
Offer to have someone from patients support network/family member present.
Allow uninterrupted time.
Employ a trained health interpreter if language barriers exist.
Find a quiet, private place.
Review key medical information from the chart.
Discussion
Sit close to the patient.
Determine what the patient and family know.
Speak slowly, deliberately and clearly.
Provide information in simple language and honestly.
Give fair warning to what will be discussed.
Provide information in small doses.
Check the patient's comprehension.
Use eye contact and body language to convey warmth, sympathy, encouragement, and/or reassurance to the patient.
Encourage the patient to express his/her feelings.
Acknowledge patients emotions with validation.
Respond to those feelings with empathy.
Discuss treatment options.
Summing up
Avoid the notion "that nothing can be done."
Convey message of hope.
Offer assistance to talk with others.
Provide information about support services.
Summarize the important information.
Arrange a time to talk again.
Document information given.

method of breaking the news, and differences in approach might be appropriate based upon individual clinician's styles and institutional setting, as well as the patient's background, education, culture, gender, age, and life situations. These recommendations are based upon clinical experience and data from the general medical, oncology, nursing, psychology, and end of life literature.

Although there is significance to the words used in delivering the prognosis, breaking the news to patients involves more than just words. Nonverbal communication is equally important as the actual words chosen. This includes facing the patient, utilizing eye contact, allowing pauses/time for patients to collect their thoughts and to formulate questions, and permitting the patient to speak without interruption. When utilizing an interpreter, one can still convey many of the nonverbal expressions of caring and sympathy. It is critical that the patient feels that you have the time to talk and listen. Avoid writing notes, reading or writing in the patient's chart, or looking elsewhere when the discussion takes place. Ensure that interruptions such as beepers, telephone calls, and physical intrusions are kept to a minimum.

Often the question of "cure in SCI" arises during this discussion. It should be recognized that there is no cure currently available for SCI and therefore no easy answers that may satisfy a patient's desire for such. In addition, there are no simple answers or treatments for the fear, anger, disappointment, depression, and mourning the patient/family may experience. However, showing empathy will help facilitate adjustment to the changes in the patient's world (157). The information should be presented at a pace the patient can follow without overwhelming the patient with details. The discussion is often compared to peeling an onion: provide an initial overview and then answer questions going into more detail depending upon the patient's tolerance level and request.

There is no truly defined appropriate time for the discussion of prognosis to take place. Often in the rehabilitation setting, this will also vary by physician, institution, the patient, and their family. Considerations should include whether or not the patient and/or family have raised questions to the physician or other staff members regarding prognosis and whether there are major differences between team and patient goals. Prognosis should be discussed before the patient and/or family are invited to a team conference where they may learn in a large group setting the current rehabilitation goals, need for permanent home modification, importance of learning the bowel and bladder program, and usefulness of assistive technology and adaptive recreational programs, as these issues will once again reflect the permanence of their condition.

Additional consideration needs to be taken when family members of an adult patient, most often parents, request that the patient not be told the negative prognosis. Discussions should take place with the family, physician, and psychologist regarding the parents' need to protect their loved one.

Driving Assessment in SCI Patients

Losing the ability to drive has an impact in many domains including social, economic, and psychological (158,159). Fortunately, individuals with SCI with levels at C5 and below have the potential to return to independent driving with the appropriate adaptive equipment. The timing for a return to driving will vary by individual, the level, and type of injury. All spinal orthoses should be discontinued. The person should be medically stable and psychologically ready to return to the road. This may require additional time if the person was injured in a motor vehicle crash.

The driving evaluation is an essential component of a comprehensive SCI program. Information on transportation should be available to all clients. Evaluation services in the United States and Canada can be located through the membership directory on the Association for Driver Rehabilitation Specialist's Web site, www.driver-ed.org. Facilities are listed by state and most include a description of the types of services offered. Vendors who belong to the National Mobility Equipment Dealers Association, www.nmeda.org, are a valuable resource to answer technical questions about equipment and the costs of vehicle modification.

A person with neurologically complete paraplegia and no additional complications will probably require mechanical hand controls and a few additional minor pieces of equipment to operate a car with an automatic transmission. If there is no expected LE return, the evaluation could occur within 3 months of injury, as there is little likelihood the equipment recommendations would change. The costs are usually less than $1,500.

For persons with tetraplegia or motor incomplete injuries, depending on their functional abilities, the cost of equipping a vehicle can be as low as $1,000 or as high as $80,000. The patient should plateau in function prior to being evaluated for driving, since any improvement in strength can mean a difference in equipment costs of thousands of dollars or the difference between requiring and not requiring equipment. It is not uncommon to wait at least 6 months to evaluate a person who is still experiencing functional return.

Predriving Assessment

The main components of the predriving assessment include a thorough history and examination, including a vision screen, physical skills, wheelchair or mobility training, and reaction time (159,160). If the individual also has a history of brain trauma, cognitive and perceptual screens should be included. The medical history includes the level and severity of the spinal injury, additional injuries such as extremity fractures or peripheral nerve damage, presence of spasticity, and history of seizures, as well as unrelated conditions such as cataracts, diabetes, and heart disease. Medications should be evaluated with attention paid to those that might cause fatigue, dizziness, altered judgment, or altered vision. The driving history should include any license restrictions, driving experience prior to the injury, and any recent at-fault motor vehicle accidents and tickets. An initial discussion of the type of vehicle the client owns and the plans to modify that vehicle are also important. If the person does not own an appropriate vehicle, it is important to wait to purchase one until all recommendations have been made.

A vision screen is performed to determine if the person can meet the state requirements, in addition to detecting other deficits that may impact driving. Tests may include acuity, contrast sensitivity, depth perception, color recognition, night vision and glare recovery, phoria, and fusion. Further evaluations of ocular motility function include fixation, saccadic eye movements, and pursuit eye movement (161). Many clinics will use vision-testing machines, which include most of the tests mentioned.

The physical skills section should include an assessment of strength of the upper and LEs, sensation, ROM for extremities and neck, sitting balance, spasticity, transfer skills, and wheelchair loading skills. If the person can ambulate and requires an assistive device such as a rolling walker or crutches, he or she should be asked about the ability to load that equipment into the car. Driving equipment predictions are made based on the physical assessment; therefore, an accurate picture of the person's abilities and deficits is crucial to driving successfully.

Strength testing should be performed in the seated position, with attention paid to the key muscles, as well as shoulder flexion, extension and abduction, horizontal adduction and adduction, and internal and external rotation. These motions provide the force needed to turn the steering wheel and to operate hand controls. Grasp strength should be measured when present, and areas of the body lacking sensation should be noted, as these areas may have to be protected from injury. For the LE, if functional strength is present, it is important to determine if the person also has sensation, particularly proprioception. If adequate proprioception is lacking, the individual may not be able to locate the pedals without looking down, thus disqualifying him or her from driving without adaptations. Reaction time and foot placement can be tested in the clinic or in the car.

Active and/or passive ROM limitations should be noted as they may affect positioning. If the person has impaired LE range due to spasticity, edema, or heterotropic ossification, it may be difficult to position the legs under the steering wheel. If there are contractures in the hand, custom orthotics may be required to interface with the steering wheel or hand controls. Cervical fusion surgery or tight neck and shoulder muscles may result in limited neck rotation, which would affect the person's ability to check traffic. This, combined with decreased active trunk rotation, may necessitate the use of additional mirrors (162).

Sitting balance is important; individuals who cannot maintain an upright position against moderate side-to-side resistance or who cannot return to an upright position without using their arms should use a chest strap or other lateral support when driving (163). Uncontrolled spasticity should be treated if it interferes with safety.

The person's ability to transfer into a car and load a wheelchair should be discussed during the clinical assessment and eventually observed in a vehicle. The LOI, weight, conditioning, and type of wheelchair will affect these skills and should be taken into account when wheelchair selection is finalized (164).

Behind-the-Wheel Assessment

The behind-the-wheel assessment involves vehicle entry and exit, operation of primary controls (i.e., steering, accelerator, and brakes), and operation of secondary controls (i.e., turn signals and gear selector). A static assessment, either in a vehicle or in the clinic, may help rule out certain equipment but it should not be used to finalize primary equipment. Only after training on the road in varied situations should the driver rehabilitation specialist determine what equipment is appropriate. Training time can range from a few hours for mechanical hand controls and standard steering to over 40 hours for joystick drivers.

Vehicle Selection

In general, an automatic transmission vehicle with power steering and power brakes is required. The only exception is a very incomplete client who has enough function in all four limbs to operate a manual transmission vehicle. Other factory options that facilitate modification include a tilt steering wheel, power windows and door locks, and possibly a power driver's seat. Air conditioning, front and rear in the case of a van, is recommended to compensate for the person's inability to regulate body temperature.

For most persons with paraplegia, an automatic transmission car is an option if there is no difficulty with transfers. If they are independent in transfers, other classes of vehicles, such as sport utility vehicles (SUVs), are also possibilities. There are transfer aides available that can raise the person up to the level of a full-size truck seat, but these are costly. If transfers or chair loading become more difficult due to shoulder pain, weight gain, medical complications, or age-related factors, then a van can be considered.

If the client cannot load his or her chair independently or chooses not to (because, for example, of the risk of staining clothes while passing the wheels and frame across the body), a loading device is an option. Most loading devices are designed to pick up a folding manual chair. Car top devices fold the wheelchair and stow it in a rooftop carrier. There are also lifts that can stow the folding chair behind the driver's seat in an extended cab three-door pickup truck. The height, width, length, and weight of the wheelchair will affect its compatibility with loading devices and vehicles (164). The person who can ambulate short distances also has the option of devices to load the chair into the trunk, in a sliding side door, or into the rear of a minivan or SUV. Some of these will even load certain power upright wheelchairs and scooters.

For most persons with tetraplegia, the choice will be a modified van. Transfers may be difficult, or they may lack the fine motor control and strength to disassemble the wheelchair to load it. Most power chairs cannot be disassembled into a car, and those that can are too heavy to be practical for routine use. For the person who uses both a manual and a power wheelchair, it is important to determine which chair is most practical for independent community use, as not every vehicle solution can be used with both. For example, access to a lowered-floor minivan requires the ability to propel up a ramp, which may be impossible for some individuals using a manual wheelchair, but easily accomplished in a power wheelchair. Even if the vehicle can be accessed with both a manual and a power wheelchair, it may not be possible to utilize a single tie-down system that would accommodate both chairs due to differences in frames and seat heights. Patients should obtain their personal wheelchair prior to starting modifications to the driver's area to ensure an appropriate fit.

C4 and higher levels

Persons with C1-4 complete tetraplegia are not able to drive, as there must be functional use of at least one extremity to operate a driving system. A person with high-level tetraplegia will most often operate a power wheelchair with a tilt or recline mechanism, and transportation equipment needs should be addressed. It is usually easier to transport persons seated in their wheelchair, which is already set up to provide the proper support, rather than in a passenger seat. A structurally modified full-size van or lowered-floor minivan will usually be required. The most common modifications to a full-size van are a lowered floor in the cargo or center seat area and/or a raised roof and doors. If possible the doorway should be tall enough to allow the wheelchair user to enter in a fully upright position. Inside the van, it is important to have at least 2 inches of head clearance. For most passengers, a lowered floor (usually 4 to 8 inches) drops their eye height to a point where they may be able to see out the side windows. A van with a raised roof alone tends to provide poor visibility as the person's head is usually above the original roofline. Depending on the seated height of the person, a combination of these modifications may be needed. A raised roof may also be chosen to allow the caregivers to stand upright when providing assistance to the wheelchair user, particularly helpful if suctioning or ICs must be performed. The primary disadvantage to a raised roof is increased overall vehicle height, which makes the vehicle difficult to fit in a garage or carport and more difficult to take into the community as it may not fit through drive-thru windows or into parking decks. It also raises the vehicle's center of gravity, affecting the handling.

Entry to a full-size van is accomplished by means of a platform lift. Lifts can be fully or semiautomatic, the latter requiring the operator to manually unfold the lift platform. A description of the lifts can be found elsewhere (161).

Smaller than full-size vans and with better gas mileage, the lowered-floor minivan has become increasingly popular. Entry is gained by use of a folding ramp that deploys from the passenger side sliding door, although a few models use a rear entry or a side under floor ramp. A lowered-floor minivan sits closer to the ground than an unmodified vehicle, and it may also be equipped with a kneeling feature, which further lowers the vehicle to decrease the angle of the ramp. The patient can be accommodated in the cargo or front passenger position if the van is equipped with a removable front passenger seat. Since the minivan has less interior space, it may be difficult for a large power chair to turn into a forward facing position; this should be attempted prior to purchase (165).

Once inside a van the passenger and wheelchair must be secured. The two primary styles of lockdowns or tie-downs are manual and automatic. There are several types of manual lockdowns but all consist of a strap system that hooks to the frame of the wheelchair. The primary advantage of a manual system is the ability to secure different chairs, which is useful if the passenger uses both a manual and power chair. Manual systems are also less costly than automatic systems. The most common automatic lockdown has two parts: one which bolts to the frame of the chair and a second which bolts to the floor of the van. The primary advantage of the automatic system is ease of use. Whichever system is chosen, it is not complete without an automotive lap and shoulder belt to secure the person to the van. Velcro belts should not be used.

C5 Level

The C5 level is the highest level of complete injury with potential to drive. The driving evaluation should be postponed until the client plateaus in strength, which can be as much as 8 months to a year from the time of injury. The same vehicle considerations mentioned previously will apply with some additional modifications specific to driving. The van will need power door openers, and the lift or ramp must be fully automatic to allow the wheelchair user to open and close the vehicle independently.

Most persons with a C5 injury will be driving from their wheelchair. Lateral stability should be carefully evaluated, as the dynamic forces affecting the body in the moving vehicle are much greater than the ones seen when operating the chair in the clinic. Options such as tapered 90-degree legrests may allow the chair to fit under the steering wheel more easily, thus allowing the person to sit closer to the wheel. A swing-away joystick may be needed to facilitate placement of primary driving controls. The driver's floor must also be lowered, making it possible to drive the wheelchair up under the steering wheel. The knees must fit under the steering wheel and not interfere with its motion.

Some persons with a C5 motor level on one side and a C4 or higher level on the other side can drive. If only one extremity is to be used, a multiaccess driving system in which the steering, accelerator, and brake are operated by a single control lever would be utilized. These systems are complex and costly. If both UEs can be used, one will perform steering and the other will operate an accelerator and brake, most often an electronic or servo hand control. If there is a difference in strength, the stronger arm is generally used for steering.

Most persons at this level will be unable to turn a standard steering wheel a full turn in each direction, even with the steering effort or force reduced. If they cannot make consistent

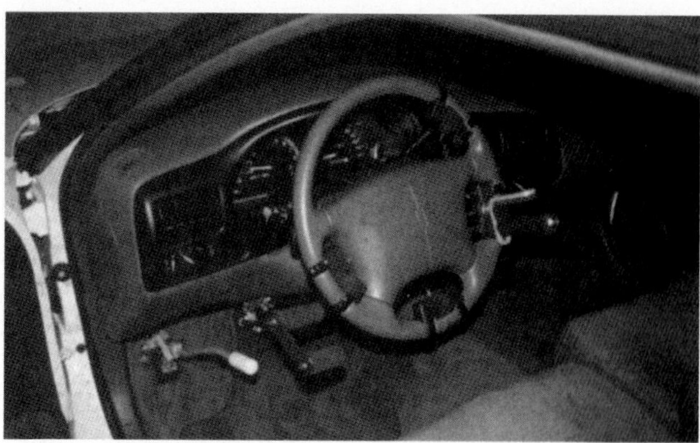

FIGURE 17.6. V-Grip orthotic.

turns at all speeds utilizing the reduced effort steering, patients will require a servo steering system. Options for steering systems are covered elsewhere (161).

A tri-pin orthotic is frequently used to keep the person's hand in contact with both the steering and hand controls (Fig. 17.6) The rear pins press on the dorsal and volar sides of the wrist with the forearm in a neutral position and the front pin rests in the web space of the hand. Wrist supports may be worn to maintain a stable wrist position in the absence of active wrist extension.

Most persons with C5 injuries will require extensive modifications of secondary controls (i.e., turn signals and gear selector). Modifications for secondary controls can be as simple as an extension on a switch or as complex as a touch pad. Touch pad systems can replace a single function or operate multiple systems through a single switch. The most complex systems control everything from gear selection to temperature controls. Simple touch pad systems may control two to eight functions. A single switch that scans several functions with auditory cues may be used to activate secondary controls that have to be accessed while in motion. Less commonly used are voice recognition systems that allow direct selection of secondary controls.

C6 Level

At the C6 level, most persons still require a van for transportation. If they cannot transfer independently, they will require the same driver's lowered floor modifications mentioned previously. If they can transfer efficiently, a six-way power driver's seat could be considered. This type of seat backs up from the steering wheel, turns 90 degrees, and can be raised or lowered to make a transfer easier. A lockdown is installed behind the seat to secure the unoccupied wheelchair.

A weak person with this LOI may still lack the active range to turn a full-size steering wheel. In this case, the same equipment mentioned in the previous section would be required. The main advantage over the C5 level is in wrist strength, as they seldom require extra wrist support. The stronger person at this level may be able to turn a full-size steering wheel but will probably need the force or effort reduced. Individuals with a C6 motor level may be able to utilize mechanical hand controls with a modified handle to provide additional wrist support; although, electronic hand controls are still needed in many cases. If reach and access are not a problem, then simple extensions for the secondary controls may be the only modifications; although, touch pads and sequencing switches are still common.

C7-8 Levels

Most persons at the C7-8 levels will have enough shoulder strength to turn the standard steering wheel and may not require reduced effort steering. If grasp strength is diminished, an orthotic, such as the tri-pin, the V-grip, or the U-grip, may be needed for steering control. The presence of triceps makes the use of mechanical hand controls for braking and acceleration appropriate. Added wrist support may be needed if the person cannot grip the handle.

In most cases, the hand controls will be mounted on the left side of the steering wheel. This allows easier activation of the turn signals with the left hand. The left hand can depress the brake while the right operates the gear selector. Most secondary controls will not require modification, although minor modifications such as switch extensions may be needed.

Some persons with these levels of injury can transfer independently. Wheelchair loading tends to be the primary difficulty as the person may lack the fine coordination and strength required for dismantling the chair and lifting it. A loading device may be utilized, but it will only be compatible with certain types of wheelchairs. If they use a power chair or cannot manage the car transfer, a van could be modified to allow driving from the wheelchair or equipped with a power driver's seat. If they transfer, their wheelchair would be locked down behind the driver's seat for safety. In a full-size van, the roof may need to be raised or the floor lowered to provide adequate head clearance for the transfer.

Paraplegia

For persons with paraplegia, standard steering will be used with the possible addition of a steering knob to make one handed turns easier. Mechanical hand controls will be used to control speed. A parking brake extension may be needed if the lever is not hand operated. A chest strap will be required for persons who do not have adequate motor return in the trunk and abdomen.

The choice of hand control style may be dictated by the available space in the driver's area rather than the hand function. A person with long legs or a small car may not have room for the lever to move far enough towards the thigh to get adequate acceleration with the push right angle style. Other systems may be required (i.e., the push twist or push rock are often used in these cases).

Vans are sometimes recommended in cases where the person uses a power wheelchair or if there are complications such as shoulder pain that limit the ability to transfer or load the chair. Power transfer seats are often used. Occasionally, an electronic hand control will be required for the very large person driving from the wheelchair if there is not enough space in the driver's area to operate mechanical hand controls.

Incomplete Injuries

Each of the clinical syndromes presents its own unique challenges. For example, a person with central cord syndrome may be able to use the existing pedals but may be unable to steer due to proximal UE weakness. If one side of the body is stronger, modifications to pedals or secondary controls may be needed. Any of the previously mentioned equipment may be appropriate for the person with an incomplete injury. It is also possible that no equipment will be needed. In this case, it is critical to test the reaction time and endurance of the LEs to support the lack of modifications. Periodic reassessment is suggested as changes to the adaptive equipment may be needed when the patient's exam improves. A formal reassessment may be required to legally remove a restriction on the driver's license for the equipment in question.

Rehabilitation for Nontraumatic Spinal Cord Injury

Nontraumatic spinal cord injury/disease (NT-SCI/D) has been a growing population and accounts for a significant percentage (39% to 60%) of patients with SCI admitted for acute rehabilitation (166,167). The most common etiologies include spinal stenosis and cancer-related compression, with infections, vascular ischemia, and multiple sclerosis occurring less frequently (167–169). Other etiologies include inflammatory disease, motor neuron disease, radiation myelopathy, syringomyelia, paraneoplastic syndrome, and vitamin B_{12} deficiency. As compared to persons with traumatic SCI, individuals with NT-SCI/D are more likely to be older, female, married, and retired. NT-SCI/D is more common than trauma in persons over 40. Persons with NT-SCI/D usually have a less severe neurological impairment as compared with traumatic SCI, as they more often present with motor incomplete (90%) lesions (170). During rehabilitation of patients with NT-SCI/D, there is a lower incidence of secondary medical complications including spasticity, orthostasis, deep vein thrombosis (DVT), pressure ulcers, AD, and wound infections (171–173). However, because cervical stenosis and neoplastic spinal cord compression have a peak incidence between the ages of 50 and 70 years, these individuals may have other premorbid medical issues that may impact their rehabilitation. No difference is noted in incidence of depression, urinary tract infections, heterotopic ossification, pain, or gastrointestinal bleeding.

The interdisciplinary model of rehabilitation has shown effectiveness for persons with NT-SCI/D (166,174). In comparison with traumatic SCI, no statistical differences were found in acute care LOS and admission to rehabilitation FIM scores. (168,170,175) Inpatient rehabilitation LOS is shorter for persons with NT injury secondary to tumors, but FIM efficiency and home discharge rates are comparable overall to traumatic SCI. Discharge to home is more likely in patients with the following characteristics: incomplete injury, married, established bowel and bladder management program, intact skin, male gender, and cognitively intact.

LONG-TERM FOLLOW-UP

Outpatient programs have recently taken on an even more important role than in previous decades because of the shortened inpatient LOS. Outpatient care should include close monitoring of the medical status, that is, bowel, bladder, skin, and respiratory management, as well as a comprehensive therapy program encompassing not only physical and occupational therapies but also psychology and vocational counseling. With the shorter LOS, there is less time to help the patient and family adjust to the disability and to address all of the obstacles present that may interfere with social, vocational, and recreational reintegration.

Long-term follow-up with the SCI specialist is extremely important (see Chapter 27). Initially, visits should occur on a monthly basis, especially while the person is attending outpatient therapy. This allows for monitoring of medical issues, reevaluation of the therapy program with updated goals, and prescription of equipment. As patients are discharged earlier, frequently medical issues that previously were experienced in the hospital now develop while at home. This includes bowel, bladder and spasticity changes, and the development of heterotopic ossification and AD. After these issues are stabilized and outpatient therapy has switched to a maintenance-type program, visits should be every 3 to 6 months through the second year. For those patients who are medically stable, yearly appointments are then recommended. The importance of these visits is to review any medical changes, monitor the neurological examination for deterioration, ensure that the equipment is being maintained, and prescribe any additional equipment that may be needed. Deterioration of the neurologic status may be secondary to a tethered cord, syringomyelia, peripheral problems such as median or ulnar nerve entrapment, or musculoskeletal complications. As a greater amount of persons with SCI are surviving longer after their injury, the importance of follow-up visits to maintain quality of life cannot be overemphasized.

At times, readmission to the rehabilitation hospital for medical or rehabilitation issues may be needed. These issues may include maintaining the proper bowel and bladder programs, skin breakdown, and awareness of the signs and symptoms of, as well as the proper treatment for, AD. In addition, many times the person with SCI may require a "refresher course" in rehabilitation techniques that can best be taught in an intensive inpatient setting. The chapter, Aging in SCI (Chapter 27), further outlines the changes over time for those with SCI.

Unfortunately, some third-party payers will not cover SCI specialists to follow the person with an SCI after the acute rehabilitation stay. This may lead to an increase in secondary SCI-specific medical complications, as issues such as heterotopic ossification, AD, spasticity, and bowel and bladder care are not commonly seen by the general practitioner. In addition, without experience regarding functional outcomes, the expenditures for equipment will often be higher.

References

1. Consortium for Spinal Cord Medicine. Early acute management in adults with spinal cord injury: a clinical practice guideline for health-care professionals. *J Spinal Cord Med* 2008;31(4):403–479.
2. Jones L, Bagnall A. Spinal injuries centres (SIC's) for acute traumatic spinal cord injury. *Cochrane Database Syst Rev* 2004;4:CD004442. doi:10.1002/14651858.CD004442.
3. Aito S, Gruppo Italiano Studio Epidemiologico Mielolesioni GISEM Group. Complications during the acute phase of traumatic spinal cord lesions. *Spinal Cord* 2003;41(11):629–635.
4. Aung TS, el Masry WS. Audit of a British Centre for spinal injury. *Spinal Cord* 1997;35(3):147–150.
5. Tator CH, Duncan EG, Edmonds VE, et al. Complications and costs of management of acute spinal cord injury. *Paraplegia* 1993;31(11):700–714.

6. DeVivo MJ, Kartus PL, Stover SL, et al. Benefits of early admission to an organised spinal cord injury care system. *Paraplegia* 1990;28(9):545–555.
7. Dalyan M, Sherman A, Cardenas DD. Factors associated with contractures in acute spinal cord injury. *Spinal Cord* 1998;36(6):405–408.
8. Wolfe DL, Hsieh JTC, Curt A, et al. Neurological and functional outcomes associated with SCI rehabilitation. *Top Spinal Cord Inj Rehabil* 2007;13(1):11–31.
9. Pagliacci MC, Celani MG, Zampolini M, et al. Gruppo Italiano Studio Epidemiologico Mielolesioni. An Italian survey of traumatic spinal cord injury. The Gruppo Italiano Studio Epidemiologico Mielolesioni study. *Arch Phys Med Rehabil* 2003;84(9):1266–1275.
10. Ragnarsson KT, Gordon WA. Rehabilitation after spinal cord injury: the team approach. *Phys Med Rehabil Clin N Am* 1992;3(4):853–878.
11. Kirshblum S, Johnston MV, Brown J, et al. Predictors of dysphagia after spinal cord injury. *Arch Phys Med Rehabil* 1999;80(9):1101–1105.
12. Final Priorities and Selection Criterion; National Institute on Disability and Rehabilitation Research (NIDRR)-Spinal Cord Injury Model Systems (SCIMS) Centers and SCIMS Multi-Site Collaborative Research Projects. A Notice by the Education Department on 06/09/2011. Federal Register / Vol. 76, No. 111 / Thursday, June 9, 2011 / Noticeshttp. URL.www.gpo.gov/fdsys/pkg/FR-2011-06-09/pdf/2011-14350.pdf
13. Consortium for Spinal Cord Medicine. Outcomes following traumatic spinal cord injury: Clinical practice guidelines for health-care professionals. *J Spinal Cord Med* 1999:23(4):289–316.
14. Devivo MJ. Sir Ludwig Guttmann Lecture: trends in spinal cord injury rehabilitation outcomes from model systems in the United States: 1973–2006. *Spinal Cord* 2007;45(11):713–721.
15. Kogos SC, DeVivo MJ, Richards SJ. Recent trends in spinal cord injury rehabilitation practices and outcome. *Top Spinal Cord Rehabil* 2004;10(2):49–57.
16. Whalley Hammell K. Experience of rehabilitation following spinal cord injury: a meta-synthesis of qualitative findings. *Spinal Cord* 2007;45(4):260–274.
17. Sliwinski MM, Druin E. Intervention priciples and position changes. In: Sisto SA, Druin E, Sliwinski MM, eds. *Spinal cord injuries: management and rehabilitation* St Louis, MO: Mosby, 2009:153–184.
18. Hanak M, Scott A. *Spinal cord injury: an illustrated guide for health care professionals*. New York, NY: Springer Publishing Co.,1983.
19. Hobson DA. Comparative effects of posture on pressure and shear at the body-seat interface. *J Rehabil Res Dev* 1992;29(4):21–31
20. Henderson JL, Price SH, Brandstater ME, et al. Efficacy of three measures to relieve pressure in seated persons with spinal cord injury. *Arch Phys Med Rehabil* 1994;75(5):535–539.
21. Burns SP, Betz KL. Seating pressures with conventional and dynamic wheelchair cushions in tetraplegia. *Arch Phys Med Rehabil* 1999;80(5):566–571.
22. Trombly CA, ed. *Occupational therapy:for physical dysfunction*. 4th ed. Baltimore, MD: Williams and Wilkins,1995.
23. Coggrave MJ, Rose LS. A specialist seating assessment clinic: changing pressure relief practice. *Spinal Cord* 2003;41(12):692–695.
24. Koontz A, Druin E. Transfer techniques. In: Sisto SA, Druin E, Sliwinski MM, eds. *Spinal cord injuries: management and rehabilitation*. St Louis, MO: Mosby, 2009:185–209.
25. de Bruin ED, Frey-Rindova P, Herzog RE, et al. Changes of tibia bone properties after spinal cord injury: effects of early intervention. *Arch Phys Med Rehabil* 1999;80(2):214–220
26. Kaplan PE, Roden W, Gilbert E, et al. Reduction of hypercalciuria in tetraplegia after weight-bearing and strengthening exercises. *Paraplegia* 1981;19(5):289–293.
27. Alekna V, Tamulaitiene M, Sinevicius T, et al. Effect of weight-bearing activities on bone mineral density in spinal cord injured patients during the period of the first two years. *Spinal Cord* 2008;46(11):727–732.
28. Biering-Sørensen F, Hansen B, Lee BS. Non-pharmacological treatment and prevention of bone loss after spinal cord injury: a systematic review. *Spinal Cord* 2009;47(7):508–518.
29. Ben M, Harvey L, Denis S, et al. Does 12 weeks of regular standing prevent loss of ankle mobility and bone mineral density in people with recent spinal cord injuries? *Aust J Physiother* 2005;51(4):251–256.
30. Kunkel CF, Scremin AM, Eisenberg B, et al. Effect of "standing" on spasticity, contracture, and osteoporosis in paralyzed males. *Arch Phys Med Rehabil* 1993;74(1): 73–78.
31. Bohannon RW. Tilt table standing for reducing spasticity after spinal cord injury. *Arch Phys Med Rehabil* 1993;74(10):1121–1122.
32. Guest RS, Klose KJ, Needham-Shropshire BM, et al. Evaluation of a training program for persons with SCI paraplegia using the Parastep 1 ambulation system: part 4. Effect on physical self-concept and depression. *Arch Phys Med Rehabil* 1997; 78(8):804–807.
33. Szollar S, Martin EM, Sartoris DJ, et al. Bone mineral density and indexes of bone metabolism in spinal cord injury. *Am J Phys Med Rehabil* 1998;77(1):28–35.
34. Kaplan, PE, Gandhavadi B, Richards L, et al. Calcium balance in paraplegic patients: influence of injury duration and ambulation. *Arch Phys Med Rehabil* 1978;59(10):447–450.
35. Ogilvie C, Bowker P, Rowley D. The physiological benefits of paraplegic orthotically aided walking. *Paraplegia.* 1993;31(2):111–115.
36. Rosenstein B, Greene WB, Herrington RT, et al. Bone density in myelomeningocele: the effects of ambulatory status and other factors. *Dev Med Child Neurol* 1987;29(4):486–494.
37. Waters RL, Lunsford BR. Energy cost of paraplegic locomotion. *J Bone Joint Surg Am* 1985;67(8):1245–1250.
38. Cerny K. Energetics of walking and wheelchair propulsion in paraplegic patients. *Orthop Clin North Am* 1978;9(2):370–372.
39. Cerny K, Waters R, HislopH, et al. Walking and wheelchair energetics in persons with paraplegia. *Phys Ther* 1980;60(9):1133–1139.
40. Rosman N, Spira E. Paraplegic use of walking braces: a survey. *Arch Phys Med Rehabil* 1974;55(7):310–314.

41. Stauffer ES, Hoffer MM, Nickel VL. Ambulation in thoracic paraplegia. *J Bone Joint Surg Am* 1978;60(6): 823–824.
42. Hussey RW Stauffer ES, Spinal cord injury: requirements for ambulation. *Arch Phys Med Rehabil* 1973;54(12): 544–547.
43. Waters RL, Yakura JS, Adkins R, et al. Determinants of gait performance following spinal cord injury. *Arch Phys Med Rehabil* 1989;70(12):811–818.
44. Waters RL, Adkins R, Yakura J, et al. Prediction of ambulatory performance based on motor scores derived from standards of the American Spinal Injury Association. *Arch Phys Med Rehabil* 1994;75(7):756–760.
45. Barbeau H, Nadeau S, Garneau G. Physical determinants, emerging concepts, and training approaches in gait of individuals with spinal cord injury. *J Neurotrauma* 2006;23(3–4):571–585.
46. Stauffer ES. Orthotics for spinal cord injuries. *Clin Orthop Relat Res* 1974;(102):92–99.
47. Nene AV, Hermens HJ, Zilvold G. Paraplegic locomotion: a review. *Spinal Cord* 1996;34(9):507–524.
48. Waters RL, Mulroy S. The energy expenditure of normal and pathologic gait. *Gait Posture* 1999;9(3):207–231.
49. Waters RL, Adkins RH, Yakura JS, et al. Motor and sensory recovery following incomplete tetraplegia. *Arch Phys Med Rehabil* 1994;75(3):306–311.
50. Waters RL, Adkins R, Yakura J, et al. Donal Munro Lecture: Functional and neurologic recovery following acute SCI. *J Spinal Cord Med* 1998;21(3):195–199.
51. Waters RL, Adkins RH, Yakura J, et al. Motor and sensory recovery following incomplete paraplegia. *Arch Phys Med Rehabil* 1994;75(1):67–72.
52. Waters RL, Yakura JS, Adkins RH, et al. Recovery following complete paraplegia. *Arch Phys Med Rehabil* 1992;73(9):784–789.
53. Kay ED, Deutsch A, Wuermser LA. Predicting walking at discharge from inpatient rehabilitation after a traumatic spinal cord injury. *Arch Phys Med Rehabil* 2007;88(6):745–750.
54. Burns SP, Golding DG, Rolle WA Jr, et al. Recovery of ambulation in motor-incomplete tetraplegia. *Arch Phys Med Rehabil* 1997;78(11):1169–1172.
55. New PW. Functional outcomes and disability after non-traumatic spinal cord injury rehabilitation: Results from a retrospective study. *Arch Phys Med Rehabil* 2005;86(2):250–261.
56. Scivoletto G, Morganti B, Ditunno P, et al. Effects on age on spinal cord lesion patients' rehabilitation. *Spinal Cord* 2003;41(8):457–464.
57. Merkel KD, Miller NE, Westbrook PR, et al. Energy expenditure of paraplegic patients standing and walking with two knee-ankle-foot orthoses. *Arch Phys Med Rehabil* 1984;65(3):121–124.
58. Bernardi M, Canale I, Castellano V, et al. The efficiency of walking of paraplegic patients using a reciprocating gait orthosis. *Paraplegia* 1995;33(7):409–415.
59. Bowker P, Messenger N, Ogilvie C, et al. Energetics of paraplegic walking. *J Biomed Eng* 1992;14(4):344–350.
60. Merati G, Sarchi P, Ferrarin M, et al. Paraplegic adaptation to assisted-walking: energy expenditure during wheelchair versus orthosis use. *Spinal Cord* 2000;38(1):37–44.
61. Franceschini M, Baratta S, Zampolini M, et al. Reciprocating gait orthoses: A multicenter study of their use by spinal cord injured patients. *Arch Phys Med Rehabil* 1997;78(6):582–586.
62. Scivoletto G, Petrelli A, Lucente LD, et al. One year follow up of spinal cord injury patients using a reciprocating gait orthosis: preliminary report. *Spinal Cord* 2000;38(9):555–558.
63. Thoumie P, Perrouin-Verbe B, Le Claire G, et al. Restoration of functional gait in paraplegic patients with the RGO-II hybrid orthosis. A multicentre controlled study. I. Clinical evaluation. *Paraplegia* 1995;33(11):647–653.
64. Hirokawa S, Grimm M, Le T, et al. Energy consumption in paraplegic ambulation using the reciprocating gait orthosis and electric stimulation of the thigh muscles. *Arch Phys Med Rehabil* 1990;71(9):687–694.
65. Kawashima N, Taguchi D, Nakazawa K, et al. Effect of lesion level on the orthotic gait performance in individuals with complete paraplegia [pubished correction appears in Spinal Cord. 2006;44(8):522]. *Spinal Cord* 2006; 44(8):487–494.
66. Massucci M, Brunetti G, Piperno R, Betti L, Franceschini M. Walking with the advanced reciprocating gait orthosis (ARGO) in thoracic paraplegic patients: energy expenditure and cardiorespiratory performance. *Spinal Cord.* 1998; 36(4): 223–227.
67. Butler PB, Major RE, Patrick JH. The technique of reciprocal walking using the hip guidance orthosis (HGO) with crutches. *Prosthet Orthot Int*1984;8(1):33–38.
68. Nene AV, Jennings SJ. Physiological cost index of paraplegic locomotion using the ORLAU ParaWalker. *Paraplegia* 1992;30(4):246–252.
69. Nene AV, Patrick JH. Energy cost of paraplegic locomotion with the ORLAU ParaWalker. *Paraplegia* 1989;27(1):5–18.
70. Nene AV, Patrick JH. Energy cost of paraplegic locomotion using the ParaWalker—electrical stimulation "hybrid" orthosis. *Arch Phys Med Rehabil* 1990;71(2):116–120.
71. Hirokawa S, Solomonow M, Barrata R, et al. Energy expenditure and fatiguability in paraplegic ambulation using reciprocating gait orthosis and electric stimulation. *Disabil Rehabil* 1996;18(3):115–122.
72. Graupe D. An overview of the state of the art of noninvasive FES for independent ambulation by thoracic level paraplegics. *Neurol Res* 2002;24(5):431–442.
73. Graupe D,Kohn KH. Functional neuromuscular stimulator for short-distance ambulation by certain thoracic-level spinal-cord-injured paraplegics. *Surg Neurol*1998;50(3):202–207.
74. Visintin M, Barbeau H. The effects of body weight support on the locomotor pattern of spastic paretic patients. *Can J Neurol Sci* 1989;16:315–325.
75. Barbeau H, Wainberg M, Finch L. Description and application of a system for locomotor rehabilitation. *Med Biol Eng Comput* 1987;25(3):341–344.
76. Barbeau H, Danakas M, Arsenault B. The effects of locomotor training in spinal cord injured subjects. *Restor Neurol Neurosci* 1993;5():81–84.
77. Barbeau H, Rossignol S. Recovery of locomotion after chronic spinalization in the adult cat. *Brain Res* 1987;412(1):84–95.

78. de Leon RD, Hodgson JA, Roy RR, et al. Locomotor capacity attributable to step training versus spontaneous recovery after spinalization in adult cats. *J Neurophysiol* 1998;79(3):1329–1340
79. de Leon RD, Tamaki H, Hodgson JA, et al. Hindlimb locomotor and postural training modulates glycinergic inhibition in the spinal cord of the adult spinal cat. *J Neurophysiol* 1999;82(1):359–369.
80. Wernig A, Müller S. Laufband locomotion with body weight support improved walking in persons with severe spinal cord injuries. *Paraplegia* 1992;30(4):229–238.
81. Wernig A, Nanassy A, Müller S. Maintenance of locomotor abilities following Laufband (treadmill) therapy in para- and tetraplegic persons: follow-up studies. *Spinal Cord* 1998;36(11):744–749.
82. Wernig A, Nanassy A, Müller S. Laufband (treadmill) therapy in incomplete paraplegia and tetraplegia. *J Neurotrauma* 1999;16(8):719–726.
83. Nymark J, DeForge D, Barbeau H, et al. Body weight support treadmill gait training in the subacute phase of incomplete spinal cord injury. *J Neurol Rehabil* 1998;12(3):119–138.
84. Maegele M, Müller S, Wernig A, et al. Recruitment of spinal motor pools during voluntary movements versus stepping after human spinal cord injury. *J Neurotrauma* 2002;19(10):1217–1229.
85. Harkema SJ. Neural plasticity after human spinal cord injury: application of locomotor training to the rehabilitation of walking. *Neuroscientist* 2001;7(5):455–468.
86. Field-Fote EC. Spinal cord control of movement: implications for locomotor rehabilitation following spinal cord injury. *Phys Ther* 2000;80(5):477–484.
87. Field-Fote EC, Tepavac D. Improved intralimb coordination in people with incomplete spinal cord injury following training with body weight support and electrical stimulation. *Phys Ther* 2002;82(7):707–715.
88. Behrman AL, Harkema SJ. Locomotor training after human spinal cord injury: a series of case studies. *Phys Ther* 2000;80(7):688–700.
89. Behrman AL, Lawless-Dixon AR, Davis SB, et al. Locomotor training progression and outcomes after incomplete spinal cord injury. *Phys Ther* 2005;85(12):1356–1371.
90. Barbeau H, Fung J. The role of rehabilitation in the recovery of walking in the neurological population. *Curr Opin Neurol* 2001;14(6):735–740.
91. Barbeau H, Pepin A, Norman KE, et al. Walking after spinal cord injury: control and recovery. *Neuroscientist* 1998;4(1):14–24.
92. Field-Fote EC, Lindley SD, Sherman AL. Locomotor training approaches for individuals with spinal cord injury: a preliminary report of walking-related outcomes. *J Neurol Phys Ther* 2005;29(3):127–137.
93. Nymark JR, Balmer SJ, Melis EH, et al. Electromyographic and kinematic nondisabled gait differences at extremely slow overground and treadmill walking speeds. *J Rehabil Res Dev* 2005;42(4):523–534.
94. Protas EJ, Holmes SA, Qureshy H, et al. Supported treadmill ambulation training after spinal cord injury: a pilot study. *Arch Phys Med Rehabil* 2001;82(6):825–831.
95. Dobkin B, Apple D, Barbeau H, et al. Weight-supported treadmill vs. over-ground training for walking after acute incomplete SCI. *Neurology* 2006;66(4):484–493.
96. Dietz V, Colombo G, Jensen L, et al. Locomotor capacity of spinal cord in paraplegic patients. *Ann Neurol* 1995;37(5):574–582.
97. Harkema SJ, Hurley SL, Patel UK, et al. Human lumbosacral spinal cord interprets loading during stepping. *J Neurophysiol* 1997;77(2):797–811.
98. Beres-Jones JA, Harkema SJ. The human spinal cord interprets velocity-dependent afferent input during stepping. *Brain* 2004;127(pt10):2232–2246.
99. Ferris DP, Gordon KE, Beres-Jones JA, et al. Muscle activation during unilateral stepping occurs in the nonstepping limb of humans with clinically complete spinal cord injury. *Spinal Cord* 2004;42(1):14–23.
100. Forrest GF, Sisto SA, Asselin PS, et al. Locomotor training with incremental changes in velocity: muscle and metabolic responses. *Top Spinal Cord Inj Rehabil* 2008;14(1):16–22.
101. Beres-Jones JA, Johnson TD, Harkema SJ. Clonus after human spinal cord injury cannot be attributed solely to recurrent muscle-tendon stretch. *Exp Brain Res* 2003;149(2):222–236.
102. Dietz V, Müller R, Colombo G. Locomotor activity in spinal man: significance of afferent input from joint and load receptors. *Brain* 2002;125(pt12):2626–2634.
103. Dobkin BH, Harkema S, Requejo P, et al. Modulation of locomotor-like EMG activity in subjects with complete and incomplete spinal cord injury. *J Neurol Rehabil* 1995;9(4):183–190.
104. Forrest GF, Sisto SA, Barbeau H, et al. Neuromotor and musculoskeletal responses to locomotor training for an individual with chronic motor complete, ASIA B spinal cord injury. *J Spinal Cord Med* 2008;31(5): 509–521.
105. Hicks AL, Adams MM, Martin Ginis K, et al. Long-term body-weight-supported treadmill training and subsequent follow-up in persons with chronic SCI: effects on functional walking ability and measures of subjective well-being. *Spinal Cord* 2005;43(5):291–298.
106. Postans NJ, Hasler JP, Granat MH, et al. Functional electric stimulation to augment partial weight-bearing supported treadmill training for patients with acute incomplete spinal cord injury: A pilot study. *Arch Phys Med Rehabil* 2004;85(4):604–610.
107. Hesse S, Uhlenbrock D. A mechanized gait trainer for restoration of gait. *J Rehabil Res Dev* 2000;37(6):701–708.
108. Hornby TG, Zemon DH, Campbell D. Robotic-assisted, body-weight-supported treadmill training in individuals following motor incomplete spinal cord injury. *Phys Ther* 2005;85(1):52–66.
109. Wirz M, Zemon DH, Rupp R, et al. Effectiveness of automated locomotor training in patients with chronic incomplete spinal cord injury: a multicenter trial. *Arch Phys Med Rehabil* 2005;86(4):672–680.
110. Field-Fote EC. Combined use of body weight support, functional electric stimulation, and treadmill training to improve walking ability in individuals with chronic incomplete spinal cord injury. *Arch Phys Med Rehabil* 2001;82(6):818–824.
111. Colombo G, Joerg M, Schreier R, et al. Treadmill training of paraplegic patients using a robotic orthosis. *J Rehabil Res Dev* 2000;37(6):693–700.

112. Colombo G, Wirz M, Dietz V. Driven gait orthosis for improvement of locomotor training in paraplegic patients. *Spinal Cord* 2001;39(5):252–255.
113. Hidler JM, Wall AE. Alterations in muscle activation patterns during robotic-assisted walking. *Clin Biomech (Bristol, Avon)* 2005;20(2):184–193.
114. Ferris DP, Gordon KE, Sawicki GS, et al. An improved powered ankle-foot orthosis using proportional myoelectric control. *Gait Posture* 2006;23(4):425–428.
115. Ferris DP, Czerniecki JM, Hannaford B. An ankle-foot orthosis powered by artificial pneumatic muscles. *J Appl Biomech* 2005;21(2):189–197.
116. Galvez JA, Budovitch A, Harkema SJ, et al. Quantification of therapists' manual assistance on the leg during treadmill gait training with partial body-weight support after spinal cord injury. *Conf Proc IEEE Eng Med Biol Soc* 2007;2007:4028–4032.
117. Aoyagi D, Ichinose WE, Harkema SJ, et al. A robot and control algorithm that can synchronously assist in naturalistic motion during body-weight-supported gait training following neurologic injury. *IEEE Trans Neural Syst Rehabil Eng* 2007;15(3):387–400.
118. Reinkensmeyer D, Aoyagi D, Emken J, et al. Robotic gait training: toward more natural movements and optimal training algorithms. *Conf Proc IEEE Eng Med Biol Soc* 2004;7:4818–4821.
119. Barbeau H, Ladouceur M, Mirbagheri MM, et al. The effect of locomotor training combined with functional electrical stimulation in chronic spinal cord injured subjects: walking and reflex studies. *Brain Res Brain Res Rev* 2002;40(1–3):274–291.
120. Wernig A. Long-term body-weight supported treadmill training and subsequent follow-up in persons with chronic SCI: effects on functional walking ability and measures of subjective well-being. *Spinal Cord* 2006;44(4):265–266.
121. Mehrohlz J Kugler J, Pohl M. Locomotor training for walking after spinal cord injury. *Cochrane Database Syst Rev* 2008;2:CD006676. doi:10.1002/14651858.CD006676.
122. Giangregorio LM, Craven BC, Webber CE. Musculoskeletal changes in women with spinal cord injury: a twin study. *J Clin Densitom* 2005;8(3):347–351.
123. Giangregorio LM, Hicks AL, Webber CE, et al. Body weight supported treadmill training in acute spinal cord injury: impact on muscle and bone. *Spinal Cord* 2005;43(11):649–657.
124. Giangregorio LM, Webber CE, Phillips SM, et al. Can body weight supported treadmill training increase bone mass and reverse muscle atrophy in individuals with chronic incomplete spinal cord injury? *Appl Physiol Nutr Metab* 2006;31(3):283–291.
125. Giangregorio LM, McCartney N. Reduced loading due to spinal-cord injury at birth results in "slender" bones: a case study. *Osteoporos Int* 2007;18(1):117–120.
126. Hicks AL, Ginis KA. Treadmill training after spinal cord injury: it's not just about the walking. *J Rehabil Res Dev* 2008;45(2):241–248.
127. Phillips SM, Stewart BG, Mahoney DJ, et al. Body-weight-support treadmill training improves blood glucose regulation in persons with incomplete spinal cord injury. *J Appl Physiol* 2004;97(2):716–724.
128. Stewart BG, Tarnopolsky MA, Hicks AL, et al. Treadmill training-induced adaptations in muscle phenotype in persons with incomplete spinal cord injury. *Muscle Nerve* 2004;30(1):61–68.
129. Sadowsky CL, McDonald JW. Activity-based restorative therapies: concepts and applications in spinal cord injury-related neurorehabilitation. Dev Disabil Res Rev 2009;15(2):112–116.
130. Harkema SJ, Forrest GF, Behrman A, et al. Improvements in functional outcome measures after human spinal cord injury from a multi-center network providing Locomotor Training. Soc Neurosci 2008 [Abstract].
131. Herman R, He J, D'Luzansky S, et al. Spinal cord stimulation facilitates functional walking in a chronic, incomplete spinal cord injured. Spinal Cord 2002;40(2):65–68.
132. Kathleen JG, Willis WT, Carhart MR, et al. Epidural spinal cord stimulation improves locomotor performance in low ASIA C, wheelchair-dependent, spinal cord-injured individuals: insights from metabolic response. Top Spinal Cord Injury Rehabil 2005;11(2): 50–63.
133. McDonald JW, Becker D, Sadowsky CL, et al. Late recovery following spinal cord injury. Case report and review of the literature. J Neurosurg 2002;97(2 Suppl): 252–265.
134. Kirshblum S, Millis S, McKinley W, et al. Late neurologic recovery after traumatic spinal cord injury. Arch Phys Med Rehabil 2004;85(11):1811–1817.
135. Cook AM, Hussey SM. *Assistive technology: principals and practice*. St Louis, MO: Mosby, 1995:5.
136. Graf M, Severe E, Holle A. Environmental control unit considerations for the person with high-level tetraplegia. *Top Spinal Cord Inj Rehabil* 1997;2(3):30–40.
137. Stiefbold G, Carolan T. Using assistive technology. In: Sisto SA, Druin E, Sliwinski MM, eds. *Spinal cord injuries: managament and rehabilitation*. St Louis, MO: Mosby, 2009:310–325.
138. Little R. Electronic aides for daily living. Phys Med Clin N Am 2010;21:33–42.
139. Wang W, Collinger JL, Perez MA, et al. Neural interface technology for rehabilitation: exploiting and promoting neuroplasticity. Phys Med Rehabil Clin N Am 2010;21(1):157–178.
140. Daly JJ, Wolpaw JR. Brain-computer interfaces in neurological rehabilitation. Lancet Neurol 2008;7(11): 1032–1043.
141. Birbaumer N, Cohen LG. Brain-computer interfaces: communication and restoration of movement in paralysis. J Physiol 2007;579:621–636.
142. Buch E, Weber C, Cohen LG, et al. Think to move: a neuromagnetic brain-computer interface (BCI) system for chronic stroke. Stroke 2008;39(3):910–917.
143. Wolpaw JR, Birbaumer N, McFarland DJ, et al. Brain-computer interfaces for communication and control. Clin Neurophysiol 2002;113(6):767–791.
144. Moritz CT, Perlmutter SI, Fetz EE. Direct control of paralysed muscles by cortical neurons. Nature 2008;456:639–642.
145. Morrow MM, Pohlmeyer EA, Miller LE. Control of muscle synergies by cortical ensembles. Adv Exp Med Biol 2009;629:179–199.

146. Eberhardt, K. Home modifications for persons with spinal cord injury. *OT Pract* 1998;3(10):24–27.
147. Kirshblum S. Fichtenbaum J. Breaking the news in spinal cord injury. *J Spinal Cord Inj Med* 2008;31(1):7–12.
148. Ditunno JF, Flanders A, Kirshblum SC, et al. Predicting outcome in traumatic spinal cord injury. In: Kirshblum S, Campagnolo DI, DeLisa JA, eds. *Spinal cord medicine*. Philadelphia, PA: Lippincott Williams & Wilkins, 2002:108–122.
149. Fallowfield LJ, Hall A, Maguire GP, et al. Psychological outcomes of different treatment policies in women with early breast cancer outside a clinical trial. *BMJ* 1990;301(6752):575–580.
150. Byock I, Corbeil YS. Caring when cure is no longer possible. In: Overcash J, Balducci L, eds. *The older cancer patient: a guide for nurses and related professionals*. New York, NY: Springer Publishing Company, 2003:193–214.
151. Salander P, Bergenheim AT, Bergstrom P, et al. How to tell cancer patients: a contribution to a theory of communicating the diagnosis. *J Psychosoc Oncol* 1999;16(2): 79–93.
152. Maguire P. Breaking bad news. *Eur J Surg Oncol* 1998;24(3):188–199.
153. Girgis A, Sanson-Fisher RW. Breaking bad news. 1: Current best advice for clinicians. *Behav Med* 1998;24(2):53–59.
154. Rosenbaum ME, Ferguson KJ, Lobas JG. Teaching medical students and residents skills for delivering bad news: a review of strategies. *Acad Med* 2004;79(2):107–117.
155. Ptacek JT, Eberhardt TL. Breaking bad news:a review of the literature. *JAMA* 1996;276(6):496–502.
156. Sher TG, Cella D, Leslie WT, et al. Communication differences between physicians and their patients in an oncology setting. *J Clin Psychol Med Settings* 1997;4(3):281–293.
157. Smith DC. *Being a wounded healer: how to heal ourselves while we are healing others*. Madison, WI: Psycho-Spiritual Publications, 1999.
158. DeJong G, Branch LG, Corcoran PJ. Independent living outcomes in spinal cord injury: Multivariate analyses. *Arch Phys Med Rehabil* 1984;65(2):66–73.
159. Monga,TN, Ostermann, HJ, Kerrigan, AJ. Driving: a clinical perspective on rehabilitation technology. In: *Physical medicine and rehabilitation: state of the art reviews*. Philadelphia, PA: Hanley & Belfus, Inc., 1997;11(1):69–92.
160. Pierce S. A roadmap for driver rehabilitation. *OT Pract* 1996;1(10):30–38.
161. Kirshblum S, Ho CH, House JG, et al. Rehabilitation of spinal cord injury. In: Kirshblum S, Campagnolo DI, DeLisa JA, eds. *Spinal cord medicine*. Philadelphia, PA: Lippincott Williams & Wilkins, 2002:275–298.
162. Harvard AB, Shipp MK. Disabilities and their implications for driver assessment and training. Ruston, LA: Louisianna Tech University, 1998.
163. Babirad J. Considerations in seating and positioning severely disabled drivers. *Assist Technol* 1989;1(2):31–37.
164. Strano CM. Physical Disabilities and their implications driving. *Work* 1997;8(3):261–266.
165. Holicky R. Big vans, minivans: pros and cons. *New Mob* 1995;6(22):50–53.
166. McKinley W. Non-traumatic spinal cord injury/disease: etiologies and outcomes. *Top Spinal Cord Inj Rehabil* 2008;14(2):1–9.
167. Gupta A, Taly AB, Srivastava A, et al. Non-traumatic spinal cord lesions: epidemiology, complications, neurological and functional outcome of rehabilitation. *Spinal Cord* 2009;47(4): 307–311.
168. McKinley WO, Conti-Wyneken AR, Vokac CN, et al. Rehabilitative functional outcome of patients with neoplastic spinal cord compression. *Arch Phys Med Rehabil*1996;77(9):892–895.
169. McKinley WO, Huang ME, Tewksbury MA. Neoplastic vs. traumatic spinal cord injury: an inpatient rehabilitation comparison. *Am J Phys Med Rehabil* 2000;79(2): 138–144.
170. McKinley WO, Tellis AA, Cifu DX, et al. Rehabilitation outcome of individuals with nontraumatic myelopathy resulting from spinal stenosis. *J Spinal Cord Med* 1998;21(2):131–136.
171. McKinley WO, Teskbury MA, Godbout CJ. Comparison of medical complications following nontraumatic and traumatic spinal cord injury. *J Spinal Cord Med* 2002;25(2):88–93.
172. New PW, Rawicki HB, Bailey MJ. Nontraumatic spinal cord injury: demographic characteristics and complications. *Arch Phys Med Rehabil* 2002;83(7):996–1001.
173. Chapman J. Comparing medical complications from nontraumatic and traumatic spinal cord injury [AAPMR abstract 26]. *Arch Phys Med Rehabil* 2000;81(9):1264.
174. Ones K, Yilmaz E, Beydogan A, et al. Comparison of functional results in non-traumatic and traumatic spinal cord injury. *Disabil Rehabil* 2007;29(15):1185–1191.
175. McKinley WO, Seel RT, Gadi RK, et al. Nontraumatic vs. traumatic spinal cord injury: a rehabilitation outcome comparison. *Am J Phys Med Rehabil* 2001;80(9): 693–699.

CHAPTER 18 ■ WHEELCHAIRS/ADAPTIVE MOBILITY EQUIPMENT AND SEATING

BRAD E. DICIANNO, MARK SCHMELER, AND BETTY Y. LIU

INTRODUCTION

The selection of an appropriate seating and mobility system is critical for the consumer with a spinal cord injury (SCI) to have optimal function. There are many factors that influence the selection of the system, including personal preference, as well as physical, medical, social, psychological, and environmental factors. A team approach is recommended to address all areas of concern for an appropriate selection. The team members should consist of the consumer and caretakers, physician, therapist, assistive technology professional, rehabilitation engineer, social worker/case manager, vocational rehabilitation counselor, and the supplier of the devices.

The consumer can become overwhelmed by the vast and ever-changing technology and the many options for seating and mobility devices. The costs of components are as varied as the variety of choices. Thus, participating in a specialty seating and wheelchair clinic has become a necessity, especially to ensure best practices and compliance with funding policies. Practitioners should be knowledgeable about the basic seating principles and available products. This chapter addresses the types, components, and principles of seating and mobility systems.

THE EVALUATION PROCESS

A mobility device assessment begins by assessing the reason for the referral and the expected outcome of the intervention. The assessment should be performed by knowledgeable and trained clinicians in a face-to-face evaluation. The team should discuss with the consumer their goals in order to prioritize importance and practicality in accordance with specific needs and lifestyle. The goals described in Table 18.1 can assist the practitioner when prescribing and justifying a seating and mobility system.

Prior to prescribing a seating and mobility system, the team must assess the consumer's abilities, functional history, medical status, accessibility issues, and postural deficits. Table 18.2 is a general but not exhaustive guideline for practitioners to follow when assessing the consumer. After a device is selected, final specifications and documentation must be completed in accordance with guidelines of the funding source. Once funding approval is obtained, the consumer usually returns to clinic for fitting and training with the device. Over time, follow-up is needed to ensure that the device continues to meet the consumer's needs and that necessary repairs are performed.

MANUAL WHEELCHAIRS

Categories of Wheelchairs

Manual wheelchairs are classified by materials used in their construction and the ability to adjust for appropriate seating and mobility. Each of these mobility systems differs in features, options, and cost. The major types of wheelchairs include the standard, lightweight, high-strength lightweight, ultra-lightweight, heavy duty, and hemi-height.

Standard wheelchairs are made of steel and weigh approximately 40 to 65 lb. They have a folding frame with a nonadjustable axle plate. The limited adjustability and lack of positioning and pressure relief options preclude prescription of these devices for an everyday wheelchair user, except in rare cases such as short-term use when the user has no positioning or pressure relief needs.

Lightweight wheelchairs are usually made of stainless steel and weigh less than 36 lb. They typically lack adjustable axles and are not recommended for the active user. Because the chair weight is fixed and both the rear wheel placement and the cross brace frame are not adjustable, active users will be limited in performance and positioning when using these wheelchairs.

Ultra-lightweight wheelchairs weigh less than 30 lb and have partial to full axle adjustment. These chairs are constructed of aluminum, titanium, or composite material and are prescribed for active users.

Some rigid frames offer the ability to adjust the seat-to-back angle for enhancing trunk stability. For the practitioner, these adjustability features are effective tools for positioning and improving mobility skills when evaluating a consumer for an appropriate seating and mobility system, especially in a novice user. The weight capacity for this wheelchair approaches 250 to 300 lb.

Heavy duty frame wheelchairs are constructed with a double cross brace–folding frame or reinforced rigid style frame for consumers who weigh more than 250 lb. The wheelchairs weigh approximately 50 to 60 lb.

Hemi-height wheelchairs vary in seat-to-floor height allowing the lower limbs to reach the floor and assist in propulsion. They usually have folding frames with swing-away footrests to allow for foot propulsion.

Manual Wheelchair Components

Frames

Earlier manual wheelchairs were not only limited in style and design but were heavier due to the chrome folding-frame. Choices

TABLE 18.1

GOALS FOR SEATING AND MOBILITY

1. Provide proper positional support to prevent/accommodate postural deformities.
2. Maximize function.
3. Enhance stability, balance, and physiological function.
4. Reduce the influences of abnormal reflexes and spasticity.
5. Ensure skin integrity through an appropriate pressure relieving system.
6. Provide a system to meet the consumer's lifestyle and environmental factors.
7. Meet the consumer's need for aesthetics and cosmesis.

expanded in the late 1970s when wheelchair athletes began to change the design and frame composition needed in lightweight wheelchairs (1). Wheelchair athletes also cultivated use of modular frames and adjustable axle plates for better performance and to address positional needs (see Table 18.3 for summary).

There are two primary types of frames: folding and rigid (Table 18.3). Folding frames have a cross (X-shaped) brace that connects the side frames and can be folded by pulling up the center of the seat (Fig. 18.1). Folding frames have more parts, are heavier, and are not as energy efficient as rigid frames due to the cross brace.

TABLE 18.2

AREAS TO ASSESS PRIOR TO PRESCRIPTION

Medical history	• Diagnosis (primary/secondary) • Past medical history including: • Cardiopulmonary status • Skin status • Orthopaedic conditions • Neurological conditions • Bowel and bladder function • Visual problems • Cognitive issues • Pain issues (i.e., shoulder) • History of falls • What alternative methods of rehabilitation have been tried • Prognosis/progression of disease
Physical examination	• Height/weight/age • Cognitive status • Cardiopulmonary endurance • Orthostasis • Active/passive ROM of joints • Strength • Sensation • Spasticity • Reflexes • Muscle tone • Balance, coordination, and trunk control • Ambulation, transfer, and fall assessment • Skin integrity • Edema
Environment	• Living situation • Accessibility • Transportation • Vocational needs
Additional technology	• Environmental control unit • Computer access
Funding	• Insurance coverage • Foundation or waiver programs • Vocational rehabilitation

Rigid frames are more energy efficient due to the lessened internal energy needed to propel fewer parts and lighter weight (Fig. 18.2). They are sometimes more difficult to transport due to the fixed size of the box frame. However, the wheels can be removed and the back can be folded down in order to be placed in a trunk or back seat of a car (Fig. 18.3). Some rigid frame designs, rather than having a box-shaped frame, have a cantilever frame in which the caster and wheel are attached by one tube on each side. This design uses less tubing and reduces overall weight.

On semiadjustable wheelchairs, the position of the rear wheels can be horizontally and/or vertically adjusted in conjunction with the caster assembly. Horizontal adjustment is usually limited in wheelchairs having folding frames but is beneficial for improving propulsion by allowing the rear wheels to be moved forward. Lowering or elevating the rear of the seat can accommodate trunk instability. Raising the axle plate will lower the rear seat, placing the consumer in a posterior tilt, or *dump*. Dump gives the user more stability in the seat and better access to the wheels for propulsion. Reasons for this type of setup are important to state in the clinical justification for an ultra-lightweight wheelchair. Another possible frame adjustment is the change of angles at the base of the wheels, or *camber*. Cambered wheels are angled outward at the base, so that the overall floor width of the chair tires is increased when compared to vertical wheels. Camber is often used by active users or wheelchair athletes to lower the center of gravity, increase stability by increasing the base of support, improve ease of turning and propulsion, and protect the fingers (since the bottom of the wheel will hit a vertical surface like a door jam before the top of the pushrim). However, excessive camber used on sports wheelchairs can also increase the overall width of the wheelchair and create environmental accessibility issues.

Performance has become the main issue in selecting an appropriate wheelchair to meet the consumer's lifestyle. In general, a rigid frame wheelchair is easier to push, has less roll resistance, and is more adjustable to meet the needs of an active user (1). Depending on the transferring ability of the user of the rigid frame, the footrest may need to accommodate the users' leg positioning. The majority of current wheelchair frames and components are constructed of strong, light materials such as aluminum, titanium, or carbon fiber, which make manual wheelchairs lighter for propulsion and more durable for everyday use.

Armrests

Armrests serve many purposes including support of the upper limbs, postural stability, and providing an anchor for transfers, repositioning, or pressure relief. The consumer's level of function, independence, lifestyle, and seating system guides selection of styles.

The two-point armrest can be either fixed or removable depending on the consumer's transferability. Fixed armrests are durable and inexpensive. The disadvantages include the need to remove the armrest for lateral or sliding board transfers, and a problem with mounting certain seating systems. Two-point armrests have several options: full or desk length, adjustable or fixed height, straight or offset, tubular, and flip-up. Full-length armrests can be used for leverage and are thus beneficial

TABLE 18.3

WHEELCHAIR OPTIONS

Wheelchair options	Advantages	Disadvantages
1. Frames:		
Folding	• Easy to transport • Absorbs uneven terrain, better for smoother ride	• Heavier • More parts • Not as durable • Limited width sizes
Rigid	• More energy efficient • Fewer parts • Lighter weight • More responsive • More durable • Smaller turning radius	• Difficult to transport • Rougher ride • Lower limb positioning concerns
2. Armrests:		
Full length	• Assists with sit to stand transfers • Upper limb positioning	• Obstacle for tabletops
Desk-length	• Improved accessibility	• Decreased arm support • Difficulty with transfers
Adjustable Height	• Upper limb positioning and support • Accessibility • Assist with transfers	• Maintenance
Fixed Height	• Less adjustments	• Poor upper limb positioning
Offset	• Decrease overall width	• Difficulty with mounting back systems
Tubular	• Ease of removal • Light weight	• Not used for weight bearing • Limited adjustment
Cantilever	• Flip back for transfers	• Do not lock in place • Difficulty with mounting back systems
3. Footrests:		
Customized foot boxes	• Accomodate orthopedic deformities, can prevent skin breakdown	• Bulky
Swing-away	• Ease of removal for transfers • Accessibility to countertops	• Added weight • Maintenance • Increases overall length • Increases turning radius
Elevating	• Positioning for lower limb orthopaedic issues or edema	• Added weight • Increases overall length • Increases turning radius • Bulky
Fixed	• Fewer parts • Increased maneuverability • Makes wheelchair lighter and more durable	• Transfer concerns • Transport issues • Lower limb limitations
4. Wheels:		
Mag	• Decreased maintenance • Durable	• Heavier
Spoke	• Light weight • Sport look	• More maintenance
X-core	• Light weight • Sport look	• Expensive • Limited type of tires used
Spinergy	• Light weight	• Expensive
Size:		
Large (24–26)	• Better upper limb positioning for propulsion	• Increases seat to floor height
Small (20,22)	• Decreased seat to floor height for ease of foot propulsion • Assist with sit to stand transfers	• Accessibility to tops of tables/desks
5. Tires:		
Pneumatic Air	• Good traction • Shock absorption	• Maintenance (flats) • Resistance due to tread
Airless	• Good traction • Maintenance free	• Harder ride • Heavier
Solid	• Ease of propulsion on level surfaces • Maintenance free	• Heavy • Slip on wet surfaces
High performance	• Ease of propulsion on level surfaces • Shock absorption	• Maintenance (flats) • Slip on wet surfaces • Poor performance on rough terrain

TABLE 18.3

WHEELCHAIR OPTIONS (*Continued*)

Wheelchair options	Advantages	Disadvantages
Kik Knobbie	• Light tread for better performance than solids • Maintenance free • Good traction on rough terrain	• Heavy • Poor shock absorption • Increased overall width • Bulky • Not good indoors
6. **Handrims:**		
Aluminum Plastic coated Projections	• Maintenance free • Enhances traction for consumers with limited grasp • Assists with propulsion	• Require good hand function • Need to maintain (cracks and cuts) • Increases overall width • Uneven placement during propulsion
Ergonomic/natural fit	• Fits hands for ease of propulsion	• More expensive
7. **Casters:**		
Large (6–8 inches)	• Better performance outdoors and on rough terrain	• Increases turning radius • Not good indoors • Limits front angle degree
Small (3–5 inches)	• Tighter turning radius • Better maneuverability	• Outdoor limitations • Decrease stability
8. **Wheel Locks:**		
Push/Pull Scissors	• Easy to operate even with limited hand function • Out of the way during propulsion	• Transfer clearance • Need good balance • Good hand function needed
High Mount Low Mount	• Easy to reach • Out of the way during propulsion and transfers	• Transfer clearance • Need good balance
9. **Back Support:**		
Sling Vinyl back	• Flexible/foldable • Hygienic • Durable	• poor trunk support
Tension Adjustable Solid Back Custom molded	• Better trunk support • Best support • Best pressure distribution	• Frequent adjustments needed • No flexibility/adjustment • Time consuming due to possible multiple fittings needed • Expensive

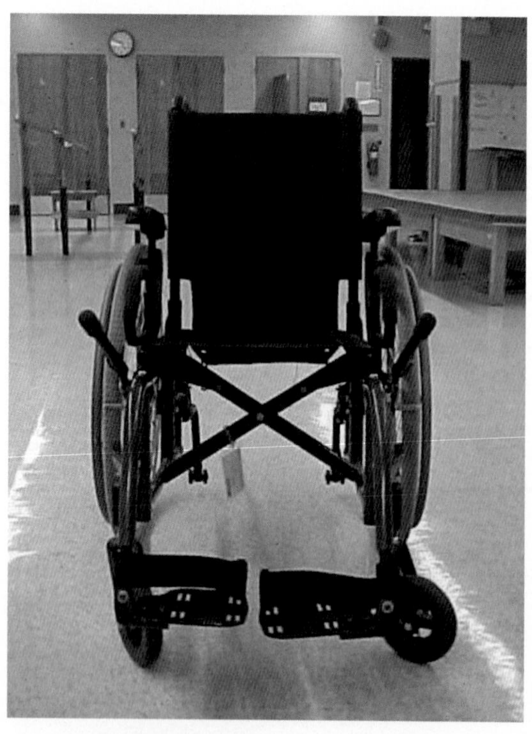

FIGURE 18.1. Folding cross brace frame.

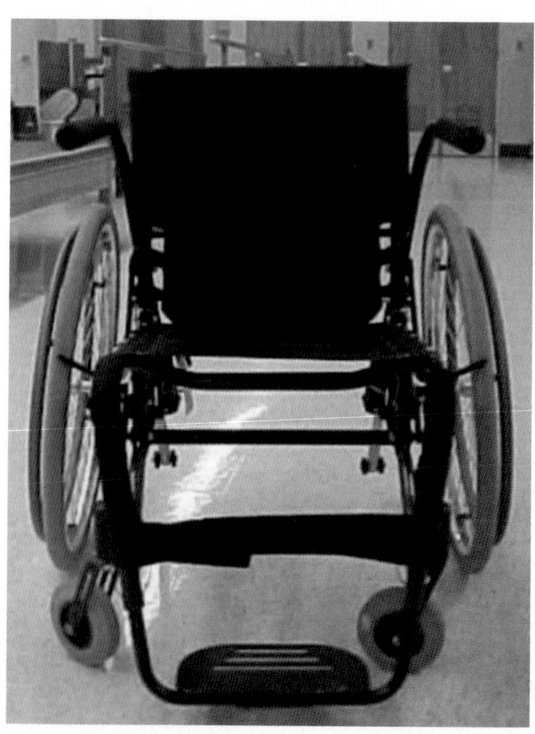

FIGURE 18.2. Rigid frame.

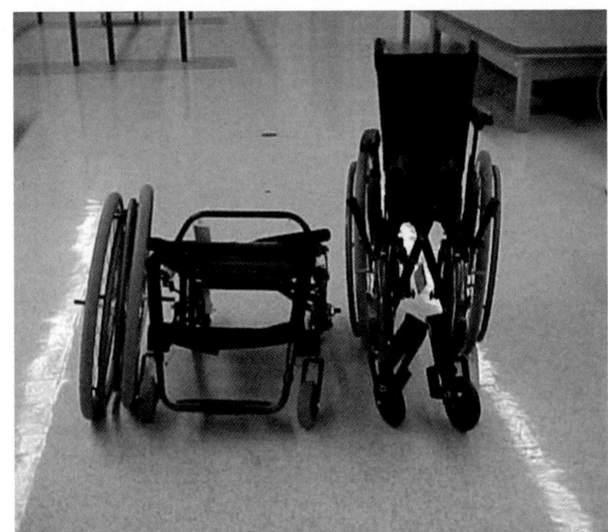

FIGURE 18.3. Rigid (on the **left**) and folding frame (on the **right**) wheelchair collapsed.

for consumers who are able to stand to transfer or ambulate. Their longer length can, however, become an obstacle for accessibility to table tops or desks. Desk length armrests extend to half of the length of the seat depth and improve accessibility but reduce full-arm support.

Height adjustment is a feature that is important to allow positioning and support of the arm and shoulder. The user can raise or lower the armrest according to his or her seat-to-elbow height. Some wheelchairs offer an offset option, which decreases the overall width of the wheelchair by wrapping around the back cane of the wheelchair. The arms may still be removed for transfers as needed. The flip-up armrest option is important for some consumers with limited hand function and strength, can permit easier transfers, and eliminates misplacing the armrest.

Tubular armrests are best for the active user who does not rely on the armrest as much for weight bearing, positioning, or stability. They are lighter in weight but generally not strong enough to provide stability for weight shifts or transfers. The tubular armrests are used for propping the arms when not propelling and are easy to swing out of the way for propulsion or transfers.

Cantilever armrests are attached to the back canes on a pivot joint and can be flipped up and out of the way. They can be used for weight bearing, positioning, and transfers. Arm troughs can be added for consumers who require additional support.

Armrests may be omitted when consumers are very active and have good trunk stability. This decreases the weight and eliminates unnecessary parts from the frame.

Footrests/Legrests

Manual wheelchairs provide lower limb support using three different types of legrests: swing-away, elevating, and fixed. This support is needed for positioning and for prevention of foot drop or other deformities. Prior to selecting the style, it is necessary to evaluate range of motion (ROM) in the limbs and muscle tone transfer ability, lifestyle, and function.

Swing-away footrests permit the consumer to swing the footrests out of the way and remove them to get closer to transfer surfaces. They favor ease of wheelchair portability and when removed reduce wheelchair weight when loading into a car. The footrest drops are available in discrete angles (60, 70, and 90 degrees), depending on the consumer's leg length (knee-to-heel), seat-to-floor height, and knee position. The closer the angle to 90 degrees, the better the turning radius, access to tables, and transfers, especially sit-to-stand transfers. The 60-degree front hangers are recommended for consumers to accommodate leg length discrepancies or knee range limitations; however, hamstring tightness needs to be assessed in a seated position, as positioning the feet further out can cause the user to slide forward in the seat and assume a compromised, slouched posture. Heel loops can attach to the footrest for positioning, and prevent the feet from falling off the legrest and impeding propulsion.

Elevating legrests are used for consumers with limited lower limb ROM, edema or spasticity, or the need to reposition the lower limbs. Careful attention needs to be paid to range of knee joint motion in a seated position, as many people have tight hamstrings. Elevating legrests are usually prescribed with a reclining backrest in order to extend the hip and remove tension on the hamstrings. Range should permit elevation of the feet above heart level in order to assist with passive management of lower extremity edema; therefore, elevating legrests typically work best with tilt-in-space and reclining backrests (2). They are also heavier and bulkier than swing-away footrests and increase the overall length of the chair. A calf pad or trough comes attached to the center of the legrest for support.

A fixed footrest cannot be removed and is most often seen on rigid frame wheelchairs. This footrest makes the frame lighter and stronger, but can make transfers and portability more difficult. While most rigid frames have nonremovable footrests, there are some that can be ordered with removable footrests as an option.

Custom footrests are sometimes needed in special consumer cases. Custom foot boxes are fabricated in cases involving postural deformity and when skin integrity may be compromised. Angle adjustable footplates permit plantar and dorsiflexion positioning with minimal inversion and eversion adjustment.

Seat and Back Upholstery and Backrests

Backrests are important for trunk support and comfortable body positioning while participating in everyday activities. A low back support may extend from the cushion to either the low lumbar spine or up to approximately 2 to 3 inches below the inferior angle of the scapula, and is best prescribed for active users with good trunk stability (i.e., clients with an injury below midthoracic level). A high back is needed for consumers who lack trunk stability. A high back supports the thoracic/lumbar spine and can range from 2 inches above the inferior angle of the scapula to the shoulder region depending on trunk stability and balance.

The standard seat and back of a manual wheelchair come with sling vinyl upholstery. Lightweight material is attached to the frame post allowing flexibility in folding for easy transport. The vinyl material is hygienic, durable, and inexpensive. Active users with good trunk control may prefer sling upholstery for ease of folding and lighter weight. The disadvantage is that sling upholstery does not provide adequate trunk support for higher level injuries and may eventually cause a hammock effect contributing to postural deformities. Tension adjustable upholstery is also an option. This upholstery has straps in the back that allow the user to tighten the back to prevent a hammock effect and improve lumbar support. Additional features such as lateral supports and a head rest can be added to a solid back. A solid back provides a firm surface for consumers who require better trunk support. Cushions with a solid bottom or insert are recommended to prevent this problem.

Some contoured backs are "off the shelf systems" with lateral supports symmetrically molded into the base. However, if consumers require more aggressive contouring or accommodation of their asymmetries, a custom-molded system is needed. This will provide the best pressure distribution and points of contact. These systems are time consuming and expensive to fabricate, but necessary for persons who are unable to sustain body position while seated.

Specialty seating can also be added and will be discussed later in the chapter.

Wheels

Wheel type and size affect the performance of the ride. The optimal reach for propelling the wheelchair is determined by the diameter of the wheel size and axle placement in relationship to the consumer's arm length and function. Wheel size and the seat-to-floor height need to be considered together. Wheel sizes vary from 20 to 26 inches, with 24 inches being the most common.

The most common types of wheels available are "mag" and spoke. Mag wheels were previously made of magnesium, but are now constructed from plastic. They are more durable and do not require maintenance, but are heavier than spoke wheels. Spoke wheels are lighter, but more care is needed to keep them tight and true. Another style seen on ultra-lightweight wheelchairs are X-core wheels, which are made of high-strength, lightweight, composite material. They are lighter than "mags" and do not require maintenance, but accept only certain high-performance tires and are more expensive. Spinergy wheels are lighter in weight than standard spoke wheels, are more durable, and require less maintenance than a standard spoke wheel, but are more expensive.

A variety of tires are currently available for wheelchair use (Table 18.3). The most common are treaded tires with the option of air or airless inserts. They provide good traction on everyday terrain, and when used with airless inserts require less maintenance. However, the ride is harder due to the solid foam insert. Other tire options include (a) high-performance tires that are air filled with minimal tread, which permit a more comfortable ride and low roll resistance, (b) Kik Tires, which are solid tires with low tread for indoor and outdoor terrain. and (c) knobby tires which give good traction on rough terrain but are bulky, increase width of the frame, and may therefore not be a good option for indoor mobility.

Handrims

Handrims, or pushrims, are located slightly lateral to each wheel and are used to enhance propulsion. They can be made from aluminum or foam/plastic coated for consumers with limited grip or hand function. Vertical or oblique projections on the rims can assist propulsion for people with limited grip. However, they are not often recommended because they increase the overall width of the chair and increase risk for injury. People with compromised grip function may need to be assessed for powered mobility as an alternative. Other pushrim options include the ergonomically designed Natural Fit Pushrim, where the space between the pushrim and wheelrim is filled and coated with a grip material to prevent fingers from getting caught, as well as to improve grip for propulsion and braking (3).

Casters

The casters are the smaller wheels in the front of the wheelchair that affect turning performance. They are available in various diameters (3 to 6, 8 inches), widths, and materials. As a general rule, the smaller the caster, the tighter the turning radius. However, smaller casters pose a problem with rougher terrain. Larger and wider casters perform better outdoors and on rougher terrain, but increase the turning radius. The materials used for casters are similar to those used for tires: pneumatic (air or airless) and solid.

The casters are attached to the wheelchair by stems and forks, which allow the casters to rotate. Suspension forks eliminate vibration and improve the smoothness of the ride.

Wheel Locks

Wheel locks act as a safety feature to stabilize the wheelchair for transfers and prevent the wheelchair from rolling. While they are sometimes called "brakes," this is somewhat of a misnomer because they lock the wheels completely. Wheel locks come in two styles depending on the consumers' hand function and balance. One style operates more easily by pushing and pulling and the other operates by a scissors action. Scissor brakes have the benefit of being out of the way during propulsion and transfers and are often prescribed for consumers having good hand function and body balance. Both styles can be mounted high or low depending on the frame construction. High mount locks are recommended for consumers who lack good trunk balance because they require minimum trunk movement to initiate. Low mount locks are appropriate for consumers with good balance, and in this case, the advantage is that the locks are out of the way during propulsion.

Additional Options

Additional wheelchair accessories that may be included in a prescription, along with their purpose, are listed in Table 18.4.

TABLE 18.4

WHEELCHAIR ACCESSORIES

Type	Purpose
Clothing Guards	To prevent clothing or skin from hitting the wheels and impeding function or causing issues with skin integrity. Some have holes to allow more easy removal.
Grade aids	Used to assist consumers when propelling up an incline. When flipped down they will allow the consumer to propel forward up an incline and prevent the wheelchair from rolling back.
Quick release wheels	Allows the consumer to remove the rims from the frame of the chair in order to disassemble for transport. An option for a quad release lever for consumers who have fine motor deficits is available.
Push handles	They attach to the canes, allowing others to assist with propulsion and negotiating environmental obstacles, i.e., curbs.
Positional belt	Attach to the frame of the wheelchair in order to maintain pelvic position and stability during propulsion.
Ventilator tray	Accommodates placement of a ventilator and battery for transport behind or underneath the frame of the wheelchair.
Antitips	Prevent the wheelchair from tipping backward especially on uneven surfaces, i.e., ramps.

Wheelchair Measurements

Figure 18.4 shows several standard wheelchair measurements. All measurements should be taken on a smooth, level surface such as a mat. To permit accurate measurement, the patient should be seated or supported in a neutral, upright posture rather than in the wheelchair. This will ensure that positioning in the new wheelchair will be optimal for preventing postural deformity and pressure sores (1).

Seat Width

Measurement of the seat width should be taken across the widest point of the hips, and incorporate clothing, braces, or orthoses. For patients who use a manual wheelchair as their primary means of mobility, the seat width should be the same as their hip width to maximize their wheel access. At times, and for functional purposes, the wheelchair seat width may be set up to 1 inch greater than the patient's measured hip width, which will permit greater independence in activities of

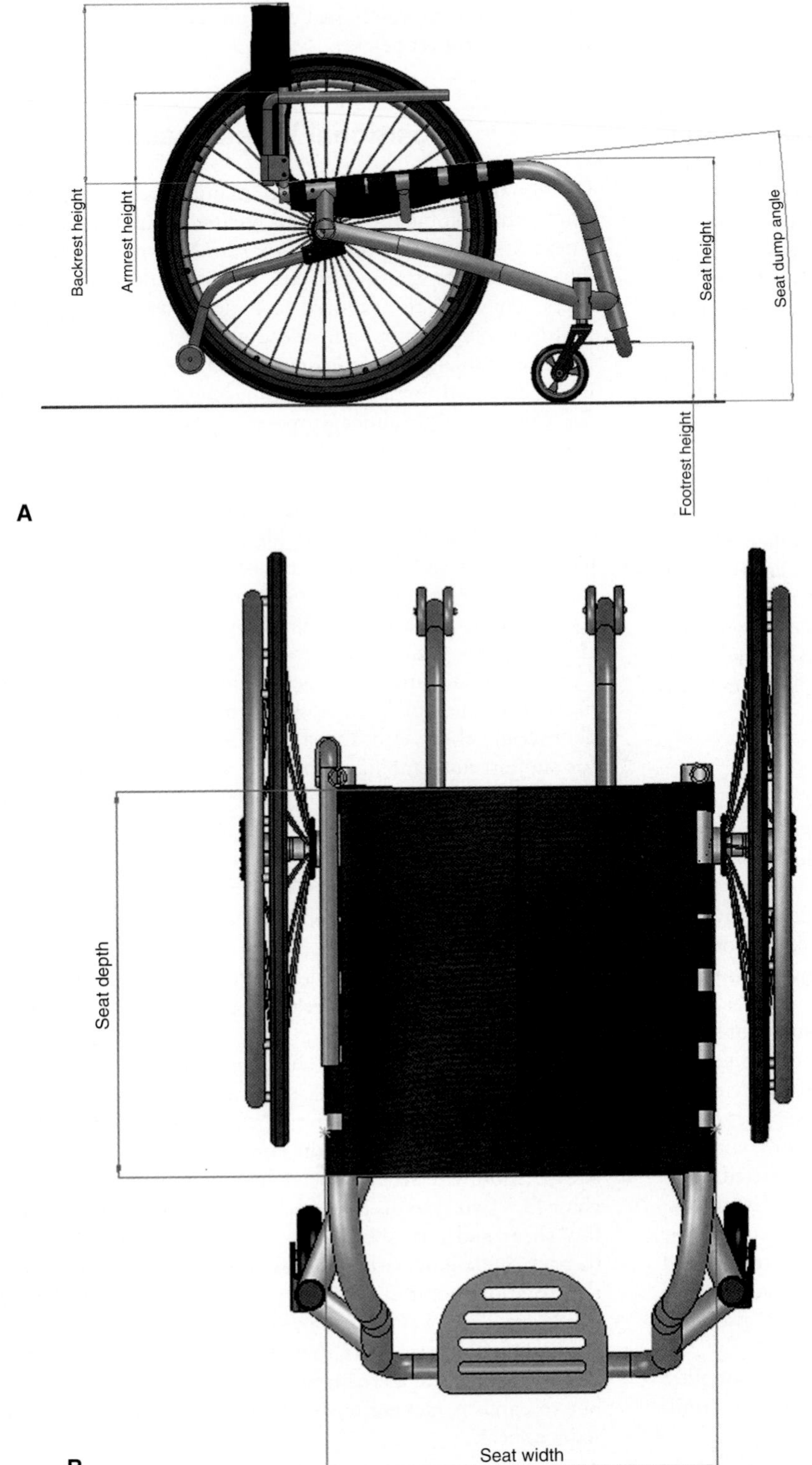

FIGURE 18.4. Measurements of a wheelchair.

daily living (ADL) or performing bladder management in their wheelchair.

If the wheelchair is too narrow, transfers will be more difficult and the patient may be more likely to develop a pressure sore in the greater trochanter area. Conversely, if the seat is too wide, truncal support is compromised leading to scoliosis, back pain, and difficulty with wheelchair propulsion. Wide seats also cause internal rotation at the shoulders, which can lead to rotator cuff impingement during propulsion.

Seat Depth

Seat depth is measured from the dorsal buttocks to the popliteal fossa and then subtracting about 2 inches from this measurement to prevent pressure in the popliteal fossa. If the backrest is cushioned, the thickness of the cushion must be considered. If a custom back is being used, it is important to measure the wheelchair seat depth from the actual position of the backrest to the front of the seat sling or pan. If the client will be propelling the manual wheelchair with his or her foot/feet, 1 to 2 inches is usually subtracted and the cushion is beveled back to allow the knee adequate flexion to propel the wheelchair.

If the seat depth is too shallow, there may be excessive hip flexion, thus increasing pressure on the ischial tuberosities.

Seat Height

Seat height is measured from the bottom of the heel of the foot or shoe to the posterior thigh. Subtract the height of the compressed seat cushion from the measurement, and then add 3 to 4 inches to allow for adequate legrest clearance. For the cushion height, it is important to consider the material: air, foam, or gel and the amount of compression that occurs when the patient is seated on it. Foam cushions compress to half their normal size; therefore, the cushion height that is subtracted is the "compressed" cushion height.

Back Support Height

The wheelchair back support height can vary depending on the capabilities and support needs of the patient. In general, the backrest should be high enough to provide good trunk support, but not inhibit movement. For very active patients with good trunk control, the backrests tend to be low and support just the lumbar spine. For better trunk support, the backrest can be extended to a point just below the inferior angle of the scapula.

To properly measure the back support, one should measure the distance from the bottom of the buttocks to the inferior angle of the scapula, and then add the "compressed" wheelchair cushion height to obtain the "true" back support height measurement. If the client has good trunk control and can propel a wheelchair, additional height can be subtracted. Caution should be taken in positioning to make sure that the client is not hyperextending the back over the back support for stability. If the patient has no upper extremity strength and poor trunk control, the back support should be just under his shoulder at the spine of the scapula. This client will also need to have a headrest for adequate support.

If the backrest is too high, it may interfere with shoulder movement. If it is too low, it will not provide adequate trunk stability.

Footrest Height

Footrest measurements should incorporate the distance from the patient's heel of the foot or shoe to the undersurface of the thigh at the popliteal fossa. Footrests are usually adjustable and should have approximately 2 inches of clearance from the floor.

Armrest Height

Armrest height should span the distance from the buttocks to the bottom of the patient's bent elbow at 90 degrees. The height of the compressed seat cushion should then be added to obtain the armrest height.

Positional Wheelchairs

Positional wheelchairs include manual reclining, tilt-in-space, and combination tilt and recline manual wheelchairs. These systems are preferred to standard and lightweight wheelchairs for those who are prone to develop pressure sores. They are also favored in patients who are unable to perform weight shifts, and those with postural deformities, balance problems, or orthostasis. A manual positional chair is not designed for self-propulsion, but is usually prescribed for a person who cannot propel a manual chair or independently operate a power chair. It is thus usually attendant propelled.

Positional manual wheelchairs weigh between 50 and 70 lb and are difficult to disassemble for transport. The recliner has the ability to fold but the type of seating system can limit this option. The tilt-in-space system permits the back canes to fold down to a box frame. However, transport for this chair requires a van, sport utility vehicle, or station wagon. Certain manufacturers will incorporate a power switch in the manual recline and/or tilt-in-space chair to facilitate independent weight shifts. A headrest and high back is recommended for support and stability, especially when performing weight shifts. Refer to Table 18.5 for the benefits and considerations of both systems.

Recline

A manual reclining wheelchair has a seat to back angle that the user can change. There are two types of recliners: semireclining and full. Semireclining wheelchairs allow up to 30 degrees of recline. A full reclining wheelchair permits to 90 degrees of recline (see Fig. 18.5).

The disadvantages of a reclining wheelchair include the weight, overall length (at least 3 inches longer), and bulk of the system. Another concern is shear of skin in the reclining position that occurs when the forces of the body are opposite to those exerted on the tissues of the buttocks by the chair (3). Two systems have been used to reduce this concern: low shear and zero shear. Low shear systems place the seat-to-back angle hinge a few inches above the seat, which alters the rotation point in reclining and lessens forward shear across the seating system. Low shear systems attach the back system to sliding mounts that move down as the system is reclined. So-called "zero-shear" systems have been developed but research is lacking on how much these systems actually reduce shear.

TABLE 18.5

WHEELCHAIR TYPES AND POWER SEATING FUNCTIONS

Type	Advantages	Disadvantages
1. **Power wheelchairs:**		
e-fix	• Easier to transport than conventional power • Two chairs in one • Lighter than power wheelchair	• Added stress on manual frame • Limited performance • Poor durability • Warranty issues
Power assist	• Two chairs in one • More easily transportable than conventional power	• Wheels are heavy • Wheels add width to frame
Transportable power	• Ability to disassemble for transport • Direct drive	• Heavy parts to transport • Limited programming • Cannot add power seat functions electronics not programmable
Conventional power	• Ability to integrate specialty controls • Programmability	• Difficult to transport
2. **Recline**	• Positioning • Easy for catheterization • Accommodate contractures when legs elevated • Comfort/rest • Manage tone • Minimize orthostasis	• Shear • May elicit extensor tone • Increases overall length
3. **Tilt-in-space**	• Pressure relief/weight shifts • Positioning • Comfort/rest • Manage tone • Minimize orthostasis • Tighter turning radius	• Urological concerns(urine back flowing during tilt when using a catheter) • Table clearance • Lap tray and communication device placement
4. **Standing**	• Pressure relief • Weight bearing • Urological benefits • Psychological benefits • Work/home accessibility	• Not appropriate for consumers with contractures, limited ROM, poor bone density • Orthostatic problems
5. **Seat elevator**	• Assist with transfers • Assist with ADLs, especially overhead when consumer has shoulder pathology • Psychological benefits • Accessibility to higher surfaces	• Adds height to chair • Tie down concerns
6. **Elevating legrests**	• Accommodate orthopaedic issues and contractures • Manage edema • Manage tone	• Add length to chair • Can interfere with transfers

Tilt-in-Space

Another option for positioning is the tilt-in-space system, in which the entire seat and back is a single unit, maintaining all seat angles (i.e., seat-to-back, seat-to-calf, and calf-to-foot). The major benefit of the tilt-in-space wheelchair is pressure relief. Many wheelchairs can tilt from 0 to 60 degrees or more. To achieve adequate pressure relief, tilt angle should be greater than 15 degrees. Although recommendations for angles vary, usually 45 degrees is recommended for pressure relief (2). In some cases, pressure relief can be optimized with a small degree of recline along with tilt. When in a tilted and reclined position, tilt should be used before recline, so that shear can be minimized when reassuming the upright position (see Fig. 18.6).

Tilt and recline can also be used for a variety of other purposes, which are more fully described elsewhere (2,4,5) and in the following section on powered wheelchairs.

Seat Elevators

Seat elevators can be added as a power seat function to power wheelchairs and even some scooters. Seat elevators raise and lower the vertical height of the seat and allow the consumer to perform ADLs above shoulder height (such as reaching cabinets) and to transfer to high or low surfaces.

Standing

Standing is described later in this chapter.

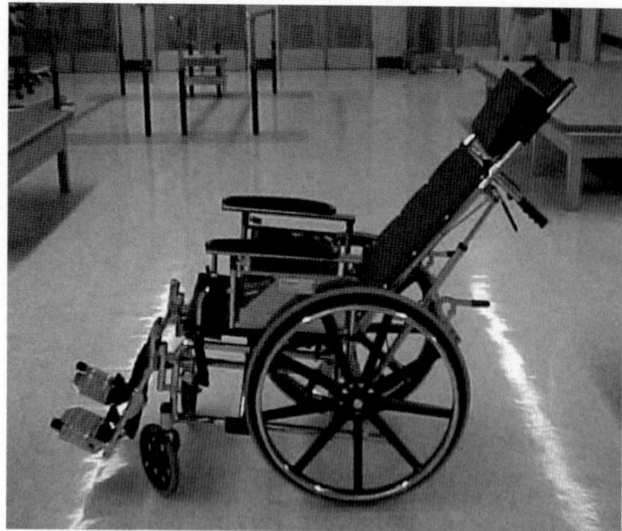

FIGURE 18.5. Recliner manual wheelchair.

POWERED MOBILITY

Powered mobility is the best option for those who cannot functionally propel an optimally configured manual wheelchair, and has been shown to improve self-care, mobility, leisure activities, and decrease reliance on others (6). Powered mobility devices have evolved significantly, with advancements achieved in construction of the bases, electronics, seating functions, and input devices. Available options include drive wheel placement, seating systems, and programming features. Consumers should play an active role in the assessment process and in selection of preferred options.

The medical justification for powered mobility should be documented to address policy and funding issues and include (a) the inability to functionally ambulate and inability to propel an optimally configured manual wheelchair due to neurological or musculoskeletal issues or risk of repetitive strain injuries; (b) the inability to maintain an upright posture during manual propulsion due to trunk instability; (c) postural deformities; (d) cardiopulmonary compromise (e) upper limb joint pain, (f) poor endurance and (g) community reentry for work, school, and/or recreation activities.

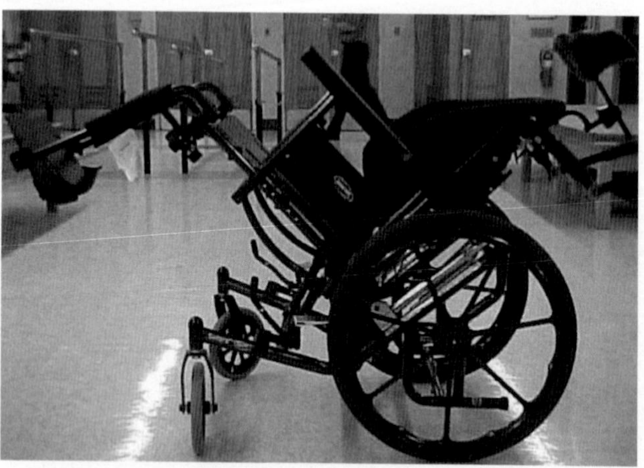

FIGURE 18.6. Tilt-in-space manual wheelchair.

The consumer should evaluate various power systems and the appropriate input devices in order to choose the optimal powered mobility system. It is necessary for the consumer to first operate the system in open terrain and then progress to tighter areas, various terrain, hallways, ramps, van access, and other environmental barriers in order to select the most appropriate system that will accommodate the consumer's lifestyle and needs.

Types of Powered Mobility

Power Add-On Units

Some consumers do not require full-time power mobility, and may be able to propel a manual wheelchair safely and functionally for short distances on a level surface. However, for extended distances and rougher terrain, propulsion can become taxing for the consumer's strength, shoulder integrity, or cardiac reserve. In these instances, a power add-on unit can be mounted to most folding and rigid frame manual wheelchairs converting the system to power or power-assisted mobility. An example of this option is the Alber E-fix Add-On Unit, which is a direct drive unit where the motors are built into the hubs of the rear wheels. A removable battery provides the power source, and the system is operated via a joystick. Limitations of the system include the significant weight added to the wheelchair by the wheels and battery. Additionally, manual wheelchair frames are typically not designed to withstand the forces of powered motors, and therefore power add-on units should only be added to manual wheelchairs that are of higher quality construction. These systems generally have very poor durability, and most active users would benefit from one of the systems described below (Table 18.5).

Another option for powered mobility is a pushrim activated power assist wheelchair (PAPAW), where the standard wheels are replaced with wheels that have gearless, brushless motors mounted in the hubs and are powered by a battery mounted inside the hub of the wheel or as an add-on unit. An entire PAPAW system weighs approximately 50 lb, excluding the wheelchair frame. When the consumer slightly strokes the pushrim, the battery provides additional power to propel the chair forward. The wheels can also be turned off to eliminate power assist. Applying backward pressure to the pushrim engages the motor-controlled brakes, which can assist in decelerating the wheelchair. When compared to manual wheelchairs with standard wheels, PAPAWs produce less strain on the shoulders (7). They are also beneficial to negotiate inclines. Due to the weight of the wheels, however, they are more difficult to lift and stow for transport. They are also difficult to maneuver over obstacles, such as curbs, and can add width to the chair.

Scooters

Unlike powered wheelchairs, scooters are designed for use by consumers who are marginal ambulators and able to independently transfer into and out of a device. A scooter has either three or four wheels, a mounted seat, and a tiller steering system.

A three-wheeled scooter is narrower and has a shorter frame than the more stable four-wheeled scooters. However, scooters have a higher center of gravity and can tip more readily than a powered wheelchair, especially on uneven surfaces. Scooters are typically better for outdoor use because they have a large turning radius. They can be disassembled for transportation stowing; however, the consumer or caregiver's ability to perform this task needs to be carefully assessed, as it is not a simple process and components can be heavy to lift.

Scooter seats are basic Captain Style seating systems; therefore, a scooter cannot satisfy complex seating needs. The seat is typically mounted on a single post permitting it to swivel for transfers. A tiller steering system is used to operate and drive the scooter. The consumer requires good upper limb dexterity and strength to steer the system. The tiller controls steering, and acceleration relies on finger control to operate a lever. The user requires good trunk control and proximal stability in order to safely operate the system. They are most appropriate for people with SCI if the user has a low-level incomplete injury, can walk short distances, and has residual sensation in the sacral region.

The main advantages of a scooter are light weight, ease of operation, cost, and the ability to disassemble for transport. For some consumers, scooters are aesthetically pleasing and more acceptable than a wheelchair.

Powered Wheelchairs

Powered wheelchairs are typically available in four different group types. Group 1 power wheelchairs have a basic configuration with a weight capacity of less than 300 lb and basic seating. They cannot accommodate complex seating or specialty controls and have limited utility for traveling long distances or outdoors. Due to inability to add power seat functions, or program or upgrade the electronics, Group 1 chairs are rarely used for people with SCI or other neuromuscular conditions, especially those with progressive impairments. Group 2 powered wheelchairs can accommodate some degree of complex seating and specialty controls, but on a limited basis. They have a larger battery capacity and can negotiate some obstacles and outdoors on a limited basis. Group 3 powered wheelchairs can accommodate multiple seat functions, complex seating needs, specialty controls, and other features commonly needed by people with SCI and other neuromuscular disorders. Group 4 powered wheelchairs can accommodate the same features as Group 3 but have added features such as larger motors, suspensions, and battery capacities that make them more appropriate for active outdoor use. Group 2, 3, and 4 powered wheelchairs are also divided into subgroups designed to accommodate different weight capacities, up to 300 lb and 301 to 450 lb (Heavy Duty), 451 to 600 lb (Extra Heavy Duty), and over 600 lb (Extra Extra Heavy Duty). At the time of this publication, Medicare and most third-party insurances cover Group 2 and 3 chairs for people with a diagnosis of SCI, but not Group 4.

Powered wheelchairs are typically not easy to disassemble and transport via a car. However, some manufacturers construct their frames to permit the batteries to be removed and the frame folded. These fall into the Group 1 category. Even with removing the batteries (which weigh ~20 lb each), the folded frame can still weigh approximately 50 lb or more due to the motor unit.

The advantages of transportable power wheelchairs include a lower cost, household and community mobility, and transport convenience. The disadvantages include weight exceeding those of manual wheelchairs, limited programming capabilities, limited durability, and inability to add power seating functions.

Conventional power wheelchairs are belt driven, which acts like a pulley system. Each wheel has a large pulley mounted around the rim to drive the wheel. The large wheels of the conventional powered wheelchairs are mounted in the front, rear, or center, and control the steering of the system (Table 18.6; Fig. 18.7). The smaller wheels are casters.

The following should be considered prior to selecting a power base:

1. Compatibility with power seating systems and specialty controls
2. How the client plans to transport the wheelchair
3. Seating options and accessories
4. A tie-down system to secure the wheelchair during transportation
5. Ground clearance needed for habitual terrain
6. Seat-to-floor heights for table or desk access
7. Battery type
8. Distances to travel on one battery charge

Powered Wheelchair Components

Many powered wheelchairs have components that are similar to and/or interchangeable with those of manual wheelchairs.

Armrests

Most powered wheelchairs use the two-point height adjustable and flip-back style in order to make transfers easier. Additional support may be needed due to the consumer's level of injury and positional requirements. Arm troughs with hand supports or wide flat arm pads are available in order to prevent subluxation of the shoulders, distribute pressure equally, and prevent contractures for those with limited or no upper

TABLE 18.6

ADVANTAGES AND DISADVANTAGES OF WHEEL PLACEMENT

Type of wheel drive	Advantages	Disadvantages
Rear wheel drive	• Greater sense of control • Greater speed • Stability	• Rear tipping is a concern on steep inclines; need to use antitips • Larger turning radius
Midwheel/center wheel drive	• Tightest turning radius • Maneuverability in tight spaces	• Less stable • Front tipping especially on rougher terrain • Not as good for consumers lacking trunk control
Front wheel drive	• Maneuverability in tight spaces • Better getting over rougher terrain	• Difficult to track in straight line • Takes more skill to operate

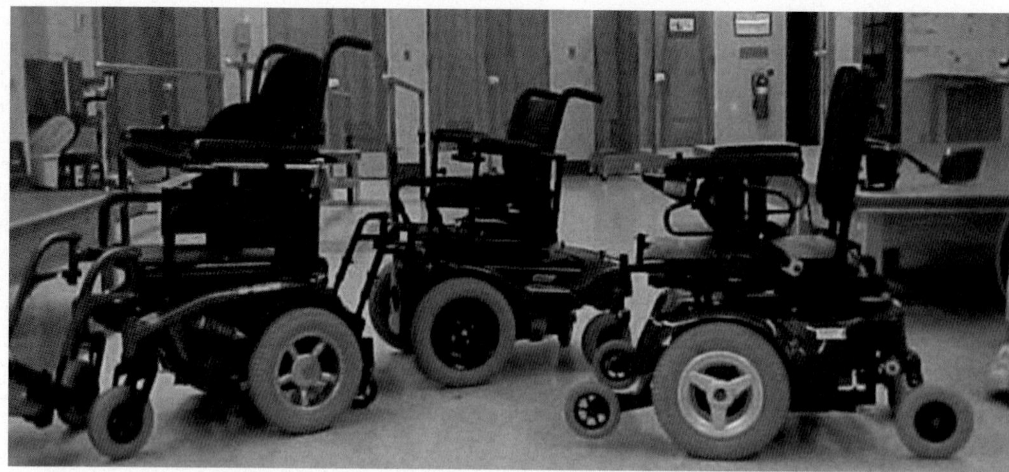

FIGURE 18.7. Positions of power base: rear wheel, midwheel, and front wheel drive.

limb movement. These contoured supports may increase the overall width of the wheelchair or interfere with armrest function to flip-back.

Legrests

Elevating legrests and smart legrests permit discrete positioning of the lower limbs. *Smart legrests* elevate and elongate forward like a telescope, maintaining the limb in an extended position. This prevents added pressure on the ischial tuberosities. The elevating legrests extend the knee joints at variable degrees depending on the needs of the consumer. They can be manual or power controlled. Additional supports using calf pads or troughs are needed with elevating legrests to maintain the limbs in the desired position. To manage edema, the legrests must be combined with power seating options in order to elevate the legs above the level of the heart.

Footrests

Standard foot supports are manufactured from composite plastic materials and lack ankle adjustability. Large plates made from metal with angle adjustable plates are available as options. Some powered wheelchairs offer a center footrest with a flip-up footplate, which shortens the overall length of the wheelchair and may be more aesthetically pleasing to the consumer.

Headrests

There are numerous types of headrests depending on the consumer's needs. When providing a tilt or recline system, a headrest must be provided to support the head and neck. A custom-contoured headrest with lateral and occipital supports can be used to correct poor head positioning, provide additional support, or accommodate other consumer's needs.

Wheels/Tires

Options for tires on powered wheelchairs often resemble those of manual chairs. Otherwise, smaller (i.e., 3 to 5 inches) casters on powered wheelchairs are more appropriate for indoor mobility or tight environments, whereas larger diameter (i.e., 6 to 8 inches) casters provide better performance for outdoor, rough, or uneven terrain. Earlier models of these wheelchairs were outfitted with rear wheels having a 20-inch diameter. However, to increase performance, manufactures are now using 10- to 14-inch diameter wheels with 2 to 4 inches widths. The smaller rear wheels have improved turning radius and traction, and it is recommended to have a solid insert in the wheels to prevent flats.

Seat and Back

Most powered wheelchairs are supplied with a solid seat pan and a specialty cushion placed upon it. The back system can be either sling upholstery or a specialty solid back, the latter being recommended by most practitioners. The sling upholstery is not appropriate when using tilt-in-space backs, as they may not be strong enough to support the consumer's weight. Solid backs come in various styles: flat, curved, contoured and molded, depending on the consumer's postural needs.

Powered Seating Functions

Powered seating functions include recline, tilt-in-space, elevating legrests, standing, and seat elevation. While a comprehensive review of these functions exceeds the scope of this chapter, they have been reviewed elsewhere (2,4,5) and are shown in Table 18.5. These features allow the user to independently change positions for many purposes including managing spasticity, pressure relief of the sitting surface (which was also described above), bladder management, balance and postural alignment, or positioning for rest or comfort. The powered seating functions can be used in combination with each other. It is important to consult with the manufacturer to determine the compatibility of these options with the wheelchair base and the overall dimensions.

Batteries

There are two types of batteries: wet cell or gel cell. Wet cell batteries store more energy, are less expensive, and require more maintenance such as cleaning. Both types of batteries are charged daily and depending on terrain, driving distance and speed, and add-ons such as ventilators, they can remain charged for up to 12 hours of use.

Accessories

A ventilator tray and a battery box are required for consumers who use a ventilator. The ventilator is usually mounted at the rear of the wheelchair with the battery underneath. The trays are usually *gimbal* style, which has a pivot point to rotate the tray outward during seating functions, or *trailer* style, which is a flat tray under the seat depending on the frame construction. The gimbal style is used with tilt and recline systems, so they do not impede the function and remain level during tilting and reclining. The ventilator tray may increase the length of the wheelchair depending on how it is mounted.

When swing-away joystick hardware is used, the user can retract the joystick to the side and back. This function gives better access to table tops, desks, and a steering wheel.

A lap tray provides support for the upper limbs and functions as a work place when a table is inaccessible. Additional accessories can be mounted on a lap tray to increase function for the user. Examples are a book holder, laptop, and communication board.

Suspension is a feature to reduce vibration, decrease wear and tear, increase the life of the frame, and improve the performance and ride of the system. Suspension can be placed within the casters, the rear wheels, or the mounting of the seating system to the base.

Integrated controls refer to the ability to plug into the wheelchair's electronics in order to operate assistive devices. Wheelchair electronics offer the ability to connect hardware to control communication devices and/or environmental control units (ECUs) through input devices that are used to operate the power base (2).

TYPES OF INPUT DEVICES

The choice of input device is crucial to operating the powered wheelchair. Selection is based upon the consumer's postural needs, the types of terrain to be traversed, and anticipated changes in user function. As these devices can be interchangeable, the latter is extremely important when addressing medical justification and approval from insurance providers.

Input devices can be classified as "proportional" or "nonproportional." *Proportional* input devices allow the speed and direction of the wheelchair to be directly proportional to the amount and direction of force. Proportional input devices provide greater control over movement of the wheelchair and speed. These systems are appropriate for consumers with fair to good strength and adequate ROM and coordination. Standard joysticks are examples of proportional controls.

Nonproportional input devices offer "all or none" signaling. Switches are an example of nonproportional control. Advanced electronics with programming adjustability permit these systems to grade responses, and to a certain extent simulate proportional control. Nonproportional input devices are used by consumers who are limited in strength, ROM, and coordination. Cognitive status should be assessed before prescribing these systems due to the need for multiple steps to scan and select functional modes.

Joysticks

A joystick input device is the most commonly used input device. Consideration needs to be given to the size, placement, mounting hardware, and accessibility. There are two types of joysticks: proportional (continuous) (see Fig. 18.8) and nonproportional (discrete). A *proportional* joystick provides 360-degree directional signal and immediately responds in the direction of the consumer's movement on the control device. A proportional joystick controls the direction and velocity of movement. A *nonproportional* joystick (discrete) is for consumers who lack motor control needed to oper-

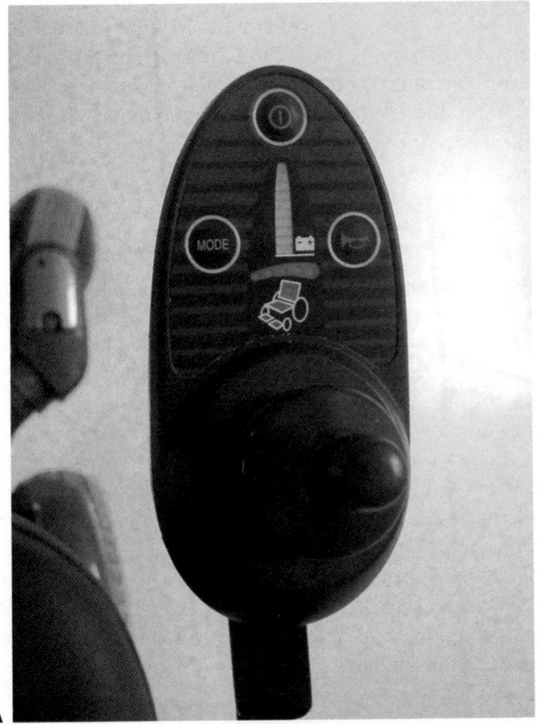

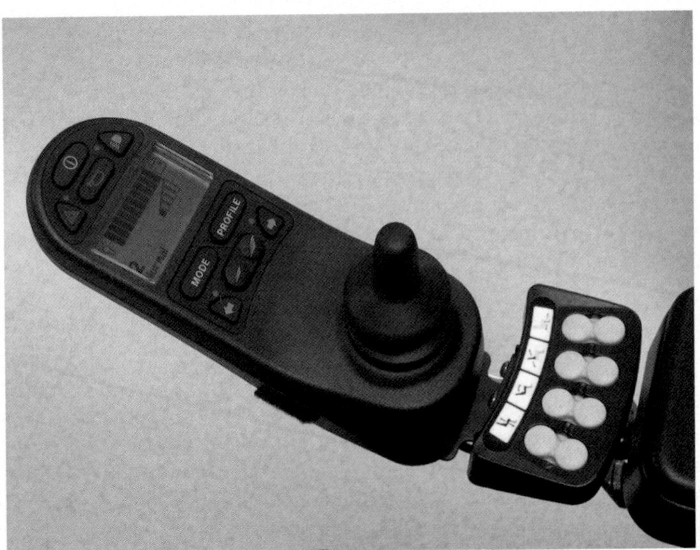

FIGURE 18.8. (A) is a basic proportional joystick and (B) shows a proportional joystick with visual display.

ate a proportional joystick but have gross motor movement. Nonproportional inputs operate in either a 4- or 8-directional mode. A 4-directional joystick will produce forward, reverse, left, and right movements. An 8-directional joystick produces movement in these four directions and their diagonals. Nonproportional input devices are either "on" or "off," and the wheelchair response is not proportional to the input. Once activated, the wheelchair will accelerate at a preset speed and stay at that speed until the switch is no longer activated.

Joysticks can be operated with the hand or any body part that has controlled and reliable function, such as a foot or a chin. The joystick can be laterally or medially mounted to the dominant side, or even midline. A goalpost device can be mounted to the joystick for consumers that have gross motor dexterity. If the consumer has consistent finger movement, a touch pad proportional joystick could be appropriate. When using this device, the consumer would place a finger in the middle of the pad and slide the finger in the desired wheelchair direction. This requires minimal movement and is a proportional input, allowing for 360-degree directional control.

When sites such as the elbow are used for controlling an input device, this typically calls for a remote proportional joystick, which is smaller than a standard proportional joystick that the user would control with the hand, has no switches activation or speed control, and is mounted to an interface.

Head control joysticks are placed at the back of the headrest on a flexible mount to allow operation using lateral rotation and flexion/extension of the neck. Lateral movement will elicit turns, and extension will drive the wheelchair forward. An additional switch is needed to provide the forward command to control reverse mode and/or power seating functions. This switch can be mounted off the headrest at a site that the consumer can activate. Head control input is appropriate for consumers who lack arm control but with spared active ROM in the cervical region and no cervical bracing or collars.

A chin control joystick is mounted in front and directly below the chin. Usually, consumers with high cervical SCI (i.e., C4 and weak C5) who are not able to independently place their hand on a joystick may benefit from a head or chin control. A small cup is used to replace the knob for better control and pressure distribution. The input works the same as a proportional hand joystick. The joystick movement directs the trajectory of the wheelchair.

A foot control joystick is mounted under a footplate on a swivel hinge, which requires intact plantar flexion, dorsiflexion, and inversion and eversion of the ankle. Most consumers who qualify for this device have an incomplete SCI (i.e., central cord syndrome), motor neuron disease, multiple sclerosis, or neuromuscular impairments effecting the upper limbs more than the lower limbs.

Breath Control (Sip and Puff)

Breath control input devices are appropriate for consumers who cannot use proportional control. Sip and Puff is controlled by a series of breaths; hard and soft sips and puffs are drawn and pushed through a straw, which is mounted to the wheelchair. The consumer can also operate power seating functions through breath control. A visual display is needed in order for the consumer to see menus. Auditory feedback is also available.

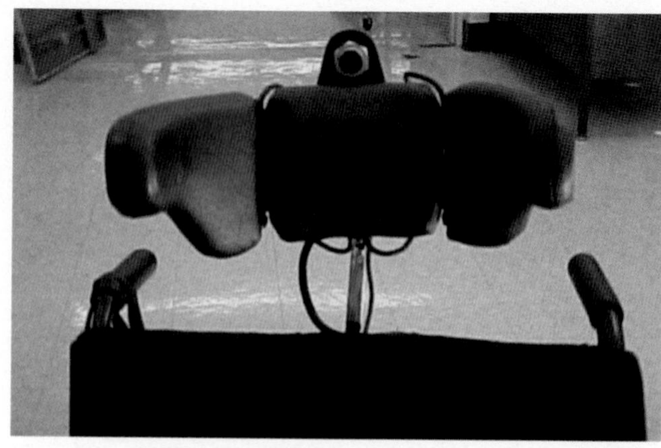

FIGURE 18.9. Head array system.

Head Array

Head array input devices are a type of nonproportional input. The head array is a three-piece padded headrest with sensors in each pad. The sensors in the wings control right and left movement, and the back pad controls forward and reverse. The sensors do not require pressure to activate. The consumer needs to move the head toward the sensor, which can be mounted anywhere in the pad to activate the switch. Different types of switches allow the consumer to switch drive modes or operate seating functions. A reset switch is needed for mode change and safety (see Fig. 18.9).

Sip and Puff/Head Array

A Sip and Puff/Head Array input device is a combination of two types of drive input devices used to obtain optimal access. Some consumers have great difficulty discriminating between hard and soft commands for breath control. This system permits any sip and puff to operate in reverse and forward drive, while the right and left direction is activated by the sensors in the lateral wings of the headrest.

Switches

There are numerous switches on the market to operate powered mobility and powered seating functions. Multiple switch input usually consists of four to five switches that are mounted in a lap tray, headrest, or at site of consistent movement to activate. Four of the switches operate the direction of the wheelchair; forward, reverse, right, and left, while the fifth switch operates the on and off mode. If power seating functions are needed more switches are added, or the switches must be toggled. More switches require greater cognitive skill to drive the wheelchair and operate ancillary functions.

Single switch input devices are usually considered a consumer's "last chance to drive." These devices are recommended for consumers who have only one controlled movement such as a finger or thumb. They require a visual scanner, which is programmed for speed with four directional arrows that light up on sequence. When the directional arrow is lit up for the desired movement, the consumer will activate the switch with his or her control. Single switch input devices can also be used to operate power seating functions.

A fiber optic switch input device involves a beam of light, which if interrupted activates a switch. This input device is ideal for consumers with very limited finger movement. The fiber optics can be mounted into a lap tray, splint, or an arm pad in order to access consistently. Optics can also be used to activate a single switch scanner for mobility and power seating functions.

Additional Features

Some joysticks can now be used for environmental control within the home or office (8). Some contain an infrared output signal for operation of a television, X-10 control for small appliances, or Bluetooth to control an on-screen keyboard.

SPECIALTY WHEELCHAIRS

Sport Wheelchairs

Sport wheelchairs for tennis, basketball, rugby, or racing are specially constructed and adjusted for the specific sport and not used as the primary wheelchair. The frames are rigid and constructed of lightweight material such as titanium or carbon fiber. Sport wheelchairs are expensive and require very specific and careful measurements for an appropriate fit. Figure 18.11 shows a racing chair with two rear wheels and wide camber. The casters are eliminated by a third wheel placed in the front.

Handcycles

Handcycles are similar to a mountain bike with gears. The gears permit the consumer to choose the most efficient gear for the grade of roadway on which they are traveling. Handcycles are available in recumbent and kneeling configurations and provide the most energy-efficient form of propulsion.

Beach, Standing, and Transport Wheelchairs

All-terrain beach wheelchairs are manually operated chairs that are used for beach transport, lounge chairs, and shallow water recreation. They require a caretaker to assist with propulsion due to the large air-filled tires in the front and rear. They are usually "one-size-fits-all" and specialized seating is not provided.

Standing is also available as a manual feature on a manual chair or as a powered feature on a powered chair (Fig. 18.10). Power standing can be used in a very select group of patients who have good ROM of joints and can tolerate standing in a therapeutic standing program. The benefits of standing include acclimation to orthostasis, ability to carry out ADLs or work duties in a more independent manner, and pressure relief. Powered wheelchairs can be driven while the user is in a standing position. However, manual wheelchairs are left stationary when in the standing position.

TRANSPORTATION CONSIDERATIONS

Manual wheelchairs, whether a rigid or folding frame, can easily be disassembled and transported by car. It is important to educate and evaluate the ability of the consumer, family member, or caretaker to disassemble and assemble the wheelchair, and move it into and from the customary transport vehicle. A car topper with a powered mechanical lift can load a folding wheelchair on the vehicle roof for transport. Trunk lifts and rear attachments that mount to a car bumper assist with transport of larger chairs or scooters.

Power-based wheelchairs pose special challenges for transportation. Even low-end folding frames that allow the batteries to be removed are still relatively heavy and not easily loaded into a car. Transport of a power wheelchair generally requires a van, a lift or ramp, and a specialized tie-down

A 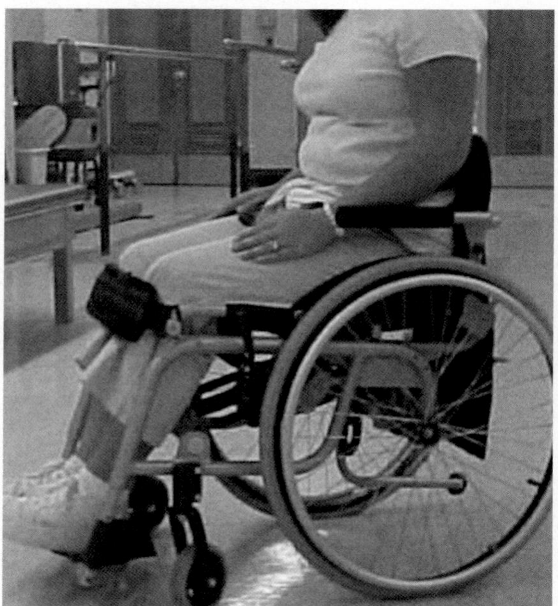

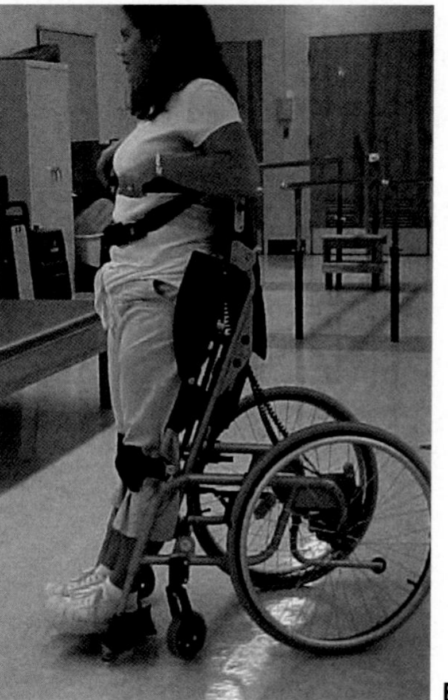 B

FIGURE 18.10. Stand-up manual wheelchair. (A) Seated position. (B) Standing position.

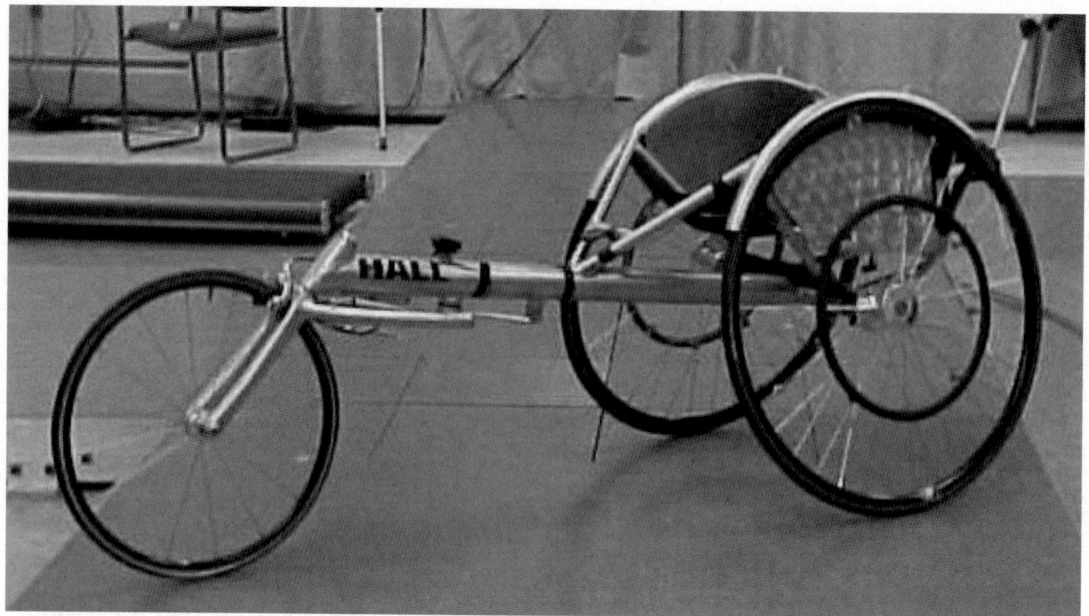

FIGURE 18.11. Racing wheelchair.

system. Important factors to consider include the combined dimensions of user and wheelchair, the internal configuration of the van for driver and passenger, the consumer's ability to drive the vehicle, and the type of lockdown system.

Accessible public transportation has improved throughout developed nations, and provides wheelchair users a newfound freedom to explore the world. Buses commonly host specialized lifts and removable seats to accommodate manual and power wheelchairs. Train stations have specific stops designated for wheelchair users with elevators to access city subways and streets. Airline travel, however, requires special consideration and preparation. Manual wheelchairs, depending on their size, can be boarded and then checked if prior arrangements are made. However, power wheelchairs are placed in the baggage compartment, and it is required that the batteries are approved for travel. Gel batteries are approved for airline transport while lead acid batteries are not. In general, the experienced traveler will remove as many parts as possible, especially the joystick and control electronics, and stow them to prevent damage during travel.

CUSHIONS AND BACKS

Cushions are considered part of the seating system and require special selection. A wide variety of cushions are currently available. Factors to consider when selecting a seating system include the consumer's motor, sensory, and functional level; skin integrity; degree of spasticity; sitting balance; postural deformities; transfer and weight shift techniques; bowel and bladder function; and cognitive status.

Cushions

Types of Surfaces

Cushions can be classified by their type of support surface: planar, contoured, and custom contoured. *Planar* systems have flat surfaces that support the body where direct body contact occurs. These are often prescribed in pediatrics, so that they continue to fit the child as he or she grows. They are also appropriate for consumers who require limited seat and body support. Their main disadvantage is the unequal distribution of pressure that comes in contact with bony prominences of the sitting surface (see Fig. 18.12).

Commercially or prefabricated contoured surfaces are made in 1-inch increments to fit the consumer. These systems can be adjusted using lateral supports and hip guides to provide proper positioning. They also distribute pressure better than planar systems due to the contour feature, especially if the consumer has minimal postural deformities. Expansion is limited with these systems and will require replacement with a larger size cushion as the consumer grows.

Custom contour molds can be fabricated on site with the use of simulators to address the consumer's position, and then sent to the shop or manufacturer to be completed. This system

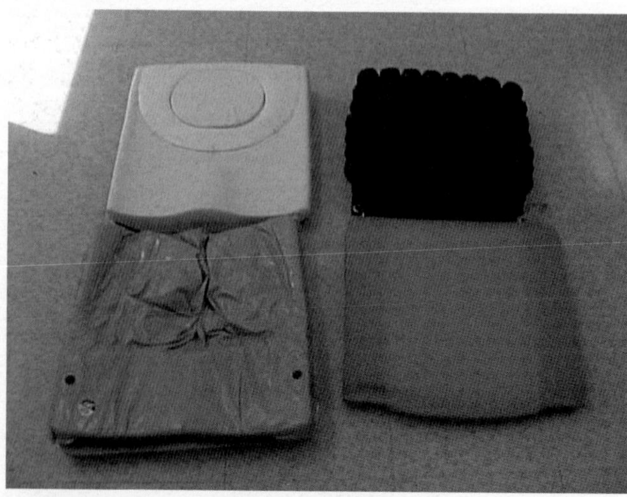

FIGURE 18.12. Cushions. From top right clockwise: air, foam with open cell, gel/foam hybrid, and foam.

TABLE 18.7

SUMMARY OF TYPES OF CUSHIONS

Types	Advantages	Disadvantages	Examples
Foam	• Inexpensive • Light weight • Easy to modify	• Short lifespan due to light and moisture • Loses resilience • Limited points of contact depending on the stiffness	T-foam Polyurethane Sunmate
Gel 1. High viscosity	• Absorbs shock • Stable seating surface • Do not change with atmospheric pressure	• Fair envelopment • Poor resilience • Limited shock absorption • Heavy	Royale Action gel
2. Low viscosity	• Good temperature regulation • Good envelopment • Good support • Absorbs shock better than high viscosity	• Poor resilience	Jay fluid pads
Air	• Good pressure relief • Light weight • Good air flow • Good resilience • Good envelopment depending on inflation	• Maintenance • Punctures • Air loss depending on temperature and altitude • Stability • Expensive	Roho Starr
Dynamic or alternating pressure cushion	• Good pressure relief	• Maintenance • Expensive	Aquila Dynamic air
Hybrid	• Good pressure relief • Good temperature regulation • Good stability and support • Good envelopment	• Fair resilience • Weight • Increased thickness • Expensive	Jay 2 Varlite

provides the greatest amount of contact surface to distribute pressure and support to accommodate or correct the consumer's posture. The main disadvantages are cost and the time-consuming process to fit the system. Consumers will require remolding if they gain weight or grow.

Properties

Table 18.7 summarizes the types of cushions with advantages and disadvantages listed for each. Cushion properties can be divided into several areas:

1. Resilience—The ability of the material to regain shape after the load has been removed.
2. Envelopment—The degree to which the consumer sinks into the cushion and it conforms to the buttocks. This promotes stability for the consumer and reduces peak pressures.
3. Shock Absorption—The ability of the cushion to prevent transmission of vibration.
4. Temperature—The ability of a cushion to absorb and dissipate heat to prevent pressure ulcers and provide thermal insulation.
5. Shear—The forces that act in parallel to the surface of the skin and cause tension on the skin and underlying tissue. It is necessary to evaluate the cushion and how the consumer moves and transfers to determine shear forces on the skin.
6. Suspension—A cutout in a specific area to eliminate pressure.
7. Weight—Manual wheelchair users should have a lighter cushion on ultra-lightweight wheelchairs. For power mobility, weight is less a concern.

Foam Cushions. Foam cushions are available in a various densities and types, but are typically inexpensive and lightweight. There are two types of cell structures for foam: open and closed cell. Open cell foam has a membrane that is interconnected with tiny holes to allow for airflow and ventilation. The main problem is absorption into the open cell, which decreases cushion life and makes it difficult to clean. Closed cell foam has an outside membrane that protects the foam but limits airflow. Life expectancy for foam cushions is approximately 6 to 12 months.

Gel Cushions. Gel cushions are characterized by viscosity. High viscosity gel will provide a more stable seating surface but less shock absorbing properties. They are heavier but provide fair envelopment and temperature regulation. Lower viscosity gels offer greater shock absorption and good envelopment, and temperature is usually not a concern. However, resilience is poor. Life expectancy is approximately 2 to 5 years.

Air Cushions. Air cushions consist of soft, flexible interconnected air cells that can be ordered in different heights (e.g., 2 or 4 inches, or combinations thereof) that allow airflow and circulation between cells. As the consumer's body shape changes or shifts, the cushion adjusts and facilitates blood flow for pressure relief and distribution. Air cushions have good resilience and envelopment, and are lightweight. However, maintenance is required to prevent over- or underinflation, punctures and air loss over time, and pressure deviations associated with temperature or altitude change. Life expectancy is approximately 2 to 5 years if cared for properly.

Hybrid Cushions. Hybrid cushions are a combination of two types of cushion material mentioned above. This combination provides good envelopment, good temperature control, postural support and stability, and optimal pressure relief. The Varlite cushion combines air and foam, contouring to the consumer's seated posture or segmentation to adjust for flexible deformities. Life expectancy is approximately 2 to 5 years.

Other Cushions. The Stimulite cushion is made of a soft, flexible form of aerospace honeycomb that contours to the body. It has open cells with perforations to facilitate airflow and evaporation. The cells are flexible to reduce shear and provide stabilization. It is extremely lightweight (~3 lb) and available in planar or contoured shape.

Alternating Pressure Cushions. All cushions discussed to this point are static cushions, which redistribute pressure over the seated position and require the consumer to perform weight shifts. Alternating pressure cushions were designed on the premise that weight-bearing surfaces can tolerate high pressures for longer periods of time if alternated with intervals of lesser pressure. These cushions have an oscillating pump to alternate pressure at preprogrammed intervals and are operated by an 8-lb battery-operated system that must be mounted to the wheelchair. If the system fails or the battery is fully discharged, the cushion will usually remain filled with air. To provide backup in cases of failure, some systems also have a 1- to 2-inch foam base.

Pressure Mapping Technology

Selection of an appropriate cushion is a challenging process, especially for consumers with a problematic skin history. Pressure mapping, which measures forces that exist between the cushion and buttocks, can be performed to measure quantitative sitting pressures with various cushions. The most common type of pressure mapping device is the multiple sensor system, which is a very thin mat having multiple sensors throughout. It is placed over the entire seating surface, measures dynamic pressure over a large surface area, and visually illustrates areas of concern. Pressure mapping is a tool that can confirm a suspected increased pressure area, compare various cushions, shorten trial time, and educate the consumer on areas of pressure that require special attention. While pressure mapping is extremely useful in making selections of cushions or equipment, or as biofeedback to train clients on how to weight shift and use their power seat functions, no specific standards of "acceptable pressures" exist.

CONCLUSION

Advancements in mobility device research and design have greatly expanded the options for patient in wheelchair seating and mobility products. This challenges the clinician to become familiar with the ever-changing products and their applications, and to be knowledgeable in basic principles of seating and mobility. It is especially important to train specialists in this clinical area in order to keep abreast of the latest seating and mobility technologies.

Seating and mobility systems are a vital part of the consumer's level of function and postural stability. A well-considered and tested mobility system will enable the consumer to become as fully independent in his or her home and community environment as his or her impairment permits. When properly prescribed and maintained, they can enhance work and community access. It is important for the consumer to play an active role in the evaluation process, and the clinic team to be advocates for the consumer in justifying the appropriate system for third-party payers. Prescribing a seating and mobility system takes commitment by specialists to address all areas of function, posture, mobility, and comfort. A seating and mobility system appropriately configured should enhance the consumer's health, function, and quality of life.

References

1. Cooper RA. *Wheelchair selection and configuration*. New York: Demos Medical Publishing, 1998.
2. Dicianno BE, Arva J, Lieberman JM, et al. RESNA position on the application of tilt, recline, and elevating legrests for wheelchairs. *Assist Technol* 2009;21(1):13–22; quiz 24.
3. Dieruf K, Ewer L, Boninger D. The natural-fit handrim: factors related to improvement in symptoms and function in wheelchair users. *J Spinal Cord Med* 2008;31(5):578.
4. Arva J, Paleg G, Lange M, et al. RESNA position on the application of wheelchair standing devices. *Assist Technol* 2009;21(3):161–168; quiz 169–171.
5. Arva J, Schmeler M, Lange M, et al. RESNA position on the application of seat-elevating devices for wheelchair users. *Assist Technol* 2009;21(2):69–72; quiz 74–75.
6. Miles-Tapping C, MacDonald LJ. Lifestyle implications of power mobility. *Phys Occup Ther Geriatr* 1995;12(4):31–49.
7. Lighthall-Haubert L, Requejo PS, Mulroy SJ, et al. Comparison of shoulder muscle electromyographic activity during standard manual wheelchair and push-rim activated power assisted wheelchair propulsion in persons with complete tetraplegia. *Arch Phys Med Rehabil* 2009;90(11):1904–1915.
8. Dicianno BE, Cooper RA, Coltellaro J. Joystick control for powered mobility: current state of technology and future directions. *Phys Med Rehabil Clin N Am* 2010 21(1):79–86.

CHAPTER 19 ■ SPINAL ORTHOSES

FREDERICK FROST AND C. RAFFI NAJARIAN

INTRODUCTION

The use of external appliances to immobilize and align the spine is described in historical literature dating to Aristotle in the fifth century BC (1,2). To this day, spinal bracing is a popular treatment modality for patients with myelopathy arising from both medical and traumatic causes. Spinal orthoses are relatively inexpensive and available worldwide. Their use in the realm of spinal pathology seems intuitive. If one can splint a fractured tibia with an external orthosis, one must certainly be able to splint a damaged spine, given enough materials and engineering expertise. Devices that are so strange and punitive in appearance simply must be medically effective. In fact, spine bracing is relatively ineffective at controlling spine motion. Even the Halo orthoses, which effectively control the overall motion of the cervical spine by using anchors fixed into the outer table of the skull, allow a substantial amount of intersegmental vertebral movement. In this light, spinal braces have a therapeutic mystique that is based upon a very limited research literature. In addition, most of the studies on bracing (employing cadavers, normal volunteers, or back pain patients) have limited relevance to spinal cord injury treatment.

As management of acute spinal injury changes, the settings in which braces are used also change. Spinal orthoses are a critical element of safe ambulance transport of injured individuals. Formerly, conservative management of spinal fractures might have placed the patient at bed rest for 6 weeks. Now, the hope is that orthoses can mitigate the adverse effects of gravity and active body movement on the healing spine and allow the patient to become active sooner after injury. For the ever-increasing number of patients who benefit from modern surgical instrumentation and stabilization of the spine, surgeons often employ bracing as an adjunct treatment, expecting that this practice will improve outcomes. Long after injury, spinal orthoses may be used to support trunk control and improve posture. For the even larger population of patients with nontraumatic myelopathy from cancer, degenerative spinal disease, and other causes, these devices may be used to reduce pain, improve spinal alignment, and augment function. While also used commonly for conditions such as low back pain and congenital scoliosis, this chapter limits its focus to the use of spinal bracing in the setting of traumatic and nontraumatic myelopathies.

Although materials, fabrication, and fitting of spinal orthoses have changed dramatically over the past three decades, the principles of treatment have not changed. Braces are designed to control motion of the spine, support the trunk, align deformities, reduce nerve root pain, and protect areas of injury or recent surgical treatment. Like orthotic devices used to treat conditions of the appendicular skeleton, most spinal braces use a "three-point pressure" mechanism (e.g., two pressure points in the front and one in back) to apply the external forces necessary to affect change in spinal posture. In this manner, the magnitude of forces applied is proportional to the distance between the corrective component of the brace and the opposing forces above and below it. Assuming that the spinal brace is correctly matched with the goals of treatment, its effectiveness will depend upon many factors including correct fit, patient compliance, and the mitigation of potential adverse side effects. Modern materials and techniques have resulted in braces that fit better, are lighter and cooler, easier to don and doff, and perhaps marginally more comfortable for the patient. Strap and closure devices are improved, and thermoplastic molding techniques allow compensation for body contours in the torso, waist, and hips. Multilayer foam products maintain stiffness while reducing pressure points with conforming skin contact surfaces. New products are latex free, allow for tracheostomy and feeding tubes, and are compatible with radiological imaging modalities. Washable pads and clear orientation markings (e.g., front, back, top, and bottom) represent important changes in design and implementation.

As spinal braces are generally designed to restrict motion of naturally mobile segments, they are uncomfortable to wear. Helping the patient set realistic expectations on this issue is an important element of promoting satisfaction and compliance. All devices, whether off-the-shelf or custom fabricated, will require fitting by a knowledgeable orthotist, but extensive postfitting modifications are more likely to thwart the effects of the brace than to add comfort. Without exception, spinal bracing is best when there is a snug fit, to reduce translational skin shear and migration of the brace as the patient changes body position. Straps and fasteners that are easily loosened and adjusted by the patient are likely to impair effectiveness. Despite the use of newer fabrication materials, these braces restrict loss of surface body heat. Excessive perspiration may result, making them difficult to wear in warm climates. The wide range of body sizes and shapes makes orthotic fitting a challenge. Persons with short necks, small chins, and sloped foreheads may be difficult to fit with cervical orthoses (COs). Those with short trunks, excessive kyphosis, obesity, or pendulous breasts will challenge the orthotist fabricating a thoracolumbar brace. For children with spinal cord injury, the spinal brace takes on an additional role. Multiple braces may be needed as the child grows, in order to minimize progressive deformity of the spine.

For most persons with traumatic spinal injury and myelopathy, axial weakness or paralysis is present, and the normal muscle and soft tissue splinting of fracture sites will be inactive or disrupted.

TABLE 19.1

ADVERSE SIDE EFFECTS OF SPINAL BRACING

Pain, discomfort, and anxiety	Brain abscess/infection from Halo pins
Dysphagia and difficulty chewing	Restriction of lung function
Osteoporosis of the spine	Psychological dependence
Axial muscle wasting	Excessive spinal motion above and below brace
Impaired balance in ambulatory patients	Restriction of movement and function
Pressure ulcers, skin breakdown, and scarring	Ingrown facial hair from chin contact
"Snaking" of spinal alignment	Cost

Nociceptive pain, which would otherwise cause volitional guarding of an injury site, is often absent. For this reason, spine surgeons commonly employ external immobilization for at least 6 weeks, and usually for 3 months. Near the end of the bracing period, patients with residual muscle function can be instructed to perform isometric muscle strengthening exercises within the brace. Providing the patient and family with reassurance and education about the rationale for brace use and clear guidelines for its proper application are crucial to optimizing adherence to a treatment plan that asks much from the patient (Table 19.1).

SPINE BIOMECHANICS

A detailed description of spine biomechanics is featured in Chapter 3. A working knowledge of normal posture and spinal motion forms the basis for prescription of spinal orthoses in pathologic states. Static external devices are inherently limited in their effectiveness because of the intrinsic triplanar flexibility of the spinal column. Restoration of anatomic lordosis in the cervical and lumbar spine through bracing may bring about abnormal alignment in rotation, and lateral forces may produce a scoliotic effect. As the vertebral anatomy changes from the cervical to sacral segments, different mechanical forces come into play. Used at all levels of the spine, braces decrease total motion. They are most effective in reducing flexion and extension and least effective in controlling rotation.

The complex biomechanics of the highly flexible cervical spine allow for support of the weight of the head and maintain crucial stability of the balance and sight sense organs. The synovial atlanto-occipital joint is primarily designed to allow flexion and extension. Lacking an intervertebral disc, the atlantoaxial (C1-2) joint accounts for as much as 50% of total cervical rotation as the atlas swivels around the odontoid. The remainder of cervical rotation is served by the lower segments. Each of the vertebrae from C3 to C7 features a similar shape. Wide anterior vertebral bodies and oblique facet joint alignment allows for movement in three planes and accommodates cervical lordosis. The greatest amount of flexion and extension in these segments is caudal, at C5-6 and C6-7, respectively. Lateral bending and axial rotation occur in concert and are greatest in the cephalad segments C2-3 and C3-4 (3). Flexibility in this area is not the only challenge for the orthotist. Above the spine, the head is heavy and round. The mobile mandible further reduces the already limited areas that allow stable brace contact. Below, the shoulders are mobile, and contact over the clavicle bones is often painful. The shorter distances in this area result in short orthotic lever arms. Although research studies that measure how orthoses restrict cervical motion employ a variety of measurement methodologies, it is clear that none of these devices are able to provide total immobilization. In real-world use outside the laboratory and in patients with varying degrees of paralysis, spinal motion is likely to be even less controlled (4) (Table 19.2).

Modern western hemisphere bracing techniques for the thoracolumbar spine date to the 17th century. French surgeon Ambroise Pare described his use of metal corsets to reduce motion and promote healing (5). The anatomy of the thoracic spine, if supported by an intact rib cage, is a remarkably stable structure that protects the thoracic cavity. The first ten rib attachments to the sternum, combined with vertical overlapping spinous processes, restrict almost all motion in the flexion and extension plane (6). Although the upper thoracic segments allow a small amount of rotation and lateral bending, the overall motion extending from T1 through T10 is quite limited. At the thoracolumbar junction, the angle of the facet joints of T10 and T11 transitions to that of the lumbar spine, from the frontal to the sagittal plane. Lacking rib attachments to the sternum, the lower thoracic segments are quite mobile. The T12-L1 disc level usually constitutes the fulcrum position between the immobile thoracic spine and the fixed sacral spine, making it susceptible to traumatic injury and degenerative spondylolisthesis. The large, weight-bearing lumbar vertebrae are articulated to allow extension and flexion, with much less lateral bending and almost no axial rotation. Although the sacral segments are fixed to the bony pelvis, the pelvis itself is quite mobile, pivoting en bloc over the hip joints. Orthotists have countered this mobility by extending fixation across the hip and adding thigh cuffs. These extensions may have a small

TABLE 19.2

EFFECTS OF CERVICAL ORTHOSES ON NORMAL CERVICAL MOTION FROM THE OCCIPUT TO THE FIRST THORACIC VERTEBRA

	Mean residual normal motion (%)		
	Flexion-extension	**Lateral bending**	**Rotation**
Normal	100	100	100
Soft collar	74.2	92.3	82.6
Philadelphia collar	28.9	66.4	43.7
SOMI brace	27.7	65.6	33.6
Four-poster brace	20.6	45.9	27.1
Yale cervicothoracic	12.8	50.5	18.2
Halo device	11.7	8.4	2.4
Minerva body jacket	14.0	15.5	0

Data from Fisher SV, et al. Spinal Orthoses in Rehabilitation. In: Braddom R, et al., eds. *Physical medicine rehabilitation.* Philadelphia, PA: Saunders, 2000.

effect in reducing motion at the lumbosacral junction, but offer little added benefit in reducing total segmental motion (7).

With only one exception, the hyperextension brace, thoracolumbar braces offer abdominal compression. The effects of this compression on the spine are inconsistent. In theory, supporting the abdominal contents should act to distract the thoracolumbar segments and reduce lumbar lordosis. In practice, studies have failed to demonstrate consistent changes in spine muscle EMG firing (in neurologically intact patients) or intra-abdominal pressures (8–11). For patients with cervical and upper thoracic spinal cord injuries and paralysis of the trunk and abdominal musculature, however, some positive effects on passive upright posture, active arm reach, and improvements in pulmonary function are associated with abdominal compression from corsets and binders (12). In this setting, trunk support through abdominal compression can be accomplished by corsets that are less restrictive and do not aim to control spinal postures.

BRACING FOR SPINAL PATHOLOGY

Interruption of normal anatomical structures by trauma or disease may render the spine unstable. In this setting, the spine is unable to protect the spinal cord and neurological elements from damage and is unable to withstand the external forces presented by gravity and daily activities without ongoing structural compromise. Even the best spinal orthoses cannot confer spinal stability. Knowledge of when and how spinal orthoses are best used includes an appreciation of when their use is inadequate. When the injured spine is unstable, the spinal brace can ***assist*** in immobilizing the injury site acting in concert with definitive conservative or surgical treatment. Bracing is also used when less serious injuries to the spinal structures occur. In this situation, the goal is to relieve pain and to improve spinal positioning in hopes of reducing angular deformities. Radiographic studies are important, but ultimately the decision on spinal stability falls to the spinal cord injury specialist, who can interpret imaging of spine trauma in the context of the full clinical picture.

The three-column concept of the spine proposed by Denis is generally accepted as the mechanical model for instability in thoracolumbar fractures, where the vast majority of spinal fractures are seen. The anterior column is comprised of the anterior longitudinal ligament and the anterior portion of the vertebral body. The middle column extends from the middle portion of the vertebral body to the posterior surface of the vertebral body, including the posterior longitudinal ligament. The posterior column includes all structures behind the posterior longitudinal ligament (pedicles, facets, spinous processes, and all ligaments) (13). An injury to the thoracolumbar spine is considered unstable if any of the following conditions are met: (a) at least a two-column injury, (b) greater than 50% collapse of the vertebral body height, (c) more than 30 degrees of kyphotic angulation, or (d) involvement of the same column in two or more adjacent spinal levels (14). In general, a fracture will be stable if the middle column is intact and unstable if it is disrupted, with only a few exceptions. Most gunshot injuries to the spine are stable, as well as injuries to the middle column of the midthoracic spine, provided that the ribcage is not injured. Occasionally, injuries to the middle column at L4 or L5 can be considered stable, if the posterior spinal elements are intact and sufficient lumbar lordosis can be maintained by an orthosis.

Over the last two decades, more frequent use of surgical instrumentation in cervical spine trauma has changed the landscape of orthotic prescription, although basic concepts regarding spinal stability remain largely unchallenged. In the cervical spine, cadaver studies by White led to a widely acknowledged method of determining the degree of structural integrity after spinal trauma (15,16). After trauma, cervical spine instability is considered when a static lateral x-ray film demonstrates sagittal plane displacement of greater than 3.5 mm or relative angulation of greater than 11 degrees. In the cervical spine, there are many unique injury patterns and situations. Many anterior wedge compression fractures are stable, provided that total angulation is not too great. Vertebral burst fractures of the cervical spine are usually unstable. Tear-drop fractures must be assessed in light of concurrent injury to the disc and posterior elements. Bilateral locked facet injuries frequently cause neurological injury and are unstable. Vertical C2 body fractures can usually be treated nonoperatively with orthoses (17).

Application of these general guidelines to children is difficult, and orthotic prescription brings special challenges. Often, young patients with ligamentous injuries are difficult to classify under the White and Punjabi criteria. In children, spinal cord injury can be seen in the setting of minimal injury to the bones and ligaments, owing to the intrinsic flexibility of the spinal column. Remarkably, many of these injuries have been demonstrated to be mechanically stable and bracing may not be necessary (18). If bone and ligament damage is found, bracing in children with spine trauma requires collateral expertise in the orthotic management of scoliosis. In younger children, bracing is employed in hopes of forestalling the progression of paralytic scoliosis, and delaying the need for surgical fusion until the child's trunk has grown to adult proportions. Children with scoliosis stemming from traumatic paralysis are usually braced when curves fall between 25 and 45 degrees, although flexible curves (those that reduce easily by postural change) as high as 80 degrees are tolerated in very young children (19–21). Similar orthotic principles are followed in children with spina bifida and myelomeningocele. Braces are commonly worn when the child is upright (22). Readers are referred to the works of Betz (23–25) and Mulcahey (26) who have outlined the important issues relevant to this group.

TAXONOMY OF SPINAL BRACING

Expansion in the orthotic industry has supported use of a remarkable number of eponyms, acronyms, and proprietary names linked to a relatively small number of brace styles. Reported by Harris, a task force of health care professionals developed a common nomenclature in order to standardize communication about these devices (27). This terminology reduces confusion by naming the body segments immobilized, and by implication, the body movements that are restricted (28). Spinal orthoses can be classified as COs, head cervical orthoses (HCOs), cervicothoracic orthoses (CTOs), thoracolumbosacral orthoses (TLSOs), lumbosacral orthoses (LSOs), and cervicothoracolumbosacral orthoses (CTLSOs). A listing of widely available and commonly prescribed braces is listed in Table 19.3.

TABLE 19.3

COMMONLY USED SPINAL ORTHOSES

Type	Common examples, eponyms, or proprietary names
Cervical orthoses	Foam collar
Head cervical orthoses	Philadelphia, Miami-J, Malibu, Aspen
Cervicothoracic orthoses	Guilford (two poster), SOMI, Yale, four poster
Head cervicothoracic orthoses	Halo, Minerva
Thoracolumbosacral orthoses	Hoke Corset, Jewett extension brace, CASH, Taylor, Knight-Taylor, clam-shell-molded body jacket, anterior molded
Lumbosacral orthoses	Chairback, Williams Flexion, Knight brace, Cybertech brace
Sacral orthoses	Trochanteric belt, sacral corset
Cervicothoracolum-bosacral orthoses	Milwaukee brace, molded body jacket with cervical extension

The Cervical Orthosis

COs provide tactile feedback, warmth, and comfort that may prove beneficial for patients with soft tissue strain (Fig. 19.1). They are inexpensive and constructed of soft polyurethane foam, with a cotton liner. These devices may serve as a kinesthetic reminder to restrict active motion. Cervical collars have minimal contact surface with the head or jaw, so they do not restrict movement of the neck in any plane (29). Their use in the spinal cord injury setting is therefore limited. They may be used temporarily for psychological reassurance in patients who have completed their course of using a more restrictive orthosis, or in postoperative patients where there is no concern of mechanical instability.

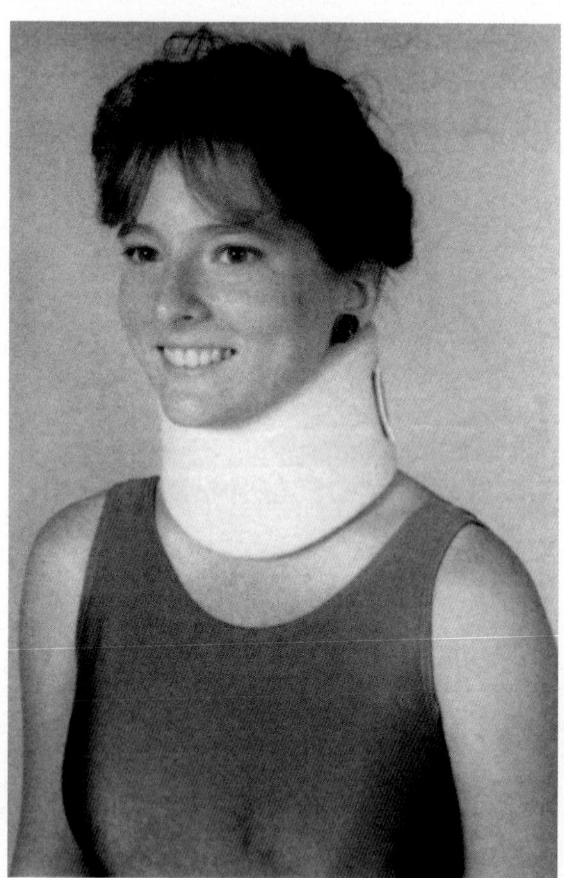

FIGURE 19.1 Soft cervical collar.

The Head Cervical Orthosis

Dozens of different models of HCOs are commercially available, and these have gained widespread use in trauma extrication and transport. All feature a firm plastic structure and molded surfaces that support the occiput and mandible. They are prefabricated, made in multiple sizes, and can accommodate tracheostomy tubes. Their caudal contact surfaces rest on the upper thorax. The Philadelphia, Miami (both from Ossur Americas Aliso Viejo, CA) (Fig. 19.2), and Aspen (Aspen Medical Products: Irvine, CA) (Fig. 19.3) collars are examples of the classic bivalve design with lateral Velcro closures. These collars are best at reducing flexion and extension but limited at restricting rotation and lateral bending. Their application serves as a visible reminder to health care providers that spinal injury is suspected or present. It has been shown that HCOs such as the Philadelphia collar do not differ from the Halo thoracic vest in their ability to restrict C1-2 sagittal motions in normal study subjects and could be used for stable odontoid fractures (30). In a study by Polin et al. (31), the healing of type II and type III odontoid fractures was no

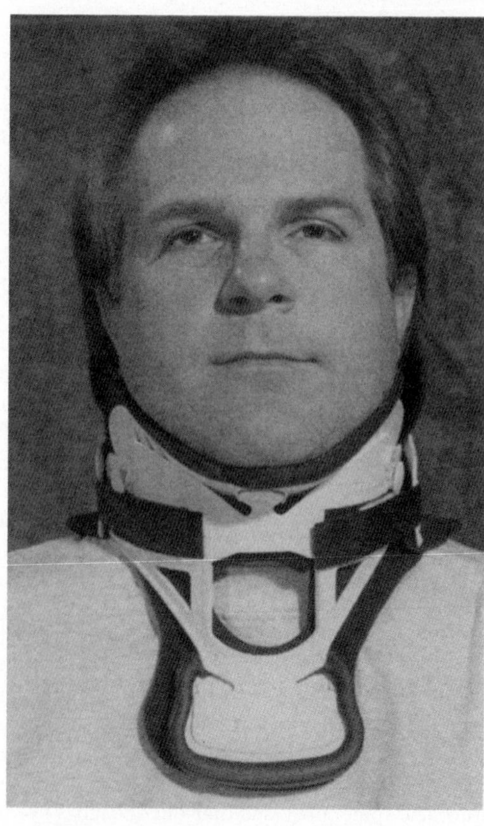

FIGURE 19.2 Miami J collar Miami Collar.

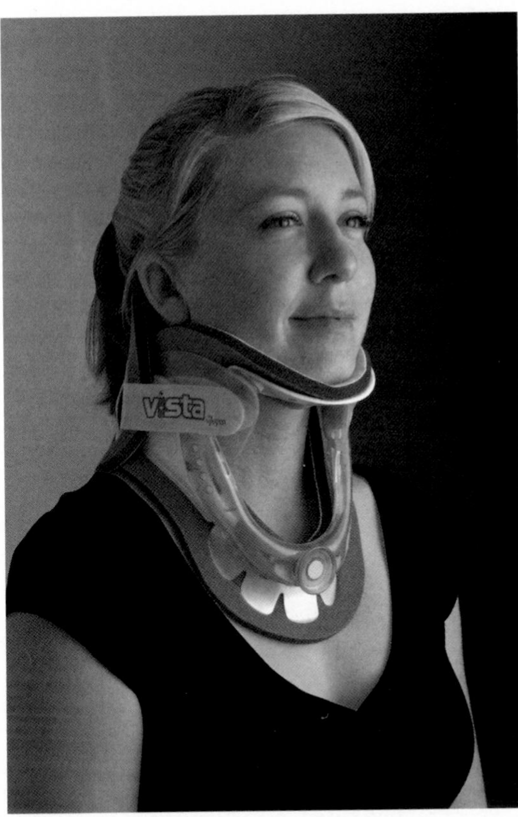

FIGURE 19.3 Aspen Vista collar. The height of the anterior chin piece is adjusted by turning the circular dial. (Aspen Medical Products: Irvine, CA.)

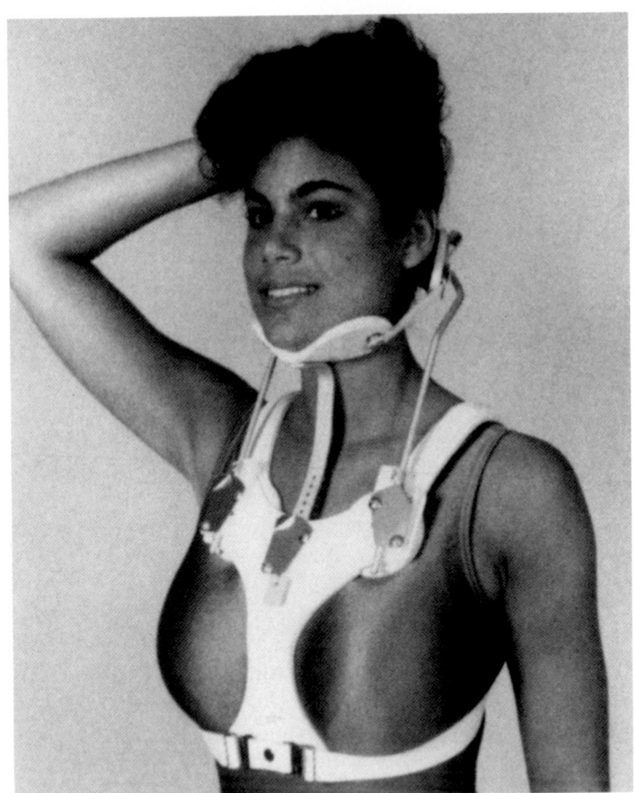

FIGURE 19.4 SOMI brace. The chin piece is sometimes removed and replaced by a forehead strap that attaches to the occipital pad. (Leimkuehler Inc., Cleveland, OH.)

different between patients who wore HCOs compared with patients who were treated with Halo devices. However, they provide inadequate support for an unstable spine when used in isolation. In severe spine injuries, they may provide limited protection on an interim basis before surgery or application of a Halo device. HCOs are commonly prescribed after midcervical spine surgery or trauma when stability is not in question or when stability has been achieved by instrumentation. In limited situations, less extensive trauma to the upper spine may heal with HCOs. In nontraumatic settings, use of HCOs is common after single-level anterior spinal fusion and instrumentation, but such bracing does not increase fusion rates or improve outcomes postoperatively (32). These collars are not benign devices. Skin problems, including chin ulcers, are common. Their use has been associated with delayed weaning in ventilator-dependent patients (33).

Cervicothoracic, Minerva, and Halo Devices

Of all external orthoses, CTOs are the most effective in reducing cervical motion. Two to four rigid struts affix support pads on the mandible, occiput, and trunk. All feature a chest piece which, in concert with increased orthotic length, provides better control over flexion and rotation. The SOMI (sternal-occipital-mandibular immobilizer) design offers several advantages in this group (Fig. 19.4). Its occipital supports bend anteriorly under the ear to attach with the chest plate. For this reason, it is easily applied with the patient lying supine and with the patient in tong traction. Control of lateral bending is limited. Restriction of flexion in the C1-3 region is good, and overall control of motion is satisfactory in the mid and lower cervical spine. This brace has been used in rheumatoid arthritis patients with atlantoaxial instability because of its ability to check unstable flexion deformity. In addition, neural arch fractures of C2, which become unstable in flexion, can be immobilized by this orthosis (34). The chin piece of the SOMI can be removed for eating by substituting a forehead strap that snaps onto the occipital support, thus converting the brace to a head cervicothoracic orthosis (HCTO).

Different styles of CTOs offer advantages based upon their component size and configuration. The Yale brace (a modified Philadelphia collar) features long fiberglass extensions that extend anteriorly and posteriorly over the thorax. The length of the brace gives it more purchase to align injuries in the lower cervical and upper thoracic spine. A high occipital pad offers greater restriction at the C1-2 region. Compared to SOMI devices, the four-poster brace features a cooler open design and broad contact pads that rest on the superior thorax, which eliminates the straps under the ribcage. It is useful in midcervical injuries where control of lateral bending and rotation is a priority. As an alternative, the aforementioned Miami and Aspen HCOs can be outfitted with thoracic attachments, extending the immobilization for persons with injuries at the cervicothoracic junction.

Highly unstable injuries to the cervical and upper thoracic spine will require the added movement restrictions imposed by HCTOs. The Halo vest is widely available and relatively easy to apply, but its effectiveness is dependent upon external fixation by pins into the outer table of the skull. The Minerva orthosis is less invasive, but requires fitting by an orthotist with great skill and experience. Both the Minerva and Halo designs offer optimal immobilization and the opportunity for the patient to remain mobile during the healing process.

The Minerva is a custom-molded, bivalved thermoplastic jacket that has full contact with the thorax, chin, and occiput. A circumferential headband immobilizes the head. Newer fabrication methods have produced a lightweight and stable brace that has several advantages (35,36). This noninvasive orthotic approach averts the risks of tong and Halo traction in agitated patients with brain injuries, mental illness, or developmental disabilities. The Minerva provides a good option for patients who cannot maintain fixation with skeletal pins, such as those with skull fractures, soft tissue injuries to the face, or excessive osteoporosis. A clinical study comparing the use of the Minerva to the Halo in patients with cervical spine trauma found that the Minerva offered improved control of angulation at all levels except C1-2 (37). It has also been used successfully in children.

For immobilization of the cervical and upper thoracic spine, Halo fixation is the most widely used and effective technique (Fig. 19.5). This system is used in a variety of situations including trauma, tumor involvement of the spine, and spinal infections (38). The Halo rings can be used for cervical distraction in the emergency setting, then attached to a thoracic vest to promote early mobilization of patients after alignment and stability is optimized (39,40). Compared to Gardner-Wells tongs, the Halo ring can be safely used with higher traction forces and offers greater stability during application of the weights (41).

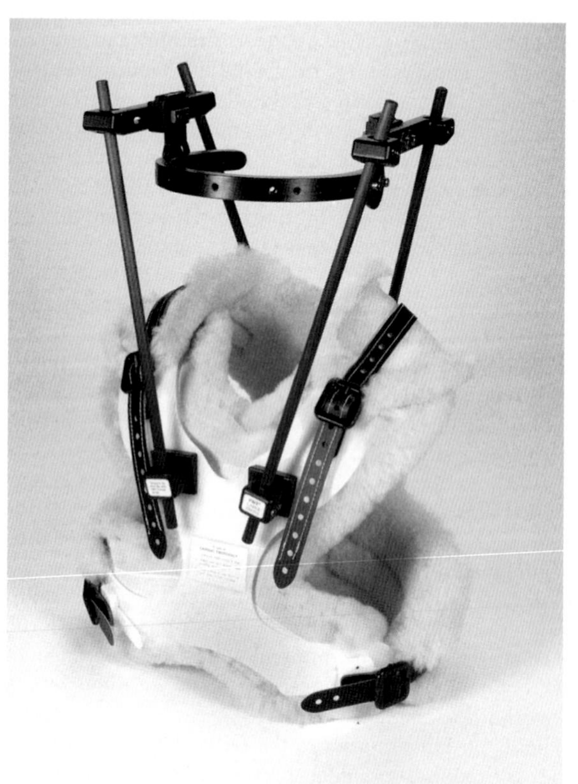

FIGURE 19.5 Halo Device (PMT Corporation Chanhassen, MN.)

The degree of spine stabilization achieved with the Halo vest has been confirmed by several methods of study (42,43). Overall free motion in all cardinal directions may be as little as 4% of normal; however, the use of the Halo is not a guarantee against poor alignment or failed bone fusion (44). Even though it offers superior spinal fixation, it is inadequate in situations where spinal trauma is severe. In patients with three-column disruption or severe facet joint damage, surgical instrumentation will be required if the goal is to mobilize the patient quickly and safely. In the active patient, the Halo is ineffective in maintaining the distraction forces needed to achieve good alignment in patients with severe bone destruction. Using the Halo in the course of daily activities, considerable paradoxical motion occurs in the midcervical region, even as overall motion (measured occiput to T1) changes very little (45). The greatest motion is at C2-3, and the least is at the cervicothoracic junction.

Although custom modifications of the Halo system have been used, most patients are fitted with prefabricated devices featuring carbon composite rings, head pins, and uprights that are designed to maximize compatibility with magnetic resonance imaging. Nylon ball joints offer freedom in three planes of adjustment and are less likely to cause unpleasant creaking and snapping during everyday movement. Several sizes of vests are available, but fit is still a challenge, especially in elderly patients with excessive kyphosis. Proper fit of the vest is a determinant of success in spine fixation. Pressure sores can develop under the vest, especially in the scapular region where routine visual inspection of the supine patient is inconvenient. The vest should give room above the shoulders to allow 90 degrees of arm abduction. Therapy staff should restrict shoulder shrug and overhead reaching exercises that may cause the vest to migrate. The vest and uprights must not be used as "handles" to move the patient.

Pin site complications are seen in up to 60% of patients (46). The most common problems are pain, pin loosening, and pin site infection. Modern pin design, with broad skull contact, may reduce the frequency of these problems. Anterior Halo pins must be inserted on the lateral third of the orbital ridge to avoid damaging the sinuses, supratrochlear, and orbital nerves. The posterior skull is thicker, and pin placement is less hazardous in this region. The target is usually 1 inch above the ear pinna, avoiding contact with the fragile ear cartilage (47). Pins are inserted with torque devices normally provided by the manufacturer. Six to eight inch-pounds of insertion torque is recommended and is usually well tolerated, even in the elderly (48). The actual forces imparted to the skull may fluctuate, as the accuracy of torque wrenches may be inconsistent, and the friction between the pin threads and the Halo affects measurement (49,50). After insertion, pin tightness is checked at 24 to 48 hours. Patients commonly report clicking and popping during the course of Halo wear. This is not necessarily a sign of pin loosening and frequent late manipulation of pins is not recommended. If necessary, tightness can be checked with a torque device, provided that resistance can be felt with gentle finger manipulation of the pin. Pins that spin freely or are seated in areas that are infected must be removed and relocated. The relocation process will change the mechanical forces of the device and is frequently associated with later pin problems (51). Routine care of the Halo pin sites involves cleansing twice daily with normal saline. The use of antiseptic cleansers has been shown to increase infection rates. These solutions change normal skin bacterial flora and retard normal healing (52). Application of ointments to the pin sites blocks normal serous drainage and may produce crusts that promote infection. Marginal erythema is common at the pin sites, although a change in local skin color or induration may herald a superficial infection that can be treated with oral antibiotics and more attentive pin care. Spread of infection to the intracranial space, pin perforation, and ring migration are recognized complications of the Halo device.

Use of the Halo has been associated with medical complications. The vest may restrict pulmonary vital capacity, and upper abdominal compression has been linked with superior mesenteric artery syndrome (53). Orthopaedic complications include avascular necrosis of the dens, degenerative changes of the facet joints, and local osteoporosis (which is reversible after brace removal) (54). During assembly and alignment of the Halo uprights, overdistraction and excessive spinal extension will cause dysphagia, especially in the elderly with kyphotic deformities (55). This problem is exacerbated by a weak cough and impaired mentation associated with pain medications. Adjustment of spinal fixation angle by experienced personnel usually relieves the problem. Over time, the neck musculature will atrophy (56). Although the Halo is relatively lightweight, it will affect static and dynamic balance. Attentive rehabilitation treatment will reduce the risk of falls and injuries linked to the use of this device (57) (Table 19.4).

TABLE 19.4

CHECKLIST FOR PATIENT TREATMENT AND EDUCATION WITH HALO ORTHOSES REHABILITATION GOALS VARY DEPENDING UPON RESIDUAL MOTOR AND SENSORY FUNCTION

Provide training throughout the patient's stay—do not teach everything 15 min before discharge
Help the patient plan for interruptions/reduction in school and work activities postdischarge
Promote liberal use of mobility devices (canes, walkers) to improve balance and safety
Expect that supine to sit mobility activities will be difficult
Encourage trials of sleeping in side-lying and prone positions
Teach special strategies for activities of daily living

- May need to don and doff clothes in the supine position
- Choose alternative clothing (e.g., slip on shoes, football jerseys, strapless bras)
- Adjust feeding activities (plate repositioning, large utensils, drinking straws)
- Find a safe method for hair washing
- Practice bathing skills before discharge (usually sponge bath in shallow water)

Develop clear indications for changing the liner to avoid overmanipulation of the device
Anticipate visual restrictions (peripheral vision, diplopia, blurred vision, eye muscle fatigue)
Instruct that extremes in ambient temperature and noisy environments may cause discomfort
Inform patients to

- AVOID driving a car
- AVOID engaging in high-velocity sport activities
- AVOID self-adjusting the screws or jacket
- AVOID use of poles for vigorous body hygiene under the jacket

Adapted from Olson B, Ustanko W, Warner S. Self care needs of patients in a halo brace. *Orthop Nurs J.* 1997;10(1):27–33.

Thoracolumbosacral Orthoses

A small number of basic styles of TLSOs are manufactured and marketed throughout the world under different names. These devices extend from the axillae to the pelvis and provide a variable degree of spinal restriction related to their materials and design. Soft cotton and canvas corsets provide abdominal compression and limited overall postural support. They have no substantial impact on spinal alignment. Although these braces are prescribed for medical treatment of back pain in able-bodied individuals, they are most often used as a balance aid in the setting of chronic thoracic spinal cord injury. The other braces, with thermoplastic or metal construction, offer restriction of spinal motion, which is most effective at the thoracolumbar junction, at the midportion of the device (58). Control of motion at the low lumbar level is minimal (8,59). None of these devices provide sufficient stabilization to allow safe, upright activity in patients with acute, unstable two- or three-column fractures. In past years, these orthoses were worn after multiple weeks of complete bed rest promoted spinal healing. Presently, they are best used in the setting of minor skeletal trauma, or as an adjunct to surgical treatment (60–62). The Jewett (Fig. 19.6) and cruciform anterior spinal hyperextension (CASH) (Fig. 19.7) braces are designed to control flexion at the thoracolumbar junction. These prefabricated, lightweight devices are used for stable vertebral compression injuries in patients without spondylolisthesis. They both offer good control of flexion and restriction motion from approximately T6 to L1. Fitted in the seated position, the brace should sit just below the sternal notch and just above the pubic bone. No control over lateral bending and rotation is offered, and abdominal compression is absent. The CASH design may be better tolerated, especially in elderly

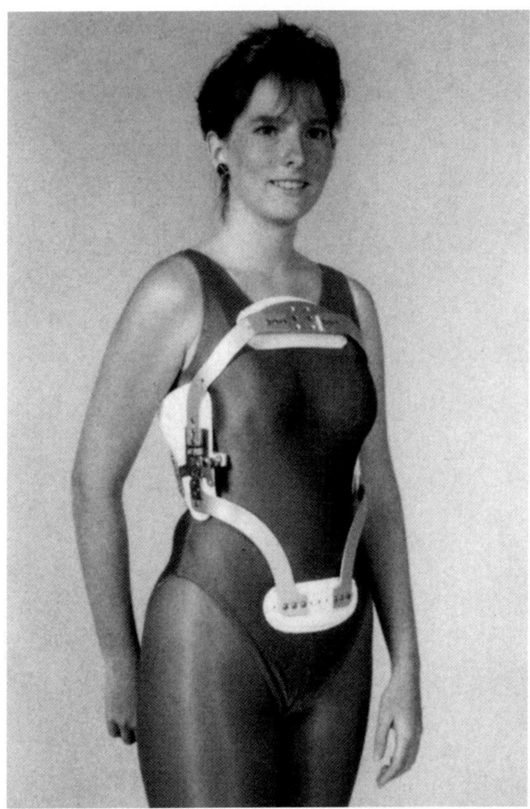

FIGURE 19.6. Jewett Brace.

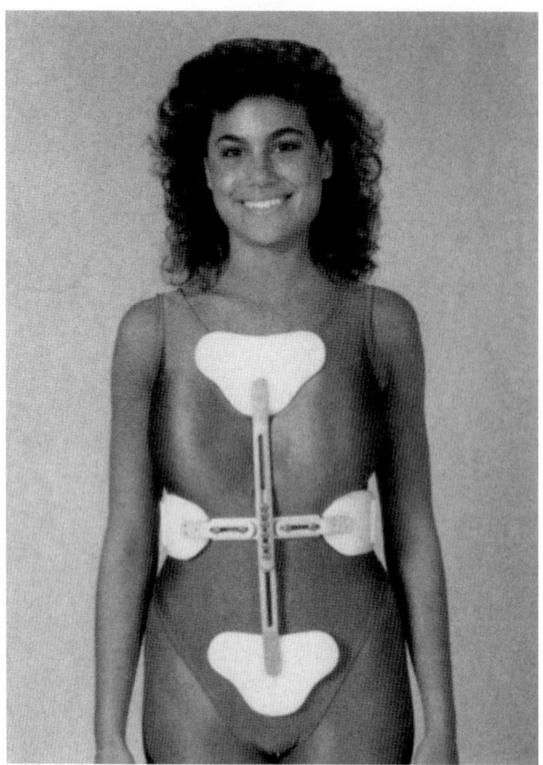

FIGURE 19.7. CASH orthosis.

or thin individuals, as it is easier to apply than the Jewett model, with less breast and axilla contact than the Jewett. Both Jewett and CASH braces feature a posterior pad in the midthoracic region.

Extension control is added to flexion control in the Taylor brace, which features aluminum paraspinal struts and an abdominal corset. Flexion is restricted by straps that course over the shoulder and through the axillae. A modification of this design, the Knight-Taylor brace (Fig. 19.8), adds inflexible lateral trunk supports and is aimed at prohibiting lateral bending. Modest control of rotation is achieved by adding rigid pads that extend vertically under the clavicles, offering an unpleasant active reminder to reduce movement. In many areas of the world where thermoplastic molding technology is not available, these braces are a mainstay of treatment.

Of all TLSOs, the total-contact molded body jacket provides the best immobilization of the thoracolumbar area (63,64) (Fig. 19.9A,B). It is fabricated from polypropylene, which has been vacuum molded around a positive cast of the patient's torso. This custom fitting provides good pressure distribution over wide areas of skin and offers relief over bony prominences, making it ideal for patients with impaired skin sensation. Its lightweight, bivalve design, and Velcro closures make donning and doffing less cumbersome. The brace is fitted over the bony pelvis and extends anteriorly to the manubrium and posteriorly to the mid-scapular region. After the patient resumes sitting activities, the brace may need to be trimmed above the pubic bone and the inguinal crease, to reduce skin irritation. Foam liners help protect the skin, and cutouts in the shell promote ventilation and can accommodate feeding tubes and ostomy sites.

After casting and fabrication, major adjustments in the molded TLSO are not feasible. Abdominal distension is often present when the cast is made and resolves as the patient becomes more active. Patients often loose weight during the course of treatment. In these cases, a replacement orthosis may be necessary to accommodate the change in body size and shape.

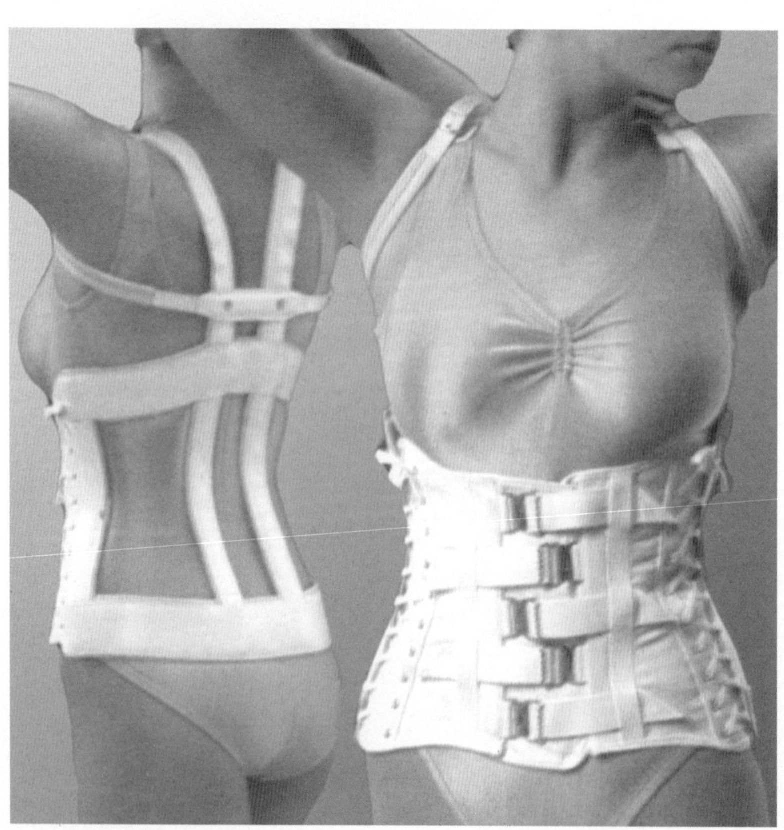

FIGURE 19.8. Knight-Taylor orthosis.

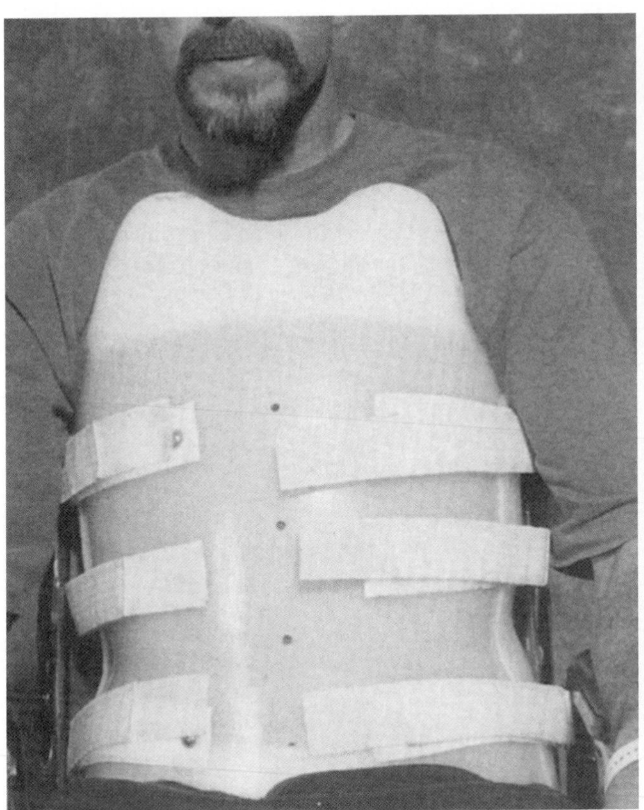

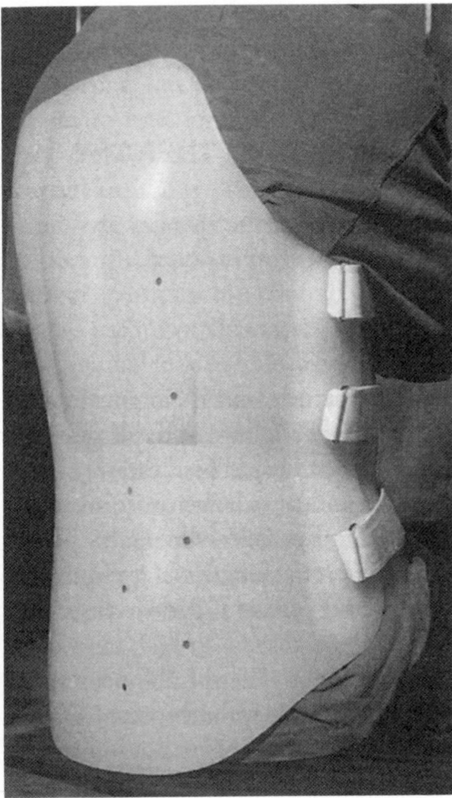

FIGURE 19.9. A: Custom thermoplastic body jacket (anterior view) (From Fig. 19.7A first edition). B: Custom thermoplastic body jacket (posterior view) (From Fig. 19.7B First Edition).

Lumbosacral and Sacral Orthoses

Like soft cervical collars, LSOs are frequently prescribed but achieve limited immobilization of the spinal column. The chairback (Fig. 19.10) and Knight braces are similar in their short profile: both use rigid posterior uprights connected to circumferential pelvic and thoracic bands. Anteriorly, there is a semirigid abdominal corset. These work best to restrict flexion and extension between L1 and L4. As with the Halo brace, studies document overall reduction in trunk motion but show limited effect on segmental motion. Most of these investigations have assessed normal volunteers, so their relevance to spinal cord injured patients may be limited. Nonetheless, research findings make the popularity of these braces even more controversial (43). For example, Norton and Brown (8) documented a paradoxical increase in spinal movement after brace application when subjects were measured in the seated position. Waters and Morris demonstrated an increase in spinal EMG activity after brace application when the patients were walking (65). The practice of prescribing these braces as kinesthetic "reminders" for the patient to restrict movement must be tempered by knowledge of their negative potential, allowing deconditioning of the trunk muscles during their use. It is possible that these devices exert a modest effect on the spine if consistent abdominal compression is gained. Modern, rigid, plastic materials combined with innovative drawstring and pulley systems (as seen in the Cybertech brace) have made abdominal compression obtainable without the inconvenience of lace hook and corset design (Fig. 19.11). The beneficial

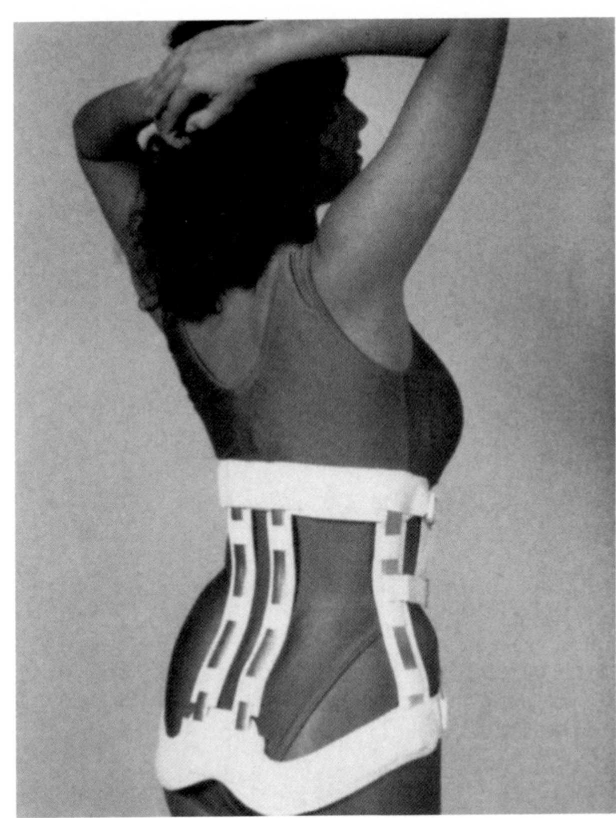

FIGURE 19.10. Chairback brace.

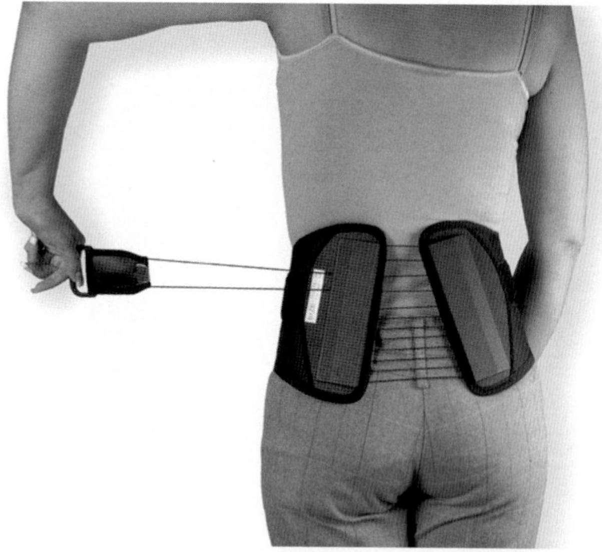

FIGURE 19.11. Cybertech lumbosacral orthosis. The posterior pulley system and pull cord cinch produces abdominal compression. The pull cord wraps to the front and attaches with Velcro. (Cybertech Medical La Verne, CA.)

effect of abdominal compression may be diminished by other factors, however. Abdominal compression may cause gastrointestinal reflux disease. These braces have also been shown to reduce pulmonary tidal volumes (66). Even in the postoperative setting, reduced loads on instrumentation hardware have yet to be demonstrated (67). There is no consistent evidence that they improve success rates of instrumented fusion or fusion in situ in the treatment of patients with spinal trauma.

Rounding out the list of LSOs is the Williams orthosis, which is designed for situations where lumbar spine extension should be avoided. Used for traumatic spondylolysis and spondylolisthesis in the lumbar spine, this brace combines a rigid posterior shell with a flexible, elastic front apron. It is useful to limit side bending and lumbar extension at end range in these patients.

Sacral orthoses (SOs) are prefabricated, compressive devices that act to maintain intra-abdominal pressure and increase kinesthetic awareness. Examples include sacral and trochanter belts and corsets. They are generally applied with perineal bands that reduce migration, and maintain alignment, so that opposing pressure can be applied to the sacral promontory. These orthoses are most commonly used to reduce pain in the setting of trauma to the bony pelvis, or for treatment of postpartum pain.

General Considerations

Taking into account the broad range of potential physical activity levels between patients, a variety of subjective factors enter into the prescription for orthoses utilization. The spinal cord medicine physician is called upon to set clear rules for the treatment staff, patient, and family about brace wear. Misunderstandings arise when different patients are given different rules for brace application from their treating physicians. One patient may be told that he or she may have his or her orthoses removed while in bed, with the head of the bed positioned below 30 degrees. The next patient may only be permitted to have his or her orthoses loosened, momentarily, for hygiene purposes. Education in this setting focuses on the fact that all spinal injuries are unique, and all spinal surgeries are unique. In the operating suite, the spine surgeon gains direct tactile and visual appreciation of the patient's level of spine stability and is the best person to judge whether the surgical fixation has enough purchase to promote healing of a stable spine.

Restrictive braces, like the Halo or TLSO body jacket, are likely to impede progress toward some higher level therapy goals. Important skills, like dressing and unlevel transfers, are often deferred until brace removal. Wheelchair prescription must be delayed. These exceptions are few, and the use of bracing should not be used as a reason to restrict early access to a spinal cord rehabilitation program. Spinal orthoses do not restrict patients from achieving important goals in the realm of medical stabilization, bowel and bladder care, strengthening of residual muscle groups, and psychosocial adjustment. These goals form the foundation of a rapid and successful discharge to the home. Even as modern spine surgery techniques reduce the need for external immobilization, spine orthoses have allowed thousands of patients to participate more actively in the rehabilitation process.

References

1. Fayssoux RS, Cho RH, Herman MJ. A history of bracing for idiopathic scoliosis in North America. *Spine* 2009;34(1):74–81.
2. Sanan A, Rengachary SS. The history of spinal biomechanics. *Neurosurgery* 1996;39(4):657–656.
3. Lucas BD. Spinal bracing. In: Licht S, ed. *Orthotics, etcetera.* New Haven, CT: Waverly Press, 1966.
4. Johnson RM, Hart DL, Simmons EF, et al. Cervical orthoses. A study comparing their effectiveness in restricting cervical motion in normal subjects. *J Bone Joint Surg Am* 1977;59(3):332–339.
5. Wolf JW, Johnson RM. Cervical orthoses. In: Bailey RW, ed. *The cervical spine.* Philadelphia, PA: JB Lippincott, 1983:54–61.
6. Andriacchi TP, Schultz AB, Belytschko TB, et al. A model for studies of mechanical interactions between the human spine and rib cage. *J Biomech* 1974;7:487.
7. Axelsson P, Johnsson R, Strömqvist B. Lumbar orthosis with unilateral hip immobilization. Effect on intervertebral mobility determined by roentgen stereophotogrammetric analysis. *Spine* 1993;18(7):876–879.
8. Brown T, Norton PL. The immobilizing efficiency of back braces; their effect on the posture and motion of the lumbosacral spine. *J Bone Joint Surg Am* 1957;39-A(1):111–139.
9. Nachemson A, Morris JM. In vivo measurements of intradiscal pressure. Discometry, a method for the determination of pressure in the lower lumbar discs. *J Bone Joint Surg Am* 1964;46:1077–1092.
10. Morris JM, Lucas DB, Bresler B. Role of the trunk in stability of the spine. *J Bone Joint Surg Am* 1961;43:327–351.
11. Calmels P, Fayolle-Minon I. An update on orthotic devices for the lumbar spine based on a review of the literature. *Rev Rhum Engl Ed* 1996;63(4):285–291.

12. Goldman JM, Rose LS, Williams SJ, et al. Effect of abdominal binders on breathing in tetraplegic patients. *Thorax* 1986;41:940–945.
13. Denis F. The three column spine and its significance in the classification of acute thoracolumbar spinal injuries. *Spine*. 1983;8(8):817–831.
14. Kern MB, Malone DG, Benzel EC. Evaluation and surgical management of thoracic and lumbar instability. *Contemp Neurosurg* 1996;18:1–8.
15. White AA III, Johnson RM, Panjabi MM, et al. Biomechanical analysis of clinical stability in the cervical spine. *Clin Orthop Relat Res* 1975;109:85–96.
16. White AA III, Panjabi MM. *Clinical biomechanics of the spine*. Philadelphia, PA: JB Lippincott, 1990:278–378.
17. German JW, Hart BL, Benzel EC. Nonoperative management of vertical C2 body fractures. *Neurosurgery* 2005;56(3):516–521.
18. Bosch PP, Vogt MT, Ward WT. Pediatric spinal cord injury without radiographic abnormality (SCIWORA). The absence of occult instability and lack of indication for bracing. *Spine* 2002;27(24):2788–2800.
19. Pang D, Sun PP. Pediatric vertebral column and spinal cord injuries. In: Winn HR, ed. *Youmans neurological surgery*. 5th ed. Philadelphia, PA: W.B. Saunders, 2004.
20. Cattell HS, Filtzer DL. Pseudosubluxation and other normal variations in the cervical spine in children. A study of one hundred and sixty children. *J Bone Joint Surg Am* 1965;47:1295–1309.
21. Komor A. Orthoses in pediatric spinal injuries. *Ortop Traumatol Rehabil* 2003;5(1):117–120.
22. Chafetz RS, Mulcahey MJ, Betz RR, et al. Impact of prophylactic thoracolumbosacral orthosis bracing on functional activities and activities of daily living in the pediatric spinal cord injury population. *J Spinal Cord Med* 2007;30(suppl 1):S178–S183.
23. Mehta S, Betz RR, Mulcahey MJ, et al. Effect of bracing on paralytic scoliosis secondary to spinal cord injury. *J Spinal Cord Med* 2004;27(suppl 1):S88–S92.
24. Sison-Williamson M, Bagley A, Hongo A, et al. Effect of thoracolumbosacral orthoses on reachable workspace volumes in children with spinal cord injury. *J Spinal Cord Med* 2007;30(suppl 1):S184–S191.
25. Dearolf WW 3rd, Betz RR, Vogel LC, et al. Scoliosis in pediatric spinal cord-injured patients. *J Pediatr Orthop* 1990;10(2):214–218.
26. Sison-Williamson M, Bagley A, Hongo A, et al. Effect of thoracolumbosacral orthoses on reachable workspace volumes in children with spinal cord injury. *J Spinal Cord Med* 2007;30(suppl 1):S184–S191.
27. Harris EE. A new orthotics terminology. *Orthot Prosthet* 1973;27:6–9.
28. Goldberg B, Hsu JD, eds. *Atlas of orthoses and assistive devices*. 3rd ed. St Louis, MO: Mosby, 1998.
29. Hartman JT, Palumbo F, Hill BJ. Cineradiography of braced normal cervical spine; comparative study of five commonly used cervical orthoses. *Clin Orthop* 1975;109:97–102.
30. Koller H, Zenner J, Hitzl W, et al. In vivo analysis of atlantoaxial motion in individuals immobilized with the halo thoracic vest or Philadelphia collar. *Spine* 2009;34(7):670–679.
31. Polin RS, Szabo T, Bogaev CA, et al. Nonoperative management of types II and III odontoid fractures: the Philadelphia collar versus the halo vest. *Neurosurgery* 1996;38:450–456.
32. Campbell MJ, Carreon LY, Traynelis V, et al. Use of cervical collar after single-level anterior cervical fusion with plate: is it necessary? *Spine* 2009;34(1):43–48.
33. Webber-Jones JE, Thomas CA, Bordeaux RE. The management and prevention of rigid cervical collar complications. *Orthop Nurs* 2002;21:19–25.
34. Hadley MN. Management of combination fractures of the atlas and axis in adults. *Neurosurgery* 2002;50(3 suppl):S140–S147.
35. Millington PJ, Ellingsen JM, Hauswirth BE, et al. Thermoplastic Minerva body jacket—a practical alternative to current methods of cervical spine stabilization. A clinical report. *Phys Ther* 1987;67(2):223–225.
36. Maiman D, Millington P, Novak S, et al. The effect of the thermoplastic Minerva body jacket on cervical spine motion. *Neurosurgery* 1989;25(3):363–367.
37. Benzel EC, Hadden TA, Saulsbery CM. A comparison of the Minerva and halo jackets for stabilization of the cervical spine. *J Neurosurg* 1989;70(3):411–414.
38. Cooper PR, Maravilla KR, Sklar FH, et al. Halo immobilization of cervical spine fractures. Indications and results. *J Neurosurg* 1979;50(5):603–610.
39. Chan RC, Schweigel JF, Thompson GB. Halo-thoracic brace immobilization in 188 patients with acute cervical spine injuries. *J Neurosurg* 1983;58(4):508–515.
40. Parry H, Delargy M, Burt A. Early mobilisation of patients with cervical cord injury using the halo brace device. *Paraplegia* 1988;26(4):226–232.
41. Hynes RJ, Koeneman EJ, et al. A biomechanical comparison of Gardner-Wells tongs and halo devices used for cervical spine traction. *Spine* 1994;19:2403–2406.
42. Johnson RM, Hart DL, Simmons EF, et al. Cervical orthoses. A study comparing their effectiveness in restricting cervical motion in normal subjects. *J Bone Joint Surg Am* 1977;59(3):332–339.
43. Woodard EJ, Benzel EC. Orthoses. In: Benzel EC, ed. *Spine surgery: techniques, complication avoidance, and management*. New York, NY: Churchill Livingstone, 1999:1363–1378.
44. Sears W, Fazl M. Prediction of stability of cervical spine fracture managed in the halo vest and indications for surgical intervention. *J Neurosurg* 1990;72(3):426–432.
45. Koch RA, Nickel VL. The halo vest: an evaluation of motion and forces across the neck. *Spine* 1978;3(2):103–107.
46. Lind B, Sihlbom H, Nordwall A. Halo-vest treatment of unstable traumatic cervical spine injuries. *Spine* 1988;13(4):425–432.
47. Fleming BC, Krag MH, Huston DR, et al. Pin loosening in a halo best orthosis; a biomechanical study. *Spine* 2000;25:1325–1331.
48. Ebraheim, J, Liu V, Patil C, et al. Evaluation of skull thickness and insertion torque at the halo pin insertion areas in the elderly: a cadaveric study. *Spine J* 2007;7(6): 689–693.
49. Whitesides TE, Mehserle WL, Hutton WC. The force exerted by the halo pin. A study comparing different halo systems. *Spine* 1992;17(10 suppl):S413–S417.

50. Kerwin GA, Chou KL, White DB, et al. Investigation of how different halos influence pin forces. *Spine* 1994;19(9):1078–1081.
51. Botte MJ, Byrne TP, Garfin SR. Application of the halo device for immobilization of the cervical spine utilizing an increased torque pressure. *J Bone Joint Surg Am* 1987;69(5):750–752.
52. Olson RS. Halo skeletal traction pin site care: toward developing a standard of care. *Rehabil Nurs* 1996;21(5): 243–246.
53. Roth EJ, Fenton LL, Gaebler-Spira DJ, et al. Superior mesenteric artery syndrome in acute traumatic quadriplegia: case reports and literature review. *Arch Phys Med Rehabil* 1991; 72(6):417–420.
54. Korovessis P, Konstantinou D, Piperos G, et al. Spinal bone mineral density changes following halo vest immobilization for cervical trauma. *Eur Spine J* 1994;3(4): 206–208.
55. Taitsman LA, Altman DT, Hecht AC, et al. Complications of cervical halo-vest orthoses in elderly patients. *Orthopedics* 2008;31:446.
56. Ono A, Amano M, Okamura Y, et al. Muscle atrophy after treatment with Halovest. *Spine* 2005;30(1): E8–E12.
57. Richardson JK, Ross AD, Riley B, et al. Halo vest effect on balance. *Arch Phys Med Rehabil* 2000;81(3): 255–257.
58. Dorski S, Buchalter D, Kahanovitz N, et al. A three dimensional analysis of lumbar brace immobilization utilizing a noninvasive technique. Proceedings of the 33rd Annual Meeting, Orthopedic Research Society, San Francisco, 1987.
59. Axelsson P, Johnsson R, Strömqvist B. Lumbar orthosis with unilateral hip immobilization. Effect on intervertebral mobility determined by roentgen stereophotogrammetric analysis. *Spine* 1993;18(7):876–879.
60. Resnick DK, Choudhri TF, Dailey AT, et al. American Association of Neurological Surgeons/Congress of Neurological Surgeons. Guidelines for the performance of fusion procedures for degenerative disease of the lumbar spine. Part 14: brace therapy as an adjunct to or substitute for lumbar fusion. *J Neurosurg Spine* 2005;2(6):716–724.
61. Giele BM, Wiertsema SH, Beelen A, et al. No evidence for the effectiveness of bracing in patients with thoracolumbar fractures. *Acta Orthop* 2009;80(2):226–232.
62. Yee AJ, Yoo JU, Marsolais EB, et al. Use of a postoperative lumbar corset after lumbar spinal arthrodesis for degenerative conditions of the spine. A prospective randomized trial. *J Bone Joint Surg Am* 2008;90(10):2062–2068.
63. Lantz SA, Schultz AB. Lumbar spine orthosis wearing. I. Restriction of gross body motions. *Spine* 1986;11(8): 834–837.
64. Fidler MW, Plasmans CM. The effect of four types of support on the segmental mobility of the lumbosacral spine. *J Bone Joint Surg Am* 1983;65(7):943–947.
65. Waters RL, Morris JM. Effect of spinal supports on the electrical activity of muscles of the trunk. *J Bone Joint Surg Am* 1970;52(1):51–60.
66. Puckree T, Lauten VA, Moodley S, et al. Thoracolumbar corsets alter breathing patterns in normal individuals. *Int J Rehabil Res* 2005;28:81–85.
67. Rohlmann A, Bergmann G, Graichen F, et al. Braces do not reduce loads on internal spinal fixation devices. *Clin Biomech* 1999;14(2):97–102.

CHAPTER 20 ■ DUAL DIAGNOSIS: TRAUMATIC BRAIN INJURY WITH SPINAL CORD INJURY

MONIFA BROOKS

INTRODUCTION

While the occurrence of a spinal cord injury (SCI) is a life-altering event for all, those who sustain a concomitant brain injury face additional challenges. The incidence of concomitant traumatic brain injury (TBI) in those with a primary SCI (dual diagnosis [DD]) is reported between 24% and 74% (1–8). The criteria used to determine the occurrence of TBI may account for the variability of reported incidence. While the majority of studies have been retrospective in fashion, these authors have utilized a number of diagnostic criteria to diagnose TBI including loss of consciousness (LOC), abnormalities on imaging studies, decreased initial Glasgow Coma Scale (GCS), presence of posttraumatic amnesia (PTA), and/or score on the cognitive domain of Functional Independence Measure (FIM). The true incidence of concomitant TBI in SCI patients may be even higher as mild TBI can easily be overlooked especially since abnormalities on imaging studies do not need to be present to establish the diagnosis.

Recalling that the spinal cord is the caudal extension of the brain, one can appreciate that any injury that affects the spinal cord may also injure the adjacent neurologic structure to which it is conjoined. An increased incidence of TBI has been associated with higher level tetraplegia, ventilator dependence, and those injured in either motor vehicle crashes or falls (1–6). Not surprisingly, falls and motor vehicle crashes are also leading causes of TBI. Those with a neurological level and an ASIA Impairment Scale (AIS) level of T1 or lower AIS D had the lowest rate. Mild TBI is the most common form of accompanying injury in those with SCI, although the higher initial mortality associated with severe TBI may skew these statistics.

DIAGNOSIS

Historical factors, such as mechanism of injury (i.e., high velocity impact), LOC, prolonged extrication and/or intubation at the scene, higher neurological level of injury, presence of PTA, and impaired initial GCS (Table 20.1) score, should alert medical personnel to the possibility of a concomitant TBI (9,10).

Other findings present either premorbidly, at the scene of injury, or during the acute hospital course, which may also suggest an underlying brain injury, include history of prior TBI, substance abuse, seizures, agitation, and respiratory insufficiency. The Model TBI System collects data on four diagnostic criteria: LOC, PTA, neuroimaging results, and GCS. Recently, Tolonen et al. (8) have proposed an algorithm to estimate both TBI presence and severity in patients with spinal cord injuries (Table 20.2). Macciocchi et al. proposed a classification system to identify mild, moderate, and severe TBI in the SCI population (Table 20.3). Utilizing these criteria, they identified the incidence of mild uncomplicated TBI as 34% in those with SCI; the incidence of mild complicated TBI was 10%, moderate TBI 6%, and severe TBI 10% (1).

The presence and duration of PTA has been shown to correlate with functional outcomes following TBI (11). The Galveston Orientation and Amnesia Test (GOAT) is utilized to assess PTA (Fig. 20.1). The test can be repeated throughout the recovery period. A score of 76 or higher on two consecutive testing sessions indicates the patient is out of PTA. The orientation log (O-log) is a ten-question scale, with each item scored 0 to 3, used to assess orientation within the rehabilitation setting (Fig. 20.2). A score of at least 25, of a possible 30, correlates with the patient being out of PTA (12). The O-log has been validated in the TBI population and can be administered serially to track changes throughout the rehabilitation process (12–15). Because it contains only 10 items, it requires less time to complete than the GOAT. There is evidence to suggest the O-log may be a better predictor of functional outcomes than the GOAT (16).

Neuroimaging often consists of an initial screening computer topography (CT) scan of the head. While this test is adequate to diagnose the presence of hemorrhage and can be performed rapidly, it may miss more subtle abnormalities. Diffuse axonal injury (DAI) typically occurs following acceleration-deceleration injuries. Magnetic resonance imaging (MRI) may reveal more subtle imaging abnormalities such as DAI, however requires more time to obtain. Newer imaging modalities including diffusion-tensor imaging may be more sensitive for detecting TBI in the SCI population (17).

Beyond initial GCS, PTA, presence of LOC, and imaging studies, neuropsychological testing can be extremely important as it may reveal subtle abnormalities, which are present with milder brain injuries (18). Unfortunately, commonly used cognitive tests, such as the Weschler Adult Intelligence Test, Thurston Word Fluency test, and the Trails Making test, require the patient be able to write or draw, which may not be possible for those with paralysis (19–21). These tests requires a skilled practitioner to administer an appropriate battery of tests to obtain valid results for each individual while accommodating the physical limitations presented by the underlying SCI.

Once the individual deficits are identified, the findings can be used to address specific deficits such as higher level executive functioning skills, which may not be apparent with less sensitive screening assessments. Precise diagnosis of cognitive impairments allows the clinical team to formulate a more specific treatment plan. Also as patients consider returning to

TABLE 20.1

GCS FOR HEAD INJURY

Eye opening	
Spontaneous	4
To loud voice	3
To pain	2
None	1
Verbal response	
Oriented	5
Confused, disoriented	4
Inappropriate words	3
Incomprehensible sounds	2
None	1
Best motor response	
Obeys	6
Localizes	5
Withdraws (flexion)	4
Abnormal flexion posturing	3
Extension posturing	2
None	1

Scores from all three domains are totaled.
GCS 13–15, Mild TBI; GCS 9–12, Moderate TBI; GCS 3–8, Severe TBI
Adapted from Teasdale G, Jennett B. Assessment of coma and impaired consciousness. A practical scale. *Lancet* 1974,2:81–84.

school and/or work where stressful environments may exacerbate deficits, it is important that patients, families, and employees/educators be aware of the potential difficulties patients may experience. Ideally, accommodations will be developed and implemented to insure the patient's successful transition to the community.

MEDICAL COMPLICATIONS

The medical challenges presented by SCI are many and detailed elsewhere in this text. However, there are medical complications posed by a concomitant brain injury that increase the complexity of clinical decision making. Medical management of problems common to the SCI population such as pain, DVT prophylaxis, spasticity, and neurogenic bladder requires special consideration in the DD patient. In addition, the physician must consider that some medications routinely used in SCI may have an impact on the recovering brain. Special care should be taken to utilize medications with minimal cognitive impact. Peripherally acting medicines are generally preferred to those with central mechanisms of action. Clinical findings in SCI individuals may have different etiologies and, as such, require different treatment in the patient with concomitant TBI.

This section will highlight the unique issues clinicians face while managing persons with DD. Table 20.4 provides an overview of select pharmacotherapy often used in this patient population.

TABLE 20.3

MACCIOCCI CLASSIFICATION OF TBI IN SCI

Severity	GCS	Clinical features
Mild uncomplicated	13–15	Clinical evidence of brain dysfunction e.g., confusion with/without LOC
Mild complicated	13–15	Above + cerebral pathology
Moderate	9–12	May or may not have cerebral pathology
Severe	<8	May or may not have cerebral pathology

LOC, loss of consciousness; cerebral pathology, contusion, hemorrhage, or skull fracture
Adapted from Macciocchi S, Seel RT, Thompson N, et al. Spinal cord injury and co-occurring traumatic brain injury: assessment and incidence. *Arch Phys Med Rehabil* 2008;89:1350–1357.

Autonomic Dysfunction

While autonomic dysfunction in those with SCI is a well-known potential complication, those with a concomitant TBI can present unique challenges to the clinician. For example, fever may represent infection, poikilothermia as a result of SCI, or dysautonomia, which occurs in TBI. Dysautonomia

TABLE 20.2

DIAGNOSTIC CRITERIA FOR CLASSIFICATION OF TBI SEVERITY BY TOLONEN ET AL.

Diagnostic criteria	Mild	Moderate	Severe
Altered level or LOC	GCS 13–15 and/or any LOC < 30 min	GCS 9–12 and/or LOC > 30 min–6 h	GCS 3–8 and/or LOC > 6 h
PTA	Any PTA < 24 h	24 h–7 d	>7 d
Neurological finding due to TBI	No findings	Transient neurological finding	Permanent neurological finding
Neuroradiological finding due to TBI	No findings	Neuroradiological TBI finding	Neuroradiological TBI finding and neurosurgical operation
Neuropsychological finding due to TBI	No neuropsychological findings, but subjective symptoms with predictable normal work and ADL performance	1–2 SD[a] in tests or limited capability in work but with normal ADL	>2 SD in tests or unable to work and permanent difficulties in ADL

[a]Worse than the normal mean in one or more neuropsychological tests.
SD, standard deviation.
Adapted from Tolonen A, Turka J, Salonen O, et al. Traumatic brain injury is under-diagnosed in patients with spinal cord injury. *J Rehabil Med* 2007;39:622–626.

Question	Error Score	Notes
What is your name?	–2 ___	Must give both first name and surname.
When were you born?	–4 ___	Must give day, month, and year.
Where do you live?	–4 ___	Town is sufficient.
Where are you now:		
a) City	–5 ___	Must give actual town.
(b) Building	–5 ___	Usually in hospital or rehab center. Actual name necessary.
When were you admitted to this hospital?	–5 ___	Date.
How did you get here?	–5 ___	Mode of transport.
What is the first event you can remember after the injury?	–5 ___	Any plausible event is sufficient (record answer)
Can you give some detail?	–5 ___	Must give relevant detail.
Can you describe the last event you can recall before the accident?	–5 ___	Any plausible event is sufficient (record answer)
What time is it now?	–5 ___	–1 for each half-hour error.
What day of the week is it?	–3 ___	–1 for each day error.
What day of the month is it? (i.e. the date)	–5 ___	–1 for each day error.
What is the month?	–15 ___	–5 for each month error.
What is the year?	–30 ___	–10 for each year error.
Total Error:		
Total Actual Score = (100 – total error) = 100 – _____ =		Can be a negative number.
76-100 = Normal / 66-75 = Borderline / <66 = Impaired		
Developed by Harvey Levin, Ph.D., Vincent M. O'Donnell, M.A., & Robert G. Grossman, M.D.		

FIGURE 20.1 The GOAT Harvey S. Levin, Ph.D., Vincent M. O'Donnell, M.A., & Robert G. Grossman, M.D. Instructions: Can be administered daily. Score of 76 or more on two consecutive occasions is considered to indicate that the patient is out of PTA.

(sometimes referred to as sympathetic storming) is more common in those with severe brain injury. It can present within the first week following brain injury and may continue for several months thereafter. Some reports have linked diffuse axonal injuries with an increased incidence of dysautonomia. The precise etiology of central dysautonomia has yet to be fully identified; however, abnormal hypothalamic function appears to be at least part of the mechanism (22,23). Aside from fever, patients may experience tachycardia, tachypnea, profuse sweating, rigidity, and/or hypertension (23,24). Tachypnea, hyperhydrosis, and rigidity are not commonly associated with autonomic dysreflexia (AD), and as such, their presence may indicate dysautonomia. Elevated blood pressure may signal the presence of AD in those with SCI at or above the T6 level. The treatment of dysreflexia is described in detail in this text (see Chapter 9). If initial interventions to treat AD do not improve the patient's BP, central dysautonomia should be considered.

Treatment options for dysautonomia include beta-blockers such as propanolol 10 mg dosed two to four times per day, calcium channel blockers, such as diltiazem 60 to 120 mg dosed four times per day, gabapentin dosed 200 to 300 mg two to three times per day, bromocriptine dosed 2.5 to 5 mg one to two times per day, benzodiazepines such as lorazepam dosed at 0.5 to 1 mg every 6 hours, and/or morphine sulfate dosed at 1 to 2 mg administered intravenously every 2 hours as needed until symptoms abate (24,25).

Thromboembolic Disease

Prophylaxis against deep vein thrombosis (DVT) is more complicated in the DD population. Given the increased incidence of DVT with the risk of a potentially fatal pulmonary embolism, those with TBI/SCI should receive chemoprophylaxis

Patient Name: Date: Time:

City									
Kind of Place									
Name of Hospital									
Month									
Date									
Year									
Day of week									
Clock Time									
Etiology/Event									
Pathology/Deficits									
Total Score									

ADMINISTRATION AND SCORING:
The Orientation Log (O-Log) is designed to be a quick quantitative measure of orientational status for use at bedside with rehabilitation inpatients. Place, time, and situational (Etiology/Event + Pathology/Deficits) domains are assessed.

Patient responses are scored according to the following criteria
3 = correct spontaneously or upon first free recall attempt
2 = correct upon logical cueing (e.g., "That was yesterday, so today must be …")
1 = correct upon multiple choice or phonemic cuing
0 = incorrect despite cueing, inappropriate response, or unable to respond

Incorrect responses should be followed by cuing at the next highest level. In the place domain, "Hospital" in any context is sufficient for Kind of Place. In the domain of time, Month, Date, Year, and Day of Week must be exact; however, Clock Time can be correct to within 30 minutes (plus or minus). Patients are allowed to look at a clock without penalty when responding to the Clock Time item. For situation, the patient must be oriented to both Etiology/Event (e.g., "What brought you into the hospital?") and Pathology/Deficits (e.g., "What kind of injuries did you have?" or "How did the stroke affect you?"). Situational responses must demonstrate awareness of head/brain injury and how the injury was sustained (e.g., MVA, fall, assault, GSW). Add scores down each column and plot total.

Adapted from Jackson WT, Novack TA, Dowler RN. Effective serial measurement of cognitive orientation in rehabilitation: the Orientation Log. *Arch Phys Med Rehabil.* 1998 Jun;79(6):718–720.

FIGURE 20.2 The orientation log.

TABLE 20.4

PHARMACOTHERAPY FOR THE PATIENT WITH DD

Medication	Common TBI indication(S)	Dosage	Potential side effects
Modafinil	Attention/arousal	100–200 mg 1–2×/d	Impaired sleep
Armodafinil	Attention/arousal	150–250 mg daily	Impaired sleep
Methylphenidate	Attention/arousal	2.5–10 mg 1–2×/d	Tachycardia/hypertension
Dextroamphetamine	Attention/arousal	5–10 mg 1–2×/d	Tachycardia/hypertension
Bromocriptine	Arousal	2.5–10 mg 1–2×/d	Hypotension
Amantidine	Arousal/fatigue	100–200 mg daily	Constipation/urinary retention
Ramelteon	Sleep	8–16 mg bedtime	
Desyrel	Sleep/agitation	25–100 mg daily	Serotonin syndrome, priapism
Risperidone	Agitation	0.25–2 mg 1–2–/d	Sedation
Quetiapine	Agitation	25–200 mg 1–3×/d	Sedation
Propanolol	Dysautonomia	5–10 mg 1–4×/d	Hypotension/bradycardia
Labetalol	Dysautonomia	20 mg IV or 100–400 mg 2×/d	Hypotension/bradycardia
Morphine	Dysautonomia	1–2 mg IV/IM	Hypotension/sedation
Gabapentin	Dysautonomia	300 mg 2–4×/d	Sedation
Lorazepam	Dysautonomia	1–2 mg IV/IM	Sedation
Escitalopram	Depression/Arousal	10–20 mg daily	Serotonin syndrome
Citalopram	Depression/Arousal	10–40 mg daily	Serotonin syndrome
Dantrolene	Spasticity/Dysautonomia	25–100 mg 2–4×/d	Weakness/abnormal liver function tests
Lioresal	Spasticity	5–20 mg 2–4×/d	Sedation/abnormal liver function tests
Tizanidine	Spasticity	2–8 mg 2–4×/d	Hypotension/abnormal liver function tests

unless contraindicated. For those with acute intracerebral hemorrhage, immediate chemoprophylaxis is generally contraindicated. However, once cessation of bleeding has been documented, prophylaxis with either low molecular weight heparin or unfractionated heparin may be initiated within 3 to 4 days (26,27). In patients for whom anticoagulation is contraindicated, placement of an inferior vena cava (IVC) filter (preferably removable) can be useful to prevent pulmonary embolism. Routine placement of IVC filters in those without a contraindication to full anticoagulation is generally not recommended (28).

While there is a paucity of literature examining the safety of full anticoagulation following intracerebral hemorrhage, there are a small number of studies indicating full anticoagulation may be restarted within 7 to 14 days of stabilization of the hemorrhage (27,28). Each case should be dealt with on an individual basis based upon consultation with the surgical referrers.

Neuroendocrine Disorders

Impaired sodium metabolism occurs secondary to abnormal pituitary function. Hyponatremia is common following TBI and may represent either the syndrome of inappropriate antidiuretic hormone (SIADH) or central salt wasting (CSW). Because serum sodium levels will be decreased in both conditions, calculating the fractional excretion of sodium (FENa) is useful to distinguish these diagnoses. The FENa is generally elevated in CSW and decreased in SIADH. Treatment of CSW includes hydration and salt replacement with salt tablets. Those with SIADH are generally treated with fluid restriction. Hypernatremia may occur as a result of diabetes insipidus and may be treated with desmopressin and/or hyposmolar fluid replacement. Care should be taken not to correct the serum sodium too rapidly as this may cause cerebral edema (29). Bushnik et al. (30) suggest growth hormone deficiency correlates with increased incidence of fatigue following brain injury.

Seizure Prophylaxis

Persons who sustain a TBI are at risk for the development of post-TBI seizures. Initial prophylaxis with antiepileptic medications is generally recommended for all patients (31–33) and should continue for 1 week for persons who do not develop early seizures and have no history of epilepsy (31,34). Early seizures are defined as those that develop within 1 week of injury. Temkin reported no increased benefit with extension of prophylaxis beyond 1 week in persons without additional risk factors for late seizures; defined as seizures that develop after 1 week of injury (31–33). The presence of an intracerebral hemorrhage, depressed skull fracture, penetrating trauma, or development of early seizures increases the risk of seizure activity. A longer duration of antiepileptic treatment may be indicated for those with additional risk factors (34).

While there are multiple medication options available for seizure prophylaxis, consideration of those with less cognitive side effects is warranted. Phenytoin that is readily available and can be administered intravenously has been shown to have a negative effect on cognitive performance and new learning (35–37). Similar negative effects on new learning have been seen with carbamazepine, valproic acid, and topiramate. Anticonvulsants with less impact on normal cognitive function such as levetiracetam or lamotrigine may be preferable (38,39–41).

Carbamazepine is most commonly used as an antiepileptic medication. Because of effects on the dopamine receptors, it may also be useful in treating agitation and restlessness (35,36). When used to modify behavior, one may use clinical benefit, rather than serum drug levels as a guide for efficacy. One should be aware of potential bone marrow suppression as a serious potential side effect and thus blood counts should be monitored. It appears to act by reducing polysynaptic responses and blocking the posttetanic potentiation. There are studies reporting a negative impact on new learning (35–37) in persons receiving carbamazepine.

It has been suggested that valproic acid's activity in epilepsy is related to increased brain concentrations of gamma-aminobutyric acid (GABA). With GABA activation, valproic acid may increase sedation and inhibit new learning, but can be useful in the treatment of agitation and restlessness (36,37). Liver function tests should be monitored as hepatotoxicity is a potential side effect of this medication.

In vitro and in vivo recordings of epileptiform activity from the hippocampus have shown that levetiracetam inhibits burst firing without affecting normal neuronal excitability, suggesting that levetiracetam may selectively prevent hypersynchronization of epileptiform burst firing and propagation of seizure activity. As such it seems to have less impact on new learning (39–41).

Attention and Arousal

Decreased levels of arousal and attention impairment are common findings in persons with TBI and can negatively impact the patient's ability to acquire new information and practice new skills. Neurostimulant medications can be helpful in improving arousal. Amphetamines have proven useful in improving attention (42–48); however, caution is required in patients with known cardiac disease. Dopaminergic medications (i.e., bromocriptine, levodopa) can also improve arousal with fewer side effects on the cardiovascular system. Impairments in attention may be addressed with both environmental and pharmacologic interventions. Minimizing environmental distractions such as utilizing smaller treatment rooms with few patients, as well as limited auditory and visual stimuli may assist brain-injured persons with maintaining attention during therapy sessions.

Methylphenidate's mode of action in humans is not completely understood, but it presumably activates the brain stem arousal system and cortex to produce its stimulant effect. It should be used with caution in those with known cardiac disease as it may cause increased blood pressure and/or tachycardia (45,48). A typical dose is 5 to 10 mg dosed once or twice daily. Side effects may include appetite suppression, insomnia, agitation, and dyskinesia. There is also the potential for abuse with this medication and therefore should be used cautiously in those with a history of substance abuse.

Modafinil has wake-promoting actions similar to sympathomimetic agents like amphetamine and methylphenidate, although the pharmacologic profile is not identical to that of sympathomimetic amines. As such, it has minimal cardiovascular effects, although it should be used with caution in those with recent myocardial infarction. The medication is generally dosed at 100 to 200 mg daily or twice daily. The precise mechanism through which modafinil promotes wakefulness is unknown. Armodafinil is similar to modafinil, however has a longer half-life. The dose is typically 150 to 250 mg given once per day. With both modafinil and armodafinil, evening dosing should be avoided to minimize insomnia.

Bromocriptine is a dopamine receptor agonist, which activates postsynaptic dopamine receptors. The dopaminergic neurons in the corpus striatum are involved in the control of motor function. Small studies have reported modest improvement in initiation and motor recovery (49–51). The medication may be initiated at 2.5 mg and titrated up to 10 mg dosed once or twice daily. Potential side effects include hypotension and akathisia.

While dopamine does not cross the blood-brain barrier, levodopa, the metabolic precursor of dopamine, does. It is presumably converted to dopamine in the brain and can improve attention and arousal. It has also been shown to stimulate motor recovery following TBI; however, the motor effect in those with DD may be limited secondary to the underlying SCI (52).

Agitation

Agitation is common in those with TBI and should be managed similarly in those with DD (53). One must be mindful to rule out potential organic causes of agitation including hypoxia, infection, electrolyte abnormalities, and medication intoxication as potential etiologies. Behavioral interventions such as redirection, limit setting, and decreasing environmental stimulation are first-line treatments. Pharmacotherapy is appropriate when behavioral modifications alone are ineffective. Measurements of agitation include the Agitated Behavior Scale (54,55) (Table 20.5). The scale can be completed by any clinician observing the patient. It records the presence or absence of 14 specific behaviors associated with agitation, thus making it an ideal tool to quantify the effectiveness of any given intervention to treat agitation.

TABLE 20.5

AGITATED BEHAVIOR SCALE

Patient _____	Period of observation:	
Observ. Environ.	From:	a.m. p.m. ___/___/___
Rater/Disc._____	To:	a.m. p.m. ___/___/___

At the end of the observation period indicate whether the behavior described in each item was present and, if so, to what degree: slight, moderate or extreme. Use the following numerical values and criteria for your ratings.

1 = **absent:** the behavior is not present.

2 = **present to a slight degree:** the behavior is present but does not prevent the conduct of other, contextually appropriate behavior. (The individual may redirect spontaneously, or the continuation of the agitated behavior does not disrupt appropriate behavior.)

3 = **present to a moderate degree:** the individual needs to be redirected from an agitated to an appropriate behavior, but benefits from such cueing.

4 = **present to an extreme degree:** the individual is not able to engage in appropriate behavior due to the interference of the agitated behavior, even when external cueing or redirection is provided.

DO NOT LEAVE BLANKS.

_____ 1. Short attention span, easy distractibility, inability to concentrate.
_____ 2. Impulsive, impatient, low tolerance for pain or frustration.
_____ 3. Uncooperative, resistant to care, demanding.
_____ 4. Violent and or threatening violence toward people or property.
_____ 5. Explosive and/or unpredictable anger.
_____ 6. Rocking, rubbing, moaning or other self-stimulating behavior.
_____ 7. Pulling at tubes, restraints, etc.
_____ 8. Wandering from treatment areas.
_____ 9. Restlessness, pacing, excessive movement.
_____ 10. Repetitive behaviors, motor and/or verbal.
_____ 11. Rapid, loud or excessive talking.
_____ 12. Sudden changes of mood.
_____ 13. Easily initiated or excessive crying and/or laughter.
_____ 14. Self-abusiveness, physical and/or verbal.
_____ **Total Score**

From Corrigan JD. Development of a scale for assessment of agitation following traumatic brain injury. *J Clin Experimental Neuropsychol* 1989;11:261–277, with permission.

In those with TBI, the acquisition of new information is often challenging. Patients may benefit from simple task repetition in therapy until the individual skills can be completed with minimal prompting from the therapist. The therapeutic environment itself may also differ, as persons with TBI may perform better in less stimulating environments (i.e., with fewer visual and auditory distractions with close supervision by the treating therapist). For those patients who continue to exhibit agitation despite behavioral interventions, pharmacotherapy may prove useful. Atypical antipsychotic medications have been successfully used to treat agitation in the brain injury population (56,57).

The precise mechanism of action of quetiapine as with other drugs having efficacy in the treatment of schizophrenia and bipolar disorder is unknown. However, it has been proposed that its mood stabilizing properties in bipolar depression and mania are mediated through a combination of dopamine type 2 (D_2) and serotonin type 2 ($5HT_2$) antagonism. Quetiapine's antagonism of histamine H_1 receptors may explain the somnolence observed with this drug, while its antagonism of adrenergic α_1 receptors may explain the orthostatic hypotension observed with this drug. Typically doses are 25 to 50 mg daily.

Risperidone is a selective monoaminergic antagonist with high affinity for the serotonin type 2 ($5HT_2$), dopamine type 2 (D_2), α_1 and α_2 adrenergic, and H_1 histaminergic receptors. It is therefore helpful in treating agitation. Risperidone has low to moderate affinity for the serotonin $5HT_{1C}$, $5HT_{1D}$, and $5HT_{1A}$ receptors, weak affinity for the dopamine D_1 and haloperidol-sensitive sigma site, and unlike haloperidol, almost no affinity for cholinergic muscarinic or β_{31} and β_{32} adrenergic receptors. This explains the relatively low incidence of extrapyramidal side effects with risperidone as compared to haloperidol (56,57). Typical doses are 0.25 to 1 mg administered once or twice daily.

Sleep Disturbance

Poor sleep is a fairly common occurrence following TBI and may exacerbate agitation (58–60). Regulation of sleep-wake cycles following TBI is critical to optimize cognitive functioning. One can employ several measures to improve sleep including maintaining daytime wakefulness/arousal, minimizing nocturnal disturbances, and appropriate medications as needed. Medications traditionally used to promote sleep in the non–brain-injured population (i.e., benzodiazepines and anticholinergics) may have negative cognitive effects on those with brain injury. Benzodiazepines in particular have been shown to adversely affect sleep architecture. In contrast to the benzodiazepines, which nonselectively bind to and activate all BZ receptor subtypes, zolpidem in vitro binds the BZ_1 receptor preferentially. The BZ_1 receptor is found primarily on the Lamina IV of the sensorimotor cortical regions, substantia nigra (pars reticulata), cerebellum molecular layer, olfactory bulb, ventral thalamic complex, pons, inferior colliculus, and globus pallidus. This selective binding of zolpidem on the BZ_1 receptor may explain the relative absence of muscle relaxant and anticonvulsant effects in animal studies as well as the preservation of deep sleep (stages 3 and 4) in human studies of zolpidem.

Serotonergic agents, such as Desyrel, have been helpful in improving sleep in those with brain injuries. In animals, Desyrel selectively inhibits serotonin uptake by brain synaptosomes and potentiates the behavioral changes induced by the serotonin precursor, 5-hydroxytryptophan. It can be helpful in treating insomnia as well as agitation and is typically dosed between 25 and 100 mg given at bedtime. Caution should be exercised in prescribing Desyrel to those taking selective serotonin reuptake inhibitor (SSRI) medications as serotonin syndrome can occur. The activity of ramelteon at the MT_1 and MT_2 receptors is believed to contribute to its sleep-promoting properties, as these receptors, acted upon by endogenous melatonin, are thought to be involved in the maintenance of the circadian rhythm underlying the normal sleep-wake cycle. It has negligible impact on cognition and thus can be quite useful in treating insomnia in those with brain injury. A typical dose would be 8 to 16 mg each evening (61).

Fatigue

Not surprisingly, with the relatively high occurrence of sleep disturbance, fatigue following brain injury can also present challenges to the rehabilitation process. Fatigue has been reported to occur in 16% to 34% of persons with moderate to severe brain injury (62). It should be noted that fatigue may be a manifestation of poor sleep, pain, depressed mood, or pituitary insufficiency. Lower quality of life scores have been correlated with fatigue in those with brain injury (63). Both patients and caretakers should be aware that fatigue symptoms may persist for years after the initial injury (64).

Interventions to optimize sleep effectively treat pain or depression, and correction of abnormal hormone levels should be instituted when appropriate. In addition to treatment of comorbidities, amantadine has been used to decrease fatigue in those with neurologic disorders. The precise mechanism of action of amantadine is not known. Data from earlier animal studies suggest that amantadine may have direct and indirect effects on dopaminergic neurons. For this reason, it can act to increase attention and arousal following TBI. The dose may start at 50 to 100 mg dosed once or twice daily. More recent studies have demonstrated that amantadine is a weak, noncompetitive NMDA receptor antagonist (65,66). Although amantadine has not been shown to possess direct anticholinergic activity in animal studies, clinically, it exhibits anticholinergic-like side effects such as dry mouth, urinary retention, and constipation. This may impact bowel and bladder care in those with DD.

Behavioral modifications can also prove useful in treating cognitive fatigue. Tasks that require prolonged mental attention may worsen fatigue symptoms (63). Utilizing pacing techniques such as planned rest breaks or alternating less demanding tasks with those requiring more concentration can be useful in maximizing cognitive function.

Depression

The prevalence of major depression in persons with TBI has been reported between 27% and 47% utilizing DSM-IV criteria (67–69). Manifestations of depression may include fatigue, sleep disturbance, poor concentration, and frustration. These symptoms can be difficult to differentiate from the behavioral changes often associated with brain injury. Given the prevalence of mood disturbance, appropriate screening of all patients is essential to facilitate early initiation of treatment. Cognitive impairments in those with DD may invalidate many of the instruments typically used to diagnose mood disturbance. The evaluation of a clinical psychologist or psychiatrist can be invaluable in distinguishing an appropriate grieving/adjustment reaction from true depression. Interventions may include psychotherapy, pharmacotherapy, and/or behavioral therapy. Fann et al. (67) reported serotoninergic antidepressants and cognitive behavioral therapy are most effective in treating depression in the brain injury population. Escitalopram is an SSRI whose mechanism of action is presumed to be linked to potentiation of serotonergic activity in the central nervous system (CNS) resulting from its inhibition of CNS neuronal reuptake of serotonin. A typical dose is 10 to 20 mg daily. In addition to improving mood, escitalopram can be useful in improving initiation and arousal (70).

The risk for depression has been reported to remain increased for up to 2 years from the time of injury, well beyond the acute rehabilitation period. (See Chapter 21 Psychological Adaptations to SCI.) It is therefore important for clinicians to continually assess patients for symptoms of mood disturbance (71). Additional psychosocial stressors such as unemployment and low socioeconomic status are also associated with increased risk of depression. To date, there is a paucity of evidenced-based medicine to clearly identify an optimal approach to treating depression in those with DD. Effective management of pain, poor sleep, and fatigue, if present, should be included in the treatment plan.

Spasticity

Spasticity may develop in both the TBI and SCI patient populations. Nonpharmacologic treatments including range of motion and positioning are enacted prior to medication trials. Generally in those with TBI, centrally acting spasticity medications that may impair new learning and/or decrease arousal levels are less desirable. However, dantrolene sodium, which acts peripherally to inhibit calcium reuptake in the sarcoplastic reticulum, is nonselective and thus may decrease strength in innervated muscles needed for functional mobility.

In those with DD and relatively focal spasticity, chemodenervation techniques can be particularly useful allowing treatment of targeted muscles without systemic side effects. For persons with motor complete SCI and predominantly lower extremity spasticity, intrathecal medication administration of Lioresal allows for smaller doses with less cognitive side effects. For those who demonstrate positive results during test dosing, moving to implantation of an intrathecal pump allows for careful and relatively quick titration of medication while monitoring closely for side effects. As with spasticity management in the non-DD population, a combination of interventions may be required for optimal treatment.

Hydrocephalus

The development of post-TBI hydrocephalus can occur at anytime following the initial injury. Symptoms can be very insidious in onset and difficult to recognize in a person with concomitant SCI. Typical symptoms associated with hydrocephalus include altered cognition, development of urinary retention or incontinence, and impaired gait secondary to balance deficits. Because many SCI patients have an underlying neurogenic bladder and are nonambulatory, these symptoms may go unnoticed. Cognitive changes may be subtle; however, if other etiologies have been eliminated, the diagnosis of hydrocephalus should be considered. The diagnosis can typically be made by CT scan. Placement of a ventricular shunt is an effective treatment.

REHABILITATION PROCESS AND FUNCTIONAL OUTCOMES

The individual with a DD presents a challenge to the rehabilitation team (72). Deficits may be seen in attention, concentration, and memory as well as interfere with new learning and problem solving. The patient may exhibit agitation, aggression, disinhibition, as well as depression. This is problematic as SCI rehabilitation requires intensive new learning, with the ability to master new skills. Compensatory techniques are needed to improve mobility and self-care skills, adapt to a new lifestyle, and reintegrate into the community. Recognizing that the TBI exists and developing a comprehensive treatment program to address the dual injury are the first steps in devising an appropriate treatment plan. Given the unique needs of this patient population, admission to a dedicated DD unit may provide the most beneficial therapeutic environment.

When attempting to teach new skills, environmental stimuli should be limited to improve attention to the desired task. Repetition of tasks can also be a useful treating tool as patients may have difficulty following complex verbal instructions. Directions should be simplified and repeated as needed. Early involvement of caregivers is also crucial as those with brain injury are likely to have difficulty instructing their care. It also allows for carryover of behavior outside of the therapeutic setting.

All members of the treating team should reinforce cognitive and behavioral therapy strategies. External cues such as memory books and timers used for weight-shift reminders are useful in improving patient autonomy. Frequent orientation should be provided during all patient encounters. Verbal redirection and limit setting should be consistent between all staff.

Following the acute rehabilitation period, an outpatient day program incorporating cognitive, physical, occupational, and vocational therapies may provide the optimal transition back to the community.

While few studies have examined the affects of TBI on outcome among individuals with SCI, greater adjustment difficulties and unmet needs were noted among person with DD (73–76). Smaller functional gains (as measured by the motor FIM) in those with DD have been reported; however, there is no significant difference in rehabilitation LOS (75). Medical morbidities may be increased. For example, there could be an increased risk of pressure ulcers due to the inability of the patient to remember to perform a pressure relief, and bladder and bowel difficulties due to the inability to perform these programs adequately.

For those with mild TBI, the majority will return to their cognitive baseline by 3 weeks postinjury. Interestingly, functional MRI revealing regional brain activity in those with TBI shows increased activation in the middle frontal gyrus, superior parietal cortex, basal ganglia, and anterior cingulate regions as compared to healthy controls. This would indicate that although cognition is improved, the brain is still working harder than usual to compensate for the effect of the brain injury. This would explain cognitive fatigue that may occur with more complex tasks (76). Approximately 15% will experience symptoms beyond 3 weeks commonly referred to as postconcussive syndrome (73).

Bradbury et al. reported increased rehabilitation costs (~170 ± 84 K for DD versus 131 ± 91 K for SCI only) and demands on clinician resources. Quality of life measures and community reintegration were also significantly lower in those with SCI and TBI as compared to those with SCI only (77). Several studies have reported greater family and personal adjustment problems in the DD population. This is not unexpected given the behavioral changes that can accompany brain injury. Given these findings, it is reasonable to conclude that this patient population may require closer clinical observation than those with SCI alone.

The unique challenges of this patient population have yet to be thoroughly researched. Going forward, as more data are available, the development of best practice guidelines may facilitate improved diagnosis and treatment of the myriad of medical, cognitive, and psychological problems faced by persons with both spinal cord and brain injury. In the interim, those with both spinal cord and TBI will continue to require the care of an interdisciplinary team dedicated to achieving the best possible outcome for patients as well as those who will care for them.

References

1. Macciocchi S, Seel RT, Thompson N, et al. Spinal cord injury and co-occurring traumatic brain injury: assessment and incidence. *Arch Phys Med Rehabil* 2008;89:1350–1357.
2. Elovic E, Kirshblum S. Epidemiology of spinal cord injury and traumatic brain injury: the scope of the problem. *Top Spinal Cord Inj Rehabil* 1999;5:1–20.
3. Brown L, Hagglund K, Bua G, et al. Spinal cord injury and concomitant traumatic brain injury. *Am J Phys Med Rehabil* 1988;67;211–216.
4. Wilmot C, Cope D, Hall K, et al. Occult head injury: its incidence in spinal cord injury. *Arch Phys Med Rehabil* 1985;66:227–231.
5. Davidoff G, Morris J, Roth E, et al. Cognitive dysfunction and mild closed head injury in traumatic spinal cord injury. *Arch Phys Med Rehabil* 1985:66:489–491.
6. Davidoff G, Thomas P, Johnson M, et al. Closed head injury in acute traumatic spinal cord injury: incidence and risk factors. *Arch Phys Med Rehabil* 1988;69:869–872.
7. Davidoff G, Morris J, Roth E, et al. Closed head injury spinal cord injured patients: retrospective study of loss of consciousness and post-traumatic amnesia. *Arch Phys Med Rehabil* 1984;l66:41–43.
8. Tolonen A, Turka J, Salonen O, et al. Traumatic brain injury is under-diagnosed in patients with spinal cord injury. *J Rehabil Med* 2007;39:622–626.
9. Watanabe T, Zafonte R, Larson E. Traumatic brain injury associated with acute spinal cord injury: risk factors, evaluation, and outcomes. *Top Spinal Cord Injury Rehabil* 1999;5:83–90.
10. Teasdale G, Jennett B. Assessment of coma and impaired consciousness. A practical scale. *Lancet* 1974,2:81–84.
11. Zafonte RD, Mann NR, Millis SR, et al. Posttraumatic amnesia: its relation to functional outcome. *Arch Phys Med Rehabil* 1997;78(10):1103–1106.
12. Jackson WT, Novack TA, Dowler RN. Effective serial measurement of cognitive orientation in rehabilitation: the Orientation Log. *Arch Phys Med Rehabil* 1998; 79(6):718–720.
13. Penna S, Novack TA. Further validation of the orientation and Cognitive Logs: their relationship to the mini-mental state examination. *Arch Phys Med Rehabil* 2007;88(10):1360–1361.
14. Alderson AL, Novack TA. Reliable serial measurement of cognitive processes in rehabilitation: the Cognitive Log. *Arch Phys Med Rehabil* 2003;84(5):668–672.
15. Novack TA, Dowler RN, Bush BA, et al. Validity of the Orientation Log, relative to the Galveston Orientation and Amnesia Test. *J Head Trauma Rehabil* 2000;15(3):957–961.
16. Frey KL, Rojas DC, Anderson CA, et al. Comparison of the O-Log and GOAT as measures of posttraumatic amnesia. *Brain Inj* 2007;21(5):513–520.
17. Wie C, Tharmakulasingam J, Crawley A, et al. Use of diffusion-tensor imaging in traumatic spinal cord injury to identify concomitant traumatic brain injury. *Arch Phys Med Rehabil* 2008;89:S85–S91.
18. Roth E, Davidoff G, Thomas P, et al. A controlled study of neuropsychological deficits in acute spinal cord injury patients. *Paraplegia* 1989;27:480–489.
19. Heilbronner RL, et al. Lateralized brain damage and performance on trail making A and B, digit span forward and backward, and TPT memory and location. *Arch Clin Neuropsychol.* 1991;6:251–258.
20. Moore AD, Stambrook M, Gill DD, et al. Factor structure of the wechsler adult intelligence scale-revised in a traumatic brain injury sample. *Can J Behav Sci.* 1993;25:605–614.
21. Pendleton MG, Heaton RK, Lehman RAW, et al. Diagnostic utility of the thurstone fluency test in neuropsychological evaluations. *J Clin Neuropsychol* 1982;4(4):307–317.
22. Baguley IJ, Heriseanu RE, Cameron ID, A critical review of the pathophysiology of dysautonomia following traumatic brain injury. *Neurocrit Care* 2008;8(2):293–300. Review.
23. Baguley IJ, Slewa-Younan S, Heriseanu RE, et al. The incidence of dysautonomia and its relationship with autonomic arousal following traumatic brain injury. *Brain Inj* 2007;21(11):1175–1181.
24. Baguley IJ, Cameron ID, Green AM, et al. Pharmacological management of Dysautonomia following traumatic brain injury. *Brain Inj* 2004;18(5):409–417.
25. Baguley IJ, Heriseanu RE, Gurka JA, et al. Gabapentin in the management of dysautonomia following severe traumatic brain injury: a case series. *J Neurol Neurosurg Psychiatry* 2007;78(5):539–541.
26. Estol CJ, Kase CS. Need for continued use of anticoagulants after intracerebral hemorrhage. *Curr Treat Options Cardiovasc Med* 2003;5:201–209.
27. J. Broderick, S. Connolly, E. Feldmann, et al. Guidelines for the Management of Spontaneous Intracerebral Hemorrhage in Adults: 2007 Update: A Guideline From the American Heart Association/American Stroke Association Stroke Council, High Blood Pressure Research Council, and the Quality of Care and Outcomes in Research Interdisciplinary Working Group: The American Academy of Neurology

affirms the value of this guideline as an educational tool for neurologists. *Stroke* 2007;38(6):2001–2023.

28. Geerts WH, Bergqvist D, Pineo GF, et al. Prevention of venous thromboembolism: American College of Chest Physicians Evidence-Based Clinical Practice Guidelines (8th Edition). College of Chest Physicians. *Chest* 2008;133(6 suppl):381S–453S.
29. Lien YH, Shapiro JI. Hyponatremia: clinical diagnosis and management. *Lien Am J Med* 2007;120(8):653–658. Review.
30. Bushnik T, Englander J, Katznelson L. Fatigue after TBI: association with neuroendocrine abnormalities. *Brain Inj* 2007;21(6):559–566.
31. Temkin NR, Dikmen SS, Winn HR. Management of head injury. Posttraumatic seizures. *Neurosurg Clin N Am* 1991;2(2):425–435. Review
32. Practice parameter: antiepileptic drug treatment of posttraumatic seizures. Brain Injury Special Interest Group of the American Academy of Physical Medicine and Rehabilitation. *Arch Phys Med Rehabil* 1998;79(5):594–597.
33. The Brain Trauma Foundation. The American Association of Neurological Surgeons. The Joint Section on Neurotrauma and Critical Care. Role of antiseizure prophylaxis following head injury. *J Neurotrauma* 2000; 17(6–7):549–553. Review.
34. Englander J, Bushnik T, Duong TT, et al. Analyzing risk factors for late posttraumatic seizures: a prospective, multicenter investigation. *Arch Phys Med Rehabil* 2003;84(3):365–73.
35. Smith KR Jr, Goulding PM, Wilderman D, et al. Neurobehavioral effects of phenytoin and carbamazepine in patients recovering from brain trauma: a comparative study. *Arch Neurol*. 1994;51(7):653–660.
36. Massagli TL. Neurobehavioral effects of phenytoin, carbamazepine, and valproic acid: implications for use in traumatic brain injury. *Arch Phys Med Rehabil*. 1991;72(3):219–226. Review.
37. Duncan JS, Shorvon SD, Trimble MR. Effects of removal of phenytoin, carbamazepine, and valproate on cognitive function. *Epilepsia* 1990;31(5):584–591.
38. Jones KE, Puccio AM, Harshman KJ, et al. Levetiracetam versus phenytoin for seizure prophylaxis in severe traumatic brain injury. *Neurosurg Focus* 2008;25(4):E3.
39. Pachet A, Friesen S, Winkelaar D, et al. Beneficial behavioral effects of lamotrigine in traumatic brain injury. *Brain Inj* 2003;17(8):715–722.
40. Daban C, Martínez-Arán A, Torrent C, et al. Cognitive functioning in bipolar patients receiving lamotrigine: preliminary results. *J Clin Psychopharmacol* 2006;26(2):178–181.
41. Gomer B, Wagner K, Frings L, et al. The influence of antiepileptic drugs on cognition: a comparison of levetiracetam with topiramate. *Epilepsy Behav* 2007;10(3):486–494.
42. Willmott C, Ponsford J. Efficacy of methylphenidate in the rehabilitation of attention following traumatic brain injury: a randomised, crossover, double blind, placebo controlled inpatient trial. *J Neurol Neurosurg Psychiatry* 2009;80(5):552–557.
43. Pavlovskaya M, Hochstein S, Keren O, et al. Methylphenidate effect on hemispheric attentional imbalance in patients with traumatic brain injury: a psychophysical study. *Brain Inj* 2007;21(5):489–497.
44. Warden DL, Gordon B, McAllister TW, et al.; Neurobehavioral Guidelines Working Group. Guidelines for the pharmacologic treatment of neurobehavioral sequelae of traumatic brain injury. *J Neurotrauma* 2006; 23(10):1468–1501.
45. Wilens TE, Hammerness PG, Biederman J, et al. Blood pressure changes associated with medication treatment of adults with attention-deficit/hyperactivity disorder. *J Clin Psychiatry* 2005;66(2):253–259.
46. Whyte J, Hart T, Vaccaro M, et al. Effects of methylphenidate on attention deficits after traumatic brain injury: a multidimensional, randomized, controlled trial. *Am J Phys Med Rehabil*. 2004;83(6):401–420.
47. Kaelin DL, Cifu DX, Matthies B.Methylphenidate effect on attention deficit in the acutely brain-injured adult. *Arch Phys Med Rehabil* 1996;77(1):6–9.
48. Alban JP, Hopson MM, Ly V, et al. Effect of methylphenidate on vital signs and adverse effects in adults with traumatic brain injury. *Am J Phys Med Rehabil* 2004; 83(2):131–137
49. Powell JH, al-Adawi S, Morgan J, et al. Motivational deficits after brain injury: effects of bromocriptine in 11 patients. *J Neurol Neurosurg Psychiatry* 1996;60(4): 416–421.
50. Whyte J, Vaccaro M, Grieb-Neff P, et al. The effects of bromocriptine on attention deficits after traumatic brain injury: a placebo-controlled pilot study. *Am J Phys Med Rehabil* 2008;87(2):85–99.
51. Passler MA, Riggs RV. Positive outcomes in traumatic brain injury-vegetative state: patients treated with bromocriptine. *Arch Phys Med Rehabil* 2001;82(3):311–315.
52. Napolitano E, Elovic EP, Qureshi AI. Pharmacological stimulant treatment of neurocognitive and functional deficits after traumatic and non-traumatic brain injury. *Med Sci Monit* 2005;11(6):RA212–RA220.
53. Lequerica AH, Rapport LJ, Loeher K, et al. Agitation in acquired brain injury: impact on acute rehabilitation therapies. *J Head Trauma Rehabil* 2007;22(3):177–183.
54. Corrigan JD. Development of a scale for assessment of agitation following traumatic brain injury. *J Clin Exp Neuropsychol* 1989;11(2):261–277.
55. Bogner JA, Corrigan JD, Bode RK, et al. Rating scale analysis of the Agitated Behavior Scale. *J Head Trauma Rehabil* 2000;15(1):656–669.
56. Silver BV, Collins L, Zidek KA. Risperidone treatment of motor restlessness following anoxic brain injury. *Brain Inj* 2003;17(3):237–244.
57. Kline AE, Massucci JL, Zafonte RD, et al. Differential effects of single versus multiple administrations of haloperidol and risperidone on functional outcome after experimental brain trauma. *Crit Care Med* 2007;35(3): 919–824.
58. Clinchot DM, Bogner J, Mysiw WJ, et al. Defining sleep disturbance after brain injury. *Am J Phys Med Rehabil* 1998;77(4):291–295.
59. Castriotta RJ, Wilde MC, Lai JM, et al. Prevalence and consequences of sleep disorders in traumatic brain injury. *J Clin Sleep Med*. 2007;3(4):349–356.
60. Fichtenberg NL, Millis SR, Mann SR, et al. Factors assoicaited with insomnia among post-acute traumatic brain injury survivors. *Brain Inj* 2000;14(7):659–667.

61. Johnson MW, Suess PE, Griffiths RR. Ramelteon: a novel hypnotic lacking abuse liability and sedative adverse effects. *Arch Gen Psychiatry* 2006;63(10):1149–1157.
62. Bushnik T, Englander J, Wright J. The experience of fatigue in the first 2 years after moderate-to-severe traumatic brain injury: a preliminary report. *J Head Trauma Rehabil* 2008;23(1):17–24.
63. Cantor JB, Ashman T, Gordon W, et al. Fatigue after traumatic brain injury and its impact on participation and quality of life. *J Head Trauma Rehabil* 2008;23(1):41–51.
64. Belmont A, Agar N, Hugeron C, et al. Fatigue and traumatic brain injury. *Ann Readapt Med Phys* 2006;49(6): 283–288, 370–374. Epub 2006 Apr 25. Review.
65. Sawyer E, Mauro LS, Ohlinger MJ. Amantadine enhancement of arousal and cognition after traumatic brain injury. *Ann Pharmacother* 2008;42(2):247–252. Epub 2008 Jan 22. Review.
66. Meythaler JM, Brunner RC, Johnson A, et al. Amantadine to improve neurorecovery in traumatic brain injury-associated diffuse axonal injury: a pilot double-blind randomized trial. *J Head Trauma Rehabil* 2002;17(4):300–313.
67. Fann JR, Hart T, Schomer KG. Treatment for depression following traumatic brain injury: a systematic review. *J Neurotrauma*. 2009;26:2383–2402.
68. Kreutzer JS, Seel RT, Gourley E. The prevalence and symptom rates of depression after traumatic brain injury: a comprehensive examination. *Brain Inj* 2001;15(7):563–576.
69. Seel RT, Kreutzer JS, Rosenthal M, et al. Depression after traumatic brain injury: a National Institute on Disability and Rehabilitation Research Model Systems multicenter investigation. *Arch Phys Med Rehabil* 2003;84(2):177–184.
70. Zafonte RD, Cullen N, Lexell J. Serotonin agents in the treatment of acquired brain injury. *J Head Trauma Rehabil* 2002;17(4):322–334. Review.
71. Perino C, Rago R, Cicolini A, et al. Mood and behavioural disorders following traumatic brain injury: clinical evaluation and pharmacological management. *Brain Inj* 2001; 15(2):139–148.
72. Sommer JL, Witkiiwicz PM. The therapeutic challenges of dual diagnosis: TBI/SCI. *Brain Inj* 2004;18: 1297–1308.
73. Richards JS, Brown L, Hagglund K, et al. Spinal cord injury and concomitant traumatic brain injury: results of a longitudinal investigation. *Am J Phys Med Rehabil* 1988;67:211–216.
74. Kreuter M, Sullivan M, Dahlof A, et al. Partner relationships, functioning, mood and global quality of life in person with spinal cord injury and traumatic brain injury. *Spinal Cord*. 1998;36;252–261.
75. Macciocchi SN, Bowman B, Coker J, et al. Effect of comorbid traumatic brain injury on functional outcome of persons with spinal cord injuries. *Am J Phys Med Rehabil* 2004;83:22–26.
76. Kohl AD, Wylie GR, Genova HM, et al. The neural correlates of cognitive fatigue in traumatic brain injury using functional MRI. *Brain Inj* 2009;23(5):420–432.
77. Bradbury CL, Wodchis WP, Mikulis DJ, et al. Traumatic brain injury in patients with traumatic spinal cord injury: clinical and economic consequences. *Arch Phys Med Rehabil* 2008;89(12 suppl):S77–S84.

CHAPTER 21 ■ PSYCHOLOGICAL IMPACT OF SPINAL CORD INJURY

JOYCE FICHTENBAUM AND STEVEN KIRSHBLUM

INTRODUCTION

Spinal cord injuries (SCIs) and disorders (SCDs), whether traumatic or nontraumatic, are life altering for all and both devastating and catastrophic for many. SCIs/SCDs impinge on physical, emotional, social, and vocational functioning. They may challenge an individual's assumptions about the environment he or she lives in, his or her physical well-being, and psychological identity (1). SCI/SCD impacts both the injured individual and his or her family. It invokes motor and sensory deficits, alters organ system function (e.g., bowel and bladder), changes mechanical and sensual aspects of sexuality, and compromises spontaneity, freedom, autonomy, and independence (2). The many physical changes are often immediate, unanticipated, severe, and permanent (3). Psychosocial stressors impose social stigma and both attitudinal and architectural barriers, while loss of freedom and spontaneity impact short- and long-term adaptation and community reintegration. A person who sustains an SCI is at risk for the "four D syndrome": dependency, depression, drug addiction, and, if married, divorce (4).

The goals of rehabilitation are to preserve residual function, prevent serious complications, and develop compensatory skills, so that injured individuals can effectively function in his or her environment (5). Individuals adjust to SCI/SCD through maximizing independence—even if at the wheelchair level, achieving optimal health, taking responsibility for their care, rebuilding a sense of control, and finding ways to fulfill their roles in life (5,6).

Increased psychosocial stress after SCI can lead to clinical syndromes and psychiatric diagnoses. These include adjustment disorders (e.g., adjustment disorder with depressed and/or anxious mood), mood disorders (e.g., major depressive disorder [MDD]), anxiety disorders (e.g., generalized anxiety disorder, social anxiety, acute and posttraumatic stress disorders [PTSDs]), grief responses, and substance abuse. Emotional sequelae that follow SCI are attributable to premorbid factors in conjunction with reactions to permanent physical and, sometimes, cognitive impairment (7).

For the purpose of this chapter, the term SCI will encompass both injury and disorders of the spinal cord unless otherwise indicated.

PSYCHOLOGICAL REACTIONS FOLLOWING SCI

The experience of SCI may be affected by prior life history, current life stressors, social relationships, financial assets, intrapsychic and personality functioning, and personal/cultural issues. As a result, transition to living with a disability is unique to each individual and usually occurs during the acute hospitalization to acute rehabilitation when awareness of the long-term implications of SCI increases. During this time, the patient and family usually transition from "please let the patient live" to "but not like this." A patient's appreciation of the challenges brought upon him or her by the injury may lead to depression or a mourning/grief reaction (1).

Depressive Disorders

Depression is not a single entity, but a spectrum of disorders that vary by duration of symptoms and degree of severity. Transient feelings of sadness are not necessarily pathological and do not require a psychiatric diagnosis. Depressive disorders include *Adjustment reactions* (e.g., adjustment reaction with depressed mood), *MDD*, and *depression not otherwise specified* (8). Adjustment reactions (with depressed and/or anxious mood or unspecified) are the most prevalent of the various depressive disorders mentioned after SCI (9). By definition, an *adjustment disorder with depressed mood* is diagnosed when the constellation of symptoms does not meet the criteria for an MDD or bereavement yet represents a maladaptive reaction to an identifiable stressor that occurs within 3 months after stressor onset and lasts no longer than 6 months (9). The reaction is indicated by impairment in occupational, social, or relationship functioning. When the stressor resolves or when a new level of adaptation occurs to a chronic stressor such as illness or SCI, the symptoms should remit (8).

Depression has received significant attention in the SCI literature. Prevalence studies report the occurrence of depressive disorders in 20% to 45% of adults with SCI and 25% to 33% of community-residing individuals with SCI (10–12). Unlike the general population, prevalence rates for *MDD* and symptom severity do not differ between men and women with SCI (13). Furthermore, depression following SCI is unpredictable by demographics or injury characteristics such as level of injury (paraplegia versus tetraplegia), severity of injury, or magnitude of functional impairments (14). A higher rate of MDD occurs in the first year following SCI with the greatest risk occurring during initial acute and rehabilitation hospitalization, followed by the 2-year mark when patients are often discharged from outpatient rehabilitation services. This highlights the importance of psychological care in both the inpatient and the outpatient rehabilitation setting (13–17). Pain, helplessness, and a lack of control are found to be predictors of a depressed mood. Pollard and Kennedy (18) found that rates of anxiety and depression remained relatively stable over a 10-year period after injury. In other words, without treatment, if persons with SCI were depressed or anxious at week 12 after injury, they remained so up to 10 years later (18).

Depression is not inevitable despite its high post-SCI incidence, and studies have shown that the majority of people who sustain an SCI adequately adjust and do not become clinically depressed (12). Depression does not necessarily occur as a direct cause of an SCI nor is it dependent on the level of injury (14). Rather, depression seems to result from problems and stressors that often follow SCI, such as unemployment and inaccessibility (19,20). Boekamp et al. (21) conceptualized a diathesis-stress model of depression after SCI, suggesting that a depressive disorder may result from interaction of biological predisposition and environmental factors that are together catalyzed by the stressors associated with the SCI.

Unlike adjustment disorders, MDD is a disabling condition. This diagnosis requires a persistent and pervasive loss of interest in other people, objects, or activities, in addition to a depressed mood lasting for more than 2 weeks. Mourning or adjustment disorders may develop into major depressive episodes with the occurrence of additional stressful events such as development of secondary conditions (e.g., heterotopic ossification) or patients' appraisal of perceived social support or degree of family conflict (22).

General risk factors for depression can be genetic, psychological, social, and environmental. They include prior history of depression, family history of depression, family history of suicide attempts, suicidal ideation, chronic pain, concurrent medical conditions, alcohol or substance abuse, poor social networking, limited financial resources, vocational difficulties, inferior living arrangements, need for personal and transportation assistance, family disruption prior to injury, and lack of social supports. Psychological risk factors for persons with acute and subacute SCI include premorbid personality traits (e.g., narcissistic and antisocial personality features and behaviors). They further take into account a preinjury history of poor coping style, poor problem-solving abilities, unresolved conflicts from previous losses or trauma, shame, hopelessness, bereavement, and having the opinion that death is better than living with an SCI (9,23).

Signs and symptoms of a major depression include mood, cognition, and behavior changes (8,9,24) (see Table 21.1). Depression is associated with poorer outcomes including longer hospital stays, fewer functional improvements, less functional independence at discharge, pressure sores, fewer social pursuits, health problems, less participation in community activities, decreased longevity, increased pain, and risk of suicide (25,26). Therefore, use of effective screening measures to identify those in need of further evaluation, diagnosis, and treatment is imperative (14).

Barriers to some customarily used depression screening and diagnostic measures are inefficiency, challenges in relating the self-report scores to MDD diagnostic criteria contained in the DSM IV, and the determination of whether somatic symptoms (sleep, appetite disturbances, and psychomotor changes) are related to the MDD or to effects of SCI. The Beck Depression Inventory, Zung Depression Rating Scale, and Center for Epidemiological Studies Depression scales are inefficient and lengthy to use as a screening measure for depression in the SCI population (14). The Ilfeld Psychiatric Symptom Index was also not found useful in the SCI population (27). By contrast, the Depression Anxiety Stress Scales-21 (28) was found to have sensitivity and clinical utility as a screening measure for both depression and anxiety when compared with the clinical interview. The Patient Health Questionnaire-9 (PHQ-9) is presently the most promising screening tool for MDD in people with SCI (14) and suggests that somatic symptoms are predictive of probable MDD rather than being symptoms of SCI. The PHQ identifies the need for further evaluation and treatment. A short form of the PHQ-9 contains the following three items: (a) "Bothered by little interest or pleasure in doing things?" (b) "Bothered by feeling down, depressed or hopeless?" and (c) "Bothered by feeling bad about yourself or that you are a failure or have let yourself or your family down?" This instrument was found to be a reasonable option as an initial screening tool (25,29).

Suicide

Motives for suicide in the general population include a genuine wish to die, escape from an intolerable situation, relieve mental distress, attract help, and influence others (7). Since 1966, suicide has been the most frequently reported type of significant event for patients in a "staffed, around-the-clock setting," including inpatient rehabilitation settings (30). Therefore, it is important to screen patients early postinjury. SCI patients are at a greater risk for suicide, with rates two to six times greater than the nondisabled population (2,31,32). Overall, suicide accounts for approximately 5% of deaths post-SCI. Risk factors include previous suicide attempts, coping style, lowered self-esteem, loss of male identity, guilt, and undiagnosed traumatic brain injury (TBI). Suicide rates are greatest in the first 5 years following injury but can occur at any time postinjury (31–33). Suicide is higher in younger age groups, especially in persons under age 25. Persons with paraplegia and with marginal injury seem to have a higher rate of suicide (31,33).

TABLE 21.1

SIGNS AND SYMPTOMS OF MAJOR DEPRESSION

Affective/mood: sadness, emptiness, demoralization, irritability, loss of interest or pleasure in activities, apathy, hopelessness, helplessness, and inappropriate shame or guilt.

Cognitive: poor attention and concentration, diminished ability to think, indecisiveness, recurrent thought of death, suicidal ideation, or self-criticality.

Behavioral/somatic: appearance that is sad or weepy, decreased attention to self-care changes in appetite, sleep, and energy levels, restlessness or agitation, being slowed down (psychomotor retardation), specific suicide plan or attempt.

While a relationship between severity of injury and "suicidality" was once hypothesized, it has not been confirmed by research (7). Assessment of "suicidality" post-SCI should include questions about suicidal ideation, plan and intent, access to lethal means, prior attempt(s), and comorbid alcohol or drug abuse (9). Risk variables include despondency, expression of shame, hopelessness, apathy, a history of family fragmentation, individual or family history of suicide attempts, alcohol abuse, active involvement in causation of injury, and preinjury depression (32).

The results of a retrospective study of 137 individuals with SCI secondary to suicide attempt indicated that the ratio of males to females was 1:1 with a mean age of 32 years (17). Schizophrenia and depression were evident in 32% and 27% of the sample, respectively, with previous attempts made by 23% of patients. In 85% of the cases, "falls" was the cause of SCI (17). Survivors of SCI secondary to attempted suicide require continued mental health follow-up, as they are at grave risk for a subsequent suicide attempt (34).

Anxiety Disorders

Anxiety disorders are less frequently studied in the SCI population than depressive disorders. Prevalence for anxiety is between 16% and 30% for the first 4 years following SCI (35). Anxiety is a perception of real or imagined worry, dread, tension, fear, and vulnerability. In the SCI population, sources of fear may include losses (i.e., independent lifestyle, finances, control, roles), medical complications, weaning from a ventilator, or anticipated difficulties of functioning in an inaccessible world where stigma and rejection occur. A salient transition from fear of death to fear of living with a disability often occurs in the acute rehabilitation setting for both patients and families. Anxiety can interfere with progress in rehabilitation and should be treated.

Acute Stress and Posttraumatic Stress Disorders

Acute stress disorder (ASD) and PTSD are anxiety diagnoses that may limit adaptation to disability. Onset of ASD occurs within 4 weeks of the traumatic event; PTSD occurs after this time (36). Stress disorders are reactions to experiencing or witnessing a traumatic event that threaten the individual with death or serious bodily injury. These include motor vehicle crashes, falls, and violence such as gunshot wounds, exposure to hideous scenes, or the vicious death or severe injury of a loved one (37).

PTSD consists of symptom clusters following trauma that includes reexperiencing, avoidance and hyperarousal reactions. To meet criteria for the diagnosis of PTSD, the person must experience sufficient symptoms in each of the following symptom clusters: (a) reexperiencing the trauma (e.g., intrusive and distressing recollections, flashbacks, and nightmares); (b) avoidance of the stimulus conditions that remind the person of the event or numbing of the individual's general responsiveness (e.g., avoiding thoughts and memories of the trauma, detachment, restricted range of affects, and a sense of foreshortened future); and (c) persistent symptoms of increased arousal (e.g., irritability, anger, difficulty sleeping, and hypervigilance). These symptoms must be present for 1 month and cause marked distress or impairment in functioning (8).

The prevalence of PTSD after SCI is estimated to range from 10% to 34% (38–40) with the rate in SCI war veterans being 44% (41). Hypothesized predictors included level of injury, type of trauma, time since injury and locus of control. Previous trauma exposure also served as a predictor of PTSD in SCI war veterans who typically experience more severe SCI-PTSD symptoms and have greater difficulty recovering from them than non–war-theater veterans (42). The relationship between level of injury and PTSD is inconclusive. Radnitz et al. (43), reported that persons with tetraplegia are less likely than those with paraplegia to experience PTSD. Chung et al. (41), however, did not find a clear relationship between level of injury and risk of PTSD. Nielson found PTSD to be related to time since injury, as well as to neurologic level (40). The number of PTSD symptoms is positively related to the development of general health problems, while external locus of control regarding their health was a variable associated with risk for the development of PTSD in SCI patients (41).

Social Phobia

Persons with SCI may develop anxiety in social situations. Fear of stigmatization and embarrassment associated with use of a wheelchair or adaptive equipment may result in the avoidance of social situations. These fears may lead to social isolation and a diagnosis of Social Phobia, or unspecified anxiety (i.e., Anxiety Disorder Not Otherwise Specified). Countermeasures to these social phobias can be taken by issuing day passes during acute rehabilitation, which serves as a social exposure technique. These passes may assist patients and families in learning to navigate newfound stressors encountered in the social world, such as people staring at them or accessibility.

Grief Reactions

Adjustment to SCI presents patients with experiences that could produce a grief reaction with a normal reactive dysphoric mood (3,24). Dysphoria is an affective state that can range from petulant to sad, and proceed to melancholy and wretched (44). It generally implies sadness, hopelessness, and helplessness (45). A transient depressed mood does not justify a diagnosis of Major Depression. Sadness, however, whether diagnostic of depression or not, impacts the patient's ability to deal with the implications, consequences, and complications of SCI (46,47).

Grief or bereavement may include feelings of depression and even vegetative symptoms, but does not usually involve prolonged functional impairment, preoccupation with worthlessness, or marked psychomotor retardation that are often concomitant with MDD. Guilt and thoughts of death are usually limited (8). Prolonged grief is diagnosed when symptoms of a grief reaction continue for longer than 6 months Symptoms of prolonged grief, previously known as *complicated grief*, include yearning for what is lost, avoiding reminders of the loss, disbelief, a sense of meaningless, bitterness/anger, emotional numbness or shock, and difficulty trusting others. Prolonged grief may accompany other diagnoses such as MDD or PTSD (8,48).

Stage theories of grief were designed to simplify and bring order to complex affective reactions. Kubler-Ross' (49) model of denial, anger, bargaining, depression, and acceptance was applied to other grieving populations including individuals with disabilities. Weller and Miller (50) presented four stages: shock, denial, anger, and depression. Denial is a normal coping mechanism used when an individual is faced with overwhelming circumstances such as a serious illness or injury. Denial is a disavowal of the injury and resultant disability. It minimizes psychic pain and can be a temporary phase or part of one's coping style (51). Patients and their families may think, "this isn't really happening," or "I know I will walk out of here" (52). Denial is often misunderstood by patients and their families, and sometimes alarms rehabilitation staff even though it may not impact short-term patient adjustment (50). Verbal disavowal of injury through denial is one way to maintain hope, and hoping to walk once again is not in itself harmful.

By contrast, adjustment to disability may be hindered by behaviors that deny the realities of SCI over a long period of time. In these cases, sustained denial may result in noncompliance with treatment recommendations or equipment prescription, and adversely impact adaptation to disability. For example, a patient who resists using powered mobility in favor of a slowly propelled manual wheelchair may be denying the severity of his or her injury or may simply be trying to sustain hope that he or she will be able to forego use of powered mobility. In these instances, hope can combat depression and anxiety, or at least make them more manageable. Conversely, it is difficult for staff; patient, and family to break through denial, and attempts to do so are often met with patient anger (47). Sustained denial and associated behavioral complications may lead to self-neglect and development of secondary medical complications such as pressure ulcers (50,53).

Anger is an outwardly directed expression of frustration with self or life situation. It is a normal reaction after SCI that accompanies increasing awareness of the consequences of injury (51,52). Hostility may be directed to health providers, family members, or nondisabled people who serve as constant reminders of their losses. Anger can accompany attempts to exert control over life events and requires resolution (50). If left untreated, it may impact patient relationships and result in alienation (50).

Bargaining during the process of rehabilitation is used to differentiate bearable outcomes. It takes many forms, changes over time, and is amenable to intervention. For example, in the inpatient setting, the desire to ambulate is often exchanged for the wish of the return of bowel and bladder function. Should neither return, independence in wheelchair propulsion and self-care of bladder and bowel may be appreciated as a tolerable outcome.

Acceptance, defined as reevaluation of life values, is related to personal growth and ability to see positive outcomes of life crisis. Acceptance is associated with less social reliance (i.e., dependent behavior) and enhanced health-related quality of life (QOL) (54,55). Some patients and their families may interpret acceptance of injury as the surrendering of hope that SCI will resolve. In these cases, use of the terms *adaptation* or *adjustment* may be more tolerable.

INTERVENTIONS

Since mental health problems affect rehabilitation, psychological services should be an integral part of the comprehensive SCI treatment team (56,57). Once depression is noted, the clinician should determine if there is a possibility that the condition is medication induced. Certain medications, for example, antiemetics (i.e., metoclopramide), glucocorticoids, anabolic steroids, histamine receptor blockers (i.e., cimetidine, ranitidine), can be the cause and may need to be discontinued or changed (9). Psychopharmacologic agents are helpful in treating neurovegetative and mood disturbance symptoms, but the cognitive, social, environmental, and interpersonal issues associated with depression and other psychological reactions are best addressed through a combination of psychotherapy and medications. Medication alone can relieve symptoms; however, a recent meta-analysis studying the effect of psychotherapy along with pharmacotherapy found a beneficial effect in favor of combined treatment over pharmacotherapy alone, with a lower dropout rate from combined treatment (58).

Psychological Counseling

Early counseling should be directed toward reducing distorted perceptions associated with development of unrealistic expectations (41). Cognitive therapy has been found to reduce symptoms of depression, with maintenance provided for up to 2 years (59–61). Cognitive behavioral therapy (CBT), a structured treatment with emphasis on education and improving problem-solving skills, is associated with positive adjustment to SCI (18). CBT has been found to significantly improve some long-term aspects of adjustment to SCI (62). Patients undergoing CBT learn to reduce their cognitive distortions such as "all-or-nothing thinking" or generalization, so that adjustment to injury becomes more achievable. Coping Effectiveness Training (CET), which emphasizes changing negative appraisals of implications of SCI to make them more manageable (63), results in positive changes in adjustment and reduction in depression and anxiety. CET is a cognitive behavioral treatment that focuses on improving skills that are already used to cope. The three parts of training include appraisal (reducing global assessment of one's situation), increasing the repertoire of coping methods, and identifying and obtaining social support under stressful conditions. The manner in which individuals first cope with injury is predictive of depression several years postinjury and, therefore, early intervention in the rehabilitation process is imperative (18).

Among other options for intervention, Pollard and Kennedy (18) reviewed *meaning-based strategies* such as "benefit finding" and "posttraumatic growth." These strategies permit an individual to view changes associated with trauma in a positive manner. They include finding a deeper meaning of themselves (e.g., self-reliance or other strengths), their relationships with others, or their understanding of life (goal setting and determination to pursue them). Posttraumatic growth involves shifting priorities about what is important in life (e.g., a sense of closeness with others), seeing availability of new opportunities that would not have been otherwise presented, stronger religious faith, and taking personal responsibility while still relying on others for assistance (18). We find that people tend to ask "why me" when their lives are disrupted by negative events, but rarely ask the same question when something positive occurs. Counseling to help patients look for positive life changes brought about by SCI is a way to foster more substantial emotional growth and adaptation to injury.

As a countermeasure to MDD, psychotherapists can teach patients active coping styles such as cognitive restructuring, emotional self-control, positive reevaluation, social support seeking, and use of problem-oriented strategies, which can lead to better adaptation and prevention against depression. When wishful thinking, which can be viewed as hope, is coupled with the use of problem-solving or solution-focused coping such as seeking advice or assistance from family and friends, behaviors can become positively adaptive (63). In contrast, use of alcohol and drugs, disengagement, wishful fantasy, escape avoidance, and unrealistic problem solving are associated with negative adjustment to SCI (18,63,64).

In sum, while not all patients experience depression following SCI, those who do can benefit from psychotherapy alone or psychotherapy together with antidepressant (AD) medication.

Pharmacological Treatment of Depression

Pharmacological intervention should be considered for patients whose mood disturbance is severe enough to interfere with their ability to perform in their rehabilitation, social, recreational, and vocational roles. The main classes of AD medications are listed in Table 21.2. Monoamine oxidase inhibitors (MAOI) are not commonly used in general (65) or in the SCI population (66), although they are effective for treatment-resistant forms of depression.

The choice of medication should be guided by anticipated safety and tolerability that aids in compliance; physician familiarity, which aids in patient education and anticipation of adverse effects; and history of prior treatments (67). Treatment failures often are caused by medication noncompliance, inadequate duration of therapy, or inadequate dosing.

The most commonly prescribed tricyclic antidepressants (TCAs) include amitriptyline (Elavil), nortriptyline (Pamelor), desipramine (Norpramin), clomipramine (Anafranil), doxepin (Sinequan), and imipramine (Tofranil). TCAs have a long record of efficacy in the treatment of depression and have the advantage of lower cost. They are less commonly prescribed because of the need to dose titrate to a therapeutic level, their adverse effect profile, and their considerable toxicity in overdose. Adverse effects largely are due to their anticholinergic and antihistaminic properties and include sedation, confusion, dry mouth, orthostasis, constipation, urinary retention, sexual dysfunction, and weight gain. Caution should be used in patients with cardiac conduction abnormalities; thus, electrocardiographic findings should be reviewed before initiating treatment and intermittently checked for QRS complex widening beyond 100 milli seconds, a sign of TCA toxicity (68).

The class of selective serotonin reuptake inhibitors (SSRIs) is currently the most commonly prescribed AD medication

TABLE 21.2

COMMONLY USED AD MEDICATION IN SCI

Medication name	Initial dosage (mg)	Therapeutic range of dosage (mg/d)
Tricyclic (TCA)		
Tertiary Amines		
Amitriptyline (Elavil)	25	50–300
Doxepin (Sinequan)	25	" "
Imipramine (Tofranil)	25	" "
Secondary Amines		
Desipramine (Norpramin)	25	50–300
Nortriptyline (Pamelor)	25	50–150
SSRI		
Citalopram (Celexa)	10	10–80
Escitalopram (Lexapro)	10	10–40
Paroxetine (Paxil)	10	20–80
Fluoxetine (Prozac)	10	20–60
Sertraline (Zoloft)	25	25–200
SNRI		
Duloxetine (Cymbalta)	30	30–120
Venlafaxine (Effexor XR)	37.5	37.5–375
Norepinephrine and dopamine reuptake inhibitors		
Bupropion (Welbutrin)	100	250–450
Bupropion SR (Welbutrin)	150	100–400
Bupropion XL	150	150–450
Serotonin antagonist and reuptake inhibitor		
Trazodone (Desyrel)	25	Insomnia: 25–200 mg qh Depression: 200–400 mg/d
Nefazodone	100	600
Serotonin antagonist	7.5	15–45 mg
Mirtazapine (Remeron)		

50 mg BID (Welbytrin) and reuptake inhibitors.
SNRI, serotonin and norepinephrine reuptake inhibitor; SSRI, selective serotonin reuptake inhibitor; TCA, tricyclic antidepressant.

(65,66). SSRIs are also effective for treatment of anxiety disorders. The most commonly prescribed SSRIs include fluoxetine (Prozac), paroxetine (Paxil), sertraline (Zoloft), citalopram (Celexa), and escitalopram (Lexapro). This group has the advantage of ease of dosing and low toxicity in overdose. Common adverse effects include GI upset, sexual dysfunction, and changes in energy level (i.e., fatigue, restlessness). Escitalopram may be superior to other ADs in the treatment of more severe depression (69) as well as anxiety, and may be at least as effective as serotonin norepinephrine reuptake inhibitors (SNRIs) while better tolerated, even in severe depression (70).

Clinicians should be aware that adverse effects including nausea or a dull headache may evolve when initiating drug treatment, which may also precede therapeutic benefits of treatment. Because these typically diminish or disappear with time, the patient should be informed that at least some of the unpleasantness of these early effects will dissipate with continued use. Jitteriness and insomnia may occur early in treatment and can be minimized by starting with doses that are lower than recommended for initial treatment. SSRIs are typically considered energizing and are usually taken once daily in the morning. With its greater tendency to cause sedation than other SSRIs, paroxetine is the exception, and is often taken at night (71). Patients should be forewarned that withdrawal from AD therapy must be slow, controlled, and supervised by a qualified health professional, especially when using paroxetine.

Combining multiple serotonergic agents should be avoided as this could precipitate serotonin syndrome; an acute, potentially fatal toxic state manifesting in mental status changes, neuromuscular signs, and automatic dysregulation. The most specific signs of excessive serotonin stimulation are clonus, hyperreflexia, agitation, diaphoresis, akathisia, and tremor (72). SSRI-induced agitation that drives suicidal behavior is most likely to occur soon after initiating treatment and constitutes a medical emergency (73). Fluoxetine is the only SSRI approved by the FDA for treatment of MDD in children and adolescents; escitalopram is approved for adolescents having more general depressive diagnoses.

SNRIs (also called "double inhibitors") are effective for depression as well as anxiety and panic disorders. The more commonly prescribed SNRIs include venlafaxine (Effexor) and duloxetine (Cymbalta). Duloxetine is approved for depression as well as diabetic peripheral neuropathy, fibromyalgia, and anxiety, and has also been used for treating urinary incontinence. Safety, tolerability, and adverse effect profiles are similar to those of the SSRIs, although SNRIs have been rarely associated with a sustained rise in blood pressure. Direct comparisons have suggested that they may be modestly more efficacious than SSRIs (74). SNRIs can be used as first-line agents, particularly in patients with significant fatigue or pain syndromes associated with the episode of depression. The SNRIs also have an important role as second-line agents in patients who have not responded to SSRIs.

Atypical ADs include bupropion (Wellbutrin), nefazodone (Serzone), mirtazapine (Remeron), and trazodone (Desyrel). The mechanism of action for bupropion is uncertain, although it seems to enhance effects of norepinephrine and dopamine. Bupropion is FDA approved for smoking cessation and commonly used for treating addictions and depression associated with excessive weight loss. The relative AD efficacy of bupropion is not significantly different from other AD drugs but is often better tolerated than SSRIs and TCAs because it is not associated with weight gain, sedation, or sexual dysfunction. Bupropion can be combined with SSRI and SNRI drugs to treat adverse sexual effects or augment their AD effects. When prescribed at higher doses, bupropion is associated with a risk of seizure, although less so for the sustained release formulation. (75) It should be prescribed with wide-ranging caution, especially in patients with a history of seizure, an elevated seizure risk, or eating disorders.

Adverse effects of SSRI and SNRIs in children are similar to those in adults. Their long-term safety, however, is unknown. Concerns that these medication can cause depressed children and adolescents to consider or attempt suicide have led to the "black box" warning on all AD labels. All children, adolescents, and adults taking AD medication should be monitored for suicidal ideation or behavior, especially in the earliest part of therapy.

Mirtazapine has potent 5-hydroxytryptamine receptor 2 (5-HT2) blocking properties and specifically counteracts SSRI-induced nonspecific stimulation of serotonin receptors. Blockade of 5-HT2 is associated with eventual shortened sleep-onset latency, increased total sleep time, and improved sleep efficiency (76). A low dose of 15 mg or less can be used for long-term treatment of insomnia, although this is not usually a first-line AD.

Trazodone is sedating and commonly used as a sleep aid rather than as a primary AD, although it is often used in combination with other AD medications. Trazodone can cause hypotension, constipation, and rarely priapism (71). Trazodone effectively induces sleep in doses of 25 to 150 mg, although it is not approved as a hypnotic; higher doses are required (150 to 600 mg) for AD effects. Nefazodone is structurally related to Trazodone, but less sedating. Its effectiveness is similar to other AD medications, but associated with less weight gain, sedation, or sexual dysfunction.

St. John's Wort (SJW) (*Hypericum perforatum*) has gained recent popularity in the United States as a treatment for mild-to-moderate depressive symptoms, although there are no reports involving use with persons with SCI. This herbal may act as an SSRI and not as an MAOI, as previously believed, although it is not recommended to combine SJW with other AD drugs or medications ordinarily contraindicated with the use of MAO inhibitors (65). Warnings for serotonin syndrome include SJW. The dosage is 300 mg three times a day with meals to prevent GI upset. A review of most non-US studies found that in a mixed population of depression, SJW is superior to placebo, similarly effective to conventional AD, and tends to have fewer adverse effects than other AD therapies apart from photosensitivity (78). If no clinical response occurs after 3 to 6 months, use of prescription medication is recommended.

The overall effectiveness of AD medications appears similar; however, there is strong evidence of differences among individual ADs with respect to onset of action and adverse effects (e.g., sexual functioning) that could affect health-related QOL and medication compliance (79,80). Since adverse effects play such an important role in medication compliance, it is important to start at a low dose and slowly titrate when prescribing these medications. Preparing the patient for early adverse effects of medications, including the apparently desirable increase in energy observed with AD treatment, will often allow them to maintain long-term compliance with therapy. Although the classes of TCAs and SSRIs do not differ in the prevalence of headache, tremor, urinary disturbance, or hypotension, TCAs are substantially more likely to induce such anticholinergic symptoms as dry mouth, constipation, dizziness, sweating, and blurred vision, and SSRIs are associated with substantially more nausea, anorexia, diarrhea, insomnia, nervousness, agitation, and anxiety (81). Drugs within a particular class may also have different tolerability. Paroxetine, for example, causes more sedation, constipation, sexual dysfunction, and weight gain than other SSRIs (71), whereas escitalopram and sertraline appear to be the best tolerated in terms of efficacy and acceptability (82). As a result of substantial serotonin reuptake blockade, second-generation ADs (SSRIs and SNRIs, such as venlafaxine) have been associated with reduced libido in both men and women, as well as genital arousal problems (erection in men and lubrication in women) and delayed or absent orgasm in up to 40% of both men and women (83). The addition of sildenafil (Viagra) or bupropion has been helpful in treating some patients with SSRI-induced sexual dysfunction. One class of drugs may even be safer than another. For example, for suicidal or impulsive patients, SSRIs are a better choice than TCAs because of their cardiac toxicity in overdose.

ADs differ in their capacity to induce weight gain. Even in low doses, tertiary amine TCAs (e.g., amitriptyline, imipramine, and doxepin) are more likely to cause weight gain than secondary amine TCAs (e.g., nortriptyline and desipramine). Bupropion is linked to the least weight gain of any AD (84). Among the SSRIs, paroxetine has the greatest potential for inducing weight gain. Mirtazapine carries a reputation for being a particularly potent appetite stimulant, although it is not clear that it is any more of a culprit than any other AD.

Side effects are by no means always problematic. For example, a TCA, trazodone, or mirtazapine can provide beneficial sedation to patients in whom insomnia figures prominently, whereas bupropion may energize a patient who is experiencing lassitude.

The goal of AD drug therapy should be to resolve significant depressive symptoms along with a complete recovery from impaired function (85). With any first-line AD medication, about 50% to 70% of patients will have a desirable treatment response (usually defined as a ≥50% decrease in depressive symptoms), although only about one-half to one-third of patients achieve full remission (65). AD therapy may require 1 to 4 weeks to produce detectable improvements, and often 6 to 12 weeks to achieve substantial benefit. For patients who do not have a satisfactory response despite optimal dosing, the two basic strategies are switching to another medication or adding a second drug.

AD medication should be continued for at least 6 months after remission of symptoms. While courses of therapy that are shorter than 6 months have been used in depressed patients with SCI, there is greater likelihood of relapse (19,65–67). If there is a relapse of symptoms, treatment for 3 years is recommended, and indefinitely after there are further recurrences. If a patient shows minimal or no response to an AD, switching to an alternative is recommended. If an SSRI is used, changing to a different SSRI can be effective; even though they have similar mechanisms of action, they may be pharmacologically dissimilar. If there is no response to two different SSRIs, switching to a different class of medication is recommended. Adding a second medication is usually helpful in cases where suboptimal response accompanies initial monotherapy. Consultation with a psychiatrist is recommended in these cases. Table 21.3 lists some general prescribing principles for the clinician to keep in mind.

When tapering AD medication, especially SSRIs and SNRIs, a gradual taper is strongly recommended to avoid discontinuation syndromes, which can include neuropsychiatric, emotional, and physical symptoms that may be confused with physical illness or depression relapse (86) The dosage should be reduced by no more than 25% per week; tapering more slowly the longer the patient has been taking the AD and the shorter the AD's half-life. For mild and transient withdrawal symptoms, reassurance may be enough; however, severe reactions may necessitate slowing the rate of taper or reinstituting the original AD dose (87). SSRI withdrawal typically starts within 3 days and can last up to 3 weeks, with symptoms including dizziness, paresthesias, tremors, anxiety, nausea, emesis, lethargy, and headache (88).

Referral to a psychiatrist should be considered if the patient fails to respond to an adequate initial AD trial (defined as a therapeutic dose of 1 or more medications for at least 8 weeks each) (89), describes a strong family history of psychiatric illness or substance abuse, portrays a labile or recurrent illness course, or provides a history consistent with past episodes of mania. Psychiatric referral should also be considered when the

TABLE 21.3

PRESCRIBING PRINCIPLES FOR AD THERAPY

1. Combining supportive counseling with pharmacological intervention is usually beneficial.
2. Inform patients of potential side effects and how they will be managed.
3. Warn patients that adverse effects will likely occur before substantial benefit, often several weeks.
4. Set realistic expectations for small, incremental improvements.
5. Choose a medication whose side-effect profile could prove of benefit to the patient, such as a sedating AD for anxiety and sleep difficulties or an activating medication for sluggishness and lack of motivation.
6. Begin with a low dose of AD and increase gradually every 5–7 d to the desired therapeutic dose, particularly if adverse effects are tolerable.
7. Avoid combining multiple serotonergic agents that could precipitate serotonin syndrome.
8. Taper gradually when discontinuing AD use to avoid discontinuation syndromes.
9. Do not abruptly discontinue use of AD, particularly SSRIs.
10. The use of AD medication should be continued for 6 to 12 mo after remission with a first episode, 3 y after a second episode, and indefinitely after ≥3 recurrences.

AD, antidepressant; SNRI, serotonin and norepinephrine reuptake inhibitor; SSRI, selective serotonin reuptake inhibitor; TCA, tricyclic antidepressant.

patient experiences only adverse effects without relief from depressive symptoms or sustains neither adverse effects nor depressive improvement. In addition, patients who have psychotic symptoms, demonstrate active suicidality, or appear to have simultaneous manic and depressive symptoms—a so-called "depressive mixed state" that is associated with an elevated risk of all forms of suicidal behavior—should also be treated by a psychiatrist (9,90,91).

Additional medications used in mood disorders can include anticonvulsant drugs, second-generation antipsychotics, and Modafinil. Anticonvulsant drugs are commonly used as mood-stabilizing drugs and include valproic acid (Depakene), divalproex sodium (Depakote), carbamazepine (Tegretol), and lamotrigine (Lamictal). Second-generation antipsychotic drugs include aripiprazole (Abilify), quetiapine (Seroquel), and risperidone (Risperdol) and are often reserved as an add-on therapy together with another AD. Buspirone (Buspar) is indicated for anxiety disorders and is often combined with AD medications to treat adverse sexual effects or augment their AD effects. Modafinil (Provigil) as well as R-modafinil (Nuvigil) have a stimulating effect that is approved for narcolepsy and excessive daytime sleepiness associated with sleep apnea. Modafinil can be used in combination with AD drugs (typically SSRIs) to augment their clinical effects and treat certain adverse effects (i.e., apathy, fatigue, and sexual dysfunction) (65). It has also been shown to improve self-esteem and self-confidence in persons with SCI (92).

Exercise and Depression

A number of clinical trials have shown that physical exercise may lead to reduction in depressive symptoms with or without medications (93,94). No study, however, in SCI has been found in this area. Having the person with SCI participating in physical activity can only serve as a helpful adjunct to treatment.

ADDITIONAL CONSIDERATIONS

Substance Abuse

Persons who drink alcohol after TBI and SCI tend not to be light or social drinkers; rather, they use alcohol on almost a daily basis (95). Substance abuse places individuals at greater risk for postinjury depression, suicide, and medical complication such as pressure ulcers (14). As a result, screening for substance abuse and appropriate referrals need to be part of the rehabilitation process (14). The CAGE is a four-question screening device for alcoholism, and is a reliable instrument for use in the SCI population (96). CAGE is an acronym for: cut down (have you ever felt that you should cut down on your drinking?), annoyed (have you ever been annoyed by others who criticize your drinking?), guilty (have you ever felt bad or guilty about drinking?), and eye opening (have you ever taken a drink first thing in the morning to steady your nerves or to get rid of a hangover?). Two or more affirmative responses suggest a higher likelihood of alcoholism. In addition, persons with SCI having higher CAGE scores have a higher incidence of medical complications (96).

Patients with SCI have substance abuse risk factors that resemble those of the general population. These include family history, concomitant psychiatric problems, and personality features and disorders. Physical, psychological, social, and vocational challenges they face after SCI may increase these risks.

Alcohol and substance abuse hamper learning and rehabilitation gains, interfere with self-care, place persons at risk for medical complications (i.e., skin breakdown), contribute to premature mortality and morbidity, and result in impulsive behavior that can reduce safety and ability to live independently (97). These risks justify a need for substance prevention and treatment programs in inpatient and outpatient rehabilitation. Individuals whose social support is limited to "drinking buddies" may feel the need to return to the drinking environment so as not to feel alone after injury and discharge back to the community. Individuals who do not drink while in inpatient rehabilitation, particularly if the injury is associated with substance abuse, believe that they will be able to quit once discharged from the hospital.

Dual Diagnosis—SCI with Concomitant TBI

SCI and TBI are commonly comorbid, and those with TBI have an increased risk for suicide (98). Cognitive decline and behavioral changes accompanying TBI adversely influence adjustment to SCI. Since SCI outcomes are affected by TBI diagnosis and severity, it is important to differentiate TBI from other sources of changes in mental status (i.e., delirium) and to evaluate and treat both diagnoses (99) (see Chapter 20 for greater detail).

Pain

Pain of musculoskeletal and neuropathic origins is prevalent after SCI and interferes with activities of daily living (78,79). Response to pain may include greater use of catastrophizing (i.e., unrealistic and negative self-evaluations) and erroneous pain-related beliefs (i.e., pain signals damage). These in turn are related to greater solicitous responses and less perceived social support, all of which are associated with poorer outcomes in the degree of pain interference, anxiety and depression, and life satisfaction (LS) (100,101) (see Chapter 26).

Since pain perception is both a cause and an effect of adjustment disorders, it requires a multidisciplinary approach to treatment that includes pharmacological, physical, and psychological intervention, and one that targets more than just pain intensity (102,103). Treatment should also focus on coping strategies, beliefs, and other psychosocial behaviors such as catastrophizing and helplessness that impact chronic pain perception and QOL (104).

OTHER ISSUES TO BE CONSIDERED IN THE SCI ADJUSTMENT PROCESS

Coping, Personality Styles, and Resilience

Coping styles are methods people use to deal with internal and external stressors and serve as mediating factors in the development of negative affective states (12). Another variable that impacts adjustment to disability is locus of control. Individuals with SCI having an internal control locus believe that their health and degree of recovery is based on their own behaviors (e.g., I developed a pressure sore because I did not pay enough attention to performing my weight shifts). People with an internal locus of control have a sense of personal control over events in their lives, have fewer medical problems, lead more active and productive lives, and are less likely to be depressed (52,105). External locus of control is the tendency to blame fate, chance, luck, or other people for life or personal events (e.g., I developed a pressure sore because the cushion was bad or my family did not remind me to do weight shifts). Persons with SCI who have external loci of control, inadequate coping mechanisms, and low perceived social support are at risk for developing psychological problems or secondary conditions when they leave the inpatient rehabilitation setting (54,56).

Extroversion and cautious management of novel situations are personality styles that commonly develop among wheelchair users after SCI. Extroversion appears to be a good prognostic indicator for adaptation even in the rehabilitation setting (64). When compared with individuals having other disabilities, persons with SCI are more likely to seek and accept assistance from others, to benefit from encouragement of health care providers, and to plan activities rather than act spontaneously (106). While many individuals with SCI believe that their relationships with family and friends support their recovery, at times, they feel overassisted in daily activities and novel situations for which they can be independent. This heightens feelings of dependency (85,107).

Resilience is a variable that has been most recently studied, and has been posited to mediate the negative reaction to death of a spouse or to acquired disability. Resilient individuals have a view that includes a belief in a just world and controllability over negative events. Resilience may buffer individuals' reactions to death and disability and may promote adjustment to the challenges imposed by SCI (108).

The Role of Hope

Martz et al. (109) reported that depression, anxiety, posttraumatic stress, and death anxiety are strong predictors of poor adaptation to SCI/SCD. Conversely, hope, a positive orientation toward future improvements, is associated with health and well-being. Regardless of the degree of recovery, 6 months postinjury, individuals can still experience hope or positive expectations for ambulation and/or recovery (110). Developing a hopeful vision of life following SCI focuses on capabilities and requires shaping expectations for life with SCI (111). The power of hope and the ability to find meaning a year after the injury (when recovery may be slowing) provide the energy and motivation to go through the process of personal growth and development throughout the lifespan (112).

Hope requires reassurance that specific scenarios of the present situation will get better. Hope and optimism are aspects of positive psychology. They permit the finding of new meaning in life and adherence to medical treatment and health-promoting behaviors. Like hope, religious belief and spirituality also assist with adjustment to chronic conditions (113).

Hope is what enables people to move from the present, which may be filled with losses, to an imagined future that is better (114). Hope is defined as a cognitive set involving a sense of agency (will) and pathways for attaining goals. Having high hope requires the delineation of clear goals and alternative ways to reach them. Low hope results from having only vague goals and uncertain routes to take to achieve them. Components of hope include (a) a realistic assessment of the threat, (b) the envisioning of alternative and setting of goals, (c) bracing for negative outcomes, (d) an assessment of internal and external resources, (e) the solicitation of mutually supportive relationships, (f) seeking signs that reinforce selected goals, and (g) a determination to endure (115). Hope should not be taken away, although the goal, the timeline set for its achievement, or change in acceptable outcomes may require modification of what one hopes over the course of rehabilitation. For example, ambulating with adaptive equipment and bracing rather than ambulating without an assistive device can be a hopeful and achievable goal in the appropriate patient. In cases where hope interferes with rehabilitation (i.e., a C4-5 patient insisting "I will not use a power wheelchair but only propel a manual chair"), discussion should take place emphasizing the risks of shoulder overuse relative to the importance of increased independence particularly over long distances.

Transition from a Sick to an Injured Role

One of the goals of acute rehabilitation is to facilitate transition from a "sick role" to the "injured or impaired role" (116). The sick role accompanies acute episodic illnesses that might require the person to forego major life responsibilities while focusing on recovery. Motivation to undergo rehabilitation therapies may be lower for those individuals who view themselves as sick. The impaired role encourages the individual to develop and maintain adaptive behaviors within the limits of impairment by maximizing residual potential and modifying life direction or methods to achieve goals.

During acute rehabilitation, individuals are exempt from fulfilling their roles at work and home. Individuals may choose to remain in the sick role upon rehabilitation discharge to relieve them of stressful decision making and duties associated with their premorbid lifestyle. Certain limitations may present themselves as attractive post-SCI. For example, a patient may use his or her injury as an excuse to not return to a job that was disliked, mundane, or resulted in little free time for family or avocations (116). These secondary gains from remaining in the sick role (such as not participating in child care or returning to work) may serve as a means of avoidance or favor monetary benefit.

Patients with SCI will often change their behaviors in an attempt to satisfy their needs with a newfound disability. In an attempt to tolerate dependency, individuals may begin to behave in a more dependent, passive, or regressive manner than explained by their level of injury. They may refuse to direct their own care or undertake the simplest tasks such as wiping their mouths after eating or pressing a button to raise the head of the bed. Psychologists can help patients differentiate "can't" from "won't" and help families by advocating that they assist when a patient truly needs their support.

Self-Neglect and Secondary Conditions

Self-neglect (117), including behaviors that range from overt and hostile to passive and inactive, can influence the success of rehabilitation, degrees of adaptation to injury, and occurrence of secondary medical conditions over the postinjury lifespan.

Noncompliance with treatment, inattentiveness to skin checks and weight shifts, departure from bowel and bladder regimens, alcohol or drug abuse, and refusal to fully participate in rehabilitation are forms of self-neglect. Self-neglect can be symptomatic of a maladjustment reaction or a depressive episode. It can also be considered "existential suicide" when the outcome will result in death. This suicidal behavior generally occurs years after the injury and is not necessarily prompted by depression or hostility, but rather expressed by a clear and active decision to refuse further medical treatment. Onset of secondary medical conditions may either ensue or result in psychological distress and depression (118–120). Referral to a mental health professional should be undertaken both to resolve these behaviors and to reestablish positive health care behaviors.

Search for Meaning, Self-Blame, and Attribution

Survival from SCI is often accompanied by a patient journey that pursues purpose or meaning in the experience. This journey attempts to place the injury in the context of one's life (121) and often begins with the question, "Why me?" Bulman and Wortman (122) reported that SCI patients gave one of six reasons for their injury: God had a reason, chance, predetermination, a personal purpose, probability, and it was deserved.

Studies of attribution for SCI reveal inconsistent patterns of responsibility and self-blame (122–124). Heinemann (2) concluded that self-blame may be adaptive shortly after injury, although it loses meaning over time. Regardless of circumstances, these attributions are highly individualized, and may vary by, or differ within patients, family members, and the treatment team.

Motivation and Compliance

Motivation is a patient personality characteristic that can be cultivated by the treatment team and enhanced by the environment (125). A desire of the patient to understand their condition, to perform self-care, and to become positively dependent is associated with high levels of motivation. Positive dependency occurs when the patient recognizes and accepts help to achieve maximum independence (126). Success rather than failure, incentives, internal inducement, and mild anxiety promote motivation and learning (127).

Compliance is the agreement between recommendations by the health care team and patient behavior (128). Compliance is related to the patient's motivation, locus of control, expectations, beliefs, values about achievable outcomes, environmental demands, and perceived ability to initiate and maintain behavioral changes in the face of multiple roles and commitments (3,128). Compliance may also be affected by comorbid conditions such as depression, substance abuse, and stress disorders (129).

Quality of Life

QOL is an all-encompassing construct used in health care that reflects emotional, social, and physical well-being, including function in performance of daily tasks. It is often used in the SCI literature and is considered "at risk" after the onset of disability. QOL is an estimation of happiness or satisfaction with subjective and objective aspects of life considered important by an individual (130). Assessment of QOL and LS have been studied in the SCI population with mixed results, largely due to sample size limitations and variable measurement tools; many were not developed for use with persons with SCI (131,132). Despite these limitations, patient-specific QOL after SCI is generally rated higher than expected. For example, persons with tetraplegia and both ventilator-assisted and independent breathing report they are glad to be alive and satisfied with their lives (106,133,134). While 78% of individuals with SCI were found to evaluate their QOL as good or excellent (135), health care professionals underestimated their QOL (136). Factors such as level of lesion, age, age at the time of injury, sex, and completeness of the lesions do not consistently correlate with lowered level of QOL (12). The ability, or perceived ability, to participate in physical activities, sports, or recreation positively impacted QOL (131,137,138). Other factors found to correlate with QOL include mood, intensity of pain, marital status, emotional support, perceived control, perceived health status, vocational and social activity, self-efficacy, and self-esteem (137–140). Injury duration, comorbid conditions, and unemployment were most consistent predictors of poor LS and health-related QOL (141–143). Environmental factors such as accessibility, mobility, transportation, need for help in the home, and health care availability need to be included in models of disability, as they are strongly related to LS. In a recent article, QOL was found to be positively associated with secondary conditions, activity, and participation limitations (144). Intervention in early phases of rehabilitation is strongly recommended for persons who rate their QOL as poor, as LS rated by persons with SCI at year 1 remains largely unchanged over the ensuing 4 years (145,146).

The concept of "the good life" is related to terms such as LS, QOL, and subjective well-being. The nature of the good life has three elements: positive connections to others, positive personal qualities (e.g., finding meaning in the disability, humor, expressing gratitude, resilience, and savoring or appreciating positive aspects of daily life), and life regulation qualities that permit individuals to regain autonomy. While some individuals have qualities that will allow them to lead the good life following acquired disability, others may benefit from psychotherapy that focuses on helping them develop these qualities (147).

Refusing Treatment

Advances in medicine have resulted in improved survival rates and life expectancy post-SCI, allowing more people with SCI to live longer lives with disability (12). As a result, the issue of whether life is worth living on life-sustaining equipment with chronic and severe SCI may increasingly arise. Staff in the rehabilitation field are discomforted when a patient on life-sustaining measures choose to die in a rehabilitation setting. Some patients have transitory thoughts of stopping treatment and may say "I don't want to live like this." Others may be more persistent when considering cessation of treatment and life termination (148). Whether or not withholding or withdrawing life sustaining is tantamount to suicide is the purview of medical ethicists and the court system, while determination of decision-making *capacity* is within the practice sphere of physicians. Psychologists, who generally assist patients with problem solving and delineation of options and alternatives, have the unique ability to guide patients through the rough and murky waters of life and death final decision. Several suggestions were made by Kirchner when a patient or proxy decides to terminate life-sustaining needs (149). Psychologists can offer balanced and unbiased information in the context of an empathic and supportive relationship. They can also address the sources of despair and suffering and question the assumptions the patient is making about life with a disability. Finally, when there is conflict, the patient should meet with caregivers and health care proxies to assist them in working through the decision making and possible conflicts of interests with their loved ones.

SOCIAL IMPLICATIONS IN SCI

In addition to the physical and emotional demands of SCI, social and family changes also occur. Social relationships after injury are subject to change and influence patients' perspectives. Social supports reinforce an injured person's self-worth, enhance independent and interdependent functioning, and assist in promoting community interactions. Adolescents and young adults often have difficulty maintaining social relationships with friends who predated their injuries. In the process, they may become uncomfortable, apathetic, or embarrassed and allow friends to drift away (5). Since poor social integration and depression are often clinically associated, counseling services should be routinely offered to individuals with SCI when they come for follow-up medical visits. In the psychotherapy setting, persons both with and without SCI can learn how to effectively communicate, counter general misperceptions regarding disability, and improve their overall social skills.

Family functioning is disrupted by SCI and may lead to the development of grief reactions or other adjustment issues for family members. The circumstances surrounding the onset of disability, the relationship of the patient to the family (child, parent, sibling, and spouse), the quality of the relationship, stage of life, and culture are important to consider when treating a family after SCI (127). Losses include deprivation of personal space and time, financial concerns, isolation, changes in relationships, loss of spontaneity, and worry about the present and the future. Age and generation of the caregivers can be factors in the amount of interpersonal support available for the patient (128). The psychological burden of living with aging family members can impact patients who are still in their 20s and 30s. As caregivers age and begin to experience both less energy and more biological dysfunction of their own, both caregiver and the injured individual may experience increased concerns regarding their ability to remain in the community when caregivers can no longer assist their needs. Aging may also influence the ability of both caregiver and patient to live independently in the community.

Spouses are often the most affected of family members after SCI, and must contend with dramatic role changes (150). Injury can lead to role confusion (i.e., becoming both spouse and attendant), role reversal (i.e., leaving a job to care for the injured spouse), and role overload (i.e., maintaining a career, childcare, and SCI caregiver responsibilities). Spouses who are also caregivers may find physical intimacy discomforting, which can lead to depression (5). Spouses with an external locus of control, limited coping strategies (e.g., use of distancing and escape avoidance), and minimal social support are at significant risk the development of severe depression, which may exceed that of their injured partners (129).Thus, family members need to be reminded to maintain their own physical, social, and emotional health. Providing them with psychological support and finding assistance from similarly situated family caregivers may prove beneficial.

POSITIVE REHABILITATION OUTCOME

In sum, the psychological and social circumstances following SCI require adjustment. Common reactions include denial, anger, bargaining, depression, and anxiety. Pollard and Kennedy (18) suggest that anxiety or depression were not related to level of injury or degree of independence. Depression and anxiety, while prevalent, do not always occur, and are otherwise amenable to treatment with medication and/or psychotherapy. Many individuals with SCI are resilient, but about 50% suffer from one emotional disorder (e.g., stress, anxiety, depression, or PTSD) and 60% suffer from two or more disorders (35). Patients in rehabilitation have to ultimately decide whether to participate in treatment, how much energy to expend in each session, how to view their current life situation, and whether they should persevere or give up (151). The roles of premorbid personality functioning, psychiatric predisposition, traits (e.g., extroversion and internal locus of control), resilience, hardiness, optimism/pessimism and coping styles cannot be discounted when discussing adjustment to disability (64,130,152,153). The way a person approaches their challenges also cannot necessarily be altered. Since attitude has an impact on SCI outcome (18) the treatment team should learn about the patient's outlook and perspective in a relatively unthreatening manner. Asking simple, matter-of-fact questions such as "wheelchair-enemy or friend?" and "do you consider ambulation with a walker and braces to be walking?" may help patients discuss their perspective on the use assistive devices or technologies. Change is difficult for many people, yet persons with SCI necessitate coping with multiple changes that present secondary from the injury. Willingness to do things differently (e.g., wheelchair sports) can be broached by asking a seemingly irrelevant question: "if you go to the movie theater to see a particular movie and that movie is all sold out, would you see a different movie or would you not see any movie at that time?" Exploring the response can open the door to a valuable discussion of their tendency to replace one activity with another, and the reason they might explore this approach or avoid it. Monitoring the change in patient's responses to these questions may help them work through the adaptation process.

A meta-analysis of rehabilitation experiences revealed several themes that patients view as important during the rehabilitation process (111). These include the ability to envision a future life of possibilities and the reintegration or merging of one's past self (i.e., interests, relationships, skill competencies) with the present situation (the injury or disability). A positive rehabilitation experience entails the following: a client-centered approach that focuses on the individuals and what they see as priorities; asking patients what they would like to learn; assisting in the development of a new life script; and preparing patients to transition from the hospital or rehabilitation setting to the world beyond. Peer counseling can provide newly injured patients with information to assist with community reintegration. Overall, allowing patients to be part of the rehabilitation team and to participate in decision making will allow for a greater sense of control (111).

This chapter has reviewed some of the many life-changing events accompanying SCI. While the recovery from injury is a process subject to lifelong change, many people deal effectively with their impairment and affirm traits and skill sets that are new and exciting. The pathway used to navigate to and through an active, satisfied, productive, and healthy lifestyle clearly resides in the coordinated efforts of the patient and the rehabilitation team.

Within the context of this journey an informed, compassionate, and well-coordinated support system will guide the patient to find meaning in their newfound life, to use behavior and cognitive skills that can enhance life quality, and to enable them to psychological grow postinjury and adapt to SCI (18,147). The treatment team should not assume that SCI always negatively impacts people, their families, and communities. Individuals with SCI do adjust and adapt. They find increases in self-esteem and self-efficacy and move on to live fulfilling lives. While it is imperative to begin to assess and treat patients' negative psychological reactions in the acute phase of their SCI/SCD, and as outpatients if they occur, we need to remember that most individuals with SCI will create a life others greatly value.

References

1. Langer KG, Depression and denial in psychotherapy of persons with disabilities *Am J Psychother* 1994;48:181–194.
2. Heinemann, AW. Spinal cord injury. In: Goreczny AJ, ed. *Handbook of health and rehabilitation psychology*. New York: Plenum Press, 1995:341–360.
3. Steins SA, Bergman SD, Formal CS. Spinal cord injury rehabilitation. Individual experience, personal adaptation, and social perspectives. *Arch Phys Med Rehabil* 1997;78:65–72.
4. Hulse L. Psychosocial health issues for individuals with spinal cord injury. *Spinal Cord Inj Psychosoc Proc* 1997;10:3–7.
5. Trieschmann R. *Spinal cord injuries: psychological, social, and vocation rehabilitation*. 2nd ed. New York: Demos Publication, 1988.
6. Peters D. Individual and family growth and development. In: Lubkin IM, ed. *Chronic illness impact and interventions*. 4th ed. Massachusetts: Jones and Bartlett, 1998:26–52.
7. Vocaturo, LC. Psychiatric sequelae of the spinal cord injured adult. In: Christian A, ed. *Medical management of adults with neurologic disabilities*. New York: Demos Medical, 2009.
8. American psychiatric Association. *Diagnostic and statistical manual of mental disorders*. 4th ed. Washington, DC: American Psychiatric Association, 1994.
9. Consortium for Spinal Cord Medicine. *Depression following spinal cord injury: a clinical practice guideline for primary care physicians*. New York: Paralyzed Veterans of America, 1998.
10. Anderson CJ, Vogel LC, Chian SK, et al. Depression in adults who sustained spinal cord injuries as children or adolescents. *J Spinal Cord Med* 2007;30(suppl 1):76–81.
11. Hancock KM, Craig AR, Dickson HG, et al. Anxiety and depression over the first year of spinal cord injury: a longitudinal study, *Paraplegia* 1993;31:349–357.
12. Craig A, Tran Y, Middleton J. Psychological morbidity and spinal cord injury: a systematic review. *Spinal Cord* 2009;47:108–114.
13. Kalpakjian CZ, Albright KJ. An examination of depression through the lens of spinal cord injury; comparative prevalence rates and severity in women and men. *Womens Health Issues* 2006;16:380–388.
14. Bombardier CH, Richards JS, Krause JS, et al. Symptoms of major depression in people with spinal cord injury: implication for screening. *Arch Phys Med Rehabil* 2004;85:1749–1756.
15. Dryden DM, Saunders LD, Rowe BH, et al. Depression following spinal cord injury. *Neuroepidemiology* 2005;25:55–61.
16. Faber RA. Depression and spinal cord injury. *Neuroepidemiology* 2005;25:53–54.
17. Kennedy P, Rogers B, Speer S, et al. Spinal cord injuries and attempted suicide: a retrospective review. *Spinal Cord* 1999;37:847–852.
18. Pollard C, Kennedy P. A longitudinal analysis of emotional impact, coping strategies and post-traumatic psychological growth following spinal cord injury: a 10-year review. *Br J Health Psychol* 2007;12:347–362.
19. Kemp BH, Kahan JS, Krause JS, et al. Treatment of major depression in individuals with spinal cord injury. *J Spinal Cord Med* 2004;27:22–28.
20. Tirch D, Radnitz CL, Bauman WA. Depression and spinal cord injury: monozygotic twin study. *J Spinal Cord Med* 1999;22(4):284–286.
21. Boekamp JR, Overholser, JC, Shubert DS. Depression following a spinal cord injury. *Int J Psychiatry Med* 1996;26:329–349.
22. Boekamp JR, Overholser JC, Schumber DSP. Depression following a spinal cord injury. *Int J Psychiatry Med* 1996;26:329–349.
23. Gill M. Psychosocial implications of spinal cord injury. *Crit Care Nurs Q* 1999;22:1–7.
24. Elliott TR, Frank R. Depression following spinal cord injury. *Arch Phys Med Rehabil* 1996;77:816–823.
25. Graves DE, Bombardier CH. Improving the efficiency of screening for major depression in people with spinal cord injury. *J Spinal Cord Med* 2008;31:177–184.
26. Furhrer MJ, Rintala DH, Hart KA, et al. Depressive symptomatology in persons with spinal cord injury who reside in the community. *Arch Phys Med Rehabil* 1993;74:255–260.
27. Campagnolo DI, Filart RA, Millis SC, et al. Appropriateness of the Ilfeld Psychiatric Symptom Index as a screening tool for depressive symptomology in persons with spinal cord injury. *J Spinal Cord Med* 2002;25:129–132.
28. Mitchell MC, Burns CR, Dorstyn DS. Screening for depression and anxiety in spinal cord injury with DASS-21. *Spinal Cord* 2008;46(8):547–551.
29. Williams RT, Heinemann AW, Bode RK, et al. Improving measurement properties of the Patient Health

Questionnaire-9 with rating scale analysis. *Rehabil Psychol* 2009;54(2):198–203.
30. Patient Safety Initiative Update. New Jersey Department of Health and Senior Services; June 6, 2008. www.nj.gov/health/ps/documents/june2008 newsletter.pdf. Accessed July 3, 2008.
31. Hartkopp A, Brønnum-Hansen H, Seidenschnur AM, et al. Suicide in a spinal cord injured population: its relation to functional status. *Arch Phys Med Rehabil* 1998;79:1356–1361.
32. Charlifue SW, Gerhart K. Behavioral and demographic predictors of suicide following traumatic spinal cord injury. *Arch Phys Med Rehabil* 1991;31:349–357.
33. DeVivo MJ, Black KJ, Richards JS, et al. Suicide following spinal cord injury. *Paraplegia* 1991;29:620–627.
34. Stanford RE, Soden R, Bartrop R, et al. Spinal cord and related injuries after attempted suicide: psychiatric diagnosis and long-term follow-up. *Spinal Cord* 2007;45:437–443.
35. Migliorini C, Tonge B, Taleporos G. Spinal cord injury and mental health. Australian and *N Z J Psychiatry* 2008;42:309–314.
36. Kaplan HI. Posttraumatic stress disorder and acute stress disorder. *Trauma Response* 1998;4:9–12.
37. Nabors NA, Meadows EA. Posttraumatic stress disorder in violence-induced spinal cord injury. *Top Spinal Cord Inj Rehabil* 1999;4:62–69.
38. Radnitz, C, Schlein IS, Walczak S, et al. The prevalence of posttraumatic stress disorder in veterans with spinal cord injury. *SCI Psychosoc Process* 1995;8:145–149.
39. Kennedy P, Evans J. Evaluation of post traumatic distress in the first 6 months following SCI. *Spinal Cord* 2001;39:381–386.
40. Nielson MS. Prevalence of posttraumatic stress disorder in persons with spinal cord injuries: a mediating effect of social support. *Rehabil Psychol.* 2003;48(4):289–295.
41. Chung MC, Preveza E, Papandreous K, et al. The relationship between posttraumatic stress disorder following pinal cord injury and locus of control. *J Affect Disord* 2006;93:229–232.
42. Radnitz CL, Schlein IS, Hsu L. The effect of prior trauma exposure on the development of PTSD following spinal cord injury. *J Anxiety Dis* 2000;14(3):313–324.
43. Radnitz CL, Hsu L, Tirch DD, et al. A comparison of posttraumatic stress disorder in veterans with and without spinal cord injury. *J Abnorm Psychol* 1998;107:676–680.
44. Zuckerman EL. The Clinician's Thesauras. 3rd ed. The Clinician's Toolbox: Pittsburgh, PA: 1993; 109.
45. Tennen H, Hall JA, Affleck G. Depression research methodologies. A review and critique. *J Pers Soc Psychol* 1995;68:870–884.
46. Widerstrom-Noga EG, Felipe-Cuervo E, Broton JG, et al. Perceived difficulty in dealing with the consequences of spinal cord injury. *Arch Phys Med Rehabil* 1999;80:580–586.
47. Scivotello G, Petrelli A, Di Lucent L, et al. Psychological investigation of spinal cord injury patients. *Spinal Cord* 1997;35:516–520.
48. Maciejewski PK, Zhang B, Block SD, et al. An empirical examination of the stage theory of grief. *JAMA* 2007;297(7):716–724.
49. Kubler-Ross E. *On death and dying*. New York: Macmillan, 1969.
50. Weller DJ, Miller PM. Emotional reactions of patient, family, and staff in acute-care period of spinal cord injury. *Soc Work Health Care* 1977;2:369–377.
51. Moore AD, Patterson DR. Psychological intervention with spinal cord injured patients: promoting control out of dependence. *Spinal Cord Inj Psychosoc Proc* 1993;6:208.
52. Bopp A, Lubkin I. Teaching. In: Lubkin IM, ed. *Chronic illness impact and interventions*. 4th ed. Boston, MA: Jones and Bartlett, 1998:343–362.
53. Silverman J. Emotional care of the cord-injured and chronically ill patient. In: Constantian M, ed. *Pressure ulcers: principles and techniques of management*. Boston, MA: Little Brown and Company, 1981.
54. Elfstrom ML, Ryden A, Kreuter M, et al. Relations between coping strategies and health-related quality of life in patients with spinal cord lesion. *Rehabil Med* 2005;37:9–16.
55. Elfstrom ML, Ryden A, Kreuter M, et al. Linkages between coping and psychological outcome in spinal cord lesioned: development of SCL-related measures. *Spinal Cord* 2002;40(1):23–29.
56. Frank RG, Elliott TR, Life stress and psychological adjustment following spinal cord injury. *Arch Phys Med Rehabil* 1987;68:344–347.
57. Hartkopp A, Bronnum-Hansen H, Seidenschnur A, et al. Suicide in a spinal cord injured population: its relation to functional status. *Arch Phys Med Rehabil* 1998;79:1356–1361.
58. Cuijpers P, Dekker J, Hollon SD, et al. Adding psychotherapy to pharmacotherapy in the treatment of depressive disorders in adults: a meta-analysis. *J Clin Psychiatry* 2009;70(9):1219–1229.
59. Craig AR, Hancock KM, Dickson HJ, et al. Long-term psychological outcomes in spinal cord injured persons: results of a controlled trial using cognitive behavior therapy. *Arch Phys Med Rehabil* 1998;79:375–377.
60. Craig AR, Hanock KM, Chang E, et al. Immunizing against depression and anxiety after spinal cord injury. *Arch Phys Med Rehabil* 1998;79:375–377.
61. Craig AR, Hancock KM, Dickson HG. Improving the long-term adjustment of spinal cord injured persons. *Spinal Cord* 1999;37:345–350.
62. Moore AD, Bombardier CH, Brown PB, et al. Coping and emotional attributions following spinal cord injury. *Int J Rehabil Res* 1994;17:39–48.
63. Kennedy P, Duff J, Evans M, et al. Coping effectiveness training reduces depression and anxiety following traumatic spinal cord injuries. *Br J Health Psychol* 2003;27:41–52.
64. Dias de Carvalho SA, Andrade MJ, Tavares MA, et al. Spinal cord injury and psychological response. *Gen Hosp Psychiatry* 1998;20:353–359.
65. Howland RH. Therapeutic armamentarium for treating depression. *Postgrad Med* 2010;122(4):66–93.
66. Smith BM, Weaver FM, Ullrich PM. Prevalence of depression diagnoses and use of antidepressant medications by veterans with spinal cord injury. *Am J Phys Med Rehabil* 2007;86:662–671.
67. Bostwick JM. A generalist's guide to treating patients with depression with an emphasis on using side effects to tailor

antidepressant therapy. *Mayo Clin Proc* 2010;85(6): 538–550.

68. Woolf AD, Erdman AR, Nelson LS, et al. Tricyclic antidepressant poisoning: an evidence-based consensus guideline for out-of-hospital management. *Clin Toxicol (Phila)*. 2007;45(3):203–233.
69. Kilts CD, Wade AG, Andersen HF, et al. Baseline severity of depression predicts antidepressant drug response relative to escitalopram. *Expert Opin Pharmacother* 2009;10(6):927–936.
70. Kornstein SG, Li D, Mao Y, et al. Escitalopram versus SNRI antidepressants in the acute treatment of major depressive disorder: integrative analysis of four double-blind, randomized clinical trials. *CNS Spectr* 2009; 14(6): 326–333.
71. Marks DM. Paris MH, Ham BJ, et at. Paroxetine: safety and tolerability issues. *Expert Opin Drug Saf* 2008; 7(6):783–794.
72. Looper KJ. Potential medical and surgical complications of serotonergic antidepressant medications. *Psychosomatics* 2007;48(1): 1–9.
73. Bostwick JM. Do SSRIs cause suicide in children? the evidence is underwhelming. *J Clin Psychol.* 2006; 62(2):235–241.
74. Papakostas GI, Thase ME, Fava M, et al. Are antidepressant drugs that combine serotonergic and noradrenergic mechanisms of action more effective than the selective serotonin reuptake inhibitors in treating major depressive disorder? A meta-analysis of studies of newer agents. *Biol Psychiatry* 2007;62(11):1217–1227.
75. Dunner DL, Zisook S, Billow AA, et al. A prospective safety surveillance study for bupropion sustained-release in the treatment of depression. *J Clin Pschiatry* 1998;59(7):366–373.
76. Thase ME. Antidepressant treatment of the depressed patient with insomnia. *J Clin Psychiatry* 1999;60(suppl 17):28–31.
77. Silber MH. Clinical practice; chronic insomnia. *N Engl J Med* 2005;353(8):803–810.
78. Linde K, Berner MM, Kriston L. St John's wort for major depression. *Cochrane Database Syst Rev* 2008;(4):CD000448.
79. Nurnberg FIG, Hensley PL, Gelenberg AJ, et al. Treatment of antidepressant-associated sexual dysfunction with sildenafil: a randomized controlled trial. *JAMA* 2003:289(1): 56–64.
80. Gartlehnar G, Hansen RA, Thieda P, DeVeaugh-Geiss AM, Gaynes BN, Krebs EE, Lux LJ, Morgan LC, Shumate JA, Monroe LG, Lohr KN. *Comparative Effectiveness of Second-Generation Antidepressants in the Pharmacologic Treatment of Adult Depression.* Comparative Effectiveness Review No.7. (Prepared by RTI International-University of North Carolina Evidence-based Practice Center under Contract No. 290-02-0016.) Rockville, MD: Agency for Healthcare Research and Quality. January 2007. Available at: www.effectivehealthcare.ahrq.gov/reports/final.cfm
81. Trindade E, Menon D, Topfer LA. et al. Adverse effects associated with selective serotonin reuptake inhibitors and tricyclic antidepressants: a meta-analysis. *Can Med Assoc J* 1998;159(10):1245–1252.
82. Cipriani A. Furukawa TA, Salanti G, et al. Comparative efficacy and acceptability of 12 new-generation antidepressants: a multiple-treatments meta- analysis. *Lancet* 2009;373(9665):746–758.
83. Segraves RT. Sexual dysfunction associated with antidepressant therapy. *Urol Clin North Am* 2007;34(4):575–579, vii.
84. Kelly K, Posternak M, Alpert JE. Toward achieving optimal response: understanding and managing antidepressant side effects. *Dialogues Clin Neurosci* 2008;10(4);409–418.
85. Rusch AJ, Kraemer HC, Suckeim HA, et al. ACNP Task Force. Report by the ACNP Task Force on response and remission in major depressive disorder. *Neuropsychopharmacology* 2006;31(9):1841–1853.
86. Maixner SM, Greden IF. Extended antidepressant maintenance and discontinuation syndromes. *Depress Anxiety* 1998;8(suppl 1):43–53.
87. Bull SA, Hu XH, Hunkeler EM, et al. Discontinuation of use and switching of antidepressants: influence of patient-physician communication. *JAMA* 2002;288(11):1403–1409.
88. Papadopoulos S. Cook AM. You can withdraw from that? the effects of abrupt discontinuation of medications. *Orthopedics* 2006;29(5):413–417.
89. Unutzer J. Clinical practice: late-life depression. *N Engl J Med.* 2007;357(22):2269–2276.
90. Timonen M, Liukkonen T. Management of depression in adults. *BMJ* 2008;336(7641):435–439.
91. Takeshima M, Kitamura T, Kitamura M, et al. Impact of depressive mixed state in an emergency psychiatry setting: a marker of bipolar disorder and a possible risk factor for emergency hospitalization. *J Affect Disord* 2008;111(1):52–60.
92. Mukai A, Costa JL. The effect of modafinil on self-esteem in spinal cord injury patients: a report of 2 cases and review of the literature. *Arch Phys Med Rehabil* 2005;86:1887–1889.
93. Mead GE, Morley W, Campbell P, et al. Exercise for depression. *Cochrane Database Syst Rev* 2009; (3): CD004366.
94. Trivedi MH, Greer TL, Grannemann BD, et al. TREAD: Treatment with exercise augmentation for depression: study rationale and design. *Clin Trials* 2006;3(3): 291–305.
95. Kolakowsky-Hayner SA, Gourley EV 3rd, Kreutzer JS, et al. Post-injury substance abuse among persons with brain injury and persons with spinal cord injury. *Brain Inj* 2002;16:583–593.
96. Tate DG. Alcohol use among spinal cord-injured patients. *Am J Phys Med Rehabil* 1993;72:192–195.
97. Heinemann AW, Hawkins D. Substance abuse and medical complications following spinal cord injury. *Rehabil Psychol* 1995;40:125–140.
98. Teasdale TW, Engberg AW. Suicide after traumatic brain injury: a population study. *J Neurol Neurosurg Psychiatry* 2001;71:436–440.
99. Macciocchi S, Seel RT, Thompson N, et al. Spinal cord injury and co-occurring traumatic brain injury: assessment and incidence. *Arch Phys Med Rehabil* 2008;89: 1350–1357.

100. Turner JA, Cardenas DD, Warms CA, et al. Chronic pain associated with spinal cord injuries: a community survey. *Arch Phys Med Rehabil* 2001;82:501–509.
101. Siddall PJ, Loeser JD, Pain following spinal cord injury. *Spinal Cord* 2001;39:63–73.
102. Budh CN, Osteraker AL Life satisfaction in individuals with a spinal cord injury and pain. *Clin Rehabil* 2007; 21:89–96.
103. Raichle KA, Hanley M, Jensen MP, et al. Cognitions, coping, and social environment predict adjustment to pain in spinal cord injury. *J Pain* 2007;8:718–729.
104. Wollaars MM, Post MW, Van Asbeck FW, et al. Spinal cord injury pain: the influence of psychologic factors and impact on quality of life. *Clin J Pain* 2007;23:383–391.
105. Trieschmann R. *Spinal cord injuries: the psychological, social, and vocational adjustment*. New York: Pergamon Press, 1980.
106. Wheeler G, Krausher R, Cumming C, et al. Personal styles and ways of coping in individuals who use wheelchairs. *Spinal Cord* 1996;34:351–357.
107. Pearcey TE, Yoshida KK, Renwick RM. Personal relationships after a spinal cord injury. *Int J Rehabil Res* 2007;30(3)209–219.
108. Bonanno GA, Wortman CB, Lehman DR, et al. Resilience to loss and chronic grief: a prospective study from preloss to 18-months postloss. *J Pers Soc Psychol* 2002;3:1150–1164.
109. Martz EM, Livneh H, Priebe M, et al. Predictors of psychosocial adaptation among people with spinal cord injury or disorder. *Arch Phys Med Rehabil* 2005;86:1182–1192.
110. Lohne V, Severinsson E. Hope during the first months after acute spinal cord injury. *J Adv Nurs* 2004;47:279–286.
111. Hammell KH. Experience of rehabilitation following spinal cord injury: a meta-synthesis of qualitative findings. *Spinal Cord* 2007;45:260–274.
112. Lohne V, Severinsson E. The power of hope: patients' experiences of hope a year after acute spinal cord injury. *J Clin Nurs* 2006;15(3)315–323.
113. Johnstone B, Glass BA, Oliver RE. Religion and disability: clinical, research and training considerations for rehabilitation professionals. *Disabil Rehabil* 2007; 29:1153–1163.
114. Snyder CR. To hope, to lose, to hope again. *J Pers Interpers Loss* 1996;1:1–16.
115. Morse JM, Doberneck B. Delineating the concept of hope. *Image J Nurs Sch* 1995;27:277–285.
116. Lewis P, Lubkin I. Illness roles. In: Lubkin IM, ed. *Chronic Illness impact and interventions*. 4th ed. Massachusetts: Jones and Bartlett, 1998:77–102.
117. Judd FK, Burrows GD. Liaison psychiatry in a spinal injuries unit. *Paraplegia* 1986;24:6–19.
118. Pope AM. Preventing secondary conditions. *Ment Retard* 1992;30:347–354.
119. Shackelford M, Farley T, Vines CL. Identifying psychosocial characteristics of adults with SCI. *Spinal Cord Inj Psychosoc Process* 1997;10:49–52.
120. Krause JS. Intercorrelations between secondary conditions and life adjustment in people with spinal cord injury. *Spinal Cord Inj Psychosoc Process* 1998; 1:3–7.
121. Thompson SC, Janigian AD. Life schemes: a framework for understanding the search for meaning. *J Soc Clin Psychol* 1988;7:260–280.
122. Bulman RJ, Wortman CB. Attributions of blame and coping in the "real world": severe accident victims react to their lot. *J Pers Soc Psychol* 1977;35:351–363.
123. Schultz, R. Decker S. Long-term adjustment to physical disability: the role of social support, perceived control, and self-blame. *J Pers Soc Psychol* 1985;48:1162–1172.
124. Nielson WR, MacDonald MR. Attributions of blame and coping following spinal cord injury: is self-blame adaptive? *J Soc Clin Psychol* 1988;4:163–175.
125. Jordan SA, Wellborn WR, Kovnick J, et al. Understanding and treating motivation difficulties in ventilator-dependent SCI patients. *Paraplegia* 1991;29:431–442.
126. Lubkin I. *Chronic Illness; impact and intervention*. 3rd ed. Boston, MA: Jones and Bartlett, 1995.
127. Redman BK. *The process of patient teaching in nursing*. 7th ed. St. Louis, MO: Mosby, 1993.
128. Blevins D, Berg J, Dunbar-Jacob J. Compliance. In: Lubkin IM, ed. *Chronic illness impact and interventions*. 4th ed. Boston, MA: Jones and Bartlett, 1998:227–257.
129. Trosper RM. Psychological factors affecting noncompliant behavior: a case study. *Spinal Cord Inj Psychosoc Process* 1998;11:70–74.
130. Glass CA, Jackson HF, Dutton J, et al. Estimating social adjustment following spinal trauma. I: who is more realistic-patient or spouse? A statistical justification. *Spinal Cord* 1997;35:320–325.
131. Taskemski T, Kennedy P, Gardner BP, et al. The association of sports and physical recreation with life satisfaction in a community sample of people with spinal cord injuries. *Neurorehabilitation* 2005;20:253–265.
132. Tate DG, Kalpakjian CZ, Forchheimer MB. Quality of life issues in individuals with spinal cord injury. *Arch Phys Med Rehabil* 2002;83(suppl 2):18–24.
133. Hall, KM, Knudsen ST, Wright J, et al. Follow-up study of individuals with high tetraplegia (C1-C4) 14 to 24 years post-injury. *Arch Phys Rehabil* 1999;80:1507–1515.
134. Bach JR, Tilton MC, Life satisfaction and well-being measures in ventilator assisted individuals with traumatic tetraplegia (C1-C4) 14 to 24 years postinjury. *Arch Phys Med Rehabil* 1994;75:626–632.
135. Weitzenkamp DA, Gerhart KA, Charlifue SW, et al. Ranking the criteria for assessing quality of life after disability: evidence for priority shifting among long-term spinal cord injury survivors. *Br J Health Psychol* 2000;5:57–69.
136. McColl MA, Charlifue S, Glass, C, et al. Aging, gender, and spinal cord injury. *Arch Phys Med Rehabil* 2004;85:363–367.
137. Lund ML, Norlund A, Bernspang B, et al. Perceived participation and problems in participation are determinant of life satisfaction in people with spinal cord injury. *Disabil Rehabil* 2007;29:1417–1422.
138. Stevens SL, Caputo JL, Fuller DK, et al. Physical activity and quality of life. *J Spinal Cord Med* 2008;31: 373–378.
139. Budh CN. Life satisfaction in individuals with a spinal cord injury and pain. *Clin Rehabil* 2007;21:89–96.

140. Dijkers MP. Correlates of life satisfaction among persons with spinal cord injury. *Arch Phys Med Rehabil* 1999;80:867–876.
141. Dowler R, Richards JS, Putzke JD, et al. Impact of demographic and medical factors on satisfaction with life after spinal cord injury: a normative study. *J Spinal Cord Med* 2001;24:87–91.
142. Veennstra LM, Hjeltnes N, Biering-Sorensen FB. Health-related quality of life in persons with long-standing spinal cord injury. *Spinal Cord* 2008;46:710–715.
143. Middleton J, Tran Y, Craig A. Relationship between quality of life and self-efficacy in persons with spinal cord injuries. *Arch Phys Med Rehabil* 2007;88:1643–1648.
144. Barker RN, Kendall MD, Amsters DI, et al. The relationship between quality of life and disability across the lifespan for people with spinal cord injury. *Spinal Cord* 2009;47:149–155.
145. Putzke JD, Barrett JJ, Richards JS, et al. Life satisfaction following spinal cord injury: long-term follow-up. *J Spinal Cord Med* 2004;27:106–110.
146. Putzke JD, Richards JS, Hicken BL, et al. Predictors of life satisfaction: a spinal cord injury cohort study. *Arch Phys Med Rehabil* 2002;83:555–561.
147. Dunn DS, Brody C. Defining the good life following acquired physical disability. *Rehabil Psychol* 2009;53(4):413–425.
148. Young JM, Browne A. Choosing death in rehabilitation. *Top Spinal Cord Inj Rehabil* 2008:13:18–29.
149. Kirschner KL. Calling it quits: When patients or proxies request to withdraw or withhold life-sustaining treatment after spinal cord injury. *Top Spinal Cord Inj Rehabil* 2008;13:30–44.
150. Weitzenkamp DA, Gerhart KA, Charlifue SW, et al. Spouses of spinal cord injury survivors: the added impact of caregiving. *Arch Phys Med Rehabil* 1997;78:822–827.
151. Gans JS. Facilitating staff/patient interaction in rehabilitation. In: Caplan B, ed. *Rehabilitation psychology desk reference*. Rockville, MD: Aspen Publications, 1987:185–218.
152. Sadok BJ, Sadok VA, Kaplan S, eds. *Sadock's comprehensive textbook of psychiatry*. 8th ed. Philadelphia, PA: Lippincott Williams & Wilkin, 2005.
153. Glass CA. The impact of home-based ventilator dependence on family life. *Paraplegia* 1993;3:93–101.

CHAPTER 22 ■ VOCATIONAL ASPECTS OF SPINAL CORD INJURY

MICHELLE A. MEADE, DEBRA J. FARRELL, AND JAMES S. KRAUSE

INTRODUCTION

Employment is an important component of meaning in the lives of individuals with disabilities, having psychological, social, and financial implications. Psychologically, employment is positively associated with life satisfaction, self-esteem, and quality of life (QOL) (1–7). Socially, it is a primary means of developing identity and forming interactions and relationships with other people. Financially, employment provides a means for supporting oneself and family and facilitates access to health care services.

Spinal cord injury (SCI) can dramatically and permanently affect key areas of a person's life—including mobility, independence, and employment. The influence that SCI exerts over these key areas is not fixed, but rather modified by both individual and environmental factors (8). These contextual factors have increasingly been recognized in models of disability, including the **International Classification of Functioning, Disability and Health** (9). For individuals with SCI, paralysis (impairments in body functions and structures) may lead to inability to walk (mobility disability), which may reduce involvement in complex life activities (participation restriction), such as meeting with close friends or engaging in employment. The relationship between impairment and participation is influenced by fixed factors such as gender, race, and pre-injury functioning, as well as modifiable factors including motivation, education, and communication skills. Many personal and environmental factors are modifiable—including products and technology, supports and relationships, attitudes and stereotypes, public/private services or policies—and these are the factors that rehabilitation professionals and disability advocates focus on.

Most individuals with SCI are motivated to work, even those with severe physical impairments. However, many, if not most, individuals with SCI are not employed. Within this chapter, we discuss the factors that serve as supports and barriers to employment for this population and provide suggestions for strategies for improving outcomes.

The goals of this chapter are to (a) describe the medical–vocational rehabilitation (VR) continuum of services after SCI, (b) provide the reader with an evidence-based understanding of basic issues associated with employment for persons with SCI, (c) increase familiarity with existing resources, policies, and programs that have been designed to support VR, and (d) provide health care professionals with practical information and suggestions that will allow them to facilitate the employment and VR process for individuals with SCI.

DEFINITION AND IMPORTANCE OF EMPLOYMENT

Individuals with disabilities, and particularly persons with SCI, have low rates of employment. While exact figures vary in the United States, the number of persons with SCI who are employed appears to range from approximately 16% to 69% (3–5,10,11). Variability between studies is attributable, in part, to differences in the definition of "employment," as well as the populations examined in each of the studies. Also, estimates for current employment rates do not include individuals who returned to work after their injuries but later discontinued employment. Although it is difficult to pinpoint the percentage who return to work (RTW) at some point after SCI, it can be estimated that for every two people who RTW and are currently working, another person will have returned to work but discontinued employment prior to age 65 (3,12).

Employment is defined as working or having a job from which one receives payment for labor or rendered services (13). Work can be regular or erratic, part time, or full time, and it can occur at home or in one's community. In much of the research literature, especially those studies using data from the National SCI Model Systems database, classification of employment is based on a single question about primary work status and answered with the categorical responses of *employed*, *unemployed*, *retired*, *homemaker*, and *student* (14). Occasionally, the time spent in paid activities from a question on the Craig Handicap Assessment and Reporting Technique is also included in analysis, and work status is further divided into part-time and full-time employment. A defined meaning for the term "unemployed" is elusive in the SCI literature, though it is better defined in the broader VR field where participants are often classified as actively seeking employment, or not (15–18). When the outcome being examined is *productive activities*, researchers generally include individuals who report being employed, students, and homemakers, and those engaging in volunteer activities (14,19,20).

Another issue that clouds our definition of work performed by persons with SCI is that of RTW versus employment. Because a significant number of individuals sustain an SCI at a young age, they may not have a work history at the time of injury. Thus, RTW is not the goal, but rather the development of job skills and vocational training, so that initial employment can occur. RTW, on the other hand, encompasses return to the same job and employer, return to the same employer in a different work capacity, finding a similar job with a different employer, or finding a new job with a different employer. There are obvious advantages for those who have the opportunity to return to the same employer as the latter circumstance sometimes requires additional job training or education. In many cases, RTW encompasses a series of carefully planned steps in returning to a full pre-injury job status.

Correlates of Employment

Employment brings significant benefits for many people with SCI. It provides a means of financially supporting one's self and family, facilitates access to health care insurance benefits and services, and serves as a means for forming and strengthening both relationships and personal identity. There is a positive relationship between employment status and QOL after SCI (1,2,5,6,10,21–23), though notably, QOL and life satisfaction are also related to education, income, and number of social and recreational activities (2,24). Individuals with SCI who are employed have been found to be more active, require fewer medical treatments, complete more years of education, perceive themselves as having fewer problems, and are more satisfied with their lives than those with SCI who are unemployed (6,22). Further, employment is associated with higher life adjustment scores while terminating employment is associated with decline in adjustment scores (5). In addition, individuals with SCI who are currently employed report greater positive feelings in life domains of economics, emotional distress, and general health, when compared with those who are chronically unemployed and those who have been employed since SCI onset but are currently unemployed (6). Despite these findings, it appears that once working, a significant percentage of individuals with SCI indicate that they would either change jobs or some aspect of their employment (e.g., duties, supervisor, or hours worked) (25).

Employment after SCI has also been associated with the positive psychological characteristics of optimism, self-esteem, and achievement orientation (26). It is not clear if these characteristics existed before employment and served as support for searching out, finding and accepting a job, or if they are developed afterwards and are then fostered by employment. There is some evidence that the benefits associated with work are only partially dependent upon work intensity (27). Part-time employment affords significant advantages over unemployment in providing both health insurance and better QOL; however, individuals who spend at least 30 hours a week in paid employment have the highest levels of benefits, including health insurance, dental insurance, sick leave, and paid vacation (27,28). While the presence (or absence) of secondary conditions may influence level/intensity of employment, for individuals with SCI working part-time still provides advantages over unemployment (27,28). Similarly, other types of productive activities have also been shown to be beneficial for health and QOL. For example, individuals with SCI who classify themselves as students report higher overall adjustment and QOL scores and fewer problems with skill deficits than individuals with SCI who report neither being students nor being employed (2,4).

PREDICTORS OF EMPLOYMENT

There are a few areas of research related to SCI that have been receiving more attention than predictors of employment status. The factors most consistently associated with current employment status after SCI are years of education (both prior to and after injury), age at injury, pre-injury occupation, injury severity, and race–ethnicity. Those who were younger at injury onset were in white-collar occupations, had less severe SCI, and are Caucasian consistently report the best outcomes. The relationships of these factors to employment have been well documented in recent reviews of the literature (29,30). For instance, Anderson and colleagues (29) identified a total of 14 factors that influenced employment after SCI, including education, type of employment, severity of the lesion, age, time since injury, sex, marital status, social support, vocational counselling, medical problems, employer attitudes, race, psychologic state, and environment. These factors obviously represent a wide variety of influences, not all of which can become the focus of interventions. Factors such as age, time since injury, and gender may best be considered *attributable differences*, as they cannot be manipulated. By contrast, *policy factors,* such as education, social support, employer attitudes, and psychological factors, are prime examples of characteristics that may become targets for interventions to improve outcomes (31,32). Policy changes have the potential to foster better outcomes when applied in a manner that improves opportunities or better utilizes and builds on individual strengths.

Fixed Characteristics

Whereas biographic, injury, and educational characteristics have been linked to employment status (i.e., employed versus unemployed), less research has addressed quality indicators of employment, such as earnings, job tenure, or job satisfaction. Two recent studies identified predictors of conditional and unconditional earnings (31,32). Conditional earnings are defined by earning levels among individuals who are employed, whereas unconditional earnings are calculated for all individuals in a cohort, including those who are unemployed and not income earning. Therefore, it is reasonable to expect that differences in unconditional earnings would be observed as a function of any characteristic for which there are fundamental differences in employment rates. Differences in conditional earnings would also indicate that the particular factor was also related to an outcome *among those who are employed.* In the first of the cited studies (31), Krause and Terza found that gender, race, and education were significantly related to conditional earnings after simultaneously controlling for multiple biographic and injury characteristics (i.e., differences among those who are employed). Differences in conditional earnings favored men ($15,946), non–African-Americans ($19,402), and those with 16 or more years of education ($35,928). In essence, these differences indicate that women, African-Americans, and those with low levels of education are likely to earn significantly less, even when employed.

It is noteworthy that several other characteristics were significantly related to both the probability of employment and unconditional earnings, including better outcomes in persons who were younger, had more years since injury, had non-cervical injuries, and were ambulatory. However, even though these characteristics lead to a greater likelihood of employment and higher unconditional earnings, among those who RTW, there was no particular advantage with regard to earnings. This seems particularly interesting for injury severity as indicated either by neurologic level or by ambulatory status. In sum, whereas those with less severe injuries were more likely to RTW, they were no more likely to earn more money.

A second study by Krause and Terza (32) expanded the methodology to include additional predictor variables related to employment, both prior to and after injury (e.g., hours per week spent working, type of employer, return to pre-injury employer). A similar pattern in differences in conditional earnings was observed for gender, race–ethnicity, and education, although the actual earnings were different due to the added statistical controls. Once again, higher earnings were observed for men ($11,317), Caucasians ($13,501), and those with a college degree ($21,751). Several additional factors related to higher conditional earnings including the number of years having worked after SCI ($1,027 per year), percentage of time having worked after SCI ($1,132 per 5% increment), and working either for the government ($24,106) or in private industry ($15,061) as opposed to being self-employed or in a family business. Again, neither indicator of injury severity is associated with differential conditional earnings.

Modifiable Factors

Education

Because of the profound relationship between education and employment, it is important to look at this variable more carefully and in conjunction with other important predictors of employment. Education is often the focus of policy decisions and targeted interventions, as it is one of the most modifiable of the variables that has been found to enhance employment outcomes.

Data from a report on the SCI Model Systems (14) identified the relationship between years of education and the percentage of individuals employed at the time of follow-up. There was a steady increase in the percentage of participants employed with each successive educational milestone, where the lowest percentage of employment (5.3%) was observed for those without a high school certificate. This figure increased to 21.5% for those with a high school certificate and more than doubled for those with an associate's degree (44.7%). The percentage increased to 60.8% for those with a 4-year degree, but increased less substantially thereafter (65.2% for those with a master's degree and 68.8% for those with a Ph.D. or M.D.).

It is particularly interesting to look at the relationship between education and employment status for those with varying severity of SCI. The same investigation of this database, grouped participants into four cohorts based on combination of neurological level of injury and the American Spinal Injury Association grade (ASIA Impairment grade), which can be used as a surrogate for neurological completeness of injury. All those without motor functional injuries (ASIA Impairment Scale [AIS] A–C) were classified in three groups according to the level of injury: C1-4, C5-8, and non-cervical. Those with ASIA D impairments were classified in a single group regardless of injury level. Employment rates increased with each successive decrease in severity of injury, ranging from a low of 13.7% for those with C1-4 (ASIA A–C) to a high of 38.7% for those with ASIA-D (C5-8 = 22.7%; Non-cervical = 28.5%) (14).

The largest gain in percentage employed for those with AIS D was noted between receiving a high school certificate and completion of an associate's degree. A somewhat similar relationship was noted for those with non-cervical injuries, although the employment percentage continued to improve through a Bachelor's degree where the outcome was almost equivalent to that of those with AIS D. For those with lower cervical injuries (C5-8), there was essentially a linear relationship between educational level and percentage employed. However, for those with the most severe injuries (C1-4, AIS A–C), the largest gain in the percentage employed was observed between a Bachelor's and a master's degree.

The primary implication of these findings is that interventions that focus on education can be targeted at much different educational milestones depending on severity of SCI. For those with less severe injuries, completion of an associate's degree may substantially enhance the employment rate. However, for those with cervical injuries, even at lower anatomical levels, the rate will continue to improve with each increasing educational milestone. Although education may be considered the great equalizer across injury severity, it is clear for those with the most severe levels of injury that employment outcomes will not be maximized without education beyond that of a master's degree.

It is also important to distinguish between educational milestones that have been reached prior to, as opposed to after, the onset of SCI. There are substantial differences in post-injury employment rates for any given level of education depending on whether the educational milestone was achieved before or after injury (33). For instance, when controlling for other factors, the odds of working after injury for those with a master's degree obtained after SCI are 10.7 times of those without a master's degree. However, the odds of post-injury employment were not statistically different for those with or without a master's degree when the degree was obtained prior to SCI onset (33). There are several possible reasons for this, including greater individual motivation among those who complete their education after their injury and/or a better fit between the certificate or degree with post-injury abilities. The study did not address the underlying factors.

Psychological Factors

Despite the primary importance of psychological factors to vocational outcomes in the general population, there has been surprisingly little work in recent years examining employment after SCI. Some factors that have been investigated include personality, interests, locus of control, and motivation.

Locus of control and work attitude were found to contribute significantly to the prediction of employment in one study conducted with 459 participants with traumatic SCI in Southeastern Australia (18). Two of three locus of control scales were significantly associated with work rate, which was defined as the portion of time spent working after injury divided by the total potential time. Chance was negatively correlated with work rate (−0.17), whereas internal was positively correlated with work rate (+0.20). Work attitude was also positively correlated with work rate (+0.26). These findings are consistent with those of an earlier study (34) that utilized a related but different outcome ("in the labor force" or "not in the labor force"). The same three psychological factors were significantly related to labor force participation. Obviously, these constructs are not highly correlated with employment, so they must be considered rather weak predictors at best.

Social support has been identified as a significant predictor of employment status and other forms of productivity following SCI (35,36). Social support may provide individuals with SCI with emotional reassurance as well as instrumental aid in various life activities. In addition, significant others may provide information and feedback about how to live independently in the community. These benefits minimize stress and increase the individual's ability to work. In a study by McShane and Karp (35), strong motivation, greater social support, and driving one's own car were predictive of having paid employment.

Anxiety, fear, and mistrust may have a significant role in the unemployment of individuals with SCI. A qualitative study of individuals with SCI from traditionally underserved backgrounds found that most (if not all) individuals who participated in focus groups and interviews—whether employed or not—seemed to acknowledge the benefits associated with working (37,38). They reported wanting to work, recognized the social and psychological benefits of work, and discussed both their frustration with being at home and their desire not to be dependent on the system. In most cases, though, these feelings and thoughts were eclipsed by a fear of losing benefits and a mistrust of the system to work with them to achieve positive outcomes.

One of the most important psychological constructs in relation to employment is vocational interest. Because the primary measure of vocational interests, the Strong Interest Inventory (39), incorporates the Holland personal typology (40), vocational interests and personality are intricately linked. The Holland theory postulates six personality types and six corresponding environments, with the match between personality and environment central to vocational choice (41–43). Rohe and associates conducted a series of studies of vocational interest among men with SCI, finding that the predominant interest pattern reflected activities that were physically challenging and often incongruent with the limitations imposed by SCI (41,42). Interests appeared to be stable over an 11-year period among those with chronic long-term SCI, even when the SCI made it practically impossible to act upon the interests (43). Because these findings are based solely on men, nearly all of whom who were Caucasian, there is no reason to believe the results would generalize to women or minorities. Nevertheless, at least for Caucasian males, there may be a strong incongruence between vocational interests and physical abilities to act upon these interests. This could contribute to the low employment rates after SCI.

Individuals with SCI from underserved populations may be more likely to be seen as having caused their own impairments, which research suggests may influence hiring decisions (44,45). These studies showed that job applicants who were perceived as being to blame for their disability are likely to receive lower ratings by employers. Thus, job applicants with disabilities resulting from a perceived internal cause are rated less favorably than applicants with disabilities deemed as external (i.e., their behavior plays little role in the development of the disability) (45). Given that research findings that traumatic injury in African-American males is often perceived as having resulted from illegal behavior (38), it seems likely that negative causal attribution with associated negative impact on hiring decisions may occur at higher rates in people with disabilities from underserved groups.

Environmental Factors

Many environmental barriers influence the ability and motivation of individuals with SCI to work. These include the portability of health insurance, financial disincentives to work, and high unemployment as well as lack of suitable jobs and compensation entitlement. Concerns about losing economic and health benefits are frequently cited reasons for not returning to work after SCI (46). These issues may be particularly salient for minorities with SCI who already mistrust that the system will work with them to achieve positive outcomes (37,38,47). Individuals with SCI express fear of losing benefits paired with a reluctance to separate from Supplemental Security Income (SSI) and Social Security Disability Insurance (SSDI) and the safety net each provides. Many individuals with SCI do not appear to be aware of the new policies and programs that may impact their ability to work without losing their health insurance, or programs such as The Ticket to Work and Work Incentives Improvement Act (TWWIIA; discussed below) or services such as benefit counseling. It is important that accurate information about these policies and programs is provided to all stakeholders in terms and methods that they can relate to.

The availability of transportation is a prominent barrier to RTW indicating the importance of having resources to facilitate work. Transportation plays an important role that can either assist or hinder the employment and community reintegration of individuals with SCI. Research has shown that addressing transportation needs, so that individuals can get to and from work, is critical for ensuring the individual's self-determination in employment, housing, and social/recreational outlets (48).

Lack of accessibility of the built environment is also a consideration and a frequently reported challenge for individuals with SCI living in the community. Persons with SCI, especially wheelchair users, often have difficulty in accessing buildings, and especially bathrooms, which limited their ability to work, participate in the community, and engage in activities with friends and families.

Despite these many perceived challenges, when actual barriers are correlated with employment status in follow-up studies, poor health was the primary factor associated with a diminished probability of RTW (49); in fact, citing economic or health disincentives at one point in time as a barrier to employment was essentially unrelated to actual employment status 4 years later. Actively looking for work and maintaining hope for RTW were associated with a greater probability of RTW.

Finally, it appears those without entitlement or compensation are more likely to RTW (50,51). The issue of compensation and entitlements should be carefully considered to avoid unilateral decisions about their negative consequences. Truthful consideration of policies and procedures that eliminate financial disincentives and focus on how employment can improve the circumstances of an individual with SCI is needed.

ROLE OF HEALTH CARE PROFESSIONALS

Health care professionals play an important role in addressing the vocational and employment issues individuals with SCI face. Collectively, they support the functional outcomes that allow those with new or exacerbated SCI conditions to pursue their vocational goals and interests, assisting with assessment and optimizing functional restoration and the development of expectations about vocational-related abilities and roles. This occurs as individuals with SCI of every level of impairment are recognized for their potential to achieve a satisfying and productive work life. In particular, the attitudes and spoken messages health care professionals and other experts convey can have a powerful effect on patients' perceptions of themselves and their abilities. One should be realistic about prognosis of injuries or conditions and should not be harsh, condescending, or overly limiting about their patients' current functional limitations or future employment opportunities.

The inpatient setting (whether acute hospitalization, inpatient rehabilitation, or long-term residential services) provides health care professionals with the opportunity to assist persons with SCI in achieving employment goals. They do so by designing and implementing evidence-based practices into their daily work. Health care professionals can engage themselves in (a) managing (and teaching the patient to manage) long-term health-related issues, (b) reducing unnecessary expenditures of patients' time and energy on self-care tasks (both in and out of the hospital), (c) assisting with prescription and acquisition of necessary equipment to simplify tasks and enhance independence at home or community re-entry, (d) identifying and implementing appropriate emotional supports or techniques, (e) identifying and facilitating adequate caregiver roles and routines, (f) providing early intervention opportunities to establish a solid, relationship with a VR counselor who can serve as a continuous link to reliable, ongoing rehabilitation services, (g) arranging access to peer counseling to share experiences with others and promote community involvement, and (h) providing mentoring opportunities for individuals with SCI that build upon the importance of giving and receiving.

A strong, ongoing partnership between the hospital and the local VR agency is recommended, as it can be a significant asset in facilitating the community re-integration and VR process of individuals with SCI (47,52). VR representatives can provide the hospital with pertinent information regarding referral, eligibility determination, employment services, and access to community resources. They may also be able to provide worker readiness sessions or conduct employment skill-building groups. The onsite availability of VR representatives provides structured opportunities for patients and their families to ask questions prior to going home or entering employment. However, community partnerships with VR agencies must be individually developed within a particular region or community and tailored to the roles and expectations of the various partners.

Having a VR representative visible within a rehabilitation program can connect patients to needed services that may promote successful employment outcomes. Prior to discharge from inpatient rehabilitation, VR representatives may meet with individuals with SCI in person to provide education and consultation regarding VR services. This marks the beginning step in establishing the "working alliance" between an individual and his or her rehabilitation counselor, a cornerstone to reaching a successful employment outcome (53). The VR agency/program may also be able to assist the individual who is preparing to re-enter the community setting and is making the transition from hospital to home. Although a patient may not be ready to RTW, the VR counselor can begin the evaluative process of determining RTW/employment readiness, and may be able to provide access to resources that may facilitate community re-entry and eventual employment or RTW.

Another important role for the health care and rehabilitation team is to make sure that the newly injured individuals with SCI get connected with the programs, benefits, and resources that may be available to support their medical treatment and continued independence. Specifically, individuals with SCI should be provided information about the two disability-based benefit programs managed by the **Social Security Administration (SSA)**—the **Social Security Disability Insurance (SSDI)** program and the **Supplemental Security Income (SSI)** program—and provided with assistance with applying if appropriate. Eligibility for these programs is based on the inability to engage in "substantial gainful activity" because of a medically determinable physical or mental impairment that has lasted or can expect to last for a continuous period of not less than 12 months. SCI, by the nature of the impairment, is one of the accepted disabilities eligible for these programs (13).

SSI monies are provided by the SSA and give a person with a disability who has very little income or resources a supportive income. The money, typically between $600 and $900 for an individual (as of 2008), is used to help pay for shelter, food, and clothing. An individual does not have to have work history to be eligible for SSI. If the individual is able to RTW, the amount SSI may be adjusted downwards as their income goes up; however, if SSI is the only income that they receive, they will always make more money working than not working. The SSI program is authorized under Title XVI of the SSA (9,13).

SSDI is a wage replacement income that pays benefits to the individual with a disability and some family members. To be eligible, the individual must be a legal resident of the United States and have obtained sufficient work credits by paying FICA taxes for a specified length of time; the number of work credits needed to qualify for SSDI depends on the age at disability onset. Individuals receiving this benefit are sometimes designated "Title II beneficiaries" (a reference to the section of the social security act that the program is authorized under) (13). The monthly disability benefit/payment is based on the social security earnings record of the insured worker. Before retirement age, disability benefits may be reduced depending on the amount that was previously earned. An individual who is already retired and collecting SSDI will not qualify for additional benefits or compensation if they become disabled. Because children and spouses of the individual with disability may also qualify for income under the individual's SSDI, working—because of associated costs such as childcare—can sometimes lead to a smaller net income for the family (54).

Individuals with SCI may also qualify for medical assistance and insurance because of their disability (and perceived inability to work). The Medical Assistance Program (**Medicaid**) is administered by states to provide medical care for public assistance recipients and medically needy persons. The program is financed by state and federal funds. An individual must meet both financial and non-financial requirements to be eligible for Medicaid. Medicaid covers a comprehensive range of services, including hospital care, doctor's visits, prescriptions, mental health services, and rehabilitative services. However, the places where these services are available from may be limited. In most states, an individual may be covered by another health insurance and still eligible for Medicaid. To apply for Medicaid and other state-funded medical programs, the individual with SCI (or their representative) should get in touch with the Department of Human (or Social) Services in their county.

Medicare is the health insurance program administered by the federal government, that covers individuals who are either of age 65 or over or who meet other criteria, including being disabled or having end-stage renal disease. An individual is only eligible for Medicare if he or she (or his or her spouse) is a citizen of the United States and worked for at least 10 years in Medicare-covered employment. Medicare is partially financed by FICA taxes and the SSA is responsible for determining Medicare eligibility and processing premium payments for the Medicare. Individuals with SCI are usually not eligible for Medicare immediately after injury; rather they become eligible after they had received SSA benefits (i.e., SSI or SSDI) for 24 months. After 24 months, SSA beneficiaries will automatically be enrolled in Medicare; if this does not happened, they should contact the SSA.

While individuals with SCI should receive information and access to these resources, it is important they recognize that (in most cases) they will be better off in RTW or becoming employed. Not only will they have increased access to resources, but the psychological importance of having a purpose and a reason to get up in the morning should not be underestimated. In addition, new policies (described in more detail below) are increasingly providing increased options and safety nets to ensure that individuals with disabilities will continue to have access to government insurance and supports and will always be better off than those not working.

COMMUNITY SETTINGS, RESOURCES, AND SUPPORTS

Successful re-entry into the community is often seen as a necessary step in optimizing the productivity and QOL of individuals with SCI. Before they can fully access either the community or employment, the individual with SCI must be able to function safely in the home within the appropriate level of provider care and support. Home evaluations may provide suggestions for altering the environment to improve activity and participation. In particular, attention should be paid to ways of minimizing the burden of self-care routines; well-planned, reliable, and efficient self-care routines are necessary to conserve the individual's time and energy and enable them to pursue work-related activities. Ultimately, individuals with SCI need to weigh out the costs of renovating a home versus relocating to another more suitable or accessible location.

The characteristics of the residential community and its accessibility, or lack thereof, should be considered well in advance of the community re-entry phase. Health care professionals and the patient should anticipate which public buildings will need to be accessed by the individual including possible work locations. If the decision is made that an individual with SCI needs to be discharged to an intermediate or long-term care residential facility, health care professionals should convey the message that community re-integration, and even employment, is still an option from this setting.

Successful access to the community requires adequate transportation (48). This can mean reliable public transportation or a personal vehicle, such as a van equipped with a lift or a car with modified driving controls. When possible, the primary mode of transportation should be determined well in advance of hospital discharge, so that adequate time can be given to acquire the vehicle or essential equipment. If a driver evaluation is indicated, the physician generally orders the evaluation during the medical rehabilitation phase. If an individual will not be performing independent driving activities for one reason or another, another reliable mode of transportation must be pursued. The health care team can provide needed assistance in acquiring information about the availability and feasibility of using public transportation resources such as special transportation services.

Centers for Independent Living can serve as valuable resources and partners for facilitating the community re-entry of individuals with SCI. The specific features of individual programs are determined by the needs of the persons served, the availability of existing community resources, the physical and social make-up of the community, and the goals of the program itself. Independent living support services can be provided by a variety of community-based programs such as self-help and information referral centers, generic service providers, transitional programs, and residential programs. At a minimum, CIL services consist of peer counseling, information and referral, independent living skills training, and advocacy. These services are primarily provided by other individuals with SCI who may or may not have professional training in those areas but who have personal experience in living with a disability.

Many CILs also offer such services as housing assistance, personal assistant training and referral, sign language interpreter referral, and community awareness programs. In addition, with the 1992 Amendments to the Rehabilitation Act, many CILs are currently placing greater emphasis on systems advocacy and consumer empowerment. Systems advocacy aims at inclusion of people with disabilities in the policy-making roles that regulate delivery of medical, social, rehabilitation, or other services. Systems advocacy may be focused at the local, state, regional, or national level depending on the nature of the underlying issue being addressed.

Vocational Rehabilitation

The primary purpose of VR is to assist and enable persons with disabilities to increase their productivity as fully integrated and contributing (taxpaying) members of society, usually through competitive employment. VR services are designed to help individuals with disabilities (including SCI) prepare for, enter into, or return to a former or new line of work within the workforce. State VR agencies under the State Department of Education have played a key role in promoting employment opportunities for persons with severe physical limitations such as those with SCI, including subsidizing their education, vocational assessment, transportation and personal care assistance costs, career development and training, job placement and by helping to purchase equipment and other resources, needed to obtain employment after SCI. State VR agencies may arrange for specialized employment services or consultations with private and not-for-profit providers who also serve the needs of individuals with disabilities.

Eligibility for services is determined on the basis of disability. An individual is not able to be deemed eligible for services until he or she leaves the hospital. Most (if not all) individuals with SCI meet the criteria for a qualified disability by the nature of their impairment. Individuals of working age (between 18 and 65 years old) who receive **SSDI or SSI** benefits are usually eligible. However, an individual does not have to already be receiving either of these benefits at the current time. If an individual with SCI has concerns about how employment may affect his or her benefits, he or she should contact a **Work**

Incentives Planning and Assistance (**WIPA**) program whose primary objective is to enable individuals with disabilities to make informed choices about work. WIPA programs in each state have incentive coordinators to provide information about how employment will directly impact the individual with SCI's benefits as well as what incentives and programs may be available to provide maximum assistance.

The first step of the VR process involves ***screening*** and ***intake***. Individuals need to make an appointment with a VR agency either through a hospital or self-referral. In most agencies, rehabilitation counselors serve as the primary case manager or coordinator of services geared toward individuals with SCI/disability within the community setting. At the initial meeting, the individual with SCI meets with a rehabilitation counselor to discuss issues related to eligibility, goals, and service options. Vocational issues may involve RTW or entry into a new career path, which may require pre-preparatory training or school.

The next step in the VR process is ***evaluation***. Assessments are conducted that examine the employability, placeability, job readiness, and functional limitations of the individual. Types of assessments include interest inventories, functional/work capacity evaluations or written medical restrictions, job task analyses, ergonomic evaluations, work tolerance screenings, and simulated work evaluations. Depending upon a person's previous work history, a transferable skills analysis may be valuable to determine what skills the individual has already acquired in previous work or school situations and ways in which such skills can be applied to a new worker role or work setting. For individuals who are already employed, assessments may include job site analysis (matching the essential functions of the job to medial/work restrictions and to the environment), assistive technology (e.g., computer hardware, software, or environmental control units), and worker readiness evaluations (functional capacity evaluation, work tolerance screening, work simulation). Assistive technology and computer adaptations, in particular, have been shown to enhance the ability of individuals with SCI to acquire or hone skills, allowing them to compete for employment (55,56).

Information gathered from these evaluations is used to assist with the development of an **Individual Plan for Employment** (IPE). The IPE will vary based upon the age, interests, goals, skills, and abilities of the person. Making an informed consumer choice (57) that is culturally sensitive (58) is an integral part of the career decision-making and goal-setting process. Informed choice places the individual at the center of the IPE and empowers the individual with SCI to make personal career choices instead of having others control or dictate one's plan for employment (59).

Formulation of the IPE should include discussion and realistic consideration of job duties and conditions imposed by the work setting environment. Once the IPE is in place and if an individual is still receiving outpatient occupational (OT) or physical therapy services, therapists can become a part of the interdisciplinary team process in assisting their patients to aim toward long-term employment skills and abilities with the great goals of fulfilling vocational and career aspirations. Therapists may be requested to support employment goals by assisting their patients to incorporate adaptive strategies that build upon essential job functions and by prescribing devices that simplify or enhance work-related tasks.

At the ***pre-employment*** step, VR services might include work hardening and reconditioning programs, job-seeking skills, job clubs, employment skills training, and job placement services. Enhancing the readiness for individuals is directly linked to the written goals of the IPE, which may include a search for conventional employment outside the home, entrepreneurial or small business development, or telecommuting to work. Telecommuting or teleworking from home can overcome many of the barriers that counteract successful employment outcomes for individuals with SCI such as fatigue factors, having a secondary medical condition (e.g., pressure ulcers), and mobility and transportation issues (60).

The next step in the VR process involves job ***acquisition or placement***. When the person with SCI has a job and is ready to enter or re-enter that setting, services are available to both the individual with SCI and their employer. Prior to employment or RTW, the VR customer service representative addresses the issues and concerns of the employer in complying with medical/work restrictions and in maintaining work and productivity standards. Services may also include disability or sensitivity training for supervisors or co-workers. The employer must consider time factors in setting up space and acquiring needed equipment. Equipment can be costly (i.e., computer hardware and software, and computer accessibility equipment) so the better prepared and well-equipped the individual, the more successful the employment outcome. ***Universally designed*** work stations are ideal and can be easily adjusted for wheelchair users, providing for proper positioning in adjusting work surfaces and adapting to the functional and anthropometric characteristics of individual users.

For persons with SCI, a good **job site assessment** is critical to the success of both the job placement and the job retention process; it is the basis on which job accommodation recommendations are made. Job site assessments may be done by an OT or a Rehabilitation Counselor who specializes in work assessment. The components typically considered include environment factors, physical factors of the work site, job tasks, productivity standards, and the overall work operation. The focus of this assessment is to determine: (a) if the employee able to perform the essential functions of his or her job with or without accommodations; and (b) what strategies or equipment are necessary to accommodate his or her performance?

Job retention services are an important part of the VR process that enable individuals with SCI to maintain employment (61). These services include (but are not limited to) worker at-risk evaluation, job site analysis and implementation of job accommodation strategies to address barriers, employer development to provide disability education to supervisors and co-workers in overcoming resistance, and job-coaching and follow-up services. **Workplace Personal Assistance Services** is one possible support that may facilitate the employment of individuals with severe disabilities (54,62). A WPA who is hired to assist with both personal needs while the individual with SCI is in the workplace (toileting, grooming, transportation, business travel) and to assist with job-related tasks (i.e., making phone calls, filing, reaching, taking notes) can greatly improve the efficiency of the individual with SCI in performing essential job duties.

The final step of the VR process is **termination** of services—that is, the point when the VR agency either declares that the case has reached a successful employment outcome or that such an outcome is deemed to be infeasible. At this point, all work supports are removed, follow-up services are concluded, and the case is placed in a *closed* status. The case may be followed for a certain period of time to collect data regarding customer satisfaction and outcomes. Once a case has reached the final step of closure, it can be re-opened if there are changes to the client's employment status or medical condition, such that they may benefit from additional assessment or services.

POLICIES, PROGRAMS, AND RESOURCES

Extensive commentary has addressed barriers to unemployment and underemployment among people with physical and cognitive disabilities, including SCI. The federal government attempted to redress these disparities by passage of the **Rehabilitation Act of 1973**. The Rehabilitation Act was designed to promote and expand employment opportunities in the public and private sectors for individuals with disabilities and to place such individuals in employment (63). This legislation authorized funding for state VR programs and supported employment services in order to increase employment opportunities and provide people with disabilities with the assistance, information, and support that they needed to obtain or retain work.

When the **Americans with Disabilities Act** (64) was passed in 1990, it represented one of the most comprehensive pieces of civil rights legislation in American history. The ADA prohibits discrimination against people with disabilities in employment, public services, public transportation, places of public accommodations (e.g., hotels and restaurants), and telecommunications. Businesses with more than 15 employees are required to make reasonable accommodations for qualified candidates with disabilities unless such accommodations would impose undue hardship. Such accommodations might include improving worksite accessibility, equipment modification, work schedule modification, or access to interpreters. The ADA defines job requirements by what is created or produced, rather than how that work is accomplished. Once these are understood, rehabilitation engineers, Occupational Therapists (OTs), and other rehabilitation specialists can work with the person with SCI and his or her employer to make creative or adaptive modifications to process or performance of activities. Modifications may realistically involve addition of equipment, changes to the work environment, or alteration in ways the work is done. While it may be debated whether the ADA has succeeded in producing such an impact (65), the prohibition of employment discrimination in the ADA only applies to *qualified* individuals with disabilities.

The **Rehabilitation Act Amendments of 1992** issued an imperative that the rehabilitation system in the United States needed to become more effective in working with diverse clients (i.e., diverse in terms of race and ethnicity) (66). The Amendments acknowledged demographic changes within the US population as well as disparities in rates of disabling conditions and services provided to minority populations by state rehabilitation agencies. The Amendments also authorized funding to provide services to increase participation in rehabilitation of underserved groups (such as persons from minority backgrounds) while requiring the development of policies and programs to increase the numbers of racial and ethnic minorities in rehabilitation careers (52,66). However, despite this landmark legislation and a resulting push for increased cultural sensitivity by state rehabilitation agencies (52), race/ethnicity remains one of the primary determinants of poorer employment outcomes among individuals with disabilities, even when factors such as educational level are controlled (68–71)and disparities in access to and quality of rehabilitation services continue to be reported. (72–76)

Through the passage of various legislative initiatives, offices and programs were established to prevent and address discrimination and disparities in employment rates for people with disabilities. One such program is **The Disability and Business Technical Assistance Centers (DBTACs), which incorporates 10 funded** regional centers established in 1991 as part of the ADA Technical Assistance Programs. The purpose of the DBTACs is to provide information, training, and technical assistance to employers, individuals with disabilities, and other entities with responsibilities under the ADA, and to facilitate program compliance and implementation.

The responsibility for enforcing legislation related to employment discrimination is charged to the **United States Equal Employment Opportunity Commission** (EEOC). When an individual feels that employment discrimination has occurred, experts suggest that the individual first try and deal directly with the employer to resolve the problem or issue (67–77). If they do not feel able to do so, or resolution with the employer cannot occur, a charge can be filed with either the EEOC or a state or local anti-discrimination agency (designated **Fair Employment Practice Agencies or FEPAs**). The U.S. EEOC shares responsibility with state and local agencies for receiving and investigating employment discrimination charges. The decision to file at an EEOC field office or FEPA is based on location, with individuals encouraged to file at the nearest agency (67). The individual making the charge (i.e., the *claimant*) can hire a lawyer to assist with and facilitate this process, but they are not obligated to do so. There is some suggestion that hiring a lawyer may increase benefits, but this may be outweighed by attorney costs. Allegations of employment discrimination may only be filed within limited time window—usually within 180 days of the alleged discriminatory action.

The **Workforce Investment Act (WIA)** was signed into law in 1998 as part of an effort to reform the nation's job training and employment programs for individuals who need specialized employment training and supports. The purpose of WIA is to increase the employment rate, job retention, and earnings of individuals who receive services through the national system of One-Stop Career Centers. The Centers were intended to unify education, vocational training, and employment programs into a single system in each community; however, individuals with disabilities originally had little success in accessing these programs.

The **Ticket to Work and Work Incentives Improvement Act of 1999 (TWWIIA)** was signed into law by President Clinton in December 1999 to meet specific employment-related needs and concerns of individuals with disabilities. TWWIIIA contains several far-reaching provisions designed to (a) eliminate structural obstacles that have required individuals to choose between working and health insurance coverage, (b) enable individuals to exercise greater autonomy in choosing service providers and obtaining rehabilitation services, and (c) lessen the dependence of individuals with disabilities on the public benefits system, with its maze of regulations and restrictions (13).

The specific provisions of TWWIIA included (a) expanded availability of health care services, including the ability to maintain Medicaid coverage while working; (b) a Ticket to Work and Self-Sufficiency Program (TWSSP), which allows consumers to exert greater choice and control of the employment services and supports they receive; and (c) the development of community-based work incentive planning and assistance programs designed to provide accurate information on work incentives for SSA beneficiaries. The TWSSP also authorized the development of programs to protect the rights of people with disabilities as they returned to work. **Protection and Advocacy for Beneficiaries of Social Security** (PABSS) Projects are funded in all 50 states and US territories to protect the rights of people with disabilities to RTW without jeopardizing their government-assisted benefits. PABSS provides free legal assistance on disability-related employment issues; however, because of limited resources, it carefully selects those cases it will pursue.

Since first enacted, the TTWSSP has been amended and updated in response to the needs and feedback of both individuals with disabilities and employment networks. In addition, the WIPA program has replaced the benefits centers developed under TWWIIA. The current work incentives that are covered in Amendments to the Social Security Act and TWWIIA include a trial work period, an extended period of eligibility for re-entitlement, tax deductions for impairment-related work expenses, extended Medicare coverage, continued payments to individuals participating in a VR or similar program, development of plans for achieving self-support, special benefits for SSI Recipients who are in paid employment despite severe medical impairment, and Medicaid eligibility for SSI recipients who work despite severe medical impairment (13). These incentives are not available to all SSA beneficiaries, so

TABLE 22.1

VOCATIONAL RESOURCES AND WEBSITES

Federal Government Disability Information Online:
http://www.disabilityinfo.gov/digov-public/public/DisplayPage.do?parentFolderId=500
A complete online guide to civil rights, benefits, housing, education, health, technology, transportation, rehabilitation, and community life. The site is managed by the U.S. Department of Labor, Office of Disability Employment Policy (ODEP) and includes a locator map that allows quick identification of state and local resources.

Directory of Independent Living Centers (CILS): http://www.virtualcil.net/cils/
A virtual site that provides a network listing and complete contact information for CILs by state. The site has an easy locator map of the United States and listings can be viewed conveniently by pointing and clicking.

Job Accommodation Network (JAN): http://www.jan.wvu.edu/_or 1-800-526-7234 (V); 1-877-781-9403 (TTY). A free service funded by the Office of Disability Employment Policy in the U.S. Department of Labor to increase the employability of people with disabilities by providing individualized worksite accommodations solutions and technical assistance regarding the ADA and other disability related legislation.

National Disability Rights Network for Client Assistance Programs (CAP): http://www.napas.org/aboutus/PA_CAP.htm or 1-202-408-9514 (V); 1-202-408-9521 (TTY).
A federally-mandated Protection and Advocacy system and Client Assistance Programs for individuals with a range of disabilities. This organization provides legal and client advocacy services to persons with disabilities throughout the U.S. Major topics include advocacy, equal opportunity, informed choice, and self-determination.

Rehabilitation Services Administration (RSA): http://www.ed.gov/about/offices/list/osers/rsa/index.html or 1-800-USA-LEARN (V); 1-800-437-0833 (TTY). This is the main site for the U.S. Department of Education, Office of Special Education and Rehabilitation Services (OSERS). The RSA administers grant programs designed to oversee employment-related services for individual with disabilities that are implemented by state VRs, with the greatest emphasis of services focused on those that are the most significantly disabled.

U. S. Department of Education State: http://www.ed.gov/about/contacts/state/index.html?src=gu
This webpage provides a locator map for identifying resources within the Department of Education within each state including contact information for state VR agencies.

Social Security Administration (SSA): http://www.ssa.gov/disability/ or 1-800-772-1213 (V); 1-800-325-0778 (TTY). This SSA site includes benefits information for individuals with disabilities including SSI and SSDI. It is equipped with a benefits screening tool to assist in determining eligibility for various benefits programs and also provides access to valuable guides, handbooks, and figures that explains the details of SSA policies and procedures.

Disability and Business Technical Assistance Center (DBTAC): http://www.adata.org/ or 1-800-949-4232 (V/TTY). This website is a national network that encompasses 10 U.S. regional ADA centers. The center specializes in providing current referrals, resources, and training services regarding the ADA to governmental agencies, employers, businesses, and individual with disabilities.

Americans With Disabilities Act (ADA) Information Line: http://www.ada.gov/ or 1-800-514-0301 (V); 1-800-514-0383 (TTY).
Provides online information regarding ADA regulations. Callers can receive live assistance from ADA specialists in answering technical questions. Also provides publications and other resource materials.

U.S. Equal Employment Opportunity Commission (EEOC): http://www.eeoc.gov/ or 1-800-669-4000 (V); 1-800-669-6820 (TTY).
The EEOC monitors equal opportunity laws and discriminatory practices as they apply to employers, particularly the federal government's Rehabilitation Act of 1973 and the Civil Service Reform Act of 1978. Other laws covered by the EEOC are the Civil Rights Act of 1964, ADA of 1990, Age Discrimination in Employment Act (ADEA), and Equal Pay Act (EPA).

it will be important for the individuals with SCI to contact a WIPA program or advocacy agency to determine supports for which they may qualify. Overall, however, these incentives and policies seem to indicate a significant investment by the federal government to facilitate employment or re-employment of individuals with disabilities.

CONCLUSIONS AND RECOMMENDATIONS

The goal of this chapter was to familiarize health care professionals with practical knowledge needed to support individuals with SCI in pursuing RTW and sustaining gainful employment. The following main points summarize our conclusions and recommendations:

- The medical–VR system is a continuum of health care and related employment services. Health care professionals, together with community-based VR professionals, play a vital role in assisting patients with SCI in reaching successful employment outcomes.
- Due to the variation and complexity of fixed, modifiable, and contextual factors affecting individuals with SCI, employment goals should be addressed through establishment of a "working alliance" between a patient and various rehabilitation professionals. Steps of the medical treatment plan should be carefully linked to the steps of the IPE to provide seamless services between the health care and vocational systems.
- Healthcare providers are encouraged to investigate resources (Table 22.1) within their own communities and to develop a method of sharing this information with patients recovering from SCI.
- Clinical practice based upon well-conceived and conducted vocational research will enhance work opportunities and outcomes for individuals with SCI.

Finally, "rehabilitation" encompasses services begin in the hospital setting and extend far into one's own community. The ability to bridge the medical and VR treatment plans by presenting information in a simplified and systematic way is a critical step in the unification of services. It is recommended that every healthcare team should have knowledge about the vocational process as a way to stay abreast of current and approved legislation, development of new vocational programs, and technological advances, all of which effectively link individuals with SCI to their vocational needs and pursuits.

ACKNOWLEDGMENTS

The authors wish to acknowledge the indirect contributions of Denise G. Tate, Ph.D. and Andrew Haig, M.D., who were the primary contributors for the previous edition of this chapter; selected information from that chapter have been included in this new one. In addition, Dr. Meade would like to extend her thanks to Drs. Brian McMahon, Allen Lewis, and Paul Wehman for their collegiality, discussion, and collaboration on many of the topics addressed in this chapter. Further support came from the National Institute on Disability and Rehabilitation Research (NIDRR), Office of Special Education and Rehabilitative Services (OSERS), Department of Education, Washington, DC, through their funding of the University of Michigan SCI Model System (H133N060032) and the Southeastern Regional Spinal Cord Injury Model System at Shepherd Center (H133N060009), Center on Health Outcomes Research and Capacity Building for Underserved Populations with SCI and TBI (H133A080064), and the UMHS-AACIL Advanced Rehabilitation Research Training Program (grants H133P090008 and H133P030004).

References

1. Crisp R. Vocational decision making by sixty spinal cord injury patients. *Paraplegia* 1992;30(6):420–424.
2. Krause JS, Anson CA. Adjustment after spinal cord injury: Relationship to participation in employment or educational activities. *Rehabil Counsel Bull* 1997;40(3):202–214.
3. Krause JS. Employment after spinal cord injury. *Arch Phys Med Rehabil* 1992;73(2):163–169.
4. Krause JS, Anson CA. Employment after spinal cord injury: relation to selected participant characteristics. *Arch Phys Med Rehabil* 1996;77(8):737–743.
5. Krause JS. Employment after spinal cord injury: Transition and life adjustment. *Rehabil Counsel Bull* 1996;39(4):244–255.
6. Krause JS. The relationship between productivity and adjustment following spinal cord injury. *Rehabil Counsel Bull.* 1990;33(3):188–199.
7. Lin KH, Chuang CC, Kao MJ, et al. Quality of life of spinal cord injured patients in Taiwan: a subgroup study. *Spinal Cord* 1997;35(12):841–849.
8. Livneh H. Person-environment congruence—a rehabilitation perspective. *Int J Rehabil Res* 1987;10(1):3–19.
9. Social Security Administration. *Supplemental Security Income (SSI)*. Vol SSA Publication No. 05-I1000. Washington, DC; 2007.
10. Krause JS. Longitudinal changes in adjustment after spinal cord injury: a 15-year study. *Arch Phys Med Rehabil* 1992;73(6):564–568.
11. Krause JS, Sternberg M, Maides J, et al. Employment after spinal cord injury: Differences related to geographic region, gender, and race. *Arch Phys Med Rehabil* 1998;79(6):615–624.
12. Krause JS. Spinal cord injury and its rehabilitation. *Curr Opin Neurol Neurosurg* 1992;5(5):669–672.
13. Social Security Administration. *2008 Red Book: A summary guide to employment supports for individuals with disabilities under the social security disability insurance and supplemental security income programs.* Vol SSA Pub. No. 64–030. Washington, DC; 2008.
14. Krause JS, Kewman D, DeVivo MJ, et al. Employment after spinal cord injury: an analysis of cases from the Model Spinal Cord Injury Systems. *Arch Phys Med Rehabil* 1999;80(11):1492–1500.
15. Athanasou JA, Brown DJ, Murphy GC. Vocational achievements following spinal cord injury in Australia. *Disabil Rehabil* 1996;18(4):191–196.
16. Murphy GC, McDonald L, McDonald S. Test-retest reliability of information about employment provided in surveys by people with spinal cord injuries. *Psychol Rep.* 1997;81(1):25–26.

17. Young AE, Murphy GC. A social psychology approach to measuring vocational rehabilitation intervention effectiveness. *J Occup Rehabil*. 2002;12(3):175–189.
18. Murphy GC, Young AE. Employment participation following spinal cord injury: relation to selected participant demographic, injury and psychological characteristics. *Disabil Rehabil* 2005;27(21):1297–1306.
19. Devivo MJ, Fine PR. Employment status of spinal-cord injured patients 3 years after injury. *Arch Phys Med Rehabil* 1982;63(5):200–203.
20. DeVivo MJ, Rutt RD, Stover SL, et al. Employment after spinal cord injury. *Arch Phys Med Rehabil* 1987;68(8):494–498.
21. Krause JS, Kjorsvig JM. Mortality after spinal cord injury: a four-year prospective study. [Erratum appears in Arch Phys Med Rehabil 1992 Aug;73(8):716]. *Arch Phys Med Rehabil* 1992;73(6):558–563.
22. Krause JS. Adjustment to life after spinal-cord injury—a comparison among 3 participant groups based on employment status. *Rehabil Counsel Bull* 1992;35(4):218–229.
23. Krause JS, Vines CL, Farley TL, et al. An exploratory study of pressure ulcers after spinal cord injury: relationship to protective behaviors and risk factors. *Arch Phys Med Rehabil* 2001;82(1):107–113.
24. Clayton KS, Chubon RA. Factors associated with the quality of life of long-term spinal cord injured persons. *Arch Phys Med Rehabil* 1994;75(6):633–638.
25. Wehman P, Wilson K, Parent W, et al. Employment satisfaction of individuals with spinal cord injury. *Am J Phys Med Rehabil* 2000;79(2):161–169.
26. Chapin MH, Kewman DG. Factors affecting employment following spinal cord injury: A qualitative study. *Rehabil Psychol* 2001;46(4):400–416.
27. Meade MA, Barrett K, Ellenbogen PS, et al. Work intensity and variations in health and personal characteristics of individuals with spinal cord injury. *J Vocational Rehabil* 2006;25(1):13–19.
28. Hess D, Meade M, Forchheimer M, et al. Psychological well-being and intensity of employment following spinal cord injury. *Top Spinal Cord Inj* 2004;9(4):1–10.
29. Anderson D, Dumont S, Azzaria L, et al. Determinants of return to work among spinal cord injury patients: a literature review. *J Vocational Rehabil* 2007;27(1):57–68.
30. Yasuda S, Wehman P, Targett P, et al. Return to work after spinal cord injury: a review of recent research. *Neurorehabilitation* 2002;17(3):177–186.
31. Krause JS, Terza JV. Injury and demographic factors predictive of disparities in earnings after spinal cord injury. *Arch Phys Med Rehabil* 2006;87(10):1318–1326.
32. Krause JS, Terza JV, Dismuke C. Earnings among people with spinal cord injury. *Arch Phys Med Rehabil* 2008;89(8):1474–1481.
33. Krause JS, Reed, KS, Obtaining Employment After Spinal Cord Injury: Relationship with Pre- and Postinjury Education. 2009; 53(1):27–33.
34. Murphy GC, Young AE, Brown DJ, et al. Explaining labor force status following spinal cord injury: the contribution of psychological variables. *J Rehabil Med* 2003;35(6):276–283.
35. Mcshane SL, Karp J. Employment following spinal-cord injury—a covariance structure-analysis. *Rehabil Psychol* 1993;38(1):27–40.
36. Decker S, Schultz R. Correlates of life satisfaction and depression in middle-aged and elderly spinal cord injured persons. *Am J Occup Ther* 1985;39:740–745.
37. Jackson M, Meade M, Ellenbogen P, et al. Perspectives on networking, cultural values, and skills among African American men with SCI: A Reconsideration of Social Capital Theory. *J Vocat Rehabil* 2006;25(1):21–33.
38. Meade M, Jackson M, Barrett K, et al. *Needs assessment of virginians with spinal cord injury: final report—findings and recommendations*. Richmond, VA: Virginia Commonwealth University, Spring 2006.
39. Harmon LW, Hansen JC, Borgen FH, et al. *Strong interest inventory: applications and technical guide*. Stanford, CA: Stanford University Press, 1994.
40. Fouad NA, Mohler CJ. Cultural Validity of Holland's Theory and the Strong Interest Inventory for Five Racial/Ethnic Groups. *J Career Assess* 2004;12(4):423–439.
41. Rohe DE, Athelstan GT. Vocational interests of persons with spinal-cord injury. *J Counsel Psychol* 1982;29(3):283–291.
42. Rohe DE, Athelstan GT. Change in vocational interests after spinal-cord injury. *Rehabil Psychol* 1985;30(3):131–143.
43. Rohe DE, Krause J. Stability of interests after severe physical disability: An 11 year longitudinal study. *J Vocat Behav* 1998;52(1):45–58.
44. Bordieri J, Drehmer D. Causal attribution and hiring recommendations for the disabled job applicants. *Rehabil Psychol* 1988;33:239–247.
45. Bordieri J, Drehmer D, Taricone P. Personnel selection bias for job applicants with cancer. *J Appl Soc Psychol* 1990;20:244–253.
46. Krause JS. Self-reported problems after spinal cord injury: Implications for rehabilitation practice. *Top Spinal Cord Inj Rehabil* 2007;12(3):35–44.
47. Meade MA, Lewis A, Jackson MN, et al. Race, employment, and spinal cord injury. *Arch Phys Med Rehabil* 2004;85(11):1782–1792.
48. West M, Hock T, Wittig K. Getting to work: training and support for transportation needs. *J Vocational Rehabil* 1998;10(2):159–167.
49. Krause JS, Pickelsimer E. Relationship of perceived barriers to employment and return to work five years later: a pilot study among 343 participants with spinal cord injury. *Rehabil Counsel Bull* 2008;51(2):118–121.
50. Engel S, Murphy GS, Athanasou JA, et al. Employment outcomes following spinal cord injury. *Int J Rehabil Res* 1998;21(2):223–229.
51. Tomassen PC, Post MW, van Asbeck FW. Return to work after spinal cord injury. *Spinal Cord* 2000;38(1):51–55.
52. Rubin SE, Roessler RT. *Foundations of the vocational rehabilitation process*. 5th ed. Austin, TX: PRO-ED, 2001.
53. Lustig DC, Stauser DR, Rice ND, et al. The relationship between working alliance and rehabilitation outcomes. *Rehabil Counsel Bull* 2002;46(1):25–33.
54. Turner E, Revell G, Brooke V. *Personal assistance in the workplace: a customer-directed guide manual*. Richmond, VA: VCU RRTC on Workplace Supports, 2001.
55. Kruse D, Krueger A, Drastal S. Computer use, computer training, and employment—outcomes among people with spinal cord injuries. *Spine* 1996;21(7):891–896.

56. McKinley W, Tewksbury MA, Sitter P, et al. Assistive technology and computer adaptations for individuals with spinal cord injury. *Neurorehabilitation* 2004;19(2):141–146.
57. Kosciulek JF. Theory of informed consumer choice in vocational rehabilitation. *Rehabil Educ* 2004;18(1):3–11.
58. Smart JF, Smart DW. Culturally sensitive informed choice in rehabilitation counseling. *J Appl Rehabil Counsel* 1997;28(2):32–37.
59. Kosciulek JF. Rehabilitation counseling with individuals with disabilities: an Empowerment framework. *Rehabil Educ* 2003;17(4):207–214.
60. Bricout JC. Using telework to enhance return to work outcomes for individuals with spinal cord injuries. *Neurorehabilitation* 2004;19(2):147–159.
61. Roessler R. Job retention services for employees with spinal cord injuries: a critical need in vocational rehabilitation. *J Appl Rehabil Counsel* 2001;32(1):3–9.
62. Turner E, Barrett JC. Providing Effective Workplace Personal Assistance Services. *PAS Facts*. Vol 3. VCU RRTC on Workplace Supports and Job Retention: Virginia Commonwealth University; 2007.
63. Rehabilitation Act of 1973: Public Law 93–112; 1973.
64. Americans with Disabilities Act of 1990.
65. Burris S, Moss K. A Road Map for ADA Title I Research. In: Blanck PD, ed. *Employment, disability, and the Americans with disabilities act: issues in law, public policy, and research*. Evanston, IL: Northwestern University Press, 2000:19–50.
66. Rehabilitation Act Amendments of 1992. Vol Public L. No. 102–569; 1992.
67. (EEOC) EEOC. www.eeoc.gov www.eeoc.gov/types/ada.html, 2008.
68. Murphy G, Brown D, Athanasou J, et al. Labour force participation and employment among a sample of Australian patients with a spinal cord injury. *Spinal Cord* 1997;35(4):238–244.
69. Hess DW, Ripley DL, McKinley WO, et al. Predictors for return to work after spinal cord injury: a 3-year multicenter analysis. *Arch Phys Med Rehabil*. 2000; 81(3):359–363.
70. James M, Devivo MJ, Richards JS. Post injury employment outcomes among african-american and white persons with spinal-cord injury. *Rehabil Psychol* 1993;38(3):151–164.
71. Young ME, Alfred WG, Rintala DH, Vocational status of persons with spinal-cord injury living in the community. *Rehabil Counsel Bull* 1994;37(3):229–243.
72. Olney MF, Kennedy J. Racial disparities in VR use and job placement rates for adults with disabilities. *Rehabil Counsel Bull* 2002;45(3):177–185.
73. Santiago AM, Villarruel FA, Leahy MJ. Latino access to rehabilitation services: evidence from Michigan. *Am Rehabil* 1996;22(1):10–17.
74. Walker S, Saravanabhavan RC, Williams V, et al. *An examination of the impact of federally supported community services and educational systems on underserved people with disabilities from diverse cultural populations*. Washington, DC: Howard University Research and Training Center for Access to Rehabilitation and Economic Opportunity, 1996.
75. Wilson K. Exploration of VR acceptance and ethnicity: a national investigation. *Rehabil Counsel Bull* 2002;45(3):168–176.
76. Wright TJ, Leung P. *Meeting the unique needs of minorities with disabilities: A report to the President and the Congress*. Washington, DC: National Council on Disability, 1993.
77. Moss K. Filing an ADA Employment Discrimination Charge: "Making It Work for You." 2000. www.mentalhealth.org/pblications/allpubs/SMA00-3471/default.asp. Published Last Modified Date. Accessed Dated Accessed. Oct 1, 2008.

CHAPTER 23 ■ SEXUAL FUNCTION AND FERTILITY AFTER SPINAL CORD INJURY

NANCY L. BRACKETT, CHARLES M. LYNNE, JENS SØNKSEN, AND DANA A. OHL

INTRODUCTION

In the United States, most spinal cord injuries (SCIs) occur to individuals between the ages of 16 and 45 years (1). Of those injured, the vast majority are male. Similar statistics are reported worldwide (2–7). As the most common causes of injury include motor vehicle accidents, violence, sports-related injuries, and falls, it has been assumed that the gender disparity is due to more men than women engaging in risk-taking behaviors. While this assumption has yet to be confirmed, some evidence suggests that hormones, rather than behavior, may contribute to the disparity. For example, it has been shown that estrogen may be neuroprotective and/or that testosterone may be neurotoxic after injury (8,9).

Although different authors use different terminology, sexual function and sexual rehabilitation after SCI focus on two important goals (10–13). One goal is the maximization and optimization of sexual function after SCI. The other goal is the adjustment or adaptation to the injury, including an understanding of the physiological changes that result from SCI. If the patient has a partner, a new physical, emotional, and logistical language of the relationship must be learned. Without a partner, these new languages must be learned as new relationships are explored and negotiated.

In many ways, societal changes over the last 20 years, combined with advancements in technology and pharmaceuticals, have improved adjustments to sexual life after SCI. A few examples are offered:

- The Americans with Disabilities Act of 1990 extended the antidiscrimination protections of the Civil Rights Act of 1964 to persons with disabilities (14).
- Aided by the popular media, today's society is often exposed to sexual issues. Evidence supporting this belief can be gleaned from students at the University of Miami. For the last 17 years, The Miami Project to Cure Paralysis Male Fertility Program has taught a class to medical students on the topic of human sexuality in people with disability. As part of this class, a volunteer panel of men and women with SCI discuss their experiences with sex, relationships, parenting, and any other issues of interest to the medical students. When the program began, students were somewhat amazed that persons with SCI could meet people, have sexual relationships, and father/conceive children. Today, these issues are not considered unusual by this group of students.
- The introduction in the late 1980s of pharmacoactive agents, which could be injected into the penis (15), and especially phosphodiesterase-5 (PDE-5) inhibitors in the late 1990s, has made information about erections widely available on the Internet.
- In 1995, a well-known actor, Christopher Reeve, sustained an SCI (16). Because of his widespread recognition, he made the life, struggles, needs, and goals of the SCI community a part of everyday life of the US public.

Christopher Reeve challenged medical researchers to listen to consumers and direct their research toward the needs of that community. Many researchers are responding. In a novel survey of the SCI community, Kim D. Anderson, Ph.D., presented a study "to determine what areas of functional recovery the SCI population would most like researchers to address in order to have a positive effect on their quality of life ...." Regaining sexual function was the highest priority among individuals with paraplegia, and the second highest priority, after regaining arm and hand function, among individuals with tetraplegia (17).

Accordingly, it is critical that the topics of sexual function and fertility be incorporated as part of any standard rehabilitation curriculum for patients, who will request this information at different times during their recovery. Some patients request information immediately after injury, whereas others may not request information for months or years after injury. It is important that caregivers, including nurses and therapists, as well as physicians, continually update their education regarding these important topics. At the very least, caregivers should be knowledgeable about professionals in their community to whom patients can be referred for this information.

SEXUAL FUNCTION IN WOMEN WITH SCI

Pelvic Innervation of Women

The pelvic nerve provides afferent innervation of the vagina, cervix, and rectum (18–20). Afferent sensory information from the genitalia to the spinal cord is relayed via the pudendal nerves (S2-4). Parasympathetic input to the genitalia is via the pelvic nerves (S2-4) and sympathetic input to the genitalia is via the hypogastric nerves (T10-L2). The hypogastric nerve conveys afferent activity from the uterus and cervix (18,20). Parasympathetic stimulation causes engorgement and swelling of the labia and clitoris, as well as vaginal lubrication. Sympathetic stimulation causes rhythmic contractions of the uterus, fallopian tubes, paraurethral glands, and pelvic floor musculature.

Although there is a low prevalence of women with SCI, several studies have addressed sexual function in this subpopulation. In women with SCI, the ability to perceive combined pinprick and sensory function in the T11-L2 dermatomes has been associated with maintenance of psychogenic genital vasocongestion (psychogenic arousal) (21–24). Reflex genital arousal has been associated with intact reflex function in the S2-4 dermatomes (25). In women with complete SCI above T6, psychogenic arousal can occur in the absence of genital vasocongestion (25). Vaginal lubrication can be diminished after SCI (26); a survey of 87 women with SCI found 48.3% reported adequate lubrication during sexual stimulation, 27.6% reported inadequate lubrication, and 24.1% were not sure. Respondents (48.3%) reported developing new areas of arousal above their level of injury, including the head, neck, and torso (27).

Some investigators have hypothesized that the vagus nerve may serve as a genital sensory pathway that bypasses the spinal cord and conveys vaginocervical afferent activity that can lead to orgasm (28). Along with other evidence, support for this idea came from women with complete SCI reporting genital sensations and orgasms (29,30). These reports were later confirmed in laboratory-based studies (31–33) and are supported by animal research showing that bilateral vagotomy abolishes vaginocervical mechanical stimulation (VCMS)-induced pupil dilation that persists after transection of the spinal cord at T7 in rats (34) or after deafferentation of all genitospinal sensory nerves known to innervate the vagina, cervix, and uterus (i.e., pelvic, pudendal, and hypogastric nerves) in rats (35). Furthermore, in women with complete interruption of the spinal cord above T10, that is, above the level of entry of all genitospinal nerves, VCMS has been shown by functional magnetic resonance imaging to activate the nucleus of the solitary tract, thus supporting a genital sensory role of the vagus nerves (28).

Sexual Activity in Women with SCI

The sexual lives of women with SCI are influenced by many emotional factors and physical limitations that may interfere with mental and physiologic sexual arousal. A review by Bughi (36) outlines some of the sexual issues experienced by women with SCI, including perceived loss of attractiveness, decreased sexual desire, fear of losing independence, muscle weakness, spasticity, spasms, tremor, contractures, and fear of losing bladder and bowel control. Medications such as codeine, tranquilizers, and antidepressants can lessen sexual desire (37).

Women with SCI reported that the primary reason for pursuing sexual activity was to fulfill a need for intimacy, and the second most commonly cited reason was to develop or maintain a relationship with a partner (27). Of respondents to an online survey, 96.9% reported they were able to have penetrative sexual intercourse and 92% had experienced vaginal penetration postinjury. Of the 8% who had not, all were women who experienced continuous chronic pain that significantly interfered with sexual activity. Factors that most often influenced difficulty with regard to intercourse were injury level (greater difficulties for cervical injuries), severe spasticity (during typical daily life), pain, spasticity, or autonomic dysreflexia (AD) during any type of sexual activity (27). Despite these limitations, more than 50% of women with SCI report weekly sexual activity (37).

A large study from centers located in Sweden, Denmark, Norway, Finland, and Iceland compared responses on a 104-item questionnaire between 545 women with SCI and 507 age-matched controls (38). Of women with SCI, 80% had engaged in sex after injury. Reasons for not wanting or not engaging in sexual activity were physical problems (such as decreased motility, problems with positioning, fear of bladder or bowel leaks), low sexual desire, low self-esteem, and feelings of being unattractive. The motivations of both groups of women (SCI and controls) to engage in sexual activity were primarily intimacy based rather than sexual. Frame of mind was important in determining receptiveness to stimulation before and during sexual activity.

Orgasm in Women with SCI

In a survey of 87 women with SCI (27), 41.4% of whom had genital sensation, 74.7% reported difficulty in becoming psychologically aroused, while 87.4% reported difficulty in becoming physically aroused. The ability to feel the buildup of sexual tension in the body was positively correlated with the presence of genital sensation, as well as the presence of AD during sexual activity. Among respondents, 82.8% had experienced orgasm preinjury and 93.1% had attempted to reach orgasm postinjury; however, only 46% reported successfully achieving orgasm after injury. Ability to achieve orgasm was associated with presence of genital sensation and spasticity (27). Women with SCI report achieving orgasm primarily through stimulation of the genitalia and breasts (37).

Assessing Sexual Dysfunction in Women with SCI

Clinicians require standard terminology to communicate effectively about spared autonomic function in persons with SCI. In 2004, the American Spinal Injury Association (ASIA) appointed a working group to develop a standard nomenclature to describe the impact of SCI on sexual functioning in women. The resulting document suggested guidelines for describing the presence of psychogenic arousal, reflex arousal, orgasm, and sexual dysfunction in women with SCI (39).

Because of the importance of preserved sensation in the T11-L2 dermatomes in predicting psychogenic arousal, and preserved sensation in the S2-5 dermatomes for predicting reflex genital arousal and orgasm, it is recommended that clinicians performing neurological examinations give special attention to evaluation of these dermatomes. Women with intact bulbocavernosus and/or anal wink reflexes should be able to experience orgasm, whereas women without S2-5 sensation or absent bulbocavernosus and anal wink reflexes should not. When based on examination and historical report, it is recommended that psychogenic arousal, reflex arousal, and orgasm each be assigned as present, possible though partially impaired, or absent (Table 23.1) (39).

Sexual dysfunction is unique from other physiological dysfunctions because alterations in response are not considered problematic unless they cause personal distress (40). It is thus recommended that sexual dysfunction be separately categorized as "present" or "absent." If present, the type of disorder (desire, arousal, orgasmic, pain) should be indicated (Table 23.1) (39).

TABLE 23.1

CHARACTERISTICS OF SEXUAL RESPONSES IN FEMALES AFTER SCI

Function	Primary response options	Subclassification
Genital arousal		
Psychogenic	Present, possible though impaired, absent	—
Reflex	Present, possible though impaired, absent	—
Orgasm	Present, possible though impaired, absent	—
Sexual dysfunction	Present, absent	Desire, arousal, orgasmic, or pain dysfunction

Genital arousal. Increased genital vasocongestion that usually manifests itself with presence of clitoral engorgement and vaginal lubrication, amongst other signs.

Orgasm. Perception of sensation of feeling good from sexual stimulation, reaching climax, after which a person with SCI feels satisfied and no longer desires further sexual stimulation. May be accompanied by an overall increase and then decrease in muscle tone.

Psychogenic genital arousal. Increased genital vasocongestion that occurs solely based on arousal in brain, e.g., through hearing, seeing, feeling, or imagining erotic thoughts.

Reflex genital arousal. Increased genital vasocongestion that occurs solely based on genital or sacral stimulation.

Sexual dysfunction. Alteration in aspect of sexual functioning that results in personal distress. If present, one should also indicate the type of disorder: desire, arousal, orgasmic, or pain.

In 2004, the ASIA appointed a working group to develop a standard nomenclature to describe the impact of SCI on sexual functioning in women. The document resulting from this work suggests guidelines for describing the presence of psychogenic arousal, reflex arousal, orgasm, and sexual dysfunction in women with SCI.

Adapted from Alexander MS, Bodner D, Brackett NL, et al. Development of international standards to document sexual and reproductive functions after spinal cord injury: preliminary report. *J Rehabil Res Dev* 2007;44:83–90.

Treating Sexual Dysfunction in Women with SCI

The role of counseling and rehabilitation programs are important components in addressing psychological issues related to sexuality after SCI. A holistic, developmental team approach to care is recommended to address the acute and long-term sexual rehabilitation needs of women with SCI. By assisting individuals through the adaptation process and promoting a positive, yet realistic self-concept, clinicians can mitigate potential problems in body image disturbances, decreased self-esteem, and gender-specific sexuality issues (38,41–43).

Several laboratory-based studies have investigated treatment of sexual dysfunction in women with SCI. In a study examining the therapeutic effects of sildenafil, 19 premenopausal women with SCI were randomly assigned to receive sildenafil (50 mg) or placebo in a double-blind, crossover design. Physiologic and subjective measures of sexual response, heart rate, and blood pressure were recorded during baseline and sexual stimulation conditions. The results showed significant increases in subjective arousal when using both drug and sexually stimulating conditions, and borderline significant ($p < 0.07$) effect of drug administration on vaginal pulse amplitude. Maximal responses occurred when sildenafil was combined with visual and manual sexual stimulation. Cardiovascular data showed modest increases in heart rate (4 to 5 beats minute) and mild decreases in blood pressure (2 to 4 mm Hg) across all stimulation conditions, consistent with the peripheral vasodilatory mechanism of the drug. Sildenafil was well tolerated and without evidence of significant adverse effects (44).

Another study examined the use of positive feedback as a means to augment sexual arousal in 37 women with SCI. Heart rate, respiratory rate, vaginal pulse amplitude, and subjective level of arousal were sampled at regular intervals during a protocol, which consisted of positive feedback or neutral feedback after periods of audiovisual erotic stimulation. Positive feedback consisted of a research assistant bringing an obviously high, but false, vaginal pulse amplitude tracing to the subject, telling her that this was her vaginal response from the last segment, that she was doing great and should continue to do the same. Neutral feedback consisted of the research assistant bringing an unremarkable tracing and telling the subject she was doing OK, but that she should try harder next time. The results showed that positive feedback increased subjective sexual arousal. Physiological responses also indicated increased responsiveness to positive feedback. Subjects with greater preservation of sensory function in the T11-L2 dermatomes, and thus a greater ability to have psychogenic genital vasocongestion, had a greater degree of genital responsiveness than subjects with minimal or no sensory preservation in those dermatomes. Overall, the findings supported the use of audiovisual feedback to augment subjective sexual arousal (24).

A similar study examined anxiety-eliciting audiovisual stimuli as a means of increasing sexual arousal in women with SCI (23). The study was based on findings in the nondisabled population showing that generalized arousal of the sympathetic nervous system elicited by preexposure to anxiety-provoking videos increased sexual responsiveness (45). The results of testing in 45 women with SCI showed that women with low sensory scores in the T11-L2 dermatomes achieved a slight increase in vaginal pulse amplitude to audiovisual erotic stimulation after anxiety preexposure than after neutral preexposure. Anxiety preexposure consisted of viewing 3 minutes of an anxiety-producing video, such as a child about to be hit by a train. Neutral preexposure consisted of viewing 3 minutes of a travelogue. Preexposure periods were followed by viewing 6 minutes of an erotic video. In contrast to women with low sensory scores in the T11-L2 dermatomes, women with SCI who maintained a high degree of preservation of sensory function in the T11-L2 dermatomes, as well as nondisabled controls, showed no specific effects of the anxiety manipulation (23).

FERTILITY IN WOMEN WITH SCI

Gender has a significant effect on fertility after SCI. Women with SCI can conceive and deliver children with nearly the same success rate as the general population (46). However, the majority of men with SCI are infertile, with only an estimated 10% retaining the ability to father children by sexual intercourse (47). These gender differences, and the disproportionate ratio of males to females with SCI, have focused the literature on reproductive function following SCI on the male gender. The medical literature on female reproductive function after SCI is scant. Testament to this paucity is the continuing practice of describing single case reports of pregnancy in women with SCI (48–50) (a practice now rarely undertaken when describing fertility outcomes in men with SCI). Because pregnant women with SCI are few in number compared to pregnant women in the general population, such cases often capture media attention (51–53).

Menstrual Function in Women with SCI

Amenorrhea is a common complication following SCI, affecting 41% to 85% of patients (36,37,54). Menstruation returns within 6 months after acute SCI in 50% of women, while 90% of women with SCI recover normal menstrual cycles within 12 months after injury (21,37,55). Menarche occurs normally in preadolescent girls with SCI (56), while women who are perimenopausal at the time of their injury may experience complete cessation of menses (36,57).

According to a review by Bughi et al. (36), the disruption of reproductive function in women with SCI is a consequence of "stress response complex" (58). Following a traumatic event, the pituitary gland displays two secretory patterns: increase of corticotrophin, prolactin, and growth hormone and decrease of luteinizing hormone (LH), follicle-stimulating hormone (FSH), and thyroid-stimulating hormone (59). The increase of corticotropin, and subsequently cortisol secretion, suppresses the pituitary response to gonadotropin-releasing hormone with subsequent decrease in LH and FSH (58). These changes occur in the first few hours or days after trauma and persist for the duration of acute critical illness, representing an adaptive response to injury (59).

Pregnancy in Women with SCI

Once normal menstruation resumes, women with SCI can become pregnant by sexual intercourse with similar success rates as the general population (60). However, pregnancy in women with SCI poses unique challenges. Reports of management issues have, to date, been anecdotal or have included only a small case series. Patients are typically placed into high risk categories due to their potential inability to detect sensations that may signal problems with the pregnancy. A comprehensive discussion of the obstetric management of women with SCI has been presented by Pereira (61). Careful management of the patient is recommended during all phases of pregnancy, including preconception, prenatal, intrapartum, and postpartum. An interdisciplinary team should monitor the patient to treat chronic SCI-related medical conditions, including asymptomatic bacteriuria, constipation, pressure ulcers, hyperthermia or hypothermia, anemia, orthostatic hypotension, and AD. Careful monitoring during labor and delivery is especially critical, as AD is most likely to occur during this period.

In women with SCI, the onset of AD during labor is intermittently timed with uterine contractions (62). A systematic review of the management of AD after SCI concluded the following: "With vaginal delivery or when caesarean delivery or instrumental delivery is indicated, adequate anesthesia (spinal or epidural if possible) is needed. There is level 4 evidence (from a single case series (63) and two observational studies (64,65)) that epidural anesthesia is preferred and may be effective for most patients with AD during labor and delivery" (66).

Skowronski and Hartman reviewed 25 years of experience at a university teaching hospital, which also housed a regional SCI center. They reported their experience with seven pregnancies in five tetraplegic women. All these women experienced recurrent UTI and episodes of AD during pregnancy, often requiring hospitalization. All pregnancies entered labor spontaneously (mean 37.9 weeks of gestation). Two required caesarian section. No serious perinatal problems were seen. Episodes of AD were managed with epidural anesthesia or sublingual nifedipine (67).

A review of studies indicated that the rate of spontaneous vaginal delivery in women with SCI was 37%, with an additional 31% of deliveries accomplished by assisted vaginal delivery, and the remaining 32% delivered by cesarean delivery. The rate of spontaneous vaginal delivery, however, is probably higher in patients whose neurological level of injury is below T6, whereas patients whose level is above T6 are more likely to develop AD and require assisted deliveries (61).

Breast feeding is possible in mothers with SCI, although a study found that women who breast fed preinjury were less likely to breast feed after injury (68). The reasons that fewer women breast feed after becoming injured are unclear but may be due to difficulties in holding the nursing infant or due to decreased milk production (46). A case of AD triggered by breast feeding has been reported (69).

The American College of Obstetrics and Gynecology has published a Committee Opinion on "Obstetric Management of Patients with Spinal Cord Injuries," which briefly addresses AD as well as a number of other issues (70). Clinically, AD may have a broad spectrum of symptoms, or even no symptoms, in the presence of significantly elevated blood pressure. Its most dangerous feature, significant hypertension, is also shared with preeclampsia, a serious complication of pregnancy and the leading cause of maternal and fetal morbidity. In women with SCI, preeclampsia and AD may be distinguished from each other by their clinical features. AD is seen in patients whose level of injury is T6 or higher. AD may occur at any time during pregnancy in response to a noxious stimulus below the level of injury. AD is usually episodic and disappears when the stimulus is treated or removed. During labor, AD may occur in conjunction with uterine contractions. With AD, hypertension is often accompanied by bradycardia, a most unusual clinical combination (65,70).

Little has been reported on the occurrence of preeclampsia in the SCI population. In the general population, preeclampsia is rare before the 20th week of pregnancy and is characterized by hypertension and proteinuria. It usually is not episodic. Multiorgan systemic involvement may be seen with liver, renal, and hematologic disturbances. There is no specific treatment except removal of the placenta, that is, delivery of the fetus as early as possible while efforts are made to stabilize the mother and hasten the maturity of the fetal lungs. Numerous tests have been described to allow early diagnosis of this condition and to identify those at risk. Unfortunately, there is still no general agreement about which tests are the most efficacious (71). It is possible that as more reliable markers of preeclampsia are discovered, they may become useful in the instance of the female patient whose neurological level of injury is T6 or rostral, and who is also suspected of being preeclamptic where the diagnosis cannot be made on clinical grounds.

Parenting by Individuals with SCI

Research on parents with SCI and their children indicates positive outcomes. For example, in a study comparing the parenting styles of 62 individuals with SCI and 62 individuals without SCI, there was no difference in the parenting factors of warmth/structure and strictness. The children in this study (ages 6 to 13) did not differ in social competence or behavior problems (72). In a study of 310 volunteers (88 mothers with SCI, 46 partners, 31 children, versus matched controls: 84 nondisabled mothers, 33 partners, 28 children), no significant differences between mothers with and without SCI in the outcomes measured, including five subscales of the Dyadic Adjustment Scale, three subscales of the Bem Sex Role Inventory, the Index of Self-Esteem, seven subscales of the McMaster Family Assessment Device, and the three subscales of the Kansas Parenting Satisfaction Scale. It was concluded that children of mothers with SCI experience characteristic individual adjustment, attitudes toward their parents, self-esteem, gender roles, and family functioning (73).

SEXUAL FUNCTION IN MEN WITH SCI

In contrast to the innate fertility capacity of most women with SCI, most men with SCI are unable to father children without medical assistance. Erectile dysfunction, ejaculatory dysfunction, and semen abnormalities are the chief contributors to this condition.

Pelvic Innervation in Men

To understand how SCI impacts on sexual dysfunction, it is important to appreciate the complex and sometimes confusing concepts of the neural regulation of the genitalia (Fig. 23.1). The sacral reflex arc of S2-4 is fundamental in neural control of erection. Autonomic (parasympathetic) fibers from neurons at this level (later identified as "lower motor neurons") originate as preganglionic fibers that enter the pelvic nerve. The pelvic nerve then enters the pelvic plexus. Postganglionic sympathetic fibers (T10-L2), via the hypogastric nerve, also enter the pelvic plexus. The cavernous nerves leave the pelvic plexus to provide autonomic innervation of the corpora cavernosa, which are important structures for erection. The dorsal nerve of the penis, via the pudendal nerve (S2-4), provides somatic sensory afferents into the reflex arc (178).

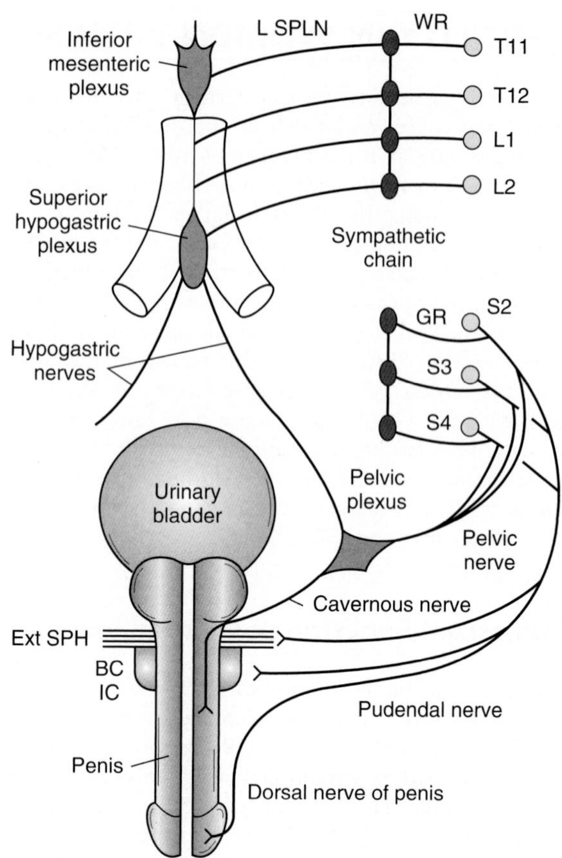

FIGURE 23.1 Pelvic innervation of the male. (Adapted from De Groat WC, Steers WD. Neuroanatomy and neurophysiology of penile erection. In: Tanagho EA, Lue TF, McClure RD, eds. Contemporary management of impotence and infertility. Baltimore, MD: Williams & Wilkins, 1988:3–27.)

Various supraspinal stimuli of the senses, such as visual, olfactory, and auditory as well as imaginative, are probably mediated via the hypothalamus, and descend to and facilitate thoracolumbar (sympathetic) outflow creating a pathway for neural input to the penis. This input, which is not dependent on the S2-4 reflex arc, is thought to be responsible for the origination of psychogenic erections (74).

Erectile Dysfunction in Men with SCI

Depending on the degree of severity and completeness of SCI, a man with an upper motor neuron (UMN) lesion (i.e., one that disrupts the spinal cord above the thoracolumbar level) will typically have preserved reflexogenic erections with minimal capacity for psychogenic erections. Lower motor neuron (LMN) lesions involving the S2-4 spinal cord segments or lesions of the conus or cauda equina involving the S2-4 efferents typically eliminate reflexogenic erections, (178) and often greatly diminish capacity to achieve psychogenic erections. It is important to note that SCIs are not always discrete lesions, and varying patterns of genital innervation and erectile capacities commonly occur. Even when erectile function is maintained, especially reflexogenic erections, they are often unreliable, of limited duration, and/or insufficiently rigid to achieve successful intercourse.

TABLE 23.2

ERECTIONS IN MEN WITH SCI

		Type of Erection	
Level of injury	% with erections	Psychogenic	Reflexogenic
Complete UMN	93	9%	95%
Incomplete UMN	99	48%	93%
Complete LMN	26	24%	12%
Incomplete LMN	90	Insufficient data	Insufficient data

UMN, upper motor neuron; LMN, lower motor neuron.
Adapted from Bors E, Comarr AE. Neurological disturbances of sexual function with special reference to 529 patients with spinal cord injury. Urol Surv 1960;10:191–222. Comarr AE. Sexual function among patients with spinal cord injury. *Urol Int* 1970;25:134–168.

Immediately after SCI, there is a period of spinal shock during which no reflex activity below the level of injury occurs. Although the period of spinal shock is variable, 80% of men with SCI will regain erectile function by one year postinjury, and the majority of these will occur in the first 6 months (75,76). The frequency and origin of erections in men with various upper and LMN lesions are summarized in Table 23.2.

Within the corpora cavernosa, a good arterial blood supply is necessary for the vascular processes that cause erection. Briefly, rapid smooth muscle relaxation of the arterioles allows rapid filling of the cavernous sinusoidal spaces, exceeding the rate of venous drainage. The expansion of the cavernous bodies causes further venous occlusion through compression of the expanding corpora by its outer container, the tunica albuginea. This process is initiated by the neurotransmitter nitric oxide crossing into the (arteriolar) smooth muscle cell. Nitric oxide activates guanyl cyclase causing the production of cyclic GMP, a potent vasodilator of the arterioles and the venous sinuses. Cyclic AMP may also act as a vasodilator. PDE-5 breaks down cyclic GMP to end the biochemical cycle (77). This knowledge has formed the basis for much of what we now know about the pharmacologic management of erectile dysfunction in men with SCI, as well as in non-SCI men with erectile dysfunction.

Treatment of Erectile Dysfunction in Men with SCI

Currently, about 80% of men with SCI will have their erectile dysfunction treated or managed with a PDE-5 inhibitor. Successful treatment in this high percent of patients is a relatively new development. For example, in their classic paper from 1960, Bors and Comarr described sexual dysfunction in all types of neurogenic disturbances, including SCI (47).Nearly 20 years passed until the first treatment for erectile dysfunction was described in men with SCI (78). This treatment, the penile prosthesis, initiated an ongoing effort to improve erectile dysfunction men with SCI.

At least five treatment alternatives are currently available to men with SCI. They include penile implants, vacuum erection devices, vasoactive intracavernosal injections, intraurethral alprostadil, and oral PDE-5 inhibitors. Topical applications of vasoactive substances to the penis, such as prostaglandin E-1 (PGE-1), minoxidil, papaverine, and nitroglycerin have been tried, but without much success or enthusiasm (77,79).

Penile Prosthesis

The penile prosthesis was the first significant treatment for erectile dysfunction to become available for men with SCI. In the mid to late 1970s, experience accumulated on the use of penile prostheses for erectile dysfunction and/or for condom catheter stability (78). As more long-term follow-up papers were published, it became clear that the prostheses produced satisfactory results in 60% to 80% of cases for erectile dysfunction and over 90% of cases for urinary management. High complication rates (15% to 20%) were also reported, especially in the earlier years with the use of noninflatable prostheses, although, complication rates with use of inflatable prostheses were lower. For example, in one series, the perforation rate for the three-piece inflatable prosthesis was 0% (80–82). In another patient series, Wilson and Delk published their experience with 1,337 consecutive implantations of inflatable penile prostheses (83). In the category of first implants, patients with diabetes had a 3% infection rate, SCI patients had a 9% infection rate, 5 of 10 patients on steroids became infected, and the infection rate for all other patients was 1%.

Vacuum Erection Device

In the mid to late 1980s, the vacuum erection device was reported to be an effective noninvasive method of managing erectile dysfunction in men with SCI (84). A vacuum created in a rigid container inserted over the penis drew blood into the penis, creating varying degrees of tumescence. A constricting ring or band was pulled tightly over the base of the penis to maintain the erection. An erection considered satisfactory for intercourse was reportedly achieved in 90% of users (84–86). When used regularly, it is the most cost-effective method of treating erectile dysfunction. Complications are usually related to the constriction band (85–87). Although fairly safe and effective, the device detracts from the already compromised spontaneity of sexual relations, is unwieldy, and for men with poor hand function requires the presence of a partner willing to be trained and participate in its use. Patients who are insensate in the genital area must be especially cautious with its use.

Intracavernous Injection

In 1982, Virag reported on the intracavernous injection of papaverine for erectile failure (88). Since that time, various combinations of vasoactive agents have been described, either alone or in combinations. These agents include papaverine, phentolamine, and alprostadil. (Alprostadil is the pharmaceutical name for PGE-1.) In general, the response rate for achieving erections has been over 90% (89–91). Currently, alprostadil is the only FDA-approved medicine for intracavernosal pharmacotherapy.

The advantage of injecting alprostadil intracavernosally is that this method works rapidly and is not dependent on the nitric oxide-PDE-5 system of maintaining high intracavernous levels of cyclic GMP (since PGE-1 stimulates higher levels of cyclic AMP, another potent vasodilator within the corpora cavernosa) (15,74,89,90). Adverse effects include hypotension, bleeding/bruising/pain/fibrosis at the injection site, and priapism, especially if the dose is not carefully titrated. As in the use of vacuum erection devices, men with poor hand function may have difficulty administering injections without help, or may be dependent on a partner who is trained and willing to give the injections.

Intraurethral Application

Alprostadil, when formulated as a small suppository (MUSE), may also be administered intraurethrally. The MUSE study group reported response rates in the 60% to 70% range (92). Subsequent reports of office procedures were disappointing, as were reports of its use in men with SCI. For example, undesirable outcomes included less than satisfactory erections, pain in the urethra, and hypotension if MUSE was not administered with a constricting band at the proximal penile shaft (93,94). Though not as efficacious as intracavernosal injection of PGE-1, administration of MUSE is less invasive and this feature may cause it to be more attractive to some patients.

PDE-5 Inhibitors

The role of nitric oxide on the production of cyclic GMP, a potent vasodilator, and PDE (which degrades cyclic GMP), has been described. Proper functioning of this system is essential for erectile function. In the mid-1990s, a report from the Pfizer Central Research Lab in the United Kingdom noted that PDE-5 seemed to be the most important of the PDE isoenzymes for inactivating cyclic GMP. They further noted that a novel oral agent, sildenafil (Viagra), was a selective inhibitor of PDE-5. Sildenafil was noted to have "suitable pharmacodynamic properties," such as a relatively short half-life, and no significant effects on heart rate and blood pressure. Further, in a clinical study of 12 patients with erectile dysfunction, it enhanced duration and rigidity of erection (95).

The Pfizer researchers felt that sildenafil held promise as "a new and effective treatment" for erectile dysfunction (95). Viagra was approved by the FDA in 1998 for the treatment of erectile dysfunction, becoming the first oral medication so designated. Also in 1998, Derry et al., (96) at the National Spinal Injury Centre, Stoke Mandeville, UK, reported on the safety and efficacy of oral sildenafil in a group of patients with SCI. A later literature review reiterated the safety and efficacy of oral sildenafil with reported improvement in erectile function in up to 94% of patients. No symptoms of AD were reported (97).

Since the introduction of Viagra, two other PDE-5 inhibitors have been approved: vardenafil (Levitra) and tadalafil (Cialis). Although less studied, they appear to have similar safety and efficacy profiles in men with SCI (98,99). Common side effects of the PDE-5 inhibitors include stuffy nose, headache, blue vision (Viagra), and back pain (Cialis). Priapism is rare. Since the PDE-5 inhibitors operate on the nitric oxide–induced cyclic GMP system, they may be less effective in men with LMN lesions where reflexogenic erections are rare. It is important to remember that PDE-5 inhibitors do not cause erections (as do intracavernosal injections) but help maintain erections via maintenance of intracavernosal levels of cyclic GMP.

PDE-5 inhibitors may be additive in their vasodilatory effects when combined with other systemic medicines commonly used for treatment of hypertension, and must therefore be used with caution in patients taking alpha adrenergic blockers. PDE-5 inhibitors are contraindicated in patients taking nitrates for angina or coronary artery disease. Since the majority of men sustaining an SCI are young with few (or no) comorbidities, the PDE-5 inhibitors have proven to be, in general, both safe and effective in this population and have become the treatment of choice for their erectile dysfunction.

Ejaculatory Function in Men with SCI

The majority of men with SCI are unable to ejaculate during sexual intercourse (100). Methods are available to improve or overcome this anejaculation, and the choice of method depends on the purpose of the ejaculation. For example, the method of penile vibratory stimulation (PVS) is available to assist ejaculation for sexual pleasure (101). If semen retrieval is required for use in assisted reproductive technologies (ARTs), additional procedures are available, including electroejaculation (EEJ), prostate massage (PM), and surgical sperm retrieval (SSR). The methods of PVS, EEJ, PM, and SSR, and the algorithms for their uses, are discussed below.

Penile Vibratory Stimulation

PVS involves placing a vibrator on the dorsum or frenulum of the glans penis (Fig. 23.2) (102). Mechanical stimulation produced by the vibrator recruits the ejaculatory reflex to induce ejaculation (103). This method is more effective in men with an intact ejaculatory reflex, that is, men with a level of injury T10 or above (88% success rate) compared to men with a level of injury T11 and below (15% success rate) (104).

Although a wide variety of devices may be used to perform PVS, not all will successfully induce ejaculation in men with SCI (102). Vibrator amplitude has been shown to be predictive of ejaculatory success. For example, studies have consistently shown that an amplitude of 2.5 mm results in higher ejaculatory success rates than in lower vibration amplitudes (105,106). This research led to the development of a device specifically engineered to induce ejaculation in men with SCI (107).

The procedure of PVS has been well described (13,102,103) and will be briefly summarized here. For safety and ease in performing PVS, the patient is usually transferred from his wheelchair to an exam table or hospital bed. If transfer is problematic, PVS may be performed in a wheelchair for those having high cervical injuries, severe pain or extreme obesity, or those wearing spinal cord stabilization devices. PVS may be administered to any man with SCI, although certain medical conditions are relatively contraindicated. Patients with severe inflammation or irritation of the glans penis should abstain from treatment, as PVS may further irritate this condition. Patients with untreated hypertension or cardiac disease should

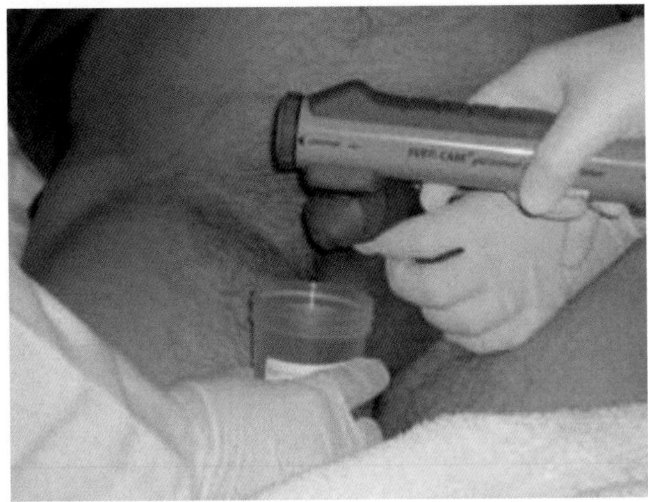

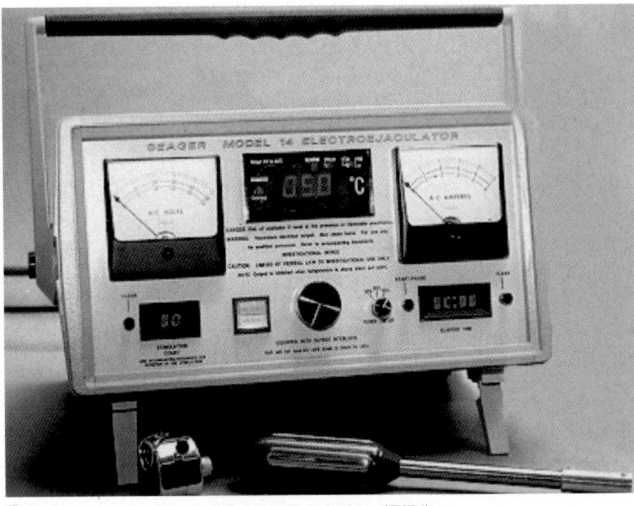

A Penile Vibratory Stimulation (PVS) B Electroejaculation (EEJ)

FIGURE 23.2 PVS and EEJ are two methods of collecting semen from anejaculatory men with SCI. In (A), an assistant holds a cup to collect semen for use in physician-ART. PVS may also be used by couples in private, as a means of sexual pleasure, or to collect semen for attempts at pregnancy by home insemination. (B) Shows the equipment used for EEJ, which can be used to successfully collect semen from the majority of men with SCI, including those who cannot respond to PVS.

also avoid this treatment, as PVS may increase blood pressure. If the patient has a penile prosthesis, PVS must be carefully monitored, because the pressure of the vibrator may push the glans onto the distal end of the prosthesis. Additionally, recently injured patients (i.e., less than 18 months) may not respond readily to PVS. PVS can provoke AD (108); therefore, patients with injury at T6 or higher should be pretreated with nifedipine, which is typically administered sublingually 15 minutes prior to stimulation onset. A dose of 20 mg is usually administered on the first trial of PVS, and adjusted on subsequent trials based on the patient's blood pressure during PVS. Blood pressure must be monitored continuously throughout the procedure. Hypotension with this nifedipine dosage is extremely rare, as most men with high-level SCI are already maximally vasodilated at rest.

The goal of PVS treatment is to activate the ejaculatory reflex in the thoracolumbar area of the spinal cord. The dorsal penile nerve must be intact (S2-4) for ejaculatory success (109). The vibrator is applied to the penis for 2 to 3 minutes or until antegrade ejaculation occurs. If no ejaculation occurs, the stimulation period is followed by a rest period of 1 to 2 minutes, and stimulation begins again. In patients who are responsive to PVS, the majority (89%) ejaculate within 2 minutes of stimulation onset (106).

If a patient is unable to ejaculate with a vibrator, additional methods may be employed to facilitate ejaculation with PVS, such as application of two vibrators (110), use of abdominal electrical stimulation in addition to PVS (111), or oral administration of Viagra prior to PVS (98).

The definition a PVS failure varies among practitioners. There is a degree of uncertainty about how many trials to administer, how many minutes per trial are optimal, or which methods, beyond use of multiple vibrators, should be tried before considering the patient or the trial a PVS failure. Studies have shown that SCI patients with a bulbocavernosus response and a hip flexor response are more likely to ejaculate with PVS than patients without these responses (112–114). In reality, the degree of effort and commitment to PVS will vary based on the skill and experience of the practitioner. Two consecutive failed PVS trials, spaced at least 1 week apart, typically define the patient as a PVS failure.

Unlike the methods of EEJ, SSR, and PM, PVS may be performed at home by selected couples. The couple should first be evaluated in a clinic prior to trying PVS at home. The evaluation should include assessment for risk of AD, assessment for optimal stimulation parameters to induce safe ejaculation in the given patient, and demonstration that the patient and/or his partner can perform the procedure properly (102).

Electroejaculation

Individuals who cannot respond to PVS are often referred for EEJ, which must be administered by a physician trained in this procedure. The method involves placement of a probe in the rectum, after which electric current delivered through the probe stimulates nerves that lead to emission of semen. The procedure of EEJ has been aptly described in the literature (100,115,116), and will be briefly summarized here.

EEJ is contraindicated for patients with inflammatory bowel disease involving the rectum, and patients on anticoagulation therapy who may have a bleeding diathesis. Rectoscopy may be performed to identify these preexisting mucosal abnormalities. The effect of EEJ on pacemakers is unknown; therefore, patients with pacemakers should be carefully considered before undergoing the procedure.

Immediately prior to EEJ, the bladder is prepared for retrograde ejaculation, which is common with EEJ (117,118). Because the acidic pH of urine is toxic to sperm, the bladder is emptied by urinary catheterization. A volume of 12 to 24 mL of buffered medium, such as sperm wash medium, may then be instilled through the catheter into the bladder. The catheterization is performed with a plastic catheter to avoid sperm adhesion commonly seen with silicone. Use of a nonspermicidal catheter lubricant is imperative.

As with PVS, EEJ can provoke AD and precautions must be taken to manage blood pressure. Recommendations for management of blood pressure during EEJ are the same as those recommended earlier in this chapter for PVS. The sole FDA-approved device for performing EEJ is the Seager Model 14 Electroejaculator (Dalzell Medical Systems, USA; Fig. 23.2). The device has a rheostat for controlling electrical delivery, and read-outs that show current delivery. A counting device tracks the number of stimulations, and a probe temperature is monitored. The device stops automatically if the temperature of the probe exceeds 38.5°C.

The patient is placed in lateral decubitus position to allow insertion of the rectal probe and collection of the semen from the urethra. The probe is inserted, so that the electrodes are just completely inside the anal verge, with electrodes facing anteriorly toward the prostate and seminal vesicles.

Electricity is delivered in a wave-like fashion. A recommended procedure is to peak at 5 V for the first stimulation, hold at that level for 5 seconds, and then abruptly turn off the current. A pause of 10 to 20 seconds is then allowed while observing muscular contractions peak and then cease. The next stimulation proceeds after complete cessation of contractions. The voltage is increased in 2.5 to 5 V increments every 1 to 2 stimulations. The procedure is stopped when further stimulations result in no more seminal emission, when the probe temperature exceeds 38.5°, or if the patient does not tolerate the procedure.

Interestingly, ejaculation during EEJ occurs during the rest period. Physiological studies of the events during EEJ suggest that peak skeletal muscular contraction may stimulate the ejaculatory reflex, and the reflex continues for several seconds after the stimulation is stopped. During the electrical rest period, rhythmic contractions of the periurethral muscles may occur, similar to normal projectile ejaculation (119). By stopping the electrical activity during emission, the external sphincter relaxes before the bladder neck relaxes, allowing for a maximum antegrade ejaculate output while limiting urine contamination of the sperm (116,119). The voltages and currents that have been reported to successfully produce ejaculation range from 5 to 25 V and 100 to 600 mA, respectively. Ten to twenty stimulations are necessary for complete emptying of the system (120).

After the procedure, the bladder is catheterized again to empty the retrograde fraction, which may be substantial in some patients. Rectoscopy is performed after the procedure to exclude injury to the rectum. Patients with complete spinal injuries can undergo EEJ without anesthesia. In men with partially preserved sensation, EEJ can cause significant discomfort, requiring conscious sedation or general anesthesia. If general anesthesia is required, the additional cost should be considered in the overall treatment plan for the couple (121).

EEJ is a highly successful procedure, with 95% resulting in ejaculation (104). The 5% failure rate can often be attributed to cases in which men with retained pelvic sensation experienced pain at low voltages (1 to 4 V) on their first trial of EEJ, and did not want to continue with further trials under sedation or general anesthesia (104).

Prostate Massage

PM has been used to collect semen from men with SCI for use in insemination (122,123). The name "prostate massage" is a misnomer because the seminal vesicles, as well as the prostate, are emptied during the procedure, which is performed by a physician who presses on these structures with a finger inserted into the patient's rectum. The rationale for performing PM is that sperm are stored in the ampulla of the vas deferens and, in men with SCI, are sequestered in the seminal vesicles as well (124). The practitioner, therefore, attempts to mechanically push the sperm out through the ejaculatory ductal system.

Surgical Sperm Retrieval

SSR is a method of retrieving sperm from reproductive tissue (Fig. 23.3). A variety of techniques may be used, including testicular sperm extraction, testicular sperm aspiration, microsurgical epididymal sperm aspiration, percutaneous epididymal sperm aspiration (PESA), and aspiration of sperm from the vas deferens (125–131). Unlike the methods discussed previously, SSR was not developed to treat anejaculation. Instead, these methods were originally developed to retrieve sperm from men without SCI who were azoospermic, that is, men with no sperm in their ejaculate.

Treating Infertility in Men with SCI

Currently, practitioners do not agree on the algorithm for administering PVS, EEJ, PM, and SSR in couples, with SCI

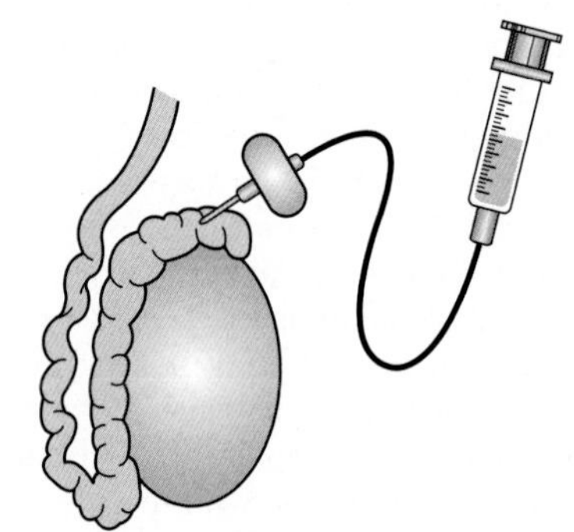

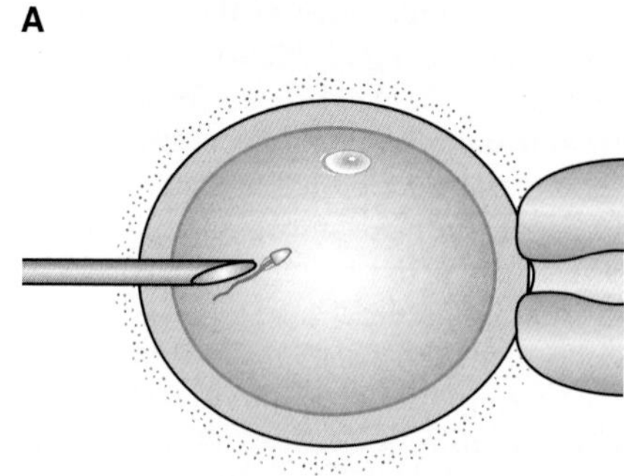

FIGURE 23.3 (A) Depicts the procedure of PESA, which is a method of SSR. In PESA, sperm are aspirated from the epididymis. In men with SCI, sperm yields obtained with any form of SSR, including PESA, are usually lower than sperm yields in the ejaculate. These low sperm yields commit the couple to ICSI in which a single sperm is injected into an egg to attempt fertilization (B). Performing SSR prior to examining the ejaculate for sperm is considered a controversial treatment.

male partners, who wish biological children. Once the ejaculate is obtained, it is examined. If the female has no medical issues that may interfere with conception or pregnancy, recommendations for ARTs depend largely on the total motile sperm count (TMSC) available. More ART options are viable with higher TMSCs. For example, the technologically simple, and relatively low-cost options of intravaginal insemination (IVI) and/or intrauterine insemination (IUI) will more likely result in pregnancy when the TMSC inseminated is above 5 million (and especially above 10 million) rather than when the TMSC inseminated is in the low millions or thousands (132).

IVI involves collecting sperm from the SCI male partner and injecting the sperm into the vagina of the female partner. The sperm must have vigorous motility to swim to the egg and inseminate. With IUI, sperm are collected from the male partner, processed to isolate the most motile sperm, and then injected into the uterus of the female partner. As with IVI, sperm inseminated during IUI must have vigorous motility to swim to the egg and inseminate.

When the TMSC is very low, more advanced and expensive ART is recommended to attempt pregnancy. The method of in vitro fertilization (IVF) involves removing sperm from the male partner and eggs from the female partner. Prior to egg retrieval, the woman is subjected to extensive hormonal manipulation to superovulate and to make her uterus receptive to implantation of an embryo. Sperm and eggs are placed in a laboratory dish where fertilization is expected to occur. Resulting embryos are injected through a catheter into the woman's uterus, where it is hoped that implantation and pregnancy will follow.

When there are not enough motile sperm to attempt fertilization by this conventional method of IVF, an advanced form of IVF may be attempted. This advanced form, termed intracytoplasmic sperm injection (ICSI), may be attempted with as few as one sperm per egg. With ICSI, the female partner is again hormonally manipulated and a single sperm is injected through a small needle into a single egg. The injected (inseminated) eggs are placed in a laboratory dish. Resulting embryos are transferred into the woman's uterus.

Research has shown that the TMSC of men with SCI is, in many cases, sufficient to attempt IVI and IUI (104). In fact, reasonable pregnancy rates by IVI or IUI have been obtained in couples with SCI male partners (121,133–136). Given the comparative ease and low cost of IVI and IUI ($200 to $600) relative to IVF and ICSI ($8,000 to $12,000), IVI and IUI should be offered to couples with SCI male partners when indicated. Unfortunately, many couples with SCI male partners are not offered or informed of IVF or IUI. Increasingly, practitioners are proceeding directly to SSR as the first option for treating anejaculation in men with SCI (104). The downside to SSR is that it usually results in a very low yield of TMSC, consequently committing the couple to ISCI, the most invasive and expensive of the ARTs.

Practitioners state that their reason for not offering IVI or IUI to couples with SCI male partners is that they (the practitioners) lack education and training in PVS and EEJ (104), procedures which were primarily developed to treat anejaculation in men with SCI. Practitioners are, however, receiving training in SSR, a relative newcomer to the armamentarium of sperm retrieval options. It is the legal and ethical responsibility of physicians to inform their patients of all treatment options for sperm retrieval and assisted conception, regardless if the physician performs the treatment (137,138). Even when a treatment is considered to have a poor prognosis, the physician must inform the patient about the option and explain why it is considered futile (139). It is recommended that practitioners evaluate the couple for IVI or IUI prior to proceeding directly to SSR. By doing so, the expensive and invasive option of ICSI may be avoided in many cases.

RESEARCH ON SEMEN QUALITY IN MEN WITH SCI

In addition to erectile dysfunction and ejaculatory dysfunction, abnormal semen quality also contributes to infertility in men with SCI. The semen quality of men with SCI is uncommon not only in the general population but also in the general male factor infertile population. The semen quality of men with SCI is characterized by normal sperm numbers, but abnormally low sperm motility and sperm viability (103,140–142). When compared to sperm from noninjured controls, sperm motility and viability are low after collection, and then decline rapidly over time (143). Because of the distinct nature of semen quality in men with SCI, research has been carried out to uncover the cause of their semen abnormalities.

Lifestyle Factors

Investigations regarding the causes of abnormal semen quality in men with SCI initially focused on factors associated with lifestyle, such as scrotal hyperthermia (144), infrequent ejaculation (145), problems associated with bladder management (146), and methods of assisted ejaculation (117). Studies showed that such factors could not entirely account for the problem. For example, scrotal temperature was similar in SCI and control subjects (144), regular ejaculation did not improve low sperm motility (142,145,147), and sperm motility remained subnormal despite improvements in bladder management (146) and methods of assisted ejaculation (118,119).

Based on this research, lifestyle factors alone could not explain the abnormal semen parameters observed in men with SCI. Investigations into secondary physiological factors also yielded negative results. For example, studies attempting to link low sperm motility to neurological level of injury, time postinjury, or age were unsuccessful (142,148). Similarly, low sperm motility was not found to be related to hormone levels (149,150) or urinary tract infections (146).

Accessory Gland Function

Other research has been carried out to determine if factors in the seminal plasma may contribute to poor semen quality in men with SCI. Seminal plasma is the fluid portion of the ejaculate, which in humans is comprised of fluids primarily from the seminal vesicles and prostate gland. Examination of seminal plasma from men with SCI shows numerous abnormalities. For example, brown-colored seminal plasma can be found in 27% of men with SCI (151). The brown color was thought to be related to semen stasis from prolonged anejaculation; however, frequent ejaculation did not eliminate the brown color. Microscopic analysis revealed that the brown color was not simply hematospermia, but instead, indicative of seminal vesicle dysfunction (151).

Additional evidence of seminal vesicle dysfunction was the finding that men with SCI have large quantities of sperm in their seminal vesicles. Because the seminal vesicles do not normally harbor large quantities of sperm, this study indicated an abnormal pattern of transport and storage of sperm in the seminal vesicles of men with SCI (124).

After the seminal vesicles, the prostate gland contributes the most fluid to the ejaculate. Studies have found evidence of prostate gland dysfunction in men with SCI. For example, compared to healthy, age-matched control subjects, prostate-specific antigen (PSA) was lower in the semen (152,153), but higher in blood serum (152) of men with SCI. This pattern of PSA expression indicates a secretory dysfunction of the prostate gland in men with SCI. Additional evidence of prostate-related abnormality is the finding of smaller prostate gland size in men with SCI compared to age-matched controls (154–156).

Additional evidence of accessory gland dysfunction in men with SCI is derived from studies showing abnormal concentrations of various biochemical substances in the semen of men with SCI versus control subjects. For example, compared to nondisabled men, men with SCI have higher concentrations of platelet-acting factor acetylhydrolase (157), reactive oxygen species (158–160), and somatostatin (in men with lesions at or above T6) (161). Conversely, the semen of men with SCI has lower levels of fructose, albumin, glutamic oxaloacetic transaminase, alkaline phosphatase (162), and TGF-beta 1 compared to the semen of nondisabled men (163).

Factors in the Seminal Plasma

Evidence of abnormal accessory gland function in men with SCI led to studies investigating the role of factors in seminal plasma as contributors to poor semen quality in these men. The studies showed that the seminal plasma of men with SCI is toxic to normal sperm. For example, when seminal plasma of men with SCI was mixed with sperm from normospermic men, a rapid and profound impairment to normal sperm motility occurs (164). Furthermore, sperm unexposed to the seminal plasma (i.e., aspirated from the vas deferens) has significantly higher motility than sperm in the ejaculate of these men (Fig. 23.4) (165). These findings introduced the concept of an abnormal seminal plasma environment as a cause of impaired sperm motility in men with SCI.

When examining the semen of men with SCI, nearly all have elevated numbers of white blood cells (166–169), a condition termed leukocytospermia. Excessive numbers of leukocytes have also been observed in the ejaculated semen and in the seminal vesicle epithelium of rats with SCI (167,170). While leukocytospermia has been associated with male infertility in the general population (171), low sperm motility in men with SCI does not seem to be caused simply by local infection of the genitourinary tract. In these men, treatment of genitourinary infections with antibiotics does not result in improved sperm motility (146).

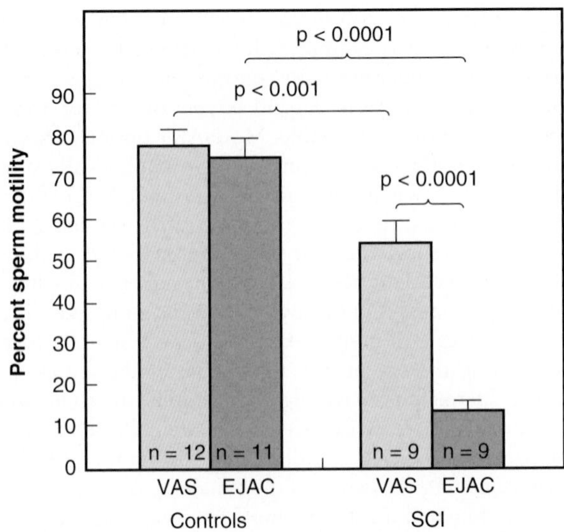

FIGURE 23.4 In able-bodied men (controls), sperm aspirated from the vas deferens had similar motility to sperm in the ejaculate. In contrast, in men with SCI, sperm aspirated from the vas deferens had significantly higher motility than sperm in the ejaculate. These results represented a major step toward understanding the source of poor sperm motility in men with SCI and elaborated the concept of an abnormal seminal plasma environment as a contributor to this problem. (Adapted from Brackett et al., ref 165). VAS, sperm aspirated from the vas deferens; EJAC, sperm in the ejaculate; SCI, subjects with spinal cord injury.

Cytokines Contribute to Low Sperm Motility in Men with SCI

When analyzing the subtypes of leukocytes in semen of men with SCI, flow cytometric analysis found large numbers of activated T lymphocytes (166), a T-cell subtype that is known to secrete cytotoxic cytokines (172). Elevated concentrations of cytokines can be harmful to sperm (167,173–175). It is possible that the activated T lymphocytes observed in semen of men with SCI are secreting cytokines that impair sperm motility. Evidence for this belief comes from studies showing elevated concentrations of specific cytokines (IL-1β, IL-6, and TNF-α) in semen of men with SCI (163), and improved sperm motility when these cytokines were neutralized (176,177).

SUMMARY

Both men and women desire sexual contact and intimacy after SCI, although SCI-related physiological changes may interfere with the enjoyment of sexual activity. Many women experience temporary amenorrhea following SCI. Once normal menstruation resumes, women with SCI can conceive via sexual intercourse, and deliver children with nearly the same success rate as women without disability. Women with SCI require careful management by an interdisciplinary team to monitor and treat medical conditions that may adversely affect health before, during, and after pregnancy.

Men with SCI experience erectile dysfunction, ejaculatory dysfunction, and semen abnormalities. One or more of these factors may interfere with sexual enjoyment or fertility.

Erectile dysfunction may be addressed using the same treatments available to the general population with impotence. These treatments include oral PDE-5 inhibitors, intracavernous or intraurethral injections of alprostadil, vacuum erection devices, and penile implants. Ejaculation for sexual pleasure can be improved with PVS. This method, as well as EEJ and PM, may be used to obtain semen from anejaculatory men with SCI. The use of SSR as the first-line treatment for anejaculation in men with SCI remains controversial.

A variety of methods may be used to assist conception in couples with SCI male partners, including IVI, IUI, and IVF, which may be performed with or without ICSI. It is recommended that the ejaculates of men with SCI be examined prior to retrieving sperm surgically. Many men with SCI have sufficient total motile sperm to warrant consideration of IVI or IUI before proceeding to the more invasive and expensive options of IVF and ICSI.

Research has investigated causes of abnormal semen quality in men with SCI. The semen profile of men with SCI is unlike that of men without disability, and men in the infertile population. Semen characteristics include normal sperm concentration, but abnormal sperm motility and viability. Simple lifestyle factors, such as elevated scrotal temperature from sitting in a wheelchair, infrequency of ejaculation, or method of bladder management cannot account for the problem. It is likely that dysfunction of the seminal vesicles and/or prostate gland lead to the presence of abnormal constituents in the seminal plasma, including elevated concentrations of leukocytes and cytokines. Such factors may contribute to poor semen quality in men with SCI.

Individuals with SCI are keenly interested in the topics of sexual function and fertility and will request information on these topics at widely variant times after injury. Clinicians who interact with couples who wish to enhance intimacy, engage in sexual activity, and bear children should be knowledgeable about current practices on these topics. Otherwise, referrals must be made to community professionals who are knowledgeable in these opportunities and can guide individuals with SCI and their partners to information on contemporary practices.

ACKNOWLEDGMENT

The authors acknowledge Emad Ibrahim, M.D., for valuable assistance in preparing the manuscript.

References

1. National SCI Statistical Center. Spinal Cord Injury—Facts and Figures at a Glance. http://www.spinalcord.uab.edu/. http://images.main.uab.edu/spinalcord/pdffiles/Facts08.pdf. Accessed Dated Accessed June 30, 2008.
2. O'Connor P. Incidence and patterns of spinal cord injury in Australia. *Accid Anal Prev* 2002;34:405–415.
3. Rathore MF, Hanif S, Farooq F, et al. Traumatic spinal cord injuries at a tertiary care rehabilitation institute in Pakistan. *J Pak Med Assoc* 2008;58:53–57.
4. Kuptniratsaikul V. Epidemiology of spinal cord injuries: a study in the Spinal Unit, Siriraj Hospital, Thailand, 1997–2000. *J Med Assoc Thai* 2003;86:1116–1121.
5. Mena Quinones PO, Nassal M, Al Bader KI, et al. Traumatic spinal cord injury in Qatar: an epidemiological study. *Middle East J Emerg Med* 2002;1:1–5.
6. Kondakov EN, Simonova IA, Poliakov IV. The epidemiology of injuries to the spine and spinal cord in Saint Petersburg, Russia. *Zh Vopr Neirokhir Im N N Burdenko* 2002;2:50–53.
7. Exner G, Meinecke FW. Trends in the treatment of patients with spinal cord lesions seen within a period of 20 years in German centers. *Spinal Cord* 1997;35:415–419.
8. Farooque M, Suo Z, Arnold PM, et al. Gender-related differences in recovery of locomotor function after spinal cord injury in mice. *Spinal Cord* 2006;44:182–187.
9. Sipski ML, Jackson AB, Gomez-Marin O, et al. Effects of gender on neurologic and functional recovery after spinal cord injury. *Arch Phys Med Rehabil* 2004;85:1826–1836.
10. Althof SE, Levine SB. Clinical approach to the sexuality of patients with spinal cord injury. *Urol Clin North Am* 1993;20:527–534.
11. Smith EM, Bodner DR. Sexual dysfunction after spinal cord injury. *Urol Clin North Am* 1993;20:535–542.
12. Elliott S. Ejaculation and orgasm: sexuality in men with SCI. *Top Spinal Cord Inj Rehabil* 2002;8:1–15.
13. Elliott S. Sexual dysfunction and infertility in men with spinal cord disorders. In: Lin V, ed. *Spinal cord medicine: principles and practice.* New York, Demos Medical Publishing, 2003:349–365.
14. The Americans with Disabilities Act. http://www.ada.gov/. Updated July 25, 2008. Accessed July 31, 2008.
15. Wyndaele JJ, de Meyer JM, de Sy WA, et al. Intracavernous injection of vasoactive drugs, an alternative for treating impotence in spinal cord injury patients. *Paraplegia* 1986;24:271–275.
16. Christopher and Dana Reeve Foundation. www.christopherreeve.org. Written and Accessed July 31, 2008.
17. Anderson KD. Targeting recovery: priorities of the spinal cord-injured population. *J Neruotrauma* 2004;21:1371–1383.
18. Berkley KJ, Hotta H, Robbins A, et al. Functional properties of afferent fibers supplying reproductive and other pelvic organs in pelvic nerve of female rat. *J Neurophysiol* 1990;63:256–272.
19. Komisaruk BR, Adler NT, Hutchison J. Genital sensory field: enlargement by estrogen treatment in female rats. *Science* 1972;178:1295–1298.
20. Peters LC, Kristal MB, Komisaruk BR. Sensory innervation of the external and internal genitalia of the female rat. *Brain Res* 1987;408:199–204.
21. Sipski ML, Alexander CJ, Rosen R. Sexual arousal and orgasm in women: effects of spinal cord injury. *Ann Neurol* 2001;49:35–44.
22. Sipski ML, Alexander CJ, Rosen RC. Physiologic parameters associated with sexual arousal in women with incomplete spinal cord injuries. *Arch Phys Med Rehabil* 1997;78:305–313.
23. Sipski ML, Rosen RC, Alexander CJ, et al. Sexual responsiveness in women with spinal cord injuries: differential effects of anxiety-eliciting stimulation. *Arch Sex Behav* 2004;33:295–302.
24. Sipski ML, Rosen R, Alexander CJ, et al. A controlled trial of positive feedback to increase sexual arousal in

women with spinal cord injuries. *NeuroRehabilitation* 2000;15:145–153.
25. Sipski ML, Alexander CJ, Rosen RC. Physiological parameters associated with psychogenic sexual arousal in women with complete spinal cord injuries. *Arch Phys Med Rehabil* 1995;76:811–818.
26. Sipski ML. Spinal cord injury: what is the effect on sexual response? *J Am Paraplegic Soc* 1991;14:40–43.
27. Anderson KD, Borisoff JF, Johnson RD, et al. Spinal cord injury influences psychogenic as well as physical components of female sexual ability. *Spinal Cord* 2007;45: 349–359.
28. Komisaruk BR, Whipple B, Crawford A, et al. Brain activation during vaginocervical self-stimulation and orgasm in women with complete spinal cord injury: fMRI evidence of mediation by the vagus nerves. *Brain Res* 2004;1024:77–88.
29. Cole TM. Sexuality and physical disabilities. *Arch Sex Behav* 1975;4:389–403.
30. Whipple.B. Female sexuality. In: Leyson J, ed. *Sexual rehabilitation of the spinal cord injured patient.* Clifton, NJ; Humana Press, 1990:19–38.
31. Komisaruk BR, Gerdes CA, Whipple B. 'Complete' spinal cord injury does not block perceptual responses to genital self-stimulation in women. *Arch Neurol* 1997;54: 1513–1520.
32. Whipple B, Komisaruk BR. Sexuality and women with complete spinal cord injury. *Spinal Cord* 1997;35:136–138.
33. Sipski M, Alexander C, Rosen R. Orgasm in women with spinal cord injuries: a laboratory assessment. *Arch Phys Med Rehabil* 1995;76:1097–1102.
34. Komisaruk BR, Bianca R, Sansone G, et al: Brain-mediated responses to vaginocervical stimulation in spinal cord-transected rats: role of the vagus nerves. *Brain Res* 1996;708:128–134.
35. Cueva-Rolon R, Sansone G, Bianca R, et al. Vagotomy blocks responses to vaginocervical stimulation after genitospinal neurectomy in rats. *Physiol Behav* 1996;60: 19–24.
36. Bughi S, Shaw SJ, Mahmood G, et al. Amenorrhea, pregnancy, and pregnancy outcomes in women following spinal cord injury: a retrospective cross-sectional study. *Endocr Pract* 2008;14:437–441.
37. Charlifue SW, Gerhart KA, Menter RR, et al. Sexual issues of women with spinal cord injuries. *Paraplegia* 1992;30:192–199.
38. Kreuter M, Siosteen A, Biering-Sorensen F. Sexuality and sexual life in women with spinal cord injury: a controlled study. *J Rehabil Med* 2008;40:61–69.
39. Alexander MS, Bodner D, Brackett NL, et al. Development of international standards to document sexual and reproductive functions after spinal cord injury: preliminary report. *J Rehabil Res Dev* 2007;44:83–90.
40. Basson R, Berman J, Burnett A, et al. Report of the international consensus development conference on female sexual dysfunction: definitions and classifications. *J Urol* 2000;163:888–893.
41. Tepper MS, Whipple B, Richards E, et al. Women with complete spinal cord injury: a phenomenological study of sexual experiences. *J Sex Marital Ther* 2001;27: 615–623.
42. Wu MY, Chan F. Psychosocial adjustment patterns of persons with spinal cord injury in Taiwan. *Disabil Rehabil* 2007;29:1847–1857.
43. Ricciardi R, Szabo CM, Poullos AY. Sexuality and spinal cord injury. *Nurs Clin North Am* 2007;42:675–684.
44. Sipski ML, Rosen RC, Alexander CJ, et al. Sildenafil effects on sexual and cardiovascular responses in women with spinal cord injury. *Urol* 2000;55:812–815.
45. Palace EM, Gorzalka BB. The enhancing effects of anxiety on arousal in sexually dysfunctional and functional women. *J Abnorm Psychol* 1990;99:403–411.
46. Sipski ML. The impact of spinal cord injury on female sexuality, menstruation and pregnancy: a review of the literature. *J Am Paraplegic Soc* 1991;14:122–126.
47. Bors E, Comarr AE. Neurological disturbances of sexual function with special reference to 529 patients with spinal cord injury. *Urol Surv* 1960;10:191–222.
48. Vanderbeke I, Boll D, Verguts JK. [Pregnancy and childbirth in a patient with a spinal cord lesion]. *Ned Tijdschr Geneeskd* 2008;152:1169–1172.
49. Osgood SL, Kuczkowski KM. Autonomic dysreflexia in a parturient with spinal cord injury. *Acta Anaesthesiol Belg* 2006;57:161–162.
50. Sosnowski S, Malewicz T, Tywoniuk J, et al. Pregnancy, labor, and puerperium in a 38-year old patient with transverse post-traumatic spinal cord injury. *Ortop Traumatol Rehabil* 2000;2:64–66.
51. KNBC.com, an NBC TV affiliate. Los Angeles, CA. Former officer paralyzed in shooting announces pregnancy. http://www.knbc.com/news/14371904/detail.html. Accessed Dated Accessed June 30, 2008.
52. Discovery Health Television Channel. Paralyzed and Pregnant. http://health.discovery.com/tv-schedules/special.html?paid=62.15276.116988.0.0.
53. MobileWomen.org. Forum for Women. http://carecure.rutgers.edu/mobilewomen/phpbb2/viewtopic.php?p=663.
54. Comarr AE. Observations on menstruation and pregnancy among female spinal cord injury patients. *Paraplegia* 1966;3:263–272.
55. Jackson AB, Wadley V. A multicenter study of women's self-reported reproductive health after spinal cord injury. *Arch Phys Med Rehabil* 1999;80:1420–1428.
56. Anderson CJ, Mulcahey MJ, Vogel LC. Menstruation and pediatric spinal cord injury. *J Spinal Cord Med* 1997;20:56–59.
57. Comarr AE. Interesting observations on females with spinal cord injury. *Med Ser J* 1966;22:651–661.
58. Liu JH. Causes of Amenorrhea. endotext.com. Published May 3, 2003. Accessed July 31, 2008. http://www.endotext.org/female/female5/femaleframe5.htm.
59. Bondanelli M, Ambrosio MR, Zatelli MC, et al. Hypopituitarism after traumatic brain injury. *Eur J Endocrinol* 2005;152:679–691.
60. Sipski ML, Alexander CJ. Sexual activities, desire and satisfaction in females pre- and post-spinal cord injury. *J Am Paraplegic Soc* 1991;14(2):72
61. Pereira L. Obstetric management of the patient with spinal cord injury. *Obstet Gynecol Surv* 2003;58:678–687.
62. McGregor JA, Meeuwsen J. Autonomic hyperreflexia: a mortal danger for spinal cord-damaged women in labor. *Am J Obstet Gynecol* 1985;151:330–333.

63. Cross LL, Meythaler JM, Tuel SM, et al. Pregnancy, labor and delivery post spinal cord injury. *Paraplegia* 1992;30:890–902.
64. Cross LL, Meythaler JM, Tuel SM, et al. Pregnancy following spinal cord injury. *West J Med* 1991;154:607–611.
65. Hughes SJ, Short DJ, Usherwood MM, et al. Management of the pregnant woman with spinal cord injuries. *Br J Obstet Gynaecol* 1991;98:513–518.
66. Krassioukov A, Warburton DE, Teasell R, et al. A systematic review of the management of autonomic dysreflexia after spinal cord injury. *Arch Phys Med Rehabil* 2009;90:682–695.
67. Skowronski E, Hartman K. Obstetric management following traumatic tetraplegia: case series and literature review. *Aust N Z J Obstet Gynaecol* 2008;48:485–491.
68. Burns AS, Jackson AB. Gynecologic and reproductive issues in women with spinal cord injury. *Phys Med Rehabil Clin N Am* 2001;12:183–199.
69. Dakhil-Jerew F, Brook S, Derry F. Autonomic dysreflexia triggered by breastfeeding in a tetraplegic mother. *J Rehabil Med* 2008;40:780–782.
70. ACOG: ACOG Committee Opinion. Obstetric management of patients with spinal cord injuries. *Obstet Gynecol* 2002;100(275):625–627.
71. Grill S, Rusterholz C, Zanetti-Dallenbach R, et al. Potential markers of preeclampsia—a review. *Reprod Biol Endocrinol* 2009;7:70
72. Rintala DH, Herson L, Hudler-Hull T. Comparison of parenting styles of persons with and without spinal cord injury and their children's social competence and behavior problems. *J Spinal Cord Med* 2000;23: 244–256.
73. Alexander CJ, Hwang K, Sipski ML. Mothers with spinal cord injuries: impact on marital, family, and children's adjustment. *Arch Phys Med Rehabil* 2002;83:24–30.
74. Monga M, Bernie J, Rajasekaran M: Male infertility and erectile dysfunction in spinal cord injury: a review. [Review] [86 refs]. *Arch Phys Med Rehabil* 1999;80:1331
75. Tsuji I, Nakajama F, Morimoto J, et al. The sexual function in patients with spinal cord injury. *Urol Int* 1961;12:270.
76. Zeitlin AB, Cottrell TL, Lloyd FA. Sexology of the paraplegic male. *Fertil Steril* 1957;8:337–344.
77. Burnett AL. Nitric oxide control of lower genitourinary tract functions: a review. *Urol* 1995;45:1071–1083.
78. Golji H. Experience with penile prosthesis in spinal cord injury patients. *J Urol* 1979;121:288–289.
79. Hairston J, Becher E, McVary K. Topical and intraurethral therapy. In: Mulcahy J, ed. *Current clinical urology: male sexual function: a guide to clinical management*. Totowa, NJ: Human Press, Inc., 2001: 225–243.
80. Kimoto Y, Iwatsubo E. Penile prostheses for the management of the neuropathic bladder and sexual dysfunction in spinal cord injury patients: long term follow up. *Paraplegia* 1994;32:336–339.
81. Dietzen CJ, Lloyd LK. Complications of intracavernous injections and penile prostheses in spinal cord injured men. *Arch Phys Med Rehabil* 1992;73:652–655.
82. Zermann DH, Kutzenberger J, Sauerwein D, et al. Penile prosthetic surgery in neurologically impaired patients: long-term followup. *J Urol* 2006;175:1041–1044.
83. Wilson SK, Delk JR. Inflatable penile implant infection: predisposing factors and treatment suggestions. *J Urol* 1995;153:659–661.
84. Nadig PW, Ware JC, Blumoff R. Noninvasive device to produce and maintain an erection-like state. *Urol* 1986;27:126–131.
85. Lloyd EE, Toth LL, Perkash I. Vacuum tumescence: an option for spinal cord injured males with erectile dysfunction. *SCI Nurs* 1989;6:25–28.
86. Zasler ND, Katz PG. Synergist erection system in the management of impotence secondary to spinal cord injury. *Arch Phys Med Rehabil* 1989;70:712–716.
87. Bensman A, Kottke FJ. Induced emission of sperm utilizing electrical stimulation of the seminal vesicles and vas deferens. *Arch Phys Med Rehabil* 1966;47:436–443.
88. Virag R. Intracavernous injection of papaverine for erectile failure. *Lancet* 1982;2:938.
89. Sidi AA, Cameron JS, Dykstra DD, et al. Vasoactive intracavernous pharmacotherapy for the treatment of erectile impotence in men with spinal cord injury. *J Urol* 1987;138:539–542.
90. Lloyd LK, Richards JS. Intracavernous pharmacotherapy for management of erectile dysfunction in spinal cord injury. *Paraplegia* 1989;27:457–464.
91. Bodner DR, Lindan R, Leffler E, et al. The application of intracavernous injection of vasoactive medications for erection in men with spinal cord injury. *J Urol* 1987;138:310–311.
92. Padma-Nathan H, Hellstrom WJ, Kaiser FE, et al. Treatment of men with erectile dysfunction with transurethral alprostadil. Medicated Urethral System for Erection (MUSE) Study Group. *N Engl J Med* 1997;336:1–7.
93. Fulgham PF, Cochran JS, Denman JL, et al. Disappointing initial results with transurethral alprostadil for erectile dysfunction in a urology practice setting. *J Urol* 1998;160:2041–2046.
94. Bodner DR, Haas CA, Krueger B, et al. Intraurethral alprostadil for treatment of erectile dysfunction in patients with spinal cord injury. *Urol* 1999;53:199–202.
95. Boolell M, Allen MJ, Ballard SA, et al. Sildenafil: an orally active type 5 cyclic GMP-specific phosphodiesterase inhibitor for the treatment of penile erectile dysfunction. *Int J Impot Res* 1996;8:47–52.
96. Derry FA, Dinsmore WW, Fraser M, et al. Efficacy and safety of oral sildenafil (Viagra) in men with erectile dysfunction caused by spinal cord injury. *Neurology* 1998;51:1629–1633.
97. Derry F, Hultling C, Seftel AD, et al. Efficacy and safety of sildenafil citrate (Viagra) in men with erectile dysfunction and spinal cord injury: a review. *Urol* 2002;60:49–57.
98. Giuliano F, Rubio-Aurioles E, Kennelly M, et al. Efficacy and safety of vardenafil in men with erectile dysfunction caused by spinal cord injury. *Neurology* 2006;66:210–216.
99. Soler JM, Previnaire JG, Denys P, et al. Phosphodiesterase inhibitors in the treatment of erectile dysfunction in spinal cord-injured men. *Spinal Cord* 2007;45:169–173.

100. Brown DJ, Hill ST, Baker HW. Male fertility and sexual function after spinal cord injury. *Prog Brain Res* 2006;152:427–439.
101. Courtois F, Charvier K, Leriche A, et al. Perceived physiological and orgasmic sensations at ejaculation in spinal cord injured men. *J Sex Med* 2008;5:2419–2430.
102. Brackett NL. Semen retrieval by penile vibratory stimulation in men with spinal cord injury. *Hum Reprod Update* 1999;5:216–222.
103. Sonksen J, Ohl DA. Penile vibratory stimulation and electroejaculation in the treatment of ejaculatory dysfunction. *Int J Androl* 2002;25:324–332.
104. Kafetsoulis A, Brackett NL, Ibrahim E, et al. Current trends in the treatment of infertility in men with spinal cord injury. *Fertil Steril* 2006;86:781–789.
105. Sonksen J, Biering-Sorensen F, Kristensen JK. Ejaculation induced by penile vibratory stimulation in men with spinal cord injuries. The importance of the vibratory amplitude. *Paraplegia* 1994;32:651–660.
106. Brackett NL, Ferrell SM, Aballa TC, et al. An analysis of 653 trials of penile vibratory stimulation on men with spinal cord injury. *J Urol* 1998;159:1931–1934.
107. FERTI CARE®personal vibrator. Multicept A/S. http://www.multicept.dk/Uk/index.htm. Accessed Dated Accessed June 30, 2008.
108. Ekland MB, Krassioukov AV, McBride KE, et al. Incidence of autonomic dysreflexia and silent autonomic dysreflexia in men with spinal cord injury undergoing sperm retrieval: implications for clinical practice. *J Spinal Cord Med* 2008;31:33–39.
109. Wieder J, Brackett N, Lynne C, et al. Anesthetic block of the dorsal penile nerve inhibits vibratory-induced ejaculation in men with spinal cord injuries. *Urology* 2000;55:915–917.
110. Brackett NL, Kafetsoulis A, Ibrahim E, et al. Application of 2 vibrators salvages ejaculatory failures to 1 vibrator during penile vibratory stimulation in men with spinal cord injuries. *J Urol* 2007;177:660–663.
111. Kafetsoulis A, Ibrahim E, Aballa TC, et al. Abdominal electrical stimulation rescues failures to penile vibratory stimulation in men with spinal cord injury: a report of two cases. *Urology* 2006;68:204–211.
112. Bird VG, Brackett NL, Lynne CM, et al. Reflexes and somatic responses as predictors of ejaculation by penile vibratory stimulation in men with spinal cord injury. *Spinal Cord* 2001;39:514–519.
113. Ohl DA, Sonksen J. Penile vibratory stimulation and electroejaculation. In: Hellstrom WJG, ed. *Male infertility and sexual dysfunction*. New York: Springer-Verlag New York, Inc., 1997:219–229.
114. Brindley GS. Reflex ejaculation under vibratory stimulation in paraplegic men. *Paraplegia* 1981;19:299–302.
115. Ohl DA, Quallich SA, Sonksen J, et al. Anejaculation and retrograde ejaculation. *Urol Clin North Am* 2008;35:211–220, viii.
116. Brackett NL, Ead DN, Aballa TC, et al. Semen retrieval in men with spinal cord injury is improved by interrupting current delivery during electroejaculation. *J Urol* 2002;167:201–203.
117. Brackett NL, Padron OF, Lynne CM. Semen quality of spinal cord injured men is better when obtained by vibratory stimulation versus electroejaculation. *J Urol* 1997;157:151–157.
118. Ohl DA, Sonksen J, Menge AC, et al. Electroejaculation versus vibratory stimulation in spinal cord injured men: sperm quality and patient preference. *J Urol* 1997;157:2147–2149.
119. Sonksen J, Ohl DA, Wedemeyer G. Sphincteric effects during penile vibratory ejaculation and electroejaculation in men with spinal cord injuries. *J Urol* 2001;165:426–429.
120. Ohl DA. Electroejaculation. *Urol Clin North Am* 1993;20:181–188.
121. Ohl DA, Wolf LJ, Menge AC, et al. Electroejaculation and assisted reproductive technologies in the treatment of anejaculatory infertility. *Fertil Steril* 2001;76:1249–1255.
122. Taylor Z, Molloy D, Hill V, et al. Contribution of the assisted reproductive technologies to fertility in males suffering spinal cord injury. *Aust N Z J Obstet Gynaecol* 1999;39:84–87.
123. Marina S, Marina F, Alcolea R, et al. Triplet pregnancy achieved through intracytoplasmic sperm injection with spermatozoa obtained by prostatic massage of a paraplegic patient: case report. *Hum Reprod* 1999;14:1546–1548.
124. Ohl DA, Menge A, Jarow J. Seminal vesicle aspiration in spinal cord injured men: insight into poor semen quality. *J Urol* 1999;162:2048–2051.
125. Craft I, Tsirigotis M. Simplified recovery, preparation and cryopreservation of testicular spermatozoa. *Hum Reprod* 1995;10:1623–1626.
126. Tsirigotis M, Pelekanos M, Beski S, et al. Cumulative experience of percutaneous epididymal sperm aspiration (PESA) with intracytoplasmic sperm injection. *J Assist Reprod Genet* 1996;13:315–319.
127. Haberle M, Scheurer P, Muhlebach P, et al. Intracytoplasmic sperm injection (ICSI) with testicular sperm extraction (TESE) in non-obstructive azoospermia—two case reports. *Andrologia* 1996;28(suppl 1):87–88.
128. Kahraman S, Ozgur S, Alatas C, et al. High implantation and pregnancy rates with testicular sperm extraction and intracytoplasmic sperm injection in obstructive and non-obstructive azoospermia. *Hum Reprod* 1996;11:673–676.
129. Craft I, Tsirigotis M, Courtauld E, et al. Testicular needle aspiration as an alternative to biopsy for the assessment of spermatogenesis. *Hum Reprod* 1997;12:1483–1487.
130. Westlander G, Hamberger L, Hanson C, et al. Diagnostic epididymal and testicular sperm recovery and genetic aspects in azoospermic men. *Hum Reprod* 1999;14:118–122.
131. Chiang H, Liu C, Tzeng C, et al. No-scalpel vasal sperm aspiration and in vitro fertilization for the treatment of anejaculation. *Urology* 2000;55:918–921.
132. Van Voorhis BJ, Barnett M, Sparks AE, et al. Effect of the total motile sperm count on the efficacy and cost-effectiveness of intrauterine insemination and in vitro fertilization. *Fertil Steril* 2001;75:661–668.
133. Biering-Sorensen F, Laeessoe L, Sonksen J, et al. The effect of penile vibratory stimulation on male fertility potential, spasticity and neurogenic detrusor overactivity in spinal cord lesioned individuals. *Acta Neurochir Suppl* 2005;93:159–163.

134. Rutkowski SB, Geraghty TJ, Hagen DL, et al. A comprehensive approach to the management of male infertility following spinal cord injury. *Spinal Cord* 1999;37:508–514.
135. Pryor JL, Kuneck PH, Blatz SM, et al. Delayed timing of intrauterine insemination results in a significantly improved pregnancy rate in female partners of quadriplegic men. *Fertil Steril* 2001;76:1130–1135.
136. Heruti RJ, Katz H, Menashe Y, et al. Treatment of male infertility due to spinal cord injury using rectal probe electroejaculation: the Israeli experience. *Spinal Cord* 2001;39:168–175.
137. Informed Consent. American Medical Association. http://www.ama-assn.org/ama/pub/category/4608.html. Accessed Dated Accessed June 30, 2008.
138. Anonymous. Elements to be considered in obtaining informed consent for ART. *Fertil Steril* 2006;86(suppl 5):S272–S273
139. Fertility treatment when the prognosis is very poor or futile. *Fertil Steril* 2004;82:806–810.
140. Linsenmeyer TA. Male infertility following spinal cord injury. *J Am Paraplegic Soc* 1991;14:116–121.
141. Denil J, Ohl DA, Menge AC, et al. Functional characteristics of sperm obtained by electroejaculation [see comments]. *J Urol* 1992;147:69–72.
142. Brackett NL, Nash MS, Lynne CM. Male fertility following spinal cord injury: facts and fiction. *Phys Ther* 1996;76:1221–1231.
143. Brackett NL, Santa-Cruz C, Lynne CM. Sperm from spinal cord injured men lose motility faster than sperm from normal men: the effect is exacerbated at body compared to room temperature. *J Urol* 1997;157:2150–2153.
144. Brackett NL, Lynne CM, Weizman MS, et al. Scrotal and oral temperatures are not related to semen quality or serum gonadotropin levels in spinal cord-injured men. *J Androl* 1994;15:614–619.
145. Laessoe L, Sonksen J, Bagi P, et al. Effects of ejaculation by penile vibratory stimulation on bladder reflex activity in a spinal cord injured man. *J Urol* 2001;166:627.
146. Ohl DA, Denil J, Fitzgerald-Shelton K, et al. Fertility of spinal cord injured males: effect of genitourinary infection and bladder management on results of electroejaculation. *J Am Paraplegic Soc* 1992;15:53–59.
147. Siosteen A, Forssman L, Steen Y, et al. Quality of semen after repeated ejaculation treatment in spinal cord injury men. *Paraplegia* 1990;28:96–104.
148. Brackett NL, Ferrell SM, Aballa TC, et al. Semen quality in spinal cord injured men: does it progressively decline post-injury? *Arch Phys Med Rehabil* 1998;79:625–628.
149. Brackett NL, Lynne CM, Weizman MS, et al. Endocrine profiles and semen quality of spinal cord injured men. *J Urol* 1994;151:114–119.
150. Naderi AR, Safarinejad MR. Endocrine profiles and semen quality in spinal cord injured men. *Clin Endocrinol* 2003;58:177–184.
151. Wieder JA, Lynne CM, Ferrell SM, et al. Brown-colored semen in men with spinal cord injury. *J Androl* 1999;20:594–600.
152. Lynne CM, Aballa TC, Wang TJ, et al. Serum and seminal plasma prostate specific antigen (PSA) levels are different in young spinal cord injured men compared to normal controls. *J Urol* 1999;162:89–91.
153. Alexandrino AP, Rodrigues MA, Matsuo T. Evaluation of serum and seminal levels of prostate specific antigen in men with spinal cord injury. *J Urol* 2004;171:2230–2232.
154. Hvarness H, Jakobsen H, Biering-Sorensen F. Men with spinal cord injury have a smaller prostate than men without. *Scand J Urol Nephrol* 2007;41:120–123.
155. Frisbie JH, Kumar S, Aguilera EJ, et al. Prostate atrophy and spinal cord lesions. *Spinal Cord* 2006;44:24–27.
156. Bartoletti R, Gavazzi A, Cai T, et al. Prostate growth and prevalence of prostate diseases in early onset spinal cord injuries. *Eur Urol* 2008;56:142–150
157. Zhu J, Brackett NL, Aballa TC, et al. High seminal platelet-activating factor acetylhydrolase activity in men with spinal cord injury. *J Androl* 2006;27:429–433.
158. Padron OF, Brackett NL, Sharma RK, et al. Seminal reactive oxygen species and sperm motility and morphology in men with spinal cord injury. *Fertil Steril* 1997;67:1115–1120.
159. de Lamirande E, Leduc BE, Iwasaki A, et al. Increased reactive oxygen species formation in semen of patients with spinal cord injury. *Fertil Steril* 1995;63:637–642.
160. Rajasekaran M, Hellstrom WJ, Sparks RL, et al. Sperm-damaging effects of electric current: possible role of free radicals. *Reprod Toxicol* 1994;8:427–432.
161. Odum L, Sonksen J, Biering-Sorensen F. Seminal somatostatin in men with spinal cord injury. *Paraplegia* 1995;33:374–376.
162. Hirsch IH, Jeyendran RS, Sedor J, et al. Biochemical analysis of electroejaculates in spinal cord injured men: comparison to normal ejaculates. *J Urol* 1991;145:73–76.
163. Basu S, Aballa TC, Ferrell SM, et al. Inflammatory cytokine concentrations are elevated in seminal plasma of men with spinal cord injuries. *J Androl* 2004;25:250–254.
164. Brackett NL, Davi RC, Padron OF, et al. Seminal plasma of spinal cord injured men inhibits sperm motility of normal men. *J Urol* 1996;155:1632–1635.
165. Brackett NL, Lynne CM, Aballa TC, et al. Sperm motility from the vas deferens of spinal cord injured men is higher than from the ejaculate. *J Urol* 2000;164:712–715.
166. Basu S, Lynne CM, Ruiz P, et al. Cytofluorographic identification of activated T-cell subpopulations in the semen of men with spinal cord injuries. *J Androl* 2002;23:551–556.
167. Garcia LI, Soto-Cid A, Carrillo P, et al. Characteristics of ejaculated rat semen after lesion of scrotal nerves. *Physiol Behav* 2007;91:120–125.
168. Aird IA, Vince GS, Bates MD, et al. Leukocytes in semen from men with spinal cord injuries. *Fertil Steril* 1999;72:97–103.
169. Trabulsi EJ, Shupp-Byrne D, Sedor J, et al. Leukocyte subtypes in electroejaculates of spinal cord injured men. *Arch Phys Med Rehabil* 2002;83:31–33.
170. Dashtdar H, Valojerdi MR. Ultrastructure of rat seminal vesicle epithelium in the acute phase of spinal cord transection. *Neurol Res* 2008;30:487–492.
171. Arata DB, Tortolero I, Villarroel V, et al. Nonsperm cells in human semen and their relationship with semen parameters. *Arch Androl* 2000;45:131–136.
172. Parham P. *The immune system*, New York: Garland Science, 2005.

173. Kocak I, Yenisey C, Dundar M, et al. Relationship between seminal plasma interleukin-6 and tumor necrosis factor alpha levels with semen parameters in fertile and infertile men. *Urol Res* 2002;30:263–267.
174. Eggert-Kruse W, Boit R, Rohr G, et al. Relationship of seminal plasma interleukin (IL) -8 and IL-6 with semen quality. *Hum Reprod* 2001;16:517–528.
175. Sikka SC, Champion HC, Bivalacqua TJ, et al. Role of genitourinary inflammation in infertility: synergistic effect of lipopolysaccharide and interferon-gamma on human spermatozoa. *Int J Androl* 2001;24:136–141.
176. Cohen DR, Basu S, Randall JM, et al. Sperm motility in men with spinal cord injuries is enhanced by inactivating cytokines in the seminal plasma. *J Androl* 2004;25: 922–925.
177. Brackett NL, Cohen DR, Ibrahim E, et al. Neutralization of cytokine activity at the receptor level improves sperm motility in men with spinal cord injuries. *J Androl* 2007;28:717–721.
178. Comarr AE. Sexual function among patients with spinal cord injury. *Urol Int* 1970;25:134–168.
179. De Groat WC, Steers WD. Neuroanatomy and neurophysiology of penile erection. In: Tanagho EA, Lue TF, McClure RD, eds. *Contemporary management of impotence and infertility*. Baltimore, MD: Williams & Wilkins, 1988:3–27.

CHAPTER 24 ■ RECREATIONAL AND THERAPEUTIC EXERCISE AFTER SPINAL CORD INJURY

MARK S. NASH, JOHN A. HORTON, RACHEL E. COWAN, AND LAURIE A. MALONE

INTRODUCTION

Recreational and therapeutic exercises serve as a cornerstone in the lives of many individuals living both with and without spinal cord injury (SCI). For those with SCI, these activities can restore or enhance function, independence, and health. Recreational exercises further provide relaxation and diversion from daily activities and challenges, while therapeutic exercises address secondary medical complications either imposed by or associated with physical deconditioning.

Unfortunately, involvement in sports, recreation, and therapeutic exercise may be limited by motor function spared after injury as well as changes in autonomic function, fuel homeostasis, temperature regulation, and motor skill. In some cases, reintegration of sports and recreation in the lives of those with SCI requires special equipment, training, and opportunities. Participation in therapeutic exercise may also require adaptive equipment and, in some instances, the use of electrical current to initiate purposeful movement of paralyzed muscles. Notwithstanding these special needs and considerations, there is considerable evidence that involvement in recreational and therapeutic exercise improves the activity, satisfaction, productivity, and health of its participants. Conversely, SCI may also increase the risks of injury and hasten the organ system deterioration as people age with their disability. Whether imprudent involvement in sports or excessive exercise creates incipient disability, orthopaedic deterioration, or neurologic dysfunction has been the topic of considerable discussion. Thus, this chapter investigates the advantages of exercise, presents authoritative recommendations regarding the preferred dose of exercise, identifies SCI-specific exercise prescription considerations, and then discusses opportunities for participation in sports and recreational activities for those with SCI. Opportunities for therapeutic exercise using voluntary and electrically stimulated exercise are examined, and benefits and risks of these therapies discussed. Information contained in this chapter will define a variety of attractive options through which persons with SCI can enhance their personal independence and life satisfaction, while not promoting injury or hastening of future disability.

THERAPEUTIC EXERCISE AND ITS BENEFITS AFTER SCI

Sedentary lifestyles and low levels of fitness are common among persons with SCI (1,2), which may explain the significant risk of cardiovascular mortality now reported for persons aging with spinal cord paralysis (3). Cross-sectional studies conducted more than 20 years ago placed persons with chronic SCI near the lowest end of the human fitness spectrum. Not only has this scenario remained essentially unchanged, more recent evidence also suggests that persons living with paraplegia have remained deconditioned and only marginally more fit than those with tetraplegia (4,5). To place the problem in perspective, nearly 25% of healthy young persons with paraplegia fail to demonstrate a level of fitness that is sufficient to maintain independence in performance of daily activities. No clinical or scientific evidence suggests that this level of fitness will improve without exercise intervention.

Many scholarly reviews published over the past decades have addressed the need for exercise in persons living with SCI (6–9). As many such individuals now face the realities of their advancing age (10), the use and potential complications of exercise in both youth and advancing years following SCI require reexamination. Of SCI survivors in the United States, more than 40% are now 45 years or older, and one in four has lived 20 or more years with disability (11). While once thought of as a "static medical condition" unaffected by the passage of time, SCI is now viewed as a "dynamic medical condition" whose needs, abilities, and limitations constantly change (12,13). These needs may be hastened or intensified by cumulative stresses imposed by decades of wheelchair propulsion, upper extremity weight bearing, and other essential repetitive activities (14,15). As fatigue, pain, weakness, joint deterioration, and even incipient neurological deficits appear (13,16), the performance of essential daily activities mastered soon after injury can again become challenging. These life challenges, and the secondary disabilities they foster, further test life adjustment, self-perception, and ability to participate in active, satisfying, productive, and rewarding pursuits (11). Prudent exercise intervention soon after SCI using well-designed exercise programs is clearly one way in which harmful effects of long-standing paralysis might be lessened.

Many forms of exercise undertaken by persons without SCI are effective for (a) increasing muscle mass, strength, and endurance; (b) reversing deconditioning and its cardiovascular (CV) disease risks; (c) lowering body fat; (d) reversing insulin resistance; and (e) attenuating the acute effects of physical stress. Regrettably, the selection of exercise activities for persons with SCI to accomplish the same goals is limited, and the consequences of imprudent exercise are more serious than those experienced by persons without disability. It is important, therefore, to identify effective and available exercise activities that reduce risks of physical dysfunction and CV diseases sustained by persons with SCI while not increasing injury risks or hastening musculoskeletal deterioration.

COMPLEX EXERCISE USING ELECTRICALLY STIMULATED CONTRACTIONS OF PARALYZED MUSCLES

Various forms of electrically stimulated exercise are used by persons with SCI. These include site-specific stimulation of the lower extremities (LE) (17,18) and upper extremities (UEs) (19–22), leg cycling (23–25), leg cycling with UE assist (hybrid cycling) (26–28), lower body rowing (29), electrically assisted arm ergometry (30), electrically stimulated standing (31,32), and electrically stimulated bipedal ambulation either without or with an orthosis (33–35) (36,37). Some of these applications can be used to strengthen muscles whose motor function is partially spared by SCI (38), while other applications use electrical current as a neuroprosthesis of the lower (33,34) and UEs (22,39,40).

Most electrical stimulation devices currently approved for use by the U.S. Food and Drug Administration (FDA) employ surface, not implanted electrical stimulation. The three most common uses of surface electrical stimulation for exercise in those with SCI include (a) site-specific electrical stimulation of individual body segments, most often the knee extensors; (b) electrically stimulated cycling either with or without UE assistive propulsion; and (c) electrically stimulated ambulation. Qualifications necessary to safely participate in exercise programs have been described (25,41), and those with lower motor neuron lesions are generally excluded from participation.

Cycling Exercise

Electrically stimulated cycling is a process by which purposeful movement is initiated by sequentially activating contractions of the bilateral quadriceps, hamstrings, and gluteus muscles (42). Sensor control from the pedal gear provides feedback to a computer microprocessor, which initiates muscle firing sequences in a synergistic pattern, and also controls electrical current output necessary to sustain muscle contraction forces and programmed pedal rates (43). Improved fitness (27,44,45) and gas exchange kinetics (46), and increased muscle mass (47) have been reported following training using electrically stimulated cycling. For those with incomplete injuries, muscle mass gains are associated with increased voluntary and electrically stimulated isometric strength and endurance (47). Two specific improvements in circulatory function have also been reported following training. First, the adaptive left ventricular atrophy reported in persons with tetraplegia is reversed following cycle training, with near normalization of cardiac mass (48). Second, LE circulation following training is significantly improved, both in the basal state and when stimulated to a hyperemic response by ischemia (49). Reversal of osteopenia has been observed by some investigators (50,51) and an increased rate of bone turnover by another (52), although the site benefiting from training is usually the lumbar spine and proximal tibia and not the distal femur that is more susceptible to fracture (51). Not all studies have found a posttraining increase in mineral density for bones located below the level of the lesion (53). Otherwise, a study examining the appearance of LE joints and joint surfaces using magnetic resonance imaging reported no degenerative changes induced by cycling and less joint surface necrosis than that previously reported in sedentary persons with SCI (54). Improved body composition favoring increased lean mass and decreased fat mass (55) and an enhancement of whole-body insulin uptake and insulin-stimulated 3-0-methyl glucose transport in the quadriceps muscle have been observed (53). The latter finding, coupled with a report of increased expression of GLUT4 transport protein (53), may be especially important for elevated numbers of persons with SCI who show patterns of insulin resistance (10,56). When combined with simultaneous UE arm ergometry, the acute CV metabolic responses are more intense, and the gains in fitness are greater than those observed with LE cycling alone (27,28).

Bipedal Ambulation

A more complex form of electrical stimulation involves activation of LE muscles to achieve bipedal ambulation. This stimulation pattern can be used as a neuroprosthesis for those with motor-complete injuries (33,34), or an assistive neuroprosthesis accompanying body weight support and pharmacological intervention for those whose muscles can weakly contract but lack strength necessary to support independent ambulation (57–60). Surface and implantable neuroprostheses for those with unspared motor function have been investigated for nearly 25 years (61,62), although the only method currently approved by the FDA uses surface electrical stimulation of the quadriceps and gluteus muscles to maintain an upright stance Sigmedics, Inc., Fairborn, OH (34). The stepping motion for this ambulation neuroprosthesis is produced by a flexor withdrawal reflex initiated by introduction of a nociceptive electrical stimulus over the ipsilateral common peroneal nerve at the fibular head. This allows the hip, knee, and ankle to move into flexion, followed by extension of the knee joint initiated by electrical stimulation to the ipsilateral quadriceps muscle group. As muscle fatigue occurs, increasing levels of stimulation can be provided using bilateral switches mounted on the handles of the rolling walker.

Walking speeds achieved during electrically stimulated ambulation are relatively slow and distances covered relatively limited (34,63). These limitations are explained by the inefficient way in which electrical current recruits muscle, as well as the need for UE stabilization to maintain upright posture. Despite the limitations of ambulation rate and distance, ambulation distances of up to one mile have been reported in some individuals following training (33,34). Interestingly, UE fitness is enhanced in persons trained by electrically stimulated ambulation, despite the targeting of lower extremities for electrically stimulated contractions (33,64). Other adaptations to training include significantly increased LE muscle mass (65), resting blood flow (66), and an augmented hyperemic response to an ischemic stimulus (66). Despite these positive benefits, no change in bone mineralization of the LE has been observed (67). Ambulation with the assistance of lower extremity electrical stimulation requires some sparing of the trunk stabilizer muscles, and these devices are thus limited for use by individuals with injuries at or below the midthoracic spine (33).

Voluntary Arm Exercise Training

There is clear evidence that UE exercise conditioning improves fitness, although the magnitude of increase depends on the level of spinal lesion and training program (68–82). It is possible for persons with low tetraplegia to train on an arm ergometer, although special measures must be taken to affix the hands to an ergometer. The maximal endurance and work capacity of those with tetraplegia do not approach their paraplegic counterparts (83). Thus, level of injury is a key determinant of the extent to which gains in fitness are achieved after SCI (84,85).

While fitness benefits of arm training are widely reported for persons with paraplegia, their performance is limited by circulatory dysfunction accompanying thoracic SCI (23,86,87). Individuals with injuries below the level of sympathetic outflow at the T1 spinal level have significantly lower stroke volumes (SVs) at rest and during exercise than able-bodied persons, which are accompanied by higher resting heart rates (HR) (88–90). The significant elevation of resting and exercise HR compensates for a lower cardiac SV imposed by any or all of the following: pooling of blood in the LE venous circuits, diminished venous return, or frank circulatory insufficiency (89,91). Additionally, higher resting catecholamine levels and exaggerated catecholamine responses to physical challenges have been reported in paraplegics with midlevel thoracic (T6) cord injuries. These resting and exercise catecholamine levels exceed those of both high-level paraplegics and healthy persons without SCI (92,93). Hypersensitivity of the supralesional spinal cord is believed to regulate this unusual adrenergic state and dynamic, which contrasts the down-regulation of adrenergic functions observed in persons with high thoracic and cervical cord lesions (92,93). To date, down-regulation of adrenergic responses to exercise has been reported after training conducted by subjects with tetraplegia (94), but not paraplegia.

An excessive cardiovascular "strain" in persons with paraplegia was first reported by Hjeltnes (86) as an exaggerated percentage of HR reserve (HRR) needed to support physical responses to work challenge. Others have since reported similar findings, and included circulatory dysregulation imposed by midthoracic paraplegia as a limiting factor in the performance of activities of daily living (90,95,96). This finding is consistent with reports in persons with paraplegia requiring higher levels of oxygen consumption to perform at the same work intensity as those without SCI (23,77,90,92,97). As the sympathetic nervous system regulates hemodynamic and metabolic changes accompanying exercise (98), the elevated oxygen consumption and HR response to work in paraplegics with injuries below T5 may be a consequence of the reported adrenergic overactivity in persons with paraplegia (92,93). Thus, while the performance of physical activities by persons with paraplegia are compromised by orthopaedic and muscular decline of the shoulder complex, they are also limited by the unique and insufficient circulatory responses imposed by thoracic SCI, by impaired work capacities, and by the excessive oxygen cost of their subpeak work.

While exercise plays an important role in reducing cardiovascular disease (CVD) risks of persons without disability, the effect of exercise on most CVD risk factors after SCI is less well defined. However, UE conditioning favorably modifies dyslipidemia in persons with SCI, especially the risk imposed by low levels of the cardioprotective HDL. These low levels have been rated by the National Cholesterol Education Program Adult Treatment Panel (NCEP ATP) II Guidelines (99) as an independent risk factor that worsens risk prognosis. Current evidence strongly supports the presence of selective dyslipidemia involving low HDL levels (less than 40 mg/dL) in up to 47% of persons with SCI (100,101). A recent study suggested that nearly two of every three young healthy persons with paraplegia would qualify for therapeutic lifestyle intervention of pharmacotherapy if properly diagnosed, although intervention on the problem of all-cause CVD after SCI remains limited (102).

Fortunately, HDL is improved by as little as 20 minutes of moderate exercise performed three times weekly in persons with SCI (76). In men with paraplegia, a 9.8% increase in HDL, a 25.95% decrease in low-density lipoprotein cholesterol (LDL), and nonsignificant decreases in TC and plasma triglycerides (TG) accompany 3 months of vigorous intensity circuit training conducted three times per week for 45 minutes at approximately 75% HR_{max} (104). The circuit-training protocol consisted of alternating resistance exercise sets and 2 minutes of low-wattage, high-cadence arm ergometry sets. De Groot et al. (103) compared similar effects of 8 weeks of high-intensity intervals (70% to 80% heart rate reserve; HRR) and low-intensity intervals (40% to 50% HRR) on lipid profiles in persons with SCI. Both groups sustained improvements in TC, HDL, LDL, TC/HDL ratios, and triglycerides, although the high-intensity group experienced a greater decrease in TC/HDL ratio and TG. De Groot et al. also reported a positive correlation between VO_2 peak and insulin sensitivity, but did not observe a change in the latter following intervention (103). Hooker et al. (76) examined the impact of low intensity (50% to 60% HRR) and moderate intensity (70% to 80% HRR) wheelchair ergometry on lipid profiles (20 minutes per session, three times weekly). VO_2 max remained unchanged in both groups, and only the moderate intensity group experienced favorable changes in lipid profiles. El-Sayed and Younesian reported an increase in HDL levels after 3 months of three times weekly arm cranking exercise at 60% to 65% VO_2 peak for 30 minutes each session (104). Overall, these studies suggest that a variety of exercise modes improve HDL profiles, and that moderate intensity exercise performed three times weekly at 40% to 59% HRR may be a minimal threshold to elicit HDL improvement in persons with SCI. Higher exercise intensities, however, are needed to obtain more robust cardiometabolic benefits, and are thus preferred when possible.

Structured exercise does not appear to be the sole pathway to CVD risk factor modification. Cross-sectional studies have linked general physical activity with more favorable lipid profiles in both paraplegia and tetraplegia. In 37 men with paraplegia, physical activity was an important determinant of TC, LDL, and HDL levels as well as TC/HDL ratios, with improved profiles associated with increasing physical activity levels (105). A separate study reported significant correlations between physical activity, fasting glucose ($r = -0.525, p < 0.05$), and HDL-C levels ($r = 0.625, p < 0.01$) in 22 men with paraplegia (106). Finally, a longitudinal study reported that persons with SCI who were physically active after discharge from rehabilitation showed greater improvements in TC and LDL than individuals reporting no activity or low physical activity levels (107). Fortunately, physical activity also appears to benefit the lipid profiles of those with higher levels of SCI, as active men with tetraplegia have higher HDL levels and lower TC/HDL ratios than sedentary men with tetraplegia (108). These results suggest general physical activity and sports participation are viable options to improve lipid profiles after SCI. Evidence from investigations of basketball, tennis, wheelchair racing, and handbiking suggests wheelchair sports elicit a training intensity sufficient to produce the described health benefits (109–113). When encouraging patients with SCI to increase their physical activity, clinicians should not overlook sports participation or unstructured exercise as effective approaches to CVD risk management.

Resistance training should be a key component of lifetime health and fitness intervention after SCI, as it offers potential to both prevent and treat shoulder pain (114) while improving or maintaining transfer and propulsion independence. Fortunately, research is increasingly focused on the benefits of resistance training, although subject injury level, training protocols, assessment techniques, and outcome measures vary widely and may influence benefits. In a study of Scandinavian men (most of whom had incomplete low thoracic lesions), a weight training program with special emphasis on the triceps (for elbow extension during crutch walking) was undertaken for 7 weeks with modest but significant increases in VO_2 max observed following training, accompanied by increased strength of the triceps brachii (115). Another study (116) examined the effects of high-intensity arm ergometry conducted at 80 rpm in subjects assigned to high intensity (70% of VO_2 peak) or low intensity (40% of VO_2 peak) for 20 or 40 minutes per session, respectively. Strength gains were limited to subjects assigned high-intensity training, and occurred only in the shoulder joint extensors and elbow flexors. Otherwise, no changes in shoulder joint abduction or adduction strengths were reported, and none of the muscles that move or stabilize the scapulothoracic articulation or chest were stronger following training.

These results suggest that arm crank exercise is less effective than resistance exercise as a training mode for UE strengthening, as it fails to target muscles most involved in performance of ADLs. While one study has reported strengthening of five subjects with paraplegia and five with tetraplegia three times weekly for 9 weeks using a hydraulic fitness machine (117), exercises were limited to four maneuvers: (a) chest press/chest horizontal row and (b) shoulder press/latissimus pull. Significant increases in VO_2 and power output measured by arm ergometry testing were observed at the conclusion of the study, although no testing was conducted that directly measured strength gain in any muscle groups undergoing training. Also, the maneuvers used for training employed concentric but not eccentric actions, which neglected the need for eccentric strength in the performance of ADLs. Another study directed their training on strengthening of the scapular muscles, although this study focused solely on the scapular retractor muscles when comparing seated rowing and a standardized scapular retraction exercise, and did so only for concentric actions (118). The authors found that higher levels of retractor activation were obtained during retro- than forward wheelchair locomotion, and suggested that rowing was effective for improving scapular retractor activity and cardiorespiratory fitness. A recent study observed lowering of subject-reported shoulder joint pain following resistance training when using elastic bands, although UE strength was not examined as a study outcome (119). Overall, we believe that greater clinical emphasis needs to be placed on strengthening of people with SCI as a technique to attenuate pain and preserve/improve function as they age with disability.

Mixed interventions including aerobic conditioning and resistance training are becoming increasingly popular and are effective at increasing both strength and CV fitness. In a mixed gender and injury level cohort, a 9-month twice-weekly exercise program (90 to 120 minutes each session) of stretching, arm ergometry, and upper body resistance training improved strength and aerobic power (120). Compared to a nonexercise control group, exercisers reported less pain, fewer depressive symptoms, greater satisfaction with their physical functioning, and higher quality of life. The exercise intervention involved a low intensity warm-up followed by gentle stretching, arm ergometry (15 to 30 minutes at 70% max heart rate), and two resistance exercises for each of the following areas: biceps, triceps, back, chest, and shoulders (two sets of each exercise at 70% to 80% of 1 repetition maximum). All effects occurred after 3 months of training and most effects continued to improve at 6 and 9 months.

Strength and aerobic improvements can both be obtained using the "circuit" training approach to integrating CV and resistance training. This approach requires as little as 45 minutes of time per session, a practical consideration that should not be overlooked when developing an exercise prescription. Jacobs and Nash (121,122) developed a 45-minute, vigorous intensity circuit program that alternates 2 minutes of high cadence low resistance arm ergometry with two resistance exercises (for each exercise 1 set of 10 repetitions at 50% to 60% 1 repetition maximum) until three sets of each exercise were completed. The resistance exercises (6 in total) included military press, horizontal rows, pectoralis (pec)dec, preacher curls, wide grip latissimus pull-down, and seated dips. Strength gains were present after as little as 4 weeks of training in 10 men with paraplegia. After 3 months of training, strength gains ranged from 12% (preacher curls) to 30% (seated dips). Aerobic conditioning likely was improved at 4 weeks, but was not assessed until month 3, at which point it had dramatically improved. Strength gains were specific to the muscles trained with no changes to the external rotators (isokinetic testing). This finding highlights the need to specifically target external rotators with resistance exercises. Clinically, these muscles are active during wheelchair propulsion (123) and body transfers (123), with weaknesses in these muscles implicated in the development of shoulder pain and dysfunction (123). Interestingly, this same circuit protocol was later demonstrated to be effective at reducing or eliminating shoulder pain in a group of middle-aged men with paraplegia (114).

CURRENT EXERCISE RECOMMENDATIONS

Given that substantial evidence indicates that regular physical activity improves morbidity and mortality, the United States Government issued the first ever Physical Activity Guidelines for Americans in 2008, which outlined types and amounts of physical activity offering substantial health benefits (Table 24.1) (124). Importantly, the recommendations both affirm that adults with disabilities should engage in regular physical activity and emphasize that persons with disabilities should avoid sedentary behavior as much as possible.

The described recommendations for adults with disabilities are similar to those for nondisabled adults and include both aerobic and strengthening components, which each confers specific health benefits. Persons with disabilities are encouraged to consult with their health care provider to determine the amounts and types of physical activity that are appropriate for their abilities. The balance of this chapter provides guidance in developing an exercise prescription for persons with SCI.

TABLE 24.1

FEDERAL GUIDELINES FOR PHYSICAL ACTIVITY IN PEOPLE WITH PHYSICAL DISABILITIES

- All adults should avoid inactivity. Some physical activity is better than none, and adults who participate in any amount of physical activity gain some health benefits.
- Adults with disabilities, who are able to, should get at least 150 min/wk (2 h and 30 min) of moderate-intensity, or 75 min (1 h and 30 min) per week of vigorous-intensity aerobic activity. Aerobic activity should be performed in episodes of at least 10 min, and preferably, it should be spread throughout the week.
- For additional and more extensive health benefits, adults should increase their aerobic physical activity to 300 min (5 h) a week of moderate-intensity, or 150 min a week of vigorous-intensity aerobic physical activity, or an equivalent combination of moderate- and vigorous-intensity activity. Additional health benefits are gained by engaging in physical activity beyond this amount.
- Adults with disabilities, who are able to, should also do muscle-strengthening activities of moderate or high intensity that involve all major muscle groups on 2 or more days per week as these activities provide additional health benefits.
- When adults with disabilities are not able to meet the above guidelines, they should engage in regular physical activity according to their abilities and should avoid inactivity.
- Adults with disabilities should consult their health care providers about the amounts and types of physical activity that are appropriate for their abilities.
- Overall, the evidence shows that regular physical activity provides important health benefits for people with disabilities. The benefits include improved cardiovascular and muscle fitness, improved mental health, and better ability to do tasks of daily life. Sufficient evidence now exists to recommend that adults with disabilities should get regular physical activity.
- In consultation with their health care providers, people with disabilities should understand how their disabilities affect their ability to do physical activity. Some may be capable of doing medium to high amounts of physical activity, and they should essentially follow the guidelines for adults. Some people with disabilities are not able to follow the Guidelines for adults. These people should adapt their physical activity program to match their abilities, in consultation with their health care providers

Exercise Authorities for Persons with SCI: Exercise is Medicine

Federal physical activity guidelines are but the most recent set of authorities that set physical activity standards. Guidelines were first issued by the American College of Sports Medicine (ACSM) during the 1990s and have since been updated (Table 24.2) (125). The ACSM and federal guidelines are very similar and can be used interchangeably.

Widespread adoption of physical activity/exercise as a part of a healthy lifestyle has been impeded by the combined effect of knowledge gaps; nonsupportive health care policies; and attitudinal, environmental, and motivational barriers. In an attempt to surmount these obstacles, a nationwide initiative, "Exercise is Medicine" was jointly launched in May 2008 by the ACSM and the American Medical Association (126). The vision of this initiative is "to make physical activity and exercise a standard part of a disease prevention and treatment paradigm in the United States." This initiative is widely supported by professional

TABLE 24.2

ACSM/AHA RECOMMENDED EXERCISE PRESCRIPTION TO MAINTAIN BODY WEIGHT AND REDUCE CHRONIC DISEASE RISK

	Aerobic exercise	
	Option 1	Option 2
Frequency:	5 d/wk	3 d/wk
Intensity:	Moderate intensity cardiovascular exercise (3–6 METs[a], 40–59% HRR/VO_2R[b], 55–69% HR_{max}[b], or 12–13 RPE[b,c])	Vigorous intensity cardiovascular exercise (>6.0 METs[a], 60–84% HRR/VO_2[b], 70–80% HR_{max}[b], or 14–16 RPE[b,c])
Time:	30 min/d (60–90 min for weight loss)	20 min/d (amount for weight loss not reported)
Type:	Any activity that achieves the above	Any activity that achieves the above
	Resistance Exercise	
Frequency:	2 d/wk	
Intensity:	Weight at which 1 set of 8–12 repetitions can be completed	
Time:	NA	
Type:	4–5 upper body exercises[d]	

A complete prescription includes aerobic exercise and resistance training. Two acceptable approaches to aerobic prescription are provided.
[a]Official intensity prescription is given in METs only.
[b]%HRR, %VO_2R, %HR_{max}, %VO_{2max}, and RPE recommendations for moderate intensity exercise are derived from separate ACSM guidelines26 and are provided for guidance purposes.
[c]RPE intensity is based on Borg's 6 to 20 RPE scale.
[d]Modified from ACSM recommendation of 8 to 10 exercises, which covers upper and lower body.
ACSM/AHA, American College of Sports Medicine and American Heart Association; METs, metabolic units; HRR, heart rate reserve; VO_2R, oxygen consumption reserve; HR_{max}, heart rate at peak VO_2; RPE, rating of perceived exertion.

societies, including the American Academy of Physical Medicine and Rehabilitation, American Physical Therapy Association, American Heart Association (AHA), and the American Osteopathic Association. A Web site–based physician toolkit (127) has been developed to facilitate exercise prescription design and implementation. Included in the kit is an algorithm to guide the prescription process and a structured prescription pad. In addition, the Web site contains links to key ACSM/AHA physical activity and public health recommendations; ACSM health, fitness, and sport position stands; and AHA scientific statements.

CURRENT EXERCISE PARTICIPATION

Although benefits of exercise are widely known and accepted for those without disability, less than 50% of nondisabled adults in the United States currently meet the Healthy People 2010 recommendations for undertaking at least 30 minutes of moderate-intensity activity on 5 or more days per week, or at least 20 minutes of vigorous-intensity activity on 3 or more days per week (128). For persons with a disability, the compliance statistics are more grim. In 1997, only 12% reported engaging in at least 30 minutes of physical activity five times weekly (128). The Healthy People 2010 goal for persons with disability is for 30% of persons with a disability to engage in at least 30 minutes of physical activity 5 days weekly. To help correct this deficiency, the U.S. Surgeon General in 2005 issued a *Call to Action to Improve the Health and Wellness of Persons with Disabilities*, which recognized the need to specifically target persons with disabilities, stressed the importance of choosing a healthy lifestyle, and provided tips for becoming physically fit (129). Rehabilitation professionals are critically positioned to take action on current initiatives by encouraging and then guiding increased physical activity and exercise among persons with SCI.

Given the known benefits of physical activity, authoritative recommendations, and best practice pursuits, incorporation of structured exercise or recreational activities into a healthy lifestyle should be standard advice from health care professionals. Unfortunately, only 18% to 42% of nondisabled patients report receiving advice to exercise from their physician (130–133). When physician advice is coupled with an exercise plan, patients are twice as likely to exercise as those who receive advice without an exercise plan (133). This level of compliance increases to three times more likely to exercise when physician advice is coupled with both an exercise plan and regular follow-up queries (133). However, not all clinicians are well versed in the design of an "exercise prescription," making effective guidance a practice challenging activity. In addition, the importance of exercise as an essential tool for treatment and prevention of chronic diseases has not always been recognized or supported by government policies and reimbursement. This has created a shortfall in global disease management that often constrains health practitioners from providing the highest standard of care and limits consumers from pursuing the most effective exercise options.

Access-related barriers are unique to persons with disabilities, and when accompanying traditional hindrances of time, knowledge, and motivation, further complicates both prescription implementation and robust exercise compliance (134,135). The so-called "all-or-nothing" approach to exercise—based upon a long-standing belief that intense, prolonged exercise is necessary to reap health benefits—may be an additional barrier to exercise adoption as a lifestyle habit. To the contrary, accumulating 30 minutes of moderate exercise in 10-minute intervals imparts significant health benefits (125). Moreover, individuals who transition from a sedentary lifestyle to low levels of fitness typically experience the largest gains in health (125). It follows that exercise interventions undertaken by deconditioned persons with SCI will result in rapid and substantial health gains.

DEVELOPING AN EXERCISE PRESCRIPTION

A physical activity/exercise prescription is developed in much the same manner as a drug prescription, which requires selection of drug type and strength, administration frequency, and duration of use. This prescription contains four elements: frequency, intensity, time, and activity type (F.I.T.T.). The current ACSM/AHA *minimum* physical activity/exercise recommendations are found in Table 24.2, and are targeted to improve or maintain health in adults under age 65. The ACSM/AHA recommendations identify minimum target levels, and that a higher dosage of exercise/physical activity will further enhance health and fitness. Highly deconditioned persons may have to begin their conditioning programs well below these levels. However, these individuals may accumulate 30 minutes of daily exercise through 10-minute sessions, an ACSM/AHA endorsed approach with proven effectiveness for conferring health benefits (125). Indeed, both the federal physical activity guidelines and these recommendations emphasize that any increase in activity will be beneficial, even if minimum target levels are not achieved. The evidence-based targets, however, are designed to maintain weight and minimize CVD risk in healthy adults, and weight loss requires longer duration than the minimum daily time required for health benefits (60 to 90 minutes versus 30 minutes). As the recommendations are not specific to persons with SCI, the balance of this section will provide SCI-relevant information to further guide the prescription process and compliance with recommended guidelines.

EXERCISE PRESCRIPTION: SPECIAL CONSIDERATIONS FOR PERSONS WITH SCI

"The art of exercise prescription is the successful integration of exercise science with behavioral techniques that result in long-term program compliance and attainment of the individual's goals" (136). The "art" of exercise prescription in SCI must address upper extremity overuse concerns and may require modifications of the general prescriptive plan to accommodate effects of lesion level on intensity targets. The following sections address these concerns, resources supporting the exercise prescription, and activity options.

Upper Extremity Pain and Injury

Upper limb injury is a serious concern for persons undertaking upper extremity exercise, as the prevalence of shoulder pain and injury is 30% to 60% after SCI (137,138). Thus, exercise prescriptions and subsequent follow-up should be preceded by a thorough upper extremity assessment. If shoulder pain is present, circuit training (139) and anterior stretching/posterior strengthening regimens (119,140) are effective treatment options. The exercise prescription can be tailored as needed to minimize pain and injury until more intense exercise is safely pursued and tolerated. This approach is consistent with recommendations for comprehensive upper limb preservation from the Consortium for Spinal Cord Medicine (141). A review of evidence-based strategies to preserve shoulder function in SCI in the Spring 2008 issue of *Topics in Spinal Cord Rehabilitation* suggests a comprehensive exercise prescription of aerobic conditioning, stretching, and strengthening will both improve CVD risk factors and help preserve upper extremity function (142).

Intensity Prescription for Injuries at T1 and Higher Levels

Persons with complete spinal cord lesions at the T1 level and higher have a blunted HR response, with a peak of approximately 120 beats per minute. This incompetent chronotropic response arises from impaired sympathetic outflow below lesion level resulting in a nonlinear relationship between exercise HR and VO_2. In these cases, HR will plateau with increasing work intensity while VO_2 continues to rise, diminishing the validity of HR_{max} or HRR methods as surrogates for fitness assessment or intensity estimation. A more accurate approach involves measurement of VO_2 peak during an arm exercise test, followed by prescription targeted at specific workloads that will elicit 60% to 80% of this value. As this method may be impractical, or provide unneeded precision for those engaging in simple recreational activity, the rating of perceived exertion (RPE) method of Borg (143) can serve as an alternative. Although Lewis et al. (144) reported that RPE is not correlated with VO_2 in persons with SCI, they did observe increasing RPE and VO_2 with increasing workload. Thus, while the relationship between RPE and VO_2 may not be linear, RPE remains a viable option for establishing the intensity component of the exercise prescriptions. A second benefit of the RPE method is that it is easily used by laypersons. A last option for intensity estimation involves use of the Centers for Disease Control and Prevention recommended talk test, which although not validated in persons with SCI, still offers a simple, easy-to-use estimate of exercise intensity (145).

Intensity Prescriptions for Injuries at T2 and Lower Levels

Injuries at and below the T2 spinal level leave the integrated sympathetic adrenergic responses to exercise stress partially intact, making the HR response closely linear with VO_2 throughout the subpeak intensity range. Exercise intensity prescriptions for individuals with T6 lesions and lower can be computed using the HRR, VO_2 reserve (VO_2R), HR_{max}, or RPE methods. We suggest using RPE, HRR, and HR_{max} methods, which can be used by laypersons after minimal instruction, a practical consideration that should not be overlooked in patient education on exercise guidelines. Clinicians should ensure their patients are competent in taking their own pulse. Both the HRR and HR_{max} methods require an estimated or measured HR_{max}. HR_{max} can be estimated by subtracting the person's age in years from 220 (220 – age) (136). Table 24.3 defines the moderate and vigorous intensity RPE and HR ranges for ages 20 to 80 years based on the age-estimated HR_{max}. HRR requires a resting HR measure (HR_{rest}). Ideally, HR_{rest} is measured immediately upon awakening in the morning. While resting pulse recorded during a typical clinical exam provides an elevated estimate of HR_{rest} that may be used for the initial prescription. The equation to establish upper and lower limits of the target range for the HRR method is as follows: upper/lower limit = HR_{max} + (intensity × HRR), where HRR= HR_{max} – HR_{rest}. Intensity is entered as a percentage of HR_{max} (i.e., 70% = 0.70). Two different intensities are used to define the upper and lower limits of the desired target range. A full description and explanation of the available methods can be found in Chapter 7 in the ACSM Guidelines for Exercise Testing and Prescription (136).

Corollary Benefits of Exercise

The 2005 Surgeon General's *Call to Action to Improve the Health and Wellness of Persons with Disabilities* provides information on becoming physically fit and emphasizes the importance of a healthy lifestyle for all persons with a disability (129). Exercise and physical activity provide benefits beyond CVD risk factor modification, further supporting the need to implement exercise prescriptions for persons with SCI. Gains in strength and fitness obtained through recreational pursuits have practical daily benefits for persons with SCI; improving mobility and facilitating greater independence, which are strongly related to quality of life (106,146–149). In addition, regular physical activity and exercise decrease pain (119,150), anxiety and depression (151,152), and improve life satisfaction (153), physical self-concept (149), and dynamic balance (154). In turn, these gains may improve a person's ability to

TABLE 24.3

TARGET HEART RATE AND RPE RANGES FOR MODERATE AND VIGOROUS ACTIVITY BASED ON AGE ADJUSTED ESTIMATED PEAK HEART RATE FOR PERSONS WITH INJURIES T2 AND BELOW

Age (y)	Moderate activity (bpm) RPE = 12–13	Vigorous activity (bpm) RPE = 14–16
20	110–140	140–160
25	107–137	137–156
30	105–133	133–152
35	102–130	130–148
40	99–126	126–144
45	96–123	123–140
50	94–119	119–136
55	91–116	116–132
60	88–112	112–128
65	85–109	109–124
70	83–105	105–120
75	80–102	102–116
80	77–98	98–112

Rate of perceived exertion (RPE) targets are applicable for all persons. RPE intensity is based on Borg's 6 to 20 scale.
bpm, beats per minute.

work, attend school, and fully engage in community life (106). Many challenging and adventurous recreation opportunities exist for persons with SCI, which are described in later portions of this chapter.

HAZARDS AND COMPLICATIONS ASSOCIATED WITH RECREATIONAL AND THERAPEUTIC EXERCISE

Complications arising from exercise are unfortunately omitted from most chapters and monographs examining the benefits of exercise in persons with SCI. Special considerations are required when designing, instituting, or performing exercise programs for persons with SCI. Some of the risks encountered will be similar to those experienced by persons without paralysis, although complications such as general overuse may be exaggerated, and their occurrence will likely compromise daily activities to a far greater extent than similar injuries arising in persons without SCI.

Trauma, Accidents, and Reinjury

Heightened awareness and prevention, better equipment, better training programs, and skilled individuals all decrease the likelihood that injury will be sustained during therapeutic exercise, sports competition, and recreation. Nonetheless, it is plausible that such participation can result in secondary injury to the spine, spinal cord, or other body parts. While no evidence suggests that activity restrictions are warranted for those with SCI, several reports have documented the various and common injuries in sports for persons with disabilities and their prevention. Although little has been documented concerning all these types of injuries among persons with SCI who participate in sports activities, it is well documented that winter skiing, hockey, and other recreational activities are associated with SCI in persons not yet so injured. Additional spinal injuries may alter the level of function for a person with an existing SCI, or may cause yet unknown effects on body systems. Given that injury to a paralyzed body has a more profound functional consequence than that in those without physical disability, and that healing rates are slower, prudence must be exercised in risking additional injury due to trauma.

Upper Extremity Injuries, Pain, and Decline

Special cautions for persons undergoing upper extremity exercise are warranted. While a single cause for shoulder pain has not been identified, many studies attribute pain to deterioration and injury resulting from insufficient shoulder strength, range, and endurance (155–158). Upper extremity pain accompanying wheelchair locomotion and other wheelchair activities reportedly interferes with functional activities including, but not limited to, UE weight bearing for transfers, high resistance muscular activity in extreme ranges of motion, wheelchair propulsion up inclines, and frequent overhead activities (157–160). All instigate or exacerbate shoulder pain (155). Several studies have reported that wheelchair propulsion and depression transfers cause the most pain and increase the intensity of existing pain more than other daily activities (81,159,160) (see Chapters 16 and 26 for a full review).

Given available evidence that wheelchair locomotion is a major source of pain and dysfunction, one might reasonably question its use as the basis for the design of an exercise training program, unless this training is both conducted using specialized equipment and specific to an athletic event in which training specificity and skill acquisition are targeted.

Immune Suppression and Infections

A spinal level–dependent immune dysfunction has been reported after SCI by various investigators (161–169). Significant depression of T- and B-cell function has been reported in persons without SCI undergoing intense and prolonged exercise (170). Further, an association has been defined between this immune deficiency and increased illness and infection susceptibility reported after athletic competitions (171). Given that persons with SCI may start with increased illness susceptibility, and experience organ system dysfunction of the lungs and bladder that provides a backdrop of chronic infection risk, intense work may worsen their immune profiles and place them at greater risk for infection. To date, a single study has examined the effects of wheelchair racing on subjects with paraplegia and found suppression of natural killer cell function and heightened levels of the stress hormone cortisol following racing, which resolved almost 24 hours after completion of exercise (172). Interestingly, the depressed NK cell function reported acutely after SCI is attenuated by moderate activity rather than complete sedentariness (165), suggesting the intensity of activity may determine whether improved or depressed immune function accompanies physical activity (171). As infection susceptibility may also be related to competition stress and overtraining just before competition (173), schedules that provide consistent training intensities and durations rather than those that escalate physical and emotional stress during preevent overtraining may decrease the likelihood of an adverse infection outcome of sports participation.

Thermal Dysregulation

Individuals with SCI often lack vasomotor and sudomotor responses below their level of injury and are thus challenged to maintain thermal stability in both hot and cold environments (174–176). It has been reported that the level of heat strain during resting heat exposure is proportional to the level of SCI (177), with tetraplegia experiencing the greatest heat strain. The interplay between lesion level, environmental conditions, exercise protocols, and thermal dysregulation remain poorly defined (177). However, it appears that persons with SCI are at increased risk for heat injury due to an inability to dissipate heat, with this effect most pronounced in hot conditions and in persons with tetraplegia (177). Interestingly, heat intolerance during exercise in absence of measurable heat gain has been reported (178). Rate of heat gain during exercise can be attenuated through local cooling to the head, chest, or feet. However, this approach does not prevent body temperature elevation (177). Thermal strain during exercise may be best countered through a combination of cooling prior to exercise and local cooling during exercise (179). Immediate postexercise cooling may be indicated for persons with tetraplegia, as their temperature continues to climb for up to 5 minutes after exercise termination. Altered sensation below the level of injury may also limit the otherwise prudent responses to numbing or freezing of tissues sometimes encountered in winter sports. Research indicates that persons with SCI may experience a net heat loss during exercise in cold weather, despite the impaired ability to dissipate heat. This is attributed to both impaired vasoconstriction in the lower limbs that hastens heat loss and the limited heat generation capacity of the upper limbs, which does not fully offset heat lost through the lower limbs and trunk. Those who participate in outdoor exercise should be especially careful to prevent hyperthermia through attention paid to hydration, local application of ice packs or cool, wet towels, cooling by combination of water spray bottles and fans, and, if possible, limiting the duration and intensity of activities performed in intemperate environments. These same considerations should be taken when exercising in an environment controlled for temperature and humidity, as overheating may still occur (180,181). Hypothermia, frostnip, and frost bite may best prevented through proper clothing and intermittent warming sessions during prolonged outdoor activities. Proper preparation to prevent and treat exercise induced hyperthermia and environmentally induced hypothermia is of extreme importance.

Autonomic Dysreflexia

Episodes of adrenergic dysregulation are common in individuals having injuries above the level of adrenal sympathetic outflow at the T6 spinal level. While these events are normally considered an uncomfortable outcome of SCI, release of catecholamine during these bouts can be considered ergogenic in those individuals whose injuries otherwise limit epinephrine and norepinephrine evolution during exercise. It should be cautioned that wheelchair racers sometimes induce dysreflexia as an ergogenic aid by intentionally obstructing urine outflow through a Foley catheter. While often referred to as "boosting" (182), such practices may be risky and should be discouraged.

Electrical Current

Several special concerns are engendered for individuals who are exercising under the control of electrical current. The foremost concern involves episodes of autonomic hyperreflexia, which can occur in individuals having injuries above the T6 spinal cord level (183,184). As the sympathetic system above this level is partially dissociated from the inhibitory influences of brain control, the nociceptive effects of electrical current may provoke a reflex adrenergic response with accompanying crisis hypertension (184–186). The recognition of these episodes, withdrawal of the offending stimulus, and the possible administration of a fast acting peripheral vasodilator may be critical in preventing serious medical complications. In such cases, prophylaxis with a slow calcium channel antagonists or alpha-$_1$-selective adrenergic antagonist may be needed (187–189). Otherwise, fracture and joint dislocation may be caused by asynergistic movement of limbs against the force imposed by either electrical stimulation or the device used for exercise (190). These activities are therefore contraindicated for individuals with severe spasticity, or spastic response to the introduction of electrical current (25). Postexercise hypotension with lost vasomotor responses to orthostatic repositioning is common in deconditioned persons with SCI (191), although these episodes can abate after upper limb training. Otherwise, skin burns may be caused by electrical stimulation, which is normally prevented through use of fresh electrodes whose surfaces are completely covered by gel conductor or moisture.

Recreational/Sports Activities

The evolution of sports for persons with disabilities is traced to Sir Ludwig Guttmann at the Stoke Mandeville Hospital in England. By involving young people who had sustained injury during World War II in sports, Sir Guttmann and his colleagues utilized sporting events as a rehabilitation tool to facilitate recovery and societal reentry. In 1948, the first Stoke Mandeville Games were held. Since that time, the evolution has been profound. In 1952, the first international competition for wheelchair athletes occurred under Stoke Mandeville sponsorship. This event sparked the formation of the International Stoke Mandeville Games Federation (subsequently called the International Stoke Mandeville Wheelchair Sports Federation, ISMWSF). In 2005, the International Wheelchair and Amputee Sports Federation (headquartered in Stoke Mandeville, Great Britain) was formed by a merger of the ISMWSF and the International Sports Federation of the Disabled.

Olympic style games for athletes with a disability, now called the Paralympic Games, were organized for the first time in Rome in 1960, with 400 athletes from 23 countries participating. In 1976, the Games in Toronto saw the inclusion of athletes with amputations and visual impairments, while the first Winter Games took place the same year in Sweden. The Paralympic Movement has continued to grow with the Paralympic Games now the pinnacle of elite sports competition for athletes from six different disability groups. For individuals with SCI, the Summer Games include 14 events and the Winter Games five events. The 2008 Beijing Summer Paralympic Games included approximately 4,000 athletes from 146 countries and the 2010 Vancouver Winter Paralympic Games approximately 1,350 athletes from 44 countries. In 2006, high-level competitions became available to a larger audience with the launching of the International Paralympic Committee (192) Internet television channel (www.paralympicsport.tv). Broadcasting 24/7 via the Internet, *ParalympicSport.TV* allows people all around the world to watch live and delayed programming, as well as Paralympic news, interviews, and event reports. This resulted in 146,683 unique viewers from 166 countries during the Beijing Summer Games and 176,350 unique viewers from 121 countries during the Vancouver Winter Games.

In addition to these high-end competitive endeavors, there are numerous opportunities for maintaining an active, healthy lifestyle. Such activities range from outdoor adventure pursuits to the more sedentary recreational activities and are all possible and increasingly available to persons with disabilities.

Recreational Activities

In the United States, the passage of the Americans with Disabilities Act of 1990 (ADA) and recently amended with changes effective January 2009 require any new public facilities to provide access for the persons with disabilities (127). The National Center on Accessibility (www.ncaonline.org), a collaborative program of Indiana University and the National

Park Service, promotes access to recreation and strives to increase awareness of inclusion of people with disabilities in parks, recreation, and tourism as mandated by the ADA and other disability legislation. In addition, the Inclusive Fitness Coalition emerged from the need to address health risks associated with a sedentary lifestyle in persons with disabilities by addressing policy, environmental, and societal issues associated with the lack of inclusion and access to physical activity (http://www.incfit.org/). The 2005 *Surgeon General's Call to Action to Improve the Health and Wellness of Persons with Disabilities* emphasizes the importance of choosing a healthy lifestyle and provides tips for getting physically fit. In 2008, the ACSM in collaboration with the National Center on Physical Activity and Disability (NCPAD) launched a specialty certification, the Certified Inclusive Fitness Trainer (193). This certification is for professionals working in the health and fitness field, and fosters full inclusion for individuals with disabilities into various exercise environments, including health club, outdoor and home-based settings.

Currently, the variety of recreational activities available to persons with disabilities is extensive, including activities spanning wheelchair dancing to downhill skiing. Whether participating in recreation for fun, structured exercise for fitness, or for competition though sports, a variety of activities are available. Common activities include fishing, bowling, golf, hand cycling, swimming, and sailing. Other less commonly imagined activities include horseback riding, mountain climbing, karate, scuba diving, water skiing, surfing, skydiving, snowboarding, and flying. Such active recreation and leisure pursuits can provide many physical and health benefits, as well as opportunities for socialization and community participation.

A rich information resource is available on the Internet identifying fun, active, healthy recreation activities. Table 24.4 lists organizations that offer recreation programs and provides their Internet addresses. Many of these activities can be pursued on a competitive as well as recreational level. The U.S. Paralympics Activity Network provides a search engine to find events and organizations across the country (http://events.usparalympics.org/). The resource links page on the Blaze Sports Web site (www.blazesports.org) provides information on a wide range of activities while the NCPAD provides information and resources to assist individuals in pursuing physical activities. These resources are supported by magazines on adapted recreation and sport including Sports 'N Spokes and Palaestra. When adaptive equipment is needed, it is typically manufactured by specialty firms. Databases that list equipment for fitness, sport, and recreation are located at www.rectech.org/equipments/index.php and www.usatechguide.org/techguide.php.

Competitive Activities

Wheelchair sports have elevated from a curiosity involving a few disabled soldiers in the 1940s, to well-established, high-performance competitive events involving thousands of athletes from all over the world. Since 1985, the Paralyzed Veterans of America (PVA) and the Department of Veterans Affairs have copresented the National Veterans Wheelchair Games (http://www1.va.gov/opa/speceven/wcg/index.asp). The Games are a multievent sports and rehabilitation program for military service veterans who use wheelchairs for sports competition due to SCI, amputation, and other neurological conditions. Attracting more than 500 athletes each year, the National Veterans Wheelchair Games is the largest annual wheelchair sports event in the world. A National Veterans Winter Sports Clinic is also offered yearly. In 2010, the inaugural Warrior Games, athletic competition for wounded, ill, and injured service members, were held through a joint effort between the U.S. Department of Defense and U.S. Olympic Committee. The Endeavor Games is a nationally recognized competition that allows all athletes with physical disabilities to participate in a multisport event.

TABLE 24.4

RECREATIONAL SPORTS—U.S. ORGANIZATIONS

Recreational sports and activities	Web site
Aerobics, Disabled Sports, USA	www.dsuas.org
American Canoe Association	www.acanet.org
Bowling, American Wheelchair Bowling Association	www.amwheelchairbowl.qpg.com
Billiards, National Wheelchair Billiards	www.nwpainc.com
Camping, National Park Services, Office of Special Programs	www.nps.gov
Disabled Sports, USA	www.dsusa.org
Flying, International Wheelchair Aviators	www.wheelchairaviators.org
Freedom's Wings International	www.freedomswings.org
Fishing, PVA	www.pva.com
Handicapped Scuba Association	www.hsascuba.com
Horseback Riding, North American Riding for the Handicapped Association	www.narha.org
Hunting, NRA Disabled Shooting Services	www.nrahq.org
POINT, Paraplegics On Independent Nature Trips	www.turningpoint1.com
Sailing, National Ocean Access Project	www.dsusa.org
Special Olympics International	www.specialolympics.org
U.S. Rowing Association	www.usrowing.org
U.S. Wheelchair Swimming, Inc.	www.wsusa.org
Water Sports, American Water Ski Association	www.usawaterski.org
Wheelchair Sports, USA	www.wsusa.org

TABLE 24.5

COMPETITIVE SPORTS—U.S. ORGANIZATIONS

Competitive sports and activities	Web site
Wheelchair Archery, USA	www.wsusa.org
Wheelchair Athletics of the USA	www.wsusa.org
National Wheelchair Basketball Association	www.nwba.org
International Wheelchair Basketball Federation	www.iwbf.org
U.S. Fencing Association	www.usfa.org
Association of Disabled American Golfers	www.toski.com/golf/adag/
American Handcycle Association	www.ushf.org
American Sled Hockey Association	www.sledhockey.org
U.S. Quad Rugby Association	www.quadrugby.com
International Wheelchair Tennis Federation	www.itftennis.org
American Wheelchair Table Tennis Association	www.wsusa.org
National Wheelchair Softball	www.wsusa.org
U.S. Wheelchair Swimming	www.usa-swimming.org
United States Wheelchair Weightlifting Federation	www.wsusa.org

More specific information regarding the goals, activities, and participatory restrictions is found on the Web sites for each organization, which are listed in Table 24.5.

Classification and Disability Categories

Athletes with disability differ widely in their impairments. Conducting competition among these different athletes is challenging with respect to making these competitions fair. The method utilized to attempt to address the relative uniqueness of these widely differing athletes is called "classification."

Originally, competitors were segregated into a disability-based classification. An example of disability type classification might be quadriplegic/C5 level versus paraplegic/T12 level. This method would not allow interimpairment competition despite relative functional similarities. This method of diagnosis-specific classification is evolving and in most cases athletes are placed in a classification based on their "functional ability." This method takes into consideration an athletes' ability to perform sport-related tasks. In doing this, people with different disabilities categories, such as cerebral palsy and/or paraplegia, are able to compete in the same event because they have similar sport-related functionality.

The process of classification is rather complex. Specially trained observers, and often a panel of evaluators, are utilized to perform this classification function. A classification is also not "set in stone." The classification is performed a number of times throughout the athlete's career and competitors may actually move into different classifications depending on their increase or decrease of functionality and/or multisystem physical decline. A small sample of classification systems and associated rules are listed below. Complete classification guidelines for all Paralympic Sports are available on their Web site (http://www.paralympic.org).

Athletics. Track classifications for the wheelchair subgroup, which includes athletes with different levels of SCI or spinal cord conditions, amputations, other musculoskeletal impairments, and congenital anomalies and nerve lesions, who meet the sport-specific minimum impairment levels, are denoted with a "T" and range from T11 to T54. Classifications for field events are denoted with an "F" ranging from F11 to F58. In both cases, a higher classification number indicates greater functional ability.

Wheelchair Basketball. Classification is based upon sport-specific tests of shooting, passing, rebounding, pushing, and dribbling, rather than a medical diagnosis or muscle function examination. There are eight classifications based upon functional ability to play wheelchair basketball (Classes 1.0, 1.5, 2.0, 2.5, 3.0, 3.5, 4.0, and 4.5), with higher classification numbers representing function. Each team is allowed to field any five-player combination such that the sum of their classification is a maximum of 14.0 points (Fig. 24.1).

Shooting. There are two categories of competition: wheelchair and standing. Athletes compete in Rifle and Pistol events from distances of 10, 25, and 50 m, in men's, women's, and mixed competitions. Shooting utilizes a functional classification system, based on existing limitations (degree of body trunk functionality, balance while seated, muscle strength, mobility of upper and lower limbs) and skills necessary in shooting. This system enables athletes with different disabilities but similar functional ability to compete together, either individually or in teams.

Swimming. Competitors have either a physical disability or visual impairment and are classified based on their functional ability to perform each stroke. In the case of swimmers with a physical disability, classification is based on several factors that is, muscle strength, movement coordination, joint range of movement, and/or limb length. The swimmers are also required to perform a practical water session in which they perform all strokes. There are 10 classes (S1 to S10) for Freestyle, Backstroke, and Butterfly, 10 classes (SM1 to SM10) for Individual Medley, and 9 classes (SB1 to SB9) for Breaststroke. The higher the class number, the greater the functional ability of the athlete.

Wheelchair Tennis. Players must have a permanent physical disability with substantial loss of function in one or both lower extremities. If due to lack of capacity a player is unable to propel the wheelchair via the wheel, then he or she may propel the wheelchair using one foot. (Note: foot cannot be

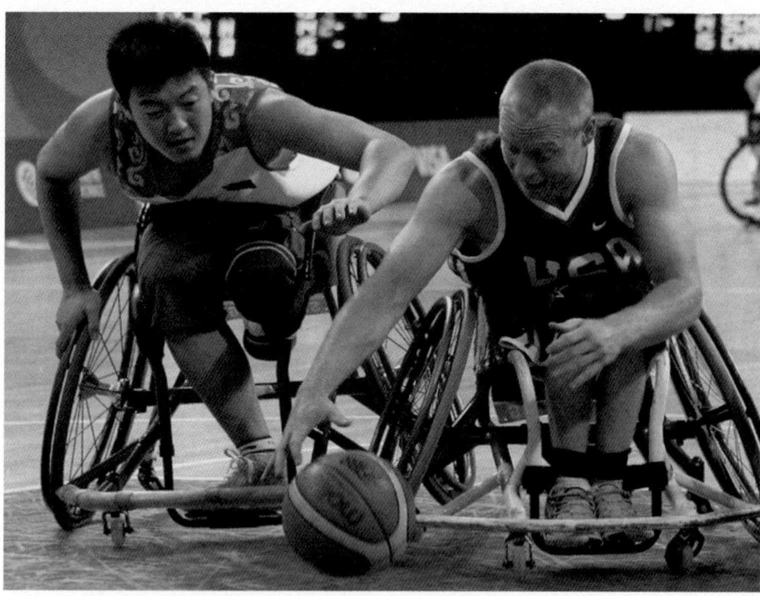

FIGURE 24.1 Wheelchair basketball (Courtesy USOC).

used during swing or service motions.) A "quad" player must also have a permanent physical disability that results in a substantial loss of function in one or both UEs. Players who have severe limitations and use a power wheelchair for everyday mobility may use a power wheelchair to play tennis.

Wheelchair Rugby. Wheelchair Rugby (also known as Quad Rugby) is a sport for quadriplegic (tetraplegic) male and female athletes. Players are classified based on functional ability and placed into one of seven groups ranging from 0.5 to 3.5 points (Fig. 24.2). The higher the class, the greater the functional ability of the player. During the game, the total value of all four players on the court for a team cannot exceed eight points. This ensures that teams must field a mix of athletes of all functional levels.

Paracycling. The competition program includes Track and Road events for individuals and teams with Sprints, Individual Pursuits, 1,000 m Time Trial, Road Races, and Road Time Trials. Paracycling sport classes include hand bike, tricycle, cycling, and tandem competition. Events are for both men and women, with the cyclists classified according to the extent of activity limitation resulting from their impairment. Impairment groups include neurological, locomotor, spinal cord lesions, and visual impairments.

Sailing. This sport is open to athletes with an amputation, cerebral palsy, blindness/visual impairment, spinal injuries, and les autres. Athletes compete in three events, which are nongender specified. The Sailing classification system is based on four factors: stability, hand function, mobility, and vision. A scoring system that assigns points based on level of ability, ranging from one (lowest level of function) to seven (highest level of function), allows athletes from different disability groups to compete together. To ensure the participation of athletes from all classes of disability, there is a maximum point count of 14, which a crew of three persons must not exceed.

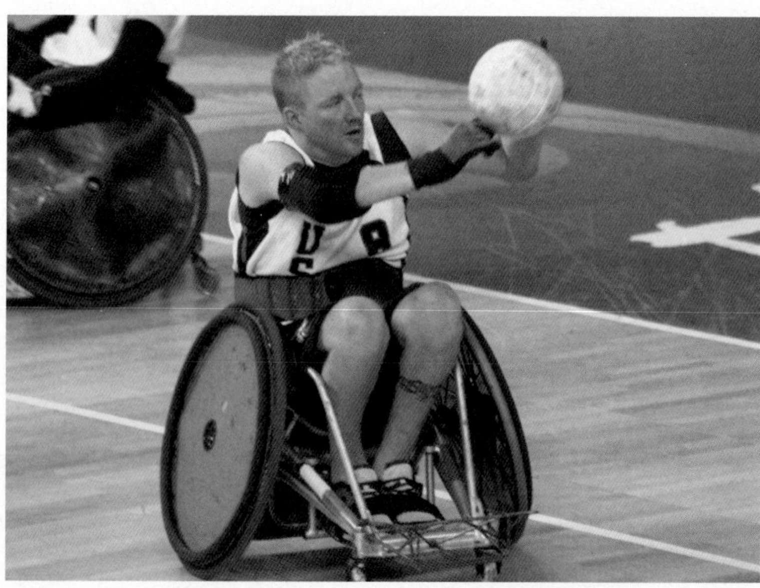

FIGURE 24.2 Quad Rugby.

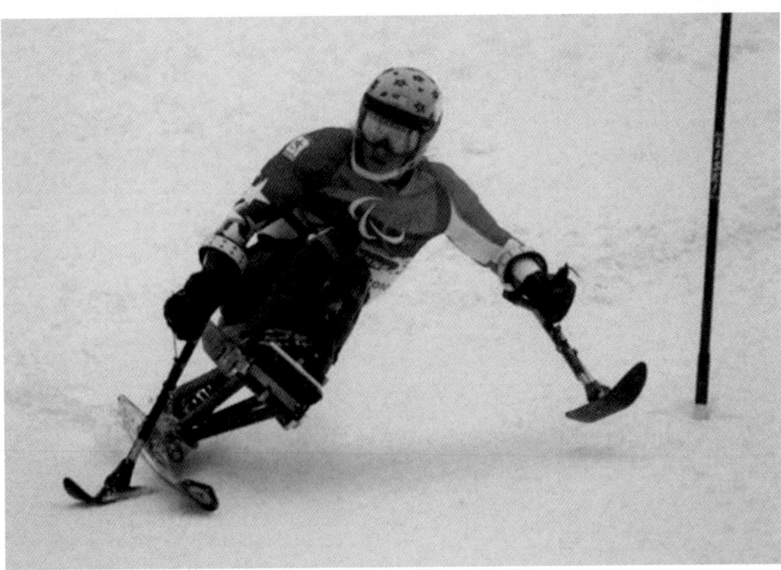

FIGURE 24.3 Alpine skiing.

This enables sailors with a more severe physical disability to take part in competition.

Table Tennis. Athletes from all disability groups (with the exception of those with blindness/visual impairment) participate and compete in Table Tennis in standing and sitting classes. Men and women compete individually, in doubles, and in team events. Athletes are classified into 11 groups depending on the skills required for the sport and their functional ability. Classes TT1 to TT10 are for athletes with a physical disability, with classes 1 to 5 competing in wheelchairs and classes 6 to 10 competing while standing.

Wheelchair Fencing. Any fencer that, due to a permanent disability, cannot fence standing as an able body fencer is eligible for wheelchair fencing. Men and women compete in events including Foil, Epée (men and women), and Sabre (men). Athletes are classified into one of five classes based on sitting balance, and arm and leg function. In wheelchair fencing, the wheelchairs are fixed in place to the ground by metal frames. The length of the playing area is decided by the fencer with the shortest arms. This person decides if the distance will be at his distance or that of his opponent. One arm/hand holds the fencing weapon, while the other arm is used to hold onto the chair when lunging and recovering.

Equestrian. Equestrian is a multidisability sport, open to athletes with a physical disability or a visual impairment, and is unique among Paralympic sports since men and women compete on the same terms and horse and rider are both declared Paralympic medal winners. Riders compete in two Dressage events: a championship test of set movements and a Freestyle Test to music. There is also a Team Test for three to four riders per team. The competitor's mobility, strength, and coordination are assessed in order to establish their classification profile. People with similar profiles are grouped into competition Grades, ranging from Grade I for the most severely impaired to Grade IV for the least impaired.

Alpine Skiing. There are five alpine skiing events on the Paralympic program: Downhill, Super-G, Super Combined, Giant Slalom, and Slalom. Paralympic competition accommodates male and female athletes with a physical disability such as spinal injury, cerebral palsy, amputation, les autres conditions, and blindness/visual impairment. Athletes compete in three categories based on their functional ability, and a result calculation system allows athletes with different impairments to compete against each other. There are thirteen classifications for athletes with a physical disability: seven for standing, three for sitting, and three for athletes with visual impairments (Fig. 24.3).

Nordic Skiing. Nordic skiing, consisting of cross-country skiing and biathlon, is open to athletes with physical disabilities that include amputation, SCI, visual impairment, and other locomotor disabilities. Athletes are classified based on activity limitation resulting from impairment, and the degree to which that impairment impacts upon sport performance. In cross-country skiing, the sport classes that include individuals with SCI compete using a sit-ski, a chair equipped with a pair of skis (Fig. 24.4).

SPORTING EQUIPMENT EVOLUTION

Improved performance has been directly linked to technological advancement in the able-bodied population. Swimming body suits, speed skating clap skates, and new materials employed for pole vaulting poles and skis, to name a few, have meant dramatic changes in performance. This link may be even stronger when it comes to the wheelchair performance spanning the past 20 years.

In the past heavy wheelchair with fixed armrests, sling seats, and hard rubber tires were used for all events. Beginning in 1967, the University of Illinois wheelchair basketball team began using pneumatic tires and lighter stainless steel "sports chairs." This resulted in two successive national championships, in part due to superior technology (194). In the late 1970s and early 1980s, Quickie Designs, Shadow, and Sopur, all began rethinking the concept of the wheelchair. Lighter, stronger and directed to sport-specific usage, these wheelchairs continue to evolve (195).

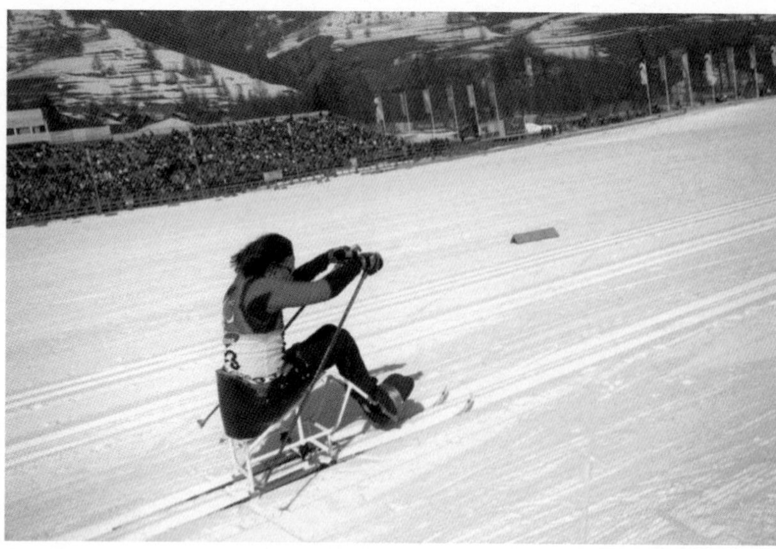

FIGURE 24.4 Nordic skiing.

Five distinct chair types are now recognized:

1. **Racing Wheelchairs**—Now almost exclusively three wheeled configuration with variable wheelbases depending on the racing event (sprint versus endurance). These custom chairs are tightly fitted to the athletes and they are positioned, generally in a kneeling position, to maximize the individual's propulsive stroke with significantly less concern for handling characteristics (Fig. 24.5).
2. **Basketball Wheelchairs**—Ultra-lightweight rigid frames with anti-tip devices in the front and sometimes the rear. These chairs use high-pressure pneumatic tires that have spoke guards in place and are mounted with significant camber. The participant is limited in the maximum seat height although positioning and securing of the athlete to the chair may benefit performance (Fig. 24.1).
3. **Tennis Wheelchairs**—A very fast sport requiring the ultimate in agility for the wheelchair user. These chairs have a single front caster with two rear wheels positioned with extreme degrees of camber to increase maneuverability and maximize lateral stability. The athlete is positioned with "pinch" causing the trunk to lean toward the thighs to enhance balance and control. The chair will often have handles to assist in leaning and reaching, and to enhance racquet power.
4. **Rugby Wheelchairs**—This sport combines elements of Basketball, Rugby, and Ice Hockey and is played by athletes with limited upper extremity function. Significant contact is permitted. Thus, rear wheels are radically cambered to increase stability and improve handling, but also help to shield the players' UEs from contact. A protective framework extends across the front of the chair to protect the lower extremities. The players are also positioned with extreme levels of "pinch" to facilitate stability and maneuverability (Fig. 24.2).
5. **Hand Cycles**—The user is in a seated position with legs extended and propels the device with a crank apparatus and gearing similar to a conventional bicycle. More akin to a recumbent bicycle, these devices provide coordinated propulsion, gearing, and steering in the same mechanisms (196) (Fig. 24.6).

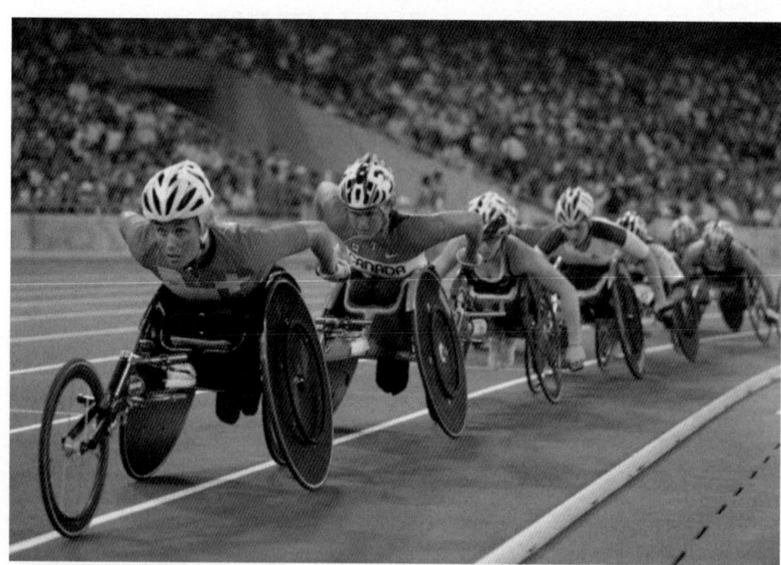

FIGURE 24.5 Example of racing wheelchair (note athlete positioning and chair configuration to maximize aerodynamics and performance).

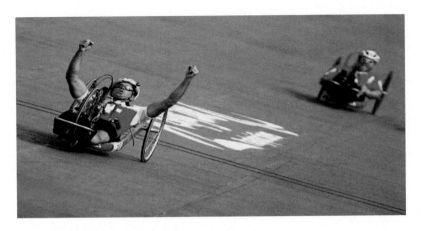

FIGURE 24.6 Handcycling.

CONCLUSIONS

Individuals living with SCI experience severe physical deconditioning, significant musculoskeletal decline, and elevated risks of all-cause cardiopulmonary and cardiometabolic diseases. Many could benefit through use of a sustained reconditioning exercise. Individuals with higher levels of cord injury may require electrical stimulation to perform exercise, which poses special restrictions on use and unique risks from participation. Nonetheless, qualified individuals benefit from chronic exercise through improved cardiovascular and musculoskeletal functions. Positive benefits of training on bone density, regulation of orthostatic tolerance, and emotions have been reported in studies with limited numbers of subjects, and require well-controlled investigations for confirmation. Individuals with spared motor control of the upper extremity can perform arm or wheelchair exercises and participate in recreational sports. Greater emphasis needs to be placed on strengthening of the upper extremity to preserve shoulder and arm functions for performance of daily living as these individuals age with their paralysis. Risks of injury or illnesses associated with imprudent exercise must be managed to ensure that the desirable benefits of physical activity can be sustained.

As in persons without disability, the challenge remains to create a lifetime commitment to the maintenance of health and a healthy lifestyle, including adequate exercise. Structure organizations are available to facilitate and foster participation in a wide range of recreational and competitive pursuits. Technological advances in wheelchair design and adaptive equipment enhance function while decreasing risk for injury. Increased participation and improved access to facilities enhance options for participating in an active lifestyle spanning leisurely activity to aggressive competition, and at any age. Health care professional should be aware of these options and recommend their adoption to afford an active, healthy, satisfied lifestyle for persons with disability from SCI.

References

1. Bauman WA, Adkins RH, Spungen AM, et al. Is immobilization associated with an abnormal lipoprotein profile? Observations from a diverse cohort. *Spinal Cord* 1999;37(7):485–493.
2. Washburn RA, Figoni SF. High density lipoprotein cholesterol in individuals with spinal cord injury: the potential role of physical activity. *Spinal Cord* 1999;37(10):685–695.
3. Berg A, Keul J, Ringwald G, et al. Physical performance and serum cholesterol fractions in healthy young men. *Clin Chim Acta* 1980;106(3):325–330.
4. Bostom AG, Toner MM, McArdle WD, et al. Lipid and lipoprotein profiles relate to peak aerobic power in spinal cord injured men. *Med Sci Sports Exerc* 1991;23(4):409–414.
5. Dearwater SR, LaPorte RE, Robertson RJ, et al. Activity in the spinal cord-injured patient: an epidemiologic analysis of metabolic parameters. *Med Sci Sports Exerc* 1986;18(5):541–544.
6. Davis GM. Exercise capacity of individuals with paraplegia. *Med Sci Sports Exerc* 1993;25(4):423–432.
7. Figoni SF. Perspectives on cardiovascular fitness and SCI. *J Am Paraplegia Soc* 1990;13(4):63–71.
8. Glaser RM. Exercise and locomotion for the spinal cord injured. *Exerc Sport Sci Rev* 1985;13:263–303.
9. Phillips WT, Kiratli BJ, Sarkarati M, et al. Effect of spinal cord injury on the heart and cardiovascular fitness. *Curr Probl Cardiol* 1998;23(11):641–716.
10. Duckworth WC, Solomon SS, Jallepalli P, et al. Glucose intolerance due to insulin resistance in patients with spinal cord injuries. *Diabetes* 1980;29(11):906–910.
11. Gerhart KA, Bergstrom E, Charlifue SW, et al. Long-term spinal cord injury: functional changes over time. *Arch Phys Med Rehabil* 1993;74(10):1030–1034.
12. Menter RR. Aging and spinal cord injury: implications for existing model systems and future federal, state, and local health care policy. In: Spinal Cord Injury: the model. Proceedings of the National Concensus Conference on Catastrophic Illness and Injury. Atlanta, GA, The Georgia Regional Spinal Cord Injury Care System, Sheperd Treatment of Spinal Injuries, Incorporated, 1990.
13. Zola IK. Toward the necessary universalizing of a disability policy. *Milbank Q*. 1989;67(suppl 2 pt 2):401–428.
14. Curtis KA, Drysdale GA, Lanza RD, et al. Shoulder pain in wheelchair users with tetraplegia and paraplegia. *Arch Phys Med Rehabil* 1999;80(4):453–457.
15. Ohry A, Shemesh Y, Rozin R. Are chronic spinal cord injured patients (SCIP) prone to premature aging? *Med Hypotheses* 1983;11(4):467–469.
16. Waters RL, Sie IH, Adkins RH. The musculoskeletal system. In: *Aging with spinal cord injury*. Demos Medical Publishing, New York, NY, 1993:53–72.

17. Figoni SF, Glaser RM, Rodgers MM, et al. Acute hemodynamic responses of spinal cord injured individuals to functional neuromuscular stimulation-induced knee extension exercise. *J Rehabil Res Dev* 1991;28(4):9–18.
18. Rodgers MM, Glaser RM, Figoni SF, et al. Musculoskeletal responses of spinal cord injured individuals to functional neuromuscular stimulation-induced knee extension exercise training. *J Rehabil Res Dev* 1991;28(4):19–26.
19. Billian C, Gorman PH. Upper extremity applications of functional neuromuscular stimulation. *Assist Technol* 1992;4(1):31–39.
20. Bryden AM, Memberg WD, Crago PE. Electrically stimulated elbow extension in persons with C5/C6 tetraplegia: a functional and physiological evaluation. *Arch Phys Med Rehabil* 2000;81(1):80–88.
21. Mulcahey MJ, Betz RR, Smith BT, et al. Implanted functional electrical stimulation hand system in adolescents with spinal injuries: an evaluation. *Arch Phys Med Rehabil* 1997;78(6):597–607.
22. Scott TR, Peckham PH, Keith MW. Upper extremity neuroprostheses using functional electrical stimulation. *Baillieres Clin Neurol* 1995;4(1):57–75.
23. Hooker SP, Greenwood JD, Hatae DT, et al. Oxygen uptake and heart rate relationship in persons with spinal cord injury. *Med Sci Sports Exerc* 1993;25(10):1115–1119.
24. Nash MS, Bilsker MS, Kearney HM, et al. Effects of electrically-stimulated exercise and passive motion on echocardiographically-derived wall-motion and cardiodynamic function in tetraplegic persons. *Paraplegia* 1995;33(2):80–89.
25. Ragnarsson KT, Pollack S, Odaniel W, et al. Clinical-evaluation of computerized functional electrical-stimulation after spinal-cord injury—a multicenter pilot-study. *Arch Phys Med Rehabil* 1988;69(9):672–677.
26. Krauss JC, Robergs RA, Depaepe JL, et al. Effects of electrical stimulation and upper body training after spinal cord injury. *Med Sci Sports Exerc* 1993;25(9):1054–1061.
27. Mutton DL, Scremin AM, Barstow TJ, et al. Physiologic responses during functional electrical stimulation leg cycling and hybrid exercise in spinal cord injured subjects. *Arch Phys Med Rehabil* 1997;78(7):712–718.
28. Raymond J, Davis GM, Climstein M, et al. Cardiorespiratory responses to arm cranking and electrical stimulation leg cycling in people with paraplegia. *Med Sci Sports Exerc* 1999;31(6):822–828.
29. Laskin JJ, Ashley EA, Olenik LM, et al. Electrical stimulation-assisted rowing exercise in spinal cord injured people. A pilot study. *Paraplegia* 1993;31(8):534–541.
30. Cameron T, Broton JG, Needham-Shropshire B, et al. An upper body exercise system incorporating resistive exercise and neuromuscular electrical stimulation (NMS). *J Spinal Cord Med* 1998;21(1):1–6.
31. Davis R, Houdayer T, Andrews B, et al. Paraplegia: prolonged closed-loop standing with implanted nucleus FES-22 stimulator and Andrews' foot-ankle orthosis. *Stereotact Funct Neurosurg* 1997;69(1–4 pt 2):281–287.
32. Triolo RJ, Bieri C, Uhlir J, et al. Implanted Functional Neuromuscular Stimulation systems for individuals with cervical spinal cord injuries: clinical case reports. *Arch Phys Med Rehabil* 1996;77(11):1119–1128.
33. Graupe D, Kohn KH. Functional neuromuscular stimulator for short-distance ambulation by certain thoracic-level spinal-cord-injured paraplegics. *Surg Neurol* 1998;50(3):202–207.
34. Klose KJ, Jacobs PL, Broton JG, et al. Evaluation of a training program for persons with SCI paraplegia using the Parastep(R)1 ambulation system: part 1. Ambulation performance and anthropometric measures. *Arch Phys Med Rehabil* 1997;78(8):789–793.
35. Kobetic R, Triolo RJ, Marsolais EB. Muscle selection and walking performance of multichannel FES systems for ambulation in paraplegia. *IEEE Trans Rehabil Eng* 1997;5(1):23–29.
36. Ferguson KA, Polando G, Kobetic R, et al. Walking with a hybrid orthosis system. *Spinal Cord* 1999;37(11):800–804.
37. Phillips CA, Gallimore JJ, Hendershot DM. Walking when utilizing a sensory feedback system and an electrical muscle stimulation gait orthosis. *Med Eng Phys* 1995;17(7):507–513.
38. Carroll SG, Bird SF, Brown DJ. Electrical stimulation of the lumbrical muscles in an incomplete quadriplegic patient: case report. *Paraplegia* 1992;30(3):223–226.
39. Dimitrijevic MM. Mesh-glove. 1. A method for whole-hand electrical stimulation in upper motor neuron dysfunction. *Scand J Rehabil Med* 1994;26(4):183–186.
40. Mulcahey MJ, Smith BT, Betz RR. Evaluation of the lower motor neuron integrity of upper extremity muscles in high level spinal cord injury. *Spinal Cord* 1999;37(8):585–591.
41. Phillips CA. Medical criteria for active physical therapy. Physician guidelines for patient participation in a program of functional electrical rehabilitation. *Am J Phys Med* 1987;66(5):269–286.
42. Glaser RM. Functional neuromuscular stimulation. Exercise conditioning of spinal cord injured patients. *Int J Sports Med* 1994;15(3):142–148.
43. Petrofsky JS, Phillips CA. The use of functional electrical stimulation for rehabilitation of spinal cord injured patients. *Cent Nerv Syst Trauma* 1984;1(1):57–74.
44. Hooker SP, Figoni SF, Rodgers MM, et al. Physiologic effects of electrical stimulation leg cycle exercise training in spinal cord injured persons. *Arch Phys Med Rehabil* 1992;73(5):470–476.
45. Hooker SP, Scremin AM, Mutton DL, et al. Peak and submaximal physiologic responses following electrical stimulation leg cycle ergometer training. *J Rehabil Res Dev* 1995;32(4):361–366.
46. Barstow TJ, Scremin AM, Mutton DL, et al. Changes in gas exchange kinetics with training in patients with spinal cord injury. *Med Sci Sports Exerc* 1996;28(10):1221–1228.
47. Scremin AM, Kurta L, Gentili A, et al. Increasing muscle mass in spinal cord injured persons with a functional electrical stimulation exercise program. *Arch Phys Med Rehabil* 1999;80(12):1531–1536.
48. Nash MS, Bilsker S, Marcillo AE, et al. Reversal of adaptive left ventricular atrophy following electrically-stimulated exercise training in human tetraplegics. *Paraplegia* 1991;29(9):590–599.
49. Nash MS, Montalvo BM, Applegate B. Lower extremity blood flow and responses to occlusion ischemia differ in

exercise-trained and sedentary tetraplegic persons. *Arch Phys Med Rehabil* 1996;77(12):1260–1265.
50. BeDell KK, Scremin AM, Perell KL, et al. Effects of functional electrical stimulation-induced lower extremity cycling on bone density of spinal cord-injured patients. *Am J Phys Med Rehabil* 1996;75(1):29–34.
51. Mohr T, Podenphant J, Biering-Sorensen F, et al. Increased bone mineral density after prolonged electrically induced cycle training of paralyzed limbs in spinal cord injured man. *Calcif Tissue Int* 1997;61(1):22–25.
52. Bloomfield SA, Mysiw WJ, Jackson RD. Bone mass and endocrine adaptations to training in spinal cord injured individuals. *Bone* 1996;19(1):61–68.
53. Hjeltnes N, Galuska D, Bjornholm M, et al. Exercise-induced overexpression of key regulatory proteins involved in glucose uptake and metabolism in tetraplegic persons: molecular mechanism for improved glucose homeostasis. *FASEB J* 1998;12(15):1701–1712.
54. Nash MS, Tehranzadeh J, Green BA, et al. Magnetic resonance imaging of osteonecrosis and osteoarthrosis in exercising quadriplegics and paraplegics. *Am J Phys Med Rehabil* 1994;73(3):184–192.
55. Hjeltnes N, Aksnes AK, Birkeland KI, et al. Improved body composition after 8 wk of electrically stimulated leg cycling in tetraplegic patients. *Am J Physiol* 1997;273 (3 pt 2):1072–1079.
56. Bauman WA, Spungen AM. Disorders of carbohydrate and lipid metabolism in veterans with paraplegia or quadriplegia: a model of premature aging. *Metabolism* 1994;43(6):749–756.
57. Barbeau H, Ladouceur M, Norman KE, et al. Walking after spinal cord injury: evaluation, treatment, and functional recovery. *Arch Phys Med Rehabil* 1999;80(2):225–235.
58. Norman KE, Pepin A, Barbeau H. Effects of drugs on walking after spinal cord injury. *Spinal Cord* 1998;36(10):699–715.
59. Remy-Neris O, Barbeau H, Daniel O, et al. Effects of intrathecal clonidine injection on spinal reflexes and human locomotion in incomplete paraplegic subjects. *Exp Brain Res* 1999;129(3):433–440.
60. Stein RB, Belanger M, Wheeler G, et al. Electrical systems for improving locomotion after incomplete spinal cord injury: an assessment. *Arch Phys Med Rehabil* 1993;74(9):954–959.
61. Graupe D, Salahi J, Kohn KH. Multifunctional prosthesis and orthosis control via microcomputer identification of temporal pattern differences in single-site myoelectric signals. *J Biomed Eng* 1982;4(1):17–22.
62. Kralj A, Bajd T, Turk R. Electrical stimulation providing functional use of paraplegic patient muscles. *Med Prog Technol* 1980;7(1):3–9.
63. Gallien P, Brissot R, Eyssette M, et al. Restoration of gait by functional electrical stimulation for spinal cord injured patients. *Paraplegia* 1995;33(11):660–664.
64. Jacobs PL, Nash MS, Klose KJ, et al. Evaluation of a training program for persons with SCI paraplegia using the Parastep 1 ambulation system: part 2. Effects on physiological responses to peak arm ergometry. *Arch Phys Med Rehabil* 1997;78(8):794–798.
65. Jaeger RJ. Lower extremity applications of functional neuromuscular stimulation. *Assist Technol* 1992;4(1):19–30.
66. Nash MS, Jacobs PL, Montalvo BM, et al. Evaluation of a training program for persons with SCI paraplegia using the Parastep 1 ambulation system: part 5. Lower extremity blood flow and hyperemic responses to occlusion are augmented by ambulation training. *Arch Phys Med Rehabil* 1997;78(8):808–814.
67. Needham-Shropshire BM, Broton JG, et al. Evaluation of a training program for persons with SCI paraplegia using the Parastep 1 ambulation system: part 3. Lack of effect on bone mineral density. *Arch Phys Med Rehabil* 1997;78(8):799–803.
68. Cowell LL, Squires WG, Raven PB. Benefits of aerobic exercise for the paraplegic: a brief review. *Med Sci Sports Exerc* 1986;18(5):501–508.
69. Davis GM, Kofsky PR, Kelsey JC, et al. Cardiorespiratory fitness and muscular strength of wheelchair users. *Can Med Assoc J* 1981;125(12):1317–1323.
70. Davis GM, Shephard RJ, Leenen FH. Cardiac effects of short term arm crank training in paraplegics: echocardiographic evidence. *Eur J Appl Physiol* 1987;56(1):90–96.
71. DiCarlo SE, Supp MD, Taylor HC. Effect of arm ergometry training on physical work capacity of individuals with spinal cord injuries. *Phys Ther* 1983;63(7):1104–1107.
72. Franklin BA. Aerobic exercise training programs for the upper body. *Med Sci Sports Exerc* 1989;21(5 suppl):141–148.
73. Franklin BA. Exercise testing, training and arm ergometry. *Sports Med* 1985;2(2):100–119.
74. Gass GC, Watson J, Camp EM, et al. The effects of physical training on high level spinal lesion patients. *Scand J Rehabil Med* 1980;12(2):61–65.
75. Hoffman MD. Cardiorespiratory fitness and training in quadriplegics and paraplegics. *Sports Med* 1986;3(5):312–330.
76. Hooker SP, Wells CL. Effects of low- and moderate-intensity training in spinal cord-injured persons. *Med Sci Sports Exerc* 1989;21(1):18–22.
77. Knutsson E, Lewenhaupt-Olsson E, Thorsen M. Physical work capacity and physical conditioning in paraplegic patients. *Paraplegia* 1973;11(3):205–216.
78. Miles DS, Sawka MN, Wilde SW, et al. Pulmonary function changes in wheelchair athletes subsequent to exercise training. *Ergonomics* 1982;25(3):239–246.
79. Pachalski A, Mekarski T. Effect of swimming on increasing of cardio-respiratory capacity in paraplegics. *Paraplegia* 1980;18(3):190–196.
80. Pollock ML, Miller HS, Linnerud AC, et al. Arm pedaling as an endurance training regimen for the disabled. *Arch Phys Med Rehabil* 1974;55(9):418–424.
81. Taylor AW, McDonell E, Brassard L. The effects of an arm ergometer training programme on wheelchair subjects. *Paraplegia*. 1986;24(2):105–114.
82. Yim SY, Cho KJ, Park CI, et al. Effect of wheelchair ergometer training on spinal cord-injured paraplegics. *Yonsei Med J* 1993;34(3):278–286.
83. DiCarlo SE. Effect of arm ergometry training on wheelchair propulsion endurance of individuals with quadriplegia. *Phys Ther* 1988;68(1):40–44.
84. Drory Y, Ohry A, Brooks ME, et al. Arm crank ergometry in chronic spinal cord injured patients. *Arch Phys Med Rehabil* 1990;71(6):389–392.

85. Hjeltnes N. Cardiorespiratory capacity in tetra- and paraplegia shortly after injury. *Scand J Rehabil Med* 1986;18(2):65–70.
86. Hjeltnes N. Oxygen uptake and cardiac output in graded arm exercise in paraplegics with low level spinal lesions. *Scand J Rehabil Med* 1979;9:107–113.
87. Hopman MT, Oeseburg B, Binkhorst RA. The effect of an anti-G suit on cardiovascular responses to exercise in persons with paraplegia. *Med Sci Sports Exerc* 1992;24(9):984–990.
88. DeBruin MIBRA. Cardiac output of paraplegics during exercise. *Int J Sports Med* 1984;5:175–176.
89. Hopman MT, Pistorius M, Kamerbeek IC, et al. Cardiac output in paraplegic subjects at high exercise intensities. *Eur J Appl Physiol* 1993;66(6):531–535.
90. Van Loan MD, McCluer S, Loftin JM, et al. Comparison of physiological responses to maximal arm exercise among able-bodied, paraplegics and quadriplegics. *Paraplegia* 1987;25(5):397–405.
91. Hopman MT, Oeseburg B, Binkhorst RA. Cardiovascular responses in paraplegic subjects during arm exercise. *Eur J Appl Physiol* 1992;65(1):73–78.
92. Schmid A, Huonker M, Barturen JM, et al. Catecholamines, heart rate, and oxygen uptake during exercise in persons with spinal cord injury. *J Appl Physiol* 1998;85(2):635–641.
93. Schmid A, Huonker M, Stahl F, et al. Free plasma catecholamines in spinal cord injured persons with different injury levels at rest and during exercise. *J Auton Nerv Syst* 1998;68(1–2):96–100.
94. Bloomfield SA, Jackson RD, Mysiw WJ. Catecholamine response to exercise and training in individuals with spinal cord injury. *Med Sci Sports Exerc* 1994;26(10):1213–1219.
95. Janssen TW, van Oers CA, van der Woude LH, et al. Physical strain in daily life of wheelchair users with spinal cord injuries. *Med Sci Sports Exerc* 1994;26(6):661–670.
96. Janssen TW, van Oers CA, Veeger HE, et al. Relationship between physical strain during standardised ADL tasks and physical capacity in men with spinal cord injuries. *Paraplegia* 1994;32(12):844–859.
97. Davis GM, Shephard RJ. Cardiorespiratory fitness in highly active versus inactive paraplegics. *Med Sci Sports Exerc* 1988;20(5):463–468.
98. Ehsani AA, Heath GW, Martin WH, et al. Effects of intense exercise training on plasma catecholamines in coronary patients. *J Appl Physiol* 1984;57(1):155–159.
99. National Cholesterol Education Program. Second Report of the Expert Panel on Detection, Evaluation, and Treatment of High Blood Cholesterol in Adults (Adult Treatment Panel II). *Circulation* 1994;89(3):1333–1445.
100. Bauman WA, Adkins RH, Spungen AM, et al. Ethnicity effect on the serum lipid profile in persons with spinal cord injury. *Arch Phys Med Rehabil* 1998;79(2):176–180.
101. Bauman WA, Spungen AM, Zhong YG, et al. Depressed serum high density lipoprotein cholesterol levels in veterans with spinal cord injury. *Paraplegia* 1992;30(10):697–703.
102. Nash MS, Mendez AJ. A guideline-driven assessment of need for cardiovascular disease risk intervention in persons with chronic paraplegia. *Arch Phys Med Rehabil* 2007;88(6):751–757.
103. de Groot PC, Hjeltnes N, Heijboer AC, et al. Effect of training intensity on physical capacity, lipid profile and insulin sensitivity in early rehabilitation of spinal cord injured individuals. *Spinal Cord* 2003;41(12):673–679.
104. El-Sayed MS, Younesian A. Lipid profiles are influenced by arm cranking exercise and training in individuals with spinal cord injury. *Spinal Cord* 2005;43(5):299–305.
105. Janssen TW, van Oers CA, van Kamp GJ, et al. Coronary heart disease risk indicators, aerobic power, and physical activity in men with spinal cord injuries. *Arch Phys Med Rehabil* 1997;78(7):697–705.
106. Manns PJ, McCubbin JA, Williams DP. Fitness, inflammation, and the metabolic syndrome in men with paraplegia. *Arch Phys Med Rehabil* 2005;86(6):1176–1181.
107. Dallmeijer AJ, van der Woude LH, Hollander AP, et al. Physical performance during rehabilitation in persons with spinal cord injuries. *Med Sci Sports Exerc* 1999;31(9):1330–1335.
108. Dallmeijer AJ, Hopman MT, van der Woude LH. Lipid, lipoprotein, and apolipoprotein profiles in active and sedentary men with tetraplegia. *Arch Phys Med Rehabil* 1997;78(11):1173–1176.
109. Abel T, Kroner M, Rojas Vega S, et al. Energy expenditure in wheelchair racing and handbiking—a basis for prevention of cardiovascular diseases in those with disabilities. *Eur J Cardiovasc Prev Rehabil* 2003;10(5):371–376.
110. Abel T, Platen P, Rojas Vega S, et al. Energy expenditure in ball games for wheelchair users. *Spinal Cord* 2008;46(12):785–790.
111. Coutts KD. Heart rates of participants in wheelchair sports. *Paraplegia* 1988;26(1):43–49.
112. Roy JL, Menear KS, Schmid MM, et al. Physiological responses of skilled players during a competitive wheelchair tennis match. *J Strength Cond Res* 2006;20(3):665–671.
113. Schmid A, Huonker M, Stober P, et al. Physical performance and cardiovascular and metabolic adaptation of elite female wheelchair basketball players in wheelchair ergometry and in competition. *Am J Phys Med Rehabil* 1998;77(6):527–533.
114. Nash MS, van de Ven I, van Elk N, et al. Effects of circuit resistance training on fitness attributes and upper-extremity pain in middle-aged men with paraplegia. *Arch Phys Med Rehabil* 2007;88(1):70–75.
115. Nilsson S, Staff PH, Pruett ED. Physical work capacity and the effect of training on subjects with long- standing paraplegia. *Scand J Rehabil Med* 1975;7(2):51–56.
116. Davis GM, Shephard RJ. Strength training for wheelchair users. *Br J Sports Med* 1990;24(1):25–30.
117. Cooney MM, Walker JB. Hydraulic resistance exercise benefits cardiovascular fitness of spinal cord injured. *Med Sci Sports Exerc* 1986;18(5):522–525.
118. Olenik LM, Laskin JJ, Burnham R, et al. Efficacy of rowing, backward wheeling and isolated scapular retractor exercise as remedial strength activities for wheelchair users: application of electromyography. *Paraplegia* 1995;33(3):148–152.
119. Curtis KA, Tyner TM, Zachary L, et al. Effect of a standard exercise protocol on shoulder pain in long-term wheelchair users. *Spinal Cord* 1999;37(6):421–429.

120. Hicks AL, Martin KA, Ditor DS, et al. Long-term exercise training in persons with spinal cord injury: effects on strength, arm ergometry performance and psychological well-being. *Spinal Cord* 2003;41(1):34–43.
121. Jacobs PL, Nash MS, Rusinowski JW. Circuit training provides cardiorespiratory and strength benefits in persons with paraplegia. *Med Sci Sports Exerc* 2001;33(5):711–717.
122. Jacobs PL, Mahoney ET, Nash MS, et al. Circuit resistance training in persons with complete paraplegia. *J Rehabil Res Dev* 2002;39(1):21–28.
123. Piscitelli JT, Parker RT. Primary care in the postmenopausal woman. *Clin Obstet Gynecol* 1986;29(2):343–352.
124. Report. PAGAC. Physical Activity Guidelines Advisory Committe. US Department of Health and Human Services, Washington DC, 2008.
125. Haskell WL, Lee IM, Pate RR, et al. Physical activity and public health: updated recommendation for adults from the American College of Sports Medicine and the American Heart Association. *Med Sci Sports Exerc* 2007;39(8):1423–1434.
126. Exercise is Medicine. http://www.exerciseismedicine.org, 2011
127. Exercise is Medicine I. Physician Toolkit. http://www.exerciseismedicine.org/documents/FULLTOOLKIT.pdf, 2011
128. U.S. Department of Health and Human Services: Office of Disease Prevention and Health Promotion—Healthy People 2010. *Nasnewsletter*. 2000;15(3):3.
129. Health USDo, Human S. The Surgeon General's Call to Action To Improve the Health and Wellness of Persons with Disabilities: U.S. Department of Health and Human Services, Office of the Surgeon General, 2005.
130. Centers for Disease C, Prevention. Prevalence of Regular Physical Acitivity Among Adults—United States 2001 and 2005. *MMWR Morb Mortal Wkly Rep* 2007;56(46):1209–1212.
131. Peek ME, Tang H, Alexander GC, et al. National Prevalence of Lifestyle Counseling or Referral Among African-Americans and Whites with Diabetes. *J Gen Intern Med*. 2008;23:1858–1864.
132. Sinclair J, Lawson B, Burge F. Which patients receive advice on diet and exercise? Do certain characteristics affect whether they receive such advice? *Can Fam Physician* 2008;54(3):404–412.
133. Weidinger KA, Lovegreen SL, Elliott MB, et al. How to make exercise counseling more effective: lessons from rural America. *J Fam Pract* 2008;57(6):394–402.
134. Rimmer JH, Riley B, Wang E, et al. Physical activity participation among persons with disabilities: barriers and facilitators. *Am J Prev Med* 2004;26(5):419–425.
135. Vissers M, van den Berg-Emons R, Sluis T, et al. Barriers to and facilitators of everyday physical activity in persons with a spinal cord injury after discharge from the rehabilitation centre. *J Rehabil Med* 2008;40(6):461–467.
136. American College of Sports M. *ACSM's guidelines for exercise testing and prescription*. Vol 6. Lippincott Williams & Wilkins, 2000:137–164.
137. Ballinger DA, Rintala DH, Hart KA. The relation of shoulder pain and range-of-motion problems to functional limitations, disability, and perceived health of men with spinal cord injury: a multifaceted longitudinal study. *Arch Phys Med Rehabil* 2000;81(12):1575–1581.
138. Subbarao JV, Klopfstein J, Turpin R. Prevalence and impact of wrist and shoulder pain in patients with spinal cord injury. *J Spinal Cord Med* 1995;18(1):9–13.
139. Nash MS, Jacobs PL, Mendez AJ, et al. Circuit resisitance training improves the atherogenic lipid profile in persons with chronic paraplegia. *J Spinal Cord Med* 2001.
140. Nawoczenski DA, Ritter-Soronen JM, Wilson CM, et al. Clinical trial of exercise for shoulder pain in chronic spinal injury. *Phys Ther* 2006;86(12):1604–1618.
141. Preservation of upper limb function following spinal cord injury: a clinical practice guideline for health-care professionals. *J Spinal Cord Med* 2005;28(5):434–470.
142. Requejo PS, Mulroy SJ, Haubert LL, et al. Evidence-based strategies to preserve shoulder function in manual wheelchair users with spinal cord injury. *Top Spinal Cord Inj Rehabil* 2008;13(4):86–119.
143. Borg G. Psychophysical bases of percieved exertion. *Med Sci Sports Exerc* 1982;14:377–381.
144. Lewis JE, Nash MS, Hamm LF, et al. The relationship between perceived exertion and physiologic indicators of stress during graded arm exercise in persons with spinal cord injuries. *Arch Phys Med Rehabil* 2007;88(9):1205–1211.
145. Foster C, Porcari JP, Anderson J, et al. The talk test as a marker of exercise training intensity. *J Cardiopulm Rehabil Prev* 2008;28(1):24–30.
146. Fujiwara T, Hara Y, Akaboshi K, et al. Relationship between shoulder muscle strength and functional independence measure (FIM) score among C6 tetraplegics. *Spinal Cord* 1999;37(1):58–61.
147. Marciello MA, Herbison GJ, Ditunno JF, et al. Wrist strength measured by myometry as an indicator of functional independence. *J Neurotrauma* 1995;12(1):99–106.
148. Noreau L, Shepard RJ. Spinal cord injury, exercise, and quality of life. *Sports Med* 1995;20(4):226–250.
149. Semerjian TZ, Montague SM, Dominguez JF, et al. Enhancement of quality of life and body satisfaction through the use of adapted exercise devices for individuals with spinal cord injuries. *Top Spinal Cord Inj Rehabil* 2005;11(2):95–108.
150. Ragnarsson KT. Management of pain in persons with spinal cord injury. *J Spinal Cord Med* 1997;20(2):186–199.
151. Coyle KA, Shank JW, Hutchins DA. Psychosocial functioning and changes in leisure lifestyle among individuals with chronic secondary health problems related to spinal cord injury. *Ther Recreation J* 1993;27:239–252.
152. Muraki S, Tsunawake N, Hiramatsu S, et al. The effect of frequency and mode of sports activity on the psychological status in tetraplegics and paraplegics. *Spinal Cord* 2000;38(5):309–314.
153. Ginis KAM, Latimer AE, McKechnie K, et al. Using exercise to enhance subjective well-being among people with spinal cord injury: the mediating influences of stress and pain. *Rehabil Psychol* 2003;48(3):157–164.
154. Bjerkefors A, Carpenter MG, Thorstensson A. Dynamic trunk stability is improved in paraplegics following kayak ergometer training. *Scand J Med Sci Sports* 2007;17(6):672–679.

155. Burnham RS, May L, Nelson E, et al. Shoulder pain in wheelchair athletes. The role of muscle imbalance. *Am J Sports Med* 1993;21(2):238–242.
156. Curtis KA, Roach KE, Applegate EB, et al. Reliability and validity of the Wheelchair User's Shoulder Pain Index (WUSPI). *Paraplegia* 1995;33(10):595–601.
157. Pentland WE, Twomey LT. The weight-bearing upper extremity in women with long term paraplegia. *Paraplegia* 1991;29(8):521–530.
158. Pentland WE, Twomey LT. Upper limb function in persons with long term paraplegia and implications for independence: part I. *Paraplegia* 1994;32(4):211–218.
159. Gellman H, Sie I, Waters RL. Late complications of the weight-bearing upper extremity in the paraplegic patient. *Clin Orthop* 1988(233):132–135.
160. Nichols PJ, Norman PA, Ennis JR. Wheelchair user's shoulder? Shoulder pain in patients with spinal cord lesions. *Scand J Rehabil Med* 1979;11(1):29–32.
161. Campagnolo DI, Bartlett JA, Keller SE, et al. Impaired phagocytosis of Staphylococcus aureus in complete tetraplegics. *Am J Phys Med Rehabil* 1997;76(4): 276–280.
162. Campagnolo DI, Keller SE, DeLisa JA, et al. Alteration of immune system function in tetraplegics. A pilot study. *Am J Phys Med Rehabil* 1994;73(6):387–393.
163. Cruse JM, Keith JC, Bryant ML, et al. Immune system-neuroendocrine dysregulation in spinal cord injury. *Immunol Res* 1996;15(4):306–314.
164. Cruse JM, Lewis RE, Bishop GR, et al. Decreased immune reactivity and neuroendocrine alterations related to chronic stress in spinal cord injury and stroke patients. *Pathobiology* 1993;61(3–4):183–192.
165. Kliesch WF, Cruse JM, Lewis RE, et al. Restoration of depressed immune function in spinal cord injury patients receiving rehabilitation therapy. *Paraplegia* 1996;34(2):82–90.
166. Nash MS. Immune responses to nervous system decentralization and exercise in quadriplegia. *Med Sci Sports Exerc* 1994;26(2):164–171.
167. Segal JL. Spinal cord injury: are interleukins a molecular link between neuronal damage and ensuing pathobiology? *Perspect Biol Med* 1993;36(2):222–240.
168. Segal JL, Brunnemann SR. Circulating levels of soluble interleukin 2 receptors are elevated in the sera of humans with spinal cord injury. *J Am Paraplegia Soc* 1993;16(1):30–33.
169. Segal JL, Gonzales E, Yousefi S, et al. Circulating levels of IL-2R, ICAM-1, and IL-6 in spinal cord injuries. *Arch Phys Med Rehabil* 1997;78(1):44–47.
170. Nieman DC, Buckley KS, Henson DA, et al. Immune function in marathon runners versus sedentary controls. *Med Sci Sports Exerc* 1995;27(7):986–992.
171. Nieman DC, Nehlsen-Cannarella SL, Markoff PA, et al. The effects of moderate exercise training on natural killer cells and acute upper respiratory tract infections. *Int J Sports Med* 1990;11(6):467–473.
172. Furusawa K, Tajima F, Tanaka Y, et al. Short-term attenuation of natural killer cell cytotoxic activity in wheelchair marathoners with paraplegia. *Arch Phys Med Rehabil* 1998;79(9):1116–1121.
173. Nash MS. The immune system. In: Whiteneck GG, Charlifue SW, Gerhart KA, et al., eds. *Aging with spinal cord injury*. New York: Demos Publications, 1993:159–182.
174. Gass GC, Camp EM, Nadel ER, et al. Rectal and rectal vs. esophageal temperatures in paraplegic men during prolonged exercise. *J Appl Physiol* 1988;64(6):2265–2271.
175. Gerner HJ, Engel P, Gass GC, et al. The effects of sauna on tetraplegic and paraplegic subjects. *Paraplegia* 1992;30(6):410–419.
176. Sawka MN, Latzka WA, Pandolf KB. Temperature regulation during upper body exercise: able-bodied and spinal cord injured. *Med Sci Sports Exerc* 1989;21(5 suppl):132–140.
177. Price MJ. Thermoregulation during exercise in individuals with spinal cord injuries. *Sports Med* 2006;36(10):863–879.
178. Yamasaki M, Kim KT, Choi SW, et al. Characteristics of body heat balance of paraplegics during exercise in a hot environment. *J Physiol Anthropol Appl Human Sci* 2001;20(4):227–232.
179. Webborn N, Price MJ, Castle PC, et al. Effects of two cooling strategies on thermoregulatory responses of tetraplegic athletes during repeated intermittent exercise in the heat. *J Appl Physiol* 2005;98(6):2101–2107.
180. Ishii K, Yamasaki M, Muraki S, et al. Effects of upper limb exercise on thermoregulatory responses in patients with spinal cord injury. *Appl Human Sci* 1995;14(3):149–154.
181. Price MJ, Campbell IG. Thermoregulatory responses of spinal cord injured and able-bodied athletes to prolonged upper body exercise and recovery. *Spinal Cord* 1999;37(11):772–779.
182. Webborn AD. "Boosting" performance in disability sport. *Br J Sports Med* 1999;33(2):74–75.
183. Bergman SB, Yarkony GM, Stiens SA. Spinal cord injury rehabilitation. 2. Medical complications. *Arch Phys Med Rehabil* 1997;78(3 suppl):53–58.
184. Comarr AE, Eltorai I. Autonomic dysreflexia/hyperreflexia. *J Spinal Cord Med* 1997;20(3):345–354.
185. Arnold JM, Feng QP, Delaney GA, et al. Autonomic dysreflexia in tetraplegic patients: evidence for alpha-adrenoceptor hyper-responsiveness. *Clin Auton Res* 1995;5(5):267–270.
186. Ashley EA, Laskin JJ, Olenik LM, et al. Evidence of autonomic dysreflexia during functional electrical stimulation in individuals with spinal cord injuries. *Paraplegia* 1993;31(9):593–605.
187. Chancellor MB, Erhard MJ, Hirsch IH, et al. Prospective evaluation of terazosin for the treatment of autonomic dysreflexia. *J Urol* 1994;151(1):111–113.
188. Steinberger RE, Ohl DA, Bennett CJ, et al. Nifedipine pretreatment for autonomic dysreflexia during electroejaculation. *Urology* 1990;36(3):228–231.
189. Vaidyanathan S, Soni BM, Sett P, et al. Pathophysiology of autonomic dysreflexia: long-term treatment with terazosin in adult and paediatric spinal cord injury patients manifesting recurrent dysreflexic episodes. *Spinal Cord* 1998;36(11):761–770.
190. Hartkopp A, Murphy RJ, Mohr T, et al. Bone fracture during electrical stimulation of the quadriceps in a spinal cord injured subject. *Arch Phys Med Rehabil* 1998;79(9):1133–1136.

191. Lopes P, Figoni SF, Perkash I. Upper limb exercise effect on tilt tolerance during orthostatic training of patients with spinal cord injury. *Arch Phys Med Rehabil* 1984;65(5):251–253.
192. Parikh A, Sochett EB, McCrindle BW, et al. Carotid artery distensibility and cardiac function in adolescents with type 1 diabetes. *J Pediatr* 2000;137(4):465–496.
193. Kanbay A, Kokturk O, Ciftci TU, et al. Comparison of serum adiponectin and tumor necrosis factor-alpha levels between patients with and without obstructive sleep apnea syndrome. *Respiration* 2008;76(3):324–330.
194. Mausser M MM. History of University of Illinois Wheelchair Sports Program.
195. Tiessen J. Lighter stronger faster: revolutionizing technology for athletes with a disability. 65–72.
196. Cooper R BMSSOT. Elite athletes with impairments in exercise and rehabilitation and medicine. Human Kinetics.

CHAPTER 25 ■ NEUROMUSCULAR ELECTRICAL STIMULATION IN SPINAL CORD INJURY

GREG NEMUNAITIS, KEVIN KILGORE, RONALD TRIOLO, RUDY KOBETIC, GRAHAM CREASEY, AND ANTHONY F. DIMARCO

INTRODUCTION

The applications of neuromuscular electrical stimulation (NMES) in spinal cord injury (SCI) can be conveniently divided into three classes, according to purpose: functional, therapeutic, or diagnostic.

1. Functional neuromuscular stimulation (FNS) is the use of NMES to activate paralyzed muscle in a precise sequence of intensity, duration, and frequency to restore muscle function. Devices or systems that provide FNS and restore muscle function are called neuroprostheses.
2. Therapeutic neuromuscular stimulation is the use of NMES to activate paralyzed muscle to prevent complications of immobility including range of motion, muscle atrophy, blood flow, pain syndromes, and muscle spasm.
3. Diagnostic neuromuscular stimulation is the use of NMES to activate muscle and assess electrodiagnostic properties of nerve and muscle, including the differentiation of upper motor neuron and lower motor neuron (LMN) paralysis, and to establish motor point locations that may be obliterated in the case of injection techniques.

This chapter focusses on the functional application of NMES in patients with traumatic SCI. The physiology of and principles of NMES as applied to nerve and muscle are reviewed. The components of NMES systems and their evolution in design are presented with emphasis on development of neuroprosthetic systems. A review of the clinical implementation of NMES systems focusses on neuroprosthetic applications for the upper extremity (UE), lower extremity (LE), trunk, respiration, and bladder. Therapeutic applications are reviewed and include cardiovascular (CV) deconditioning, muscle atrophy, osteoporosis, pressure ulcer, and deep venous thrombosis. Finally, perspectives on the future developments and directions are presented.

PHYSIOLOGY OF NEUROMUSCULAR ELECTRICAL STIMULATION

Excitation of Nervous Tissue by Neuromuscular Electrical Stimulation

Fundamental to the practical application of NMES is direct activation of the peripheral nerve rather than the muscle. Thus, the anterior horn cell, axon, neuromuscular junction, and muscle fiber must be intact for NMES to work. Furthermore, direct activation of muscle is not practical due to the large current and charge required for depolarization. The threshold for direct muscle fiber excitation is about 100 to 1,000 times higher than the threshold for nerve stimulation (1). Therefore, it is unlikely that direct muscle stimulation is a factor in any of the electrical stimulation (ES) paradigms described in this chapter.

The action potential of the nerve produced by NMES is identical to the action potential produced by natural means with the same "all or none" response described by Henry P. Bowditch in 1871 (2). The all or nothing response is the principle that defines that the force of muscle contraction is not dependent on the size of the stimulus, but rather the strength of the stimulus above the threshold potential. If the stimulus is of any strength above membrane threshold, the nerve will depolarize and all muscle fibers innervated by the nerve will fire. The stimulus threshold of any neuron is inversely proportional to the diameter of the neuron. Large-diameter neurons, which have the lowest threshold for stimulation, are activated first, followed by smaller neurons down to the smallest C-fiber (1,3). This property of NMES is called the reverse recruitment order. Note this is in reverse order of the Henneman's size principle (4), whereby smaller motor units are recruited before large motor units during progressive activation of muscle.

The stimulus current diminishes as a function of the distance from the stimulating electrode (1,5). Therefore, neurons furthest away from an electrode are least likely to receive stimulation at a level above threshold. Although FNS systems are often described as involving stimulation of a "muscle," this is, in fact, referring to stimulation of the nerves innervating the muscle, resulting in muscle contraction.

Muscle Response to Neuromuscular Electrical Stimulation

Muscle fibers are divided into groups depending on their contractile properties. At one end of the spectrum are the fast-twitch glycolytic fibers, which generate high levels of force, but fatigue rapidly (5,6). At the other end of the spectrum are the slow-twitch oxidative fibers, which generate lower forces, but are fatigue resistant (5,6). Fatigue resistance is a key requirement for most NMES applications involving the skeletal muscle. Therefore, recruitment of slow-twitch, fatigue-resistant fibers is most desirable for NMES. However, because large fibers have lower threshold for stimulation, large rapidly fatiguing fibers are recruited preferentially by NMES. Furthermore, disuse atrophy tends to convert slow-twitch fibers to rapidly fatiguing fast-twitch fibers (7,8). Fortunately, muscle atrophy and the concomitant change in fiber type can be reversed with chronic NMES through development of more fatigue-resistant muscle fibers (9–13). Human studies have demonstrated that cyclic NMES of paralyzed muscles can increase muscle bulk, joint force (14,15), and muscle endurance (16–18). All current neuroprosthetic applications use some form of muscle conditioning, which is patterned after these studies. The effects of NMES on muscle physiology are presented in detail in the section describing therapeutic applications.

Successful stimulation of muscle for functional purposes requires that the LMN is intact. In cases of SCI, there is frequently some damage to the LMN pool at the level of the injury (19). If most or all of the LMNs to a particular muscle are damaged, then the muscle will be unexcitable and it will not be possible to obtain functional levels of force with NMES. NMES-mediated exercise will not reverse atrophy in fibers where the LMN has been damaged. Patients with extensive LMN damage, from disease or trauma (i.e., amyotrophic lateral sclerosis, poliomyelitis, or brachial plexus injury), are not likely to benefit.

Varying the stimulus pulse amplitude, duration, and frequency modulates NMES-mediated muscle force generation. A single stimulus pulse delivered to a nerve above its threshold will generate an action potential with a corresponding muscle twitch. When repeated pulses are delivered to a nerve, the muscle twitch response will begin before the previous twitch is complete, leading to a summation phenomenon. At higher frequencies, the contractions fuse leading to tetany. While smooth tetanic contractions are desirable for NMES applications, a higher frequency of stimulation also leads to more rapid fatigue. Thus, in order to maintain both smooth contraction and maximum possible fatigue resistance, the ideal stimulation frequency ranges between 12 and 16 Hz for UE applications and 18 and 25 Hz for LE applications.

As the duration or amplitude of a stimulus pulse is increased, the stimulus threshold will be reached for neurons farther away from the stimulating electrode leading to activation of more neurons and greater force generation. This spatial summation resulting from modulating the duration or amplitude of a stimulus pulse is the principal means of modulating muscle force in NMES. Although a decision to choose duration versus amplitude to modulate force is primarily a function of circuit design, modulating the duration appears to require less charge transfer per stimulus for a given force level (20).

Force output with NMES is also dependent on factors uncontrolled by stimulation parameters. Movement of the stimulating electrode with respect to the target nerve during passive movement or muscle contraction can substantially change recruitment curve characteristics (21,22). Muscles have inherent length-tension characteristics, so that even at a constant level of recruitment, there will be changes in the force generated by the muscle contractile elements as a function of the length of the muscle for a given application. Changes in the tendon moment arm as a function of joint angle will also alter the torque output even if the tension on the tendon is kept constant. Finally, because the stimulus field is not limited by anatomical boundaries, a single electrode in a given muscle is likely to recruit motor units from other muscles. Muscle selectivity of stimulation is highest for implanted electrodes and lowest for surface electrodes. In most functional applications, it is desirable to isolate the recruitment to single muscles or muscle groups.

Safe Stimulation of Living Tissue

The parameters for safe stimulation and materials for safe electrodes used in implanted systems have been experimentally established (1). Improper stimulation can result in electrochemical changes in the electrode material, leading to corrosion or dissolution of metal ions. Strong negative charge on the electrode can result in hydrogen formation at the electrode. In addition, reactions at the electrode can cause changes in pH, which can result in tissue necrosis. To prevent this occurrence, balanced biphasic stimulation should always be used with intramuscular (IM) stimulation. The balancing pulse (typically an anodic pulse) balances the charge injected into the tissue and greatly reduces the potential for damage. Despite detrimental reactions that can occur, safe stimulation can be achieved at current levels that are sufficient to stimulate muscles at functionally useful levels.

Tissue damage from NMES is related to the charge per unit area of stimulation, not the voltage of the stimulus. The critical parameters for safe stimulation are current amplitude and electrode-tissue contact area. It is therefore safer to use constant current stimulation for electrodes within muscle or nerve tissue because it provides better control of the charge density. When constant voltage stimulation is used, the current densities are uncontrolled and can become very high if the resistance of the electrode-tissue interface is high. Therefore, stimulus current should always be regulated for electrodes located within living tissue.

There are other factors to consider when transcutaneous electrodes are used. The electrode-tissue contact area is generally not constant as electrodes often pull away from the skin, which significantly decreases the electrode-tissue contact area. When constant current stimulation is used, this will lead to high current densities, which can burn the underlying tissue. When using constant voltage stimulation, the increased resistance will result in decreased current delivered to the tissue. Although this may be safer, it results in variations in the stimulation delivered to the muscle, thus changing the force output. No matter which type of stimulation is used, it is important to maintain good contact between the electrode and skin. Even with good skin contact, transcutaneous NMES may still result in warming and reddening of the skin and, in certain conditions, burning of the tissue. The warming and reddening of the skin are due to the increase in circulation and is generally benign. If the current densities are too high, burning of the tissue can occur, even with good electrode-skin contact. Transcutaneous stimulation should be used with caution and with frequent examination of the skin when applied to patients with impaired sensation or cognition.

IM electrodes eliminate the hazard of direct skin reaction to the applied stimulus, but still have a risk of muscle tissue damage if the stimulus is improperly applied. Safe stimulus levels for balanced biphasic stimulation have been established at a minimum of 0.4 $\mu C/mm^2$ (1). Therefore, maximum stimulus levels depend upon the stimulating surface area of the electrode. Percutaneous IM electrodes used for many neuromuscular applications have surface areas of approximately 10 mm^2 (1). Safe stimulation parameters with this type of electrode are biphasic pulses with an amplitude of 20 mA and a pulse duration of 200 μs. Frequencies are typically in the range of 10 to 50 Hz, although frequency is not a factor in adverse tissue response to stimulation. IM NMES using these parameters has been applied for human use for over 15 years without any evidence of muscle damage (23).

Most forms of direct nerve stimulation use a nerve cuff electrode that encompasses the nerve trunk. Nerve tissue damage can occur through the same electrochemical mechanism as muscle tissue damage, but it can also occur through mechanical movement of the cuff relative to the nerve. In addition, tissue growth around nerve cuff electrodes can result in compression of the nerve and therefore secondary damage (24). Despite these potential problems, nerve cuffs have been used safely in many applications (25–27). Stimulation of nerves typically requires about one tenth of the current necessary for IM stimulation.

Secondary tissue damage as a result of infection at the electrode site has been studied. Kilgore analyzed 238 electrodes that had been implanted as part of an upper-limb neuroprosthesis. Each electrode had been implanted at least 3 years, with a maximum implantation time of over 16 years; with only one electrode infection reported (28).

SYSTEM COMPONENTS AND EVOLUTION IN DESIGN

The user of any neuroprosthesis must have a way to communicate his or her intent to the device in order to select, activate, or directly control the resulting limb movement. This command input can take any number of forms, spanning simple switch closures and timer settings to more complicated sequences of EMG activity from muscles still under volitional control (29,30). Once the user delivers a command to the system, the device must process the input, which could be interpreted differently depending on the prior history of stimulation, the current state of device, or the status of the limb. After the command processor unambiguously recognizes the intent of the user, the neuroprosthesis must respond. The control processor selects the appropriate stimulation channels as well as their relative timing, intensity, and frequency. These parameters are then used by the stimulus delivery subsystem to generate the stimulation waveforms and deliver current via the cables, leads, and electrodes that interface with the body. Optionally, the user can be made aware of what the system is doing through cognitive feedback of the state of the device via displays, warning lights, or audio tones. The majority of clinically applied FNS systems operate "open loop," that is, they are unresponsive to the environment and do not automatically correct for errors that arise between the intended and executed motions of the limbs. Sensors have been employed experimentally to feed kinematic information (joint angles, contact forces, etc.) back to the controller. Such "closed loop" systems require a sensor processor to monitor the actions of the limbs and allow the control processor to adjust stimulus levels automatically without conscious input from the user. Finally, the user can be informed of the orientation and state of his or her body (rather than the state of the device) through substitute sensory feedback. In this scheme, sensor signals are used to modulate tactile stimulation to sensate areas, or provide other indications of the status of the limbs and joints and their interaction with the environment (31,32).

FNS systems can be completely external to the body, in which case no foreign material is introduced into the body and only the stimulating current crosses the skin boundary. When subsystems are implanted (e.g., the electrodes and/or stimulus delivery circuitry), communication must be maintained with components of the system remaining outside of the body. This can be done by direct percutaneous connection, or via radio frequency (RF), inductive or optical links. In the latter cases, nothing crosses the skin except energy, reducing the likelihood of infection accompanying percutaneous connections, and reducing the burden of donning and doffing common to external controllers. Implanting components of the system requires additional circuitry (transmitters and receivers) to maintain the communication pathways between components, and may increase the complexity of the design. In spite of the required surgery, implantable systems offer advantages of placing the stimulating electrodes in close proximity to nerves, thus greatly increasing the selectivity and efficiency of activation while reducing the activation current. For long-term clinical application, implanted systems such as these provide major advantages over other systems including improved convenience, cosmesis, reliability, and consistency (33).

Electrodes used for FNS applications are classified according to the location of their stimulating surfaces. They are usually designed to activate nerves in the periphery, but increasing attention is being paid to developing new technologies to stimulate the spinal cord, motor cortex, or other regions of the brain. Most clinically available electrodes fall into three broad classes: transcutaneous electrodes applied to the skin, muscle-based electrodes, and nerve-based electrodes. Alternatively, lead wires connecting the electrodes to the stimulus generating circuitry are described by the course they take and the tissues through which they pass. Electrode leads can be classified as external, percutaneous, or implanted. All transcutaneous electrodes use external leads, while muscle- and nerve-based electrodes can be connected to either percutaneous or implanted lead wires.

Transcutaneous electrodes deliver electrical charge to the motor nerve through the skin. They are applied to the surface of the skin over the "motor point," the location exhibiting the best contraction from the target muscle at the lowest levels of stimulation. NMES with transcutaneous electrodes offers several distinct advantages: (a) the electrodes are generally easy to apply and remove, (b) the stimulation technique is noninvasive and therefore reversible (i.e., the position of the electrodes can be readily changed to elicit optimal stimulated responses), (c) are easily learned and applied in the clinic, and (d) the electrodes and stimulators are relatively inexpensive and commercially available. Stimulation with transcutaneous electrodes is the most widely used technique for therapeutic applications (34), and has been successfully employed to produce standing, stepping, and grasping motions and to assist with respiratory function (33,35–37).

In spite of their apparent convenience when applied individually in small numbers, transcutaneous electrodes have several disadvantages: (a) they tend to activate any nerve beneath them, making it difficult to produce an isolated contraction of a single muscle, (b) daily doffing and donning can complicate use, especially if electrode positions vary slightly from day to day, producing different stimulated responses, and (c) multiple electrode systems rapidly become impractical as the number of stimulus channels required for function increases and connecting multiple electrodes becomes cumbersome. Large currents may be required to drive sufficient charge through the skin and intervening tissues between the electrode and the peripheral nerve. In many cases, cutaneous pain receptors are excited, and patients with preserved or heightened sensation may find it difficult to tolerate transcutaneous stimulation at the levels required to produce a strong motor response.

Muscle-based electrodes bypass both the high resistance of the skin and cutaneous sensory fibers. Because their stimulating surfaces lie closer to the motor nerve branches of the target muscles, they provide a means to produce more efficient contractions (i.e., with smaller currents) while more selectively activating than transcutaneous electrodes. For these reasons, muscle-based electrodes are preferable for situations that require independent control of several isolated muscles. The stimulating tips of IM electrodes reside within the muscle tissue and generally include a barbing mechanism to resist movement until encapsulation occurs. Depending on their intended application, IM electrodes can be introduced either percutaneously (14,38) or in an open surgical procedure (39). In addition to their selectivity, low current requirements, and ease of implantation, IM electrodes allow access to deep nerves that are difficult to approach transcutaneously. When used with percutaneous leads, they can also be easily removed and provide a means for producing strong repeatable contractions on either an acute or longer term basis. Early movement away from the target nerve within the first 6 weeks postimplantation (before encapsulation is complete) can result in altered stimulated responses and is the most frequently observed failure of these devices (40). Epimysial electrodes are sutured directly to the epimysium or fascia to eliminate this early movement and provide immediate and permanent fixation. Because they are surgically installed, they are used almost exclusively with implanted stimulators, but have also been connected to percutaneous leads (41).

Nerve-based electrodes have a more intimate contact with neural structures than muscle-based electrodes, and therefore require even less current to produce a contraction. They are typically used as epineural electrodes, which are sutured to the connective tissue surrounding a motor nerve; cuff electrodes, which envelope the nerve; and penetrating intraneural probes, which are still laboratory-based investigational tools. Epineural and nerve cuff designs have both been employed as stimulating electrodes in FNS systems to restore motor function in SCI and stroke (27,42). Cuff electrodes have also been configured to record from afferent nerves in attempts to utilize the natural sensors in the body to provide feedback signals to control and adjust the stimulation (43). Nerve cuff electrodes have been widely used in humans for phrenic pacing, or to stimulate the peroneal nerve to produce dorsiflexion in individuals with hemiplegia.

Electrodes are connected to stimulating or recording circuitry through lead wires. Percutaneous leads have been designed to connect chronically indwelling IM and epimysial electrodes to circuitry external to the body while maintaining a barrier to infection. The leads are made of multiple strands of insulated stainless steel that are helically wound to form a thin, flexible cable of small enough diameter for the tissue to heal around as it exits the skin. The helical configuration converts bending motions to torsional stresses in the coils of the lead, providing mechanical resistance to fracture due to metal fatigue. The open coils also promote tissue ingrowth and assist with fixation. A thin layer of endothelial cells proliferates around the coils near the skin surface at sufficient depth to provide a barrier to infection.

Although they facilitate donning and doffing of neural prosthesis by eliminating the need to apply individual electrodes and simplifying connecting to other electronic components, percutaneous leads require continual attention from the user. They must be cleaned, dressed, and properly inspected and maintained. These leads are subject to breakage at areas of high shear stress, such as where they cross fascial planes. Although they can remain functional for years without infection or complication, percutaneous leads are usually reserved for acute and subacute applications and are generally considered to be ill-suited for long-term clinical use.

Implanted leads can be of larger dimensions than percutaneous lead wires because they need to be more robust and resistant to failure, and are not required to cross the skin. One popular configuration consists of two insulated stranded stainless steel cables wound in tandem and enclosed in an elastomer sheath to prevent ingrowth, provide mechanical stability, and allow the leads to slide through the tissues between the electrode and the implanted stimulating circuitry (44). To allow repair or revision of implanted FNS systems, provisions have been made in several designs to isolate system subcomponents from each other via high reliability implantable connectors (45). In-line connectors permit the surgical removal and repositioning of individual electrodes with minimal dissection and without extensive exposure of larger implanted circuit packages. These designs reduce the risk of infection and minimize the likelihood of damage to other implanted components during maintenance procedures. Implantable electronic components can also be designed as passive devices, which derive their power from the RF signals that provide communication channels to external command or control processors. Systems utilizing this configuration eliminate the need for additional surgery to replace internal batteries.

Alternative leadless systems of distributed single-channel micromodular implanted stimulators are also under development (46). Each of these small, glass-enclosed capsules contains an individually addressable receiver and stimulus delivery circuit. Multiple single-channel stimulators can be inserted with a cannula, and controlled by a single external radio frequency transmitter. The potential advantages of this design approach include elimination of percutaneous or implanted lead wires and connectors and the possible reduction of the invasiveness of the surgery required for installation. Disadvantages include the necessity for a large transmitting coil and increased power requirements if the modular receiver/stimulators are not concentrated at a single location but distributed at multiple motor points. The design also presupposes that the neuroprosthesis user will not require any additional reconstructive surgery to correct acquired deformities, which is often the case after prolonged paralysis. The practicality of this approach over more conventional pacemaker-like neuroprosthetic systems remains to be determined.

UPPER EXTREMITY NEUROPROSTHESES

FNS has been used to provide grasp and release for individuals with tetraplegia (33,47–49). The objectives of these systems are to reduce the need of individuals to rely on assistance from others, reduce the need for adaptive equipment, reduce the need to wear braces or other orthotic devices, and reduce the time it takes to perform tasks. Typically, patients use the neuroprosthesis for such tasks as eating, personal hygiene, writing, and office tasks.

The majority of UE neuroprostheses have been targeted for individuals with C5 and C6 motor levels. For these patients, the provision of grasp opening and closing using FNS provides a distinct functional benefit. At the C4 motor level, control of elbow flexion and shoulder stability must be provided by stimulation of the biceps and/or brachialis, or by a mechanical or surgical means. FNS has been used to a limited extent by these individuals, but there are no clinically deployed systems for this population to date. For individuals with C7 or C8 motor level function, there are other surgical options such as tendon transfers to provide similar levels of function, and FNS is not commonly used.

When used as an upper limb neuroprosthesis, ES is delivered to intact LMNs as earlier described, and is not used to directly activate denervated muscle. For C5 and C6 injuries, the muscles most likely to sustain LMN damage are the wrist extensors. Peckham and Keith (50) found that between 80% and 100% of the muscles necessary for grasp had sufficient intact innervation to generate functional levels of force. In many cases, other paralyzed muscles can be used to substitute for the function (51). FNS can be applied at any time postinjury, but it is typically applied after neurological stability has been achieved. Joint contractures must be corrected or functional ability will be limited. Spasticity must be under control. Individuals who are motivated and desire greater independence are the best candidates for neuroprostheses. In addition, most current neuroprosthetic systems still require assistance in donning the device, so it is necessary for the individual to have good attendant support.

All existing UE neuroprosthetic systems consist of a stimulator that activates the muscles of the forearm and hand, an input transducer, and control unit. The control signal for grasp is derived from an action for which the user has retained voluntary control, which can include joint movement (47,52–56), muscle activity (57–61), respiration (62), or voice control (47,48,63). A coordinated stimulation pattern is developed so that the muscles are activated in a sequence that produces a functional grasp pattern. Two basic grasp patterns are generally provided for functional activities: lateral pinch and palmar prehension (64). Other grasp patterns have been described for use in neuroprostheses, including a "pinch grip" between the index and thumb (65) and "parallel extension grasp" with finger extension and thumb abduction (66). The user typically has control over grasp opening and closing, but does not have direct control over the activation of each muscle. This design simplifies the control required by the user.

Clinically Evaluated Applications

Two fundamental designs for neuroprosthetic systems are currently utilized in tetraplegia; transcutaneous systems using surface-based electrodes and implanted neuroprostheses. Transcutaneous systems are generally indicated for muscle conditioning, whereas implanted systems are indicated for long-term functional use.

Transcutaneous Neuroprosthesis

Nathan (48,49) from BeerSheva, Israel, has developed a splint that incorporates transcutaneous electrodes for grasp, called the NESS H200 (Bioness, Inc., Santa Clarita, CA). The brace fixes the wrist in neutral, making it applicable primarily to C5 level individuals who do not have a tenodesis grasp. A clinical study of the Handmaster was performed that studied subjects with C5/C6 tetraplegia (49). After 2 weeks of muscle conditioning using the stimulator and 6 to 12 weeks of functional training, functional performance was assessed in at least four tasks that included pouring water from a can, opening a jar, opening a bottle, and inserting and removing a video tape. The four subjects were independently able to perform at least two tasks using the Handmaster that they could not perform without assistance when using their hand with a splint. Three of the subjects demonstrated improvement in pouring from a can and opening a bottle. Other improved tasks included shaving, putting on socks, and handling a hammer. However, in this group, only one subject continued to use the Handmaster at home. Another study by Alon et al. (67) demonstrated similar results, indicating significant muscle conditioning, but with few subjects utilizing the device long-term for function. The Handmaster has the European Community (CE) Mark in Europe and is approved by the Food and Drug Administration (FDA) as a therapeutic device in the United States. The University of Toronto has also developed a similar surface stimulation-based system and has demonstrated similar therapeutic benefit from the stimulation (68).

Implanted Neuroprosthesis

An implanted UE neuroprosthesis was first developed in 1986 by Peckham and colleagues in Cleveland and is now known as the FreeHand System (Fig. 25.1) (23,33). The FreeHand System consists of eight implanted electrodes and an implanted receiver-stimulator unit (44), providing lateral and palmar grasp to persons with C5 and C6 tetraplegia. A RF inductive link provides communication and power to the implant receiver-stimulator. The proportional control of grasp opening and closing is achieved using shoulder motion, which is measured using an externally worn joystick on the chest and shoulder (53). The FreeHand System has FDA approval in the United States and the CE Mark as a neuroprosthesis providing hand function for SCI.

A multicenter study was conducted to evaluate the safety, effectiveness, and clinical impact of the implanted neuroprosthesis on 50 individuals with tetraplegia (33,69). The inclusion criteria for study participants included traumatic SCI resulting in motor complete tetraplegia at the C5 or C6 levels; at least 1 year postinjury; and demonstrated innervation of key muscles of the forearm and hand, or their substitutes, as indicated by a grade 4 response to transcutaneous ES. Key muscles tested include the thumb abductors, adductors, flexors and extensors, and finger flexors and extensors. Exclusion criteria included cardiac pacemaker; history of chronic systemic infection or illness that increased surgical risk; uncontrolled spasticity; extensive and irreversible contractures in UE joints; diabetes; immune disease; heart disease or cardiac arrhythmia; and breast masses with a high probability of being cancerous.

Paralyzed muscle excitability was evaluated using transcutaneous stimulation applied to each muscle in the forearm and hand. Each candidate underwent a 1-month muscle conditioning program using transcutaneous stimulation to build muscle strength. Candidates received the implanted neuroprosthesis in a 4- to 6-hour surgical procedure that included placement of all eight electrodes and, in almost all cases, concomitant surgical procedures such as tendon transfers or joint arthrodeses (51). Postoperatively, the treated arm was immobilized in a cast for 3 weeks to allow electrode encapsulation and wound healing. After cast removal, muscle conditioning

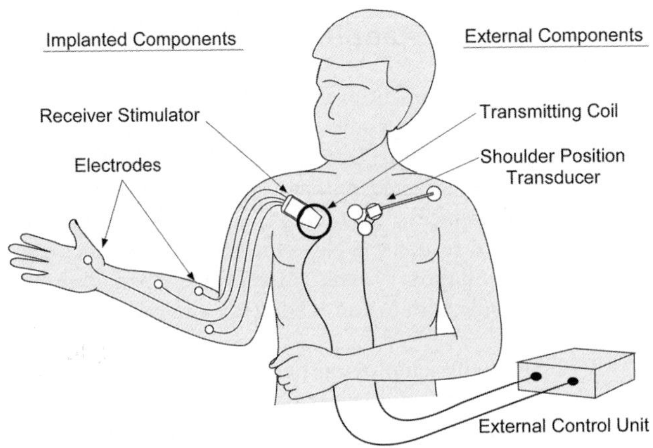

FIGURE 25.1 Freehand in BW.

using the neuroprosthesis was initiated to build fatigue resistance in the muscles. After approximately 4 weeks of daily muscle conditioning at home, training and evaluation using the neuroprosthesis was performed during a 1- to 3-week inpatient stay. Follow-up studies were performed at 6 months and 1 year postimplant.

The neuroprosthesis produced increased pinch force in all patients. In a test of grasp and release ability using six objects of different size and weight (70,71), 49 of the 50 participants (98%) moved at least one more object with the neuroprosthesis than they could without it. The direct impact of the neuroprosthesis in the performance of activities of daily living (ADL) was tested in 28 patients (72). Each participant was tested while performing 6 to 15 tasks, which included eating with a fork, drinking from a glass, writing with a pen, dialing a phone, using a computer diskette, and brushing teeth. Every participant received training both with and without the neuroprosthesis to achieve their maximum independence using each method. If necessary, participants were provided with splints or adaptive equipment to perform the task. Therefore, the independence provided by the neuroprosthesis was directly compared to the maximum independence that could be provided by any other means. All participants improved in independence in at least one task, and 78% were more independent using the neuroprosthesis in at least three tasks tested. All participants preferred to use the neuroprosthesis in at least one task tested and 27 (96%) preferred to use the neuroprosthesis in at least three tasks tested. Satisfaction and daily utilization of the neuroprosthesis at home was measured through surveys and device data logging (73). More than 90% of the participants were satisfied with the neuroprosthesis, and most used it regularly. Follow-up surveys indicate that usage patterns were maintained at least 4 years postimplant.

Current Research in Upper Extremity Neuroprostheses

Current research in the application of neuroprosthetics to the UE in SCI includes the provision of additional function through the stimulation of more muscles, evaluation of new methods of control, new technological advancements, and the development of systems for C4 and higher level SCI.

Additional Function

First-generation neuroprosthetic systems focused on the provision of grasp and release, but it has been shown that stimulation of additional muscles can provide even more function. Overhead reach can be provided by stimulation of the triceps muscle, and subjects can combine triceps activation with stimulated grasp function to gain improved functional abilities (48,74–76). Stimulation of the pronator quadratus muscle can develop adequate pronation that can be opposed by voluntarily generated supination (77). Stimulation of the finger intrinsic muscles can improve grasp function (78).

New Control Methods

A number of alternative methods for controlling a neuroprosthesis have been pursued. The use of wrist position to control grasp has been shown to be a better method of control for some patients when compared to control of grasp using shoulder position (56). Activation of voluntary antagonists has been used to control elbow angle and forearm supination/pronation (76,77). The use of the myoelectric signal from either forearm or neck muscles has been shown to be a viable method of control (56,57,59,60,61,79). Methods of obtaining cortical signals for neuroprosthetic control are also being pursued (80).

Second-Generation Implanted Neuroprostheses

Second-generation neuroprostheses have been developed that are based on the success of the Freehand System and take advantage of the technological advances from the 1990s. Clinical implementation of two configurations of the second-generation system have been initiated, including a system having 10 stimulus channels with an implanted joint angle sensor (81), and a system having 12 stimulus channels with two channels of myoelectric signal acquisition (82). This latter system is currently undergoing clinical studies, and is known as the Implantable Stimulator-Telemeter ("IST-12") System (61).

The myoelectrically controlled IST-12 neuroprosthesis provides control of grasp, forearm pronation, and elbow extension for individuals with tetraplegia. A key feature of this system, shown in Fig. 25.2, is the implantation of both the control and the stimulation source, which reduced the external components by 50% compared to the Freehand System. Results from the first three subjects to receive this system show that each demonstrated functional improvement in at least five different ADL, such as eating, writing, and reaching objects from an overhead shelf (61). Each subject was able to utilize the device at home. The use of myoelectric control in neuroprostheses allows considerable flexibility in the control algorithms, allowing them to be tailored to each individual subject. The elimination of the need for an externally mounted control source is extremely desirable and makes system use much simpler.

Application to C3/C4 SCI

Neuroprosthetic applications for high-level tetraplegia have been clinically demonstrated (48,62,63,66,83,84). Transcutaneous or percutaneous stimulation has been used to provide hand and elbow motion. Braces are used to support the shoulder. User control of both hand and arm function is provided through voice command, sip-puff control, facial myoelectric signal, head movement, or voluntary shoulder movements. Functional ability has been demonstrated in activities such as eating, drinking, and writing.

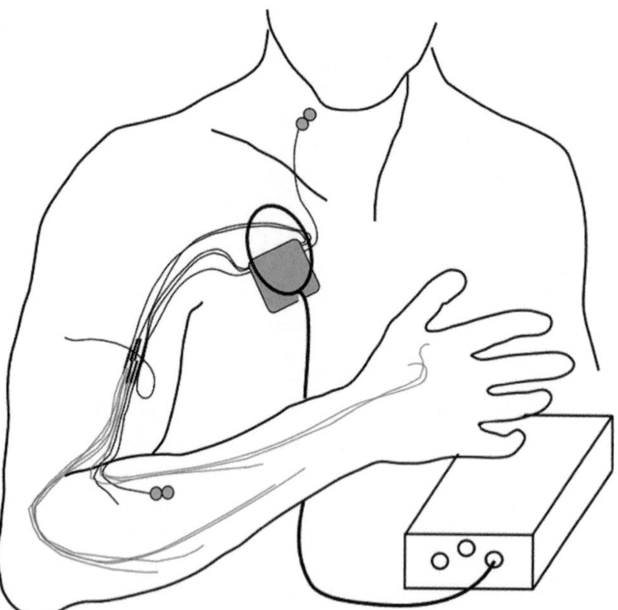

FIGURE 25.2 Second-generation implanted hand neuroprosthesis, the IST-12. This neuroprosthesis consists of an implanted device capable of twelve channels of stimulation and two channels of myoelectric signal recording. The external components included the transmit/receive coil that is taped on the chest, and an external control unit. Myoelectric signals are used to control grasp opening and closing, and can be obtained from any two muscles under voluntary control.

LOWER EXTREMITY AND TRUNK NEUROPROSTHESES

FNS with or without bracing can provide or enhance an individual's ability to exercise, stand, transfer, walk, climb stairs, or maintain controlled seated posture depending on the extent of their paralysis from thoracic or low cervical SCI (85–87).

Exercise, Standing, and Transfers

Standing with FNS has been achieved with relatively simple systems consisting of two to six channels of transcutaneous stimulation (88,89). Electrodes can be easily applied to the skin over the targeted muscles; however, daily variation in electrode placement can adversely affect the repeatability of the stimulated responses. Nevertheless, multichannel transcutaneous stimulation systems have provided standing and stepping in people with SCI in laboratory and clinical settings (36,90,91).

LE FNS systems employing percutaneous IM electrodes have also been successful in providing standing with ability to do one-handed reaching tasks (92) and walking by individuals with paraplegia (40,93). Percutaneous approaches to most muscles of the LE have been defined, allowing the generation of more complex movements than with transcutaneous stimulation alone (94). Based on the results of studies involving stimulation via surface and percutaneous electrodes, totally implanted pacemaker-like neuroprostheses for standing after SCI have been defined and successfully undergone initial clinical testing (95,96). For long-term clinical application, implanted systems provide major advantages over transcutaneous and percutaneous stimulation including improved convenience, cosmesis, reliability, and repeatability (33).

An individual with sensory-incomplete tetraplegia SCI (C6-ASIA B) is shown in Fig. 25.3 using the described implanted standing system. The implanted components of the standing and transfer system include an eight-channel receiver-stimulator (44) with in-lead connectors (45) to epimysial (97) or surgically implanted IM (39) electrodes shown in Fig. 25.3. Surgically implanted IM electrodes, which can be introduced through minimally invasive techniques, are being utilized more frequently in implanted systems. These approaches reduce the surgical time and dissection required to implant epimysial electrodes, which need to be sutured to targeted muscle at the

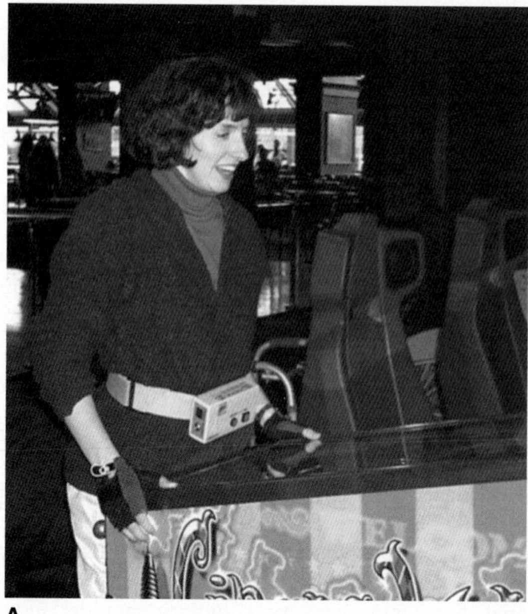

A

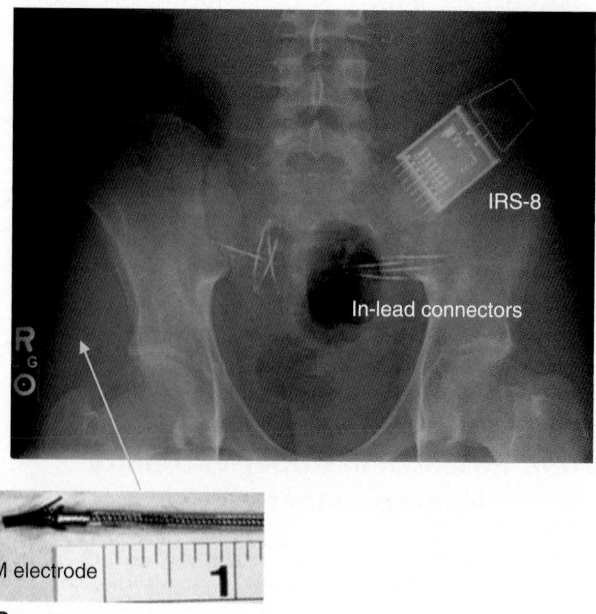

B

FIGURE 25.3 An individual with SCI using implanted standing system for recreation (**A**). The implanted components of a standing system are shown in (**B**).

nerve entry point. In a single surgical procedure, electrodes are bilaterally implanted in the vastus lateralis, semimembranosus, or posterior portion of the adductor magnus, and gluteus maximus, and at L1/L2 spinal level to activate the lumbar spinal roots for the erector spinae muscles. After 2 weeks of restricted activity followed by 8 weeks of progressive resistance and endurance exercise with the implanted FNS system, patterns of stimulation are constructed for the sit-to-stand and stand-to-sit transitions for users to progress from standing in parallel bars to a walker, to standing pivot transfers and swing-through gait. Balance training includes stand-to-retrieve tasks and releasing a hand to manipulate the controls of a wearable external control unit that provides power and command information to the implanted receiver/stimulator through an inductive link established via a transmitting coil placed on the surface of the skin above the implant.

The wearable external controller is programmed via a clinical interface suitable for use by nontechnical personnel (98,99). Users or their assistants interact with the FES system through switches mounted on the external controller, worn on a ring, or attached to the walking aid. To stand, a single activation of a switch ramps up the stimulation sequence to the trunk, hip, and knee extensors that raises the body from a seated position into standing. The stimulation level is maintained to brace the body against collapse while the hands are used for balance (100) until the user initiates the stand-to-sit pattern where stimulation is slowly ramped down to lower the body into sitting.

Stepping can be achieved with 16 channels of stimulation through the addition of a second implant to activate the hip flexors and ankle dorsiflexors (101,102). To date, a total of 18 such surgically implanted neuroprostheses for standing or stepping have been successfully installed at MetroHealth Medical Center and the Cleveland Department of Veterans Affairs Medical Center, as well as collaborating institutions in a multicenter Phase III clinical trial (103). Long-term follow-up for at least 2 years has been completed on 14 subjects, indicating that stimulation thresholds are stable and internal components are reliable (104,105). The stimulated responses of the knee, hip, and trunk extensors are sufficiently strong and fatigue resistant to complete various functional activities ranging from standing transfers to working at a counter. The amount of practice and training, body size, hip and trunk extensor strength, and quadriceps endurance appear to be important influences on standing duration, which can vary from 3 to greater than 40 minutes. Average elapsed standing time for users of the implanted neuroprostheses exceeds 10 minutes with a median time approximating 4 minutes, an interval sufficient for completing simple mobility and reaching activities.

All LE FNS systems still require assistive devices such as walkers or crutches to use the UE for additional support and balance. The magnitude of the upper body support can be quite small—on the order of 10% of body weight or less routinely produced by a single extremity without undue exertion (106)—thus freeing the other hand to perform reaching tasks or other functions. The metabolic energy consumption during standing with FNS is less than three times the rate of standing in a nondisabled individual (107), and close to that of standing with knee-ankle-foot orthoses (108,109). Energy costs are due primarily to stimulation of the large LE muscles since UE effort to maintain standing balance is minimal. Upper body effort to maintain standing is directly related to the postural alignment achieved by the stimulated extension moments produced at the hip and trunk. Maintaining balance automatically and minimizing high levels of continuous stimulation to provide hands free supported standing—even for the brief periods of time—has been an elusive goal and is still an active area of research.

Users and their assistants report a preference for FNS-assisted transfers over conventional methods when moving to and from high surfaces, while conventional pivot or sliding transfers were still the method of choice for level transfers (110). Transfers to heights otherwise impossible to perform by conventional lifting transfers require only moderate effort or assistance when using the neuroprosthesis.

FNS-Only Systems for Ambulation

Transcutanous FNS systems achieve standing by activating the quadriceps bilaterally to extend the knees (111) with or without simultaneous activation of the gluteal muscles to extend the hips (112). Stepping is produced by maintaining activation to the quadriceps of the stance leg while initiating a flexion withdrawal through surface stimulation of afferent sensory fibers to trigger a spinal reflex arc that causes hip, knee, and ankle flexion in the contralateral limb (113–115). To complete the step, activation of the knee extensors on the swing leg is initiated while the reflex is still active and flexing the hip. The stimulus producing the flexion reflex is then removed, leaving the user in double-limb support with bilateral quadriceps stimulation. A system of this type has received FDA approval and has been commercially available (Parastep, Sigmedics, Inc. Northfield, IL) for standing and stepping (36,37). Complicating issues with such surface stimulation systems include active flexion generated by the rectus femoris when the quadriceps are activated, making it difficult to maintain the erect posture. In addition, not all patients exhibit a flexion withdrawal reflex that is strong or repeatable enough to be used for stepping, and when available it tends to habituate with repeated activation thus limiting the number of steps.

The energy expenditure required for experienced users to walk distances up to 200 ft with the Parastep system has been reported to be approximately equivalent to a 1.5 mi walk at 3 mi/h for a nondisabled adult (116). The Physiological Cost Index (PCI), which is the ratio of change in heart rate from baseline (beats/meter or b/m) to steady-state velocity (m/min) has been used as a measure of energy cost during normal walking (117) as well as ambulating with transcutaneous stimulation. The PCI (b/m) has been shown to be an indicator of energy costs in disabled individuals (118) and applied as a measure of gait efficiency with different assistive devices after SCI (119). A wide range of walking performances were observed in five fully trained Parastep users with physiological cost indices ranging from 2.3 to 6.3 b/m, and at speeds of 5 to more than 24 m/min (120). These values are comparable to those reported for persons with paraplegia walking in a reciprocating gait orthosis, or RGO (121). Just as with other upright mobility devices for individuals with SCI, walking with the Parastep system is slower and less energy efficient than normal walking, which exhibits a PCI ranging between 0.11 and 0.51 b/m (with a mean of 0.21) at self-selected speeds. However, Parastep provides reasonable upright mobility at velocities and energy costs that appear to be within the physiological capacities of people with paraplegia (122). With energy costs similar to long leg braces, transcutaneous FNS systems may be better suited in providing physical benefits of exercise than as a daily mode of ambulation (123–126).

An increasing proportion of traumatic SCI is resulting in neurologically incomplete lesions (127). With the help of FNS, many of these individuals can become functional walkers, since some of their motor, sensory, and proprioception function has been preserved. But the high variability of the incomplete SCI population requires caution in the application of FNS (128). Voluntary strength has been shown to improve with voluntary exercise and therapy augmented by ES. In these cases, increased stride length and reduced PCI during walking have been achieved. Alternatively, the quality of stimulated responses can improve while volitional function remains unchanged, necessitating a neuroprosthetic application of FNS. In some patients, an exaggerated extensor tone can provide safe standing, but they are unable to initiate a step. In these patients, peroneal stimulators may be useful to inhibit extensor tone and help initiate a step (129,130). To improve posture, hip abductors, hamstrings, and trunk extensors are included in stimulation patterns as needed (131).

More recently, FNS systems utilizing implanted stimulator telemeters (IST-12) with 12 channels of stimulation and 2 channels of EMG recording have improved mobility function in individuals with incomplete SCI (Fig. 25.4). These individuals can usually stand but cannot initiate a step with one or both legs because of weakness or excessive extensor tone (132). These FNS systems can be tailored to the needs of individuals to correct their individual gait deficits with stimulation and to synchronize stimulation with activities of their own muscles. The recorded EMG from spared or partially paralyzed muscles are recorded by the implant, transmitted to an external controller for processing, and used to initiate stepping or modulate walking cadence (133). Thus, the desire to initiate a step or change walking speed is intimately under the user's control and integrated with their voluntary motor patterns without the need for external switches.

Multichannel implanted systems for walking after motor-complete paraplegia have also been reported to provide standing and swing-through gait (42,134). In individuals with complete paralysis, implanted electrodes have been used for personal mobility functions such as transfers, standing, one-handed reaching, forward, side and back stepping, and stair ascent and descent. This approach involves individual activation of a number of muscles (typically 16 or more) rather than the use of synergistic patterns such as the flexion withdrawal reflex or extensive bracing. Complex LE motions for walking (93) have been synthesized by activating up to 48 channels of stimulation using chronically indwelling helically coiled fine wire IM electrodes with percutaneous leads under the control of a programmable microprocessor-based external stimulator (135). Some well-trained subjects were able to repeatedly walk 300 m at 0.5 m/s using this system (136). Two individuals have used FNS systems with percutaneous electrodes for exercise and walking for more than 20 years (137). All components are worn by the user, freeing them from cabling to a walker or other assistive device. Freely articulating ankle foot orthosis are used to protect the ligaments and structures of the foot and ankle. The quality of the motions produced by FNS with this system depended on the availability, strength and endurance of paralyzed muscles, the ability of the therapist or engineer to specify patterns of stimulation for ambulation, and the subject's experience with the device.

Hybrid Systems Combining FNS and Orthoses

One method to achieve ambulation after SCI involves combining FNS with conventional bracing (87,138–141). The energy required to operate these hybrid systems is less than that

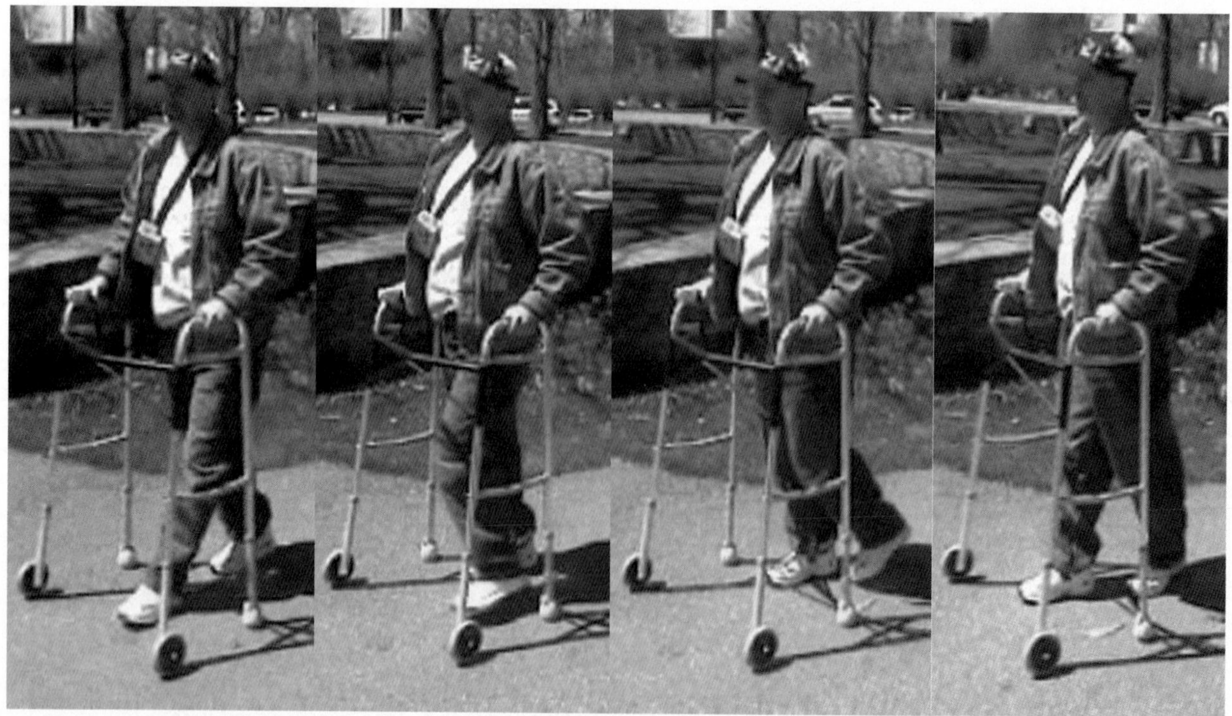

FIGURE 25.4 An individual with incomplete SCI (C6-ASIA D) using an implanted FNS system for a limited community ambulation.

required when using braces alone, but increases rapidly with walking speed. At slow to moderate speeds, energy consumption for both modes of walking is still less than that required with FNS alone. However, energy consumption for FNS walking decreases as walking speed increases, suggesting that as velocities approach normal the differences between walking modalities will be minimized or reversed (with brace walking requiring more energy than FNS). The energy saving effect of hybrid systems is primarily due to their ability to constrain the motions of the joints, reduce the degrees of freedom of movement, and provide mechanical stability. For static activities such as quiet standing, individuals with paraplegia can assume a stable posture with little or no muscular exertion by locking the knees and hips of the brace, thus avoiding the fatigue associated with continuous stimulation. FNS is quite effective at generating large propulsive forces through activation of the LE muscles, which reduces the UE exertion required for walking in conventional braces. Combining FNS and bracing in a hybrid orthosis takes advantage of the positive aspects of each technology and minimizes the potential shortcomings (142,143).

The Louisiana State University Reciprocating Gait Orthosis (LSU-RGO) hybrid system consists of a four-channel transcutaneous stimulator and a flexible copolymer electrode cuff that locates and maintains the transcutaneous electrodes over the rectus femoris and hamstrings. Since walking is accomplished with the knees locked in full extension, stimulating the hamstrings extends the hip, and flexes the contralateral hip through the action of the reciprocating mechanism. Conversely, the rectus femoris is used to actively flex the hip, rather than extend the knee, and assists with contralateral hip extension via the reciprocating mechanism. Rectus femoris and contralateral hamstrings are simultaneously activated to initiate a step upon the depression of a walker-mounted switch. Hybrid systems of this type have been fitted to more than 50 patients with complete or incomplete thoracic or low-level cervical injuries at LSU and collaborating centers. Similar systems employing a hip-guidance orthosis or alternative reciprocating mechanism have been devised and tested in various centers in North America and Europe (144). Follow-up studies on RGO-based hybrid orthoses showed that up to 41% of system recipients used it for gait (145), while 66% used it for exercise (146).

Development of hybrid orthoses for walking in paraplegia is primarily motivated by the need to improve hip and trunk stability and forward progression. The simplest hybrid system utilizes a reciprocating gait orthosis for support against gravity via mechanical locks at the joints. Stimulation assists in moving the user into stance and powering the reciprocal motion during walking (147). Other hybrid systems use the brace to provide mechanical support at only certain times in the gait cycle. With the joints passively locked by gravity, the stimulation switches off and is only reactivated when the joint becomes unstable. In this way, stimulation duty cycle is reduced and the onset of fatigue can be delayed (148). A third type of hybrid system regulates joint position with a controllable friction brake (149), hand-controlled mechanical joint locks (150), or with externally powered joint actuators (151). Recently, a hybrid orthosis based on a modified RGO has been developed with a variable constraint hip mechanism utilizing a hydraulic system to reciprocally couple the hips or individually lock/unlock the hips (152). This hybrid system powers the motion of the limbs via an implanted FNS system, and provides the hip and trunk stability of an RGO while allowing the hip motion required for increasing step length with speed and for ascending or descending stairs which are impossible to navigate with conventional bracing.

Hybrid systems are reliable and simple to implement in clinical environments with orthotic and prosthetic fabricating capacity. Standing with the knee joints of the brace locked allows all stimulation to be removed, thus postponing the onset of fatigue. The orthotic components of these systems may also protect the insensate joints and osteoporotic bones of users with long-standing SCI from possible damage resulting from the loads applied during weight bearing and ambulation. However, the bracing employed by hybrid systems can potentially encumber individuals in the execution of ADL for which they were not designed. For example, locking the knees can hinder the completion of more complex movements useful for personal mobility, such as stair climbing. Similarly, the thoracic component can prohibit lateral bending and trunk rotation while sitting in the wheelchair. The devices are usually worn outside the clothing, and donning, doffing, and cosmetic aspects are similar to conventional braces.

Oxygen consumption (VO_2), heart rate, and ambulation velocity with an RGO alone, and with a hybrid FNS-RGO system, have been documented. In a single-subject case study, a hybrid FES-RGO system reduced PCI values and increased speed as compared to braces alone (112). The addition of FNS to the reciprocating orthosis appeared to decrease mean PCI from 2.55 to 1.54 b/m at average self-selected velocities of approximately 24 and 25 m/min, respectively. These results are at the upper limits of performance observed for the Parastep system (120) and for the RGO alone (121), but the statistical significance of any apparent differences cannot be determined and care should be taken when comparing the results (122).

In a well-controlled study comparing VO_2 during ambulation with the LSU-RGO and the hybrid FNS-RGO system, six subjects with comparable experience in using each device experienced a 16% lower energy consumption at walking speeds ranging from 0.1 to 0.4 m/s when using the hybrid FNS-RGO system (153). Rate of energy consumption similarly increased with walking speed for both RGO-only and hybrid systems. When expressed in terms of energy consumed per meter walked, a similar 16% to 18% reduction in energy costs were observed with the hybrid system at velocities slower than the self-selected pace of 21 m/min although these advantages diminished rapidly with increasing walking speed (142). As reported with use of the Parastep system, energy costs are still considerably larger than those reported for nondisabled ambulation, indicating that hybrid systems may also be most useful as an effective mode of exercise for individuals with SCI (148,154), rather than a means of mobility.

FNS for Seated Postural Control

In seated nonparalyzed individuals, the center of pressure (COP) is controlled by synergies involving muscles of the leg, pelvis, hip, and trunk (155). In individuals with SCI, paralysis of these muscles makes it more difficult to maintain a balanced posture, decreases the range within which the COP can be actively moved, and decreases the acceleration with which sitting posture can be changed (156,157). Trunk instability after SCI due to paralysis of the abdominal and back muscles responsible for maintaining erect sitting posture leads to a "C"-shaped kyphotic posture with flattened lumbar spine and posterior pelvic tilt (158–160). This sitting posture is statically stable and effectively shifts the center of gravity of the trunk backwards within the base of support to avoid loss of balance. However, this passive kyphotic sitting posture can cause back pain, rotator cuff injury, and other chronic health problems due to increased pressure on the vertebral disks (161,162) or poor mechanics when using manual wheelchairs (163,164). A flexed or kyphotic posture in the sitting position resulting from paralysis can also limit rib cage and lung expansion during inhalation and therefore restrict ventilation (165,166). The resultant drop in ventilatory volumes can lead to retention of secretions with accompanying atelectasis and pneumonia (167–170). Individuals with lower level SCI can adopt a number of compensatory strategies to maintain sitting balance utilizing preserved voluntary actions of the latissimus dorsi and ascending part of the trapezius (158,171). Such options are not available to individuals with higher level lesions.

Because of lack of trunk control, bimanual reach is particularly difficult for individuals with low-cervical and thoracic SCI because one hand is always needed to maintain balance to prevent falling and to return to upright sitting. In this segment of the population, reaching depends more on the ability to control the trunk than the UEs, since proximal arm and shoulder strength are minimally affected. When both arms are extended to work bimanually, the forearms or elbows are often used for support, further limiting workspace volume. Loss of stability during reaching can also lead to falls from the wheelchair. Thus, the ability to control body position can profoundly affect the stability of wheelchair users, which can significantly reduce the possibility of falling or tipping (172).

Paralysis of the trunk musculature also has an effect on wheelchair propulsion efficiency (173,174). When compared with individuals with lower injuries, individuals with higher level injuries compensate for trunk instability by a more backward position on the push rim at the start of the push phase (175). There is also a well-documented and significant increase of trunk forward lean with fatigue, which individuals without volitional trunk control cannot adopt, thereby restricting their available options for optimizing propulsion performance (176–178).

A consistent change in seated posture can be achieved by FNS activation of the lumbar trunk extensors (erector spinae) and hip extensors (gluteus maximus and hamstring muscles). Stabilizing the trunk through stimulation of the paraspinal muscles can result in a significant increase in forward and upward shifts in seated workspace volume, and cause a significant anterior rotation of the pelvis to restore a more natural lumbar curve during sitting (179). Thus, application of FNS can allow individuals with SCI to reach farther and manipulate heavier objects, as well as improve efficiency of manual wheelchair propulsion by stabilizing the hips and trunk (180). Controlled lateral bending can also be achieved by activation of quadratus lumborum and gluteus maximus, to provide further adjustments to seated posture (181). The variation in seated posture possible with FNS can be used to provide active pressure relief, provide trunk stability during the execution of manual tasks and ADL, or improve respiratory function. By correcting kyphotic posture, FNS can allow the voluntary muscles of respiration to be more effective and facilitate increases in forced expiratory volume, and vital capacity (182).

For individuals with tetraplegia, stimulation of the gluteal, paraspinal, and quadratus lumborum muscles can maintain erect seated posture in the wheelchair and reduce the reliance on belts, straps, or specialized seating adaptations. Application of FNS to the hip and trunk muscles can provide users with the ability to regain an erect sitting position from a fully flexed or laterally bent position without the need for personal assistance or use of the UEs (Fig. 25.5). Furthermore, seated stability in terms of the ability to withstand anteriorly directed disturbances increases significantly when the hip and trunk muscles were activated, suggesting that the stability offered by hip and trunk stimulation may ultimately decrease the likelihood of accidental falls.

Bed turning for individuals with tetraplegia can also be facilitated by FNS to the trunk muscles. Stiffening the spine with stimulation allows the torso to rotate axially as a rigid unit, thus permitting the pelvis to follow the rotation of the shoulders to complete the turning maneuver with the use of a simple leg strap. The addition of a flexor withdraw reflex to the trunk stimulation can enable a user to flex the hip and knee without the leg strap and accomplish the turn without assistance or any adaptive equipment other than the FNS system (182).

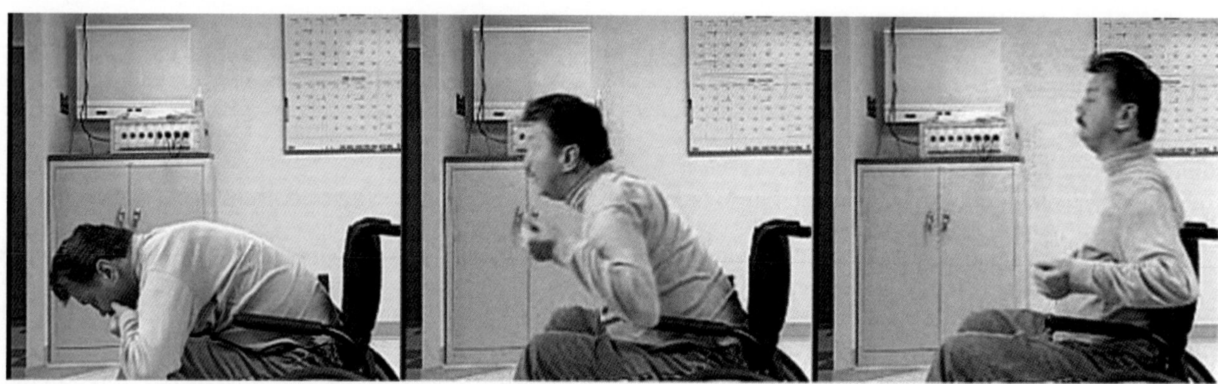

FIGURE 25.5. Bilateral stimulation of the trunk and hip muscles (erector spinae, quadratus lumborum, and gluteus maximus) allows an individual with a C4-5 ASIA A injury to independently resume an upright seated posture from a fully flexed position.

Summary

FNS systems for seated postural control and LE mobility enhance wheelchair stability and maneuverability, and permit persons with SCI to overcome physical and architectural barriers near their wheelchairs. Exercise, standing, standing transfers, and one-handed reaching are all possible with relatively simple transcutaneous or surgically implanted FNS systems without extensive external bracing. The functional impact of these FNS neuroprosthetic applications on the ability to complete ADL is still an active area of research. It is clear from preliminary work; however, that exercise, standing, and walking with FNS can improve tissue viability and overall health, facilitate standing transfers by eliminating the heavy lifting and lowering required by an assistant, and allow selected individuals with SCI to regain access to objects, places, and opportunities impossible or exceedingly difficult from the wheelchair. FNS can augment and extend the function of the wheelchair and may prove to be a valuable option to enhance the well-being and independence of persons with disabilities. All of this can be achieved with reliable implanted components that maximize cosmesis, personal convenience, and long-term use. To date, walking with FNS after complete paralysis from SCI appears to be a promising form of exercise, rather than an alternative to wheelchair locomotion, while in those with partial paralysis FNS can increase the level of independence from physiologic or household to limited community ambulation. In individuals with complete paralysis, a hybrid orthosis combining electromechanically controlled bracing and FNS has the potential to significantly improve function of either bracing or FNS alone by providing greater bracing stability and the ability to move the body to stand up, walk, and climb stairs provided by the power of their own paralyzed muscles. To date, the metabolic energy currently required to walk with FNS is too high to make it a truly practical alternative to the wheelchair for long distance transportation over level surfaces, although this remains a worthwhile and achievable long-term goal.

BLADDER NEUROPROSTHESES

SCI above the sacral segments often results in hyperreflexia of the bladder and external sphincter. Bowel function is also impaired, with constipation, difficulty in evacuation and occasional reflex incontinence of stool. Patients with suprasacral cord lesions can have ES applied to the surviving sacral nerves or nerve roots to improve bladder and bowel function. The technique has been used by more that 3,000 patients in over 20 countries during the last 3 decades to produce effective micturition, and to improve bowel function (183–190). An implantable stimulator is clinically available for this purpose from the manufacturer, Finetech Medical Ltd., in England. Following a multicenter clinical trial in the United States, the stimulator received FDA approval as a Humanitarian Use Device in 1998.

Micturition

Contraction of the bladder can be produced by electrical activation of the parasympathetic (PS) preganglionic efferent neurons whose cell bodies are in the sacral segments of the spinal cord and whose axons usually travel in the S3 and sometimes S4 or S2 anterior roots and nerves. These axons are closely accompanied for much of their course by somatic efferent axons to the external sphincter and pelvic floor. The latter axons, being of larger diameter than the PS axons, have a lower threshold for electrical activation, and it is therefore difficult to produce contraction of the bladder without contraction of the external sphincter. However, micturition can be produced by the technique of poststimulus voiding, during which smooth muscle of the bladder relaxes more slowly than the striated muscle of the external sphincter. Bladder pressure can be built up by a series of bursts of ES, each lasting a few seconds, and maintained between the bursts; the external sphincter contracts strongly during bursts but relaxes rapidly for a few seconds between bursts, allowing urine to flow. It was initially thought by some that the intermittent contraction of the sphincter during voiding might produce harmful pressures in the bladder leading to ureteric reflux or hydronephrosis, but these concerns have not been borne out in long-term follow-up.

Continence

The major cause of incontinence in subjects with suprasacral SCI continues to be bladder hyperreflexia. Large doses of anticholinergic medication as well as botulinum toxin injections, while useful for reducing bladder contraction, can also reduce the effects of ES. Capsaicin and resiniferatoxin have been investigated for their potential to reduce detrusor hyperreflexia by blocking sensory nerve input, though this has not yet reached clinical practice. Research is in progress evaluating reflex inhibition of the bladder by ES of large afferent neurons in the sacral dermatomes, a process known as neuromodulation, which shows some benefit in nondisabled subjects with urge incontinence (191,192). However, the most dramatic abolition of reflex incontinence can be produced by surgical division of the sacral sensory nerve roots, and since the mid-80s this procedure, known as posterior rhizotomy, has increasingly been combined with implantation of an electrical stimulator intended to stimulate the motor roots for micturition. The rhizotomy typically increases bladder capacity and compliance, and reduces the risk of damage to the upper urinary tracts by lowering the pressure at which urine is stored in the bladder; it may even result in some improvement in reflux or hydronephrosis if these have already occurred. It also abolishes spasticity of the external urethral and anal sphincters and abolishes the autonomic hyperreflexia and potentially dangerous rises in blood pressure that can otherwise result from sacral afferent input when the bladder or bowel is distended. However, it also abolishes other potentially useful sacral reflexes, such as reflex erection and reflex ejaculation, as well as sacral sensation and orgasm from sacral stimulation if these were preserved after the SCI. Reflex erection is not always effective after SCI, and many subjects resort to injection of papaverine or prostaglandins into the corpora cavernosa, external erection aids, or implanted penile prostheses. Reflex ejaculation too is not always effective but seminal emission can now be produced from a high proportion of men with SCI by rectal probe electrostimulation, and other techniques for obtaining viable sperm are available. These alternative techniques for assisting with erectile function or fertility can still be used after posterior rhizotomy, and the implant itself may produce erection when S2 roots are stimulated, an effect that appears to be potentiated by oral sildenafil. A decision about posterior rhizotomy should therefore be made on an individual case basis. However, the advantages of posterior rhizotomy are such that it is generally carried out when a bladder stimulator is implanted, thereby improving both micturition and continence.

Candidate Selection

Micturition by ES requires intact PS efferent neurons to the bladder. The function of these neurons can be demonstrated by the presence of reflex bladder contractions when performing a cystometrogram; it is desirable to show a pressure rise of at least 35 cm H_2O in a woman and 50 cm H_2O in a man. Other sacral reflexes such as ankle tendon reflexes, the bulbocavernosus reflex, anal skin reflex, and reflex erection are confirmatory of intact sacral segments. Subjects with complete cord lesions are most suitable for ES and rhizotomy but some subjects with incomplete lesions can also have the procedures if selected with care. Subjects can be implanted at any time after reaching neurological stability. They should also have a degree of emotional and social stability. Frequent urinary tract infection (UTI), incontinence in spite of anticholinergic medication, and problems with catheters are further indications.

Female paraplegics with persistent reflex incontinence are often particularly grateful for the continence produced by posterior rhizotomy, because of the lack of satisfactory urine collecting devices for women. Males with paraplegia and tetraplegia at lower spinal levels often wish to dispense with a urine collection bag, whereas males with higher tetraplegia may choose to continue to wear a condom collection device. If a tetraplegic male plans to use condom drainage with ES, it is wise to check preoperatively that the condom can be retained satisfactorily. Tetraplegic females who wish to use the stimulator for micturition should have a method of collecting urine voided through the urethra. It is wise to evaluate the urogenital system for any other complications such as stones, strictures, or diverticula and to treat these concurrently. It is also advisable to discuss options for sexual function and to offer a trial of various techniques for erectile function.

Technique

Electrodes may be placed either intradurally on the sacral anterior nerve roots in the cauda equine, via a lower lumbar laminectomy, or extradurally on the mixed sacral nerves in the sacral canal via a laminectomy of S1-3. The intradural approach has been more widely used in Europe but extradural electrodes are usually used in the United States. Intraoperative ES and recording of bladder pressure is used to confirm the identity of the nerves supplying the bladder. Leads from the electrodes are subcutaneously tunneled to a radioreceiver/stimulator placed under the skin of the abdomen or chest, and powered and controlled by a battery-powered remote operated by the patient.

The posterior rhizotomy is best performed intradurally where the sensory and motor roots can be more easily separated. If intradural electrodes are being implanted, the rhizotomy can be performed at the cauda equina. If extradural electrodes are used, the rhizotomy is usually performed at the conus medullaris through a separate laminectomy, though it can also be accomplished within the lower end of the dural sac.

Postoperative urodynamic studies are used to guide the setting of stimulus parameters to give an acceptable voiding pressure and rate and pattern of flow. The patient can usually be discharged with a working device within a week of surgery. The stimulus program should be checked between 1 and 3 months after the operation since the response of the bladder may change with repeated use; thereafter, review is recommended at least annually, monitoring lower and upper urinary tract function.

Clinical Outcomes

The majority of patients with an implanted bladder stimulator use it routinely for producing micturition four to six times per day. Residual volume in the bladder following implant-driven micturition is usually less than 60 mL. and often less than 30 mL (189). A substantial decrease in symptomatic UTI has been reported by many groups following the use of the implant (184,189,193,194). In a series of 20 subjects in Cleveland, the average postvoid residual volume with the stimulator was 22 ± 14 mL and the median number of urine infections decreased from 7 to 1 per year (195).

Continence is achieved in over 85% of patients (196,197). This is largely attributable to the abolition of detrusor hyperreflexia and increase in bladder compliance that follow posterior sacral rhizotomy. Approximately 10% to 15% of patients report some stress incontinence of urine following implantation of the stimulator and posterior rhizotomy (199); although it is not always clear whether this stress incontinence results from the abolition of spasticity in the external urethral sphincter. However, being of small volume, it is usually more manageable than reflex incontinence, which may require a change of clothing, and is managed in some subjects by low-level stimulation to activate the external urethral sphincter and not the bladder. Urodynamic studies show that there are substantial increases in bladder capacity and compliance following the abolition of reflex bladder contraction by posterior rhizotomy (199,200). Typically, bladder capacity is greater than 400 mL with a storage pressure less than 40 cm water. Voiding pressure can be controlled by adjusting the parameters of the ES (183,184,193,200,201).

Several centers in Europe have followed patients long-term, particularly with regard to the upper tracts (185,189,200). This experience indicates that bladder trabeculation, ureteric reflux, and hydronephrosis tend to decrease in patients who undergo implantation and posterior rhizotomy. It appears likely in these patients that any harmful effects from transient high pressure during micturition are outweighed by the beneficial effects of low pressure storage of urine during the majority of each day. There also is a reduction in the incidence of autonomic dysreflexia due to the interruption of afferent fibers from the bladder, lower bowel, and the perineum by posterior sacral rhizotomy. This outcome is particularly beneficial to tetraplegic males formerly dependent on an indwelling catheter prone to blockage from frequent infection. The ability to micturate on demand and improved continence of urine both contribute to a reduction in use of intermittent and indwelling catheterization. In a series in Cleveland, 18 of 20 subjects became catheter free (195). Most users become free of urine collection bags but some male tetraplegics with impaired ability to handle clothing or a urine bottle choose to continue to wear a condom drainage system for convenience. Reduction of UTI results in substantially less use of antibiotics. The abolition of detrusor hyperreflexia by posterior rhizotomy allows patients to discontinue anticholinergic medication, which in turn reduces constipation and other side effects such as a dry mouth, blurred vision, and drowsiness.

Regular stimulation of the sacral PS nerves contributes to transport of stool through the distal colon into the rectum, and most users report a reduction in constipation and need for laxatives and stool softeners. Some users are able to defecate by a pattern of intermittent stimulation similar to that used for micturition but with longer intervals between bursts of stimulation to allow passage of stool. However, most patients also check with a finger in the rectum whether there is stool remaining after this procedure and if so, remove it manually. The frequency of bowel emptying increases toward the preinjury pattern and the overall time spent on bowel management is greatly reduced. In the Cleveland series, the time spent on bowel emptying was reduced by 75% (195).

Studies in Europe indicate that the use of the implanted stimulator together with posterior sacral rhizotomy results in substantial savings in the cost of bladder and bowel care, particularly from reduction in supplies needed for bladder care, medications, and visits to physicians for management of complications (202). In the United States, interviews by a life care plan analyst with patients between 6 months and 6 years after implantation and rhizotomy indicated a sixfold reduction in the costs of bladder and bowel care, predicting that savings in bladder and bowel care would equal the cost of purchasing and implanting the stimulator after approximately 5 years, and thereafter be expected to result in progressive savings to the health care payer (203).

Complications

Infection of these implants is rare, occurring in 1% of the first 500 implants. Infection is usually introduced at surgery or through a subsequent break in the skin. A technique of coating the implants with antibiotics was introduced in 1982 and can reduce the infection rate (204). Technical faults in the implanted equipment are uncommon, occurring on average once every 19.6 implant-years (190). The most common site for system failure is the cable that connects the electrode to the stimulator, which are sometimes mechanically damaged by compression against a rib but can usually be repaired under local anesthesia.

Summary and Conclusions

NMES can produce effective micturition in selected patients with suprasacral spinal cord lesions, greatly reducing UTIs and the use of catheters and medications. The improved micturition and reduced infection may also improve continence; though at present reflex incontinence can be more dramatically reduced by performing posterior rhizotomy. Stimulation can also reduce constipation and produce defecation in some patients, reducing the need for laxatives and stool softeners. The technique is safe and reliable and can reduce costs of bladder and bowel care after SCI.

RESPIRATORY MUSCLE STIMULATION

Respiratory muscle paralysis is common in persons with SCI. Since the respiratory muscles are innervated by spinal roots spanning a broad range of the spinal levels located between the upper cervical and upper lumbar regions, most cases of SCI adversely impact respiratory muscle function to some degree (205–211). With an understanding of the innervations of the major and accessory respiratory muscles, the respiratory consequences of a specific SCI level become readily apparent (see Chapter 10).

The major inspiratory muscles include the diaphragm, which is innervated by spinal roots C3-5 that form the phrenic nerves, and inspiratory intercostal muscles, primarily innervated by spinal roots located at T1-6. Since the diaphragm is the primary inspiratory muscle, resting ventilation can be comfortably maintained with rhythmic contraction of this muscle alone. Consequently, persons with injuries below the C3-5 roots and intact phrenic motoneuron function are able to breathe spontaneously. Conversely, persons with injuries compromising phrenic motoneuron function in the mid-cervical spinal cord or injuries that interrupt pathways between the respiratory centers in the medulla (high cervical SCI) have paralysis of virtually all of their inspiratory muscles and are dependent upon some form of artificial ventilatory support.

The major expiratory muscles include the abdominal muscles, innervated by spinal roots T4-L2 and expiratory intercostal muscles, innervated primarily by spinal roots T6-12. These muscles are important for cough generation, an important defense mechanism necessary for airway clearance and to prevent respiratory tract infections and atelectasis. Persons with significant expiratory muscle paralysis are usually dependent upon some artificial form of airway clearance management including suctioning, cough assist maneuvers and/or use of other devices, and are at increased risk for the development of pneumonia.

In most instances of SCI, the spinal cord above and below the level of injury are intact. These latter regions of the spinal cord and associated neuromuscular apparatus, therefore, are amenable to electrical and magnetic stimulation techniques to restore function. In this chapter, conventional and investigational techniques to restore inspiratory and expiratory function are reviewed.

Inspiratory Muscle Stimulation: Diaphragm Pacing

Fifteen to twenty percent of patients with acute cervical SCI suffer from respiratory failure on initial presentation (212). Fortunately, the majority of these patients are eventually able to breathe spontaneously. Nonetheless, a substantial number (~4% to 5%) develop chronic respiratory insufficiency requiring some form of mechanical ventilatory support (213).

While lifesaving, mechanical ventilation is associated with substantial morbidity and mortality. Major side effects of mechanical ventilation include increased risk of respiratory tract infections, reduced mobility, difficulty with speech, physical discomfort, and embarrassment associated with dependence on the ventilator with attached tubing, and significant patient and caregiver anxiety associated with fear of disconnection (209,212,214–217). In contrast, artificial ventilation produced by diaphragm pacing eliminates many of these problems and provides a more natural form of breathing (218–220).

Since the initial development of diaphragm pacing more than 30 years ago, this technique has matured into a clinically accepted modality for the management of trauma-induced ventilator-dependent tetraplegia. While the specific clinical benefits vary somewhat between patients, most report better speech, improved level of comfort, reduced anxiety and embarrassment, increased mobility and greater sense of well-being restoration of olfaction (388), and overall health when compared to mechanical ventilation (Table 25.1).

Available Stimulation Devices

There are two basic configurations of diaphragm pacing systems, which include conventional systems that are totally implantable and activated by RF transmission, and the more recently developed IM diaphragm pacing system that incorporates a percutaneous system in which the electrode wires emanate through the skin.

Conventional Pacing Devices. Each of these devices has a similar basic configuration. The stimulating electrodes (generally placed by thoracotomy), RF receivers, and attached wiring comprise the internal components. A RF transmitter, wires, and antenna comprise the external components. The stimulating electrodes are implanted on each phrenic nerve, typically in the thorax. Wires tunneled subcutaneously connect each of the electrodes to a corresponding RF receiver, both of which are implanted in an easily accessible area over the anterior portion of the thorax. External antennas connect to the transmitter, which generate a RF signal that is inductively coupled to the implanted receivers. The signal is demodulated by the receivers converting it to electrical signals, which are delivered to the stimulating electrodes in contact with the phrenic nerves.

There are three commercially available systems, the technical characteristics of which are presented in Table 25.2. The Avery system (Avery Laboratories Inc., Commack, New York, USA) has FDA approval in the United States and is available worldwide (221). Monopolar electrodes are used most commonly but bipolar electrodes are also available and recommended in patients with cardiac pacemakers (25,221). The Atrotech system (Atrotech OY, Tampere, Finland) is commercially available in most developed countries but is no longer available in the United States. The Atrotech device employs a four-pole electrode system and stimulation paradigm that reduces the stimulation frequency of individual axons to about one fourth of that with unipolar stimulation. This technique is purported to lessen the risk of fatigue, enhance transformation of muscle fibers to more fatigue-resistant Type I fibers, and shorten the reconditioning process (222–224). The MedImplant system (MedImplant Biotechnisches Labor, Vienna, Austria) has limited availability, predominantly in Austria and Germany. This system utilizes a four electrode array positioned around each nerve (225). As with the Atrotech device, only a portion of the nerve is stimulated, and consequently, only a portion of the diaphragm is activated at any given time. This form of sequential stimulation is also thought to reduce the incidence of fatigue compared to monopolar stimulation (226).

TABLE 25.1

POTENTIAL BENEFITS OF DIAPHRAGM PACING

A. Improved quality of life
  1. Greater comfort level
    a. Elimination of pull of ventilator tubing
    b. Negative pressure breathing
  2. Improved speech
  3. Increased mobility
    a. Easier bed/chair transfer
    b. Easier transport outside the home
  4. Restoration of olfactory sensation
  5. Reduced anxiety and embarrassment
    a. Elimination of fear of ventilator disconnection
    b. Daytime closure of tracheostomy
    c. Elimination of ventilator and attached tubing
    d. Elimination of ventilator noise
  6. Subjective sense of more normal breathing
    a. Engagement of breathing muscles
    b. More physiologic negative pressure breathing
B. Reduced overall costs
  1. Reduction or elimination of ventilator supplies
  2. Reduced level of trained caregiver support

Intramuscular Diaphragm Pacing System. The phrenic nerve motor roots can also be activated by placement of electrodes directly into the body of the diaphragm via laparoscopy (Synapse Biomedical, Oberlin, Ohio, USA) (227–231). Four laparoscopic ports are necessary to provide access to the abdominal cavity for visualization, insufflation of the abdominal cavity, diaphragm mapping, and insertion of the implant tool (Fig. 25.6) (227–229,232–234). Specially designed surgical tools are necessary to implant two IM electrodes into each hemidiaphragm near the phrenic nerve motor points (227–231). A mapping procedure is necessary to determine optimal electrode placement (228,229,232). By this technique, ventilatory support can be maintained in ventilator-dependent tetraplegics with success rates similar to those of conventional phrenic nerve stimulation (228,229,237,238). This method has significant advantages, however, in that laparoscopy is less invasive than thoracotomy (239) and can be performed on an outpatient basis or overnight observational stay significantly reducing costs (228). In addition, this procedure does not require manipulation of the phrenic nerve, virtually eliminating the risk of phrenic nerve injury. A significant limitation, however, is that this is a percutaneous system with electrode wires exiting the skin. The Synapse system is now commercially available in the United States and Europe. The technical characteristics of this device are provided in Table 25.2.

Investigational Devices

Combined Phrenic Nerve and Intercostal Muscle Stimulation. A significant percentage of persons with tetraplegia have damage

TABLE 25.2

TECHNICAL FEATURES OF PHRENIC NERVE PACING SYSTEMS

	Conventional			Intramuscular
	Manufacturer			
	Avery biomedical devices[a]	Atrotech OY	Medimplant	Synapse biomedical
Implanted components				
Receiver	Model I-110A (Monopolar)	RX44-27-2		
Specifications	Model I-110 (Bipolar)			
	30 (diam) × 8	44 (diam) × 6	56 × 53 × 14	
Size (mm)	2	2	1	
	E-377-05 (Monopolar) E-325 (Bipolar)	TF 4-40 (Quadripolar)	(Quadripolar)	Peterson Electrode (Monopolar)
Number needed to provide bilateral stimulation	2	2	8	2–4
Electrodes				
Specifications				
Number needed to provide bilateral stimulation				
External Components				
Transmitter (stimulus generator)	Mark IV[b]	PX 244 V2.1	Medimplant 8-channel stimulator	NeuRx RA/4
Size (mm)	146 × 140 × 25	185 × 88 × 28	170 × 130 × 51	150 × 80 × 40
Transmitter/battery weight (kg)	0.54	0.45 + 0.6 (12V) 0.45 + 0.045 (9V)	1.42	0.26
Battery life (h)	400	160–320 (12V) 8 (9V)	24	500
Parameters				
Rate (breaths/min)	6–28	8–35	5–60	8–18
Inspiratory period (s)	1.0–2.8	0.5–4		0.8–1.5
Amplitude (mA)	0–10	0–6	0–4	5–25
Pulse width (ms)	160–1,000	200	100–1,200	20–200
Pulse interval (ms)	25–130	10–100		20–250
Sigh possible	Yes	Yes	Yes	Yes
	Amplitude	Amplitude and frequency	Amplitude	Pulse width
Ramp				
Antenna	902A	TC 27-250/80	RF transmission coil	

[a]Formerly known as Avery Laboratories, Inc.
[b]The Mark IV supersedes all earlier versions manufactured by Avery Laboratories. Most patients implanted with earlier models have been upgraded to the Mark IV.
Reprinted from American Paraplegia Society. DiMarco AF, Onders RP, Ignagni A, et al. Inspiratory muscle pacing in spinal cord injury: case report and clinical commentary. *J Spinal Cord Med* 2006;29:95–108, with permission.

to one or both of the phrenic motoneuron pools in the spinal cord and/or phrenic rootlets and are therefore not candidates for diaphragm pacing (240–242). Large inspired volumes can also be achieved, however, by activation of the inspiratory intercostal muscles. This technique requires epidural placement of electrodes on the ventral surface of the upper thoracic spinal cord via laminotomy incisions to stimulate the ventral roots. In initial clinical trials, stimulation of the intercostal muscles alone in patients with absent diaphragm function resulted in inspired volumes that were similar in magnitude to those achieved from activation of a single hemidiaphragm (240). Inspired volume generation was sufficient to maintain ventilatory support, however, for only a few hours. In subsequent clinical trials in tetraplegic individuals with unilateral diaphragm function, stimulation of the intercostal muscles in combination with unilateral phrenic nerve stimulation has been shown to be successful in providing long-term ventilatory support (241).

Side effects of intercostal muscle stimulation include mild flexion of both hands and contraction of the muscles of the upper torso, which are well tolerated (240,241). Intercostal muscle pacing therefore may be a useful adjunct to increase inspired volume production in persons having suboptimal inspired volume production with phrenic nerve pacing alone.

This technique has received approval by the FDA through an Investigational Device Exemption, but is not commercially available.

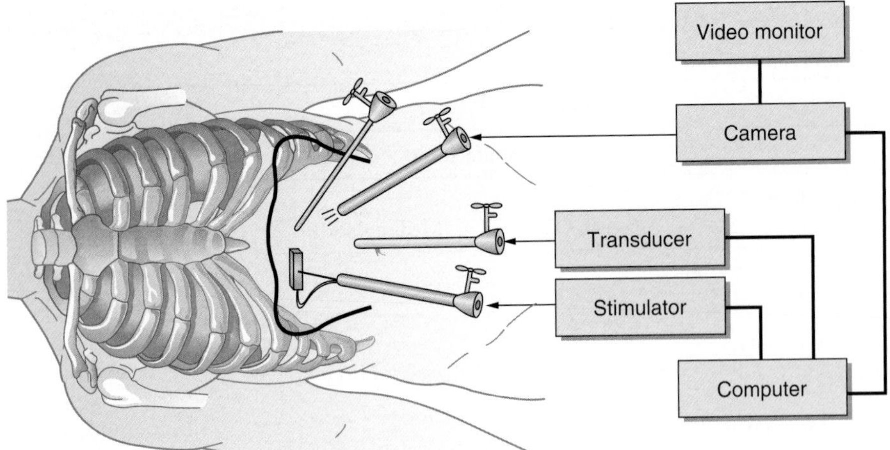

FIGURE 25.6 Schematic illustration of laparoscopic implant materials required for implantation of IM diaphragm electrodes. Four laparoscopic ports are necessary to provide access to the abdominal cavity. Ports are necessary for visualization, insufflation of the abdominal cavity, diaphragm mapping and insertion of the electrode implant tool. (Reprinted from American Thoracic Society. DiMarco AF, Onders RP, Kowalski KE, et al. Phrenic nerve pacing in a tetraplegic patient via intramuscular diaphragm electrodes. *Am J Respir Crit Care Med* 2002;166:1604–1606, with permission.)

Patient Evaluation and Assessment

Individuals considered for diaphragm pacing should be free of significant lung disease or primary muscle disease since these conditions will preclude successful pacing (25,243–246). After careful evaluation, some patients with sufficient inspiratory muscle strength may be better suited for noninvasive means of ventilator assistance (247,248) such as intermittent mouth positive pressure ventilation (248).

A thorough evaluation of phrenic nerve function is mandatory for all potential candidates undergoing any type of diaphragm pacing (25,220,228). Phrenic nerve function can be assessed by measurements of nerve conduction times (249,250). This test is performed by applying ES at the posterior border of the sternocleidomastoid muscles at the level of the cricoid cartilage to stimulate the phrenic nerves. Diaphragmatic action potentials are monitored by surface electrodes positioned between the seventh and ninth intercostal spaces. Phrenic nerve conduction times can be determined by measuring the time interval between the applied stimulus and onset of the compound muscle action potential. Mean onset latency is 7 to 9 milliseconds in normal adults (249,250). However, mild prolongation of conduction times (up to 14 milliseconds) does not preclude successful pacing (245). Other indicators of adequate phrenic nerve function include diaphragm descent of at least 3 to 4 cm during supramaximal tetanic stimulation (25,251) and transdiaphragmatic pressures of approximately 10 cm H_2O with single shock stimulation to either phrenic nerve (252).

While the success of pacing is dependent upon technical considerations, psychosocial conditions are also important (228,238,251). Prior to any technical assessment, evaluation of the motivation of the patient and family members is critical. Diaphragm pacing is most likely to be successful in home situations in which the candidate and family members are anxious to improve the overall health, mobility, social interaction, and occupational potential of the patient. The subject should also have a thorough understanding of the potential benefits that can be reasonably achieved with pacing techniques.

Implementation and Pacing Schedules

The various surgical techniques to implant electrodes and achieve diaphragm pacing have been described in detail (25,228–231,243–245,253–255) and will therefore not be discussed in this chapter. Pacing is usually initiated approximately 2 weeks following surgery to allow time for healing of surgical wounds and resolution of inflammation and edema around the electrode sites (25). Due to atrophy, the diaphragm must be gradually reconditioned to improve strength and endurance. During the initial trials of diaphragm pacing, minute ventilation (product of inspired volume and respiratory rate) necessary to maintain normal values for pCO_2 (35 to 45 mm Hg) should be determined over 5 to 10 minutes periods. Respiratory rate (stimulus train rate) should be set between 8 and 14 b/m. Tidal volume should be adjusted by altering stimulation frequency (pulses per second) to achieve the desired level of ventilation. Stimulus frequency should be set at the lowest possible level and should not exceed 20 Hz. Further adjustments of respiratory rate and tidal volume can be made for patient comfort.

There are no definitive guidelines in terms of specific pacing schedules to achieve full-time ventilatory support, which should be the ultimate goal in each subject. The overall objective is to transition from mechanical ventilation to diaphragm pacing as quickly as possible but without the development of diaphragm fatigue (220,228,229,244,256). Utilizing the above mentioned stimulus parameters, continuous bilateral diaphragm pacing is initially provided until significant reductions are experienced in inspired volume generation (monitored every 5 to 10 minutes) or oxygen saturation, or patient discomfort is observed related to air hunger. Pacing is then initiated for a somewhat shorter time period (~5 min) every hour during the day for the first week. This assessment is repeated weekly and a new pacing schedule is applied accordingly. After full-time pacing is achieved during waking hours, pacing is provided during sleep. While the conditioning phase may take 8 to 10 weeks or longer, it is possible to achieve full-time support in some subjects within 4 weeks. Most subjects cap the tracheostomy tube while pacing during the day. During sleep, however, the tracheostomy is usually left open or capped with a valve such as the Passy-Muir device, which allows airflow through the tracheostomy. Higher levels of stimulation may be required in the sitting compared to the supine posture due to the shorter diaphragm length and higher resting lung volume. This can be alleviated to a significant degree, however, by use of a snug fitting abdominal binder that reduces the change in abdominal girth.

Patient Outcomes

In subjects with ventilator-dependent tetraplegia having intact phrenic nerve function, diaphragm pacing is clearly an effective means of providing ventilatory support, with significant advantages over mechanical ventilation (228,237,243,244). The actual success rates of diaphragm pacing are difficult to determine as most subjects have undergone this technique at locations where patient numbers were small (258–260). Moreover, technology was still in development at centers where the outcome of diaphragm pacing was evaluated in previous large series. These results, therefore, are not applicable to systems available today.

There is evidence that improved electrode and receiver design is associated with a low incidence of pacer malfunction and high success rates when applied in appropriate candidates. In a study of 45 tetraplegics who underwent diaphragm pacing with the Atrotech system since 1990, approximately 50% of adult subjects were able to maintain full-time ventilatory support and at least 75% were able to pace throughout the day (214). In a separate study, long-term follow-up of 14 tetraplegics who used bilateral low frequency stimulation with the Avery system recorded using the device successfully for as long as 15 years with a mean use of 7.6 years (258).

Conceivably, diaphragm pacing may improve life expectancy in subjects with tetraplegia. Mechanical ventilation is associated with a high incidence of respiratory tract infections, which may be reduced with diaphragm pacing. Moreover, the mechanical problems associated with the mechanical ventilator, tubing, and tracheostomy are eliminated. In the absence of studies controlling for age at injury and comorbid illness, however, this issue remains an open question.

Complications and Side Effects

Technical developments and clinical experience have markedly reduced the incidence of complications and adverse effects associated with diaphragm pacing (224). With careful subject selection, appropriate use of stimulus parameters, adequate monitoring, and proper use of stimulus paradigms, the rate of complications is low. Nonetheless, complications do arise and appropriate precautions must be taken and remedial action instituted promptly, as the outcome of pacemaker failure can be catastrophic.

A variety of factors may result in inadequate ventilatory support. While loss of battery power is the most common cause of system failure, this is easily prevented by routine maintenance involving regular battery changes and adherence to recharging schedules. Low battery alarms are also present to alert caregivers. Breakage of the external antenna wire at stress points either near the connection to the transmitter or more commonly at the connection to the receivers can also occur. Receiver failure was a common occurrence with older systems (220,244,261,262) but is much less frequent with current systems due to improvement in housing materials. With conventional diaphragm pacing, iatrogenic injury to the phrenic nerve may occur during implantation but can be prevented by meticulous dissection technique (263). Also, following implantation, adverse tissue reaction and scar tissue formation can lead to gradual reduction in inspired volume generation and may require surgical intervention (220,241,244). Increases in airway resistance due to secretions or decrements in respiratory system compliance due to atelectasis will also result in reductions in inspired volume generation. Removal of secretions either by suctioning or by other means usually results in prompt improvement in respiratory system mechanics. A more serious, but fortunately less common complication is the development of infection of the implanted materials, which necessitates removal of all implanted components (220,224,264).

In a follow-up study of 64 subjects who underwent diaphragm pacing with the Atrotech system (average pacing duration of 2 years), the incidence of electrode and receiver failures were low at 3.1% and 5.9%, respectively (214), values that are lower than previously reported with monopolar-bipolar systems (265). Additionally, none of the tetraplegic subjects in this group developed infection of the implanted materials (209).

Although there are some reports of successful tracheostomy closure following institution of diaphragm pacing, these are very uncommon (226). The state of wakefulness is associated with synchronous activation of the upper airway muscles and diaphragm during pacing. During sleep, however, there is reduced activation of the upper airway dilator muscles and a greater tendency toward asynchronous upper airway muscle contraction resulting in the development of upper airway obstruction, a form of obstructive sleep apnea (213,257,266). In general, therefore, subjects undergoing diaphragm pacing require a patent tracheostomy for nocturnal use.

Since exposure of the pacing system to strong magnetic fields can lead to phrenic nerve injury, magnetic resonance imaging (MRI) scanning is contraindicated in subjects with diaphragm pacers. Electrotherapeutic devices that generate strong RF fields could interfere with the pacing device and should also be avoided.

In children, paradoxical motion of the rib cage may be substantial due to its high compliance, resulting in reduced inspired volume generation (220,267). Since compliance of the rib cage musculoskeleton gradually decreases between 10 and 15 years of age, the performance of the pacing system can be expected to improve over time. Since the diaphragm in small children has a very small percentage of Type I fatigue-resistant fibers, a much longer period of conditioning may be required to achieve full-time ventilatory support compared to adults.

Expiratory Muscle Stimulation

Current airway management techniques include mechanical suctioning, manually assisted cough, use of the mechanical insufflation/exsufflation device, and other methods. Most individuals with SCI find these techniques uncomfortable, cumbersome, embarrassing, and of limited effectiveness. Moreover, despite their use, respiratory complications remain a major cause of morbidity and mortality in SCI (215,216,268,269).

Generation of an effective cough via restoration of expiratory muscle function by means of stimulation techniques has several important potential benefits (Table 25.3). Theoretically, engagement of the expiratory muscles to produce cough would provide a more natural and effective means of secretion removal. Most currently employed mechanical methods primarily achieve evacuation of secretions from the upper airway, whereas an assisted cough may result in clearance of

TABLE 25.3

POTENTIAL BENEFITS OF EXPIRATORY MUSCLE STIMULATION TO RESTORE COUGH

A. Reduction in incidence of respiratory tract infections
B. Improved comfort level
1. Greater ease in raising secretions
C. Reduced level of trained caregiver support
D. Reduced anxiety and embarrassment
1. Elimination of need for suctioning or use of other mechanical devices
2. Possible closure of tracheostomy
E. Improved sense of well-being and overall health
F. Reduced overall costs
1. Reduction and/or elimination of suction supplies and cost of other mechanical devices
2. Reduction in hospitalization rate

more distal airways. It is possible; therefore, that restoration of a cough generated by stimulation techniques would result in a reduction in the incidence of respiratory complications including pneumonia, bronchitis, and atelectasis. Other benefits might include reduction or elimination of caregiver requirements for secretion management, greater comfort and ease in raising secretions, greater mobility, and reduction in the level of anxiety and embarrassment associated with current methods of airway management. Reductions in the need for trained personnel, suction supplies, and other equipment should also result in an overall lessening in cost.

The expiratory muscles can be stimulated by several different methods, including high-frequency magnetic stimulation, surface abdominal muscle stimulation and ES applied in the region of the lower thoracic spinal cord. It should be noted that cough is a complex reflex with several components, including an initial inspiration and subsequent glottis closure followed by expiratory muscle contraction. Most persons with SCI are able to control their upper airway and inspiratory muscles and lack only the ability to contract their expiratory muscles. It is possible for these individuals to be trained to activate their expiratory muscles in phase with the other components of the cough reflex. Regarding subjects on mechanical ventilation, the ventilator can be used to generate the inspiratory component of the reflex.

Magnetic stimulation requires placement of a stimulating coil over the mid portion of the back (T9-10 level) to activate the neural pathways innervating the expiratory muscles (270,271). When applied in nondisabled subjects, this method results in the generation of large positive airway pressures and expiratory flow rates, and has the advantage of being noninvasive (270,271). In studies performed in tetraplegics, however, airway pressures and flow rates were not significantly different than those generated during spontaneous efforts (271). Muscle atrophy most likely contributed to these low values, and would improve with conditioning. Practical application of this method is limited, however, by the fact that the device is large, requires an external power source, and is not easily portable. Other disadvantages include the potential for significant heat to be generated at the stimulating coil and secondary risk for thermal injury. Also, the presence of large amounts of adipose tissue may interfere with successful stimulation due to the greater distance between the stimulating coil and motor roots. Nonetheless, this device may have application in selected individuals.

The expiratory muscles can also be noninvasively stimulated by electrodes placed directly over the surface of the abdominal wall (272–274). In nondisabled subjects, ES of electrodes with large surface areas results in the generation of large airway pressures (275). In subject with SCI, however airway pressure generation is substantially smaller. Practical application of this method is limited by the fact that repeated application of electrodes to the skin surface may prove to be quite tedious and cumbersome, and potentially lead to irritation and skin breakdown. Again, the presence of significant adipose tissue may also interfere with optimal expiratory muscle activation due to the high electrical resistance of fatty tissue.

Spinal cord stimulation (SCS) involves the placement of electrodes on the dorsal surface of the lower thoracic spinal cord via laminotomy incisions in the region of the T9, T11, and L1 spinal levels. Electrode wires are connected to a RF receiver placed over the anterior chest wall. Like conventional inspiratory muscle pacing devices, stimulation is applied by activating a small portable external control box connected to a rubberized transmitter placed over the implanted receiver (Fig. 25.7). This method results in marked activation of the internal intercostal and abdominal muscles and generation of airway pressures and peak flow rates in the range of those achieved by nondisabled subjects during a maximal cough effort. The mean changes in airway pressure and peak airflow rates generated in an initial study group of nine subjects are shown in Fig. 25.8. Single site stimulation at the T9, T11, and L1 spinal

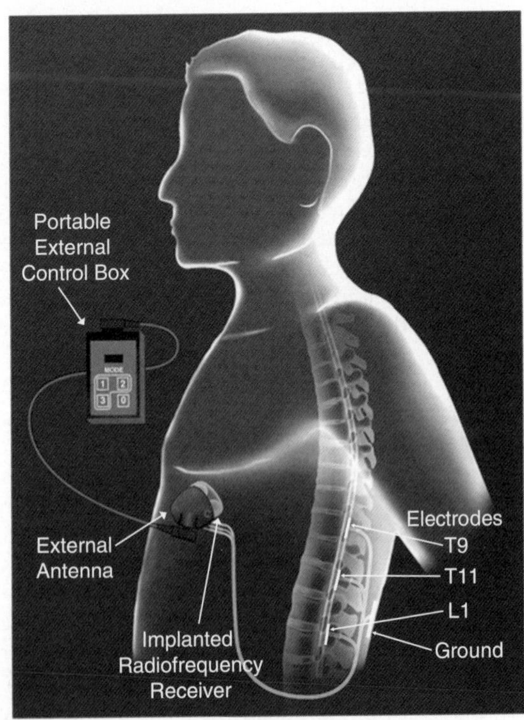

FIGURE 25.7 ES system. (Reprinted from Elsevier. DiMarco AF, Kowalski KE, Geertman RT, et al. Lower thoracic spinal cord stimulation to restore cough in patients with spinal cord injury: results of an NIH Sponsored Clinical Trial. Part I: methodology and effectiveness of expiratory muscle activation. *Arch Phys Med Rehabil* 2009;90:717–725, with permission.)

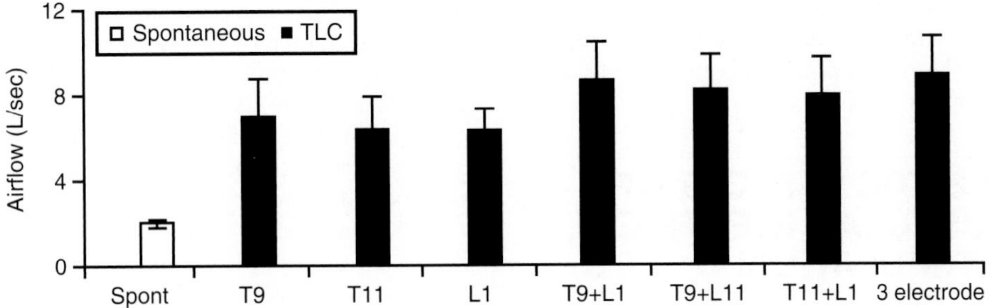

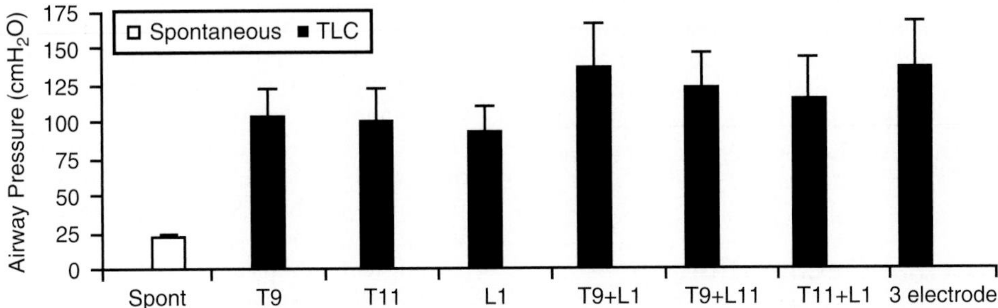

FIGURE 25.8 Mean peak airflow rates (**upper panel**) and mean airway pressures (**lower panel**) during SCS at the T9, T11, and L1 spinal levels alone and in combinations at TLC. Mean spontaneous airway pressure and peak expiratory flow rates are shown for comparison (empty bars). Large airway pressures and peak airflow rates of similar magnitude were generated during SCS during single site stimulation. Combined stimulation of two sites, however, resulted in significantly greater airway pressures and peak airflow rates ($p < 0.05$, for each). There were no significant differences in either peak airflow rates or airway pressure generation between any two sites. Combined stimulation of three sites did not result in further increases in these parameters. (Reprinted from Elsevier. DiMarco AF, Kowalski KE, Geertman RT, et al. Lower thoracic spinal cord stimulation to restore cough in patients with spinal cord injury: results of an NIH Sponsored Clinical Trial. Part I: methodology and effectiveness of expiratory muscle activation. *Arch Phys Med Rehabil* 2009;90:717–725, with permission.)

levels at total lung capacity (TLC) resulted in large airway pressures and peak airflow rates in the range of 100 cm H_2O and 6 to 7 L/s, respectively. Combined stimulation of two sites resulted in significantly greater pressures and airflow rates of approximately 125 cm H_2O and 8 L/s, respectively. Combined stimulation of three sites did not further increase the magnitude of these parameters (276a).

Major advantages of this technique are that the device is portable and allows the individual to generate a cough on demand. In addition, effects of stimulation are highly reproducible and can be repeatedly used without the development of muscle fatigue (276b). In a pilot clinical trial this method has provided significant short-term benefits in terms of airway management including greater ease in raising secretions, reductions in the need for caregiver assistance and reductions in the incidence of pneumonia (277,278). Mobility is also enhanced, since the need for trained caregiver assistance while traveling with family or for recreational activities may be eliminated (277,278). A limitation of the SCS application in people with lower thoracic SCI involves coincident activation of the paraspinal and upper leg muscles causing some straightening of the back and leg jerks. This movement is well tolerated without pain or discomfort. Moreover, significant movement can be reduced or eliminated by mild reduction in stimulus amplitude. In some subjects, initiation of SCS is associated with increases in blood pressure and reductions in pulse rate. Following acclimatization to ES over several weeks, this response completely resolves such that the frequent application of stimulation elicits no hemodynamic responses (277). Finally, SCS does not result in either bowel or bladder leakage.

Future Directions

Diaphragm pacing systems have some limitations and require further refinement. First, many subjects with ventilator-dependent tetraplegia cannot be offered diaphragm pacing due to partial or complete injury to one of the phrenic nerves. Moreover, in carefully screened subjects, the success rate in terms of achieving full-time ventilatory support is only approximately 50% (224,232). ES of the intercostal/accessory muscle group in concert with diaphragm pacing in subjects with only single phrenic nerve function would increase the pool of persons eligible for pacing, and possibly enhance the success rate of individuals with inadequate ventilation by bilateral diaphragm pacing alone (240,241,279,280). Further investigation is needed to coordinate paced breaths with the respiratory drive, as this would serve to improve speech cadence, match ventilation with metabolic demand and eliminate the need for tracheostomy. Finally, the development of fully implantable systems would eliminate the need for the application of materials on the body surface and eliminate the risk of decoupling between the transmitter and receiver.

While considerable progress has been made in preliminary studies to restore an effective cough mechanism, further validation studies are necessary. Additionally, minimally invasive techniques using wire electrodes which can be placed through a small needle incision are under development. This type of system would reduce the risk of potential complications and increase physician and user acceptance.

THERAPEUTIC EFFECTS OF NEUROMUSCULAR ELECTRICAL STIMULATION

Persons with SCI are at risk for developing multiple complications of immobility including CV deconditioning, muscle atrophy, joint contractures, pressure ulcers, osteoporosis, and thromboembolic disease. Most of these complications are directly related to a loss of normal somatic and autonomic nervous system function, a sedentary lifestyle and limited exercise capacity. With the development and availability of NMES mediated exercise equipment, a number of these conditions may be prevented or treated (281). This section reviews the efficacy of NMES mediated exercise in preventing and treating these disorders.

Cardiovascular Deconditioning

Heart disease is a leading cause of death in individuals after SCI (214,282,283). Alterations in CV physiology after SCI include hypotension (284–287), reduced stroke volume (288–292), impaired cardiac output (288–292), decrease in VO_2 (293,294), and an impaired autonomic response to exercise (284–286,295,296). These abnormalities lead to lower exercise and physical work capacity. In the presence of a sedentary lifestyle, these factors may contribute to obesity, glucose intolerance, a reduction of high-density lipoprotein (HDL) (297–299), an increment of low-density lipoprotein (LDL) (297,298), and an elevation of C-reactive protein (300–302) resulting in the development of diabetes and metabolic syndrome and creating an increased risk for cardiovascular disease (CVD) (301–309). However, as in nondisabled persons, exercise for persons with SCI can increase the level of HDL and decrease serum total cholesterol and LDL levels (154,288–290,310). Among wheelchair athletes, indices of CV function such as VO_2, cardiac output and stroke volume are significantly higher than those of sedentary SCI individuals (311–313). Thus, in view of the increased risk factors for CVD, the aging population, and positive benefits of exercise, an aggressive cardiac prevention program is appropriate for persons with SCI. Until recently, exercise options for persons with SCI were limited to UE ergometry. However, the therapeutic effects of UE ergometry are limited by venous pooling in the LEs and abdomen, which decreases preload, stroke volume and cardiac output, resulting in UE ischemia, inefficient energy expenditure, early fatigue, and the potential for UE musculoskeletal injury. Through the development of LE NMES-mediated exercise systems, improved CV performance can be achieved.

The acute CV effects of NMES therapy can be demonstrated with LE NMES-mediated exercises alone or in combination with UE exercises. NMES-mediated nonergometry LE exercises increase stroke volume and cardiac output, and decrease total peripheral resistance in persons with paraplegia (314–319). NMES of the LE in combination with rowing is associated with higher VO_2 than rowing alone (320,321). Similarly, NMES-mediated leg cycle ergometry in combination with arm ergometry is associated with significantly higher peak VO_2 and stroke volume than arm ergometry alone (322–327). These acute CV effects in response to NMES-mediated exercises of the LE likely result from increased venous return associated with skeletal muscle pump, as well as decrease in total peripheral resistance (315,316,327,328).

CV training effects can be achieved with NMES-mediated leg cycle ergometry, leg cycle ergometry in combination with arm crank ergometry and with LE neuroprosthetic systems. LE stress testing after training with NMES-mediated leg cycle ergometry demonstrates significant increases in peak VO_2, pulmonary ventilation, heart rate and cardiac output, and significant decreases in total peripheral resistance compared to pretraining status (329,330). Hybrid training protocols that combine leg cycle and arm crank ergometry are associated with even higher posttraining peak VO_2 than leg cycle ergometry training alone (331,332) Similarly, training programs with ambulation neuroprostheses systems increase peak VO_2 (125,333–335), increase HDL (336,337), and reduce total cholesterol and LDL compared to pretraining levels (154). Training with NMES-mediated leg cycle ergometry is also associated with reversal of left ventricular atrophy reported in persons with tetraplegia (338).

With the aging of the spinal cord population and increasing incidence and survival of older individuals with SCI, CV fitness is becoming more relevant in the long-term management of persons with SCI. As in nondisabled persons, exercise among persons with SCI is associated with acute changes in CV indices that translate into substantial training effect. These training effects include increased peak VO_2, stroke volume and cardiac output in response to stress testing, improvements in serum total cholesterol, HDL and LDL levels, and reversal of left ventricular atrophy. It is likely that these training effects, if maintained, will lead to prevention of CVD in the long term with concomitant decreases in associated morbidity and mortality and overall improvements in quality of life. While these postulated long-term benefits remain to be demonstrated in future controlled trials, it appears prudent to include CV fitness programs for persons with SCI as part of their ongoing rehabilitation management.

Muscle Atrophy

Disuse atrophy develops over weeks and predominantly affects Type I muscle fibers, leading to conversion to easily fatigable Type II muscle fibers (339,340). Conversely, chronic NMES produces characteristic histochemical and morphologic changes in paralyzed muscles after SCI. Chronic low frequency (10 Hz) IM NMES converts Type II fiber to more fatigue resistant Type I fiber (341,342) with concomitant increases in strength and endurance (9,14). At higher frequencies of stimulation employed by most commercially available transcutaneous NMES systems, fiber conversion from Type II to Type I is modest (343) or minimal (344). However, further evaluation of the Type II muscle fibers with ATPase technique demonstrates significant increase in the number of Type IIa fibers (345), which are characterized by fast-twitch contractility with intermediate fatigability. Consistent with this observation, evaluation of myosin heavy chain (MHC) composition of single fibers by sodium dodecyl sulfate-polyacrylamide gel electrophoresis before and after NMES training demonstrates significant increase in the expression of MHC of the type seen in Type IIa fibers (346). While studies generally report increases in the population of more fatigue resistant fiber types after NMES therapy, observations on change in fiber size are inconsistent. Some studies report significant increases in the size of all fiber types (344,347), while others report no changes (343,345).

With the induction of these histochemical and morphologic changes, training with NMES partially reverses muscle atrophy among persons with chronic SCI, prevents atrophy when used in the subacute phase of recovery, and increases muscle performance. Computed topography evaluations demonstrate significant increases in the cross-sectional area of LE muscles after NMES-mediated ergometry (348–351) and nonergometry (347) training programs. MRI evaluation of persons with tetraplegia within 1 year of their injury also demonstrates significant increases in cross-sectional area of the quadriceps femoris muscles after NMES nonergometry training. This increase is comparable to cross sectional area at 6 weeks postinjury (352). Finally, muscle biopsy studies of individuals with SCI involved in a long-term FES program showed almost complete anatomic reversal of muscle atrophy and degeneration (353). In recognition of the likelihood that total reversal of muscle atrophy is not achievable, prevention of atrophy is a reasonable strategy. In a controlled study, 26 persons with SCI were assigned to control, NMES-mediated isometric contractions or NMES-mediated cycle ergometry. After 3 and 6 months of training, only NMES-mediated ergometry prevented loss of lower limb and gluteal lean body mass. After 6 months of training, NMES-mediated ergometry also prevented loss of total lean body mass (354). Corresponding to the changes in muscle bulk, significant improvements in muscle strength and endurance are observed after NMES-mediated ergometry (16,349,350) and nonergometry (355,356) training programs.

In summary, NMES-mediated LE exercise programs facilitate the conversion of Type IIb fibers to more fatigue resistant Type IIa or Type I fibers, partially reverse muscle atrophy among persons with chronic SCI, prevent atrophy early after SCI, and increase overall stimulated muscle strength and endurance. The histochemical changes and improvements in muscle performance have significant ramifications on the candidacy of SCI survivors for the various neuroprostheses programs. With respect to secondary complications, it remains uncertain whether partial reversal of muscle atrophy is sufficient to be clinically useful. In view of the inherent difficulty in completely reversing muscle atrophy, the efficacy of NMES-mediated exercises in preventing atrophy should be further investigated in controlled trials prior to formulating recommendations.

Pressure Ulcers

The incidence of pressure ulcer formation is reported to be as high as 34% in individuals with acute SCI prior to discharge from the hospital (357) and as high as 32% 20 years postdischarge (358). ES is one of only two treatment modalities recommended by the Agency for Health Care Policy and Research for treatment of pressure ulcers that are unresponsive to traditional therapies (359).

ES has been shown to directly facilitate healing (360,361) by improving blood flow (126,362,363) and tissue oxygenation (364,365). ES has also been shown to relieve interface pressures over bony surfaces (365,366), increase muscle bulk (367), and provide for effective weight relief through intermittent gluteal muscle percutaneous stimulation (368,369). These findings support the view that chronic use of NMES may have a quantifiable benefit on tissue health and prevention of the development of pressure ulcers (see Chapter—for details).

Osteoporosis

The loss of mechanical stimuli in the form of muscle contraction and the lack of weight bearing due to SCI commonly results in sublesional osteoporosis (370,371). It has been shown that as much as 50% of bone mineral content may be lost after the first 3 years of paralysis (372). Pathologic fractures follow the progression of osteoporosis, with annual incidence of long-bone fracture in the LE estimated to be 4% to 7% (373). The National SCI Database found that 14% of individuals with SCI reported fractures at 5 years; 28% at 10 years; and 39% at 15 years postinjury (374). A Veterans Affairs Medical Center reported that 34% of their male patients had a fracture after SCI (375). A number of preventive measures such as application of electric fields and pharmacological interventions have been suggested, but efficacy remains to be elucidated. Since disuse osteoporosis occurs due to unloading, it is thought that an exercise program may prevent or reverse the bone loss. ES of the sciatic nerve of rats prevents suspension-induced osteopenia (376). In humans, a program of weight bearing and strengthening appears to decrease hypercalciuria (377). However, the effect on osteoporosis is uncertain.

In view of the relationship between loading and loss of bone mass, exploration of NMES-mediated exercises for reversal or prevention of osteoporosis is reasonable. While initial experience with NMES-mediated leg cycle ergometry (348,378) and leg extension exercises (355) demonstrated no evidence of reversal of osteoporosis, NMES-mediated exercises have more recently shown a decreased rate of bone loss (355,379) and that leg cycle ergometry has the potential to reverse disuse osteoporosis (380–382). The phenomenon appears to be dose dependent with reversal of osteoporosis observed at higher intensity regimen (381–383) and loss of effect at lower intensities (382). More recently, Shields completed a study of unilateral electric stimulation in subjects with SCI for more than 3 years. Compressive loads delivered to the tibia were estimated to be at 1.5 times body weight. At the conclusion of the study, peripheral quantitative computed tomography revealed that trabecular bone mineral density at the distal tibia was 31% higher than observed in the untrained limb (384) (see Chapter—for details).

Emerging data demonstrate the feasibility of NMES-mediated exercises in reducing the rate of bone loss, and in certain cases partially reversing disuse osteoporosis. However, in view of the dynamic nature of bone loss after SCI, controlled designs should be employed to confirm the above observations. The study population should be more narrowly defined with respect to chronicity and the level of the lesion. The aims of the controlled trials should be to confirm the therapeutic effect and elucidate the most appropriate prescriptive parameters including type of NMES-mediated exercises, loading parameters, power output goals, duration of exercise sessions, number of sessions per week, and total duration of exercise. Long-term follow-up should document not only changes in bone density but incidence of fractures as well. The role of ambulation neuroprosthetic systems in preventing or reversing osteoporosis should also be rigorously evaluated. In view of the axial loading, ambulation neuroprosthetic systems theoretically have greater potential than nonaxial loading systems for preventing and reversing osteoporosis.

Deep Venous Thrombosis

The incidence of deep vein thrombosis (DVT) after SCI varies from 49% to 100% in the first 12 weeks, with the first 2 weeks posing the greatest period of risk (385). NMES of the LE is associated with increased venous flow (315,370,328) and enhanced systemic fibrinolytic activity in persons with SCI (386). NMES with low-dose subcutaneous (SQ) heparin is associated with significantly lower incidence of DVT among acute SCI patients than low-dose SQ heparin alone or saline placebo (387). A similar study with low molecular weight heparin in conjunction with external pneumatic compression or NMES suggested superior outcomes with the combination therapy using NMES (385). However, these studies have small sample sizes and results should be confirmed in larger studies involving multiple centers. Furthermore, the stimulation can be painful for those with incomplete lesions, and autonomic dysreflexia may occur for those with lesions above T6.

CONCLUSION

The principal goal of the rehabilitation management of persons with SCI is to improve function, maximize independence, and enhance the quality of health and life. NMES systems bypass the injured central nervous system circuitry to activate neural tissue and contract muscles to improve these domains. Recent advances in clinical medicine and biomedical engineering have made the clinical implementation of NMES systems to enhance the mobility and function of paralyzed person more feasible. Hand neuroprosthesis systems can significantly enhance the UE ADLs of persons with tetraplegia. Several LE systems, with and without bracing, are being investigated to assist functional transfers and standing, and to a lesser degree for ambulation in persons with paraplegia. Trunk FNS systems have improved stability for persons with paraplegia and tetraplegia permitting a more functional reach. Bladder FNS system can provide catheter-free micturition for persons with either paraplegia or tetraplegia. Breathing FNS systems allow individuals with tetraplegia to be ventilator free. Cough FNS systems have allowed individuals with tetraplegia the safe removal of tracheostomy tubes because they no longer need suctioning. NMES systems are available to prevent or treat various complications of immobility including CV deconditioning, muscle atrophy, osteoporosis, decubitus ulcers, and deep vein thrombosis.

After decades of development, the clinical utility of NMES systems is finally becoming realized. However, in view of the dynamic nature of the present health care environment, the future of NMES technology is still difficult to predict. By necessity, scientists and clinicians must continue to explore new ideas and improve upon the present systems. Components will be smaller, more durable, and more reliable. The issues of cosmesis and ease of donning and doffing will require systems to be fully implantable. Control issues will remain central, and the implementation of cortical control will dictate the nature of future generations of neuroprosthetic systems. Consumers will direct future developments. In the present health care environment where cost has become an overwhelming factor in the development and implementation of new technology, the consumer will become one of technology's greatest advocates. Finally, the usual drive toward greater complexity will be tempered by the practical issues of clinical implementation where patient and clinician acceptances are often a function of a tenuous balance between the "burden and cost" associated with using a system and the system's impact on the user's quality of life.

ACKNOWLEDGMENTS

This work was supported in part by grants from the National Institutes of Child Health and Human Development, the National Institutes of Neurological Diseases and Strokes, the US Army Medical Research and Materiel Command of the Department of Defense, the US Food and Drug Administration, the Rehabilitation Research & Development Service of the US Department of Veterans Affairs, and the National Institute of Disability and Rehabilitation Research of the US Department of Education.

CONFLICT OF INTEREST

Dr. DiMarco is a founder of and has a significant financial interest in Synapse BioMedical, Inc., a manufacturer of diaphragm pacing systems. He holds patents on spinal cord stimulation to restore cough.

References

1. Mortimer JT. Motor prostheses. In: Brookhart JM, Mountcastle VB, eds. *Handbook of physiology—the nervous system II*. Bethesda, MD: American Physiological Society, 1981:155–187.
2. Bowditch, Henry P. Über die Eigenthümlichkeiten der Reizbarkeit, welche die Muskelfasern des Herzens zeigen. *Berichte über die Verhandlungen der Königlich-Sächsischen Gesellschaft der Wissenschaften zu Leipzig: Mathematisch-Physische Klasse* 1871;23: 652–689.
3. McNeal R. Analysis of a model for excitation of myelinated nerve. *IEEE Trans Biomed Eng* 1976;23:329–337.
4. Henneman E. Relation between size of neurons and their susceptibility to discharge. *Science* 1957;126:1345–1347.
5. Burke RE. Motor units: anatomy, physiology, and functional organization. In: Brookhart JM, Mountcastle VB, eds. *Handbook of physiology—the nervous system II*. Bethesda, MD: American Physiological Society, 1981:345–422.
6. Sweeney JD. Skeletal muscle response to electrical stimulation. In: Reilly JP, ed. *Electrical stimulation and electropathology*. New York, Cambridge University Press, 1992:391–398.

7. Riley DA, Allin EF. The effects of inactivity, programmed stimulation, and denervation of the histochemistry of skeletal muscle fiber types. *Exp Neurol* 1973;40:391–398.
8. Burnham R, Martin T, Stein R, et al. Skeletal muscle fibre type transformation following spinal cord injury. *Spinal Cord* 1997;35(2):86–91.
9. Peckham PH, Mortimer JT, Marsolais EB. Alteration in the force and fatigability of skeletal muscle in quadriplegic humans following exercise induced by chronic electrical stimulation. *Clin Orthop* 1976;114:326–334.
10. Brown WE, Salmons S, Whalen RG. The sequential replacement of myosin subunit isoforms during muscle type transformation induced by long term electrical stimulation. *J Biol Chem* 1983;258(23):14686–14692.
11. Gordon T, Tyreman N, Rafuse VF, et al. Fast-to-slow conversion following chronic low-frequency activation of medial gastrocnemius muscle in cats. I. Muscle and motor unit properties. *J Neurophysiol* 1997;77(5):2585–604.
12. Salmons S, Sréter FA. Significance of impulse activity in the transformation of skeletal muscle type. *Nature* 1976;263(5572):30–34.
13. Sutherland H, Jarvis JC, Kwende MM, et al. The dose-related response of rabbit fast muscle to long-term low-frequency stimulation. *Muscle Nerve* 1998;21(12):1632–1646.
14. Marsolais E, Kobetic R. Functional walking in paralyzed patients by means of electrical stimulation. *Clin Orthop* 1983;175:39–36.
15. Kagaya H, Shimada Y, Sato K, et al. Changes in muscle force following therapeutic electrical stimulation in patients with complete paraplegia. *Paraplegia* 1996;34:24–29.
16. Gerrits HL, de Haan A, Sargeant AJ, et al. Altered contractile properties of the quadriceps muscle in people with spinal cord injury following functional electrical stimulated cycle training. *Spinal Cord* 2000;38(4): 214–223.
17. Gerrits HL, Hopman MT, Sargeant AJ, et al. Effects of training on contractile properties of paralyzed quadriceps muscle. *Muscle Nerve* 2002;25(4):559–567.
18. Mohr T, Andersen JL, Biering-Sørensen F, et al. Long-term adaptation to electrically induced cycle training in severe spinal cord injured individuals. *Spinal Cord* 1997;35(1):1–16.
19. Peckham PH, Mortimer JT, Marsolais EB. Upper and lower motor neuron lesions in the upper extremity muscles of tetraplegics. *Paraplegia* 1976;14:115–121.
20. Crago PE, Peckham PH, Thrope GB. Modulation of muscle force by recruitment during intramuscular stimulation. *IEEE Trans Biomed Eng* 1980;27:679–684.
21. Grandjean PA, Mortimer JT. Recruitment properties of monopolar and bipolar epimysial electrodes. *Ann Biomed Eng* 1986;14:53–66.
22. Kilgore KL, Peckham PH, Keith MW, et al. Electrode characterization for functional application to upper extremity FNS. *IEEE Trans Biomed Eng* 1990;37:12–21.
23. Keith MW, Peckham PH, Thrope GB, et al. Implantable functional neuromuscular stimulation in the tetraplegic hand. *J Hand Surg [Am]* 1989;14:524–530.
24. Naples GG, Mortimer JT, Scheiner A, et al. A spiral nerve cuff electrode for peripheral nerve stimulation. *IEEE Trans Biomed Eng* 1988;35:905–916.
25. Glenn WWL, Phelps ML. Diaphragm pacing by electrical stimulation of the phrenic nerve. *Neurosurgery* 1985;17:974–984.
26. Kim JH, Manuelidis EE, Glen WW, et al. Diaphragm pacing: histopathological changes in the phrenic nerve following long-term electrical stimulation. *J Thorac Cardiovasc Surg* 1976;72:602–608.
27. Waters R, McNeal D, Faloon W, et al. Functional electrical stimulation of peroneal nerve for hemiplegia. *J Bone Joint Surg* 1985;67:792–793.
28. Kilgore KL, Peckham PH, Keith MW, et al. The durability of implanted electrodes and leads in upper extremity neuroprostheses. *J Rehabil Res Dev* 2003;40(6):457–468.
29. Kralj A, Bajd T. *Functional electrical stimulation: standing and walking after spinal cord injury*. Boca Raton, FL: CRC Press, 1989.
30. Graupe D. EMG pattern analysis for patient-responsive control of FES in paraplegics for walker-supported walking. *IEEE Trans Biomed Eng* 1989;36:711–719.
31. Chizeck HJ, Kobetic R, Marsolais EB, et al. Control of functional neuromuscular stimulation systems for standing and locomotion in paraplegics. *Proc IEEE* 1988;76:1155–1165.
32. Crago PE, Chizeck HJ, Neuman MR, et al. Sensors for use with functional neuromuscular stimulation. *IEEE Trans Biomed Eng* 1986;33:256–268.
33. Kilgore KL, Peckham PH, Keith MW, et al. An implanted upper-extremity neuroprosthesis. Follow-up of five patients. *J Bone Joint Surg Am* 1997;79:533–541.
34. Benton LA, Baker LL, Bowman BR, et al. Functional electrical stimulation: a practical clinical guide. Downey, CA: Ranchos Los Amigos Medical Center, 1981.
35. Bajd T, Kralj A, Turk R, et al. The use of a four channel electrical stimulator as an ambulatory aid for paraplegic patients. *Phys Ther* 1983;63:1116–1120.
36. Graupe D, Kohn K. *Functional electrical stimulation for ambulation by paraplegics*. Malabar, FL: Krieger Publishing Co., 1994.
37. Gallien P, Brissot R, Eyssette M, et al. Restoration of gait by functional electrical stimulation for spinal cord injured patients. *Paraplegia* 1995;33:660–664.
38. Handa Y, Hoshimiya N, Iguchi Y, et al. Development of percutaneous intramuscular electrode for multichannel FES system. *IEEE Trans Biomed Eng* 1989;36:706–710.
39. Memberg W, Peckham PH, Keith MH. A surgically implanted intramuscular electrode for an implantable neuromuscular stimulation system. *IEEE Trans Rehabil Eng* 1994;2:80–91.
40. Scheiner A, Polando G, Marsolais EB. Design and clinical application of a double helix electrode for functional electrical stimulation. *IEEE Trans Biomed Eng* 1994;41:425–431.
41. Waters RL, Campbell JM, Nakai R. Therapeutic electrical stimulation of the lower limb by epimysial electrodes. *Clin Orthop* 1988:44–52.
42. Holle J, Frey M, Gruber H, et al. Functional electrostimulation of paraplegics. Experimental investigations and first clinical experience with an implantable stimulation device. *Orthopaedics* 1984;7:1145–1160.
43. Haugland MK, Hoffer JA, Sinkjaer T. Skin contact force information in sensory nerve signals recorded by implanted cuff electrodes. *IEEE Trans Rehabil Eng* 1994;2:18–28.

44. Smith B, Peckham PH, Keith MW, et al. An externally powered, multichannel implantable stimulator for versatile control of paralyzed muscle. *IEEE Trans Biomed Eng* 1987;34(7):499–508.
45. Letechipia JE, Peckham PH, Gazdik M, et al. In-line lead connector for use with implanted neuroprosthesis. *IEEE Trans Biomed Eng* 1991;38:707–709.
46. Cameron T, Loeb GE, Peck RA. Micromodular implants to provide electrical stimulation of paralyzed muscles and limbs. *IEEE Trans Biomed Eng* 1997;44:781–790.
47. Handa Y, Hoshimiya N. Functional electrical stimulation for the control of the upper extremities. *Med Prog Technol* 1987;12:51–63.
48. Nathan RH, Ohry A. Upper limb functions regained in quadriplegia: A hybrid computerized FNS system. *Arch Phys Med Rehabil* 1990;71:415–421.
49. Snoek GJ, Ijzerman MJ, in't Groen FACG, et al. Use of the NESS Handmaster to restore hand function in tetraplegia. *Spinal Cord* 2000;38:244–249.
50. Peckham PH, Keith MW. Motor prostheses for restoration of upper extremity function. In: Stein RB, Peckham PH, Popovic DB, eds. *Neural prostheses: replacing motor function after disease or disability*. New York: Oxford University Press, 1992:162–190.
51. Keith MW, Kilgore KL, Peckham PH, et al. Tendon transfers and functional electrical stimulation for restoration of hand function in spinal cord injury. *J Hand Surg [Am]* 1996;21:89–99.
52. Buckett JR, Peckham PH, Thrope GB, et al. A flexible, portable system for neuromuscular stimulation in the paralyzed upper extremity. *IEEE Trans Biomed Eng* 1988;35:897–904.
53. Johnson MW, Peckham PH. Evaluation of shoulder movement as a command control source. *IEEE Trans Biomed Eng* 1990;37:876–885.
54. Perkins TA, Brindley GS, Donaldson ND, et al. Implant provision of key, pinch and power grips in a C6 tetraplegic. *Med Biol Eng Comput* 1994;32:367–372.
55. Scott TR, Peckham PH, Keith MW. Upper extremity neuroprostheses using functional electrical stimulation. In: Brindley GS, Rushton DN, eds. *Baillieres clin neurol*. Vol. 4. London, UK: Bailliere Tindall, 1995:57–75.
56. Hart RL, Kilgore KL, Peckham PH. A comparison between control methods for implanted FES hand-grasp systems. *IEEE Trans Rehabil Eng* 1998;6:208–218.
57. Vodovnik L, Long C, Reswick JB, et al. Myo-electric control of paralyzed muscles. *IEEE Trans Biomed Eng* 1965;12:169–172.
58. Peckham PH, Mortimer JT, Marsolais EB. Controlled prehension and release in the C5 quadriplegic elicited by functional electrical stimulation of the paralyzed forearm musculature. *Ann Biomed Eng* 1980;8:369–388.
59. Saxena S, Nikolic S, Popovic D. An EMG-controlled grasping system for tetraplegics. *J Rehabil Res Dev* 1995;32:17–24.
60. Solomonow M, Barrata R, Shoji H, et al. The myoelectric signal of electrically stimulated muscle during recruitment: An inherent feedback parameter for a closed-loop control scheme. *IEEE Trans Biomed Eng* 1986;33:735–745.
61. Kilgore KL, Hoyen HA, Bryden AM, et al. An implanted upper extremity neuroprosthesis utilizing myoelectric control. *J Hand Surg* 2008;33A:539–550.
62. Hoshimiya N, Naito A, Yajima M, et al. A multichannel FES system for the restoration of motor functions in high spinal cord injury patients: a respiration-controlled system for multijoint upper extremity. *IEEE Trans Biomed Eng* 1989;36:754–760.
63. Handa Y, Handa T, Nakatsuchi Y, et al. A voice-controlled functional electrical stimulation system for the paralyzed hand. *Iyodenshi To Seitai Kogaku* 1985;23:292–298.
64. Peckham PH, Thrope G, Buckett JR, et al. Coordinated two mode grasp in the quadriplegic initiated by functional neuromuscular stimulation. In: Campell RM, ed. *IFAC control aspects of prosthetics and orthotics*. Oxford, UK: Pergamon Press, 1983.
65. Nathan RH. Control strategies in FNS systems for the upper extremities. *Crit Rev Biomed Eng* 1993;21:485–568.
66. Handa Y, Handa T, Ichie M, et al. Functional electrical stimulation (FES) systems for restoration of motor function of paralyzed muscles—versatile systems and a portable system. *Front Med Biol Eng* 1992;4:241–255.
67. Alon G, McBride K. Persons with C5 or C6 tetraplegia achieve selected functional gains using a neuroprosthesis. *Arch Phys Med Rehabil* 2003;84(1):119–124.
68. Popovic MR, Thrasher TA, Adams ME, et al. Functional electrical therapy: retraining grasping in spinal cord injury. *Spinal Cord* 2006;44(3):143–151.
69. Peckham PH, Keith MW, Kilgore KL, et al. Efficacy of an implanted neuroprosthesis for restoring hand grasp in tetraplegia: a multicenter study. *Arch Phys Med Rehabil* 2001;82:1380–1388.
70. Wuolle KS, Van Doren CL, Thrope GB, et al. Development of a quantitative hand grasp and release test for patients with tetraplegia using a hand neuroprosthesis. *J Hand Surg [Am]* 1994;19:209–218.
71. Smith BT, Mulcahey MJ, Betz RR. Quantitative comparison of grasp and release abilities with and without functional neuromuscular stimulation in adolescents with tetraplegia. *Paraplegia* 1996;34:16–23.
72. Bryden AM, Kilgore KL, Keith MW, et al, Assessing activity of daily living performance after implantation of an upper extremity neuroprosthesis. *Top Spinal Cord Inj Rehabil* 2008;13(4):37–53.
73. Wuolle KS, Van Doren CL, Bryden AM, et al. Satisfaction and usage of a hand neuroprosthesis. *Arch Phys Med Rehabil* 1999;80:206–213.
74. Grill JH, Peckham PH. Functional neuromuscular stimulation for combined control of elbow extension and hand grasp in C5 and C6 quadriplegics. *IEEE Trans Rehabil Eng* 1998;6:190–199.
75. Bryden AM, Memberg WD, Crago PE. Electrically stimulated elbow extension in persons with C5/C6 tetraplegia: a functional and physiological evaluation. *Arch Phys Med Rehabil* 2000;81:80–88.
76. Crago PE, Memberg WD, Usey MK, et al. An elbow extension neuroprosthesis for individuals with tetraplegia. *IEEE Trans Rehabil Eng* 1998;6:1–6.
77. Lemay MA, Crago PE, Keith MW. Restoration of pronosupination control by FNS in tetraplegia—experimental and biomechanical evaluation of feasibility. *J Biomech* 1996;29:435–442.
78. Lauer RT, Kilgore KL, Peckham PH, et al. The function of the finger intrinsic muscles in response to electrical stimulation. *IEEE Trans Rehab Eng* 2009;7(1):19–26.

79. Knutson JS, Hoyen HA, Kilgore KL, et al. Simulated neuroprosthesis state activation and hand position control using myoelectric signals from wrist muscles. *J Rehabil Res Dev* 2004;41(3B):461–472.
80. Vaughan TM, Heetderks WJ, Trejo LJ, et al. Brain-computer interface technology: a review of the Second International Meeting. *IEEE Trans Neural Syst Rehabil Eng* 2003;11(2):94–109.
81. Peckham PH, Kilgore KL, Keith MW, et al. An advanced neuroprosthesis for restoration of hand and upper arm control employing an implantable controller. *J Hand Surg* 2002;27A(2):265–276.
82. Peckham PH, Knutson JS. Functional electrical stimulation for neuromuscular applications. *Annu Rev Biomed Eng* 2005;7:327–360.
83. Betz RR, Mulcahey MJ, Smith BT, et al. Bipolar latissimus dorsi transposition and functional neuromuscular stimulation to restore elbow flexion in an individual with C4 quadriplegia and C5 denervation. *J Am Paraplegia Soc* 1992;15:220–228.
84. Bryden AM, Kilgore KL, Kirsch RF, et al. An implanted neuroprosthesis for high tetraplegia. *Top Spinal Cord Inj Rehabil* 2005;10(3):38–52.
85. Jaeger RJ. Lower extremity applications of functional neuromuscular stimulation. *Assist Technol* 1992;4(1):19–30.
86. Marsolais EB, Kobetic R. Functional electrical stimulation for walking in paraplegia. *J Bone Joint Surg [Am]* 1987;69(5):728–733.
87. Marsolais EB, Kobetic R, Chizeck HJ, et al. Orthoses and electrical stimulation for walking in complete paraplegics. *J Neuro Rehabil* 1991;5:13–22.
88. Jaeger RJ, Yarkony GM, Roth EJ. Rehabilitation technology for standing and walking after spinal cord injury. *Am J Phys Med Rehabil* 1989;68(3):128–133.
89. Yarkony GM, Roth EJ, Cybulski GR, et al. Neuromuscular stimulation in spinal cord injury: Restoration of functional movement of the extremities. *Arch Phys Med Rehabil* 1992;73(1):78–86.
90. Jaeger RJ, Yarkony GM, Smith RM. Standing the spinal cord injured patient by electrical stimulation: refinement of a protocol for clinical use. *IEEE Trans Biomed Eng* 1989;36(7):720–728.
91. Yarkony GM, Jaeger RJ, Roth E, et al. Functional neuromuscular stimulation for standing after spinal cord injury. *Arch Phys Med Rehabil* 1990;71(3):201–206.
92. Triolo RJ, Bieri C, Uhlir J, et al. Implanted FNS systems for assisted standing and transfers for individuals with cervical spinal cord injuries. *Arch Phys Med Rehabil* 1996;7(11):1119–1128.
93. Kobetic R, Marsolais EB. Synthesis of paraplegic gait with multichannel functional neuromuscular stimulation. *IEEE Trans Biomed Eng* 1994;2:66–67.
94. Marsolais EB, Kobetic R. Implantation technique and experience with percutaneous intramuscular electrodes in the lower extremities. *J Rehabil Res Dev* 1986;23(3):1–8.
95. Davis R, Eckhouse R, Patrick JF, et al. Computer-controlled 22-channel stimulator for limb movement. *Acta Neurochir* 1987;39S:117–120.
96. Donaldson N, Rushton D, Tromans T. Neuroprostheses for leg function after spinal cord injury. *Lancet* 1997;350(9079):711.
97. Akers JM, Peckham PH, Keith MW, et al. Tissue response to chronically stimulated implanted epimysial and intramuscular electrodes. *IEEE Trans Rehabil Eng* 1997;5(2):207–220.
98. Buckett J, Triolo R, Ferencz D, et al. A wearable controller for clinical studies involving multi-implant FNS systems. *J Spinal Cord Inj* 1998;21:179.
99. Vrabec T, Triolo R, Uhlir J, et al. A clinical interface for control and evaluation of FNS systems, 2nd National Meeting VA Rehabilitation Research and Development Service, Washington, DC, 2000:187.
100. Triolo RJ, Bogie K. Lower extremity applications of functional neuromuscular stimulation after spinal cord injury. *Topics in SCI Rehabil* 1999;5:44–65.
101. Sharma M, Marsolais EB, Polando G, et al. Implantation of a 16-channel functional electrical stimulation walking system. *Clin Orthop* 1998;347:236–242.
102. Kobetic R, Triolo RJ, Uhlir JP, et al. Implanted functional electrical stimulation system for mobility in paraplegia: a follow-up case report. *IEEE Trans Rehabil Eng* 1999;7(4):390–398.
103. Davis JA, Triolo RJ, Uhlir JP, et al. Preliminary performance of a surgically implanted neuroprosthesis for standing and transfer. *J Rehabil Res Dev* 2001;38(6): 609–617.
104. Uhlir JP, Triolo RJ, Davis JA, et al. Performance of epimysial stimulating electrodes in the lower extremities of individuals with spinal cord injury. *IEEE Trans Neural Syst Rehabil Eng* 2004;12(2):279–287.
105. Davis JA, Triolo RJ, Uhlir JP, et al. Surgical technique for installing an 8-channel neuroprosthesis for standing. *Clin Orthop Relat Res* 2001;385:237–252.
106. Moynahan M. Postural responses during standing in subjects with spinal-cord injury. *Gait Posture* 1995;3: 156–165.
107. Miller P, Kobetic R, Lew R. Energy costs of walking and standing using functional electrical stimulation. Proceedings, 13th Annual RESNA Conference, Washington, DC, 1990:155–156.
108. Barnette N, Lamitie H. *A comparison of energy expenditure between KAFO and FNS standing in adolescents with spinal cord injuries.* Glenside, PA: Department of Physical Therapy, Beaver College, 1991.
109. Forrest GP, Smith TC, Triolo RJ, et al. Energy cost of the Case Western Reserve standing neuroprosthesis. *Arch Phys Med Rehabil* 2007;88(8):1074–1076.
110. Bieri C, Rohde L, Danford GS, et al. Development of a new assessment of effort and assistance in standing pivot transfers with FES. *J Spinal Cord Med* 2004;27(3): 226–235.
111. Bajd T, Kralj A, Turk R. Standing up of a healthy subject and a paraplegic patient. *J Biomech* 1982;15(1):1–10.
112. Isakov E, Mizrahi J, Najenson T. Biomechanical and physiological evaluation of FES-activated paraplegic patients. *J Rehabil Res Dev* 1986;23(8):9–19.
113. Kralj A, Bajd T, Turk R, et al. Gait restoration in paraplegic patients: a feasibility demonstration using multichannel surface electrode FES. *J Rehabil Res Dev* 1983;20(1):3–20.
114. Kralj A, Bajd T, Turk R. Enhancement of gait restoration in spinal injured patients by functional electrical stimulation. *Clin Orthop Relat Res* 1988;233:34–43.

115. Kralj AR, Bajd T. *Functional electrical stimulation: standing and walking after spinal cord injury*. Boca Raton, FL: CRC Press Inc., 1989:123–138.
116. Graupe D, Kohn K. Clinical results and observations over 12 years of FES-based ambulation. In: *Functional electrical stimulation for ambulation by paraplegics*. Malabar FL: Kreiger Publishing Co., 1994:136.
117. MacGregor J. The evaluation of patient performance using long-term ambulatory monitoring technique in the domiciliary environment. *Physiotherapy* 1981;67(2):30–33.
118. Rose J, Gamble JG, Medeiros J, et al. Energy cost of walking in normal children and those with cerebral palsey: comparison of heart rate and oxygen uptake. *J Pediatr Orthop* 1989;9(3):276–279.
119. Isakov E, Douglas R, Berns P. Ambulation using the reciprocating gait orthosis and functional electrical stimulation. *Paraplegia* 1992;30(4):239–245.
120. Winchester P, Carollo JJ, Habasevich R. Physiologic cost of reciprocal gait in FES assisted walking. *Paraplegia* 1994;32(10):680–686.
121. Bowker P, Messenger N, Ogilvie C, et al. Energetics of paraplegic walking. *J Biomed Eng* 1992;14(4):344–350.
122. Chaplin E. Functional neuromuscular stimulation for mobility in people with spinal cord injuries. The Parastep I System. *J Spinal Cord Med* 1996;19(2):99–105.
123. Klose KJ, Jacobs PL, Broton JG, et al. Evaluation of training program for persons with SCI paraplegia using the Parastep 1 Ambulation system: part 1. Ambulation performance and anthropometric measures. *Arch Phys Med Rehabil* 1997;78(8):789–793.
124. Guest RS, Klose KJ, Needham-Shropshire BM, et al. Evaluation of a training program for persons with SCI paraplegia using the Parastep 1 ambulation system: part 4. Effect on physical self-concept and depression. *Arch Phys Med Rehabil* 1997;78(8):804–807.
125. Jacobs PL, Nash MS, Klose KJ, et al. Evaluation of a training program for persons with SCI paraplegia using the Parastep 1 ambulation system: part 2. Effects on physiological responses to peak arm ergometry. *Arch Phys Med Rehabil* 1997;78(8):794–798.
126. Nash MS, Jacobs PL, Montalvo BM, et al. Evaluation of a training program for persons with SCI paraplegia using the Parastep 1 ambulation system: part 5. Lower extremity blood flow and hyperemic responses to occlusion are augmented by ambulation training. *Arch Phys Med Rehabil* 1997;78(8):808–814.
127. Bedbrook GM. A balanced viewpoint in the early management of patients with spinal injuries who have neurological damage. *Paraplegia* 1985;23(1):8–15.
128. Bajd T, Kralj A, Turk R, et al. FES rehabilitative approach in incomplete SCI patients. Proceedings, 9th Annual RESNA Conference, Minneapolis, MN, 1986:316–318.
129. Bajd T, Kralj A, Stefancic M, et al. Use of functional electrical stimulation in the lower extremities of incomplete spinal cord injured patients. *Artif Organs* 1999;23(5):403–409.
130. Kralj A, Bajd T, Kvesic Z, et al. Electrical stimulation of incomplete paraplegic patients. Proceedings, 4th Annual RESNA Conference. Washington, DC, 1981:226–228.
131. Granat MH, Ferguson AC, Andrews BJ, et al. The role of functional electrical stimulation in the rehabilitation of patients with incomplete spinal cord injury—observed benefits during gait studies. *Paraplegia* 1993;31(4):207–215.
132. Hardin E, Kobetic R, Murray L, et al. Walking after incomplete spinal cord injury using implanted FES system: a case report. *J Rehabil Res Dev* 2007;44(3):333–346.
133. Dutta A, Kobetic R, Triolo RJ. Ambulation after incomplete spinal cord injury with EMG-triggered functional electrical stimulation. *IEEE Trans Biomed Eng* 2008;55(2):791–794.
134. Brindley GS, Polkey CE, Rushton DN. Electrical splinting of the knee in paraplegia. *Paraplegia* 1979;16(4):428–437.
135. Borges G, Ferguson K, Kobetic R. Development and operations of portable and laboratory electrical stimulation systems for walking in paraplegic subjects. *IEEE Trans Biomed Eng* 1989;36(7):798–800.
136. Triolo R, Kobetic R. The next step: artificial walking. In: Rose J, Gamble JG, eds. *Human walking*. Baltimore, MD: Williams & Wilkins, 2006:209–222.
137. Agarwal S, Kobetic R, Nandurkar S, et al. Functional electrical stimulation for walking in paraplegia: 17-year follow-up of 2 cases. *J Spinal Cord Med* 2003;26(1):86–91.
138. Granat MH, Heller BW, Nicol DJ, et al. Improving limb flexion in FES gait using the flexion withdrawal response for the spinal cord injured person. *J Biomed Eng* 1993;15(1):51–56.
139. Solomonow M, Baratta RV, Hirokawa S, et al. The RGO generation II: muscle stimulation powered orthosis as a practical walking system for paraplegics. *Orthopaedics* 1989;12(10):1309–1315.
140. Solomonow M. Biomechanics and physiology of a practical functional neuromuscular stimulation powered walking orthosis for paraplegics. In: Stein RB, Peckham PH, Popovic DP, eds. *Neural prostheses: replacing motor function after disease or disability*. New York: Oxford University Press, 1992:202–232.
141. Kantor C, Andrews BJ, Marsolais EB, et al. Report on a conference on motor prostheses for workplace mobility of paraplegic patients in North America. *Paraplegia* 1993;31(7):439–456.
142. Schwirlich L, Popovich D. Hybrid orthoses for deficient locomotion. Proceedings, Advances in External Control of Human Extremities. Dubrovnik, Yugoslavia, 1984. Vol. VII. ISTN: 23–32.
143. Andrews BJ, Baxendale RH, Barnett R, et al. Hybrid FES orthosis incorporating closed loop control and sensory feedback. *J Biomed Eng* 1988;10(2):189–195.
144. McClelland M, Andrews BJ, Patrick JH, et al. Augmentation of the Oswestry Parawalker orthosis by means of surface electrical stimulation: gait analysis of three patients. *Paraplegia* 1987;25(1):32–38.
145. Franceschini M, Baratta S, Zampolini M, et al. Reciprocating gait orthosis: a multicenter study of their use by spinal cord injured patients. *Arch Phys Med Rehabil* 1997;78(6):582–586.
146. Solomonow M, Aguilar E, Reisin E, et al. Reciprocating gait orthosis powered with electrical muscle stimulation (RGO II). Part I: performance evaluation of 70 paraplegic patients. *Orthopedics* 1997;20(4):315–324.

147. Petrofsky JS, Phillips CA, Douglas R, et al. A computer-controlled walking system: The combination of an orthosis with functional electrical stimulation. *J Clin Eng* 1986;11:121–133.
148. Andrews BJ, Baxendale RH, Barnett R, et al. A hybrid orthosis for paraplegics incorporating feedback control. *Proc 9th Symp ECHE*, 1997;297–311.
149. Goldfarb M, Durfee W. Design of a controlled-brake orthosis for FES-added gait. *IEEE Trans Rehab Eng* 1996;4(1):13–24.
150. Popovic DB, Schwirtlich L. Design and evaluation of the self-fitting modular orthosis (SFMO). *IEEE Trans Rehabil Eng* 1993;1:165–174.
151. Popovic DB. Functional electrical stimulation for lower extremities. In: Stein RB, Peckham PH, Popovic DB, eds. *Neural prostheses, replacing motor function after disease or disability*. New York: Oxford University Press, 1992;233–251.
152. To CS, Kobetic R, Schnellenberger JR, et al. Design of a variable constraint hip mechanism for a hybrid neuroprosthesis to restore gait after spinal cord injury. *IEEE/ASME Trans Mechatronics* 2008;13(2):197–205.
153. Hirokawa S, Grimm M, Le T, et al. Energy consumption in paraplegic ambulation using the reciprocating gait orthosis and electrical stimulation of the thigh muscles. *Arch Phys Med Rehabil* 1990;71(9):687–694.
154. Solomonow M, Reisin E, Aguilar E, et al. Reciprocating gait orthosis powered with electrical muscle stimulation (RGO II). Part II: medical evaluation of 70 paraplegic patients. *Orthopedics* 1997;20(5):411–418.
155. Schobert H. *Orthopädie des sitzens*. Berlin: Springer-Verlag, 1989.
156. Seelen HAM, Potten YJM, Drukker J, et al. Development of new muscle synergies in postural control in spinal cord injured subjects. *J Electromyogr Kinesiol* 1998;8(1):23–34.
157. Seelen HAM, Potten YJM, Huson A, et al. Impaired balance control in paraplegic subjects. *J Electromyogr Kinesiol* 1997;7:149–160.
158. Andersson GBJ, Winters D. Role of muscle in postural tasks: spinal loading and postural stability. In: Winters JM, Woo SLY, eds. *Multiple muscle systems*. New York: Springer-Verlag, 1990:377–395.
159. Chaffin DB, Andersson GBJ. *Occupational biomechanics*. New York: John Wiley and Sons Inc., 1991.
160. Hobson DA, Tooms RE. Seated lumbar/pelvic alignment. A comparison between spinal cord-injured and non-injured groups. *Spine* 1992;17(3):293–298.
161. Andersson GBJ, Ortengren R. Lumbar disc pressure and myo-electric back muscle activity during sitting. II. Studies on an office chair. *Scand J Rehabil Med* 1974;6(3):91–108.
162. Andersson GBJ, Oretengren R, Machemson AL, et al. The sitting posture: an electro-myographic and discometric study. *Orthop North Am* 1975;6(1):105–20.
163. Rintala DH, Loubser PG, Castro J, et al. Chronic pain in a community-based sample of men with spinal cord injury: prevalence, severity, and relationship with impairment, disability, handicap, and subjective well-being. *Arch Phys Med Rehabil* 1998;79(6):604–14.
164. Curtis KA, Drysdale GA, Lanza RD, et al. Shoulder pain in wheelchair users with tetraplegia and paraplegia. *Arch Phys Med Rehabil* 1999;80(4):453–457.
165. Baydur A, Adkins R, Milic-Emili J. Lung mechanics in individuals with spinal cord injury: effects of injury level and posture. *J Appl Physiol*2001;90(2):405–411.
166. Klefbeck B, Mattsson E, Weinberg J. The effect of trunk support on performance during arm ergometry in patients with cervical cord injuries. *Paraplegia* 1996;34(3):167–172.
167. Bellamy R, Pitts RW, Stauffer ES. Respiratory complications in traumatic quadriplegia. *J Neurosurg* 1973;39(5):596–600.
168. Carter RE. Respiratory aspects of spinal cord injury management. *Paraplegia* 1987;25(3):262–266.
169. Kiwerski J. Respiratory problems in patients with high lesion quadriplegia. *Int J Rehabil Res* 1992;15(1):49–52.
170. Reines HD, Harris RC. Pulmonary complications of acute spinal cord injuries. *Neurosurgery* 1987;21(2):193–196.
171. Potten YJM, Seelen HAM, Drukker J, et al. Postural muscle responses in the spinal cord injured persons during forward reaching. *Ergonomics* 1999;42(9):1200–1215.
172. Kirby RL, Sampson MT, Thoren AV, et al. Wheelchair stability: effect of body position. *J Rehab Res Dev* 1995;32(4):367–372.
173. Newsam CJ, Mulroy SJ, Gronley JK, et al. Temporal-spatial characteristics of wheelchair propulsion. *Am J Phys Med Rehabil* 1996;75(4):292–299.
174. Newsam CJ, Rao SS, Mulroy SJ, et al. Three-dimensional upper extremity motion during wheelchair propulsion in men with different levels of spinal cord injury. *Gait Posture* 1999;10(3):223–232.
175. Dallmeijer AJ, van der Woude LH, Veeger HE, et al. Effectiveness of force application in manual wheelchair propulsion in persons with spinal cord injuries. *Am J Phys Med Rehabil* 1998;77 (3):213–221.
176. Rodgers MM, Gayle GW, Figoni SF, et al. Biomechanics of wheelchair propulsion during fatigue. *Arch Phys Med Rehabil* 1994;75(1):85–93.
177. Sanderson DJ, Sommer HJ. Kinematic features of wheelchair propulsion. *J Biomech* 1985;18(6):423–9.
178. Rodgers MM, Keyser RE, Gardner ER, et al. Influence of trunk flexion on biomechanics of wheelchair propulsion. *J Rehab Res Dev* 2000;37(3):283–295.
179. Kukke S, Triolo RJ. The effects of trunk stimulation on bimanual seated workspace. *IEEE Trans Neural Syst Biomed Eng* 2004;12(2):117–185.
180. Yang Y, Koontz A, Triolo R, et al. Surface electromyography activity of trunk muscles during wheelchair propulsion. *Clin Biomech* 2006;21(10):1032–1041.
181. Triolo R, Boggs L, Bryden A, et al. Implanted electrical stimulation of the trunk for seated postural stability and functional mobility after cervical SCI. Proceedings 12th Annual Conference of the International FES Society, Nov 2007, Philadelphia PA.
182. Triolo RJ, Boggs L, Miller M, et al. Implanted electrical stimulation of the trunk for seated postural stability and function after cervical SCI. *Arch Phys Med Rehabil* 2009;90(2):340–347.
183. Arnold EP, Gowland SP, MacFarlane MR, et al. Sacral anterior root stimulation of the bladder in paraplegia. *Aust N Z J Surg* 1986;56:319–324.
184. Brindley GS, Polkey CE, Rushton DN, et al. Sacral anterior root stimulators for bladder control in

paraplegia: the first 50 cases. *J Neurol Neurosurg Psychiatry* 1986;49:1104–1114.
185. Robinson LQ, Grant A, Weston P, et al. Experience with the Brindley anterior sacral root stimulator. *Br J Urol* 1988;62:553–557.
186. Brindley GS, Rushton DN. Long-term follow-up of patients with sacral anterior root stimulator implants. *Paraplegia* 1990;28:469–475.
187. Creasey GH, Grill JH, Korsten M, et al. An implantable neuroprosthesis for restoring bladder and bowel control to patients with spinal cord injuries: a multi-center trial. *Arch Phys Med Rehabil* 82;1512–9, 2001.
188. Creasey GH. Emptying the neurogenic bladder by electrical stimulation. In: Corcos J, Schick E, eds. *Textbook of the neurogenic bladder*. 1st ed. London, Martin Dunitz, Taylor & Francis Group, 2004:536–545.
189. Van Kerrebroeck PE, Koldewijn EL, Debruyne FM. Worldwide experience with the Finetech-Brindley sacral anterior root stimulator. *Neurourol Urodyn* 1993;12:497–503.
190. Brindley GS. The first 500 patients with sacral anterior root stimulator implants: general description. *Paraplegia* 1994;32:795–805.
191. Bosch JL, Groen J. Sacral (S3) segmental nerve stimulation as a treatment for urge incontinence in patients with detrusor instability: results of chronic electrical stimulation using an implantable neural prosthesis. *J Urol* 1995;154:504–507.
192. Ishigooka M, Hashimoto T, Hayami S, et al. Electrical pelvic floor stimulation: a possible alternative treatment for reflex urinary incontinence in patients with spinal cord injury. *Spinal Cord* 1996;34:411–415.
193. Madersbacher H, Fischer J, Ebner A. Anterior sacral root stimulator (Brindley): Experience especially in women with neurogenic urinary incontinence. *Neurourol Urodyn* 1988;7:593–601.
194. Colombel P, Egon G. Electrostimulation of the anterior sacral nerve roots. *Ann Urol Paris* 1991;25:48–52.
195. Creasey G. Restoration of bladder, bowel, and sexual function. *Top Spinal Cord Rehabil* 1999;5:21–32.
196. Madersbacher H, Fischer J. Anterior sacral root stimulation and posterior sacral root rhizotomy. *Akt Urol* 1993;24(Suppl):32–35.
197. Van Kerrebroeck PE, Koldewijn EL, Rosier PF, et al. Results of the treatment of neurogenic bladder dysfunction in spinal cord injury by sacral posterior root rhizotomy and anterior sacral root stimulation. *J Urol* 1996;155:1378–1381.
198. Egon G, Barat M, Colombel P, et al. Implantation of anterior sacral root stimulators combined with posterior sacral rhizotomy in spinal injury patients. *World J Urol* 1998;16:342–349.
199. MacDonagh RP, Forster DM, Thomas DG. Urinary continence in spinal injury patients following complete sacral posterior rhizotomy. *Br J Urol* 1990;66:618–622.
200. Van Kerrebroeck PEV, Kolewijn EL, Wijkstra H, et al. Urodynamic evaluation before and after intradural posterior sacral rhizotomies and implantation of the Finetech-Brindley anterior sacral root stimulator. *Urodinamica* 1992;1:7–12.
201. Cardozo L, Krishnan KR, Polkey CE, et al. Urodynamic observations on patients with sacral anterior root stimulators. *Paraplegia* 1984;22:201–209.
202. Wielink G, Essink-Bot ML, van Kerrebroeck PE, et al. Sacral rhizotomies and electrical bladder stimulation in spinal cord injury. 2. Cost-effectiveness and quality of life analysis. Dutch Study Group on Sacral Anterior Root Stimulation. *Eur Urol* 1997;31:441–446.
203. Creasey GH, Dahlberg JE. Economic consequences of an implanted neural prosthesis for bladder and bowel management. *Arch Phys Med Rehabil* 82;1520–5, 2001.
204. Rushton DN, Brindley GS, Polkey CE, et al. Implant infections and antibiotic-impregnated silicone rubber coating. *J Neurol Neurosurg Psychiatry* 1989;52:223–229.
205. Carter RE. Experience with high tetraplegia. *Paraplegia* 1979;17:140–146.
206. Carter RE. Experience with ventilator dependent patients. *Paraplegia* 1993;31:150–153.
207. DeVivo MJ, Ivie CS III. Life expectancy of ventilator-dependent persons with spinal cord injuries. *Chest* 1995;108:226–232.
208. McMichan JC, Michel L, Westbrook PR. Pulmonary dysfunction following traumatic quadriplegia: recognition, prevention and treatment. *JAMA* 1980;243:528–531.
209. Shavelle RM, DeVivo MJ, Strauss DJ, et al. Long-term survival of persons ventilator dependent after spinal cord injury. *J Spinal Cord Med* 2006;29:511–519.
210. Whiteneck G. Long-term outlook for persons with high quadriplegia. In: Whiteneck G, Alder C, Carter RE, et al., eds. *The management of high quadriplegia*. New York, NY: Demos Publications, 1989:353–361.
211. Wick AB, Menter RR. Long-term outlook in quadriplegic patients with initial ventilator dependency. *Chest* 1986;90:406–410.
212. Spinal cord injury: facts and figures at a glance 2008. The National Spinal Cord Injury Statistical Center, University of Alabama, Birmingham, AL. www.spinalcord.uab.edu.
213. Carter RE, Donovan WH, Halstead L, Wilkerson MA. Comparative study of electrophrenic nerve stimulation and mechanical ventilatory support in traumatic spinal cord injury. *Paraplegia* 1987;25:86–91.
214. DeVivo MJ, Stover SL. Long-term survival and causes of death. In: Stover SL, DeLisa JA, Whiteneck GG, eds. *Spinal cord injury: clinical outcomes from the model systems*. Gaithersburg MD: Aspen Publishers, 1995:289–316.
215. Frankel HL, Coll JR, Charlifue SW, et al. Long-term survival in spinal cord injury: a fifty year investigation. *Spinal Cord* 1998;36:266–274.
216. Hartkopp A, Bronnum-Hansen H, Seidenschnur AM, et al. Survival and cause of death after traumatic spinal cord injury: a long-term epidemiological survey from Denmark. *Spinal Cord* 1997;35:76–85.
217. Whiteneck GG, Charlifue SW, Frankel HL, et al. Mortality, morbidity, and psychosocial outcomes of persons spinal cord injured more than 20 years ago. *Paraplegia* 1992;30:617–630.
218. Chae J, Triolo RJ, Kilgore KL, et al. Neuromuscular electrical stimulation in spinal cord injury. In: Kirshblum S, Campagnolo DI, DeLisa JA, eds. *Spinal cord medicine*. Philadelphia, PA: Lippincott Williams & Wilkins, 2002:360–388.
219. Chen CF, Lien IN. Spinal cord injuries in Taipei, Taiwan, 1978–1981. *Paraplegia* 1985;23:364–370.

220. Glenn WW, Brouillette RT, Dentz B, et al. Fundamental considerations in pacing of the diaphragm for chronic ventilatory insufficiency: a multi-center study. *Pacing Clin Electrophysiol* 1988;11:2121–2127.
221. Dobelle WH, D'Angelo MS, Goetz BF, et al. 200 cases with a new breathing pacemaker dispel myths about diaphragm pacing. *ASAIO J* 1994;40:M244–M252.
222. Baer GA, Talonen PP, Shneerson JM, et al. Phrenic nerve stimulation for central ventilatory failure with bipolar and four-pole electrode systems. *Pacing Clin Eletrophysiol* 1990;19:1061–1072.
223. Talonen PP, Baer GA, Hakkinen V, et al. Neurophysiological and technical considerations for the design of an implantable phrenic nerve stimulator. *Med Biol Eng Comput* 1990;28:31–37.
224. Weese-Mayer DE, Silvestri JM, Kenny AS, et al. Diaphragm pacing with a quadripolar phrenic nerve electrode: an international study. *Pacing Clin Electrophysiol* 1996;19:1311–1319.
225. Thoma H, Gerner H, Holle J, et al. The phrenic pacemaker: substitution of paralyzed functions in tetraplegia. *ASAIO Trans* 1987;33:472–479.
226. Mayr W, Bijak M, Girsch W, et al. Multichannel stimulation of phrenic nerves by epineural electrodes. *ASAIO J* 1993;39:M729–M735.
227. Aiyar H, Stellato TA, Onders RP, et al. Laparoscopic implant instrument for the placement of intramuscular electrodes in the diaphragm. *IEEE Trans Rehabil Eng* 1999;7:360–371.
228. DiMarco AF, Onders RP, Ignagni A, et al. Phrenic nerve pacing via intramuscular diaphragm electrodes in tetraplegic subjects. *Chest* 2005;127:671–678.
229. DiMarco AF, Onders RP, Kowalski KE, et al. Phrenic nerve pacing in a tetraplegic patient via intramuscular diaphragm electrodes. *Am J Respir Crit Care Med* 2002;166:1604–1606.
230. Nochomovitz ML, DiMarco AF, Mortimer JT, et al. Diaphragm activation with intramuscular stimulation in dogs. *Am Rev Respir Dis* 1983;127:325–329.
231. Peterson DK, Nochomovitz ML, DiMarco AF, et al. Intramuscular electrical activation of the phrenic nerve. *IEEE Trans Biomed Eng* 1986;33:342–352.
232. Onders RP, DiMarco AF, Ignagni AR, et al. Mapping the phrenic nerve motor point: the key to a successful laparoscopic diaphragm pacing system in the first human series. *Surgery* 2004;136:819–826.
233. Peterson DK, Nochomovitz ML, Stellato TA, et al. Long-term intramuscular electrical activation of the phrenic nerve: efficacy as a ventilatory prosthesis. *IEEE Trans Biomed Eng* 1994;41:1127–1135.
234. Peterson DK, Nochomovitz ML, Stellato TA, et al. Long-term intramuscular electrical activation of the phrenic nerve: safety and reliability. *IEEE Trans Biomed Eng* 1994;41:1115–1126.
235. Schmit BD, Mortimer JT. The effects of epimysial electrode location on phrenic nerve recruitment and the relation between tidal volume and interpulse interval. *IEEE Trans Rehabil Eng* 1999;7:150–158.
236. Schmit BD, Stellato TA, Miller ME, et al. Laparoscopic placement of electrodes for diaphragm pacing using stimulation to locate the phrenic nerve motor points. *IEEE Trans Rehabil Eng* 1998;6:382–390.
237. Elefteriades JA, Quin JA, Hogan JF, et al. Long-term follow-up of pacing of the conditioned diaphragm in quadriplegia. *Pacing Clin Electrophysiol* 2002;25:897–906.
238. Sarnoff SJ, Hardenberg E, Whittenberger JL. Electrophrenic respiration. *Am J Physiol* 1948;155:1–9.
239. Paw P, Sackier JM. Complications of laparoscopy and thoracoscopy. *J Intensive Care Med* 1994;9:290–304.
240. DiMarco AF, Supinski GS, Petro J, et al. Evaluation of intercostal pacing to provide artificial ventilation in quadriplegics. *Am J Respir Crit Care Med* 1994;150:934–940.
241. DiMarco AF, Takaoka Y, Kowalski KE. Evaluation of intercostal and diaphragm pacing to provide artificial ventilation in tetraplegics. *Arch Phys Med Rehabil* 2005;86:1200–1207.
242. Oo T, Watt JWH, Soni BM, et al. Delayed diaphragm recovery in 12 patients after high cervical spinal cord injury. A retrospective review of the diaphragm status of 107 patients ventilated after acute spinal cord injury. *Spinal Cord* 1999;37:117–122.
243. Glenn WWL, Hogan JF, Loke JS, et al. Ventilatory support by pacing of the conditioned diaphragm in quadriplegia. *N Engl J Med* 1984;310:1150–1155.
244. Glenn WWL, Phelps ML, Elefteriades JA, et al. Twenty years experience in phrenic nerve stimulation to pace the diaphragm. *Pacing Clin Electrophysiol* 1986;9:780–784.
245. Glenn WW, Sairenji H. Diaphragm pacing in the treatment of chronic ventilatory insufficiency. In: Roussos C, Macklem PT, eds. *The thorax: lung biology in health and disease*. Vol. 29. New York: Marcel Dekker, 1985:1407–1440.
246. Oliven A. Electrical stimulation of the respiratory muscles. In: Cherniack NS, Altose MD, Homma I, eds. *Rehabilitation of the patient with respiratory disease*. New York: Mc-Graw-Hill, 1999:535–542.
247. Bach JR, Alba AS. Management of chronic alveolar hypoventilation by nasal ventilation. *Chest* 1990;97:52–57.
248. Bach JR, Alba AS. Noninvasive options for ventilatory support of the traumatic high level tetraplegic patient. *Chest* 1990;98:613–619.
249. MacLean IC, Mattioni TA. Phrenic nerve conduction studies: a new technique and its application in quadriplegic patients. *Arch Phys Med Rehabil* 1981;62:70–73.
250. McKenzie DK, Gandevia SC. Phrenic nerve conduction times and twitch pressures of the human diaphragm. *J Appl Phsiol* 1985;58:1496–1504.
251. DiMarco AF. Diaphragm pacing in patients with spinal cord injury. *Top Spinal Cord Inj Rehabil* 1999;5:6–20.
252. Miller JM, Moxham J, Green M. The maximal sniff in the assessment of diaphragm function in man. *Clin Sci (London)* 1985;69:91–96.
253. Glenn WWL, Hogan JF. *Technique of transthoracic placement of phrenic nerve electrodes for diaphragm pacing*. Chicago, IL: Film Library, American College of Surgeons, 1982.
254. Glenn WW, Hogan JF, Phelps ML. Ventilatory support of the quadriplegic patient with respiratory paralysis by diaphragm pacing. *Surg Clin North Am* 1980;60:1055–1078.
255. Judson JP, Glenn WWl. Radio-frequency electrophrenic respiration: Long-term application to a patient with primary hypoventilation. *JAMA* 1968;203:1033–1037.

256. Nochomovitz ML, Hopkins M, Brodkey J, et al. Conditioning of the diaphragm with phrenic nerve stimulation after prolonged disuse. *Am Rev Respir Dis* 1984;130:685–688.
257. Hunt CE, Brouillette RT, Weese-Mayer DE, et al. Diaphragm pacing in infants and children. *Pacing Clin Electrophysiol* 1988;11:2135–2141.
258. Fodstad H. The Swedish experience in phrenic nerve stimulation. *Pacing Clin Electrophysiol* 1987;10: 246–251.
259. Hunt CE, Matalon SV, Thompson TR, et al. Central hypoventilation syndrome: experience with bilateral phrenic nerve pacing in 3 neonates. *Am Rev Respir Dis* 1978;118:23–28.
260. Tibballs J. Diaphragmatic pacing: an alternative to long-term mechanical ventilation. *Anaesth Intensive Care* 1991;19:597–601.
261. Glenn WWL, Holcomb WG, Hogan JF, et al. Diaphragm pacing by radiofrequency transmission in the treatment of chronic ventilatory insufficiency: present status. *J Thorac Cardiovasc Surg* 1973;66:505–520.
262. Ilbawi MN, Idriss FS, Hunt CE, et al. Diaphragmatic pacing in infants: techniques and results. *Ann Thorac Surg* 1985;40:323–329.
263. Elefteriades JA, Quin JA. Diaphragm pacing. *Chest Surg Clin N Am* 1998;8:331–357.
264. Weese-Mayer DE, Morrow AS, Brouillette RT, et al. Diaphragm pacing in infants and children. A life-table analysis of implanted components. *Am Rev Respir Dis* 1989;139:974–979.
265. Vanderlinden RG, Epstein SW, Hyland RH, et al. Management of chronic ventilatory insufficiency with electrical diaphragm pacing. *Can J Neuro Sci* 1988;15:63–67.
266. Glenn WWL, Gee JB, Cole DR, et al. Combined central alveolar hypoventilation and upper airway obstruction. Treatment by tracheostomy and diaphragm pacing. *Am J Med* 1978;64:50–60.
267. Weese-Mayer DE, Hunt CE, Brouillette RT, et al. Diaphragm pacing in infants and children. *J Pediatr* 1992;120:1–8.
268. DeVivo MJ, Krause JS, Lammertse DP. Recent trends in mortality and causes of death among persons with spinal cord injury. *Arch Phys Med Rehabil* 1999;80: 1411–1419.
269. Kiwerski JE. Factors contributing to the increased threat of life following spinal cord injury. *Paraplegia* 1993;31:793–799.
270. Kyroussis D, Polkey MI, Mills GH, et al. Simulation of cough in man by magnetic stimulation of the thoracic nerve roots. *Am J Respir Crit Care Med* 1997;156,1696–1699.
271. Lin VWH, Hsieh C, Hsiao IN, et al. Functional magnetic stimulation of the expiratory muscles: a noninvasive and new method for restoring cough. *J Appl Physiol* 1998;84:1144–1150.
272. Jaeger RJ, Langbein EW, Kralj A. Augmenting cough by FES in tetraplegia: a comparison of results at three clinical centers. *BAM* 1994;4:195–200.
273. Jaeger RJ, Turba RM, Yarkony GM, et al. Cough in spinal cord injured patients. A comparison of three methods to produce cough. *Arch Phys Med Rehabil* 1993;74: 1358–1361.
274. Lee BB, Boswell-Ruys C, Butler JE, Gandevia SC. Surface functional electrical stimulation of the abdominal muscles to enhance cough and assist tracheostomy decannulation after high-level spinal cord injury. *J Spinal Cord Med* 2008;31:78–82.
275. Lim J, Gorman RB, Saboisky JP, et al. Optimal electrode placement for noninvasive electrical stimulation of human abdominal muscles. *J Appl Physiol* 2007;102:1612–1617.
276a. DiMarco AF, Kowalski KE, Geertman RT, Hromyak DR. Lower thoracic spinal cord stimulation to restore cough in patients with spinal cord injury: results of a National Institutes of Health-sponsored clinical trial. Part I: methodology and effectiveness of expiratory muscle activation. *Arch Phys Med Rehabil* 90:717–725, 2009.
276b. DiMarco AF, Kowalski KE, Geertman RT, et al. Lower thoracic spinal cord stimulation to restore cough in patients with spinal cord injury: results of a National Institutes of Health-sponsored clinical trial. Part II: clinical outcomes. *Arch Phys Med Rehabil* 90:726–732, 2009
277. DiMarco AF, Kowalski KE, Geertman RT, et al. Spinal cord stimulation: a new technique to produce an effective cough in patients with spinal cord injury. *Am J Respir Crit Care Med* 2006;173:1386–1389.
278. DiMarco AF, Kowalski KE, Geertman RT, et al. Lower thoracic spinal cord stimulation to restore cough in patients with spinal cord injury: results of a National Institutes of Health-sponsored clinical trial. Part II: clinical outcomes. *Arch Phys Med Rehabil* 90:726–732, 2009
279. DiMarco AF, Altose MD, Cropp A, et al. Activation of intercostal muscles by electrical stimulation of the spinal cord. *Am Rev Respir Dis* 1987;136:1385–1390.
280. DiMarco AF, Budzinska K, Supinski GS. Artificial ventilation by means of electrical activation of intercostal/ accessory muscles alone in anesthetized dogs. *Am Rev Respir Dis* 1989;139:961–967.
281. Ragnarsson KT. Functional electrical stimulation after spinal cord injury: current use, therapeutic effects and future directions. *Spinal Cord* 2008;46(4):255–274.
282. Myers J, Lee M, Kiratli J. Cardiovascular disease in spinal cord injury: an overview of prevalence, risk, evaluation, and management. *Am J Phys Med Rehabil* 2007;86(2):142–152.
283. Garshick, E, Kelly A, Cohen SA, et al. A prospective assessment of mortality in chronic spinal cord injury. *Spinal Cord* 2005;43:408–416.
284. Teasell RW, Malcom J, Arnold O, et al. Cardiovascular consequences of loss of supraspinal control of the sympathetic nervous system after spinal cord injury. *Arch Phys Med Rehabil* 2000;81:506–506.
285. Blood pressure management after spinal cord injury *Neurosurgery* 2002;(3Suppl) 50:S58–S62.
286. Blackmer J. Orthostatic Hypotension in spinal cord injured patients. J Spinal Cord Med 1997;20:212–217.
287. Claydon VE, Steeves JD, Krassioukov A. Orthostatic hypotension following spinal cord injury: understanding clinical pathophysiology. *Spinal Cord*. 2006;44(6):341–351.
288. Phillips WT, Kiratli BJ, Sarkati M, et al. Effect of spinal cord injury on the heart and cardiovascular fitness. *Curr Probl Cardiol* 1988;23:641–720.
289. Washburn RA, Figoni SF. Physical activity and chronic cardiovascular disease prevention in spinal cord injury:

a comprehensive literature review. *Top Spinal Cord Injury Rehabil* 1998;3:16–32.

290. Jacobs PL, Nash MS. Exercise recommendations for individuals with spinal cord injury. *Sports Med* 2004;34:727–751.
291. Ditor DS, Macdonald MJ, Kamath MV, et al. The effects of body-weight supported treadmill training on cardiovascular regulation in individuals with motor-complete SCI. *Spinal Cord* 2005;43(11):664–673.
292. Thijssen DH, Ellenkamp R, Smits P, et al. Rapid vascular adaptations to training and detraining in persons with spinal cord injury. *Arch Phys Med Rehabil* 2006;87(4):474–481.
293. Coutts KD, Rhodes EC, McKenzie DC. Maximal exercise responses of tetraplegics and paraplegics. *J Appl Physiol* 1983;55:479–482.
294. Ellenberg M, MacRitchie M, Franklin B, et al. Aerobic capacity in early paraplegia: implications for rehabilitation. *Paraplegia* 1989;27:261–268.
295. Drory Y, Ohry A, Brooks ME, et al. Arm crank ergometry in chronic spinal cord injured patients. *Arch Phys Med Rehabil* 1990;71:389–392.
296. Figoni SF. Exercise responses and quadriplegia. *Med Sci Sports Exerc* 1993;25:433–441.
297. Dallmeijer AJ, van der Woude LH, van Kamp GJ, et al. Changes in lipid, lipoprotein and apolipoprotein profiles in persons with spinal cord injuries during the first 2 years post-injury. *Spinal Cord* 1999;37(2):96–102.
298. Bauman WA, Spungen AM. Disorders of carbohydrate and lipid metabolism in veterans with paraplegia or quadriplegia: a model of premature aging. *Metabolism* 1994;43(6):749–756.
299. Bauman WA, Spungen AM, Zhong YG, et al. Depressed serum high density lipoprotein cholesterol levels in veterans with spinal cord injury. *Paraplegia* 1992;30(10):697–703.
300. Frost F, Roach MJ, Kushner I, et al. Inflammatory C-reactive protein and cytokine levels in asymptomatic people with chronic spinal cord injury. *Arch Phys Med Rehabil* 2005;86(2):312–317.
301. Lee MY, Myers J, Hayes A, et al. C-reactive protein, metabolic syndrome, and insulin resistance in individuals with spinal cord injury. *J Spinal Cord Med* 2005;28:20–25.
302. Guerrero-Romero F, Rodriguez-Moran M. Relation of C-reactive protein to features of the metabolic syndrome in normal glucose tolerant, impaired glucose tolerant, newly diagnosed type 2 diabetic subjects. *Diabetes Metab* 2003;29:65–71.
303. Bauman WA, Kahan NN, Grimm DR, et al: Risk factors for atherogenesis and cardiovascular autonomic function in persons with spinal cord injury. *Spinal Cord* 1999;37:601–616.
304. Manns PJ, McCubbin JA, Williams DP. Fitness, inflammation, and the metabolic syndrome in men with paraplegia. *Arch Phys Med Rehabil* 2005;86:1176–1181.
305. Bauman WA, Spungen AM. Metabolic changes in persons with spinal cord injury. *Phys Med Rehabil Clin N Am* 2000;11:109–40.
306. Demirel S, Demirel G, Tukek T, et al. Risk factors for coronary heart disease in patients with spinal cord injury in Turkey. *Spinal Cord* 2001;39:134–138.
307. Maruyama Y, Mizuguchi M, Yaginuma T, et al. Serum leptin, abdominal obesity and the metabolic syndrome in individuals with chronic spinal cord injury. *Spinal Cord* 2008;46(7):494–499.
308. Liang H, Mojtahedi MC, Chen D, et al. Elevated C-reactive protein associated with decreased high-density lipoprotein cholesterol in men with spinal cord injury. *Arch Phys Med Rehabil* 2008;89(1):36–41.
309. Bauman WA, Spungen AM. Coronary heart disease in individuals with spinal cord injury: assessment of risk factors. *Spinal Cord* 2008;46(7):466–476.
310. Brenes G, Dearwater S, Shapera R, et al. High density lipoprotein cholesterol concentrations in physically active and sedentary spinal cord injured patients. *Arch Phys Med Rehabil* 1986;67:445–450.
311. Okuma H, Ogata H, Hatada K. Transition of physical fitness in wheelchair marathon competitors over several years. *Paraplegia* 1989;27:237–243.
312. Zwiren LD, Bar-Or O. Responses to exercise of paraplegics who differ in conditioning level. *Med Sci Sports* 1975;7:94–98.
313. Price DT, Davidoff R, Balady GJ. Comparison of cardiovascular adaptations to long-term arm and leg exercise in wheelchair athletes versus long-distance runners. *Am J Cardiol* 2000;85(8):996–1001.
314. Figoni SF. Perspectives on cardiovascular fitness and SCI [published erratum appears in *J Am Paraplegia Soc* 1991;14(1):21]. *J Am Paraplegia Soc* 1990;13:63–71.
315. Thomas AJ, Davis GM, Sutton JR. Cardiovascular and metabolic responses to electrical stimulation-induced leg exercise in spinal cord injury. *Methods Inf Med* 1997;36:372–375.
316. Raymond J, Davis GM, Bryant G, et al. Cardiovascular responses to an orthostatic challenge and electrical-stimulation-induced leg muscle contractions in individuals with paraplegia. *Eur J Appl Physiol* 1999;80:205–212.
317. Fornusek C, Davis GM. Cardiovascular and metabolic responses during functional electric stimulation cycling at different cadences. *Arch Phys Med Rehabil* 2008;89(4):719–25.
318. Raymond J, Davis GM, van der Plas M. Cardiovascular responses during submaximal electrical stimulation-induced leg cycling in individuals with paraplegia. *Clin Physiolol Funct Imaging* 2002;22(2):92–98.
319. Stoner L, Sabatier MJ, Mahoney ET, *Dudley GA, McCully KK*. Electrical stimulation-evoked resistance exercise therapy improves arterial health after chronic spinal cord injury. *Spinal Cord* 2007;45(1):49–56.
320. Laskin JJ, Ashley EA, Olenik LM, et al. Electrical stimulation-assisted rowing exercise in spinal cord injured people. A pilot study. *Paraplegia* 1993;31:534–541.
321. Wheeler GD, Andrews B, Lederer R, et al. Functional electric stimulation [ndash]assisted rowing: increasing cardiovascular fitness through functional electric stimulation rowing training in persons with spinal cord injury. *Arch Phys Med Rehabil* 2002;83:1093–1099.
322. Raymond J, Davis GM, Fahey A, et al. Oxygen uptake and heart rate responses during arm vs combined arm/electrically stimulated leg exercise in people with paraplegia. *Spinal Cord* 1997;35:680–685.
323. Phillips WT, Burkett LN. Augmented upper body contribution to oxygen uptake during upper body

exercise with concurrent leg functional electrical stimulation in persons with spinal cord injury. *Spinal Cord* 1998;36:750–755.
324. Raymond J, Davis GM, Climstein M, et al. Cardiorespiratory responses to arm cranking and electrical stimulation leg cycling in people with paraplegia. *Med Sci Sports Exerc* 1999;31:822–828.
325. Hooker SP, Figoni SF, Rodgers MM, et al. Metabolic and hemodynamic responses to concurrent voluntary arm crank and electrical stimulation leg cycle exercise in quadriplegics. *J Rehabil Res Dev* 1992;29:1–11.
326. Raymond J, Davis GM, Clarke J, et al. Cardiovascular responses during arm exercises and orthostatic challenge in individuals with paraplegia. *Eur J Appl Physiol* 2001;85(1–2):89–95.
327. Thijssen DH, Heesterbeek P, van Kuppevelt DJ, et al. Local vascular adaptations after hybrid training in spinal cord-injured subjects. *Med Sci Sports Exerc* 2005;37:1112–1118.
328. Phillips W, Burkett LN, Munro R, et al. Relative changes in blood flow with functional electrical stimulation during exercise of the paralyzed lower limbs. *Paraplegia* 1995;33:90–93.
329. Hooker SP, Figoni SF, Rodgers MM, et al. Physiologic effects of electrical stimulation leg cycle exercise training in spinal cord injured persons. *Arch Phys Med Rehabil* 1992;73:470–476.
330. Hooker SP, Scremin AM, Mutton DL, et al. Peak and submaximal physiologic responses following electrical stimulation leg cycle ergometer training. *J Rehabil Res Dev* 1995;32:361–366.
331. Krauss JC, Robergs RA, Depaepe JL, et al. Effects of electrical stimulation and upper body training after spinal cord injury. *Med Sci Sports Exerc* 1993;25:1054–1061.
332. Mutton DL, Scremin AM, Barstow TJ, et al. Physiologic responses during functional electrical stimulation leg cycling and hybrid exercise in spinal cord injured subjects. *Arch Phys Med Rehabil* 1997;78:712–718.
333. Carvalho DC, de Cassia Zanchetta M, Sereni JM, et al. Metabolic and cardiorespiratory responses of tetraplegic subjects during treadmill walking using neuromuscular stimulation and partial body weight support. *Spinal Cord* 2005;43:400–405.
334. Carvalho DC, Chiquet A Jr. Energy expenditure during rest and treadmill gait training in quadriplegic subjects. *Spinal Cord* 2005;43:658–63.
335. Carvalho DC, Martins CL, Cardoso SD, et al. Improvement of metabolic and cardiorespiratory responses through treadmill gait training with neuromuscular electrical stimulation in quadriplegic subjects. *Artif Organs* 2006;30:56–63.
336. Nash MS, Jacobs PL, Mendez AJ, et al. Circuit resistance training improves the atherogenic lipid profiles of persons with chronic paraplegia. *J Spinal Cord Med* 2001;24(1):2–9.
337. Szlachcic Y, Adkins RH, Adal T, et al. The effect of dietary intervention on lipid profiles in individuals with spinal cord injury. *J Spinal Cord Med* 2001;24(1):26–29.
338. Nash MS, Bilsker S, Marcillo AE, et al. Reversal of adaptive left ventricular atrophy following electrically-stimulated exercise training in human tetraplegics. *Paraplegia* 1991;29:590–599.
339. Burnham R, Dearwater S, Stein R, et al. Skeletal muscle fibre type transformation following spinal cord injury. *Spinal Cord* 1997;35:86–91.
340. Thomas CK, Zaidner EY, Calancie B, et al. Muscle weakness, paralysis, and atrophy after human cervical spinal cord injury. *Exp Neurol* 1997;148:414–423.
341. Peckham PH, Mortimer JT, Van Der Meulen JP. Physiologic and metabolic changes in white muscle of cat following induced exercise. *Brain Res* 1973;50:424–429.
342. Pette D, Muller W, Leisner E, et al. Time dependent effects on contractile properties, fibre population, myosin light chains and enzymes of energy metabolism in intermittently and continuously stimulated fast twitch muscles of the rabbit. *Pflugers Arch* 1976;364:103–112.
343. Martin TP, Stein RB, Hoeppner PH, et al. Influence of electrical stimulation on the morphological and metabolic properties of paralyzed muscle. *J Appl Physiol* 1992;72:1401–1406.
344. Chilibeck PD, Jeon J, Weiss C, et al. Histochemical changes in muscle of individuals with spinal cord injury following functional electrical stimulated exercise training. *Spinal Cord* 1999;37:264–268.
345. Greve JM, Muszkat R, Schmidt B, et al. Functional electrical stimulation (FES): muscle histochemical analysis. *Paraplegia* 1993;31:764–770.
346. Andersen JL, Mohr T, Biering-Sorensen F, et al. Myosin heavy chain isoform transformation in single fibres from m. vastus lateralis in spinal cord injured individuals: effects of long-term functional electrical stimulation (FES). *Pflugers Arch* 1996;431:513–518.
347. Neumayer C, Happak W, Kern H, et al. Hypertrophy and transformation of muscle fibers in paraplegic patients. *Artif Organs* 1997;21:188–190.
348. Pacy PJ, Hesp R, Halliday DA, et al. Muscle and bone in paraplegic patients, and the effect of functional electrical stimulation. *Clin Sci* 1988;75:481–487.
349. Ragnarsson KT. Physiologic effects of functional electrical stimulation-induced exercises in spinal cord-injured individuals. *Clin Orthop* 1988:53–63.
350. Sloan KE, Bremner LA, Byrne J, et al. Musculoskeletal effects of an electrical stimulation induced cycling programme in the spinal injured. *Paraplegia* 1994;32:407–415.
351. Scremin AM, Kurta L, Gentili A, et al. Increasing muscle mass in spinal cord injured persons with a functional electrical stimulation exercise program. *Arch Phys Med Rehabil* 1999;80:1531–1536.
352. Dudley GA, Castro MJ, Rogers S, et al. A simple means of increasing muscle size after spinal cord injury: a pilot study. *Eur J Appl Physiol* 1999;80:394–396.
353. Kern H, Rossini K, Carraro U, et al. Muscle biopsies show that FES of denervated muscles reverses human muscle degeneration from permanent spinal motoneuron lesion. *J Rehabil Res Dev* 2005;42(3 Suppl 1):43–53.
354. Baldi JC, Jackson RD, Moraille R, et al. Muscle atrophy is prevented in patients with acute spinal cord injury using functional electrical stimulation. *Spinal Cord* 1998;36:463–469.
355. Rodgers MM, Glaser RM, Figoni SF, et al. Musculoskeletal responses of spinal cord injured individuals to functional neuromuscular stimulation-induced knee extension exercise training. *J Rehabil Res Dev* 1991;28:19–26.

356. Sabatier MJ, Stoner L, Mahoney ET, et al. Electrically stimulated resistance training in SCI individuals increases muscle fatigue resistance but not femoral artery size or blood flow. *Spinal Cord* 2006;44(4):227–233.
357. National Spinal Cord Injury Statistical Center, University of Alabama at Birmingham, 2006 Annual Statistical Report, July, 2006.
358. Yarkony GM, heinemann AW. Pressure ulcers. In: Stover SL, Delisa JA, Whiteneck GG, eds. *Spinal cord injury: clinical outcomes from the model systems*. Gathersburg, MD: Aspen Publishing, 1995.
359. Bergstrom N, Bennett MA, Carlson CE, et al. Treatment of pressure ulcers. Clinical Practice Guidelines No 15. Rockville Md: US Department of Health and Human Services, Agency for Health Care Policy and Research, 1994.
360. Griffin JW, Tooms RE, Mendius RA, et al. Efficacy of high voltage pulsed current for healing of pressure ulcers in patients with spinal cord injury. *Phys Ther* 1991;71(6):433–442.
361. Feedar JA, Kloth LC, Gentzkow GD. Chronic dermal ulcer healing enhanced with monophasic pulsed electrical stimulation. *Phys Ther* 1991;71(9):639–649.
362. Gerrits HL, de Haan A, Sargeant AJ, et al. Peripheral vascular changes after electrically stimulated cycle training in people with spinal cord injury. *Arch Phys Med Rehabil* 2001;82(6):832–839.
363. Levine SP, Kett RL, Gross MD, et al. Blood flow in the gluteus maximus of seated individuals during electrical muscle stimulation. *Arch Phys Med Rehabil* 1990;71(9):682–686.
364. Liu LQ, Nicholson GP, Knight SL, et al. Interface pressure and cutaneous hemoglobin and oxygenation changes under ischial tuberosities during sacral nerve root stimulation in spinal cord injury. *J Rehabil Res Dev* 2006;43(4):553–564.
365. Bogie KM, Triolo RJ. Effects of regular use of neuromuscular electrical stimulation on tissue health. *J Rehabil Res Dev* 2003;40(6):469–475.
366. Liu LQ, Nicholson GP, Knight SL, et al. Pressure changes under the ischial tuberosities of seated individuals during sacral nerve root stimulation. *J Rehabil Res Dev* 2006;43(2):209–218.
367. Seib TP, Price R, Reyes MR, et al.The quantitative measurement of spasticity: effect of cutaneous electrical stimulation. *Arch Phys Med Rehabil.* 1994;75(7):746–750.
368. Bogie KM, Wang X, Triolo RJ. Long-term prevention of pressure ulcers in high-risk patients: a single case study of the use of gluteal neuromuscular electric stimulation. *Arch Phys Med Rehabil* 2006;87(4):585–591.
369. Levine SP, Kett RL, Cederna PS, et al. Electric muscle stimulation for pressure sore prevention: tissue shape variation. *Arch Phys Med Rehabil* 1990;71(3):210–215.
370. Garland DE, Stewart CA, Adkins RH, et al. Osteoporosis after spinal cord injury. *J Orthop Res* 1992;10:371–378.
371. Chen B, Stein A. Osteoporosis in acute spinal cord injury. *Top Spinal Cord Inj Rehabil* 2003;9:26–35.
372. Eser P, Frotzler A, Zehnder Y, et al. Relationship between the duration of paralysis and bone structure: a pQCT study of spinal cord injured individuals. *Bone* 2004;34(5):869–880.
373. Ragnarsson KT, Sell GH. Lower extremity fractures after SCI: A retrospective study. *Arch Phys Med Rehabil* 1981;62:418–423.
374. Jones LM, Legge M, Goulding A. Intensive exercise may preserve bone mass of the upper limbs in spinal cord injured males but does not retard demineralization of the lower body. *Spinal Cord* 2002;40: 230–235.
375. Lazo MG, Shirazi P, Sam M, et al. Osteoporosis and risk of fracture in men with spinal cord injury. *Spinal Cord* 2001;39:208–214.
376. Wei CN. Does electrical stimulation of the sciatic nerve prevent suspension-induced changes in rat hindlimb bones? *Jpn J Physiol* 1998;48:33–37.
377. Kaplan RE, Roden W, Gilbert E, et al. Reduction of hypercalciuria in tetraplegia after weight-bearing and strengthening. *Paraplegia* 1981;19:289–293.
378. Leeds EM, Klose KJ, Ganz W, et al. Bone mineral density after bicycle ergometry training. *Arch Phys Med Rehabil* 1990;71:207–209.
379. Hangartner TN, Rodgers MM, Glaser RM, et al. Tibial bone density loss in spinal cord injured patients: effects of FES exercise. *J Rehabil Res Dev* 1994;31: 50–61.
380. BeDell KK, Scremin AME, Perell KL, et al. Effects of functional electrical stimulation-induced lower extremity cycling on bone density of spinal cord-injured patients. *Am J Phys Med Rehabil* 1996;75:29–34.
381. Bloomfield SA, Mysiw WJ, Jackson RD. Bone mass and endocrine adaptations to training in spinal cord injured individuals. *Bone* 1996;19:61–68.
382. Mohr T, Podenphant J, Biering-Sorensen F, et al. Increased bone mineral density after prolonged electrically induced cycle training of paralyzed limbs in spinal cord injured man. *Calcif Tissue Int* 1997;61: 22–25.
383. Dudley-Javoroski S, Shields RK. Muscle and bone plasticity after spinal cord injury: review of adaptations to disuse and to electrical muscle stimulation. *J Rehabil Res Dev* 2008;45(2):283–96.
384. Shields RK, Dudley-Javoroski S. Musculoskeletal plasticity after acute spinal cord injury: effects of long-term neuromuscular electrical stimulation training. *J Neurophysiol* 2006;95(4):2380–2390.
385. Merli GJ, Crabbe S, Paluzzi RG, et al. Etiology, incidence, and prevention of deep vein thrombosis in acute spinal cord injury. *Arch Phys Med Rehabil* 1993;74:1199–1205.
386. Katz RT, Green D, Sullivan T, et al. Functional electrical stimulation to enhance systemic fibrinolytic activity in spinal cord injury patients. *Arch Phys Med Rehabil* 1987;68:423–426.
387. Merli GJ, Herbison GJ, Ditunno JF, et al. Deep vein thrombosis: prophylaxis in acute spinal cord injured patients. *Arch Phys Med Rehabil* 1988;69:661–664.
388. Adler D, Gonzalez-Bermejo J, Duguet A, et.al. Diaphragm pacing restores olfaction in tetraplegia. *Eur Respir* 2009;34:365–370.

CHAPTER 26 ■ NEUROPATHIC PAIN AFTER SPINAL CORD INJURY

EVA G. WIDERSTRÖM-NOGA

CHAPTER OVERVIEW

This chapter focuses on the persistent pain types that occur after a spinal cord injury (SCI) with a specific emphasis on the neuropathic pain. Because there is a current and strong emphasis on a mechanism-based classification for pain in general (1,2), as well as after SCI (3), this chapter discusses basic mechanisms of neuropathic pain, pain assessment and classification, and treatment approaches to the neuropathic pain types after SCI. Musculoskeletal pains are covered in chapter 16.

Problem

Chronic pain is a serious consequence of SCI that is associated with lower general health and well-being, and with higher levels of depression (4). Because some of the pain types that occur after an SCI can be both persistent and severe, there is a risk for significant psychosocial impact (5,6) and a substantially reduced quality of life (7).

Despite best efforts, chronic pain associated with SCI is not consistently relieved by currently available treatments (8–10). Therefore, individuals with SCI continue to experience pain long after their initial injury (11,12). Indeed, pain relief, together with issues related to occupational and sexual activities, has been identified in a large multicenter study (13) as a significant and unmet need after SCI.

Prevalence

The prevalence of SCI-related pain varies among studies primarily due to methodological differences including diverse assessment criteria and classification schemes (14). Interestingly, several large scale studies that have investigated the prevalence of persistent pain conditions after SCI show remarkably similar rates ranging from 66% to 79% (4,15–21).

Classification of Pain

One important goal of SCI pain classification is to differentiate between nociceptive and neuropathic pain types since they usually require different treatment strategies. Unfortunately, there is no diagnostic measure available that can accurately diagnose neuropathic pain after SCI. This is not only a problem after SCI but has been recognized as a general problem in pain research and in clinical pain management. Therefore, the International Association for the Study of Pain (IASP) recently proposed a revision of the current pain terminology. While neuropathic pain is currently defined as "Pain initiated or caused by a primary lesion or dysfunction in the nervous system" (22), Treede et al. (23) suggested to omit "dysfunction" from this definition and define neuropathic pain as "Pain arising as a direct consequence of a lesion or disease affecting the somatosensory system." Because of the difficulty of diagnosing pain as being either neuropathic or non-neuropathic, these authors proposed a grading system of "definite," "probable," and "possible" neuropathic pain. For the diagnosis of "definite" neuropathic pain, the following criteria were proposed: (a) a pain distribution consistent with injury to the peripheral nervous system (PNS) or the central nervous system (CNS); (b) a history of an injury or disease affecting the PNS or CNS; (c) abnormal sensory signs within the body area corresponding to the injured component of the CNS or PNS; and (d) a diagnostic test confirming a lesion or disease in these structures. Although these criteria can usually be applied to SCI-related pain, the differentiation between neuropathic and nociceptive pain may be more difficult when pain is located below the lesion level and the injury is incomplete. In these cases, abnormal sensory signs may not contribute to the diagnosis of neuropathic pain, since sensory abnormalities will be present regardless of whether pain is nociceptive or neuropathic (24).

SCI Pain Taxonomy

There are currently several classification systems available that aim to provide a framework for the different types of pain that people experience following an SCI (25–28). These were recently reviewed by an SCI pain consensus group sponsored by the National Institute on Disability and Rehabilitation Research (NIDDR) in the Office of Special Education and Rehabilitation Services, US Department of Education (29). Due to the fact that the underlying mechanisms of SCI-related pain are incompletely known, a mechanisms-based SCI pain taxonomy needs to be updated when new knowledge becomes available. The most recently published version is included in the International SCI Basic Pain Data Set (ISCIBPDS) (30). The ISCIBPD includes an SCI pain classification as part of a more general pain assessment and integrates aspects of earlier SCI pain taxonomies.

The most frequently used SCI pain classification is the IASP taxonomy (Table 26.1) (31), which first classifies pain

TABLE 26.1

INTERNATIONAL ASSOCIATION FOR THE STUDY OF PAIN TAXONOMY

Broad type (Tier 1)	Broad system (Tier 2)	Specific structures/pathology (Tier 3)
Nociceptive	Musculoskeletal	Bone, joint, muscle trauma or inflammation. Mechanical instability. Muscle spasm. Secondary overuse syndromes.
	Visceral	Renal calculus, bowel, sphincter dysfunction, etc. Dysreflexic headache
Neuropathic	Above level	Compressive mononeuropathies. Complex regional pain syndromes
	At level	Nerve root compression (including cauda equina) Syringomyelia Spinal cord trauma/ischaemia (transitional zone, etc.) Dual level cord and root trauma (double lesion syndrome)
	Below level	Spinal cord trauma/ischemia (central dysesthesia syndrome, etc.)

as either nociceptive or neuropathic (Tier 1). In Tier 2, further differentiation of these two subgroups of pain is made. Nociceptive pain is differentiated into either musculoskeletal or visceral, and neuropathic pain is categorized into above, at, and below level pain. The last and third Tier defines the structural causes underlying the specific pain when this information is available. "Good" (78%) agreement between raters in differentiating pain into neuropathic or nociceptive pain was reported by Putzke and collegues (Putzke JD, Richards JS, Ness T, Kezar L. Interrater reliability of the International Association for the Study of Pain and Tunks' spinal cord injury pain classification schemes. Am J Phys Med Rehabil. 2003;82:437-440).

TABLE 26.2

BRYCE/RAGNARSSON SCI PAIN TAXONOMY

Location		Type	Etiologic subtype
Above level	Nociceptive	1	Mechanical/musculoskeletal
		2	Autonomic dysreflexia
		3	headache
			Other
	Neuropathic	4	Compressive neuropathy
		5	Other
At level	Nociceptive	6	Mechanical/musculoskeletal
		7	Visceral
	Neuropathic	8	Central
		9	Radicular
		10	Compressive neuropathy
		11	CRPS
Below level	Nociceptive	12	Mechanical/musculoskeletal
		13	Visceral
	Neuropathic	14	Central
		15	Other

From Bryce TN, Ragnarsson KT. Pain after spinal cord injury. *Phys Med Rehabil Clin N Am* 2000;11(1):157–168.

The Bryce/Ragnarsson SCI Pain taxonomy (Table 26.2) (26) is a three-tiered taxonomy similar to the IASP pain taxonomy. The primary difference between the two taxonomies is that the two first tiers are reversed, that is, *first* the location of pain relative to injury is defined and *second* a differentiation into a neuropathic or nociceptive subcategory is made. It is important to note that in this classification, "at level" encompasses five dermatomes including two levels below and two levels above the neurological level of injury (NLI). "Above the level" therefore starts at two dermatomes rostral to the NLI and "below the level," two levels distal to the NLI. Psychometric examination of Tier 1 and 2 classification indicated "very good" (84 and 86% agreement, respectively) inter-rater reliability (32).

The Cardenas SCI Pain taxonomy (25) divides pain into two categories, that is, neurologic and musculoskeletal. The neurologic category is differentiated into SCI pain, transition zone pain, radicular pain, and visceral pain, and the musculoskeletal pain is divided into mechanical spine pain and overuse pain. The test–retest reliability of the Cardenas taxonomy is supported (33) with kappa values indicating "good"(68%) agreement.

The SCI pain classification section of the ISCIBPDS is similar to the IASP and Bryce/Ragnarsson SCI pain taxonomies, in that a differentiation into nociceptive or neuropathic pain categories is made. The pain classification within the ISCIBPDS will be discussed in more detail below in the context of the other elements of the ISCIBPDS (see also Tables 26.3–26.7). The ISCIBPDS in its entirety has been reviewed and endorsed by major SCI and pain organizations with a significant interest in SCI, and is now part of the National Institute of Neurological

TABLE 26.3

THE ISCIPBDS FORM

Date of data collection: YYYY/MM/DD
Have you had any pain during the last 7 d including today: ❑ No ❑ Yes
If yes, how many different pain problems did you have? ❑ 1; ❑ 2; ❑ 3; ❑ 4; ❑ ≥5
Please describe your *three* worst pain problems:

Pain locations/sites	R	M	L	Type of pain	Intensity and temporal pattern of pain
(can be more than one, so check all that apply): right (R), midline (M), or left (L)				(check all that apply)	
Head **Neck/shoulders** throat neck Shoulder				**Nociceptive** ❑ Musculoskeletal ❑ Visceral ❑ Other	**Average pain intensity in the last week:** 0 = no pain; 10 = pain as bad as you can imagine ❑ 0; ❑ 1; ❑ 2; ❑ 3; ❑ 4; ❑ 5; ❑ 6; ❑ 7; ❑ 8; ❑ 9; ❑ 10 **Date of onset:** YYYY/MM/DD **Number of days with pain in the last 7 d including today:**
Arms/hands upper arm elbow forearm wrist hand/fingers				**Neuropathic** ❑ At-level ❑ Below-level ❑ Other **❑ Unknown**	❑ none; ❑ 1; ❑ 2; ❑ 3; ❑ 4; ❑ 5; ❑ 6; ❑ 7; ❑ unknown **How long does your pain usually last:** ❑ ≤ 1 min; ❑ > 1 min but < 1 h; ❑ ≥ 1 h but < 24 h; ❑ ≥ 24 h;
Frontal torso/genitals chest Abdomen pelvis/genitalia					❑ constant or continuous; ❑ unknown **When during the day is the pain most intense:**
Back upper back lower back **Buttocks/hips** buttocks hip anus					❑ morning (06.01–12.00); ❑ afternoon (12.01–18.00); ❑ evening (18.01–24.00); ❑ night (00.01–06.00); ❑ unpredictable; pain is not consistently more intense at any one time of day
Upper legs/thighs **Lower legs/feet** knee shin calf ankle foot/toes					

Please note that the time period during the last week applies to all pain interference questions.

How much do you limit your activities in order to keep your pain from getting worse?
Not at all ❑ 0 - ❑ 1 - ❑ 2 - ❑ 3 - ❑ 4 - ❑ 5 - ❑ 6 Very much

How much has your pain changed your ability to take part in recreational and other social activities?
No change ❑ 0 - ❑ 1 - ❑ 2 - ❑ 3 - ❑ 4 - ❑ 5 - ❑ 6 Extreme change

How much has your pain changed the amount of satisfaction or enjoyment you get from family-related activities?
No change ❑ 0 - ❑ 1 - ❑ 2 - ❑ 3 - ❑ 4 - ❑ 5 - ❑ 6 Extreme change

In general, how much has pain interfered with your day-to-day activities in the last week?
No interference ❑ 0 - ❑ 1 - ❑ 2 - ❑ 3 - ❑ 4 - ❑ 5 - ❑ 6 Extreme interference

In general, how much has pain interfered with your overall mood in the past week?
No interference ❑ 0 - ❑ 1 - ❑ 2 - ❑ 3 - ❑ 4 - ❑ 5 - ❑ 6 Extreme interference

In general, how much has pain interfered with your ability to get a good night's sleep?
No interference ❑ 0 - ❑ 1 - ❑ 2 - ❑ 3 - ❑ 4 - ❑ 5 - ❑ 6 Extreme interference

Are you using or receiving any *Treatment* for your pain problem: ❑ No ❑ Yes

TABLE 26.4

THE ISCIBPDS: BACKGROUND QUESTIONS, NUMBER OF PAIN PROBLEMS, AND PAIN LOCATION

Items	Instructions
Date of data collection	This purpose for collecting this information is to relate these data to others collected in the same individual at various time points.
Have you had any pain during the last 7 d including today?	This question evaluates any present, chronic, and intermittent pain. The 7-d interval was chosen to capture both constant and intermittent pain. This question can also be used as Basic Pain Question in other questionnaires, i.e., a gate question to the ISCIBPDS.
If yes, how many different pain problems do you have?	This question is asked to determine how many different pain problems a person perceives that he or she has experienced during the last 7 d. A "pain problem" is defined by the person himself as a pain that has a specific quality and character. A pain problem can be located in one area or extend over several areas. Persons who experience SCI-related pain can usually differentiate between different pain problems (88).
Description of the three worst pain problems	In this question, each person is asked to describe the three worst pain problems they are currently experiencing. The description provided is limited to 3 problems because most people with SCI experience 3 or fewer pain problems (88). In addition, describing more than 3 different simultaneous pain problems may induce errors in the data collection due to assessment burden.
Location(s) of pain	This question concerns the location of pain and is based on each individual's perception of where his or her pain is located. The division into pain areas is based on a pain drawing originally described by Margolis et al. (183). This has been recalculated into 8 body areas (184): (a) head; (b) neck/shoulders; (c) arms/hands; (d) frontal torso/genitals; (e) back; (f) buttocks/hips; (g) upper legs/thighs; and (h) lower legs/feet. Within each pain area, further divisions into more precise locations can be made. Please note that pain may be experienced in more than one pain area. The descriptions of the pain locations are meant to be based on each individual's perception of the location of pain. Therefore, the delineations of these areas are not defined with precise anatomical landmarks. Several locations may be given for each pain problem, e.g., neck and either shoulders, or pain in the abdomen extending into the buttocks and thighs areas and further down to the feet.

TABLE 26.5

THE ISCIBPDS: PAIN CLASSIFICATION

Pain type	Description
Nociceptive *Musculoskeletal*	Pain above, at or below the NLI, in a region where there is some preserved sensation. Generated by nociceptors in muscles and joints and may be described as "dull" or "aching" pain related to movement, tenderness upon palpation, pain relief in response to anti-inflammatory medications or evidence of skeletal pathology on imaging. *Examples include spinal fractures, muscular injury, shoulder overuse syndromes, and muscle spasms.*
Nociceptive *Visceral*	Pain in the thorax or abdomen and generated in visceral structures. This pain may be described as "dull," "aching" or "cramping" and due to known visceral pathology or dysfunction, e.g., infection or obstruction. *Examples include urinary tract infection, ureteric calculus and bowel impaction.* A neuropathic pain diagnosis may be considered if no evidence of visceral pathology or positive response to treatments targeting such pathology.
Nociceptive *Other*	Nociceptive pain that do not fall into the musculoskeletal or visceral categories. These pains may be directly related to SCI (e.g., pressure areas and dysreflexic headache) or unrelated to SCI (e.g., migraine). This category provides a classification for nociceptive pains that are not specifically related to SCI.
Neuropathic *At-level*	Pain located anywhere within the dermatome of the level of neurological injury and three dermatomes below this level and may be described as "burning," "electric" or "shooting." Sensory abnormalities such as allodynia or hyperalgesia within the painful area are common. The pain may be unilateral or bilateral. Neuropathic pain associated with cauda equina injury is radicular in nature and defined as *At-level* pain regardless of distribution.
Neuropathic *Below-level*	Pain located in the region more than three dermatomes below the NLI. This pain may be described as "burning," "electric" or "shooting" and may have a diffuse, regional distribution. Sensory abnormalities such as allodynia or hyperalgesia may be present. If the neuropathic pain is present both at and below the level of injury and the patient is unable to distinguish two separate pain problems, both At-level (Neuropathic) and Below-level (Neuropathic) can be checked. If two separate pains are distinguishable, the two pain types, i.e., *At-level (Neuropathic)* and *Below-level (Neuropathic)* are classified as two different pains.
Neuropathic *Other*	Pain located above, at or below the NLI but not caused directly by a lesion or disease affecting the spinal cord or nerve roots. *Examples include post-herpetic neuralgia, pain associated with diabetic neuropathy, central post stroke pain, and compressive mononeuropathies.*
Unknown	Pain that cannot be classified into the categories listed above.

TABLE 26.6

THE ISCIBPDS: PAIN INTENSITY AND TEMPORAL PATTERN

Items	Instructions
Average pain intensity in the last week	The 7 d time frame was selected to balance the need to assess pain over a long enough epoch to capture usual pain, against the need to keep the time frame short enough to maximize recall accuracy. This question uses a 0–10 NRS (ranging from 0 = "No pain" to a maximum of 10 = "Pain as bad as you can imagine") of average pain intensity for each of the pain problems.
Date of onset.	This variable specifies the date when each pain problem started.
Number of days with pain in the last 7 d including today.	This variable specifies the total number of days with pain during the last 7 d, including today.
How long does your pain usually last?	This question concerns the duration of pain and the response categories range from "1 min or less" to "constant or continuous." The duration of pain can be defined when a specific pain follows a predictable pattern. If no predictable pattern for a specific pain exists, the answer "unknown" is given
When is the pain most intense?	This question identifies the diurnal peak in pain intensity. The response categories are "morning," "afternoon," "evening," "night," and "unpredictable."

Disorders and Stroke's SCI Common Data Elements http://www.commondataelements.ninds.nih.gov/SCI.aspx. However, additional revisions of the SCI pain taxonomy and psychometric studies are underway for the purpose of standardization, facilitating collaborations, research, and ultimately the clinical management of SCI-related pain.

MULTIDIMENSIONAL PAIN ASSESSMENT

Since persistent pain, regardless of type, depends on multiple pathophysiological mechanisms and a variety of psychosocial factors, a comprehensive pain evaluation should, in addition to a clinical examination, include characteristics of pain, sensory status, and relevant psychosocial factors. In contrast to many other chronic pain populations, persons with SCI often experience several concomitant types of pain, each with specific clinical characteristics (20) and potentially differing origins. Therefore, it is important to evaluate each pain separately since the diagnosis and the treatment strategy may differ between various types of pain.

Symptoms

The diagnosis of neuropathic pain is complex and includes in addition to positive sensory signs (e.g., allodynia or hyperalgesia) or negative signs (e.g., sensory deficits) a combination of self-reported symptoms, such as "burning" or "electric" pain qualities (34). There are several self-report methods available that are useful in clinical or research settings as part of the neuropathic pain diagnosis. For example, the Neuropathic Pain Symptom Inventory (NPSI) (35) assesses temporal aspects, quality, and severity of pain rated on a numerical rating scale (NRS). The NPSI includes questions about the severity of specific *spontaneous* pain qualities (i.e., "burning," "squeezing," "pressure," "electric," or "stabbing"), pain *evoked* by various stimuli (i.e., "brushing," "pressure," or "cold"), and other abnormal *spontaneous* sensations (i.e., "pins and needles," or "tingling"). The validity of the questions included in the NPSI and the potential usefulness across various neuropathic pain populations is supported by other research indicating that "burning," "electric shocks," "numbness," and "pins and needles" are some of the most common descriptors used by persons who experience neuropathic pain (36). The Neuro-

TABLE 26.7

THE ISCIBPDS: PAIN INTERFERENCE QUESTIONS

Items	Instructions
How much do you limit your activities in order to keep your pain from getting worse? *How much has your pain changed your ability to take part in recreational and other social activities?* *How much has your pain changed the amount of satisfaction or enjoyment you get from family-related activities?* *In general, how much has pain interfered with your day-to-day activities in the last week?* *In general, how much has pain interfered with your overall mood in the past week?* *In general, how much has pain interfered with your ability to get a good night's sleep?*	The answers to the interference questions are scaled from 0–6 and refer to pain interference experienced during the previous week.

pathic Pain Scale (NPS) (37) is another instrument that appears to be particularly useful in the differentiation of neuropathic and non-neuropathic pain in patients with heterogeneous pain (38). It includes ratings of pain intensity and unpleasantness, pain quality ("sharp," "dull," "sensitive," "hot," "cold," and "itchy pain"), and spatial qualities ("deep" and "surface" pain). Each item is rated on a NRS ranging from 0 = "no pain" or "not (sensation/item)" to 10 = "the most (descriptor) pain sensation imaginable." Each item can be scored separately to define treatment effects on specific symptoms, or the items can be added to create an average score to determine a more general treatment effect. This scale also includes a description of the temporal aspects of pain (constant, constant with fluctuations, or intermittent). Similarly, the Leeds Assessment of Neuropathic Symptoms and Signs (LANSS) (39) is a seven-item instrument designed to differentiate between neuropathic and non-neuropathic pain. The LANSS consists of two parts, that is, a self-report part including five questions, and a sensory examination. The questions are designed to define specific neuropathic symptoms of: (a) Dysesthesia (i.e., Does your pain feel like strange, unpleasant sensations in your skin?); (b) Autonomic dysfunction (i.e., Does your pain make the skin in the painful area look different from normal?); (c) Evoked pain (Does your pain make the affected skin abnormally sensitive to touch?); (d) Paroxysmal pain (Does your pain come on suddenly and in bursts for no apparent reason when you are still?); and (e) Thermal quality (Does your pain feel as if the skin temperature in the painful area has changed abnormally?). All these questions are answered "yes" or "no." The sensory examination includes simple bedside measures to examine allodynia (lightly stroking with cotton wool) and hypo/hyperalgesia (mechanical pinprick threshold) of the painful site in comparison with a non-painful site. The psychometric properties of pain assessment methods including instruments specifically designed to differentiate between neuropathic and nociceptive pain were recently reviewed by an SCI pain consensus group sponsored by the NIDDR (29). The recommended measures for evaluating change in neuropathic pain and differentiating between neuropathic and nociceptive pain were the NPS (37) and the LANSS (39).

Another way to approach the problem of pain differentiation is data driven and based on statistical grouping of pain characteristics (40). The idea is to statistically group self-reported clinical pain characteristics of pain to produce specific symptom and signs profiles or clinical pain *phenotypes*. For example, a combination of burning, tingling, pricking, shooting, and freezing spontaneous pain, and evoked pain, has previously been shown to differentiate between neuropathic and non-neuropathic pain in 618 patients with neuropathic pain (diabetic neuropathic pain, idiopathic neuropathic pain, or post-herpetic neuralgia) or nociceptive pain (osteoarthritis pain or low back pain) (41). Diagnostic sensitivity and specificity for such methods have been reported to be adequate for heterogeneous neuropathic pain types (42). Although there is evidence that specific neuropathic pain symptom profiles exist also in persons with SCI (43), the psychometric properties of such profiles have not been conclusively determined in this population. One of difficulties after SCI is that some of the sensory qualities (e.g., "cold," "sensitive," "tingling") commonly used in differentiation of pain type in other neuropathic pain conditions may not be related specifically to pain but to the sensory abnormalities resulting from the injury itself. The diagnosis of neuropathic pain after SCI is therefore complicated and more research is needed to determine the most appropriate variables for diagnosing neuropathic pain after SCI.

Sensory Signs

Quantitative sensory testing (QST) is a psychophysical method that can be used to quantify sensory signs associated with pain (44). Due to the increasing interest in a mechanism-based assessment of pain (45), QST is used in clinical pain research both as an outcome measure and to determine the underlying mechanisms of pain (46,47). Measurement of detection thresholds for tactile stimuli, including von Frey monofilaments and vibration, can help assess large-fiber and dorsal column–mediated function, while the measurement of thermal detection and pain thresholds assess the integrity of small-fiber and spinothalamic tract–mediated function. An interesting aspect of QST is that it facilitates the comparisons with basic research studies, since these studies usually utilize behavioral, evoked nociceptive responses as outcome measures. Although QST may potentially be a very useful diagnostic and outcome measure after SCI, it is recognized that only limited validity and reliability data are available for the SCI neuropathic pain population (48), and therefore further research is needed (29). Despite these limitations, a comprehensive pain evaluation including both QST and self-report of pain symptoms is currently the most promising way to determine specific pain phenotypes that may be linked to underlying mechanisms.

Psychosocial Factors

The biospsychosocial model of pain includes a dynamic interaction between biological factors, psychological status, and social and cultural factors (49). While biological mechanisms initiate, maintain, and modulate pain after SCI, psychological factors influence the perception of pain, and social factors can modulate the individual's behavior in response to these perceptions. Only a few clinical treatments reduce the severity of pain in a limited number of individuals with SCI (50,51), and no treatments are currently available that can completely relieve neuropathic pain after SCI (52,53). Therefore, the majority of people with SCI may have to live with some degree of pain. This fact emphasizes that personal characteristics related to adaptation and coping skills are crucial for optimal quality of life after SCI (54).

People living with an SCI have many aspects of their life altered by their injury. An important determinant for quality of life following SCI is successful independent living (55). This may include having control over one's life, having a satisfying social function such as being employed and being minimally dependent on others for daily life activities. Therefore, people with SCI who experience persistent pain are more likely to have a diminished quality of life (4) since persistent pain further decreases independent living by interfering with daily activities, including social activities and work (56,57). Indeed, *greater* life satisfaction following SCI has been shown to be related to higher levels of education, income, employment, and social/recreational activities, whereas medical complications are often related to *lower* satisfaction with life (58–60).

Affective Distress

Affective distress, such as depressed mood, anxiety, and anger, is closely related to the experience of chronic pain in a variety of heterogeneous populations (61). However, the causality in these relationships is not clear (62,63). After an SCI, greater psychological distress and excessive fatigue has been reported by individuals who experience persistent pain (13). Similarly, anxiety and depression have been found to exhibit strong relationships with severity of pain as well as with pain interference (64). A recent study (65) identified three different psychosocial subgroups associated with SCI-related chronic pain. Two of the three subgroups, *Dysfunctional* with higher levels of pain severity and life interference (LI); and *Adaptive Copers* with lower levels of pain severity and LI closely resembled subgroups observed in multiple heterogeneous chronic pain populations. However, a third subgroup unique to the SCI population, that is, the *Interpersonally Supported,* reported high levels of perceived positive support from significant others in response to pain in combination with intimate interpersonal support and lower degree of pain interference and affective distress, despite moderately high pain severity. This subgroup had opposite characteristics compared to the interpersonally distressed subgroup observed in other chronic pain samples (66).

Social Support

Although greater levels of social support may encourage healthy behaviors such as improved adherence to treatment and more adaptive coping, the relationship between pain-related interpersonal responses and both pain severity and treatment outcome is complex (67). For example, low levels of social support have been associated with persistent pain, and suggested to moderate the relationship between stress and affective distress in persons with SCI (68). In contrast, solicitous spouse behaviors and responses have been associated with both increased pain severity and disability in heterogeneous pain populations, (69) and with depression and pain interference after SCI (70). Perceived negative responses from significant others have also been reported to be related to more pain and disability (71). This suggests that the relationship between social support and impact of pain may not be simply linear but may be influenced by multiple factors.

Cognitive Factors

The relationship between cognitive factors, such as catastrophizing thoughts (i.e., irrational thoughts that something is far worse than it actually is) and negative pain beliefs, and impact of pain after SCI was recently examined (72). The authors of that study found that catastrophizing thoughts and negative pain beliefs were related to greater pain interference and poorer mental health. Similarly, another study in individuals with SCI identified a relationship between lower pain intensity and greater levels of internal locus of control (i.e., the belief that one's actions determine various health-related factors such as pain relief) and adaptive coping, and less catastrophizing thoughts (4).

Pain beliefs, including the extent to which an individual believes that his pain can be internally controlled (i.e., controlled by himself), may be influenced not only by the type of pain but also by various other medical and psychosocial issues. For example, after an SCI, locus of control has been shown to be related to many important issues, such as long-term adjustment (73), coping (74), psychological distress (75), and physical disability (76). In addition, Boschen and colleagues (115) found that internal locus of control influenced not only quality of life but also productivity, satisfaction with performance of daily activities, and community integration. Using the Multidimensional Pain Inventory (MPI)-SCI (77), in which life control is evaluated specifically with reference to pain, both severity of spontaneous pain (65) and frequency of evoked pain (78) were related to decreased perceptions of life control. Importantly, the perception of life control can be reinforced and it has been shown that education regarding medical complications improved sense of control after SCI (79). This is consistent with the observation that education, if part of a multidisciplinary pain management program, can reduce the severity of neuropathic pain after SCI (80). Therefore, it is important to determine to what extent cognitive factors may influence the pain experience, so that these factors may be addressed in pain management strategies that aim to reduce the influence of negative cognitions, and enhance the sense of control and adaptive coping (81).

THE INTERNATIONAL SPINAL CORD INJURY BASIC PAIN DATA SET

The International Spinal Cord Injury Basic Pain Data Set (ISCIBPDS) is a result of a collaborative effort by members of the International Spinal Cord Society, the American Spinal Injury Association, the International Association for the Study of Pain, and the American Pain Society. The ISCIBPDS (30) was developed to provide a simple, multidimensional, standardized pain assessment for individuals with SCI. The underlying idea was that comparable sets of outcome measures in clinical practice and in clinical trials would facilitate collaboration, translation of basic research, interpretation, and the application of results to improve the clinical management of SCI-related pain.

The ISCIBPDS collects a minimal amount of pain information, and can thus be used in the daily practice of health care professionals with expertise in SCI. In addition, the assessment proposed in the ISCIBPDS is intended for use across various settings and countries and several language versions are being produced. Although the intent of the data set is to evaluate each separate pain problem, it may also be used to evaluate the most significant or "worst" pain problem if there are time constraints. The overall purpose of the ISCIBPDS concurs with the purpose and vision of the International Spinal Cord Injury Data Sets (82) and should be used in combination with data in the International SCI Core Data Set (83), which includes information on date of birth and injury, gender, the cause of spinal cord lesion, and neurological status.

Background of the ISCIBPDS

The Initiative on Methods, Measurement, and Pain Assessment in Clinical Trials (IMMPACT) group recommended that clinical pain trials designed to evaluate the effectiveness of a therapy should consider including a core set of outcomes (84,85), and suggested that the assessment of pain severity, and physical and emotional functioning was needed to capture the multidimensional nature of pain. However, it was also recognized that other assessment domains might be useful in specific pain populations. This is particularly relevant for the SCI population where a decrease in physical function may be more related to the physical impairments of the injury per se rather than specific to pain. Therefore, a decrease in function specifically due to pain, that is, pain interference should be assessed in this population (86). The questions of the ISCIBPDS are based upon the domains recommended by IMMPACT but adapted to consider the special issues related to SCI (i.e., several simultaneous different pain problems, physical impairments, etc.). The utility and validity of a self-report version of the ISCIBPDS items and scales that measure pain interference, intensity, site(s), frequency, duration and timing (time of day of worst pain) was recently demonstrated (87).

The items of the ISCIBPDS are collected on a one-page form (Table 26.3). The specific variables and their use and rationale for inclusion in the ISCIBPDS are detailed below and in (Tables 26.4–26.7).

Background Questions, Number of Pain Problems, and Pain Location

Information is collected regarding specific characteristics of each pain problem including location, intensity, and temporal pattern (Table 26.4). Each person is required to describe the three worst pain problems he or she is currently experiencing (within the last 7 days). The reasons for this are twofold. First, most people with SCI experience three or fewer pain problems (88). Second, describing the details of more than three different simultaneous pain problems may induce errors in the data collection.

SCI Pain Classification

The ISCIBPDS includes a classification of six different types of pain (Table 26.5). While it incorporates elements of the classification schemes used in previous SCI pain taxonomies (25,26,28,31), it is primarily based upon the IASP taxonomy (see Table 26.1). The categories of the ISCIBPDS are intended to cover all persistent pain types that a person with SCI may experience, including pain that is not directly caused by the SCI. The ISCIBPDS encompasses the following pain types: (a) Musculoskeletal (Nociceptive); (b) Visceral (Nociceptive); (c) Other (Nociceptive); (d) At-level (Neuropathic); (e) Below-level (Neuropathic); and (f) Other (Neuropathic). If it is not possible to classify the pain into one of these categories, "Unknown" should be used.

One important distinction of the taxonomy proposed in the ISCIBPDS compared the IASP taxonomy (31) is that the ASIA Impairment Scale (89) is used as an integral part of the SCI pain classification to define the pain location relative to the NLI. Another divergence from the IASP taxonomy is that nociceptive pains that are uncommon or not directly related to SCI, and not categorized as musculoskeletal or visceral pains, are classified as "Other (Nociceptive)." Neuropathic pain is divided into "at or below" neuropathic pain categories, which is consistent with both the IASP (Table 26.1) and the Bryce/Ragnarsson (Table 26.2) taxonomies. Similarly, one neuropathic pain type was added, that is, Other (Neuropathic), in order to classify neuropathic pain not directly associated with a lesion or disease affecting the spinal cord or nerve roots. The category, "unknown," was proposed for pain that did not fall into one of the categories listed above.

Pain Intensity and Temporal Pattern

Pain intensity is the most widely used domain assessed in research and clinical settings. Several different rating scales have proven to be valid for assessing pain intensity, including the NRS, the Verbal Rating Scale, and the Visual Analogue Scale. However, the 0 to 10 NRS has the most strengths and fewest weaknesses of available measures (90). Moreover, the 0 to 10 NRS has been recommended by the IMMPACT consensus group for use in pain clinical trials (85), and by a NIDDR-sponsored consensus group regarding SCI-related pain (29).

Temporal characteristics of pain are important to evaluate since these provide information regarding the pain type and the burden of pain that the patient experiences. It has been shown that constancy is a factor that significantly contributes to making a pain particularly disturbing after SCI (88). The temporal factors listed in Table 26.6 are evaluated in the ISCIBPDS, and include questions regarding the onset of pain and daily variations in pain severity.

The ISCIBPDS includes a rating of pain intensity and items concerning the temporal pattern of pain (Table 26.6).

Pain Interference

The IMMPACT group suggested that measures of physical and emotional functioning including pain interference were important domains to evaluate in clinical pain trials (85). Consistent with these recommendations, the ISCIPDS includes a section regarding pain interference, which is the extent that pain negatively affects or hinders an individual's daily activities (Table 26.7). Pain interference is an important and sensitive (86) outcome in clinical SCI pain trials. In a recent study, a high level of pain interference was significantly predictive of a particular pain being viewed as "most disturbing" (88). This section of the ISCIBPDS contains three items from the LI subscale of the MPI-SCI version (77) evaluating impact of pain on activities in general and on recreational, social, and family-related activities, and three items specifically asking about pain interference with general activities, mood, and sleep.

The eight-item MPI-SCI LI subscale is a recommended measure for assessing pain interference after SCI (29). The psychometric properties of the LI have been established for the SCI chronic pain population (60,86) and include convergent construct validity, that is, high correlation ($r = 0.61$) with a measure of a similar construct such as the Pain Disability Index (91), and excellent reliability, that is, internal consistency ($r = 0.90$) and test–retest ($r = 0.81$) values. To reduce patient burden, only three of the eight LI items were included in the ISCIBPDS. These were selected based on high factor loadings, that is, high correlations between these items and the eight-item LI subscale (77). The internal consistency of these three items was 0.80 and test–retest was 0.78. Three additional pain interference items were included in the ISCIBPDS to obtain measures of overall pain interference and interference with mood and sleep since these were not assessed by the LI subscale (Table 26.7).

Treatments

A single question addresses whether the patient is receiving treatment for pain: Are you using or receiving any treatment for your pain problem? The question is answered with a "yes" or a "no." A "yes" is intended to lead into a treatment module, which is under development for an extended SCI pain data set. By "treatment" is meant any prescribed or non-prescribed medical, surgical, psychological, or physical treatment that the patient is using or receiving for pain the last 7 days to alleviate his/her pain/pains. This variable may include chronic and intermittent drug treatment, physical therapy, relaxation training, nerve blocks, etc.

Recommendations for Use

The ISCIBPDS is designed to be useful across various settings and applications. Therefore, the ISCIBPDS committee has provided the following recommendations for its use: (a) *Clinical SCI practice*: It is recognized that health care professionals may have limited time to collect patient information. If this is the case, only the worst pain (rather than all pain types than an individual may experience) can be evaluated, in order to significantly reduce the time required to collect this information. Similarly, although clinically important, the interference questions can be considered optional; (b) *Clinical SCI trials*: The ISCIBPDS should be used in its entirety as a general measure of SCI-related pain; and (c) For clinical trials specifically focusing on *SCI-related pain*, the ISCIBPDS is intended to be used as a general basic measure in combination with other appropriate pain measures to facilitate comparisons between research studies. The ISCIBPDS is part of the NIH/NINDS Common Data Elements: "to provide a foundation of variables that are common across studies in order to increase the efficiency and consistency of data collection and to facilitate data sharing."

MECHANISMS-BASED UNDERSTANDING OF NEUROPATHIC PAIN AFTER SCI

The neuropathic pains experienced after SCI are heterogeneous with differing mechanistic origins (92) that may be influenced by genetic background (93–96). There is a growing knowledge base regarding the pathophysiological mechanisms at the spinal, thalamic, and cortical levels (3) involved in causing, exacerbating, and sustaining SCI-related neuropathic pain (97–101). However, the translation of this research into effective treatments for patients is hampered by several factors. One of the primary problems is that the underlying mechanisms of neuropathic pain and their relationship with specific signs and symptoms observed in the patient are incompletely understood (33,93,102). Interestingly, research suggests that specific pathophysiological mechanisms may cause unique combinations of sensory signs and symptoms such as burning pain, thermal, or mechanical hyperalgesia (93,103). Thus, standardized assessment of clinical pain phenotypes including both the measurement of pain symptoms and sensory signs may help to bridge the gap between the clinical presentation of neuropathic pain in people with SCI and pain-generating mechanisms, and thus provide a basis for mechanisms-based treatments (104).

MECHANISMS OF NEUROPATHIC PAIN

Clinical Research Findings

Clinical research studies indicate that sensory signs assessed with QST, suggestive of neuronal hyperexcitability in combination with impaired spinothalamic mediated function, are associated with the presence of neuropathic pain after SCI (105,106). Two primary mechanisms, that is, central disinhibition and central sensitization (3,107), are hypothesized to cause hyperexcitability of both spinal and supraspinal neurons.

In the patient with SCI and neuropathic pain, signs of decreased spinothalamic-mediated function include impaired thermal perception or elevated thermal pain thresholds (105,106,108). In contrast, allodynia (pain caused by a stimulus that is normally not painful, such as light touch), hyperalgesia (exaggerated pain sensation in response to a painful stimulus), or wind-up pain (pain triggered by the repetition of a non-painful stimulus) in painful skin areas at or below the level of injury, may be interpreted as signs of neuronal hyperexcitability (109,110). A recent study by Wasner et al. (111) provided further evidence for a relationship between intact spinothalamic afferents projecting through the injured part of the spinal cord and the presence of neuropathic pain below the level of injury in complete patients. In this study, the authors hypothesized that hyperactivity in spinothalamic neurons was caused by a cascade of events initially triggered by a chronic inflammatory response due to the degeneration of lesioned neighboring neurons. The inflammation would activate microglia resulting in a release of excitatory substances causing spontaneous activity in spinothalamic neurons. The findings of Wasner et al. (111) concur with another study (48), which found that lower thermal pain thresholds (indicating spinothalamic dysfunction) in painful areas were significantly related to greater perceived neuropathic pain severity. Thus, a significant body of clinical research suggests that neuropathic pain is associated with neuronal hyperexcitability and/or spinothalamic impairment and that this is an important clinical sign, which may indicate specific underlying mechanisms of neuropathic pain.

Basic Research Findings

The damage or loss of neuronal tissue following an SCI can induce reorganization at multiple levels in the CNS. Basic research has demonstrated that lesions in the anterolateral spinothalamic tract combined with lesions in the gray matter cause allodynia and hyperalgesia in animals (112,113). Similarly, other research studies indicate that spontaneous and evoked pain behaviors may be caused by lesions in the spinal gray matter and hyperexcitable and hyperactive neurons in the dorsal horn of the spinal cord (114,115). Other research studies show significant plastic changes in parallel with the development of neuropathic pain and these include changes in expression of ion channels, neurotransmitters, receptors and activation of microglia, and structural changes including sprouting of primary afferents (for recent reviews see (116,117)).

Ion Channels

Various neurochemical changes have been suggested to generate neuropathic SCI-related pain. For example, up-regulated expression of sodium channel Nav1.3 has been observed both within centrally projecting spinal cord dorsal horn neurons and within thalamic neurons along the spinothalamic tract after an SCI (118). The up-regulation of sodium channels causes an increase in neuronal activity that is associated with pain-related behaviors in animals. The authors of this study suggested that these hyperexcitable spinal and thalamic neurons may potentially both generate and amplify pain caused by other mechanisms.

Neurotransmitters

Several neurochemical and neurotoxic changes are hypothesized to contribute to the development of neuropathic pain and hyperexcitability of spinal neurons. For example, the excitatory amino acid glutamate is suggested to exert excitotoxic actions on both spinal and descending inhibitory control systems involving γ-aminobutyric acid resulting in hyperexcitability (119,120). Similarly, injury to serotonin (5-HT) containing descending endogenous pain modulatory neurons from the raphe nuclei, also results in a loss of inhibitory control and pain (121).

Inflammation

Inflammatory and immune activations play important roles in the generation and maintenance of chronic neuropathic pain after SCI (122). Several studies show that SCI result in significant activation of microglia in the spinal cord as well as the thalamus and that this activation is associated with pain-related behaviors (123,124). Specifically, glial cells in the dorsal root ganglion and spinal dorsal horn produce and release pro-inflammatory cytokines and neuroactive substances that can increase the excitability of neurons. For example, tumor necrosis factor-alpha, an inflammatory cytokine with both growth stimulating and inhibitory properties, has been suggested to contribute both to the development of neuropathic below-level pain and to mechanical allodynia (125,126). This is further supported by research showing that Wallerian degeneration following a peripheral axon injury contributes to the development of neuropathic pain by producing cytokines and nerve growth factors (NGFs) (127). NGF is thought to regulate the expression of neuropeptides such as substance P and calcitonin gene-related peptides (CGRPs), which may cause both mechanical hyperalgesia and increased responsiveness of spinal Wide Dynamic Range neurons (55). Recently, Carlton et al. 2009 (128) suggested that a combination of peripheral and central sensitization, and glial activation in the uninjured cervical cord underlies above-level neuropathic pain. Importantly, activation of microglia can be inhibited and pain behaviors reduced (123,129) and may therefore provide a potential avenue for the treatment of the neuropathic pain after SCI.

Structural Changes

Neuronal plasticity including sprouting of low threshold non-nociceptive sensory fibers, and increased numbers of nociceptive neurons terminating on central neurons may also be related to the development of neuropathic pain. For example, deafferentation and sprouting of spinal CGRPs and substance P containing neurons play an important role in the increase in excitability of central neurons (120,130). Crown et al. (131) provided further support for spinal plasticity after injury by demonstrating that activation of intracellular signaling cascades previously associated with long-term potentiation and memory mechanisms were associated with the development of chronic neuropathic pain in rats with SCI.

Brain Imaging

Plastic changes induced by an SCI are also possible in the brain. For example, work by Hubscher and Johnson (132) indicated that neurons in specific regions of the thalamus undergo significant changes in responsiveness following a severe SCI. They concluded that the resulting hypersensitivity was part of a general central reorganization process that caused a multitude of sensory disturbances after SCI. Consistent with basic research, evidence for changes in central structures in human subjects who experience neuropathic pain after SCI has been provided by Pattany et al. (133). In this study, metabolite concentrations were assessed in the right and left thalami in people with SCI and chronic pain using non-invasive Magnetic Resonance Spectroscopy (MRS). The advantage of MRS is the stability of the signals analyzed (134). Therefore, when changes in biochemistry are found, they are presumed to reflect long-term plasticity. Several metabolites can be quantified with this method. *N*-acetyl aspartate (NAA) is a free amino acid thought to be localized in neurons and neuronal processes in the mature brain. NAA is commonly thought of as a neuronal marker but may also reflect neuronal dysfunction (135). Another metabolite of interest is *myo*-inositol (Ins), which is often considered a glial marker. Ins is suggested to act as an organic osmolyte, with a major role in the volume and osmoregulation of astrocytes (135). Evidence suggesting that neuropathic pain after SCI may cause functional reorganization in supraspinal structures such as the cortex and the thalamus is supported by the observation that pain intensity was significantly correlated with low NAA and high Ins concentrations in persons with SCI and neuropathic pain (133). The low levels of NAA were hypothesized to be related to a decreased function of inhibitory neurons in the thalamic region, whereas higher concentrations of Ins were hypothesized to reflect gliosis. Although significant atrophy in thalamic gray matter was demonstrated in a study by Apkarian et al. (136), a smaller MRI study in nine patients with mostly nociceptive back pain by Schmidt-Wilcke et al. (137) suggested that chronic pain may be associated with an increase in thalamic gray matter rather than a decrease. The authors of the latter study compared their results with the study by Apkarian et al. (136) and suggested that the differences between the two studies may have been due to differences in the participants' pain problems. For example, the study by Apkarian et al. (136) included 26 persons with chronic back pain of both neuropathic and nociceptive origin, whereas patients with signs of neuropathic pain were not included in the Schmidt-Wilcke study. Further evidence for supraspinal changes associated with SCI-related neuropathic pain was presented in a recent study by Wrigley et al. (138). In that study, significant relationships were obtained between degree of somatosensory reorganization in the S1 cortical area and intensity of pain. Thus, it appears that some metabolic changes may primarily be associated with neuropathic pain types.

Diffusion tensor imaging (DTI) is an imaging method used to determine the integrity of white matter nervous tissue (139). The tissue microstructure significantly influences water diffusion and therefore provides a unique method of assessing the orientation and integrity of neural fibers. Two primary indices are used to quantify mobility of water in white matter, that is, Fractional Anisotropy (FA) and Mean Diffusivity (MD). MD is a measure of the average molecular motion independent of any tissue directionality and is affected by cellular size and integrity (140,141). A reduction in MD suggests more restrictive tissue barriers, such as neuronal sprouting, cellular proliferation, and tumor formation without edema. As a contrast, an increase in MD suggests decreased tissue barriers associated with edema, demyelination, cell death, and axonal loss (142). FA is one of the most used measures (140) and reflects the degree of alignment of cellular structures within fiber tracts, as well as their structural integrity. Thus, DTI is a method that holds significant potential for further understanding of structural integrity of the nociceptive system and thus the mechanistic basis for pain.

Only one study has examined the utility of DTI in examining the relationship between persistent neuropathic pain following SCI and changes in regional brain anatomy and connectivity using DTI (143). This study demonstrated significant changes in regional brain anatomy (MD) in 12 people with SCI-related neuropathic pain compared to pain-free controls. The anatomical changes were located in pain-related regions as well as in regions of the classic reward circuitry (nucleus accumbens and orbitofrontal, dorsolateral prefrontal, and posterior parietal cortices). DTI has also been used in central pain conditions to determine the integrity of the corticospinal and the thalamocortical tracts (TCT) in humans with central post-stroke pain (144). In these 17 subjects, lesions to the TCT were confirmed by imaging and it was found that lower delineation of the TCT was significantly associated with poorer pain relief in response to transcranial magnetic stimulation of the motor cortex. These authors suggested that severe impairment of thalamic nuclei and the TCT may cause hyperexcitability in the thalamus and cortex counteracting the effect of the transcranial stimulation.

Based on these and other studies, it is reasonable to assume that chronic neuropathic pain causes specific changes in the thalamus and other brain regions involved with pain that are related to the perceived severity of neuropathic pain. Thus, supraspinal mechanisms may be future therapeutic targets for persistent neuropathic pain following SCI. Utilizing imaging methods in neuropathic pain research will facilitate the translation of basic research and expand the understanding of the role of brain mechanisms associated with neuropathic pain.

TREATMENT OF PERSISTENT PAIN AFTER SCI

Although there has been significant progress toward mechanisms-based treatments, there are still significant barriers to applying this approach to SCI-related neuropathic pain. This fact is reflected in the large number of people with SCI who continue to experience persistent pain (11,12). Because the biopsychosocial model of pain identifies psychological and social factors as major contributors to the pain experience, a comprehensive treatment strategy targeting neuropathic SCI-related pain should consider including important psychosocial factors. Increased knowledge regarding the relationships between underlying mechanisms and the clinical presentation of neuropathic pain including relevant psychosocial factors is needed to improve pain management for those who live with SCI-related neuropathic pain.

Pharmacological Treatments

Although many pharmacological treatments relieve neuropathic pain in general, few treatments consistently relieve neuropathic pain after SCI. Clinical trials in this population show that pain relief is mostly ineffective (52). Recent reviews (145,146) provide some evidence for the effectiveness of anticonvulsants including gabapentin and pregabalin, for intravenous analgesics including lidocaine and ketamine, and for non-pharmacological interventions such as neurostimulation and cognitive approaches to reduce the severity and impact of pain. However, this evidence is limited with few studies appropriately powered, highlighting the need for large-scale trials including individuals with SCI and neuropathic pain (147).

The two most widely used pharmacological treatment strategies used to relieve neuropathic pain in the general population include antidepressants and anticonvulsants (148). The pain relieving effects of these two agents are based on different mechanisms of action. The effects of tricyclic antidepressants are thought to be mediated by enhancing endogenous modulatory systems that involve neurotransmitters such as serotonin and norepinephrine (149). Clinical trials involving tricyclic antidepressants suggest that approximately 60% to 70% of people with heterogeneous neuropathic pain report at least moderate reductions in pain with these agents (18). However, a problem with older tricyclic antidepressants, such as imipramine and amitriptyline, is the presence of significant side effects that may hinder effective dosing (150). Several clinical trials using tricyclic antidepressants have shown significant relief of neuropathic pain in diverse chronic pain populations (e.g., post-herpetic neuralgia, diabetic neuropathy) (149,151,152). The newer generation of antidepressants with a balanced serotonin–norepinephrine reuptake inhibition is designed to cause fewer side effects than the older tricyclic antidepressants, and a study conducted in patients with neuropathic cancer pain (124) suggested that venlafaxine hydrochloride induced dose-dependent pain relief. To date only two larger, randomized controlled trials have examined the effects of antidepressant medication on neuropathic pain in persons with SCI. One study (153) found no significant pain relieving effect of amitriptyline compared to active placebo. However, Rintala and colleagues (51) found that amitriptyline was effective in reducing neuropathic pain intensity in the participants who had significant depressive symptomatology.

The analgesic effects of anticonvulsants are thought to be mediated by suppression of aberrant electrical activity throughout the nervous system (154). Anticonvulsants have been shown to be effective in several types of neuropathic pain conditions, such as carbamazepine in trigeminal neuralgia (155), gabapentin in diabetic peripheral neuropathy (156), and post-herpetic neuralgia (157). Two randomized, controlled trials and an observational study in persons with SCI show beneficial results for anticonvulsants for neuropathic pain (158–160).

Similarly, one multicenter trial concluded that pregabalin was more effective than placebo in relieving neuropathic pain after SCI and improving sleep, anxiety, and overall patient status (50). Pain relief with pregabalin compared to placebo control was also demonstrated in another study including 40 persons with SCI and neuropathic pain (161). The pain relieving effects of other anticonvulsants such as lamotrigine (162) and topiramate (163) have also been tested with some success in SCI pain populations. For recent detailed reviews of clinical pharmacological pain trials in SCI, see Finnerup et al. (53), Baastrup and Finnerup (164), Siddall (52), and Teasell et al. (145).

The analgesic properties of another class of pharmacological agents, sodium channel blockers (i.e., lidocaine), have also been examined in persons experiencing SCI-related neuropathic pain. Loubser and Donovan (165) showed that lidocaine delivered into the subarachnoid space significantly relieved SCI-related pain. Similarly, Attal et al. (166) examined the effects of intravenous lidocaine in persons with either stroke- or SCI-related pain and showed a significant reduction in pain intensity and in mechanical allodynia and hyperalgesia, but no reduction of thermal allodynia and hyperalgesia. These results support the idea that different types of sensory abnormalities may represent different underlying mechanisms. However, oral administration of mexilitine, which is structurally similar to lidocaine, does not appear to reduce SCI-related neuropathic pain (164). Another study in a small group of persons with SCI used intravenous administration of ketamine, an *N*-methyl *D*-aspartate (NMDA) receptor antagonist, and demonstrated a significant reduction of SCI-related neuropathic pain (167). The results from this study support the hypothesis that underlying mechanisms of neuropathic pain include central sensitization via activation of NMDA receptors.

Another option for neuropathic pain management is opioid receptor agonists. However, oral administration of opioids seems to result only in minimal pain relief, often accompanied by dose-dependent adverse effects such as constipation. A randomized controlled clinical trial using intravenous morphine (168) in persons with neuropathic pain after stroke or SCI showed a reduction in the intensity of brush-evoked allodynia but no significant effect on spontaneous pain. Similarly, intravenous administration of alfentanil, a mu-opioid receptor agonist in nine individuals with SCI and neuropathic pain caused a significant decrease in both spontaneous and evoked pain (167). Although these studies suggest that opioids effectively reduce pain after SCI when administered intravenously, this mode of administration may not be suitable for long-term treatment.

Nonpharmacological Treatments

Many non-pharmacological treatments are available for the treatment of SCI-related neuropathic pain. These include surgery as well as non-invasive treatments including physical therapies. When neuropathic pain is caused by a peripheral nerve compression, tethering of nerve roots or the spinal cord and syringomyelia, surgical methods including stabilization of the spine, decompression and un-tethering of nerve roots may be effective. Similarly, thermo-coagulation of hyperactive nerve cells in the dorsal horn by dorsal root entry zone (DREZ) lesioning has produced relief in some patients with SCI and neuropathic pain (169–171). Pain relieving effects of spinal cord and deep brain stimulation in persons with SCI have also been suggested (172), although these therapies do not appear to provide long-lasting effects. Other non-invasive therapies, such as transcranial motor cortex stimulation, have shown inconclusive results with regard to relief of SCI-related neuropathic pain (173).

Many types of non-pharmacological treatment interventions with minimal side effects are frequently used to treat SCI-related neuropathic pain. For example, recent studies suggest that treatments like acupuncture, TENS, and massage may be helpful for some people with neuropathic pain (174–176). The biopsychosocial approach to the management of pain aims to increase individual coping skills to improve quality of life (49). Therefore, treatment strategies that include cognitive behavioral components directed toward enhancing a person's coping ability and adaptation to pain are important components of a multidisciplinary management of pain after SCI (80,81,177).

The Patient Perspective

Several studies have investigated the self-reported use of treatments and amount of pain relief in people with SCI and chronic pain (8–10,174). The weakness with most of these studies is that the effects on specific pain types are usually not specified and, therefore, it is difficult to interpret the results. However, the advantage of survey studies is that they provide the persons own perspective regarding the pain relieving effects of various treatments in the context of daily life rather than in a clinical trial setting.

Most of these studies consistently report that the most common medications used to relieve pain after SCI include NSAIDs, acetaminophen, and opioids, followed closely by anticonvulsants, antispasmodics, and sedatives. Understandably, the reported frequencies of use, however, vary somewhat among studies probably due to diverse settings. Although opioids are considered less effective for relief of neuropathic pain than nociceptive pain (178,179), opioids are frequently prescribed and perceived as one of the most useful medications by many persons with SCI-related chronic pain (9,10,180). Because it cannot be determined from these studies which type of pain is being treated, it is possible that opioids primarily reduce the severity of nociceptive components of pain, rather than purely neuropathic. A study by Norrbrink and Lundeberg (180) concurs with this idea and showed that those with neuropathic pain types achieved less pain relief with opioids.

Massage and other physiotherapeutic interventions (e.g., application of heat, cold, TENS) are among the most common non-pharmacological methods used to relieve pain after SCI (8–10,174,181). Overall physiotherapeutic interventions were perceived as providing "considerable to complete" pain relief in 50% of an SCI sample (78), with pain relief often lasting hours to days (10). Similarly, marijuana is frequently viewed by respondents as an effective way to obtain pain relief. A survey study showed that 32% of a sample of 117 had used marijuana to reduce pain at least some time during the course of their SCI and 23% were currently using it at the time of study (10). However, a recent small clinical trial in SCI showed no pain relieving effect on neuropathic pain below the level of injury of the oral cannabinoid, dronabinol, compared to active placebo (182). Thus, these types of therapies may be useful as adjunct treatments to pain medication for a significant proportion of people, even long after they sustained their SCIs.

CONCLUSION

Neuropathic pain is a serious consequence that affects many people after an SCI. Severe, chronic pain regardless of type can significantly interfere with daily activities and reduce quality of life. Unfortunately, currently available treatments rarely relieve SCI-related neuropathic pain. The complex clinical presentation with multiple simultaneous pains and variable psychosocial impact strongly suggest a significant need for individually tailored mechanism-based treatment approaches that include psychosocial interventions.

Although basic research studies suggest that multiple mechanisms are responsible for the development of neuropathic pain after SCI, there is a significant knowledge gap regarding how to determine the specific underlying pathophysiological causes in persons with SCI. Bridging this gap would facilitate translation of basic research findings into the clinic and thus the development of more effective treatments. Large-scale multicenter clinical trials including individuals with SCI and neuropathic pain are limited and urgently needed. This requires standardized and generalizable pain evaluation protocols and pain classification systems that can be used to define specific pain phenotypes and to evaluate treatment outcome. The ISCIBPDS is consistent with this goal and assesses pain symptoms, pain type, and psychosocial impact. However, in order to move toward mechanisms-based treatments that can provide a link between basic and clinical research, more comprehensive assessments protocols that incorporate sensory assessments and various biomarkers are necessary.

References

1. Woolf CJ, Max MB. Mechanism-based pain diagnosis: issues for analgesic drug development. *Anesthesiology* 2001;95(1):241–249.
2. Finnerup NB, Sindrup SH, Jensen TS. Chronic neuropathic pain: mechanisms, drug targets and measurement. *Fundam Clin Pharmacol* 2007;21(2):129–136.
3. Finnerup NB, Jensen TS. Spinal cord injury pain—mechanisms and treatment. *Eur J Neurol* 2004;11(2):73–82.
4. Wollaars MM, Post MW, Brand N. Spinal cord injury pain: the influence of psychologic factors and impact on quality of life. *Clin J Pain* 2007;23(5):383–391.
5. Richards JS, Meredith RL, Nepomuceno C, et al. Psychosocial aspects of chronic pain in spinal cord injury. *Pain* 1980;8(3):355–366.
6. Summers JD, Rapoff MA, Varghese G, et al. Psychosocial factors in chronic spinal cord injury pain. *Pain* 1991;47(2):183–189.
7. Middleton J, Tran Y, Craig A. Relationship between quality of life and self-efficacy in persons with spinal cord injuries. *Arch Phys Med Rehabil* 2007;88(12):1643–1648.
8. Warms CA, Turner JA, Marshall HM, et al. Treatments for chronic pain associated with spinal cord injuries: many are tried, few are helpful. *Clin J Pain* 2002;18(3):154–163.
9. Widerstrom-Noga EG, Turk DC. Types and effectiveness of treatments used by people with chronic pain associated with spinal cord injuries: influence of pain and psychosocial characteristics. *Spinal Cord* 2003;41(11):600–609.
10. Cardenas DD, Jensen MP. Treatments for chronic pain in persons with spinal cord injury: A survey study. *J Spinal Cord Med* 2006;29(2):109–117.
11. Cruz-Almeida Y, Martinez-Arizala A, Widerstrom-Noga EG. Chronicity of pain associated with spinal cord injury: A longitudinal analysis. *J Rehabil Res Dev* 2005;42(5):585–594.
12. Jensen MP, Hoffman AJ, Cardenas DD. Chronic pain in individuals with spinal cord injury: a survey and longitudinal study. *Spinal Cord* 2005;43(12):704–712.
13. Kennedy P, Lude P, Taylor N. Quality of life, social participation, appraisals and coping post spinal cord injury: a review of four community samples. *Spinal Cord* 2006;44(2):95–105.
14. Yezierski RP. Pain following spinal cord injury: the clinical problem and experimental studies. *Pain* 1996;68(2–3):185–194.
15. Stormer S, Gerner HJ, Gruninger W, et al. Chronic pain/dysaesthesiae in spinal cord injury patients: results of a multicentre study. *Spinal Cord* 1997;35(7):446–455.
16. Widerstrom-Noga EG, Felipe-Cuervo E, Broton JG, et al. Perceived difficulty in dealing with consequences of spinal cord injury. *Arch Phys Med Rehabil* 1999;80(5):580–586.
17. Turner JA, Cardenas DD, Warms CA, et al. Chronic pain associated with spinal cord injuries: a community survey. *Arch Phys Med Rehabil* 2001;82(4):501–509.
18. Finnerup NB, Johannesen IL, Sindrup SH, et al. Pain and dysesthesia in patients with spinal cord injury: a postal survey. *Spinal Cord* 2001;39(5):256–262.
19. Rintala DH, Loubser PG, Castro J, et al. Chronic pain in a community-based sample of men with spinal cord injury: prevalence, severity, and relationship with impairment, disability, handicap, and subjective well-being. *Arch Phys Med Rehabil* 1998;79(6):604–614.
20. Siddall PJ, McClelland JM, Rutkowski SB, et al. A longitudinal study of the prevalence and characteristics of pain in the first 5 years following spinal cord injury. *Pain* 2003;103(3):249–257.
21. Rintala DH, Holmes SA, Fiess RN, et al. Prevalence and characteristics of chronic pain in veterans with spinal cord injury. *J Rehabil Res Dev* 2005;42(5):573–584.
22. Merskey H. Classification of chronic pain, description of chronic pain syndromes and definitions of pain terms. Seattle, WA: IASP Press, 1994.
23. Treede RD, Jensen TS, Campbell JN, et al. Neuropathic pain: redefinition and a grading system for clinical and research purposes. *Neurology* 2008;70(18):1630–1635.
24. Finnerup NB, Sorensen L, Biering-Sorensen F, et al. Segmental hypersensitivity and spinothalamic function in spinal cord injury pain. *Exp Neurol* 2007;207(1):139–149.
25. Cardenas DD, Turner JA, Warms CA, et al. Classification of chronic pain associated with spinal cord injuries. *Arch Phys Med Rehabil* 2002;83(12):1708–1714.
26. Bryce TN, Ragnarsson KT. Pain after spinal cord injury. *Phys Med Rehabil Clin N Am* 2000;11(1):157–168.
27. Siddall PJ, Taylor DA, Cousins MJ. Classification of pain following spinal cord injury. *Spinal Cord* 1997;35(2):69–75.
28. Donovan WH, Dimitrijevic MR, Dahm L, et al. Neurophysiological approaches to chronic pain following spinal cord injury. *Paraplegia* 1982;20(3):135–146.

29. Bryce TN, Budh CN, Cardenas DD, et al. Pain after spinal cord injury: an evidence-based review for clinical practice and research. Report of the National Institute on Disability and Rehabilitation Research Spinal Cord Injury Measures meeting. *J Spinal Cord Med* 2007;30(5): 421–440.
30. Widerstrom-Noga E, Biering-Sorensen F, Bryce T, et al. The international spinal cord injury pain basic data set. *Spinal Cord* 2008;46(12):818–823.
31. Siddall PJ, Yezierski RP, Loeser JD. Pain following spinal cord injury: clinical features, prevalence, and taxonomy. International Association for the Study of Pain Newsletter 2000;3:3–7.
32. Bryce TN, Dijkers MP, Ragnarsson KT, et al. Reliability of the Bryce/Ragnarsson spinal cord injury pain taxonomy. *J Spinal Cord Med* 2006;29(2):118–132.
33. Hansson P. Neuropathic pain: clinical characteristics and diagnostic workup. *Eur J Pain* 2002;6(suppl A):47–50.
34. Attal N, Fermanian C, Fermanian J, et al. Neuropathic pain: are there distinct subtypes depending on the aetiology or anatomical lesion? *Pain* 2008;138(2):343–353.
35. Bouhassira D, Attal N, Fermanian J, et al. Development and validation of the Neuropathic Pain Symptom Inventory. *Pain* 2004;108(3):248–257.
36. Crawford B, Bouhassira D, Wong A, et al. Conceptual adequacy of the neuropathic pain symptom inventory in six countries. *Health Qual Life Outcomes* 2008;6:62.
37. Galer BS, Jensen MP. Development and preliminary validation of a pain measure specific to neuropathic pain: the Neuropathic Pain Scale. *Neurology* 1997;48(2): 332–338.
38. Fishbain DA, Lewis JE, Cutler R, et al. Can the neuropathic pain scale discriminate between non-neuropathic and neuropathic pain? *Pain Med* 2008;9(2):149–160.
39. Bennett M. The LANSS Pain Scale: the Leeds assessment of neuropathic symptoms and signs. *Pain* 2001;92(1–2): 147–157.
40. Victor TW, Jensen MP, Gammaitoni AR, et al. The dimensions of pain quality: factor analysis of the Pain Quality Assessment Scale. *Clin J Pain* 2008;24(6):550–555.
41. Dworkin RH, Jensen MP, Gammaitoni AR, et al. Symptom profiles differ in patients with neuropathic versus non-neuropathic pain. *J.Pain* 2007;8(2):118–126.
42. Bennett MI, Attal N, Backonja MM, et al. Using screening tools to identify neuropathic pain. *Pain* 2007;127(3): 199–203.
43. Cruz-Almeida Y, Felix ER, Martinez-Arizala A, et al. Pain symptom profiles in persons with spinal cord injury. *Pain Med* 2009;10(7):1246–1259.
44. Lindblom U. Analysis of abnormal touch, pain, and temperature sensation in patients. In: Hansson P, Lindblom U, eds. *Touch, temperature, and pain in health and disease: mechanisms and assessments. progress in pain research and management*. Seattle, WA: IASP Press, 1994:63–84.
45. Cruccu G, Anand P, Attal N, et al. EFNS guidelines on neuropathic pain assessment. *Eur J Neurol* 2004;11(3):153–162.
46. Rolke R, Magerl W, Campbell KA, et al. Quantitative sensory testing: a comprehensive protocol for clinical trials. *Eur J Pain* 2006;10(1):77–88.
47. Maier C, Baron R, Tolle TR, et al. Quantitative sensory testing in the German Research Network on Neuropathic Pain (DFNS): somatosensory abnormalities in 1236 patients with different neuropathic pain syndromes. *Pain* 2010;150(3):439–450.
48. Felix ER, Widerstrom-Noga EG. Reliability and validity of quantitative sensory testing in persons with spinal cord injury and neuropathic pain. *J Rehabil Res Dev* 2009;46(1):69–83.
49. Turk DC. Biopsychosocial perspective on chronic pain. In: Gatchel R, Turk DC, eds. *Psychological approaches to chronic pain management: a clinician's handbook*. New York: Guilford Press, 1996:3–33.
50. Siddall PJ, Cousins MJ, Otte A, et al. Pregabalin in central neuropathic pain associated with spinal cord injury: a placebo-controlled trial. *Neurology* 2006;67(10):1792–1800.
51. Rintala DH, Holmes SA, Courtade D, et al. Comparison of the effectiveness of amitriptyline and gabapentin on chronic neuropathic pain in persons with spinal cord injury. *Arch Phys Med Rehabil* 2007;88(12):1547–1560.
52. Siddall PJ. Management of neuropathic pain following spinal cord injury: now and in the future. *Spinal Cord* 2009;47(5):352–359.
53. Finnerup NB, Otto M, Jensen TS, et al. An evidence-based algorithm for the treatment of neuropathic pain. *Med Gen Med* 2007;9(2):36.
54. Haythornthwaite JA, Benrud-Larson LM. Psychological aspects of neuropathic pain. *Clin J Pain* 2000;16 (2 suppl):S101–S105.
55. Harker WF, Dawson DR, Boschen KA, et al. A comparison of independent living outcomes following traumatic brain injury and spinal cord injury. *Int J Rehabil Res* 2002;25(2):93–102.
56. Ravenscroft A, Ahmed YS, Burnside IG. Chronic pain after SCI. A patient survey. *Spinal Cord* 2000;38(10): 611–614.
57. Widerstrom-Noga EG, Felipe-Cuervo E, Yezierski RP. Chronic pain after spinal injury: interference with sleep and daily activities. *Arch Phys Med Rehabil* 2001;82(11):1571–1577.
58. Vogel LC, Klaas SJ, Lubicky JP, et al. Long-term outcomes and life satisfaction of adults who had pediatric spinal cord injuries. *Arch Phys Med Rehabil* 1998;79(12): 1496–1503.
59. Anderson CJ, Vogel LC. Employment outcomes of adults who sustained spinal cord injuries as children or adolescents. *Arch Phys Med Rehabil* 2002;83(6):791–801.
60. Widerstrom-Noga EG, Cruz-Almeida Y, Martinez-Arizala A, et al. Internal consistency, stability, and validity of the spinal cord injury version of the multidimensional pain inventory. *Arch Phys Med Rehabil* 2006;87(4): 516–523.
61. Banks SM, Kerns RD. Explaining high rates of depression in chronic pain: a diathesis-stress framework. *Psychol Bull* 1996;119(1):95–110.
62. Romano JM, Turner JA. Chronic pain and depression: does the evidence support a relationship? *Psychol Bull* 1985;97(1):18–34.
63. Gamsa A. Is emotional disturbance a precipitator or a consequence of chronic pain? *Pain* 1990;42(2):183–195.
64. Nicholson PK, Nicholas MK, Middleton J. Spinal cord injury-related pain in rehabilitation: a cross-sectional study of relationships with cognitions, mood and physical function. *Eur J Pain* 2009;13:511–517.

65. Widerstrom-Noga EG, Felix ER, Cruz-Almeida Y, et al. Psychosocial subgroups in persons with spinal cord injuries and chronic pain. *Arch Phys Med Rehabil* 2007; 88(12):1628–1635.
66. Turk DC, Rudy TE. Toward an empirically derived taxonomy of chronic pain patients: integration of psychological assessment data. *J Consult Clin Psychol* 1988; 56(2):233–238.
67. McCracken LM. Social context and acceptance of chronic pain: the role of solicitous and punishing responses. *Pain* 2005;113(1–2):155–159.
68. Rintala DH, Hart KA, Priebe MM. Predicting consistency of pain over a 10-year period in persons with spinal cord injury. *J Rehabil Res Dev* 2004;41(1):75–88.
69. Romano JM, Turner JA, Jensen MP, et al. Chronic pain patient-spouse behavioral interactions predict patient disability. *Pain* 1995;63(3):353–360.
70. Stroud MW, Turner JA, Jensen MP, et al. Partner responses to pain behaviors are associated with depression and activity interference among persons with chronic pain and spinal cord injury. *J Pain* 2006;7(2):91–99.
71. Cano A, Weisberg JN, Gallagher RM. Marital satisfaction and pain severity mediate the association between negative spouse responses to pain and depressive symptoms in a chronic pain patient sample. *Pain Med* 2000;1(1):35–43.
72. Hanley MA, Raichle K, Jensen M, et al. Pain catastrophizing and beliefs predict changes in pain interference and psychological functioning in persons with spinal cord injury. *J Pain* 2008;9(9):863–871.
73. Boschen KA, Tonack M, Gargaro J. Long-term adjustment and community reintegration following spinal cord injury. *Int J Rehabil Res* 2003;26(3):157–164.
74. Chan RC, Lee PW, Lieh-Mak F. The pattern of coping in persons with spinal cord injuries. *Disabil Rehabil* 2000;22(11):501–507.
75. Craig A, Hancock K, Chang E, et al. The effectiveness of group psychological intervention in enhancing perceptions of control following spinal cord injury. *Aust N Z J Psychiatry* 1998;32(1):112–118.
76. Macleod L, Macleod G. Control cognitions and psychological disturbance in people with contrasting physically disabling conditions. *Disabil Rehabil* 1998;20(12):448–456.
77. Widerstrom-Noga EG, Duncan R, Felipe-Cuervo E, et al. Assessment of the impact of pain and impairments associated with spinal cord injuries. *Arch Phys Med Rehabil* 2002;83(3):395–404.
78. Widerstrom-Noga EG, Turk DC. Exacerbation of chronic pain following spinal cord injury. *J Neurotrauma* 2004;21(10):1384–1395.
79. Cardenas DD, Hoffman JM, Kelly E, et al. Impact of a urinary tract infection educational program in persons with spinal cord injury. *J Spinal Cord Med* 2004;27(1):47–54.
80. Norrbrink BC, Kowalski J, Lundeberg T. A comprehensive pain management programme comprising educational, cognitive and behavioural interventions for neuropathic pain following spinal cord injury. *J Rehabil Med* 2006;38(3):172–180.
81. Jensen MP, Turner JA, Romano JM. Changes after multidisciplinary pain treatment in patient pain beliefs and coping are associated with concurrent changes in patient functioning. *Pain* 2007;131(1–2):38–47.
82. Biering-Sorensen F, Charlifue S, DeVivo M, et al. International Spinal Cord Injury Data Sets. *Spinal Cord* 2006;44(9):530–534.
83. DeVivo M, Biering-Sorensen F, Charlifue S, et al. International Spinal Cord Injury Core Data Set. *Spinal Cord* 2006;44(9):535–540.
84. Turk DC, Dworkin RH, Allen RR, et al. Core outcome domains for chronic pain clinical trials: IMMPACT recommendations. *Pain* 2003;106(3):337–345.
85. Dworkin RH, Turk DC, Farrar JT, et al. Core outcome measures for chronic pain clinical trials: IMMPACT recommendations. *Pain* 2005;113(1–2):9–19.
86. Cruz-Almeida Y, Alameda G, Widerstrom-Noga EG. Differentiation between pain-related interference and interference caused by the functional impairments of spinal cord injury. *Spinal Cord* 2009;47(5):390–395.
87. Jensen MP, Widerstrom-Noga E, Richards JS, et al. Reliability and validity of the International Spinal Cord Injury Basic Pain Data Set items as self-report measures. *Spinal Cord* 2010;48(3):230–238.
88. Felix ER, Cruz-Almeida Y, Widerstrom-Noga EG. Chronic pain after spinal cord injury: what characteristics make some pains more disturbing than others? *J Rehabil Res Dev* 2007;44(5):703–716.
89. Marino RJ, Barros T, Biering-Sorensen F, et al. International standards for neurological classification of spinal cord injury. *J Spinal Cord Med* 2003;26(suppl 1): S50–S56.
90. Jensen MP, Karoly P. *Self-report scales and procedures for assessing pain in adults*. New York: Guilford Publications, 2001.
91. Chibnall JT, Tait RC. The Pain Disability Index: factor structure and normative data. *Arch Phys Med Rehabil* 1994;75(10):1082–1086.
92. Siddall PJ, Loeser JD. Pain following spinal cord injury. *Spinal Cord* 2001;39(2):63–73.
93. Costigan M, Scholz J, Woolf CJ. Neuropathic pain: a maladaptive response of the nervous system to damage. *Annu Rev Neurosci* 2009;32:1–32.
94. Foulkes T, Wood JN. Pain genes. *PLoS.Genet* 2008; 4(7):e1000086.
95. Tegeder I, Costigan M, Griffin RS, et al. GTP cyclohydrolase and tetrahydrobiopterin regulate pain sensitivity and persistence. *Nat Med* 2006;12(11):1269–1277.
96. Diatchenko L, Slade GD, Nackley AG, et al. Genetic basis for individual variations in pain perception and the development of a chronic pain condition. *Hum Mol Genet* 2005;14(1):135–143.
97. Yamamoto T, Katayama Y, Hirayama T, et al. Pharmacological classification of central post-stroke pain: comparison with the results of chronic motor cortex stimulation therapy. *Pain* 1997;72(1–2):5–12.
98. Jorum E, Warncke T, Stubhaug A. Cold allodynia and hyperalgesia in neuropathic pain: the effect of *N*-methyl-*D*-aspartate (NMDA) receptor antagonist ketamine—a double-blind, cross-over comparison with alfentanil and placebo. *Pain* 2003;101(3):229–235.
99. Jensen TS. Anticonvulsants in neuropathic pain: rationale and clinical evidence. *Eur J Pain* 2002;6(suppl A): 61–68.
100. Deumens R, Joosten EA, Waxman SG, et al. Locomotor dysfunction and pain: the scylla and charybdis of fiber sprouting after spinal cord injury. *Mol Neurobiol* 2008;37(1):52–63.

101. Hulsebosch CE, Hains BC, Crown ED, et al. Mechanisms of chronic central neuropathic pain after spinal cord injury. *Brain Res Rev* 2009;60:202–213.
102. Jensen TS, Baron R. Translation of symptoms and signs into mechanisms in neuropathic pain. *Pain* 2003; 102(1–2): 1–8.
103. Woolf CJ, Salter MW. Neuronal plasticity: increasing the gain in pain. *Science* 2000;288(5472):1765–1769.
104. Widerstrom-Noga EG, Finnerup NB, Siddall PJ. A biopsychosocial perspective on a mechanisms-based approach to pain assessment and treatment of pain following spinal cord injury. *J Rehabil Res Dev*. 2009;46:1–12.
105. Defrin R, Ohry A, Blumen N, et al. Characterization of chronic pain and somatosensory function in spinal cord injury subjects. *Pain* 2001;89(2–3):253–263.
106. Finnerup NB, Johannesen IL, Fuglsang-Frederiksen A, et al. Sensory function in spinal cord injury patients with and without central pain. *Brain* 2003;126(pt 1):57–70.
107. Boivie J, Leijon G, Johansson I. Central post-stroke pain—a study of the mechanisms through analyses of the sensory abnormalities. *Pain* 1989;37(2):173–185.
108. Eide PK, Jorum E, Stenehjem AE. Somatosensory findings in patients with spinal cord injury and central dysaesthesia pain. *J Neurol Neurosurg Psychiatry* 1996; 60(4):411–415.
109. Finnerup NB, Johannesen IL, Bach FW, et al. Sensory function above lesion level in spinal cord injury patients with and without pain. *Somatosens Mot Res* 2003; 20(1):71–76.
110. Eide PK. Pathophysiological mechanisms of central neuropathic pain after spinal cord injury. *Spinal Cord* 1998;36(9):601–612.
111. Wasner G, Lee BB, Engel S, et al. Residual spinothalamic tract pathways predict development of central pain after spinal cord injury. *Brain* 2008;131(pt 9):2387–2400.
112. Vierck CJ Jr, Light AR. Effects of combined hemotoxic and anterolateral spinal lesions on nociceptive sensitivity. *Pain* 1999;83(3):447–457.
113. Vierck CJ Jr, Siddall P, Yezierski RP. Pain following spinal cord injury: animal models and mechanistic studies. *Pain* 2000;89(1):1–5.
114. Yezierski RP, Park SH. The mechanosensitivity of spinal sensory neurons following intraspinal injections of quisqualic acid in the rat. *Neurosci Lett* 1993;157(1):115–119.
115. Hao JX, Kupers RC, Xu XJ. Response characteristics of spinal cord dorsal horn neurons in chronic allodynic rats after spinal cord injury. *J Neurophysiol* 2004;92(3): 1391–1399.
116. Hulsebosch CE, Hains BC, Crown ED, et al. Mechanisms of chronic central neuropathic pain after spinal cord injury. *Brain Res Rev* 2009;60(1):202–213.
117. Yezierski RP. Spinal cord injury pain: spinal and supraspinal mechanisms. *J Rehabil Res Dev* 2009; 46(1):95–107.
118. Hains BC, Johnson KM, Eaton MJ, et al. Serotonergic neural precursor cell grafts attenuate bilateral hyperexcitability of dorsal horn neurons after spinal hemisection in rat. *Neuroscience* 2003;116(4):1097–1110.
119. Wiesenfeld-Hallin Z, Aldskogius H, Grant G, et al. Central inhibitory dysfunctions: mechanisms and clinical implications. *Behav Brain Sci* 1997;20(3):420–425.
120. Gwak YS, Nam TS, Paik KS, et al. Attenuation of mechanical hyperalgesia following spinal cord injury by administration of antibodies to nerve growth factor in the rat. *Neurosci Lett* 2003;336(2):117–120.
121. Hains BC, Everhart AW, Fullwood SD, et al. Changes in serotonin, serotonin transporter expression and serotonin denervation supersensitivity: involvement in chronic central pain after spinal hemisection in the rat. *Exp Neurol* 2002;175(2):347–362.
122. DeLeo JA, Yezierski RP. The role of neuroinflammation and neuroimmune activation in persistent pain. *Pain* 2001;90(1–2):1–6.
123. Hains BC, Waxman SG. Activated microglia contribute to the maintenance of chronic pain after spinal cord injury. *J Neurosci* 2006;26(16):4308–4317.
124. Zhao P, Waxman SG, Hains BC. Modulation of thalamic nociceptive processing after spinal cord injury through remote activation of thalamic microglia by cysteine cysteine chemokine ligand 21. *J Neurosci* 2007; 27(33):8893–8902.
125. Peng XM, Zhou ZG, Glorioso JC, et al. Tumor necrosis factor-alpha contributes to below-level neuropathic pain after spinal cord injury. *Ann Neurol* 2006;59(5):843–851.
126. Wieseler-Frank J, Maier SF, Watkins LR. Glial activation and pathological pain. *Neurochem Int* 2004;45(2–3): 389–395.
127. George A, Buehl A, Sommer C. Wallerian degeneration after crush injury of rat sciatic nerve increases endo- and epineurial tumor necrosis factor-alpha protein. *Neurosci Lett* 2004;372(3):215–219.
128. Carlton SM, Du J, Tan HY, et al. Peripheral and central sensitization in remote spinal cord regions contribute to central neuropathic pain after spinal cord injury. *Pain* 2009;147:265–276.
129. Tan AM, Zhao P, Waxman SG, et al. Early microglial inhibition preemptively mitigates chronic pain development after experimental spinal cord injury. *J Rehabil Res Dev* 2009;46(1):123–133.
130. Christensen MD, Hulsebosch CE. Spinal cord injury and anti-NGF treatment results in changes in CGRP density and distribution in the dorsal horn in the rat. *Exp Neurol* 1997;147(2):463–475.
131. Crown ED, Ye Z, Johnson KM, et al. Increases in the activated forms of ERK 1/2, p38 MAPK, and CREB are correlated with the expression of at-level mechanical allodynia following spinal cord injury. *Exp Neurol* 2006;199(2):397–407.
132. Hubscher CH, Johnson RD. Chronic spinal cord injury induced changes in the responses of thalamic neurons. *Exp Neurol* 2006;197(1):177–188.
133. Pattany PM, Yezierski RP, Widerstrom-Noga EG, et al. Proton magnetic resonance spectroscopy of the thalamus in patients with chronic neuropathic pain after spinal cord injury. *Am J Neuroradiol* 2002;23(6):901–905.
134. Apkarian AV, Bushnell MC, Treede RD, et al. Human brain mechanisms of pain perception and regulation in health and disease. *Eur J Pain* 2005;9(4):463–484.
135. Govindaraju V, Young K, Maudsley AA. Proton NMR chemical shifts and coupling constants for brain metabolites. *NMR Biomed* 2000;13(3):129–153.
136. Apkarian AV, Sosa Y, Sonty S, et al. Chronic back pain is associated with decreased prefrontal and thalamic gray matter density. *J Neurosci* 2004;24(46):10410–10415.

137. Schmidt-Wilcke T, Leinisch E, Ganssbauer S, et al. Affective components and intensity of pain correlate with structural differences in gray matter in chronic back pain patients. *Pain* 2006;125(1–2):89–97.
138. Wrigley PJ, Press SR, Gustin SM, et al. Neuropathic pain and primary somatosensory cortex reorganization following spinal cord injury. *Pain* 2009;141(1–2):52–59.
139. Beaulieu C. The basis of anisotropic water diffusion in the nervous system—a technical review. *NMR Biomed* 2002;15(7–8):435–455.
140. Basser PJ, Pierpaoli C. Microstructural and physiological features of tissues elucidated by quantitative-diffusion-tensor MRI. *J Magn Reson B* 1996;111(3):209–219.
141. Pierpaoli C, Jezzard P, Basser PJ, et al. Diffusion tensor MR imaging of the human brain. *Radiology* 1996;201(3):637–648.
142. Iannucci G, Rovaris M, Giacomotti L, et al. Correlation of multiple sclerosis measures derived from T2-weighted, T1-weighted, magnetization transfer, and diffusion tensor MR imaging. *Am J Neuroradiol* 2001;22(8):1462–1467.
143. Gustin SM, Wrigley PJ, Siddall PJ, et al. Brain anatomy changes associated with persistent neuropathic pain following spinal cord injury. *Cereb Cortex* 2010;20(6):1409–1419.
144. Goto T, Saitoh Y, Hashimoto N, et al. Diffusion tensor fiber tracking in patients with central post-stroke pain; correlation with efficacy of repetitive transcranial magnetic stimulation. *Pain* 2008;140(3):509–518.
145. Teasell RW, Mehta S, Aubut JA, et al. A systematic review of pharmacologic treatments of pain after spinal cord injury. *Arch Phys Med Rehabil* 2010;91(5):816–831.
146. Siddall PJ. Management of neuropathic pain following spinal cord injury: now and in the future. *Spinal Cord* 2009;47(5):352–359.
147. Attal N, Mazaltarine G, Perrouin-Verbe B, et al. Chronic neuropathic pain management in spinal cord injury patients. What is the efficacy of pharmacological treatments with a general mode of administration? (oral, transdermal, intravenous). *Ann Phys Rehabil Med* 2009;52(2):124–141.
148. Sindrup SH, Jensen TS. Efficacy of pharmacological treatments of neuropathic pain: an update and effect related to mechanism of drug action. *Pain* 1999;83(3):389–400.
149. Magni G. The use of antidepressants in the treatment of chronic pain. A review of the current evidence. *Drugs* 1991;42(5):730–778.
150. Ansari A. The efficacy of newer antidepressants in the treatment of chronic pain: a review of current literature. *Harv Rev Psychiatry* 2000;7(5):257–277.
151. Onghena P, Van HB. Antidepressant-induced analgesia in chronic non-malignant pain: a meta-analysis of 39 placebo-controlled studies. *Pain* 1992;49(2):205–219.
152. Max MB, Culnane M, Schafer SC, et al. Amitriptyline relieves diabetic neuropathy pain in patients with normal or depressed mood. *Neurology* 1987;37(4):589–596.
153. Cardenas DD, Warms CA, Turner JA, et al. Efficacy of amitriptyline for relief of pain in spinal cord injury: results of a randomized controlled trial. *Pain* 2002;96(3):365–373.
154. Dickenson AH, Matthews EA, Suzuki R. Neurobiology of neuropathic pain: mode of action of anticonvulsants. *Eur J Pain* 2002;6(suppl A):51–60.
155. Campbell FG, Graham JG, Zilkha KJ. Clinical trial of carbazepine (tegretol) in trigeminal neuralgia. *J Neurol Neurosurg Psychiatry* 1966;29(3):265–267.
156. Backonja M, Beydoun A, Edwards KR, et al. Gabapentin for the symptomatic treatment of painful neuropathy in patients with diabetes mellitus: a randomized controlled trial. *JAMA* 1998;280(21):1831–1836.
157. Rowbotham M, Harden N, Stacey B, et al. Gabapentin for the treatment of postherpetic neuralgia: a randomized controlled trial. *JAMA* 1998;280(21):1837–1842.
158. Putzke JD, Richards JS, Kezar L, et al. Long-term use of gabapentin for treatment of pain after traumatic spinal cord injury. *Clin J Pain* 2002;18(2):116–121.
159. Tai Q, Kirshblum S, Chen B, et al. Gabapentin in the treatment of neuropathic pain after spinal cord injury: a prospective, randomized, double-blind, crossover trial. *J Spinal Cord Med.* 2002;25(2):100–105.
160. Levendoglu F, Ogun CO, Ozerbil O, et al. Gabapentin is a first line drug for the treatment of neuropathic pain in spinal cord injury. *Spine (Phila Pa 1976.)* 2004; 29(7):743–751.
161. Vranken JH, Dijkgraaf MG, Kruis MR, et al. Pregabalin in patients with central neuropathic pain: a randomized, double-blind, placebo-controlled trial of a flexible-dose regimen. *Pain* 2008;136(1–2):150–157.
162. Finnerup NB, Sindrup SH, Bach FW, et al. Lamotrigine in spinal cord injury pain: a randomized controlled trial. *Pain* 2002;96(3):375–383.
163. Dinoff BL, Richards JS, Ness TJ. Use of topiramate for spinal cord injury-related pain. *J Spinal Cord Med* 2003;26(4):401–403.
164. Baastrup C, Finnerup NB. Pharmacological management of neuropathic pain following spinal cord injury. *CNS Drugs* 2008;22(6):455–475.
165. Loubser PG, Donovan WH. Diagnostic spinal anaesthesia in chronic spinal cord injury pain. *Paraplegia* 1991; 29(1):25–36.
166. Attal N, Gaude V, Brasseur L, et al. Intravenous lidocaine in central pain: a double-blind, placebo-controlled, psychophysical study. *Neurology* 2000;54(3):564–574.
167. Eide PK, Stubhaug A, Stenehjem AE. Central dysesthesia pain after traumatic spinal cord injury is dependent on *N*-methyl-*D*-aspartate receptor activation. *Neurosurgery* 1995;37(6):1080–1087.
168. Attal N, Guirimand F, Brasseur L, et al. Effects of IV morphine in central pain: a randomized placebo-controlled study. *Neurology* 2002;58(4):554–563.
169. Friedman AH, Nashold BS Jr. DREZ lesions for relief of pain related to spinal cord injury. *J Neurosurg* 1986; 65(4):465–469.
170. Edgar RE, Best LG, Quail PA, et al. Computer-assisted DREZ microcoagulation: posttraumatic spinal deafferentation pain. *J Spinal Disord* 1993;6(1):48–56.
171. Falci S, Best L, Bayles R, et al. Dorsal root entry zone microcoagulation for spinal cord injury-related central pain: operative intramedullary electrophysiological guidance and clinical outcome. *J Neurosurg* 2002;97 (2 suppl):193–200.

172. Cioni B, Meglio M, Pentimalli L, et al. Spinal cord stimulation in the treatment of paraplegic pain. *J Neurosurg* 1995;82(1):35–39.
173. Previnaire JG, Nguyen JP, Perrouin-Verbe B, et al. Chronic neuropathic pain in spinal cord injury: efficiency of deep brain and motor cortex stimulation therapies for neuropathic pain in spinal cord injury patients. *Ann Phys Rehabil Med* 2009;52(2):188–193.
174. Norrbrink BC, Lundeberg T. Non-pharmacological pain-relieving therapies in individuals with spinal cord injury: a patient perspective. *Complement Ther Med* 2004;12(4):189–197.
175. Nayak S, Shiflett SC, Schoenberger NE, et al. Is acupuncture effective in treating chronic pain after spinal cord injury? *Arch Phys Med Rehabil* 2001;82(11):1578–1586.
176. Rapson LM, Wells N, Pepper J, et al. Acupuncture as a promising treatment for below-level central neuropathic pain: a retrospective study. *J Spinal Cord Med* 2003;26(1):21–26.
177. Molton IR, Graham C, Stoelb BL, et al. Current psychological approaches to the management of chronic pain. *Curr Opin Anaesthesiol* 2007;20(5):485–489.
178. Arner S, Meyerson BA. Lack of analgesic effect of opioids on neuropathic and idiopathic forms of pain. *Pain* 1988;33(1):11–23.
179. McQuay HJ. Neuropathic pain: evidence matters. *Eur.J Pain* 2002;6(suppl A):11–18.
180. Norrbrink BC, Lundeberg T. Use of analgesic drugs in individuals with spinal cord injury. *J Rehabil Med* 2005;37(2):87–94.
181. Heutink M, Post MW, Wollaars MM, et al. Chronic spinal cord injury pain: pharmacological and non-pharmacological treatments and treatment effectiveness. *Disabil Rehabil.* 2011;33(5):433–440.
182. Rintala DH, Fiess RN, Tan G, et al. Effect of dronabinol on central neuropathic pain after spinal cord injury: a pilot study. *Am J Phys Med Rehabil* 2010;89(10):840–848.
183. Margolis RB, Chibnall JT, Tait RC. Test-retest reliability of the pain drawing instrument. *Pain* 1988; 33(1):49–51.
184. Widerstrom-Noga EG, Felipe-Cuervo E, Yezierski RP. Relationships among clinical characteristics of chronic pain after spinal cord injury. *Arch Phys Med Rehabil* 2001;82(9):1191–1197

CHAPTER 27 ■ AGING IN SCI

AMITABH JHA AND SUSAN CHARLIFUE

INTRODUCTION

Emergency, acute, and rehabilitation treatments have advanced to the benefit of people with spinal cord injuries (SCIs) allowing them to survive the early years after injury in greater numbers (1–4). Advances in the availability of long-term health interventions, as well as the monitoring and even prevention of secondary conditions in the later years, further benefit people with SCI, who are often aging into their 60s, 70s, and beyond. The benefits of long, productive lives, however, come with challenges faced by all aging individuals, not only the physical decline that naturally occurs but also issues related to psychological changes with age, alterations in living situations and family structure, and the potential depletion of many social and economic resources. Adding SCI-specific issues to these challenges has the potential to further complicate the aging process.

This chapter describes the latest insights into issues of aging with SCI and offers suggestions for minimizing effects of aging in this group. First, an update of SCI mortality and life expectancy is presented, demonstrating the growing numbers of people facing various consequences of the aging process. Next, the impact of SCI and aging on both physical and psychosocial health is described, reviewing specific effects by body system. The chapter concludes with thoughts on the future of SCI and aging.

Mortality and Life Expectancy

Patterns in causes of death following SCI have undergone substantial change, as reported by a variety of studies. Renal failure and urinary tract complications were once reported to be the leading causes of death, (5–9) but this is no longer the case. More recently, respiratory complications primarily contribute to deaths in people with tetraplegia (10–16) and heart disease and cancer among those with paraplegia (12–14,17–20). With these changing patterns in the cause of death, it appears likely that many of the more recent causes are the culmination of chronic conditions encountered by individuals with SCI who are living longer and thus have a greater risk of exposure to the natural consequences of human aging.

While life expectancy for individuals with SCI is still lower than that for the general population, there are numerous indicators that survival has improved (21). Specifically, several studies demonstrate that survival is influenced by level and severity of injury (22–25), as well as by age at injury (26,27) and decade of injury (3,28–30). In general, individuals with higher injury level, with more neurologically complete lesions, and who are injured at older ages have higher mortality rates. With improvements in emergency and rehabilitative services, as well as ongoing medical management of health issues after injury, life expectancy in the more recent decades showed overall some improvement. Specifically, although first-year mortality rates showed steady improvement over time, long-term survival since 1982 has not improved (2,4). Nonetheless, data appear to indicate that individuals with SCI can live many years with disability, though they may be at greater risk to encounter chronic health conditions typically associated with aging. In addition, many of these aging-associated conditions may lead to death, especially when complicated by SCI. With these factors in mind, it is critical that clinicians understand the practical issues and mechanisms of human aging in general, in order to better address the consequences of these processes after SCI.

Organ System Effects of Aging in SCI

The cumulative effect of injury over many years of survival likely will result in the development of secondary complications, which may become increasingly prevalent with longer duration of impairment. This likelihood, in fact, has been confirmed in several studies describing health complications associated with aging and SCI (31–33).

The Gastrointestinal System

Several reviews have described the consequences of the aging process on gastrointestinal (GI) physiology and function in the general population (34). Within the esophagus, there is an age-related deterioration of function after the age of 40 (35). Although there are conflicting reports, the general consensus is that aging is associated with modest slowing of gastric emptying (36) as well as diminished acid secretion (37). While the small bowel shows little if any specific change related to aging, the colon and rectum exhibit diminished motility and an increase in diverticular disease (48).

Surveys of individuals with SCI have documented a variety of GI complications and functional changes that accompany the aging process, which may necessitate additional assistance with activities of daily living (ADL) (38,39). While some have speculated on increased rates of gastroesophageal reflux disease in those with SCI, a recent study confirmed the previously reported prevalence of 22% to 27% (40–42). Gastric motility changes may be implicated in chronic abdominal distention in long-term SCI; however, the underlying cause of gastric dilatation remains poorly understood (43).

Research indicates that gallstone disease is approximately seven times more prevalent in the SCI population than in the general population (44), having been found at autopsy in 29% of SCI subjects compared to a 4% incidence in nondisabled matched controls (45). It does not appear that the risk of gallstones is solely related to aging in SCI (46), but clinicians should be aware of the increased incidence of this condition when evaluating abdominal complaints in long-term medical follow-up. A recent report examining the prevalence and natural history of gallstones in people with SCI concluded that, while there was an increased risk for the development of gallstones, the risk of biliary complications was not of sufficient magnitude in this group to warrant prophylactic cholecystectomy (47).

In the GI system, colorectal function is significantly altered by SCI and would be expected to be a prominent source of problems in the aging SCI population. In particular, constipation is a frequently reported problem in numerous SCI studies regardless of age, but when coupled with generalized aging, it is likely to be more prevalent in older or longer-injured individuals with SCI (48). A longitudinal study of people more than 20 years postinjury in the United Kingdom showed that 42% had difficulties with constipation, while 27% reported problems with fecal incontinence, and 35% had GI pain (31,39). Even greater prevalence of constipation and fecal incontinence have been reported elsewhere (67% and 85%, respectively) (49). Furthermore, megacolon may be associated with being over 50 years of age with SCI or 10 years postinjury (50). Colonic transit time is known to be prolonged in persons with SCI, especially in the left colon and rectum (51,52). This slowing of distal gut motility correlates with the common report of constipation in this population.

The most profound alteration in GI physiology resulting from SCI is the loss of volitional control over bowel emptying, which can have substantial consequences on daily functions. The neurogenic bowel requires adopting a specific, individualized evacuation regimen that utilizes a variety of reflex stimulation maneuvers, laxatives, and dietary interventions. Constipation manifested by difficulties in producing reflex bowel evacuation is commonly the result of anorectal dyssynergia or inadequate rectal expulsive force due to SCI gut motility impairment (52). Primary treatment is predicated on a detailed assessment of the bowel routine, with suggestions for alterations based on common sense "return to basics." Many individuals with SCI may have chosen excessively long intervals between bowel programs for their convenience, although a healthier option is to maintain a bowel program frequency of daily or every other day evacuation. Regardless of the regimen selected, a consistent schedule that fits with the changing needs and the lifestyle of the individual aging with SCI is recommended (53). It is further recommended that laxative and enema use be avoided or kept to a minimum and, when necessary, suppository use should be supplemental to digital stimulation and evacuation. In persons with refractory bowel dysfunction characterized by excessively long duration of bowel program or frequent fecal incontinence, new cost-effective options are showing promise, including transanal irrigation techniques (54–56). Finally, when other methods no longer are effective or manageable, the performance of an elective colostomy may significantly improve quality of life (QOL) (57,58) (see Chapter 11 for additional details).

Hemorrhoids are also a common complication in those with chronic SCI, with a majority of people reporting the condition and accompanying periodic rectal bleeding (41). Topical therapy may suffice for minor symptomatic lesions, but banding is commonly required on more severe hemorrhoids. Operative hemorrhoidectomy can generally be avoided, but may be necessary in the most severe refractory cases with abundant hemorrhoid tissue and recurrent major bleeding.

While there is no current evidence to suggest that persons with SCI are at added risk for colon cancer, it is reasonable to assume that this population is at similar risk to the general population for this common cancer. Therefore, periodic SCI follow-up should include screening for colorectal cancer (43,59). Because of the frequent presence of hemorrhoids, rectal prolapse, and other distal rectal pathology common to those aging with SCI, fecal occult blood may not be a reliable screening tool. SCI survivors in the at-risk age group should therefore be screened periodically by endoscopy. The reported high frequency of GI problems in the aging SCI population warrants specific attention to bowel symptoms during routine follow-up, as well as emphasis on education regarding bowel program performance and a bowel-friendly diet.

The Genitourinary System

Normal aging in the general population is accompanied by diminished bladder capacity and urethral compliance, as well as an increase in uninhibited detrusor contractions and residual bladder volumes (60–62). Aging is also associated with a gradual decline in kidney function characterized by a decrease in glomerular filtration rate and renal plasma flow (63,64). Age-related changes in medication use, altered circadian rhythm, and diurnal output of urine can result in an increase in nocturia (64). Furthermore, elderly individuals appear to be at increased risk for urinary tract infections (UTIs), presumably related to the decline in immune function, postmenopausal changes, increased postvoid residual urine volumes, and prostatic disease (65–67).

Disruption of genitourinary (GU) function following SCI is characterized by loss of volitional control over micturition as well as loss of coordination of detrusor and sphincter reflexes that commonly results in sphincter/detrusor dyssynergia and elevated lower urinary tract pressure. This ultimately leads to hypertrophy of the detrusor muscle and decreased bladder compliance. Over time, the cumulative effect of these changes can lead to hydronephrosis and upper tract deterioration (68).

While SCI-related alterations in urinary tract physiology pose significant risks to health, urinary tract complications that were formerly the leading cause of death in SCI now account for between 3.8% and 5.4% of mortality in this population (69,70). Reduction in mortality from urinary tract complications is likely due to advances in urologic management and the availability of various antibiotics. It should be noted, however, that urological complications continue to be common (22,71,72) and UTIs are among the most frequent reasons for rehospitalization in the years following SCI (73,74). There is also a demonstrated decline with age in renal function as gauged by estimated creatinine clearance, serum creatinine, and serum urea (75).

Certain urinary complications seem to be associated with the method of bladder management, and may worsen with aging. Most studies have documented higher rates of UTI, bladder stones, and bladder cancer associated with the use of indwelling catheter management. In those who are managed with indwelling catheters, the routine use of anticholinergic medication may improve health outcomes (76,77). The use of long-term intermittent catheterization may increase an individual's risk for developing urethral strictures and epididymitis, two complications that have been found to increase with the number of years on intermittent catheterization (78).

Bladder cancer is one of the few neoplasms for which incidence is increased by the presence of SCI (79–82), although findings to the contrary have been reported (83,84). Bladder management technique is implicated in one study, which showed that indwelling catheter management resulted in a fourfold higher risk for development of bladder cancer than non–indwelling catheter methods of management (85). However, a recent study suggested that the neurogenic bladder, not the indwelling catheter, may be the risk factor for bladder cancer (86). Additional risk factors for the development of bladder cancer that derive from SCI include irritation to the bladder from recurrent UTIs and bladder stones (85,87,88), with the diagnosis of cancer being made approximately 20 years postinjury. It appears as though malignant degeneration requires the chronic cumulative effects of various risk factor exposure (e.g., recurrent infections, indwelling catheter management, urinary tract stones, cigarette smoking, etc.). Persons with SCI who develop bladder carcinoma typically present with hematuria; however, as hematuria commonly occurs with UTI, bladder stones, and catheter change, this sign alone is not a reliable indicator of bladder cancer in the SCI population. The clinical approach for care of the aging urinary tract should be based on prevention and early detection. Individuals with SCI should be educated regarding the fundamentals of bladder management in an effort to reduce the risk of recurrent UTI. Adequate hydration, hygienic bladder management technique, and routine urologic follow-up should be stressed, and smoking cessation programs should also be strongly encouraged.

Bladder tumors are commonly metastatic and invasive at the time of diagnosis in persons with SCI, and the importance of identifying and utilizing effective screening methods cannot be underestimated. Urine cytology and biochemical markers of urinary tract malignancy are problematic in that they have high false-positive rates, possibly due to concomitant UTIs and related hematuria. While some have questioned the effectiveness of screening cystoscopy to detect these tumors in chronically catheterized spinal cord individuals, most clinicians feel that this method remains the best option for early detection of bladder cancer in persons with SCI (87,89,90). Because of the risk of chronic prostatitis related to recurrent UTI, it is reasonable to speculate that there may be some added risk of prostate cancer in males with chronic SCI. To date, there is no compelling evidence that such an association exists. In fact, one study found that there was a lower incidence of carcinoma of the prostate in those individuals who were more disabled, suggesting that, at the very least, there is no *added* risk of this cancer associated with SCI (91). Nonetheless, it has been demonstrated that when prostate cancer is diagnosed in men with SCI, it is usually at a more advanced grade and stage (92). Deaths from prostate cancer in SCI are more common than previously reported, but this is more likely due to improved survival and longevity (93). Nonetheless, males aging with SCI should be considered at risk and be provided with the same age-specific prostate cancer screening that is recommended for the general population (see Chapter 13 for further details).

The Nervous System

Studies of general population aging have documented a number of changes referable to the nervous system, including diminished strength and reaction time, loss of vibratory sense, decreased fine coordination and agility, loss of muscle mass, diminished deep tendon reflexes, and a deterioration of station and gait (94–99). Research has demonstrated a continuous neuronal loss with aging in the spinal cord (100). Neuronal loss appears to result from a decline in cervical cord fractional anisotropy that starts early in life, but is dramatically accelerated in individuals over the age of 50 (101). This finding indicates that an alteration of cord tissue geometry is present with aging, likely as a consequence of a loss of nerve fiber alignment in the cords of elderly people. The clinical or functional significance of these changes for those with SCI is unclear.

Individuals aging with SCI demonstrate several nervous system changes, with one study showing 12% of subjects reporting some degree of sensory loss while 21% complained of increasing motor deficits over the years (102). While it is tempting to speculate that age-related dropout of anterior horn cells and loss of myelinated tracts may contribute to these reported symptoms, verification of this mechanism awaits further study.

Surveys of chronic SCI survivors have shown a high incidence of upper extremity (UE) entrapment neuropathies, with up to 63% of people with paraplegia showing evidence of this problem on electrodiagnostic testing and symptom survey (103,104). Individuals with SCI are at risk for nerve entrapments in the UEs by virtue of their repetitive hand contact with the wheelchair rim (105). Positioning of the wrist during critical transfer and pressure relief maneuvers may also be contributory. While most clinicians have felt that the incidence of significant entrapment increases with duration of injury, this association has not been conclusively proven, and underlying processes such as posttraumatic syringomyelia must be considered. The most frequent site of involvement is the median nerve at the wrist, but ulnar nerve entrapments at the elbow and wrist are also common. The treatment approach should include an assessment of the mechanics of ADL and mobility activities to determine the underlying sources of repetitive trauma. Activity modification may result in a resolution of symptoms in some cases. Although many individuals may not be able to completely eliminate offending activities from their daily routines, education regarding "wrist conservation" can have a beneficial effect for some individuals. Wrist splinting should also be offered as a means of reducing repetitive trauma and extremes of wrist flexion and extension, which are known to contribute to carpal tunnel symptomology. Corticosteroid injection therapy has been tried as an additional conservative measure for persons with carpal tunnel syndrome but has commonly been of only temporary benefit. When conservative measures have failed to produce symptomatic relief in people with significant entrapments, surgical release of the transverse carpal ligament is commonly recommended. Patients undergoing this surgery should anticipate a period of activity restriction after the surgery, which may necessitate a temporary increase in personal care assistance. Advances in surgical technique, including the percutaneous endoscopic approach to transverse carpal ligament section, have reduced the duration of postoperative activity restriction. Ulnar entrapments at the wrist may prompt consideration of surgical treatment, although these neuropathies are usually successfully treated in persons with SCI using activity and equipment modification, and as such, rarely require surgical intervention.

Neurologic deterioration in chronic SCI is most commonly the result of progressive posttraumatic cystic myelopathy (106–108). This condition, also referred to as posttraumatic syringomyelia, is characterized by the progressive enlargement of a cystic cavity originating at the site of injury and extending in either a cephalad or caudal direction in the spinal cord. More recently, progressive cystic myelopathy has been expanded to include progressive noncystic or myelomalacic myelopathies, which are both felt to respond to surgical intervention (109). The signs and symptoms of this late progressive neurologic deterioration include loss of motor and sensory function, increased spasticity, late onset neurological pain, increased autonomic dysreflexia, increased sweating and the development of a variable, positional Horner syndrome. The diagnosis is confirmed by the combination of typical history and physical findings accompanied by the magnetic resonance imaging abnormality of an enlarging syrinx or myelomalacic spinal cord. The onset of this neurologic complication may vary from several months to several decades after injury, but most commonly occurs within the first 5 to 10 years postinjury. The underlying mechanism of the progressive spinal cord pathology appears to be related to arachnoid scarring that interferes with spinal fluid flow and spinal cord mobility. When neurologic deterioration is progressive, surgical treatment including untethering of the arachnoid scar and, in some cases, shunting of cyst cavity fluid, is indicated (108,110). Because of the potential for late neurologic change in all patients with SCI, periodic assessment of motor and sensory function as well as a neurological review of systems should be included in periodic follow-up. Signs or symptoms of neurologic deterioration should result in appropriate electrodiagnostic and imaging studies (108,111) (see Chapter 16 for details).

The Musculoskeletal System

Aging is the major risk factor for osteoarthritis (OA), which is the single most debilitating disease in elderly individuals (112,113). Because OA occurs in tissues with little capacity for repair (114), the continued degenerative loss will result in subsequent functional limitations. OA is also a common cause of pain, which is the most common manifestation of the disease (115). In addition to pain, in its advanced state, OA can result in a loss of active and passive range of motion (116). Osteoporosis is also a common accompaniment to the aging process, being most commonly associated with postmenopausal elderly women but also occurring in aging men (117).

Surveys have documented that UE pain is reported by more than 50% of SCI survivors (118). Not only is there a positive association between shoulder pain and age, but this condition occurs at a younger age in those with SCI compared to the general population (119). UE discomfort is most commonly experienced during transfers, wheelchair propulsion, and pressure relief maneuvers. Acromioclavicular degenerative changes may be seen on x-ray but plain radiographs are commonly of little value in the assessment of shoulder pain in these individuals. Arthrography, MRI imaging, and ultrasound have better diagnostic yield and commonly show impingement syndromes, tendinopathies, and rotator cuff tears in both symptomatic and asymptomatic individuals with SCI reporting shoulder pain (120–122). When individuals with SCI present with shoulder pain, conservative management should include a review of daily activities and mobility mechanics that may result in suggestions for activity modification in an effort to avoid pain-causing maneuvers (123). Many individuals with overuse syndrome at the shoulders have a muscular imbalance across the glenohumeral joint, with anterior musculature development significantly greater than posterior to the shoulder. An exercise regimen specifically designed to address the posterior shoulder girdle may reestablish muscular balance across the joint and thus restore optimal glenohumeral geometric relationships (118). When conservative measures fail, surgery for impingement or rotator cuff tears has been suggested. While operative treatment has produced successful outcome in some patients, postoperative rehabilitation may be difficult and prolonged, considering the shoulder activity restrictions commonly utilized after such procedures. Patients contemplating operative treatment for impingement or rotator cuff tears should also anticipate a prolonged but temporary impact on independence, with additional personal care assistance commonly required (124,125).

Osteoporosis due to paralysis and disuse is commonly felt to be the underlying risk factor for pathologic fractures following SCI. Studies have documented an extremity fracture rate of over 30% for individuals followed several decades (126). Lower extremity osteoporosis develops rapidly in the first postinjury year, with about one third of the original bone mass being lost by 16 months postinjury before relative stability is achieved (127). Several interventions have been proposed to limit further bone loss and even enhance bone growth, including standing, functional electrical stimulation (FES), and treatment with bisphosphonates; however, these do not provide long-term prevention of osteoporosis and protection from fracture risk. There is evidence that high-volume FES cycling induces some bone formation at the distal femur, although other areas of the lower extremities do not show the same benefit (128). Furthermore, preliminary trials of pamidronate showed some promise (129) but more recent evidence suggested less efficacy in preventing bone loss (130).

Because of both the frequency of musculoskeletal complaints in this population as well as increased fracture risk, SCI clinicians should incorporate a thorough symptom review and examination as a part of periodic reassessment. Modifications to equipment, posture, and the ways in which individuals perform functional activities may be necessary as they age. Periodic bone density evaluations may be warranted, particularly for menopausal women with SCI.

The Integument

Normal aging of the skin results in atrophy and changes in the histologic structures that comprise the dermis (131). The epidermis thins and dermal ridges flatten, making the skin less resistant to shearing forces (132), and resulting in a greater likelihood of epidermal detachment and blister formation. Decreased vascularity and sweating may also add to the risk of thermal injury.

Persons with SCI are known to be at risk for skin trauma that results in pressure ulcers. Immobility, lack of sensory protection, and spasticity all contribute to the common occurrence of skin sores in this population. Analysis of National Institute on Disability and Rehabilitation Research Model Spinal Cord Injury Systems data from the United States showed a statistically significant increase in the average number of pressure ulcers from 5 to 20 years of follow-up (133). The Model Systems data also showed the incidence of pressure ulcers increasing from 15% at 1 year postinjury to nearly 30% at 20 years postinjury (72). More recent evidence suggests that the incidence of pressure ulcers is increasing (134). A Canadian study showed similar findings, with the hazards ratio for developing pressure ulcers increasing each year postinjury (33).

The clinical approach to management of skin sores after SCI is primarily prevention through patient education regarding skin protection, pressure relief, hygiene, and routine surveillance. Conservative treatment of pressure sores is commonly effective if promptly initiated and diligently performed. The basic principles of pressure relief, debridement, and asepsis are still the foundation of successful conservative management (135,136). Anecdotal clinical experience and published data suggest that vacuum-assisted wound closure may be beneficial in clearing drainage and promoting wound healing (137). Large and deep skin sores will commonly require myocutaneous flap closure. Local infection will require treatment with appropriate antibiotics and deep wounds should raise the suspicion of contiguous osteomyelitis. In such cases, a bone biopsy should be performed for the purposes of diagnosis and identification of the causative organisms in order to guide antibiotic therapy. Chronic open skin sores of long duration have been associated with the development of Marjolins ulcer and the development of squamous carcinoma in the sore. Because of the high frequency of skin sore occurrence in the chronic SCI population, periodic assessment should include a thorough evaluation of the integument and reinforcement of skin sore prevention education (see Chapter 14 for details).

The Immune System

Research on normal aging in the immune system has shown age-related decline of immune function with increased risk of infection (138,139). It is suggested that immunosenescence is likely influenced by multiple factors including the pathogen load that individuals are exposed to throughout their lives (140). In addition, while aging is a major risk factor for infection, it has been suggested that infection may also contribute to the aging process (141). Of note is that UTIs are more prevalent in the elderly than in younger adults (141). The function of the immune system is also known to be influenced by factors such as depression, deterioration of social support systems, pain, and the influence of medications (142).

Studies of individuals with SCI have shown evidence of diminished immune function in those with tetraplegia manifested by impaired bacterial phagocytosis, while those with paraplegia with lesions at or below T-10 showed no loss of phagocytic function (143). The British study of aging with SCI showed a dramatic increase in UTIs among those aged 60 and over and a slight increase in frequency of infection between the 10 and 30th postinjury year (31). It appears safe to assume that persons aging with SCI will have more likelihood of immune impairment than their nondisabled counterparts. Studies have suggested that exercise and rehabilitation therapies are associated with improved cellular immunity in persons with SCI (144,145). Clearly, with the high incidence of urinary infection in SCI and the increase of these infectious processes with aging, advances in immunological assessment and treatment hopefully will yield therapies that can improve immune defenses in these individuals.

The Respiratory System

Studies of aging in the general population have shown a number of changes that result in a gradual loss of respiratory system function with advancing years (146,147). Loss of lung and chest wall compliance is accompanied by a decrease in the number of alveoli. There is a progressive loss of vital capacity as well as centrally mediated respiratory drive. Sleep disordered breathing is also more prevalent among the elderly, particularly males, likely as a result of age-related increases in body weight, loss of upper airway muscle tone, and other factors that operate on the ventilator control system (148–150).

SCI is associated with respiratory complications, both in the immediate postinjury period and during long-term follow-up (33,72). Individuals with neurologically complete tetraplegia are at highest risk, followed by those with incomplete tetraplegia and paraplegia. Older age at the time of injury is also associated with a higher risk of respiratory complications (33). The combined effects of SCI and older age are likely to pose a significant risk for respiratory tract complications such as pneumonia and atelectasis, as well as sleep disordered breathing. This is particularly concerning as the leading causes of rehospitalization and death in people with both acute and chronic SCI are respiratory disorders (15). Studies have investigated the incidence of respiratory tract morbidity in persons aging with SCI. In a study of 834 persons followed at one of two British SCI centers who were at least 20 years postinjury, the incidence of pneumonia and atelectasis was found to increase with age (going from 1.6% in the less than 30 years of age group to 5.4% in the over 60 years of age group), but not with duration of injury (31). Model Systems data reveal similar findings, with pneumonia incidence increasing from 1.5% per year in the 16 to 30 year age group to 8.2% in the over 76-year-old group (151). Thus, it would appear that within the time frames studied, the risk of respiratory complications is associated with the age of the patient rather than their duration of injury.

Several studies have documented a higher rate of sleep disordered breathing in individuals with SCI, noted within weeks of injury and continuing in the follow-up years, with prevalence ranging from 25% to 53% (152–155). Interestingly, the level of impairment does not appear to be the main contributing factor, and increased abdominal girth, neck circumference, and duration of injury also do not consistently identify those at greater risk of sleep apnea.

What should these findings mean to clinicians? An appreciation of the respiratory risk of aging SCI patients should lead to heightened surveillance for changes in function. Periodic assessments should include measurement of vital capacity, especially in those with cervical levels of injury who are at the highest risk (156). Persons with SCI who have respiratory impairment should receive pneumococcal vaccination as well as yearly influenza immunization. Diagnosis and treatment of sleep disordered breathing may also be indicated in symptomatic individuals (157). Obese individuals should be encouraged to lose weight in order to reduce the risk of further respiratory compromise that may accompany overweight. Smoking cessation programs should be offered to all smokers as a means to further lessen the risk of respiratory complications. Exercise may benefit respiratory capacity as well. When the individual with SCI presents with community-acquired pneumonia, clinicians are encouraged to adopt a more aggressive treatment approach, including hospitalization, mobilizing pulmonary secretions via manually assisted coughing and mechanical cough assistance, and prompt administration of antibiotics (15). In spite of these efforts, those with borderline respiratory reserve may face the prospect of aging-related respiratory failure due to the combined effects of gradual functional decline and development of respiratory complications such as pneumonia. In these circumstances, difficult choices regarding the acceptance of mechanical ventilatory support will need to be made.

The Cardiovascular System

Cardiovascular diseases (CVDs) are the most common causes of death in the United States among both men and women of all racial and ethnic groups (158). Age is the most important risk factor for manifest ischemic heart disease, but the contribution of other risk factors is significant (159). Atherosclerosis in humans appears to develop gradually, usually in the absence of any known disease, and is often exacerbated by genetic and environmental factors (160,161). In addition to these changes, there are a number of age-related alterations in the structure and function of the heart and blood vessels. Physical inactivity, common in older individuals, also is associated with cardiovascular deconditioning (160).

Heart disease is known to be one of the leading causes of death in long-term SCI, now causing more than 20% of deaths (28,69,70). In a study of long-term SCI survivors, the risk of developing CVD was associated with both level and completeness of injury (162). Although a number of SCI studies have documented abnormalities of glucose and lipid metabolism as well as other risk factors for the development of CVD (163–165), a report from the Agency for Healthcare Research and Quality concluded that there was insufficient evidence to suggest that adults with SCI are at greater risk of carbohydrate and lipid disorders, nor did it support the use of different thresholds to define or treat lipid abnormalities in this population (166). While the published literature may not be conclusive, it is possible that cardiovascular risk in SCI is underestimated (166) and heightened surveillance is prudent.

People with SCI tend to have a lipid profile characterized by low HDL, although total cholesterol and LDL are not significantly different from matched nondisabled controls (167). With regard to insulin resistance, it has been suggested that diabetes is an independent risk factor for mortality in people with SCI (69). A study of male veterans with SCI found 22% to be diabetic when using oral glucose tolerance testing as the diagnostic standard compared to 6% in nondisabled control subjects (164). While 82% of the control subjects had normal glucose tolerance, only 50% of those with paraplegia and 38% of those with tetraplegia had normal testing. Changes in body composition, which are common in SCI, may contribute to impaired glucose metabolism (165). Spinal injured individuals typically have a reduction of lean muscle mass and a corresponding increase of fat mass. In addition, the diminished activity level of people with SCI may also contribute to insulin resistance and lowered HDL (see Chapter 12).

The described alterations in lipid and glucose metabolism indicate that people with SCI may have an elevated risk of coronary heart disease and other manifestations of CVD. As for the general population, periodic assessment of risk factors such as blood lipids, glucose, weight, blood pressure, dietary habits, smoking, activity level, and alcohol consumption may help identify modifiable risk factors. Individuals should be encouraged to follow a diet that limits intake of saturated fats and cholesterol. Weight management should be promoted and incorporated into nutritional counseling. When adverse lipid profiles require pharmacological management, compliance with medication regimens should be encouraged (168). As evidence suggests that FES may improve arterial function and metabolic profiles in people with SCI (169,170), exercise and a general increase in physical activity may prove beneficial. Finally, smoking cessation programs should be aggressively promoted.

SCI and Aging—Psychosocial Aspects

Physical changes of aging in people with SCI are often accompanied by changes in an individual's satisfaction with life and degree of community integration. Unlike physical aging, these aspects of a person's life may improve. In addition, when potential problems do arise, much can be done to intervene and delay, modify, or eliminate potential negative consequences. Investigating these issues provides a complex, often confusing picture, as so many interrelated factors are involved. Consideration must be given not only to the physical and potential cognitive changes associated with aging but also to the highly individualized psychological adjustment to these changes. Economic factors, environmental barriers and facilitators, cultural issues, and changes in intimate and more remote social relationships may also affect, or be affected by physiological aging. Consideration of these multiple factors in the evaluation of individuals aging with SCI is critical in order to understand the thorough contextual basis that underlies this complex phenomenon.

Independence

Declining function is one of the many consequences of aging. As people grow older, many experience a loss of physical independence resulting from diminished muscle strength, decreased sensory acuity, slowed reflexes, decreased coordination, inadequate aerobic capacity, and lower energy levels (171–177). These and other chronic conditions, as well as injuries, can limit an individual's ability to carry out the predominant social role expected of a person at a given age, whether that role involves attending school, working, or living independently. Data from the National Center for Health Statistics showed that nearly 20% of the civilian community-dwelling population of the United States aged 55 to 64 and more than 34% of those aged 65 and older reported some degree of activity limitation (178).

The presence of some form of activity limitation is almost inevitable from the onset of SCI. This is not a static condition, however, and aging may magnify issues of dependency as needs, abilities, and limitations change over time. Three main issues appear to be of concern to people aging with SCI: their overall health, ability to remain independent, and their ability to sustain a satisfying lifestyle (179). Research has indicated that some of these concerns may be well founded. In a study of British individuals with SCI for 20 or more years' duration, increasing age was a significant predictor of functional decline. The average age when additional functional assistance was first needed was 49 years for those with tetraplegia and 54 years for those with paraplegia (180). Functional decline or decreasing physical independence has been identified as an adverse outcome of long-term SCI, with one study showing 22% of participants reporting a decline over a 3-year time span (181). In another investigation, there were significant cross-sectional and longitudinal increases in the need for assistance among older individuals (182).

Fortunately, preserving functional ability and maintaining independence are areas that are amenable to intervention, either through changing the manner in which certain activities are accomplished, such as transfers, or by using adaptive equipment. Even when assistance from others is necessary, this can be incorporated into an individual's life in such a way that optimizes independence for the person with SCI. Although often limited by physical status, independence is still intellectually realistic, even as the person ages with SCI. This allows the individual with SCI to make decisions and be the director in all health and care-related issues such as having the power to hire, train, and even fire helpers.

Stress, Depression, and Perceived Quality of Life

Changes in the level of independence that accompanies the aging process have been shown to be consistently related to reports of health, stress, depression, and declining QOL (172,183). However, research has shown that to assume older people experience more stress than younger individuals may not be entirely accurate. Aldwin and colleagues evaluated stress and coping using a sample of 1,065 men who participated in the longitudinal Normative Aging Study. Their study found age differences in the types of problems reported, with health and "general hassles" being reported as problems more often with increasing age, but also a trend for the older groups to rate their problems as less stressful (184).

Stress and poor health have been linked with depression in older individuals (185). The consequences of depression in later life can be quite serious, as mental and physical health of older individuals are often inseparable (186,187). Specifically, prospective cohort studies have demonstrated compelling evidence that psychosocial factors such as depression are independent, etiological and prognostic factors for coronary heart disease (188,189).

In spite of the many reports of increasing depression with age, there is evidence that perceived QOL is not necessarily worse for older individuals (190). Often used interchangeably with concepts such as life satisfaction, happiness, and well-being, QOL is multidimensional, and includes biological, psychological, interpersonal, social, economic, and cultural dimensions. For some individuals, QOL may be determined by financial security; for others, maintaining health or having good relationships with others are determinants of life satisfaction. Often, it is not aging, in and of itself that is associated with lower perceived QOL. Maintaining good health, social support, and participation in activities have been found to be more predictive of higher QOL (190) and a person's sense of contentment has been suggested as an underlying factor of life satisfaction (191).

Studies of stress, depression, and QOL in people aging with SCI generally support findings in the general aging literature. Gerhart and colleagues (192) found no significant differences in perceived stress by age, duration of injury, gender, or severity of impairment among a group of British individuals aging with SCI. In fact, there was a tendency toward less stress in older individuals. Although there was no evidence of a strong relationship between stress and medical outcomes, there was a clear relationship between stress and other psychosocial outcomes, particularly depressive symptomatology, life satisfaction, and QOL.

Of all the possible psychosocial outcomes, depression has received a great deal of attention by researchers studying SCI. Clearly, depression is common among individuals with SCI (193,194) and is greater for those who are older and who have been injured longer (195). There are inconsistencies, however, in reports of life satisfaction for people aging with SCI, with some studies indicating that life satisfaction is not necessarily negatively impacted by aging (182), while others find mixed patterns of change over time (196,197). The variation in these findings may best be explained by the differences in how older and younger individuals assess QOL. Nonetheless, in general, it does appear that individuals with SCI maintain relatively good and reportedly stable life satisfaction over time—even after many years of living with SCI (198). Clearly, identifying the potential multitude of underlying factors that might contribute to declines in perceived QOL, increased stress, or depressive symptoms is a difficult task. To effectively understand these phenomena, health care providers must not only assess the physical health and well-being of the individual aging with SCI but also the psychological status, social situation, and environment, as all have an impact on successful aging.

Family Issues

SCI can have a far-reaching impact on family members, friends, and others in the community close to the individual, particularly when that person requires physical assistance. It has been suggested that nearly 70% of people with SCI will receive some form of assistance and support from family members (199). In addition, evidence suggests that SCI survivors' need for help increases as they age (180). Related to this issue is the fact that many SCI caregivers are also aging, and are faced with their own age-related health issues. Potentially, poor health of the caregiver can have negative consequences for the recipient of that assistance, and with the advancing age of both, these consequences are likely to be magnified. Therefore, the physical and emotional health of family members, particularly if they provide personal assistance services to their loved one with SCI, also need to be addressed during routine follow-up. Detecting potential difficulties as early as possible and offering appropriate interventions such as seeking occasional respite care or utilizing home health agency assistance can help families maintain a positive focus on issues other than caregiving.

Another aspect of caregiving relates to the person with SCI's willingness and ability to adapt to needing more assistance. There is evidence that assistance provided by a caregiving spouse is not always positively perceived by the recipient, and increasing age is a significant predictor of negative reactions to receiving assistance (200). This may be of particular concern for those individuals with SCI who, having been independent when younger, begin to need assistance as they age. The new need for help can be difficult to accept, as maintaining independence is important to people aging with SCI. Beneficial strategies include encouraging people with SCI to prioritize those activities that are most time consuming, difficult, or tedious, as those such as dressing, tub transfers, or bowel programs can be delegated to others,. This can enable them to preserve energy and use it to engage in desired personal and social activities.

Role Changes

SCI often requires that families make adjustments in which home and work activities are done by whom. The differential distribution of day-to-day tasks after injury may add to an imbalance in perceived equality of family members, making it difficult to maintain family relationships (201,202). Conversely, some studies have noted that the ability to form new or maintain existing relationships actually improves after SCI (203,204). Role functions that may have changed early postinjury are not likely to be static. As people with SCI age and forfeit some degree of independence, further adjustments in the distribution of tasks may be needed. This particularly impacts those who previously had been able to assume the majority of familial responsibility after their injuries and find themselves becoming more dependent with age. Clinicians can be of best service to people with SCI and their families by being aware that this type of role-related stress in a relationship can ultimately have a detrimental impact on the health of both the caregiver and care recipient.

Environmental Issues

Not all issues for the person aging with SCI are focused on physical or psychosocial changes that may occur as time passes. An important and often overlooked factor is the environment. Environmental factors such as architecture, attitudes, and policies may place restrictions on the degree to which people with disabilities can fully participate in society. Conversely, it is possible that these environmental factors may also remove barriers and thus facilitate an individual's societal participation.

Studies in the general population have suggested that environmental as well as personal factors have significant effects on the QOL and activity level of older individuals living independently in the community (205,206). Access to resources, the ability to move about in the community, attitudes of others, and the impact of public policies all may be altered for people as they age. This can be even more pronounced in those aging with a disability such as SCI. Recent research has shown that significant differences exist between people with and without disabilities in terms of both the frequency with which they encountered environmental barriers and the magnitude of the problems those barriers created (207). Of interest, however, is that a large US study showed that a group of individuals with SCI aged 50 and older report encountering *fewer* environmental barriers than do individuals aged 20 to 49 (208). Different factors may account for this finding. First, older individuals with SCI, who might have encountered a variety of environmental barriers when younger or more newly injured, may have made adjustments to their lives in order to avoid or minimize such barriers. Thus, as they age, they are less likely to encounter some of the environmental barriers that older individuals without disabilities may face. Second, older individuals with SCI may be less likely to be as mobile in their communities and spend more time at home, thus not encountering external barriers as often. Whether or not adjustments to avoid environmental barriers are enhancements to QOL is unclear. It is recommended, therefore, that exploration of perceived and real environmental barriers be included as part of long-term follow-up. If in fact identified barriers are perceived as minimally limiting to both activity and QOL, they are unlikely to have an overall negative impact for the individual aging with SCI. If identified barriers do, however, act to diminish a person's perceived health, QOL, or life satisfaction, then addressing these barriers and seeking ways to eliminate or minimize their impact is warranted.

TABLE 27.1

EXAMPLE GUIDELINES FOR AGING WITH SCI

General health maintenance	SCI specific
Things to do monthly Women: breast self-examination Men: testicular self-examination	**Things to Do Daily** Self skin checks
Things to do every 1–2 y Checkup with health care provider Fecal occult blood test (A) Mammography, ages 40 and older (A) Digital rectal exam and Prostate Specific Antigen (PSA), beginning at age 75 (A) Comprehensive eye examination, age 55 and older (B)	**Things to do every 1–2 y** Check weight and blood pressure Flu immunization, especially T8 and higher
Things to do every 2–3 y Complete blood count with biochemistry survey Clinical breast cancer exam (A) Gynecological exam and Pap test (C)	**Things to do at least every 2–3 y with SCI specialist/team[a]** Full history and physical review with physician[a] Urologic assessment—upper and lower tracts[a,b] Assess equipment and posture[a] Assess range of motion, contractures, function[a] Full skin evaluation[a]
Things to do every 5 y CT colonography (A) Screening sigmoidoscopy (A) Full lipid panel, beginning at age 35/45 (C) Things to do every 10 y Tetanus booster (D) Colonoscopy (A)	**Things to do at least every 5 y with SCI specialist/team** Motor and sensory testing Review changes in life situation, including coping, adjustment, life satisfaction Assess lung function (FEV_1/FVC) Things to do every 10 y Pneumococcal pneumonia vaccination at earliest opportunity, especially for T8 and higher

Recommendations may vary by different organizations and by age, ethnicity, family history, and other factors.
[a]Assessments done annually for the first 3 to 5 years after injury, until health established.
[b]Do annually for the first 3 years after any major change in urologic management.
Sources: A, American Cancer Society; B, Prevent Blindness America; C, US Preventive Services Task Force (also http://www.ahrq.gov/clinic/pocketgd08/gcp08s1.htm); D, Centers for Disease Control and Prevention, 2009.

Anticipating the Future

As more people with SCI survive into their later years, the community of health care providers is faced with new challenges to facilitate the successful aging of these individuals. Increasing liaisons with gerontologists and other professionals with an expertise in aging is increasingly important to the SCI rehabilitation community.

If aging with SCI is to be effectively managed, strategies to minimize conditions and complications that occur with aging should be identified and implemented as early as possible. This process involves routine clinical follow-up, continuing education for both clinicians and individuals aging with SCI, and further research. The first critical component involves systematic surveillance by an experienced SCI team in order to identify potential problems at their earliest onset. A recommended follow-up regimen is shown in Table 27.1.

Ongoing education for the clinician involves learning about the physical, psychological, social, and environmental consequences of aging and their potential impact on people with SCI. Education for the person with SCI is widely enhanced via electronic access to information. Unfortunately, much of this easily accessible information is inaccurate and potentially damaging. Encouraging an open atmosphere of questions and answers will help guide people with SCI through the maze of information, and is critical to ensure that the best practices are adopted. Stressing the need for continued rehabilitation or equipment modifications will also be valuable as physical needs and independence change over time. Finally, research efforts to understand the complexity of aging with SCI will need to continue with larger, more representative study samples.

Aging needs to be viewed without prejudice as simply another step along the continuum of life with SCI—equal in importance to milestones of initial rehabilitation, returning to work, developing relationships, and engaging in other life activities. In doing so, the likelihood of successfully managing the myriad of changes that will be encountered by both the clinician and the person with SCI will be greatly enhanced.

References

1. Waters RL, Apple DF, Meyer PR. Emergency and acute management of spine trauma. In: Stover SL, DeLisa JA, Whiteneck GG, eds. *Spinal cord injury: clinical outcomes from the model systems*. Gaithersburg, MD: Aspen Publishers, 1995;56–78.
2. DeVivo MJ, Krause JS, Lammertse DP. Recent trends in mortality and causes of death among persons with spinal cord injury. *Arch Phys Med Rehabil* 1999;80:1411–1419.
3. Strauss DJ, Devivo MJ, Paculdo DR, et al. Trends in life expectancy after spinal cord injury. *Arch Phys Med Rehabil* 2006;87:1079–1085.
4. DeVivo MJ. Sir Ludwig Guttmann lecture: trends in spinal cord injury rehabilitation outcomes from model systems in the United States: 1973–2006. *Spinal Cord* 2007;45:713–721.
5. Tribe CR. Causes of death in the early and late stages of paraplegia. *Paraplegia* 1963;1:19–47.
6. Barber KE, Cross RR Jr. The urinary tract as a cause of death in paraplegia. *J Urol* 1952;67:494–502.
7. Dietrick RB, Russi S. Tabulation and review of autopsy findings in fifty-five paraplegics. *J Am Med Assoc* 1958;166:41–44.
8. Nyquist RH, Bors E. Mortality and survival in traumatic myelopathy during nineteen years, from 1946 to 1965. *Paraplegia* 1967;5:22–48.
9. Whiteneck GG, Charlifue SW, Frankel HL, et al. Mortality, morbidity, and psychosocial outcomes of persons spinal cord injured more than 20 years ago. *Paraplegia* 1992;30:617–630.
10. Carter RE. Experiences with high tetraplegics. *Paraplegia* 1979;17:140–146.
11. Kiwerski J, Weiss M, Chrostowska T. Analysis of mortality of patients after cervical spine trauma. *Paraplegia* 1981; 19:347–351.
12. Frisbie JH, Kache A. Increasing survival and changing causes of death in myelopathy patients. *J Am Paraplegia Soc* 1983;6:51–56.
13. DeVivo MJ, Kartus PL, Stover SL, et al. Cause of death for patients with spinal cord injuries. *Arch Intern Med* 1989;149:1761–1766.
14. DeVivo MJ, Black KJ, Stover SL. Causes of death during the first 12 years after spinal cord injury. *Arch Phys Med Rehabil* 1993;74:248–254.
15. Burns SP. Acute respiratory infections in persons with spinal cord injury. *Phys Med Rehabil Clin N Am* 2007; 18:203–216, v–vi.
16. Lidal IB, Snekkevik H, Aamodt G, et al. Mortality after spinal cord injury in Norway. *J Rehabil Med* 2007; 39:145–151.
17. Samsa GP, Patrick CH, Feussner JR. Long-term survival of veterans with traumatic spinal cord injury. *Arch Neurol* 1993;50:909–914.
18. Le CT, Price M. Survival from spinal cord injury. *J Chronic Dis* 1982;35:487–492.
19. Charlifue SW, Gerhart KA. Behavioral and demographic predictors of suicide after traumatic spinal cord injury. *Arch Phys Med Rehabil* 1991;72:488–492.
20. DeVivo MJ, Black KJ, Richards JS, et al. Suicide following spinal cord injury. *Paraplegia* 1991;29:620–627.
21. DeVivo MJ, Stover SL. Long-term survival and causes of death. In: Stover SL, DeLisa JA, Whiteneck GG, eds. *Spinal cord injury: clinical outcomes from the model systems*. Gaithersburg, MD: Aspen Publishers, Inc., 1995.
22. Vaidyanathan S, Soni BM, Gopalan L, et al. A review of the readmissions of patients with tetraplegia to the Regional Spinal Injuries Centre, Southport, United Kingdom, between January 1994 and December 1995. *Spinal Cord* 1998;36:838–846.
23. Yeo JD, Walsh J, Rutkowski S, et al. Mortality following spinal cord injury. *Spinal Cord* 1998;36:329–336.
24. McColl MA, Walker J, Stirling P, et al. Expectations of life and health among spinal cord injured adults. *Spinal Cord* 1997;35:818–828.
25. Strauss D, DeVivo M, Shavelle R, et al. Economic factors and longevity in spinal cord injury: a reappraisal. *Arch Phys Med Rehabil* 2008;89:572–574.
26. Alander DH, Parker J, Stauffer ES. Intermediate-term outcome of cervical spinal cord-injured patients older than 50 years of age. *Spine* 1997;22:1189–1192.
27. Shavelle RM, DeVivo MJ, Paculdo DR, et al. Long-term survival after childhood spinal cord injury. *J Spinal Cord Med* 2007;30:S48–S54.

28. DeVivo MJ, Ivie CS. Life expectancy of ventilator-dependent persons with spinal cord injuries. *Chest* 1995;108:226–232.
29. Frankel HL, Coll JR, Charlifue SW, et al. Long-term survival in spinal cord injury: a fifty year investigation. *Spinal Cord* 1998;36:266–274.
30. Shavelle RM, DeVivo MJ, Strauss DJ, et al. Long-term survival of persons ventilator dependent after spinal cord injury. *J Spinal Cord Med* 2006;29:511–519.
31. Whiteneck GG, Charlifue SW, Frankel HL, et al. Mortality, morbidity, and psychosocial outcomes of persons spinal cord injured more than 20 years ago. *Paraplegia* 1992;30:617–630.
32. Whiteneck GG, Charlifue SW, Gerhart KA, et al., eds. *Aging with spinal cord injury*. New York, NY: Demos Medical Publishers, 1993.
33. Hitzig SL, Tonack M, Campbell KA, et al. Secondary health complications in an aging Canadian spinal cord injury sample. *Am J Phys Med Rehabil* 2008;87:545–555.
34. Bhutto A, Morley JE. The clinical significance of gastrointestinal changes with aging. *Curr Opin Clin Nutr Metab Care* 2008;11:651–660.
35. Gregersen H, Pedersen J, Drewes AM. Deterioration of muscle function in the human esophagus with age. *Dig Dis Sci* 2008;53:3065–3070.
36. Kuo P, Rayner CK, Horowitz M. Gastric emptying, diabetes, and aging. *Clin Geriatr Med* 2007;23:785–808, vi.
37. Hall KE, Proctor DD, Fisher L, et al. American Gastroenterological Association Future Trends Committee report: effects of aging of the population on gastroenterology practice, education, and research. *Gastroenterology* 2005;129:1305–1338.
38. Liem NR, McColl MA, King W, et al. Aging with a spinal cord injury: factors associated with the need for more help with activities of daily living. *Arch Phys Med Rehabil* 2004;85:1567–1577.
39. Menter R, Weitzenkamp D, Cooper D, et al. Bowel management outcomes in individuals with long-term spinal cord injuries. *Spinal Cord* 1997;35:608–612.
40. Singh G, Triadafilopoulos G. Gastroesophageal reflux disease in patients with spinal cord injury. *J Spinal Cord Med* 2000;23:23–27.
41. Stone JM, Nino-Murcia M, Wolfe VA, et al. Chronic gastrointestinal problems in spinal cord injury patients: a prospective analysis. *Am J Gastroenterol* 1990;85:1114–1119.
42. Silva CB, Martinez JC, Yanagita ET, et al. The repercussions of spinal cord injury on the action of the diaphragmatic crura for gastroesophageal reflux containment. *Spine* 2008;33:2892–2897.
43. Cosman BC, Stone JM, Perkash I. The gastrointestinal system. In: Whiteneck GG, Charlifue SW, Gerhart KA, et al., eds. *Aging with Spinal Cord Injury*. New York, NY: Demos Publications, 1993.
44. Xia CS, Han YQ, Yang XY, et al. Spinal cord injury and cholelithiasis. *Hepatobiliary Pancreat Dis Int* 2004;3:595–598.
45. Apstein MD, Dalecki-Chipperfield K. Spinal cord injury is a risk factor for gallstone disease. *Gastroenterology* 1987;92:966–968.
46. Rotter KP, Larrain CG. Gallstones in spinal cord injury (SCI): a late medical complication? *Spinal Cord* 2003;41:105–108.
47. Moonka R, Stiens SA, Resnick WJ, et al. The prevalence and natural history of gallstones in spinal cord injured patients. *J Am Coll Surg* 1999;189:274–281.
48. Faaborg PM, Christensen P, Finnerup N, et al. The pattern of colorectal dysfunction changes with time since spinal cord injury. *Spinal Cord* 2008;46:234–238.
49. Valles M, Vidal J, Clave P, et al. Bowel dysfunction in patients with motor complete spinal cord injury: clinical, neurological, and pathophysiological associations. *Am J Gastroenterol* 2006;101:2290–2299.
50. Harari D, Minaker KL. Megacolon in patients with chronic spinal cord injury. *Spinal Cord* 2000;38:331–339.
51. Menardo G, Bausano G, Corazziari E, et al. Large-bowel transit in paraplegic patients. *Dis Colon Rectum* 1987;30:924–928.
52. Nino-Murcia M, Stone JM, Chang PJ, et al. Colonic transit in spinal cord-injured patients. *Invest Radiol* 1990;25:109–112.
53. Consortium for Spinal Cord Medicine. *Neurogenic bowel management in adults with spinal cord injury*. Washington, DC: Clinical Practice Guidelines, 1998.
54. Del Popolo G, Mosiello G, Pilati C, et al. Treatment of neurogenic bowel dysfunction using transanal irrigation: a multicenter Italian study. *Spinal Cord* 2008;46:517–522.
55. Christensen P, Andreasen J, Ehlers L. Cost-effectiveness of transanal irrigation versus conservative bowel management for spinal cord injury patients. *Spinal Cord* 2009;47:138–143.
56. Christensen P, Bazzocchi G, Coggrave M, et al. A randomized, controlled trial of transanal irrigation versus conservative bowel management in spinal cord-injured patients. *Gastroenterology* 2006;131:738–747.
57. Hocevar B, Gray M. Intestinal diversion (colostomy or ileostomy) in patients with severe bowel dysfunction following spinal cord injury. *J Wound Ostomy Continence Nurs* 2008;35:159–166.
58. Rosito O, Nino-Murcia M, Wolfe VA, et al. The effects of colostomy on the quality of life in patients with spinal cord injury: a retrospective analysis. *J Spinal Cord Med* 2002;25:174–183.
59. Johnston MV, Diab ME, Chu BC, et al. Preventive services and health behaviors among people with spinal cord injury. *J Spinal Cord Med* 2005;28:43–54.
60. Resnick NM, Yalla SV. Aging and its effect on the bladder. *Semin Urol* 1987;5:82–86.
61. Madersbacher S, Pycha A, Klingler CH, et al. Interrelationships of bladder compliance with age, detrusor instability, and obstruction in elderly men with lower urinary tract symptoms. *Neurourol Urodyn* 1999;18:3–15.
62. Pfisterer MH, Griffiths DJ, Schaefer W, et al. The effect of age on lower urinary tract function: a study in women. *J Am Geriatr Soc* 2006;54:405–412.
63. Esposito C, Plati A, Mazzullo T, et al. Renal function and functional reserve in healthy elderly individuals. *J Nephrol* 2007;20:617–625.
64. Kujubu DA, Aboseif SR. An overview of nocturia and the syndrome of nocturnal polyuria in the elderly. *Nat Clin Pract Nephrol* 2008;4:426–435.
65. Liang SY, Mackowiak PA. Infections in the elderly. *Clin Geriatr Med* 2007;23:441–456, viii.

66. Htwe TH, Mushtaq A, Robinson SB, et al. Infection in the elderly. *Infect Dis Clin North Am* 2007;21:711–743, ix.
67. Truzzi JC, Almeida FM, Nunes EC, et al. Residual urinary volume and urinary tract infection—when are they linked? *J Urol* 2008;180:182–185.
68. Madersbacher G, Oberwalder M. The elderly para- and tetraplegic: special aspects of the urological care. *Paraplegia* 1987;25:318–323.
69. Garshick E, Kelley A, Cohen SA, et al. A prospective assessment of mortality in chronic spinal cord injury. *Spinal Cord* 2005;43:408–416.
70. National Spinal Cord Injury Statistical Center. The 2007 Annual Statistical Report for the Spinal Cord Injury Model Systems. Birmingham, AL: University of Alabama, 2007.
71. Cardenas DD, Hoffman JM, Kirshblum S, et al. Etiology and incidence of rehospitalization after traumatic spinal cord injury: a multicenter analysis. *Arch Phys Med Rehabil* 2004;85:1757–1763.
72. McKinley WO, Jackson AB, Cardenas DD, et al. Long-term medical complications after traumatic spinal cord injury: a regional model systems analysis. *Arch Phys Med Rehabil* 1999;80:1402–1410.
73. Savic G, Short DJ, Weitzenkamp D, et al. Hospital readmissions in people with chronic spinal cord injury. *Spinal Cord* 2000;38:371–377.
74. Haisma JA, van der Woude LH, Stam HJ, et al. Complications following spinal cord injury: occurrence and risk factors in a longitudinal study during and after inpatient rehabilitation. *J Rehabil Med* 2007;39:393–398.
75. Drake MJ, Cortina-Borja M, Savic G, et al. Prospective evaluation of urological effects of aging in chronic spinal cord injury by method of bladder management. *Neurourol Urodyn* 2005;24:111–116.
76. Bennett N, O'Leary M, Patel AS, et al. Can higher doses of oxybutynin improve efficacy in neurogenic bladder? *J Urol* 2004;171:749–751.
77. O'Leary M, Erickson JR, Smith CP, et al. Effect of controlled-release oxybutynin on neurogenic bladder function in spinal cord injury. *J Spinal Cord Med* 2003;26:159–162.
78. Ku JH, Jung TY, Lee JK, et al. Influence of bladder management on epididymo-orchitis in patients with spinal cord injury: clean intermittent catheterization is a risk factor for epididymo-orchitis. *Spinal Cord* 2006;44:165–169.
79. Melzak J. The incidence of bladder cancer in paraplegia. *Paraplegia* 1966;4:85–96.
80. El-Masri WS, Fellows G. Bladder cancer after spinal cord injury. *Paraplegia* 1981;19:265–270.
81. Kaufman JM, Fam B, Jacobs SC, et al. Bladder cancer and squamous metaplasia in spinal cord injury patients. *J Urol* 1977;118:967–971.
82. Stonehill WH, Dmochowski RR, Patterson AL, et al. Risk factors for bladder tumors in spinal cord injury patients. *J Urol* 1996;155:1248–1250.
83. Pannek J. Transitional cell carcinoma in patients with spinal cord injury: a high risk malignancy? *Urology* 2002;59:240–244.
84. Subramonian K, Cartwright RA, Harnden P, et al. Bladder cancer in patients with spinal cord injuries. *BJU Int* 2004;93:739–743.
85. Groah SL, Weitzenkamp DA, Lammertse DP, et al. Excess risk of bladder cancer in spinal cord injury: evidence for an association between indwelling catheter use and bladder cancer. *Arch Phys Med Rehabil* 2002;83:346–351.
86. Kalisvaart JF, Katsumi HK, Ronningen LD, et al. Bladder cancer in spinal cord injury patients. *Spinal Cord* 2010;48(3):257–261.
87. Yang CC, Clowers DE. Screening cystoscopy in chronically catheterized spinal cord injury patients. *Spinal Cord* 1999;37:204–207.
88. Castillo CM, Ha CY, Gater DR, et al. Prophylactic radical cystectomy for the management of keratinizing squamous metaplasia of the bladder in a man with tetraplegia. *J Spinal Cord Med* 2007;30:389–391.
89. Navon JD, Soliman H, Khonsari F, et al. Screening cystoscopy and survival of spinal cord injured patients with squamous cell cancer of the bladder. *J Urol* 1997;157:2109–2111.
90. Shokeir AA. Squamous cell carcinoma of the bladder: pathology, diagnosis and treatment. *BJU Int* 2004; 93:216–220.
91. Frisbie JH, Binard J. Low prevalence of prostatic cancer among myelopathy patients. *J Am Paraplegia Soc* 1994;17:148–149.
92. Scott PAS, Perkash I, Mode D, et al. Prostate cancer diagnosed in spinal cord-injured patients is more commonly advanced stage than in able-bodied patients. *Urology* 2004;63:509–512.
93. Wyndaele JJ, Iwatsubo E, Perkash I, et al. Prostate cancer: a hazard also to be considered in the ageing male patient with spinal cord injury. *Spinal Cord* 1998;36:299–302.
94. Shaffer SW, Harrison AL. Aging of the somatosensory system: a translational perspective. *Phys Ther* 2007;87: 193–207.
95. Lauretani F, Bandinelli S, Bartali B, et al. Axonal degeneration affects muscle density in older men and women. *Neurobiol Aging* 2006;27:1145–1154.
96. Pathy M. The central nervous system: clinical presentation and management of neurologic disorders in old age. In: Brocklehurst JC, ed. *Textbook of geriatric medicine and gerontology*. Edinburgh, UK: Churchill-Livingstone, 1985.
97. Hatzitaki V, Amiridis IG, Arabatzi F. Aging effects on postural responses to self-imposed balance perturbations. *Gait Posture* 2005;22:250–257.
98. Olafsdottir H, Yoshida N, Zatsiorsky VM, et al. Elderly show decreased adjustments of motor synergies in preparation to action. *Clin Biomech (Bristol, Avon)* 2007;22:44–51.
99. Olafsdottir H, Zhang W, Zatsiorsky VM, et al. Age-related changes in multifinger synergies in accurate moment of force production tasks. *J Appl Physiol* 2007;102: 1490–1501.
100. Cruz-Sanchez FF, Moral A, Tolosa E, et al. Evaluation of neuronal loss, astrocytosis and abnormalities of cytoskeletal components of large motor neurons in the human anterior horn in aging. *J Neural Transm* 1998;105: 689–701.
101. Agosta F, Lagana M, Valsasina P, et al. Evidence for cervical cord tissue disorganisation with aging by diffusion tensor MRI. *Neuroimage* 2007;36:728–735.

102. Lammertse DP. The Nervous System. In: Whiteneck GG, Charlifue SW, Gerhart KA, et al., eds. *Aging with spinal cord injury*. New York, NY: Demos Publications, 1993.
103. Gellman H, Sie I, Waters RL. Late complications of the weight-bearing upper extremity in the paraplegic patient. *Clin Orthop Relat Res* 1988;233:132–135.
104. Davidoff G, Werner R, Waring W. Compressive mononeuropathies of the upper extremity in chronic paraplegia. *Paraplegia* 1991;29:17–24.
105. Boninger ML, Cooper RA, Baldwin MA, et al. Wheelchair pushrim kinetics: body weight and median nerve function. *Arch Phys Med Rehabil* 1999;80:910–915.
106. Edgar R, Quail P. Progressive post-traumatic cystic and non-cystic myelopathy. *Br J Neurosurg* 1994;8:7–22.
107. Falci S, Holtz A, Akesson E, et al. Obliteration of a post-traumatic spinal cord cyst with solid human embryonic spinal cord grafts: first clinical attempt. *J Neurotrauma* 1997;14:875–884.
108. Falci SP, Lammertse DP, Best L, et al. Surgical treatment of posttraumatic cystic and tethered spinal cords. *J Spinal Cord Med* 1999;22:173–181.
109. Falcone S, Quencer RM, Green BA, et al. Progressive post-traumatic myelomalacic myelopathy: imaging and clinical features. *Am J. Neuroradiol* 1994;15(4):747–754.
110. Lee TT, Arias JM, Andrus HL, et al. Progressive post-traumatic myelomalacic myelopathy: treatment with untethering and expansive duraplasty. *J Neurosurg* 1997;86:624–628.
111. Bursell JP, Little JW, Stiens SA. Electrodiagnosis in spinal cord injured persons with new weakness or sensory loss: central and peripheral etiologies. *Arch Phys Med Rehabil* 1999;80:904–909.
112. Bos SD, Slagboom PE, Meulenbelt I. New insights into osteoarthritis: early developmental features of an ageing-related disease. *Curr Opin Rheumatol* 2008;20:553–559.
113. Taniguchi N, Carames B, Ronfani L, et al. Aging-related loss of the chromatin protein HMGB2 in articular cartilage is linked to reduced cellularity and osteoarthritis. *Proc Natl Acad Sci U S A* 2009;106:1181–1186.
114. van der Kraan PM, van den Berg WB. Osteoarthritis in the context of ageing and evolution. Loss of chondrocyte differentiation block during ageing. *Ageing Res Rev* 2008;7:106–113.
115. Keen HI, Wakefield RJ, Grainger AJ, et al. An ultrasonographic study of osteoarthritis of the hand: synovitis and its relationship to structural pathology and symptoms. *Arthritis Rheum* 2008;59:1756–1763.
116. Millett PJ, Gobezie R, Boykin RE. Shoulder osteoarthritis: diagnosis and management. *Am Fam Physician* 2008;78:605–611.
117. Burger H, de Laet CE, van Daele PL, et al. Risk factors for increased bone loss in an elderly population: the Rotterdam Study. *Am J Epidemiol* 1998;147:871–879.
118. Consortium for Spinal Cord Medicine. Preservation of upper limb function following spinal cord injury: a clinical practice guideline for health-care professionals. *J Spinal Cord Med* 2005;28:434–470.
119. Alm M, Saraste H, Norrbrink C. Shoulder pain in persons with thoracic spinal cord injury: prevalence and characteristics. *J Rehabil Med* 2008;40:277–283.
120. Escobedo EM, Hunter JC, Hollister MC, et al. MR imaging of rotator cuff tears in individuals with paraplegia. *AJR Am J Roentgenol* 1997;168:919–923.
121. Bayley JC, Cochran TP, Sledge CB. The weight-bearing shoulder. The impingement syndrome in paraplegics. *J Bone Joint Surg Am* 1987;69:676–678.
122. Brose SW, Boninger ML, Fullerton B, et al. Shoulder ultrasound abnormalities, physical examination findings, and pain in manual wheelchair users with spinal cord injury. *Arch Phys Med Rehabil* 2008;89:2086–2093.
123. Boninger ML, Koontz AM, Sisto SA, et al. Pushrim biomechanics and injury prevention in spinal cord injury: recommendations based on CULP-SCI investigations. *Rehabil Res Dev* 2005;42:9–19.
124. Robinson MD, Hussey RW, Ha CY. Surgical decompression of impingement in the weightbearing shoulder. *Arch Phys Med Rehabil* 1993;74:324–327.
125. Goldstein B, Young J, Escobedo EM. Rotator cuff repairs in individuals with paraplegia. *Am J Phys Med Rehabil* 1997;76:316–322.
126. Frisbie JH. Fractures after myelopathy: the risk quantified. *J Spinal Cord Med* 1997;20:66–69.
127. Garland DE, Stewart CA, Adkins RH, et al. Osteoporosis after spinal cord injury. *J Orthop Res* 1992;10:371–378.
128. Frotzler A, Coupaud S, Perret C, et al. High-volume FES-cycling partially reverses bone loss in people with chronic spinal cord injury. *Bone* 2008;43:169–176.
129. Nance PW, Schryvers O, Leslie W, et al. Intravenous pamidronate attenuates bone density loss after acute spinal cord injury. *Arch Phys Med Rehabil* 1999;80:243–251.
130. Bauman WA, Wecht JM, Kirshblum S, et al. Effect of pamidronate administration on bone in patients with acute spinal cord injury. *J Rehabil Res Dev* 2005;42:305–313.
131. Fenske NA, Lober CW. Structural and functional changes of normal aging skin. *J Am Acad Dermatol* 1986;15:571–585.
132. Callaghan TM, Wilhelm KP. A review of ageing and an examination of clinical methods in the assessment of ageing skin. Part I: cellular and molecular perspectives of skin ageing. *Int J Cosmet Sci* 2008;30:313–322.
133. Charlifue S, Lammertse DP, Adkins RH. Aging with spinal cord injury: changes in selected health indices and life satisfaction. *Arch Phys Med Rehabil* 2004;85:1848–1853.
134. Chen Y, DeVivo MJ, Jackson AB. Pressure ulcer prevalence in people with spinal cord injury: age-period-duration effects. *Arch Phys Med Rehabil* 2005;86:1208–1213.
135. Yarkony GM. Aging skin, pressure ulcerations, and spinal cord injury. In: Whiteneck GG, Charlifue SW, Gerhart KA, et al., eds. *Aging with spinal cord injury*. New York, NY: Demos Publications, 1993.
136. Consortium for Spinal Cord Medicine Clinical Practice Guidelines. Pressure ulcer prevention and treatment following spinal cord injury: a clinical practice guideline for health-care professionals. *J Spinal Cord Med* 2001;24(suppl 1):S40–S101.
137. Vicario C, de Juan J, Esclarin A, et al. Treatment of deep wound infections after spinal fusion with a

vacuum-assisted device in patients with spinal cord injury. *Acta Orthop Belg* 2007;73:102–106.
138. Weksler ME. Immune senescence. *Ann Neurol* 1994;35(suppl):S35–S37.
139. Ershler WB. Biomarkers of aging: immunological events. *Exp Gerontol* 1988;23:387–389.
140. Pawelec G, Derhovanessian E, Larbi A, et al. Cytomegalovirus and human immunosenescence. *Rev Med Virol* 2009;19:47–56.
141. Gavazzi G, Krause KH. Ageing and infection. *Lancet Infect Dis* 2002;2:659–666.
142. Nash MS, Fletcher MA. The immune system. In: Whiteneck GG, Charlifue SW, Gerhart KA, et al., eds. *Aging with spinal cord injury*. New York, NY: Demos Publications, 1993.
143. Campagnolo DI, Bartlett JA, Chatterton RJ, et al. Adrenal and pituitary hormone patterns after spinal cord injury. *Am J Phys Med Rehabil* 1999;78:361–366.
144. Kliesch WF, Cruse JM, Lewis RE, et al. Restoration of depressed immune function in spinal cord injury patients receiving rehabilitation therapy. *Paraplegia* 1996;34:82–90.
145. Nash MS. Immune responses to nervous system decentralization and exercise in quadriplegia. *Med Sci Sports Exerc* 1994;26:164–171.
146. Wilmot CB, Hall KM. The respiratory system. In: Whiteneck GG, Charlifue SW, Gerhart KA, et al., eds. *Aging with spinal cord injury*. New York, NY: Demos Publications; 1993.
147. Katial R, Zheng W. Allergy and immunology of the aging lung. *Clin Chest Med* 2007;28:663–672, v.
148. Martinez D. Effects of aging on peripheral chemoreceptor CO2 response during sleep and wakefulness in healthy men. *Respir Physiol Neurobiol* 2008;162:138–143.
149. Eckert DJ, Malhotra A. Pathophysiology of adult obstructive sleep apnea. *Proc Am Thorac Soc* 2008;5:144–153.
150. Wolkove N, Elkholy O, Baltzan M, et al. Sleep and aging: 1. Sleep disorders commonly found in older people. *Can Med Assoc J* 2007;176:1299–1304.
151. Menter RR, Hudson LM. Effects of age at injury and the aging process. In: Stover SL, DeLisa JA, Whiteneck GG, eds. *Spinal cord injury: clinical outcomes from the model systems*. Gaithersburg, MD: Aspen Publishers, Inc., 1995: 272–288.
152. Short DJ, Stradling JR, Williams SJ. Prevalence of sleep apnoea in patients over 40 years of age with spinal cord lesions. *J Neurol Neurosurg Psychiatry* 1992;55:1032–1036.
153. Burns SP, Little JW, Hussey JD, et al. Sleep apnea syndrome in chronic spinal cord injury: associated factors and treatment. *Arch Phys Med Rehabil* 2000;81: 1334–1339.
154. Consortium for Spinal Cord Medicine. Respiratory management following spinal cord injury: a clinical practice guideline for health-care professionals. *J Spinal Cord Med* 2005;28:259–293.
155. Leduc BE, Dagher JH, Mayer P, et al. Estimated prevalence of obstructive sleep apnea-hypopnea syndrome after cervical cord injury. *Arch Phys Med Rehabil* 2007; 88:333–337.
156. Lanig IS, Peterson WP. The respiratory system in spinal cord injury. *Phys Med Rehabil Clin N Am* 2000; 11:29–43, vii.
157. Burns SP, Rad MY, Bryant S, et al. Long-term treatment of sleep apnea in persons with spinal cord injury. *Am J Phys Med Rehabil* 2005;84:620–626.
158. Lloyd-Jones D, Adams R, Carnethon M, et al. Heart disease and stroke statistics—2009 update: a report from the American Heart Association Statistics Committee and Stroke Statistics Subcommittee. *Circulation* 2009;119:e21–e181.
159. Ferdinandy P, Schulz R, Baxter GF. Interaction of cardiovascular risk factors with myocardial ischemia/reperfusion injury, preconditioning, and postconditioning. *Pharmacol Rev* 2007;59:418–458.
160. Ragnarsson KT. The cardiovascular system. In: Whiteneck GG, Charlifue SW, Gerhart KA, et al., eds. *Aging with spinal cord injury*. New York, NY: Demos Publications, 1993:73–92.
161. Arnett DK, Baird AE, Barkley RA, et al. Relevance of genetics and genomics for prevention and treatment of cardiovascular disease: a scientific statement from the American Heart Association Council on Epidemiology and Prevention, the Stroke Council, and the Functional Genomics and Translational Biology Interdisciplinary Working Group. *Circulation* 2007;115:2878–2901.
162. Groah SL, Weitzenkamp D, Sett P, et al. The relationship between neurological level of injury and symptomatic cardiovascular disease risk in the aging spinal injured. *Spinal Cord* 2001;39:310–317.
163. Brenes G, Dearwater S, Shapera R, et al. High density lipoprotein cholesterol concentrations in physically active and sedentary spinal cord injured patients. *Arch Phys Med Rehabil* 1986;67:445–450.
164. Bauman WA, Spungen AM. Disorders of carbohydrate and lipid metabolism in veterans with paraplegia or quadriplegia: a model of premature aging. *Metabolism* 1994;43:749–756.
165. Bauman WA, Kahn NN, Grimm DR, et al. Risk factors for atherogenesis and cardiovascular autonomic function in persons with spinal cord injury. *Spinal Cord* 1999;37:601–616.
166. Wilt TJ, Carlson KF, Goldish GD, et al. Carbohydrate and lipid disorders and relevant considerations in persons with spinal cord injury. *Evid Rep Technol Assess (Full Rep)*. 2008;163:1–95
167. Liang H, Chen D, Wang Y, et al. Different risk factor patterns for metabolic syndrome in men with spinal cord injury compared with able-bodied men despite similar prevalence rates. *Arch Phys Med Rehabil* 2007;88:1198–1204.
168. Dyson-Hudson TA, Nash MS. Guideline-driven assessment of cardiovascular disease and related risks after spinal cord injury. *Top Spinal Cord Inj Rehabil* 2009;14(3):32–34
169. Davis GM, Hamzaid NA, Fornusek C. Cardiorespiratory, metabolic, and biomechanical responses during functional electrical stimulation leg exercise: health and fitness benefits. *Artif Organs* 2008;32:625–629.
170. Zbogar D, Eng JJ, Krassioukov AV, et al. The effects of functional electrical stimulation leg cycle ergometry training on arterial compliance in individuals with spinal cord injury. *Spinal Cord* 2008;46:722–726.
171. Bear-Lehman J, Albert SM, Burkhardt A. Cutaneous sensitivity and functional limitation. *Top Geriatr Rehabil* 2006;22:61–69.

172. Couture M, Lariviere N, Lefrancois R. Psychological distress in older adults with low functional independence: a multidimensional perspective. *Arch Gerontol Geriatr* 2005;41:101–111.
173. Rejeski WJ, Fielding RA, Blair SN, et al. The lifestyle interventions and independence for elders (LIFE) pilot study: design and methods. *Contemp Clin Trials* 2005;26:141–154.
174. Song J, Chang RW, Dunlop DD. Population impact of arthritis on disability in older adults. *Arthritis Rheum* 2006;55:248–255.
175. Collins K, Rooney BL, Smalley KJ, et al. Functional fitness, disease and independence in community-dwelling older adults in western Wisconsin. *WMJ* 2004;103:42–48.
176. Tanaka H. Habitual exercise for the elderly. *Fam Community Health* 2009;32:S57–S65.
177. Arnett SW, Laity JH, Agrawal SK, et al. Aerobic reserve and physical functional performance in older adults. *Age Ageing* 2008;37:384–389.
178. National Center for Health Statistics, ed. *Health, United States, 2006 with Chartbook on trends in the health of Americans*. Hyattsville, MD: US Department of Health and Human Services, 2006.
179. McColl MA, Rosenthal C. A model of resource needs of aging spinal cord injured men. *Paraplegia* 1994;32:261–270.
180. Gerhart KA, Bergstrom E, Charlifue SW, et al. Long-term spinal cord injury: functional changes over time. *Arch Phys Med Rehabil* 1993;74:1030–1034.
181. Gerhart KA, Charlifue SW, Weitzenkamp DA, et al. Aging with spinal cord injury. *Am Rehabil* 1997;23:19–25.
182. Charlifue SW, Weitzenkamp DA, Whiteneck GG. Longitudinal outcomes in spinal cord injury: aging, secondary conditions, and well-being. *Arch Phys Med Rehabil* 1999;80:1429–1434.
183. Gitlin LN, Hauck WW, Dennis MP, et al. Depressive symptoms in older African-American and white adults with functional difficulties: the role of control strategies. *J Am Geriatr Soc* 2007;55:1023–1030.
184. Aldwin CM, Sutton KJ, Chiara G, et al. Age differences in stress, coping, and appraisal: findings from the Normative Aging Study. *J Gerontol B Psychol Sci Soc Sci* 1996;51:P179–P188.
185. Jorm AF, Windsor TD, Dear KB, et al. Age group differences in psychological distress: the role of psychosocial risk factors that vary with age. *Psychol Med* 2005;35:1253–1263.
186. McGuire LC, Strine TW, Vachirasudlekha S, et al. The prevalence of depression in older U.S. women: 2006 behavioral risk factor surveillance system. *J Womens Health (Larchmt)* 2008;17:501–507.
187. Lee Y, Park K. Does physical activity moderate the association between depressive symptoms and disability in older adults? *Int J Geriatr Psychiatry* 2008;23:249–256.
188. Rafanelli C, Roncuzzi R, Milaneschi Y, et al. Stressful life events, depression and demoralization as risk factors for acute coronary heart disease. *Psychother Psychosom* 2005;74:179–184.
189. Frasure-Smith N, Lesperance F. Recent evidence linking coronary heart disease and depression. *Can J Psychiatry* 2006;51:730–737.
190. Lachman ME, Rocke C, Rosnick C, et al. Realism and illusion in Americans' temporal views of their life satisfaction: age differences in reconstructing the past and anticipating the future. *Psychol Sci* 2008;19:889–897.
191. Fisher BJ. Successful aging, life satisfaction, and generativity in later life. *Int J Aging Hum Dev* 1995;41:239–250.
192. Gerhart KA, Weitzenkamp DA, Kennedy P, et al. Correlates of stress in long-term spinal cord injury. *Spinal Cord* 1999;37:183–190.
193. Kemp BJ, Kahan JS, Krause JS, et al. Treatment of major depression in individuals with spinal cord injury. *J Spinal Cord Med* 2004;27:22–28.
194. Dryden DM, Saunders LD, Rowe BH, et al. Depression following traumatic spinal cord injury. *Neuroepidemiology* 2005;25. 25:55–61, 55–61. Epub 2005 Jun 2008.
195. Krause JS, Kemp B, Coker J. Depression after spinal cord injury: relation to gender, ethnicity, aging, and socioeconomic indicators. *Arch Phys Med Rehabil* 2000;81:1099–1109.
196. Krause JS, Broderick L. A 25-year longitudinal study of the natural course of aging after spinal cord injury. *Spinal Cord* 2005;43:349–356.
197. Krause JS, Coker JL. Aging after spinal cord injury: A 30-year longitudinal study. *J Spinal Cord Med* 2006;29:371–376.
198. Charlifue S, Gerhart K. Changing psychosocial morbidity in people aging with spinal cord injury. *NeuroRehabilitation* 2004;19:15–23.
199. Nosek MA. Personal assistance: key to employability of persons with physical disabilities. *J Appl Rehabil Couns* 1990;21:3–8.
200. Newsom JT, Schulz R. Caregiving from the recipient's perspective: negative reactions to being helped. *Health Psychol* 1998;17:172–181.
201. Holicky R, Charlifue S. Ageing with spinal cord injury: the impact of spousal support. *Dis Rehabil* 1999;21:250–257.
202. Chan RC. How does spinal cord injury affect marital relationship? A story from both sides of the couple. *Disabil Rehabil* 2000;22:764–775.
203. Kreuter M. Spinal cord injury and partner relationships. *Spinal Cord* 2000;38:2–6.
204. Pearcey TE, Yoshida KK, Renwick RM. Personal relationships after a spinal cord injury. *Int J Rehabil Res* 2007;30:209–219.
205. Levasseur M, St-Cyr Tribble D, Desrosiers J. Meaning of quality of life for older adults: Importance of human functioning components. *Arch Gerontol Geriatr* 2008;49:91–100.
206. Freedman VA, Grafova IB, Schoeni RF, et al. Neighborhoods and disability in later life. *Soc Sci Med* 2008;66:2253–2267.
207. Whiteneck GG, Harrison-Felix CL, Mellick DC, et al. Quantifying environmental factors: a measure of physical, attitudinal, service, productivity, and policy barriers. *Arch Phys Med Rehabil* 2004;85:1324–1335.
208. Whiteneck G, Meade MA, Dijkers M, et al. Environmental factors and their role in participation and life satisfaction after spinal cord injury. *Arch Phys Med Rehabil* 2004;85:1793–1803.

CHAPTER 28 ■ SURGICAL RESTORATION OF THE HAND IN TETRAPLEGIA: TENDON TRANSFERS

ALLAN E. PELJOVICH, ANNE M. BRYDEN, AMY BOHN, AND MICHAEL W. KEITH

INTRODUCTION

The genesis of applying surgical techniques to improve hand and arm function in people with spinal cord injury (SCI) coincided with Dr. Eric Moberg's work in the early 1970s (1–6). While previous reports of hand surgery for tetraplegia exist, it was Eric Moberg who revolutionized the approach to surgical treatment (1). Dr. Moberg recognized that individuals with paralysis preferred not to draw additional attention to themselves; therefore, often spurning orthotics of various forms, including functional hinge splints (7). And, at a time when rehabilitation centers were fostering the development of stiff, hooked hands (and many still do), Dr. Moberg recognized that these individuals preferred the same supple, soft hands that their able-bodied counterparts took for granted. Finally, like Hanson and Franklin (8) recognized in 1974, many paralyzed individuals wanted more attention focused on hand and arm function than they were receiving at rehabilitation centers around the world. Armed with these observations, Moberg began applying the surgical technique of tendon transfers, already used to restore lost function from peripheral nerve injury, to individuals with tetraplegia. He created the "key pinch procedure," which allowed individuals to use lateral pinch with strength and advocated to restore elbow extension using the posterior deltoid as a donor motor. Moberg's original techniques have since been modified, and newer ones have been developed as dedicated surgeons interested in caring for these individuals have advanced the science that he spawned.

Surgical restoration of the hand and upper extremity in tetraplegia currently stands as its own clinical and scientific discipline. There are hundreds of research publications dedicated to the subject; and, the nature of the research spans a wide spectrum from basic science projects focusing on neuromuscular physiology and the mathematical modeling of tendon transfers to surgical issues such as surgical criteria/goals/techniques, to clinical outcomes research. New concepts in restoration such as functional electrical stimulation (FES) have been developed from this growing discipline. There is also an international group of surgeons and therapists dedicated to the discipline that have been meeting throughout the globe on a regular basis since 1979 (9). This group developed the surgery-specific classification system for tetraplegia (10).

We believe conceptually, that in order to aid the patient in the long run, treatment directed to the hand and upper extremity should begin early in the acute phase of care; and that this treatment extends beyond traditional concepts of exercise, splinting, and braces. True rehabilitation of the tetraplegic hand should be thought of as the judicious application of nonoperative and operative interventions tailor-made to the particular patient to maximize their function bearing in mind their global psychosocial and medical state. This chapter updates the reader on the current status of tendon transfer restoration in the setting of tetraplegia.

BACKGROUND

While tetraplegia is defined as the impairment from an injury to any of the cervical segments of the spine, the extent of disability is primarily determined from the specific functional level of the injury (11). The fifth cervical spinal cord segment is not only the most common injured level in tetraplegia but also the most common level injured in all SCI (14.9%) (12,13). The next two most commonly injured levels are also in the cervical spine, namely the C4 and C6 segments, with both amounting to about 24% of all SCI. The remaining cervical segments comprise about 12% of all SCI. Most tetraplegic patients retain at least the ability to flex their elbows and some can extend their wrists; but most do not retain voluntarily elbow extension, wrist flexion, or finger control. Factors that influence functional ability include whether the injury is neurologically "complete," if any cognitive impairment exists (brain injury), the age of the patient, any other upper extremity injury, the presence of uncontrolled spasticity, contractures that limit mobility, and/or depression (14).

Intuitively, the level of function and independence improves as the level of injury moves distal and patients retain more function. High-level tetraplegia, with functional levels, from C2-4 generally have no movement of the arms short of some shoulder elevation. They have some control of their neck muscles, and are likely ventilatory support–dependent depending on the actual functional level of injury. Patients who retain voluntary innervation in the C5 myotome can flex their elbows, and retain functional deltoid control. They are able to feed themselves, and perhaps even groom themselves with the aid of special adaptive equipment attached to their wrists and hands. At the C6 level, a patient can voluntarily extend their wrists, and as such, can, with the aid of adaptive equipment, be independent in grooming, bathing, driving, and preparing a simple meal. At the C7 level, patients retain use of their triceps, and perhaps the ability to extend their fingers. These patients may be able to perform all the previous activities, and be fairly efficient in daily living tasks. Importantly, if the triceps is of sufficient strength, they may be able to independently transfer themselves provided they have voluntary control of most of their shoulder musculature; therefore, can live alone with the aid of special hand and environmental adaptive equipment.

These individuals also retain strong wrist flexion that is particularly useful in propelling a manual wheelchair. With the exception of this latter patient, patients with higher cervical level injuries usually require an able-bodied attendant nearly most of the time to help with their daily activities. While this is an oversimplified and generalized view of function based upon level of injury, it should be readily apparent that any treatment or intervention that improves a level of function, for example, C5-6, would result in a dramatic improvement in both function and independence (15–19).

Persons who sustain an SCI are often young, usually otherwise healthy, whose impact extends into their personal life, with sound data indicating lower rates of marriage and higher rates of divorce among SCI patients (12,20). The results of modern SCI care and management have improved the quality of life and life expectancy. However, any intervention that can improve a patient's functional ability will have a tremendous positive impact that will extend beyond activities they can perform. To this end, Hanson and Franklin studied SCI patients to determine what they perceived as their greatest functional losses (8). Among both tetraplegic patients (76%) and caregivers (64%), the restoration of hand and upper extremity function was considered the most important function to be restored. These concepts have been reinforced in recent study, where patients continue to place great importance in improving hand and upper extremity function among the various components of SCI rehabilitation (21–23). Robert Waters, a surgeon from Ranchos Los Amigos, noted "...the greatest potential for improvement of quality of life lies in rehabilitation and maximal restoration of upper extremity function" (24). Clearly, attention should be directed to rehabilitating the hand and upper extremity as part of a more global approach to treating patients with tetraplegia.

THINKING ABOUT RESTORATION—RECONCILING GOALS AND PATHOPHYSIOLOGY

An individual learns to use their hands and arms as they recover from SCI with a combination of therapy, orthotics, and creative strategizing. Early therapy helps to maintain joint mobility and maximize the strength, endurance, and the balance of voluntary muscles. Orthotics are initially used to help "mold" the resting hand positions needed for tenodesis grasp, namely intrinsic plus fingers with wrist extension and extended fingers with wrist flexion. There are a variety of commercially available orthotics to aid individuals with both position and functioning. The primary problem with these is that most individuals do not use them and generally prefer to be brace free (7). These functional orthotics also usually require assistance donning and doffing. While electrical stimulation implants have been described, these are currently not available for implantation. Finally, over the course of months, and perhaps even longer, individuals learn to use their arms to accomplish tasks beyond what they would seem capable of doing. For example, it is common for the layperson observing an individual with tetraplegia to be easily fooled into concluding that the individual has functional triceps muscle, control of forearm rotation, and pinch—when, in fact, they are lacking in these functions but have found ways to compensate. Simply stated, despite excellent nonoperative management, individuals with tetraplegia remain severely impaired when one considers the able-bodied upper extremity.

The great difficulty in executing a surgical plan is that it is not possible with currently available techniques to completely restore upper extremity function to the able-bodied state. This is because surgery cannot reanimate the paralyzed muscles or reconnect the lost communication between the brain and the peripheral nervous system below the level of the injury. Upper extremity function must be distilled into its most fundamental elements to maximize gains from limited options. Once we understand how the arm and hand functions, we can then plan a reconstructive strategy. Surgical strategies rely primarily on tendon transfer–based restoration; with some research centers performing FES neuroprosthesis-based restoration.

A tendon transfer procedure is one in which a functioning muscle and its tendon are detached from its normal insertion and rerouted into a different muscle that helps perform the function that needs restoration. In this way, when the donor muscle contracts, it will now power a new and desired motion. For tendon transfer–based restoration, the number of functions and joints that can be restored is directly proportional to the distal level of injury as more muscles are left under voluntary control as the injury moves toward the thoracic spine. Compromise and creativity form the basis of planning surgery for a particular individual; but, there are traditional compromises and priorities that exist based upon experience gained in treating individuals with paralysis of all forms.

Understanding the Elements of Upper Extremity Function—Goals of Reconstruction

The upper extremity performs the act of physically manipulating our environment. In a sense, the hand is the universal "tool" for manipulation, and the shoulder, elbow, and forearm provide the mode of transporting the hand in space and positioning it for function. Better mobility, stability, and strength of the shoulder and elbow confer a large potential workspace for the hand. Elbow extension is extremely important and can translate to functional abilities such as self-care, hygiene, wheelchair propulsion, and transferring—critical to creating functional independence (25). Manipulation of the hand is dependent upon the functional capacity of the hand and wrist.

In order to maximize the work space available for the hand, elbow, and shoulder, maintaining full range of motion (ROM) must be a priority in good rehabilitation care. For the individual with traumatic tetraplegia, both the transport function and the manipulation function are severely compromised. The average patient with tetraplegia (C5/6 level injury) retains shoulder mobility and elbow flexion, but elbow extension is deficient. Restoration of elbow extensor function is often a priority for surgical intervention in these individuals.

The basis for hand function in most individuals is the wrist tenodesis effect, the key to which is strong wrist extension. Wrist extension activates the natural tenodesis grasp pattern and serves as the foundation upon which finger function is activated and restored (Fig. 28.1). Surgical restoration of hand function, in fact, builds upon the provision or presence of the wrist tenodesis pinch and grasp. When it comes to manipulation of

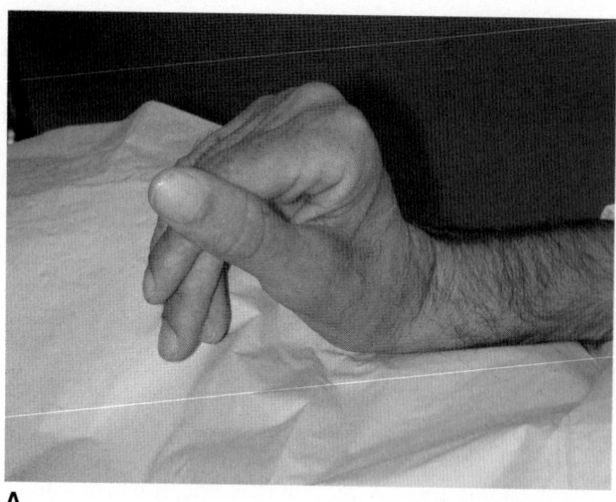

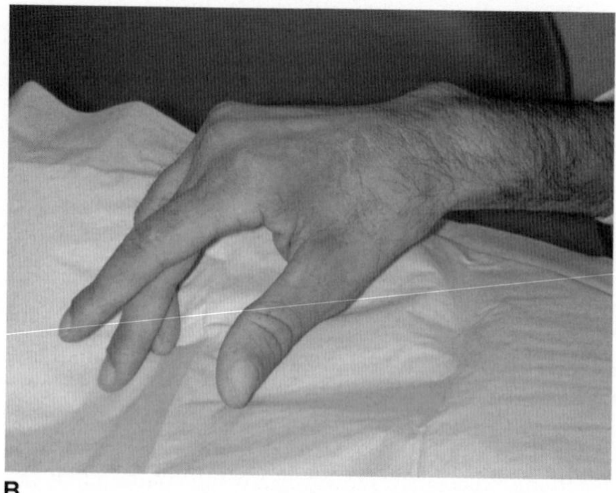

FIGURE 28.1 Clinical photograph of the wrist tenodesis effect. (**A**) As the individual extends his or her wrist, the fingers and thumb assume a flexed lateral pinch posture due to the passive properties of the extrinsic digital flexors. (**B**) In wrist flexion, the passive properties of the extrinsic extensor create extension of the fingers and thumb to release a held object.

objects, it is necessary to make some compromises with regard to desired outcomes. Regarding finger function, while it would be ideal to restore all the different grasp patterns, we apply subconsciously in our daily activities, previous study has demonstrated that lateral pinch, not opposition or tip pinch, and palmar grasp are utilized most commonly (26). Since lateral pinch is used more often for activities of daily living (ADL), this form of grasp is prioritized over palmar grasp when both cannot be restored (27). A limitation to surgical restoration is that to date, sensation cannot be restored (28).

The fundamental functions to be restored, in order of priority, include elbow extension, wrist extension, lateral pinch and release, and palmar grasp and release (4,5,9,16,17,24,26,29–33). Current surgical techniques and technology do not allow reliable restoration of shoulder function as of yet, and therefore, patients with motor levels proximal to C5 are rarely candidates for surgery. By example of the most common levels of injury in tetraplegia, C5-6 injury, the typical individual retains shoulder function, elbow flexion, and possibly strong wrist extension. In such individuals, the priority in tendon transfer–based restoration would be restoration of elbow extension, lateral pinch (if brachioradialis [BR] is available for transfer), and possibly palmar grasp (if extensor carpi radialis longus [ECRL] is available for transfer). In a patient with C4 level tetraplegia, tendon transfer–based restoration of the upper extremity is not yet possible. At the same time, if the individual has a C7 level of injury, elbow extension usually does not require restoration, and more elegant procedures for lateral pinch and grasp can be applied.

Organizing Tetraplegic Individuals into Discrete Groups

Several classification systems have been formulated to characterize the patterns of neurological injury to understand the impairment and disability (9–11,18,19,30,34,35). Calculating the difference between what an individual lacks functionally with concepts of reconstructive strategies allows for the formulation of a plan. Classification systems simplify the heterogeneity of SCI into discrete groups.

Classification systems based upon the anatomic level of injury alone are too ambiguous as the zone of cord injury and the functional consequences is not precisely concordant with the skeletal anatomic level of the injury. Instead, most classification systems turn to the functional level of injury as health care providers understood that gross motor functions confer important prognostic information. Since the innervation of the hand and upper extremity, from spinal roots C4 through T1, proceeds in a fairly ordered and segmental pattern from proximal to distal (Table 28.1), predictions of functional loss, and retention are fairly reliable once the functional level of the injury is understood. The classification system most commonly used in traumatic SCI, the International Standards for Neurological Classification of Spinal Cord Injury (ISNCSCI) that includes the ASIA Impairment Scale (AIS), is based upon this functional level, and distinguishes the completeness of the injury and the motor and sensory integrity of the extremities (11). In this system, the most distal myotome with British Medical Research Council (BMRC) strength of at least 3, with the motor levels rostral graded as normal, is the motor level. The motor grade of 3 was chosen because it is unambiguous while motor grades 4 and 5 are more difficult to be differentiated when examiners of varying strength confront persons with varying strength.

While useful for the general examination and classification of SCI, the ISNCSCI and the AIS classification is not precise enough from the standpoint of hand reconstruction. Patients with preserved myotomes can still vary in terms of the number of motors (muscle groups) with voluntary innervation. For example, a C5 patient, defined by at least grade 3 elbow flexion, may or may not have a strong voluntary BR; and, a C6 patient, defined by at least grade 3 wrist extension, may or may not have a strong voluntary extensor carpi radialis brevis (ECRB). From the standpoint of surgical restoration, these differences are very significant and was the impetus for the International Classification of Tetraplegia (ICT) created in 1984 in Giens, France, during an international meeting of hand surgeons devoted to the care of tetraplegic patients (35). Since that time, the classification system has undergone some modification, and its present form is shown in Table 28.2 (10). The classification has two components: a sensory and a motor category. The sensory category is simplified to whether an

TABLE 28.1

SEGMENTAL UPPER EXTREMITY INNERVATION BY MYOTOME

C5	C6	C7	C8	T1
Biceps				
Brachialis				
BR				
Supinator				
	ECRL			
	ECRB			
	PT			
		Flexor carpi radialis brevis		
		Triceps		
		Extensor dig. communis		
		Extensor dig. quinti		
		Extensor carpi ulnaris		
		Extensor indicis propius		
		EPL		
		Pronator quadratus		
			FDP	
			FPL	
			Flexor carpi ulnaris	
			Lumbricals	
			Flexor dig. sublimis	
			Thenar muscles	
			AdP	
				Interossei
				Hypothenar M.
C5	C6	C7	C8	T1

Adapted from Zancolli E. *Structural and dynamic basis of hand surgery.* 2nd ed. Philadelphia, PA: JB Lippincott, 1979.

individual has intact two-point discrimination in the thumb and index finger, critical to lateral pinch, or not. The presence of intact sensation (two-point discrimination less than10 mm) in the index finger and thumb is called "cutaneous," and the absence of good sensation is labeled "ocular." The latter refers to the reality that individuals with impaired discrimination sensation will need to visually monitor their grasp function since they lack higher order ability to "imagine" the object in their hand as they turn away to perform some other task.

TABLE 28.2

INTERNATIONAL CLASSIFICATION FOR SURGERY OF THE HAND IN TETRAPLEGIA (ICT)

Group	Muscle at grade 4 strength
1	BR
2	ECRL
3	ECRB
4	PT
5	FCR (flexor carpi radialis)
6	EDC and finger extensors
7	EPL and thumb extensors
8	Finger flexors
9	All except intrinsics
0	Exceptions
T+ or T−	Triceps at grade 4

Sensory testing for two-point discrimination.
O, ocular feedback only; Cu, presence 10 mm static two-point discrimination of the index finger and thumb.
Revised in Cleveland Ohio 1998 at the 6th International Conference on Surgical Rehabilitation of the Upper Limb in Tetraplegia.
McDowell C, Moberg E, House J. The second international conference on surgical rahabilitation of the upper limb in tetraplegia (quadriplegia). *J Hand Surg* 1986;11A:604–608.

For the motor classification, a muscle grade of 4 is considered functional, rather than a 3 as in the International Standards examination, since donor muscles often lose some degree of strength as it is tasked to mobilize a joint it was not designed for after transfer. This information (those muscles with a strength of ≥4) supplies the physician with the number of "candidate" donor muscles eligible for tendon transfer. The ICT is currently the accepted classification used by most surgeons performing hand surgery in patients with tetraplegia. A correlation of the ICT with the motor levels can be seen in Table 28.3.

Who Qualifies for Surgery?—Establishing Criteria for Hand and Upper Extremity Reconstruction

Only with a thorough evaluation of an individual with tetraplegia at various points in time can one determine the appropriate goals of rehabilitation and reconstruction (5,7,13,16–19, 24,30,32,36–41). The health care provider must develop a relationship with the individual patient and together they can discuss goals and desires for the procedure. Consideration for rehabilitation, especially surgical intervention, requires that the patient and primary caregivers

TABLE 28.3

ICT WITH CORRESPONDING INTERNATIONAL STANDARDS MOTOR LEVELS

ICT	International standards—Motor level
Group 0—No muscles for transfer	C5—Elbow Flexors
Group 1—BR Group 2—ECRL Group 3—ECRB Group 4—PT	C6—Wrist Extensors
Group 5—Flexor Carpi Radialis Group 6—Finger extensors	C7—Elbow Extensors
Group 7—EPL Group 8—Finger Flexors Group 9—Lacks only intrinsics	C8—Finger Flexors

ICT, International Classification for Surgery of the hand in tetraplegia; ECRL, extensor carpi radialis longus; ECRB, extensor carpi radialis brevis.

understand the reconstructive options, their risks and benefits. Surgery, for example, means that for a period of time, the individual will be more impaired as their arm is temporarily immobilized and then only progressively "given back" to them as they undergo therapy. Individuals must have a good support system in place to assist them through what is a trying time for themselves and their assistants/family.

There are other considerations that must be considered as practical to the success of any restorative program (5,7,13,16–19,24,30,32,36–41). A person must be motivated to improve and be cooperative throughout the postoperative phase of rehabilitation. Similarly, the individual's general medical condition and cognition must be stable enough in order to undergo a potentially lengthy surgery, and not interfere with the postoperative rehabilitation program. The success of restorations requires continual effort on the part of the individual both physically and mentally; otherwise, they may lose the benefits of any surgical reconstruction. Then, too, if the person or surgeon is too overly optimistic about the results of surgery, the individual will lose the motivation to continue rehabilitation, and may be worse off for it. Recent studies have explored the reasons that individuals choose surgery and the likelihood of success. Individuals are more likely to pursue surgical restoration if they feel they have the time to devote to the recovery process, and if they have specific goals and functions they want to achieve (42,43). Clearly, the decision to undergo surgical restoration must not be taken lightly.

There are also important physical criteria to establish. As many of the restorative procedures involve the transfer of voluntary muscles to more effective insertions (tendon transfers), the prerequisites to successful procedures must exist including supple joints, and sufficient strength of the donor muscle. A patient who is allowed to develop joint contractures in their hands, wrists, forearms, elbows, and shoulders will be a poor candidate for a complete restorative program that includes surgical reconstruction or even a splinting program. A muscle that is spastic and difficult to control with therapy or medication cannot serve as a useful donor. Patients should be easily transferable to a wheelchair and have good trunk support and adequate seating, so that they can stay seated in order to take full advantage of any use of their upper extremities.

These criteria have been established through years of experience, and remain a useful tool in guiding clinicians to distinguish which patients will have a good chance of success through surgical restoration. The evidence suggests that desirable postsurgical outcomes are achieved when the individual is able to meet these strict psychosocial and physical criteria (44,45).The chronic phase of SCI is when neurological recovery is considered complete, and this is the earliest that surgical restoration should be performed (26,44). It is commonly accepted that by 1 year post injury, those with complete SCI are likely to make no significant additional neurologic improvement. Recent evidence, however, suggests that from a surgical point of view, individuals with complete traumatic tetraplegia plateau at an average of 6 months following injury (46). In those individuals with an incomplete injury, however, recovery may continue longer than 1 year. When serial assessments confirm that the individual has reached a plateau, and the individual is motivated to undergo the procedure, then surgical intervention may be appropriate.

The decision to undertake surgical restoration should be a deliberate and structured process. The fact is that not all individuals are good candidates for surgery. Individuals already satisfied with their level of function, those without specific goals, and those who lack family support are not going to experience successful surgical outcomes (43). Studies indicate that between 50% and 60% of all individuals with tetraplegia will meet criteria for tendon transfer–based surgical restoration (4,47), and 13% of individuals will meet criteria for surgical restoration using implantable FES systems (when they are available) (37). Individuals with tetraplegia have impairments and conditions that are specific to the individual that must be considered in the process of surgical decision making.

SURGERY

The current standard surgical approach to reconstructing hand and arm function in SCI relies on the tendon transfer technique. The early conceptualization of tendon transfers to augment upper extremity function in SCI was largely influenced by experiences with individuals with residual deficits from poliomyelitis (48,49). Using the tendon transfer approach, the function of a paralyzed muscle is restored by substituting a strong muscle (the "donor muscle") over which the individual has voluntary control. The tendon of a nearby donor muscle is detached from its normal insertion and sewn into the muscle that the intervention is meant to restore (Fig. 28.2). An effective donor muscle must have sufficient voluntary strength (a manual muscle test grade of ≥4 [since it can = 4 also]). Ideal donor muscles are redundant such that their loss does not compromise function. For example, the biceps brachii muscle makes a suitable donor muscle for a paralyzed triceps muscle provided the brachialis muscle is still under voluntary control. Usually a function, like finger flexion, is distilled to the activity of one muscle, that is, the flexor digitorum profundus (FDP). When the patient "learns" to isolate the contraction of the transferred muscle, the fingers flex.

Together with other ancillary procedures, tendon transfer procedures represent the core of traditional reconstruction of the upper extremity in tetraplegia. Basic principles for tendon transfers are followed in order to realize successful reconstruction (50,51):

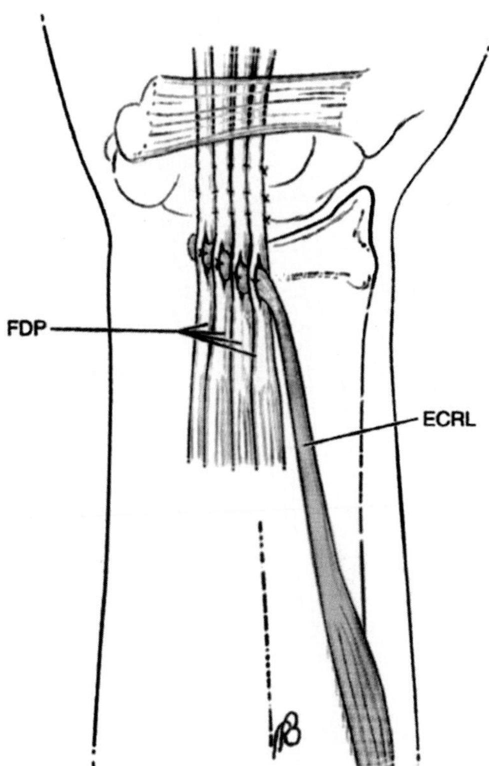

FIGURE 28.2 Illustration of a tendon transfer procedure. In this diagram, the tendon of the ECRL has been detached from its normal insertion on the dorsal base of the index metacarpal, mobilized, and then transposed into the volar forearm compartment around the radial side of the forearm. The tendon is then weaved into the four tendons of the FDP and secured with sutures. Just distal to the transfer, the four FDP tendons have been sutured together, such that all four fingers will flex simultaneously when the individual contracts the ECRL (Peljovich 2002, p. 562).

1. Supple joints with at least a functional arc of passive motion are necessary for mobility. A transfer will not restore mobility to a contracted joint.
2. The donor muscle must have sufficient inherent strength to perform the "new" task that is required of it.
3. Comparable excursion and force of contraction between the transfer with the muscle it is to replace should be present or provided (52). The term excursion is another way of expressing the amount of muscle shortening that is measured during its contraction. For example, the flexor carpi ulnaris muscle is a strong wrist flexor with a potential excursion of 4.2 cm (52). While it could be a suitable wrist extensor, it would function as a poor choice for finger flexion since the extrinsic finger flexor muscles normally shorten 6 to 8 cm to make a complete fist.
4. Synergy, whenever possible will facilitate re-education. In this setting, synergy refers to joint motions synchronized during functional activity that is, wrist extension usually occurs with finger flexion during grasp. Transferring the ECRB to the FDP takes advantage of synergy. (The biceps to triceps transfer for elbow extension is a notable exception.)
5. The transfer should traverse a healthy bed of tissue to minimize scarring.
6. Stabilization of a joint, whenever a single transfer spans across multiple joints increases its efficacy and efficiency, as has been clearly demonstrated with BR transfers (53,54). The power of a transfer is otherwise lost as its force is dispersed over multiple joints. For example, stabilizing the interphalangeal (IP) joint of the thumb increases the pinch force of a BR to flexor pollicis longus (FPL) transfer through the thumb's metacarpophalangeal (MCP) joint.
7. A straight line of pull from the donor motor to the recipient tendon will minimize lost strength from the transfer. The potential force of the transfer follows simple geometric principles, so the greatest force of pull occurs when the donor muscle's fibers are in a straight line to its insertion point. The great angle the donor muscle takes with respect to its fiber orientation, the more potential force is lost to "out of plane" pull.
8. The morbidity from loss of the donor motor should be none or minimal.
9. Anticipate secondary motions based upon the vector of pull of the donor muscle. For example, the BR can be routed into the FPL in such a way as to create secondary pronation, if so desired (55).

As previously discussed, the functions to be restored must be prioritized based upon the number of donor muscles available, and individuals with tetraplegia have only a limited number of suitable donor muscles. As such, each donor muscle's usefulness must be maximized to achieve as much function as possible. Ancillary surgical procedures are combined with tendon transfers to optimize what can be achieved and to allow the tendon transfer to recreate function. Tendon transfers are often combined with joint stabilization procedures such as arthrodeses or tenodeses to minimize the number of joints a donor muscle activates. For example, in order for thumb pinch to be effective, the pulp of the thumb needs to contact the side of the flexed index finger. The BR is often transferred into the FPL to recreate the pinch pattern. If the IP joint of the thumb is not stabilized, then when the individual contracts the BR both the MCP joint and the IP joint will flex and may miss the side of the index finger. By stabilizing the IP joint, only the MCP joint will flex and now the pulp of the straight IP joint will contact the index finger. This is accomplished by a soft tissue procedure that keeps the IP joint fairly straight during contraction. Using this same example, the carpometacarpal (CMC) joint of the thumb is often fused in the opposition position, so that when the thumb flexes, it always goes directly the side of the flexed index finger near its distal interphalangeal joint. Such ancillary procedures help the transfers become more effective. In other cases, passive tendon transfers, or "tenodeses," are used in place of tendon transfers. An example is "powering" finger extension by attaching the extensor tendons into a bone proximal to the wrist (radius), so that wrist flexion produces greater finger extension than would be provided by the static properties of the more elastic muscle. These passive transfers are not powered by the muscles themselves, but by the tension placed upon them as the joints they cross move; as opposed to active tendon transfers where the power is derived from the donor muscle's voluntary contraction.

Reliable Donor Muscles and Their Traditional Uses

The specific tendon transfers performed in tetraplegia reconstruction have been distilled over decades of accrued experience and research. While the International Classification lists the number of potential donor muscles in the forearm that can be used for transfer, not all are used. Certain functions and muscles are never sacrificed. With experience, the surgeon learns which donor motors to use and which to spare, which transfers work well and which do not.

Which Motors (Muscles) Should be Preserved

Extensor Carpi Radialis Brevis

Since wrist extension is critical to tenodesis function that forms the foundation of hand restoration, a wrist extensor is only a suitable donor motor when there are at least two under voluntary control and of sufficient strength. Wrist extension is never sacrificed when performing hand restoration for individuals with tetraplegia. Only individuals who are ICT ≥ 3 have a wrist extensor that can be sacrificed as a donor muscle.

The different force vectors of the ECRL and ECRB confer different motions (56). The ECRL, with its insertion radial to the center of the wrist on the base of the index metacarpal, produces radial deviation along with wrist extension. The ECRB, on the other hand, with its central insertion on the base of the long finger metacarpal, produces wrist extension with minimal radial/ulnar deviation, a more balanced and desirable motion. When transferring one of two strong and voluntary wrist extensors, the ECRL is chosen to restore either lateral pinch or palmar grasp depending on the patient's ICT. Similarly, when restoring wrist extension, the ECRB is the preferred recipient (15,24,30,31).

Flexor Carpi Radialis

In patients with an ICT ≥ 5, the FCR is of sufficient strength to be considered a potential donor motor. With an increasing number of available donor motors, significant gains in function through tendon transfers could be realized (16). Zancolli and House, however, have recommended to preserve the FCR (17,39,57,58), since the presence of an active, voluntary wrist flexor improves the finger tenodesis extension as well as preventing wrist extension contractures by improving wrist balance. Voluntary wrist flexion is also helpful in patients who use a manual wheelchair, and for weight shifts to prevent pressure sores. We do not currently use the FCR as a donor motor when presented with the uncommon ICT ≥ 5 person desiring surgical restoration.

Reliable Donor Muscles and Their Traditional Uses

Deltoid

One of the original tendon transfers applied in individuals with tetraplegia involved utilizing the posterior portion of the deltoid muscle to restore elbow extension, and the deltoid to triceps transfer remains a gold standard operation (Fig. 28.3) (2). All persons with motor levels of C5 or higher (ICT ≥ 1) will retain a strong voluntary deltoid in the absence of peripheral nerve injury. The usefulness and reliability of the transfer was well known clinically prior to biomechanical

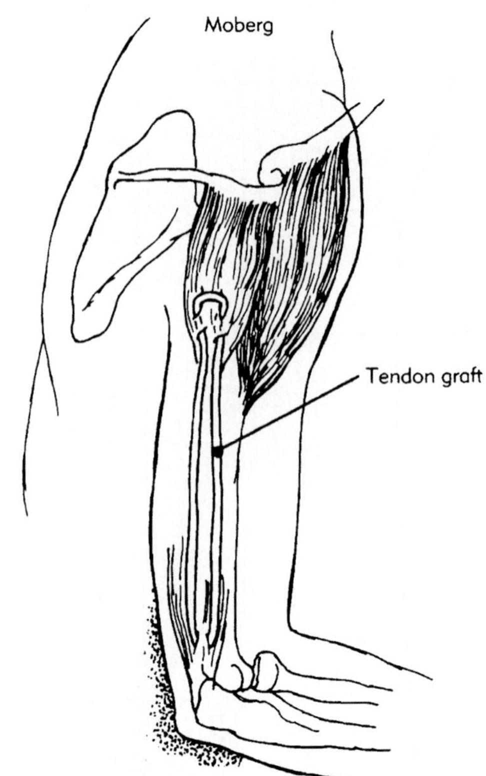

FIGURE 28.3 Illustration of Posterior Deltoid to Triceps Transfer. This particular graphic demonstrates the procedure as initially described by Moberg. The posterior deltoid is detached from its insertion onto the proximal humerus. A tendon graft, the tibialis anterior tendon in the illustrating, is used to bridge the distance from the deltoid to the triceps tendon. There are various other methods designed to bridge the distance as well. (Leclercq C, Hentz VR, Kozin SH, et al. Reconstruction of elbow extension. *Hand Clin* 2008;24:185–201, vi.)

analysis (36,59–63). As studies demonstrate, the deltoid muscle is able to only generate approximately 20% of the potential maximum isometric tension of the triceps muscle it is substituting for; but, has such a long excursion and an ability to maintain tension over a such large percentage of that excursion that it serves as a suitable donor (64–66). The ability to maintain a consistent strong "pull" while the muscle fibers shorten more than makes the deltoid transfer a reliable and predictable operation. While obtaining antigravity strength elbow extension is typical, the limited strength of the deltoid as a donor makes it more difficult to obtain strength for weight transfers—and this is borne out in clinic study. Extensive analysis has supported the need to maintain a strict and extended postoperative therapeutic regimen to help the transfer succeed (67,68).

Biceps

Strong elbow flexion (ICT ≥ 1; Motor level at or below C5) translates to the presence of voluntary and strong biceps, brachialis, and BR. In 1954, Friedenberg first described using the biceps muscle to restore elbow extension a patient with poliomyelitis and one with traumatic tetraplegia (69). Then, two publications in 1999 advanced the clinical efficacy of utilizing the biceps as a donor motor to restore elbow extension in the setting of tetraplegia (70,71). Although a nonsynergist transfer, both studies found that patients were able to learn how to

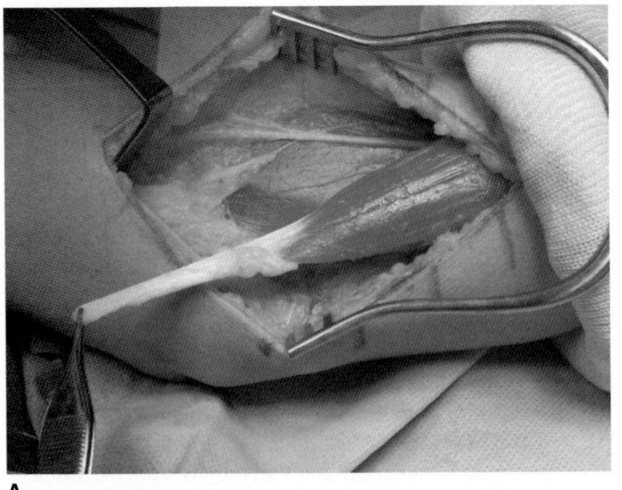
A

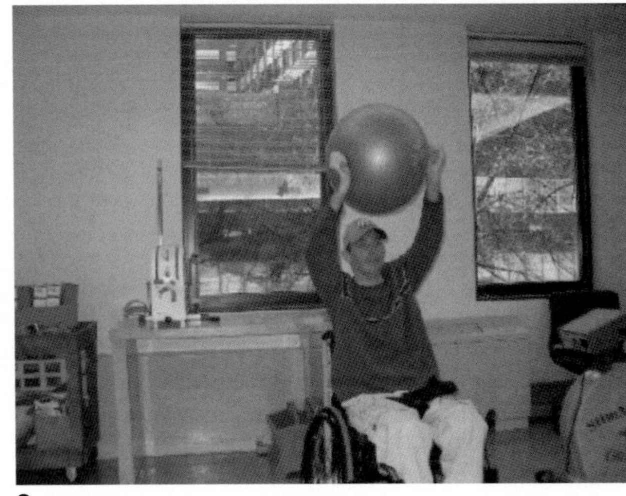
C

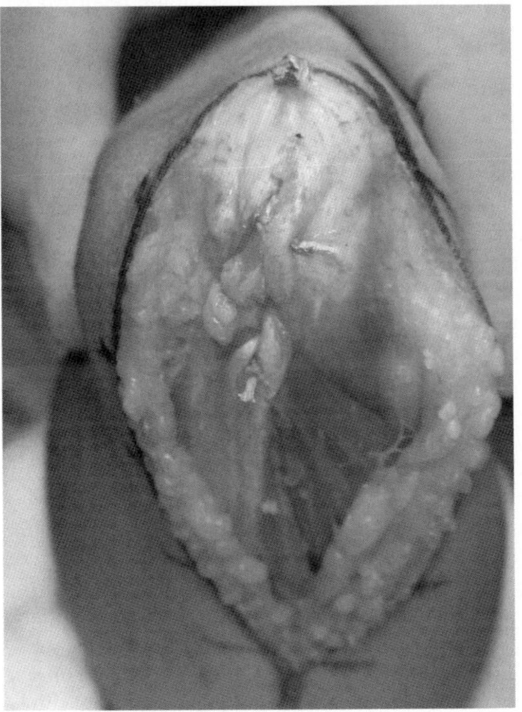
B

FIGURE 28.4 Example of biceps to triceps transfer. (A) The biceps tendon is detached and the tendon and muscle are both mobilized via an anterior incision. (B) The biceps is then routed around the medial side of the upper arm, deep to the ulnar nerve, and then weaved into the triceps tendon and anchored directly into the bone of the olecranon process. This intra-operative photograph illustrates the posterior surface of the arm with the elbow superior and the shoulder inferior. The tendon of the biceps is woven into the triceps tendon and secured with multiple sutures. (C) Example of an individual's ability to raise their arms following the procedure.

isolate the biceps contraction in order to activate the transfer, the postoperative regimen was simpler, and that the postoperative elbow extension strength was superior to antigravity strength. Since the brachialis is the primary elbow flexor, the biceps can be spared as a donor motor without sacrificing meaningful elbow flexion strength; but, it is critical to ensure that the brachialis is functional prior to the transfer. Revol et al. measured a loss of elbow flexion strength of up to 47% in their study, but also noted that patients were not dissatisfied with that loss (70,71). Individuals also lose some supination strength (a function of the biceps brachii), but this may actually be desirable to prevent supination contractures, and help balance a forearm in someone that does not have strong voluntary pronation function. The biceps has gained wide acceptance for use as an elbow extension donor muscle (Fig. 28.4). A more recent comparative study found that the biceps transfer provided more elbow extension strength compared to a posterior deltoid transfer (72).

Brachioradialis

The BR is the most readily available and versatile muscle for reconstructive transfers in tetraplegia (Fig. 28.5). Because it functions secondarily as an elbow flexor, and since most patients who are C5 have a strong biceps brachii and brachialis, the BR is commonly sacrificed with minimal deficit to the patient. It is truly the workhorse donor muscle in tetraplegia surgery. By mobilizing the muscle during a transfer, its potential excursion can be increased from its native 41.7 mm to upwards of 77.9 mm making it a useful mimic for most of the extrinsic forearm muscles (52,54,73). The BR also contracts

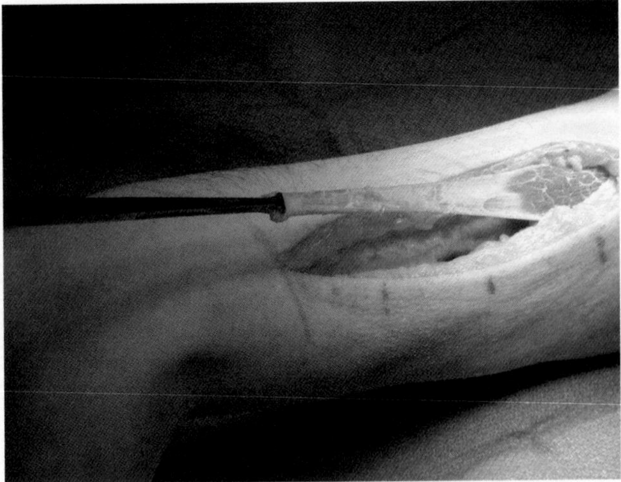

FIGURE 28.5 The BR muscle is dissected in this clinical photograph. Its tendon has been released from its insertion on the radial side of the distal radius, and it is mobilized from its various fibrous connections to surrounding tissues, tendons, and muscles. By mobilizing this muscle from its insertion to near its origin, its potential excursion during contracture can reach over 7 cm, making it a useful donor motor. Since its innervation comes from the radial nerve proximal to the elbow, the muscle can be mobilized this extensively safely.

with near maximal strength over a long portion of its total excursion, allowing it to maintain a strong and consistent pull (31). In fact, a variety of tendon transfers using the BR have been described: BR to ECRB for wrist extension, BR to FDP for palmar grasp, BR to FPL for lateral pinch, BR for adduction opponensplasty, and BR to extensor digitorum communis (EDC)/extensor pollicis longus (EPL) for finger and thumb extension (19,34,39,74–77).

Extensor Carpi Radialis Longus

The ECRL is available for transfer whenever there is a strong ECRB (ICT ≥ 3). We commonly transfer the ECRL to a synchronized FDP to restore palmar grasp. We initially create a "reverse cascade" such that all fingers flex simultaneously and equally as advocated by Hentz (38,78–80). The transfer is synergistic for wrist extension and finger flexion. The line of pull around the radial border of radius creates secondary forearm supination. The ECRL can alternatively be routed through the interosseous membrane between the radius and ulna if secondary supination is not desired in a particular individual's case. Other common uses for the ECRL that have been described include transfer to the FPL for lateral grasp, the EDC/EPL for finger extension, and for intrinsic reconstruction (15,16,19,29–32,38,39,57,81,82).

Pronator Teres

House has had favorable experience with transfer of the PT into the FPL since the early 1970s without adverse effects on Pronation (83). Zancolli also favors transfer of the PT, especially to the FCR, placing emphasis on the restoration of active wrist flexion to stabilize the wrist in patients with strong wrist extension, and to improve the finger tenodesis effect (18,58). In addition, we have not observed, nor have we seen reported, cases of supination contractures occurring in patients with ICT ≥ 2 when the PT is used as a donor muscle.

TETRAPLEGIA HAND RECONSTRUCTION—THE COMMON TENDON TRANSFERS

General Principles of Postsurgical Care

Traditionally, the upper extremity is placed in a bulky, but durable plaster splint and then converted to a cast as necessary over the next few weeks to protect the transfers while they heal. If multiple procedures are performed simultaneously, that is, elbow extension and pinch and/or grasp restoration, all appropriate joints are immobilized. During this period of immobilization, it is essential to maintain ROM of the joints that are not casted, as well as that of the extremity that did not undergo surgery. Education for individuals and the families and caregivers should focus on signs of infection, proper positioning, and precautions. The individual should be instructed on how to perform transitions and transfer for mobility and adaptations that need to be made for ADL, wheelchair mobility, and weight shifts.

Cast removal occurs approximately 3 to 4 weeks after surgery. When the cast is removed, the therapist should identify what muscles are involved in tendon transfer and understand functional purpose. Emphasis should be placed on educating the patient and family regarding what motions are to be avoided and demonstrate how to position or hold the extremity while out of cast or splint.

Therapy after cast removal emphasizes protective splinting, scar mobilization, retrograde massage, and active ROM (re-education activities). To protect the tendon transfer and to prevent the development or reoccurrence of deformity, protective splints are fabricated to position the extremity in the appropriate position. Splints are lined with thin foam to protect insensate areas.

Retrograde massage (for edema control) and scar mobilization are performed prior to active ROM exercises. Retrograde massage may be used for edema reduction. Scar mobilization is initially performed along the perimeter of the incision, and when the incision is well healed, it is performed over the surgical site at least twice daily. Active ROM exercises and muscle re-education focuses on retraining the individual how to use the donor muscle in its new function. There are many alternative techniques available to assist with training for individuals who may have difficulty learning how to perform the new function and include biofeedback or surface electrical stimulation that may be incorporated into the training program. Early practice of functional skills will aid in the retraining process.

More recently, therapy protocols have begun incorporating early mobilization instead of casting for 3 to 4 weeks. Individuals are still kept in a protective splint or brace, but the protective device is removed several times a day for mobilization and tendon transfer retraining. This is possible due to the strength of the techniques that coapt the donor tendon into the recipient muscle/tendon. Such techniques have been studied with regard to the deltoid to triceps transfer, and the lateral pinch transfer (84,85). In both studies, early mobilization protocols resulted in better mobility and strength of transfer. More importantly perhaps, the earlier return to function allowed therapists to gain a "head start" on training individuals on ADL, thereby reducing the postoperative down time—a huge issue for individuals deciding on whether to proceed with surgery (42).

Elbow Extension

Moberg initially stressed the importance of restoring active elbow extension for the individual with tetraplegia. From a technical perspective, restoring elbow extension also improves the outcomes of more distal tendon transfers employed to restore hand function (4). Restoring elbow extension does more than allowing the individual to power their hand away from them, it also confers intrinsic stability to the elbow joint through the provision of moment forces in all of the joint's axes of motion. Moberg emphasized the beneficial effect of restoring elbow stability on the functional outcome of procedures that use either the BR or ECRL for muscle transfers (5). Brys and Waters found that pinch strength following BR-to-FPL tendon transfer increased by 150% when the elbow could be stabilized (53). Today, two surgical procedures are utilized to restore active elbow extension: these are the posterior deltoid to triceps transfer and the bicep-to-triceps transfer.

Posterior Deltoid to Triceps Transfer

Restoring elbow extension using the deltoid as a donor muscle remains the traditional procedure used since it was first described by Moberg in 1975 (2). In this procedure, the function of the triceps is restored by using the posterior one-third to one-half of the posterior deltoid as a donor muscle. The intrinsic biomechanics of the deltoid muscle provide more than sufficient excursion for elbow extension, but can only generate 20% to 50% of the average triceps force (86). This is consistent with the observed outcomes of the procedure in that it rarely provides more than good antigravity strength (61,62,87). There are two aspects of the posterior deltoid to triceps procedure that merit mentioning. The relatively short size of the gross muscle requires a bridging tissue graft to allow attachment into the triceps (4,5,60,65,66), and, requires a very demanding postsurgical rehabilitation protocol to avoid stretching and weakening (68). Newer postsurgical protocols that include early mobilization of the transfer results in improved elbow mobility and elbow extension strength (84).

Postoperative Therapy. Following surgery, the upper extremity is placed in a long arm cast with the elbow in no more than 20 degrees of flexion and with the wrist and hand mobile (2,88). While the patient is in bed, the arm is elevated to prevent edema, and the shoulder is positioned in 30 degrees of abduction. Passive ROM of the shoulder should begin after surgery, with shoulder flexion and shoulder abduction limited to 90 degrees and horizontal adduction to midline. No lifting under the axilla area should occur. All these restrictions are intended to avoid shoulder positions that could stretch the graft during the early postsurgical period.

The cast is removed 3 to 4 weeks after surgery, unless an early motion protocol is utilized. A hinged elbow orthosis is used to further protect the tendon transfer and to prevent overstretching or rupture of the tendon transfer. Initially, the orthosis is locked in 0 degrees of extension for the first week and is worn at all times, except during therapy and skin checks. The hinged orthosis is progressed 15 degrees of flexion per week, provided that active motion to full elbow extension is present (2,88,90). The therapist increases flexion only when it is certain that full range of elbow extension is present. If the individual demonstrates a restriction in the extension ROM, then it is better to maintain the brace position and increase strength prior to increasing allowable flexion. When the hinged orthosis is advanced to 15 degrees of flexion (during day wear), a static elbow extension brace is fabricated for nighttime wear. When the dial-hinge elbow orthosis reaches 90 degrees of flexion for 1 week, the brace is discontinued.

Therapy initially focuses on successful activation of the tendon transfer. In order to achieve elbow extension successfully via the tendon transfer, the shoulder is positioned in 90 degrees of abduction, and the individual is cued to pull the shoulder back (horizontal abduction). It is important to ensure that the individual is not substituting with external rotation and the use of gravity to complete elbow extension. The active ROM of elbow extension continues in this gravity-eliminated plane. As the individual progresses, strengthening activities in all planes of motion are added to the therapy. Active elbow flexion beyond the limits of the orthosis is avoided until 12 weeks after surgery, at which time retraining in performing transitions, transfers, and wheelchair propulsion may be considered. A soft splint to avoid elongation of the tendon is worn at night for a total of 6 months. The tendon transfer will continue to strengthen and become more useful for a year or more after surgery.

Biceps to Triceps Transfer

The first published description of using biceps brachii to provide elbow extension appeared in 1954 (69). This procedure has gained momentum as an alternative to the deltoid to triceps transfer, and in some centers, it has become the primary mode of surgically restoring elbow extension (70–72). Research indicates that the biceps proves as strong if not stronger than the deltoid as a donor for elbow extension (70,72). And, while a couple of reports have noted a loss of elbow flexion strength (a smaller reduction is also noted with the deltoid tendon transfer), the functional gains associated with the provision of strong elbow extension more than compensate for the reduction in elbow flexion strength (71,72).The advantages of this transfer include the ability to surgically insert the tendon of the biceps directly into the triceps tendon and the olecranon insertion (which requires a less demanding rehabilitation protocol), and it is performed in less time than the deltoid tendon transfer. Ironically, and in apparent contradiction to the tenets of tendon transfer principles, this transfer is not synergistic.

Postoperative Therapy. After surgery, the upper extremity is placed in a long-arm cast, with the elbow fixed in no more than 20 degrees of flexion. While the individual is in bed, the arm is elevated to prevent edema, and the shoulder is positioned in 30 degrees of abduction. Passive ROM exercises for the shoulder should begin after surgery and is limited to 90 degrees of shoulder flexion and shoulder abduction.

The cast is removed 3 to 4 weeks after surgery. Again, if an early motion protocol is utilized, the casting period is shortened to 1 to 2 weeks. A dial-hinge elbow orthosis is used to further protect the tendon transfer and prevent overstretching or rupture of the tendon transfer. Initially, the orthosis is locked at 0 degrees of extension for the first week and worn at all times except for therapy and skin checks. The hinged orthosis is progressed 15 degrees of flexion per week provided that active motion to full elbow extension is present without substitution. When the hinged orthosis is advanced to 15 degrees of flexion (day wear), a static elbow extension brace is fabricated for nighttime wear. When the dial-hinge elbow orthosis reaches 90 degrees of flexion for 1 week, the brace is discontinued.

Therapy initially focuses on successful activation of the tendon transfer. In order to achieve elbow extension successfully by the tendon transfer, the shoulder is positioned in 90 degrees of abduction and the individual is cued to supinate the forearm. It is important to ensure that the individual is not substituting external rotation and the use of gravity to complete elbow extension. The active ROM of elbow extension continues in this gravity-eliminated plane. As the individual progresses, strengthening should take place in all planes of motion. Active elbow flexion beyond the limits of the orthosis is avoided until 12 weeks after surgery, at which time mobility transfers and wheelchair propulsion may be considered. A soft splint to avoid elongation of the tendon is worn at night for a total of 6 months. The tendon transfer will continue to strengthen and become more useful for a year or more after surgery.

Wrist Extension

Moberg pointed out that in individuals with higher levels of injury, namely those who fall under International Classification 0 or 1, voluntary wrist extension is either absent or weak; therefore, the primary goal of surgical restoration of the hand is the provision of wrist extension (2). If this can be achieved, then an automatic/passive lateral tenodesis pinch can be constructed with a series of secondary procedures to augment the strength of natural tenodesis pinch. For weak ICT 1 individuals, the BR is the donor muscle into the ECRB. In order to optimize this transfer, the surgeon must free the BR of its intermuscular fascial connections to create the necessary excursion for wrist extension. Strong ICT 1 individuals, and all those with higher grades, do not require this transfer. In our experience, this provides sufficient stability to the wrist, so that a patient no longer requires a universal wrist cuff, but rarely creates enough wrist extension to power an effective tenodesis pinch and grasp.

Lateral Pinch

The active lateral pinch provides the ability to secure small objects with useful force. The result is the enhancement ADL functions, including self-catheterization, writing, feeding, etc. Conceptually, pinch/grasp can be understood as four phases: (a) object acquisition, (b) pinch/grasp, (c) hold/manipulation, and (d) object release (28). The functional outcome of the surgical restoration procedure requires the coordination of precise digital motions, so that all phases of the pattern can be accomplished. In the case of lateral pinch, object acquisition depends upon the thumb extending sufficiently (EPL, extensor pollicis brevis, and abductor pollicis longus [APL]) with gravity powered wrist flexion. A secure grasp is best achieved as the thumb moves into opposition (abductor pollicis brevis [APB]) and firmly rests against the index finger with force (FPL, adductor pollicis [AdP], index flexors, index intrinsics). The grasp must be secure enough, so that the individual can maintain it with minimal fatigue while an object is handled, and then he/she must be able to easily release the object.

In most individuals with C5-6 tetraplegia, the number of muscles remaining under voluntary control is insufficient to replace the many paralyzed hand and forearm muscles. Therefore, the challenges of this procedure are to recreate a meaningful pinch, as well as achieve precise digital positioning by distilling this complex set of motions into its most fundamental elements. This can all be achieved with one tendon transfer using the BR to FPL transfer. Active pinch reconstruction requires full voluntary wrist extension, so this procedure is only performed in strong ICT 1 in which wrist extension strength is grade 3.

Since only one of the four phases of pinch is actually restored with a tendon transfer, ancillary procedures are employed. Object acquisition is insured as long as the thumb is in opposition. If the patient lacks this naturally with tenodesis (most do), then the CMC joint of the thumb is fused in opposition. While leaving the CMC joint alone preserves greater mobility and "opening" for lateral pinch, the pinch strength is increased when the CMC joint is fused (91). An effective pinch is best reconstructed when the pulp of the thumb rests against the flexed index finger when the wrist is in extension. The BR to FPL transfer will work through all the joints of the thumb, namely the CMC, MCP, and IP. Unless the individual has voluntary thumb extension (ICT ≥ 7) then the tendency will be for both the MCP and IP joint to flex when the BR is contracted (the CMC is often already fused). In this scenario, either the tip of the thumb contacts the index finger or it misses altogether—neither is ideal. So, the IP joint of the thumb is stabilized with a passive tendon transfer that maintains the suppleness of the joint but insures that the thumb pulp will rest against the side of the index finger. If natural tenodesis finger/thumb extension is insufficient for releasing an object, then the thumb and finger extensors can be tenodesed to the dorsum of the radius bone to generate a stronger extension force, albeit passively, when the wrist drops into flexion. House demonstrated that all the components of lateral pinch reconstruction can be achieved with a single surgical procedure (92). This combination of procedures and its recent modifications from the original "key-pinch" procedure devised by Moberg, is the currently favored intervention (4,38,44,93).

In individuals with weak or absent wrist extension where the BR will be required to augment it, only a passive lateral pinch is possible. By "tying" or tenodesing the FPL into the radius, wrist extension generates greater tension on the muscle during wrist extension generating greater pinch force than natural tenodesis alone could provide. The ancillary procedures to position the thumb for ideal pinch position are still performed. The passive lateral pinch procedure is rarely performed since the BR to wrist extensor transfer rarely creates sufficient wrist extension to power finger/thumb tenodesis.

In individuals having ICT motor scores of 3 or greater, there are even more options. More elegant reconstructions are possible since there are more potential donor muscles available to the surgeon: BR, ECRL, and PT. In addition to the provision of pinch, powered palmar grasp can be reconstructed for a truly functional hand. The ECRL is typically reserved to power finger flexion; therefore, the BR and PT are usual donor muscles that could be used to create active lateral pinch. House devised two methods of reconstructing thumb pinch in these stronger individuals: one method used FPL activation via tendon transfer and thumb CMC fusion for strength as just described, the other used FPL activation via tendon transfer and another tendon transfer creating opposition for precision/dexterity using the BR (92). In the latter technique, named the adduction opponensplasty, the BR powers opposition using the ring finger flexor digitorum superficialis (FDS) tendon weaved into the APB, and the PT powers the FPL. It is most common to apply the adduction opponensplasty when the surgeon is performing a bilateral reconstruction in which one thumb is reconstructed for strength and the other for dexterity (92). Other reports have described various methods of achieving thumb position without the need for CMC fusion (94). Thumb extension, if needed, is achieved either with a tenodesis procedure or by using BR to power digital extension. Thumb IP stabilization remains an important part of the procedure in order to create an effective pinch platform on the flexed index finger.

Postoperative Therapy

Following the surgical procedure for restoration of passive lateral pinch, the arm is immobilized for 3 to 4 weeks in 90 degree elbow flexion, 20 degree wrist extension, and flexion of the thumb and index MCP joints. The arm is elevated to limit edema while the individual is in bed. Shoulder ROM exercises continue on the surgical side, with no limitations. Following cast removal, a dorsal splint is fabricated to position the wrist in 20 degrees of extension, with the thumb and index MCP joints in flexion. It is not necessary to splint the elbow; however, to protect the BR tendon transfer, activities involving high stress (hooking of the arm around wheelchair) should be avoided. The first 2 weeks of rehabilitation should concentrate on scar mobilization and on successful voluntary activation of the tendon transfer. In order to activate the passive pinch, the forearm is positioned in a neutral position and the individual is instructed to bend the elbow.

When the individual is consistently activating the tendon transfer, practice is continued with the elbow positioned at different angles of flexion. In addition, functional activities are initiated when the individual is consistently able to activate the tendon transfer. When practicing grasp activities, the objects to be grasped should be of small diameter so as not to stretch out the FPL tenodesis pattern. The thumb should be positioned between the index and middle finger during functional tasks to avoid resistive pinch until 8 to 10 weeks after surgery. Wrist flexion angle should not exceed the angle that is passively available, nor should thumb extension exceed what is passively available. At 8 weeks post surgery, wrist extension should be approaching presurgical range. At this time, strengthening of the transfer may occur by adding resistance to wrist extension exercises. A daytime splint is worn until the individual demonstrates consistent activation of the tendon transfer, good control of wrist extension, and sufficient ROM to allow placement of the thumb pad against the fingers. This usually occurs 3 to 4 weeks after cast removal. Nighttime splinting is continued indefinitely to ensure optimal posture of the hand.

Palmar Grasp

Palmar grasp allows the individual to manipulate larger objects than they would be capable with pinch alone. Cans, bottles, bags, and the like become easily accessible items individuals can manipulate. Lateral pinch is normally reconstructed in the place of palmar grasp in strong ICT 1 and 2 individuals since it is a more useful grasp pattern. Some individuals might prefer palmar grasp in place of lateral pinch, but we have not found that. The presence of sufficient donor muscles results in the ability to reconstruct both lateral pinch and palmar grasp (ICT ≥ 3). In general, the results of the procedure may be better in individuals with lower levels of injury (IC ≥ 4) (44).

As with the lateral pinch, palmar grasp requires the coordinated motions of a variety of joints that are synchronized with wrist motion. Also, like lateral pinch, compromises are made. In the able-bodied hand, there is much coordination between the extrinsic forearm muscles and the intrinsic hand muscles during palmar grasp and release. Both these muscle groups work in concert to create normal digital flexion and extension, with the intrinsic muscles being largely responsible for MCP flexion and IP extension (95). Many individuals with tetraplegia have a hand posture of MCP extension, with partial flexion of the IP joints of the fingers and thumb (intrinsic minus hand position); therefore, some capacity for MCP flexion during grasp improves strength (96). Object acquisition requires that the fingers extend to be able to wrap around the desired object. Unlike lateral pinch, finger extension must be powered in order to avoid longer term finger flexion contractures ($3 \leq$ ICT ≤ 6) if one relied on natural tenodesis to balance powered finger flexion. This is usually accomplished by tenodesing the finger extensors and occasionally by powering them with a tendon transfer. The problem is that the nature of the postsurgical rehabilitation requires that these procedures be accomplished in two surgeries: one to create the finger extension and one for the flexion (two-staged procedures are discussed below). Finger flexion is achieved by powering the action of the FDP, which flexes all of the IP joints of the fingers. Powering the FDP via tendon transfer is usually achieved with the ECRL as the donor muscle, as opposed to the BR or PT since it is both synergistic and a good match for the FDP. Since one donor muscle cannot singlehandedly restore the independent digital motion of all the fingers, the ECRL is weaved into all four tendons of the FDP to create an all-in-one grasp pattern. The FDP tendons are first prepared for the transfer by coapting them to each other such that, with active wrist extension, all four fingers are synchronized to flex level to each other (reverse cascade FDP synchronization). The ECRL is then weaved into the FDP mass proximal to the synchronization sutures. If the MCP joints do not flex sufficiently with wrist extension naturally, then restoration of intrinsic muscle function may also be considered in a select group of individuals (97). This is to maximize the large object acquisition ability of the transfer. Careful presurgical examination helps identify the individual's specific tenodesis grasp pattern. Two techniques are available to mimic intrinsic function. One method involves using the FDS tendons to passively bring the MCP joints into flexion with wrist extension. The other method uses a tendon graft but has the added advantage of helping to create PIP extension if preoperative examination shows the individual to have a drooped PIP joint that does not passively extend during wrist extension (92).

Postoperative Therapy

After the surgical procedure for restoration of active lateral pinch and active grip, the arm is casted for 3 to 4 weeks with the elbow fixed at a flexion of 90 degrees. The arm is elevated to limit edema while the individual is in bed. Shoulder ROM exercises should continue with no limitations while in the arm is in the cast. If the active grip procedure was performed, then the volar surface of the fingers should not be casted, but supported with a strap. Beginning the day after surgery, the strap is removed at least two times per day, and the individual should gently activate the grip transfer. This is done in an effort to decrease the risk of adhesions.

After cast removal, a dorsal-based splint is fabricated to position the wrist in 20 degrees of extension, with the thumb aligned for lateral pinch, and MCP joints of digits are fixed at 90 degrees of flexion. The splint is worn at all times during the first week after cast removal, except for therapy and skin checks. The splint may be discontinued during light ADL (eating, grooming, writing, etc.) when the individual is able to do the following: verbalize an understanding of postsurgical precautions, demonstrate awareness of restrictions (see below) during therapy activities, and demonstrate the ability to consistently activate all transferred muscles. The splint can be used for night wear only when the individual demonstrates consistent control/activation of the tendon transfer without substitution, demonstrates functional range in the restored joint, and demonstrates an understanding of postsurgical precautions. As a general guideline, splints are changed to a night wear–only schedule approximately 2 to 3 weeks after cast removal. The Kirschner (K)-wire for IP is removed 3 to 4 weeks post surgery if it was used to help protect the passive transfer to help stabilize the IP joint. However, if a CMC fusion was performed, then the individual will wear a protective thumb splint until the CMC K-wire is removed (wrist support during day may be discontinued if the above guidelines are met). The CMC fusion is x-rayed at week 8 post surgery, and if healed, the K-wire is removed at that time.

General precautions following the surgical procedure are as follows: no forced wrist extension beyond the available passive range, and no forced thumb extension beyond the available passive range, no forced thumb flexion beyond the available passive range, no heavy weight bearing for at least 6 to 8 weeks after surgery. After that time, the surgeon's evaluation may determine that heavy weight bearing may be initiated. Manual wheelchair propulsion and transferring should be added when the surgeon discerns that criteria have been met.

Therapy initially focuses on scar management and successful activation of the tendon transfer. In order to achieve active pinch and grip, the positioning will depend on which muscles have been transferred. Activation of pinch function will be the initial focus. If the BR was transferred to the FPL, in order to activate pinch function, the wrist is positioned in neutral and the forearm in a pronated position. The individual is then cued to activate the BR by bending the elbow toward the mouth. If the pronator teres (PT) was transferred to the FPL, the wrist and forearm are positioned in neutral (Fig. 28.6) and the individual is cued to pronate the forearm. In either case, the therapist will want to be certain that the appropriate muscles are being activated and that the individual is not substituting wrist extension to perform or enhance the motion. Once the individual is successful in activating the lateral pinch, training for activation of grip in initiated.

In order to activate the grip, the forearm is positioned in neutral and the individual is cued to extend the wrist in the radial direction. Training the active ROM of both the pinch and grip continues in the gravity-eliminated plane until the individual is able to perform each consistently. Once the activation of the pinch and grip is consistent, the individual must learn to activate the tendon transfer in multiple planes as well as coactivate these functions with other procedures that may have been done at the same time. Early incorporation of light functional activities should be stressed. The activities should be of interest to the individual and should include different elbow and wrist motions and levels of resistance to increase strength. As a general guideline, light ADL should begin 2 to 3 weeks after cast removal. Functional activities that generate high forces and resistance, such as manual wheelchair propulsion and transfers, should be added when the surgeon has determined that criteria have been met.

Two-stage Procedures

All of the previous mentioned transfers can easily be accomplished in one single operation, and typically are. The exception is when palmar grasp is reconstructed along with lateral pinch in individuals lacking voluntary finger extension

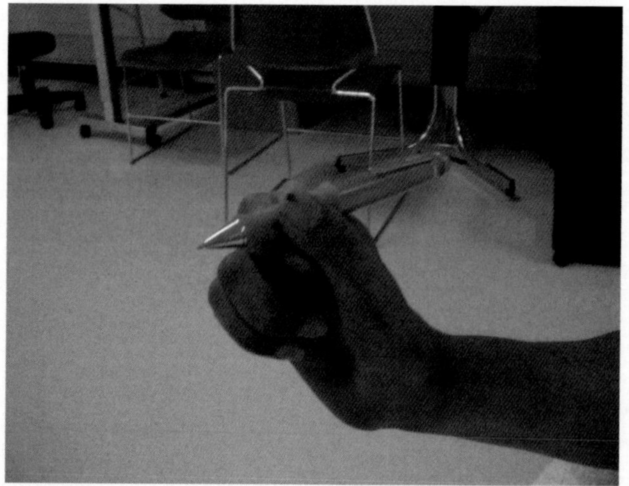

A

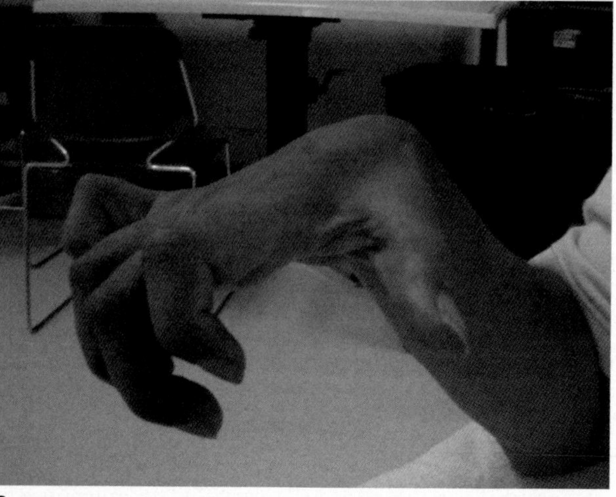

B

FIGURE 28.6. These clinical photographs demonstrate the (A) grasp and (B) release phases of the lateral pinch following tendon transfer reconstruction. This individual powers his pinch using a PT to FPL transfers. His thumb CMC joint opposition was secured using a BR-mediated FDS ring opponensplasty. Notice how his thumb rests against his index holding a pen. The IP joint is stabilized using the FPL split transfer to keep the joint from hyperflexing when activated by the PT.

($3 \leq$ ICT ≤ 6). The inevitable finger flexion contractures that result from powering the FDP without balancing it with powered finger extensors would limit the effectiveness of the procedure. Unlike lateral pinch, where the IP joint of the thumb is stabilized to prevent the very same problem in one operation, balance of finger flexion and extension cannot be achieved in one operation. This is because the rehabilitative protocols for extensor reconstruction contradict those for flexion. This must be accounted for in the preoperative planning and in discussions with the patient. On more than one occasion, only lateral pinch has been restored in patients ICT > 3 because the individual was not willing to deal with the extended recovery, even if the long-term outcomes would be more favorable with both pinch and grasp reconstructed.

The surgical procedures for restoration of finger flexion and extension are performed 2 to 6 months apart, depending on how the wounds heal and how supple the tendon transfers are at the time of second stage. There are two original descriptions for this sequence, one in which the flexors are reconstructed first and the other in which the extensors are reconstructed first (92,97). Extensor phase reconstruction involves extensor activation (EDC and EPL) passively by tenodesis or by tendon transfer to the EPL, APL, and EDC (IC ≥ 4) using a number of donor muscles (18,44,58,97,98). An intrinsic plasty is typically performed during the extensor phase. The thumb is treated by an CMC arthrodesis (if opponensplasty is not performed) or APL tenodesis (if opponensplasty is performed). The flexor phase consists of transferring the ECRL tendon to power the FDP muscle after synchronizing the FDP and transferring the PT or BR to power the FPL muscle (depending upon what is done during the extensor phase and how the thumb is to be reconstructed) along with the other elements of the lateral pinch procedure. Variations using alternative tendon transfers and alternative ordering of the surgical procedures have been described and illustrate the importance of individualizing the surgical plan to fit the candidate's needs (18,19,44,45,97,98).

Postoperative Therapy

Stage I (Extensor Stage). The individual is casted for 3 to 4 weeks. After cast removal, during the first 2 weeks of therapy, the focus is on active ROM of the wrist flexors to facilitate passive tenodesis opening or to initiate passive motion of the BR. In addition, passive ROM exercises of the proximal and distal IP joint are performed. These exercises are performed with the wrist positioned in extension to avoid stretching the tendon transfers. Muscle re-education of the BR muscle and active range-of-motion exercises for the ECRL are initiated during the sixth week after surgery, and by week 8, strengthening activities are performed.

Stage II (Flexor Stage). When full wrist flexion is obtained, typically between 7 and 10 weeks after surgery for the extensor stage, the flexor stage reconstruction is performed. The rehabilitation for this stage is the same as the active pinch and grip section.

Putting It All Together

The previous section reviewed the various methods in which various components of hand and arm reconstruction are performed. This section reviews how surgical planning for a particular individual tends to work, and place the restorative ladder into perspective. In general, as the ICT grade improves, the number of strong voluntary donor muscles in the forearm available for transfer increases. While any individual who lacks voluntary elbow extension qualifies for an elbow extension reconstruction, the number of donor muscles limits the possibilities for hand reconstruction. An individual with SCI who is ICT 0 does not meet the criteria for tendon transfer reconstruction of the hand, and only if they have a particularly strong deltoid or biceps could they undergo an elbow extension transfer. For these higher level injuries, the only reconstructions are conducted at research centers utilizing FES or potentially nerve transfers in the future. At ICT 1, the only individuals who could qualify for an active pinch or grasp transfer need to have antigravity wrist extension (BMRC 3/5—does not move the grade to ICT 2); otherwise, only a wrist extension transfer and possibly a subsequent passive pinch or grasp transfer is possible. It is when the individual is ICT 2, is there definitive ability to perform an active pinch or grasp transfer in concert with an elbow extension transfer; and, it is when these hand reconstructions are powered by tendon transfers that they become more effective (44,45,99). As stated earlier, lateral pinch is usually prioritized over palmar grasp. As the IC motor scores improve, and more than two donor muscles are available without sacrificing wrist extension (IC ≥ 3), both lateral pinch and palmar grasp can be reconstructed. Tendon transfer procedures are typically prioritized to create power, that is, flexion for pinch and grasp, with extension provided by passive tenodesis if necessary. As the IC motor score improves to a score of 4 or greater and more donor muscles become available, both flexion and extension can be powered without requiring tenodeses; or, a more dextrous adductor opponensplasty can be utilized in the reconstruction of lateral pinch. And, as the levels continue to increase, some functions, like digital extension, no longer require reconstruction.

Many individuals also desire reconstruction of both upper extremities. There are no fundamental differences in surgical strategy when reconstructing both limbs, but there are a few considerations. One such consideration regards the method used to restore lateral pinch in ICT ≥ 4. In such individuals, where the useful donors include BR, ECRL, and PT, there is variability in thumb reconstruction without compromising the ability to restore palmar grasp and release. In one alternative, the thumb CMC joint is treated with an arthrodesis, which confers strength, and frees one of the donor muscles to some other function such as powered finger extension. In the other alternative, an opponensplasty is created for the thumb to add dexterity. The FDS of the ring finger is typically detached and inserted into the APB muscle to recreate thumb palmar abduction and opposition, and standard technique used in able-bodied individuals with median nerve palsy. Since the flexor is paralyzed in individuals with tetraplegia, this transfer is then powered by transferring the BR into the FDS of the ring finger, leaving the PT to power FPL. Finger extension is achieved through passive tenodesis. So, an individual with ICT ≥ 4 tetraplegia may chose the opponensplasty for their dominant arm, and the arthrodesis for strength in their nondominant arm. A second consideration in bilateral reconstructions includes logistical timing of surgery. We generally allow patients to choose whether they want such reconstructions performed in one surgery, or in a staged fashion. For those who choose the former, rarely, they must understand

TABLE 28.4

SURGICAL ALGORITHM BY ICT LEVEL

IC Muscle Level	Surgical Goals (typical)
1	Elbow extension[a]; Wrist extension; Tenodesis-based lateral pinch
2	Elbow extension; Lateral pinch[b]
3	Elbow extension; Lateral pinch; Consider palmar grasp[c]
4	Elbow extension; Lateral pinch; Palmar grasp; Consider single vs. two-stage procedure
5	May not require elbow extension transfer; Lateral pinch; Palmar Grasp; single vs. two stage
6	Same as above
7	Will not require elbow extension transfer; Lateral pinch and palmar grasp in single stage
8	May need lateral pinch; May not require palmar grasp procedure
9	Intrinsic restoration only[d]
X	Assess needs on individual basis

[a]Elbow extension—biceps or deltoid as donor to triceps.
[b]Lateral pinch—BR or PT as donor to FPL. Thumb CMC undergoes arthrodesis or opponensplasty (IC ≥ 4).
[c]Palmar grasp—ECRL as donor to FDP.
[d]Intrinsic restoration—FDS lasso versus House tenodesis (consider with any palmar grasp).
Adapted from Peljovich AE. Tendon transfers for restoration of active grasp. In: Kozin SH, ed. *Atlas of the hand clinics*. Philadelphia, PA: W.B. Saunders, 2002:79–96.

and the surgeon must ensure that adequate resources exist to help the individual during an extremely dependent state where both arms are restricted for up to 2 to 3 months. For individuals who choose staged procedures, more commonly, the delay between each arm is often chosen with regard to their resource availability and personal desires. The spectrum here varies considerably and includes people who want everything completed before they "move on," to those who have one arm operated on, then wait, by example, until the end of the next school year or work cycle before proceeding with the second arm reconstruction. The final consideration regards the influence of thumb/index sensation on these decisions. Individuals without good sensation of their thumb and index finger usually require "eyes on" use of the hand during activities. Individuals without adequate sensation will not be able to easily and independently manipulate objects in both hands simultaneously and they need to be aware of this. But, if patients have appropriate goals, and feel that having increased function in both hands will help them, then we would proceed with bilateral reconstruction in the setting of inadequate peripheral sensation. A detailed list of surgical procedures by ICT level is illustrated in Table 28.4.

OUTCOMES

A well-selected, comprehensive program of hand and upper extremity rehabilitation will have a reliably beneficial impact on patients' lives. These benefits can and have been measured in terms of improved strength of grasp and pinch, increased number of different daily living activities that can be performed independently and brace free, including bowel/bladder care, and decreased need for both orthotics/braces and full-time assistant care. The impact that these improvements confer onto the quality of life has been inferred by the high rates of satisfaction, the improved "comfort" level in the community, and the number of patients who develop personal interests including vocations, education, and hobbies. The greatest benefit may be upon the patients' psyche, with dramatic improvements in their self-image, confidence, and overall quality of life. As stated by Sterling Bunnell many years ago, "... if you have nothing, a little is a lot...." (5)

Measuring the impact of a comprehensive, tailored approach to restoration of upper extremity function in the person with tetraplegia is critical for determining the benefits to patients, which ultimately affects the decision-making process for health care resource allocation. Historically, outcomes of reconstructive procedures have been measured in terms of grasp and pinch strength and ADL performance. As early as 1972, authors reported results from surgical restoration that extended beyond simply measuring voluntary motion that was not previously available (16). House found that patients improved in their ability to function, including bowel and bladder care (39,57). In 1983, Lamb and Chan reported that of the 41 patients with greater than 7-year follow-up, 83% experienced good to excellent regarding improved function (32). They noted both a change from being completely dependent, especially with regard to bowel/bladder care; and, that hand restoration facilitated the development of personal interests and hobbies. Seventy-five percent of individuals undergoing lateral-pinch reconstruction were able to self-catheterize, which translated to improved urinary status and quality of life (100). In Freehafer's experience with treating 68 patients, none were worse, and only 4 remained unimproved (15). Ejeskar and Dahloff noted improvements in 35 of 43 patients (29). In 1992, Mohammed et al. (82), presented their results of surgical restoration using tendon transfers in a heterogeneous group of 57 patients, with 84% reporting an improved quality of life. About two-thirds noted independence in eating, writing and typing, using a telephone, and improvements in self-care. The long-term benefit of surgery was confirmed in this same group of patients when they were re-evaluated

10 years later (101). Lo et al. (102) in 1998, found that all of the nine patients with C6 motor level tetraplegia benefited from surgical reconstruction both objectively and subjectively, and would have the surgery again. Paul et al. (62), reported that in addition to improvements in ADL, many were able to become brace free. Two recent studies exploring long-term outcomes of reconstruction confirm that both patient satisfaction and positive functional benefits persist with little evidence of any deterioration (103,104).

A newer set of research studies are beginning to provide surgeon's insight into the actual technical aspects of these procedures. Mulcahey et al. (72), compared two popular procedures for restoring elbow extension and determined that the transfer of the biceps is a viable alternative to the posterior deltoid to restore this function. Murray et al. (105) examined the influence of elbow angle on transfers of the BR to restore wrist extension, concluding that altering surgical tensioning can improve wrist extension when the elbow is flexed. Additional work by Lieber et al., proposes improved surgical outcomes through the use of an intraoperative technique for measuring sarcomere length to facilitate the length setting process of the transferred muscle (106). Such study may soon help surgeons make intraoperative decisions regarding technical issues such as tensioning a tendon transfer to create a specific, desired effect (107,108).

BARRIERS

Recent studies unfortunately continue to demonstrate underutilization of resources and treatment (47,109–111). The reasons appear multifactorial. There seem to be too few surgeons and physiatrists paying attention to the hand and upper extremity. The traditional pillars of SCI rehabilitation that most centers exclusively emphasize, that is, bowel/bladder care, skin care, and ambulation, seem difficult to "break" into. Since this surgery is practiced in numbers only in a few centralized SCI model centers, and only sporadically elsewhere, most surgeon trainees are not exposed or trained in these techniques. In part, there is a lack of interest and interdisciplinary associations between surgeons and physiatrists. In part, misconceptions persist that people with SCI tend to be noncompliant with treatment and lack the resources and support to carry out rehabilitative protocols in an outpatient setting. Physicians also seem to be under the impression that third-party payers do not reimburse for treatment of the hand and upper extremity in the setting of SCI. None of these reasons bear out—the reality is just the opposite of perception.

CONCLUSION

In only a few decades since the first model, spinal cord system facilities first developed, our knowledge of and ability to care for spinal cord injuries has grown exponentially. While tendon transfer surgery cannot recreate the able-bodied hand, it does improve arm and hand function that translates into increased independence, a treasured benefit to individuals living with SCI. Surgically restoration of hand and upper extremity function in individuals with tetraplegia is an important arm of SCI management; and, should be considered one of the pillars of treatment along with skin care, bowel/bladder care, sexual function, ambulation, and psychosocial community reintegration.

References

1. Moberg E. Fingers were made before forks. *Hand* 1972;4:201–206.
2. Moberg E. Surgical treatment for absent single-hand grip and elbow extension in quadriplegia. Principles and preliminary experience. *J Bone Joint Surg [Am]* 1975;57:196–206.
3. Moberg E. Reconstructive hand surgery in tetraplegia, stroke, and cerebral palsy: some basic concepts in physiology and neurology. *J Hand Surg [Am]* 1976;1:29–34.
4. Moberg E. *The upper limb in tetraplegia: a new approach to surgical rehabilitation*. Stuttgart, Germany: Georg Thieme Publishers, 1978.
5. Moberg E. Helpful upper limb surgery in tetraplegia. In: Hunter J, Schneider L, Mackin E, Bell J, eds. *Rehabilitation of the hand*. St. Louis, MO: The CV Mosby Co., 1978.
6. Moberg E. Surgical rehabilitation of the upper extremity in quadriplegics. *Handchirurgie* 1980;12:151–153.
7. Wuolle KS, Doren CLV, Bryden AM, et al. Satisfaction with and usage of a hand neuroprosthesis. *Arch Phys Med Rehabil* 1999;80:206–213.
8. Hanson RW, Franklin MR. Sexual loss in relation to other functional losses for spinal cord injured males. *Arch Phys Med Rehabil* 1976;57:291–293.
9. McDowell C, Moberg E, Graham-Smith A. International conference on surgical rehabiitation of the upper limb in tetraplegia. *J Hand Surg* 1979;4A:387–90.
10. LeClercq C, McDowell C. Fourth international conference on surgical rehabilitation of the upper limb in tetraplegia. *Ann Chir Main Membre Superievr* 1991;10:258–260.
11. International Standards for Neurological Classification of Spinal Cord Injury. Revised 2000. Reprinted 2008. Chicago, IL: American Spinal Injury Association.
12. Spinal Cord Injury: Facts and Figures at a Glance—June 2006 [Website]. Birmingham, UK: National Spinal Cord Injury Statistical Center, 2006.
13. Peckham PH, Creasey GH. Neural prostheses: clinical applications of functional electrical stimulation in spinal cord injury. *Paraplegia* 1992;30:96–101.
14. Whiteneck G, Tate D, Charlifue S. Predicting community reintegration after spinal cord injury from demographic and injury characteristics. *Arch Phys Med Rehabil* 1999;80:1485–1491.
15. Freehafer AA, Kelly CM, Peckham PH. Tendon transfer for the restoration of upper limb function after a cervical spinal cord injury. *J Hand Surg [Am]* 1984;9:887–893.
16. Lamb DW, Landry RM. The hand in quadriplegia. *Paraplegia* 1972;9:204–212.
17. Zancolli E. *Structural and dynamic basis of hand surgery*. Philadelphia, PA: JB Lippincott Co., 1968.
18. Zancolli E. Surgery for the quadriplegic hand with active, strong wrist extension preserved. A study of 97 cases. *Clin Orthop* 1975:101–113.
19. Zancolli E. *Structural and dynamic basis of hand surgery*. 2nd ed. Philadelphia, PA: JB Lippincott, 1979.
20. *Spinal cord injury*: *The facts and figures*. Birmingham, UK: The University of Alabama at Birmingham; 1986.

21. Anderson KD. Targeting recovery: priorities of the spinal cord-injured population. *J Neurotrauma* 2004;21:1371–1383.
22. Snoek GJ, IJzerman MJ, Hermens HJ, et al. Survey of the needs of patients with spinal cord injury: impact and priority for improvement in hand function in tetraplegics. *Spinal Cord* 2004;42:526–532.
23. Snoek GJ, IJzerman MJ, Post MW, et al. Choice-based evaluation for the improvement of upper-extremity function compared with other impairments in tetraplegia. *Arch Phys Med Rehabil* 2005;86:1623–1630.
24. Waters RL, Sie IH, Gellman H, et al. Functional hand surgery following tetraplegia. *Arch Phys Med Rehabil* 1996;77:86–94.
25. Hoyen H, Gonzalez E, Williams P, et al. Management of the paralyzed elbow in tetraplegia. *Hand Clin* 2002;18:113–133.
26. Keith M, Lacey S. Surgical rehabilitation of the tetraplegic upper extremity. *J Neuro Rehabil* 1991;5:75–87.
27. Boelter L, Keller A, Taylor C, et al. Studies to determine the functional requirements for hand and arm prosthesis. Final report to the National Academy of Sciences. University of California, Los Angeles, CA: National Academy of Sciences; 1947. Report No.: Contract VA M-21223.
28. Peljovich AE. Tendon transfers for restoration of active grasp. In: Kozin SH, ed. *Atlas of the hand clinics.* Philadelphia, PA: W.B. Saunders, 2002:79–96.
29. Ejeskar A, Dahllof A. Results of reconstructive surgery in the upper limb of tetraplegic patients. *Paraplegia* 1988;26:204–208.
30. Freehafer A, Peckham P, Keith M. Surgical treatment for tetraplegia: upper limb. In: Chapman M, ed. *Operative orthopaedics*. Philadelphia, PA: JB Lippincott, 1988:1459–1467.
31. Freehafer AA, Peckham PH, Keith MW. New concepts on treatment of the upper limb in the tetraplegic. Surgical restoration and functional neuromuscular stimulation. *Hand Clin* 1988;4:563–574.
32. Lamb DW, Chan KM. Surgical reconstruction of the upper limb in traumatic tetraplegia. A review of 41 patients. *J Bone Joint Surg [Br]* 1983;65:291–298.
33. Moberg E. The present state of surgical rehabilitation of the upper limb in tetraplegia. *Paraplegia* 1987;25:351–356.
34. Freehafer A, Vonhaam V. Tendon transfer to improve grasp after injuries of the the cervical spinal cord. *J Bone Joint Surg* 1974;56A:951–959.
35. McDowell C, Moberg E, House J. The second international conference on surgical rahabilitation of the upper limb in tetraplegia (quadriplegia). *J Hand Surg* 1986;11A:604–608.
36. DeBenedetti M. Restoration of elbow extension in the tetraplegic patient using the Moberg technique. *J Hand Surg* 1979;4:86–89.
37. Gorman PH, Wuolle KS, Peckham PH, et al. Patient selection for an upper extremity neuroprosthesis in tetraplegic individuals. *Spinal Cord* 1997;35:569–573.
38. Hentz VR, Hamlin C, Keoshian LA. Surgical reconstruction in tetraplegia. *Hand Clin* 1988;4:601–607.
39. House JH, Gwathmey FW, Lundsgaard DK. Restoration of strong grasp and lateral pinch in tetraplegia due to cervical spinal cord injury. *J Hand Surg [Am]* 1976;1:152–159.
40. Keith MW, Peckham PH, Thrope GB, et al. Implantable functional neuromuscular stimulation in the tetraplegic hand. *J Hand Surg [Am]* 1989;14:524–530.
41. Peckham P, Keith M, Freehafer A. Restoration of functional control by electrical stimulation in the upper extremity of the quadriplegic patient. *J Bone Joint Surg* 1988;70:144–148.
42. Hay-Smith J, Whitehead L, Keeling S. Getta a good grip on it: people with quadriplegia making decisions about upper limb surgery. In: Tenth International Meeting on Surgical Rehabilitation of The Tetraplegic Upper Limb, Paris, 2010.
43. Tournebise H, Allieu Y. What are elements that help a quadriplegic to decide to have surgery of the upper limb. In: Tenth International Meeting on Surgical Rehabilitation of The Tetraplegic Upper Limb, Paris, 2010.
44. Hentz VR, Leclercq C. *Surgical rehabilitation of the upper limb in tetraplegia.* London, UK: W.B. Saunders, 2002.
45. Peljovich AE, Kucera K, Gonzalez E, et al. Rehabilitation of the hand and upper extremity in tetraplegia. In: Mackin EJ, Callahan AD, Osterman AL, et al., eds. *Rehabilitation of the hand and upper extremity.* 5th ed. St. Louis, MO: Mosby, 2002.
46. Peljovich AE, Candia J, Kalmer S, et al. Achieving neurological stability in complete traumatic tetraplegia. In: Tenth International Meeting on Surgical Rehabilitation Of the Tetraplegic Upper Limb, Paris, France, 2010.
47. Curtin CM, Gater DR, Chung KC. Upper extremity reconstruction in the tetraplegic population, a national epidemiologic study. *J Hand Surg [Am]* 2005;30:94–99.
48. Moberg E. The new surgical rehabilitation of arm-hand function in the tetraplegic patient. *Scand J Rehabil Med Suppl* 1988;17:131–132.
49. Moberg EA, Lamb DW. Surgical rehabilitation of the upper limb in tetraplegia. *Hand* 1980;12:209–213.
50. Brand P. *Clinical mechanics of the hand.* St. Louis, MO: Mosby; 1985.
51. Green D. Radial nerve palsy. In: Green D, Hotchkiss R, Pederson W, eds. *Green's operative hand surgery.* 4 ed. New York: Churchill Livingstone, 1999:1481–1496.
52. Brand P, Beach R, Thompson D. Relative tension and potential excursion of the muscles in the forearm and the hand. *J Hand Surg* 1981;6:209–219.
53. Brys D, Waters RL. Effect of triceps function on the brachioradialis transfer in quadriplegia. *J Hand Surg [Am]* 1987;12:237–239.
54. Freehafer AA, Peckham PH, Keith MW, et al. The brachioradialis: anatomy, properties, and value for tendon transfer in the tetraplegic. *J Hand Surg [Am]* 1988;13:99–104.
55. Ward SR, Peace WJ, Friden J, et al. Dorsal transfer of the brachioradialis to the flexor pollicis longus enables simultaneous powering of key pinch and forearm pronation. *J Hand Surg [Am]* 2006;31:993–997.
56. Smith AG. Early complications of key grip hand surgery for tetraplegia. *Paraplegia* 1981;19:123–126.
57. House JH, Shannon MA. Restoration of strong grasp and lateral pinch in tetraplegia: a comparison of two methods of thumb control in each patient. *J Hand Surg [Am]* 1985;10:22–29.

58. Zancolli E. Functional restoration of the upper limb in traumatic quadriplegia. In: *Structural and dynamic basis of hand surgery*. 2nd ed. Philadelphia, PA: JB Lippincott, 1979:229–262.
59. Bryan RS. The Moberg deltoid-triceps replacement and key-pinch operations in quadriplegia: preliminary experiences. *Hand* 1977;9:207–214.
60. Castro-Sierra A, Lopez-Pita A. A new surgical technique to correct triceps paralysis. *Hand* 1983;15:42–46.
61. Mennen V, Boonzaier A. An improved technique of posterior deltoid to triceps transfer in tetraplegia. *J Hand Surg Br* 1991;16:197–201.
62. Paul SD, Gellman H, Waters R, et al. Single-stage reconstruction of key pinch and extension of the elbow in tetraplegic patients [see comments]. *J Bone Joint Surg Am* 1994;76:1451–1456.
63. Raczka R, Braun R, Waters R. Posterior deltoid-to-triceps transfer in quadriplegia. *Clin Orthop* 1984;187: 163–167.
64. Friden J, Lieber RL. Quantitative evaluation of the posterior deltoid to triceps tendon transfer based on muscle architectural properties. *J Hand Surg [Am]* 2001;26: 147–155.
65. Lacey S, Wilber R, Peckham P, et al. The posterior deltoid to triceps transfer, a clinical and biomechanical assessment. *J Hand Surg* 1986;11:542–547.
66. Rabischong E, Benoit P, Benichou M, et al. Length-tension relationship of the posterior deltoid to triceps transfer in C6 tetraplegic patients. *Paraplegia* 1993;31:33–39.
67. Friden J, Ejeskar A, Dahlgren A, et al. Protection of the deltoid-to-triceps tendon transfer repair sites. In: XVII International Society of Biomechanics, Calgary, 1999:598.
68. Friden J, Ejeskar A, Dahlgren A, et al. Protection of the deltoid to triceps tendon transfer repair sites. *J Hand Surg [Am]* 2000;25:144–149.
69. Friedenberg Z. Transposition of the biceps brachii for triceps weakness. *J Bone Joint Surg* 1954;36:656–658.
70. Kuz J, Van Heest A, House J. Biceps-to-triceps transfer in tetraplegic patients; report of the medial routing technique and follow-up of three cases. *J Hand Surg* 1999;24:161–172.
71. Revol M, Briand E, Servant J. Biceps-to-triceps transfer in tetraplegia: the medial route. *J Hand Surg* 1999;24B: 235–237.
72. Mulcahey MJ, Lutz C, Kozin SH, et al. Prospective evaluation of biceps to triceps and deltoid to triceps for elbow extension in tetraplegia. *J Hand Surg [Am]* 2003;28: 964–971.
73. Lieber R, Jacobson M, Fazeli B, Abrams R, Botte M. Architecture of selected muscles of the arm and forearm: Anatomy and implications for tendon transfer. *J Hand Surg* 1992;17A:787–798.
74. Bunnell S. *Instructional course lectures, american academy of orthopaedic surgeons*. Ann Arbor, MI: J. W. Edwards, 1949.
75. Freehafer AA, Mast WA. Transfer of the brachioradialis to improve wrist extension in high spinal-cord injury. *J Bone Joint Surg Am* 1967;49:648–652.
76. Lipscomb P, Elkins EC, Henderson ED. Tendon transfers to restore function of hands in tetraplegia, especially after fracture-dislocation of the sixth cervical vertebra on the seventh. *J Bone Joint Surg* 1958;40A:1071–1080.
77. Waters R, Moore KR, Graboff SR,et al. Brachioradialis to flexor pollicis longus tendon transfer for active lateral pinch in the tetraplegic. *J Hand Surg [Am]* 1985;10:385–391.
78. Hentz V, House J, McDowell C, et al. Rehabilitation and surgical reconstruction of the upper limb in tetraplegia: An update. *J Hand Surg* 1992;17A:964–967.
79. Hentz VR. Historical background and changing perspectives in surgical reconstruction of the upper limb in quadriplegia. *J Am Paraplegia Soc* 1984;7:36–38.
80. Hentz VR, Brown M, Keoshian LA. Upper limb reconstruction in quadriplegia: functional assessment and proposed treatment modifications. *J Hand Surg [Am]* 1983;8:119–131.
81. House JH, Comadoll J, Dahl AL. One-stage key pinch and release with thumb carpal-metacarpal fusion in tetraplegia. *J Hand Surg [Am]* 1992;17:530–538.
82. Mohammed K, Rothwell A, Sinclair S, et al. Upper limb surgery for tetraplegia. *J Bone Joint Surg* 1992;74B:873–879.
83. McDowell C, House J. Tetraplegia Chapter 52. In: Green D, Hochkiss R, Pederson WC, eds. *Green's operative hand surgery*. 4th ed. London, UK: Churchill Livingstone; 1998:1588–1606.
84. Friden J. Early active training of deltoid to triceps transfers: a controlled study. In: Xth International Meeting on Surgical Rehabilitation of The Tetraplegic Upper Limb, Paris, 2010.
85. Wangdell J, Reinholdt C, Friden J. Enhanced post operative training after grip reconstruction facilitates return to critical functions. In: Xth International Meeting on Surgical Rehabilitation of The Tetraplegic Upper Limb, Paris, 2010.
86. Friden J, Albrecht D, Lieber RL. Biomechanical analysis of the brachioradialis as a donor in tendon transfer. *Clin Orthop Relat Res* 2001;383:152–161.
87. Dunkerley AL, Ashburn A, Stack EL. Deltoid triceps transfer and functional independence of people with tetraplegia. *Spinal Cord* 2000;38:435–441.
88. Freehafer A, Kelly C, Peckham H. Planning tendon transfers in tetraplegia: "Cleveland Technique." In: Hunter J, Schneider L, Mackin E, eds. *Tendon surgery in the hand*. St. Louis, MO: The CV Mosby Co., 1987:506–515.
89. Bryden A, Wuolle K, Frost F. Training of tetraplegic persons with new upper extremity tendon transfers: a cost-sensitive program. *J Am Paraplegia Soc* 1994;17:230.
90. Freehafer AA, Peckham PH, Keith MW. New concepts in the treatment of the upper limb in tetraplegia: surgical restoration and functional neuromuscular stimulation. In: Tubiana AR, ed. *The hand*. Philadelphia, PA: W.B. Saunders, 1991:564–574.
91. Teissier J, Fattal C, Lumens D, et al. Arthrodesis or conservation of the carpometacarpal joint when constructing a key-grip in tetraplegic patients: a comparative study on 40 key grips. In: Xth International Meeting on Surgical Rehabilitation of The Tetraplegic Upper Limb, Paris, 2010.
92. House JH. Reconstruction of the thumb in tetraplegia following spinal cord injury. *Clin Orthop* 1985:117–128.
93. Rieser TV, Waters RL. Long-term follow-up of the Moberg key grip procedure. *J Hand Surg [Am]* 1986;11: 724–728.

94. Kelly CM, Freehafer AA, Peckham PH, et al. Postoperative results of opponensplasty and flexor tendon transfer in patients with spinal cord injuries. *J Hand Surg [Am]* 1985;10:890–894.
95. Smith R. Chapter 12 Intrinsic muscles of the finger: Function, dysfunction and surgical reconstruction. In: *AAOS intructional course lectures*. St. Louis, MO: CV Mosby, 1975:200–220.
96. McCarthy CK, House JH, Van Heest A, et al. Intrinsic balancing in reconstruction of the tetraplegic hand. *J Hand Surg [Am]* 1997;22:596–604.
97. Zancolli E, Zancolli E. Tetraplegies traumatiques. In: Tubiana R, ed. *Traite' de Chirurgie de la Main*. Paris, France: Masson, 1991.
98. Zancolli E, Zancolli EJ. Surgical reconstruction of the upper limb in middle-level tetraplegia. In: Tubiana R, ed. *The hand*. Vol. 4. Philadelphia, PA: WB Saunders Co.; 1993:548–563.
99. Allieu Y. General indications for functional surgery of the hand in tetraplegic patients. *Hand Clin* 2002;18:413–421.
100. Guinet A, Rech C, Even-Schneider A, et al. Self-catheterization acquisition after hand reanimation protocols in C5-C7 tetraplegic patients. In: Xth International Meeting on Surgical Rehabilitation of The Tetraplegic Upper Limb, Paris, 2010.
101. Rothwell AG, Sinnott KA, Mohammed KD, et al. Upper limb surgery for tetraplegia: a 10-year re-review of hand function. *J Hand Surg [Am]* 2003;28:489–497.
102. Lo IK, Turner R, Connolly S, et al. The outcome of tendon transfers for C6-spared quadriplegics. *J Hand Surg [Br]* 1998;23:156–161.
103. Carles A, Vincenti P, Floris L, et al. Evaluation of the long term results of functional surgery of the upper limbs in tetraplegic individuals. In: Xth International Meeting on Surgical Rehabilitation of The Tetraplegic Upper Limb, Paris, 2010.
104. Snoek GJ, Bongers-Janssen H, Nene A. Long term patient satisfaction after reconstructive upper extremity surgery to improve arm-hand function in tetraplegia. In: Xth International Meeting on Surgical Rehabilitation of The Tetraplegic Upper Limb, Paris, 2010.
105. Murray WM, Bryden AM, Kilgore KL, et al. The influence of elbow position on the range of motion of the wrist following transfer of the brachioradialis to the extensor carpi radialis brevis tendon. *J Bone Joint Surg Am* 2002;84A:2203–2210.
106. Lieber RL, Friden J. Implications of muscle design on surgical reconstruction of upper extremities. *Clin Orthop Relat Res* 2004;419:267–279.
107. Lieber RL, Murray WM, Clark DL, et al. Biomechanical Properties of the Brachioradialis Muscle: Implications for Surgical Tendon Transfer. *J Hand Surg [Am]* 2005; 30:273–282.
108. Murray WM, Hentz VR, Friden J, et al. Variability in surgical Technique for Brachioradialis Tendon Transfer. *J Bone Joint Surg Am* 2006;88A:2009–2016.
109. Bryden AM, Wuolle KS, Murray PK, et al. Perceived outcomes and utilization of upper extremity surgical reconstruction in individuals with tetraplegia at model spinal cord injury systems. *Spinal Cord* 2004;42: 169–176.
110. Curtin CM, Hayward RA, Kim HM, et al. Physician perceptions of upper extremity reconstruction for the person with tetraplegia. *J Hand Surg [Am]* 2005;30:87–93.
111. Curtin CM, Wagner JP, Gater DR, et al. Opinions on the treatment of people with tetraplegia: contrasting perceptions of physiatrists and hand surgeons. *J Spinal Cord Med* 2007;30:256–262.
112. Leclercq C, Hentz VR, Kozin SH, et al. Reconstruction of elbow extension. *Hand Clin* 2008;24:185–201, vi.

CHAPTER 29 ■ PEDIATRIC SPINAL CORD DISORDERS

LAWRENCE C. VOGEL, RANDAL R. BETZ, AND MARY JANE MULCAHEY

This chapter reviews spinal cord disorders in children and adolescents, including spinal cord injuries (SCIs), myelomeningocele, and hydrosyringomyelia. Although these disorders are not limited to the pediatric population, the clinical presentation and management of children and adolescents with these spinal cord disorders are distinctive because of the impact of growth and development. Both SCI and myelomeningocele share many of the same manifestations related to spinal cord dysfunction, namely paralysis, sensory loss, and bladder, bowel and sexual dysfunction. Children with both disorders also experience similar complications as a result of growth, such as scoliosis and hip dysplasia. However, myelomeningocele has many distinguishing features because of associated brain abnormalities and its onset in utero, resulting in cognitive and behavioral abnormalities and congenital malformations, such as clubfeet, respectively.

The general principles in caring for children and adolescents with spinal cord disorders are fundamentally different compared to adults with similar impairments. Care for pediatric spinal cord disorders must be family centered because of the central role of parents and family for a child or adolescent (1). Because of the growth and development inherent to childhood, care must be developmentally based and be responsive to the dynamic changes that occur with growth. Children and young adolescents need developmentally appropriate programming with compatible physical and philosophical characteristics, including recreation therapy and child life. In contrast, older adolescents benefit from an adolescent approach rather than a more traditional pediatric or adult setting.

Anticipatory guidance, a term used to refer to the education of children and parents about future implications of a disability, is critical to successful transition throughout each developmental stage and ultimately into adulthood. Anticipatory guidance must be provided in a developmentally sensitive manner in order to prepare them for potential complications and transitions, such as sexual development and functioning or progression from ambulation in the young and energetic child to wheelchair mobility in the older child or adolescent.

Transition into adulthood is a major goal in caring for children and adolescents with spinal cord disorders (2,3). Transition planning must be initiated early in childhood and intensify as they become adolescents. A preeminent goal for children and adolescents with spinal cord disorders is that they have satisfying and productive lives as independently functioning adults in society. Transition encompasses many spheres of functioning, including independent living, employment, financial resources, socialization, and health care (4). From the time of diagnosis, even if present at birth, parents need to be reassured that their child has the potential to be an independently functioning adult. Parents, health care providers, and other adults significantly involved with the child must foster these expectations for the child's future. As a result, these expectations will become ingrained into the child and adolescent's life, assuring a more successful transition into adulthood.

An example of the importance for transition planning to begin at an early age for children is the central role that employment has in adult life, including life satisfaction (5,6). Adults with childhood onset SCI are employed less frequently compared to the general population, and employment is significantly associated with life satisfaction. Compared to the general population, children and adolescents with SCI have significantly less prevocational experiences (7). The fact that young adults with pediatric-onset SCI are employed less often than their able-bodied peers highlights the need to address transitional issues more aggressively and at younger ages. Despite the tendency for parents to exclude children with spinal cord disorders in typical childhood chores, they should be expected to have age-appropriate chores, similar to their peers (7,8). As they grow older, they must be involved in developmentally appropriate prevocational and vocational activities that will prepare them for adult employment (7,9).

Provision of comprehensive primary care, including preventive medicine, health care maintenance, and management of intercurrent illnesses, for children and adolescents with spinal cord disorders is frequently neglected and overshadowed by tertiary care needs (10). In addition to the standard childhood immunizations, children and adolescents with spinal cord disorders should receive the pneumococcal vaccine and annual influenza vaccinations.

Sexuality issues must also be addressed in a developmentally appropriate manner. Sexuality is often overlooked in children and adolescents with spinal cord disorders. Sexuality issues common to all children and adolescents as well as spinal cord disorder–specific areas must be addressed. This is particularly important because children and adolescents with disabilities tend to be "infantalized" or treated as asexual beings.

SPINAL CORD INJURIES

The manifestations and complications of SCI in children and adolescents are unique because of distinctive anatomic and physiologic features and growth and development, characteristic of the pediatric population (11–13). Aspects of pediatric SCI that are a consequence of childhood include SCIs without radiologic abnormalities (SCIWORA), upper cervical injuries, birth injuries, lap-belt injuries, and delayed onset of neurological deficits. The interaction between growth and development and the manifestations and complications of SCI are responsible for many of the unique features of pediatric SCI. As a result of growth, there is a high incidence of scoliosis and hip dislocation in individuals who sustained their SCI prior to puberty. Development helps to explain why the untrainable toddler becomes the model patient during the early years of school and then the noncompliant adolescent with pressure ulcers, urinary tract infections (UTIs), and substance abuse. SCI can impact growth, as reflected by failure of paralyzed limbs to grow normally. Impaired mobility resulting from the SCI limits the ability of youth to explore their environment, resulting in psychosocial, educational, and vocational disadvantages and delays.

Epidemiology

Approximately 3% to 5% of cases of traumatic SCI occur in individuals younger than 15 years of age and if one includes birth to 20 years of age the incidence increases to 20% (14–20). Similar to adults with SCI, males more commonly sustain SCI than females during adolescence. However, the preponderance of males becomes less marked as age of injury decreases, such that females equal males in those 3 years of age and younger (21). Similar to the experience of adults with SCI, a higher percentage of minorities are affected by SCI (21). The life expectancy of children and adolescents with SCI is a function of neurological level and category (21–23). The less severe the SCI, in respect to level and category, the longer the expected survival.

Neurological level and degree of completeness vary as a function of age (21,22). Among children who sustained their SCI when they are 8 years of age or younger, 70% are paraplegic and approximately two-thirds have complete lesions. In contrast, approximately 50% of older children, adolescents, or adults are paraplegic and approximately 50% have complete lesions. In addition, younger children are more likely to have upper cervical injuries and less likely to have C4-6 injuries. Among children who sustained their SCI prior to 13 years of age, 8.2% to 9.6% have C1-3 lesions compared to 4.3% to 4.5% of those injured as adolescents. In contrast, approximately 25% of those injured prior to 13 years of age had C4-5 lesions compared to 47% to 50% of those injured as adolescents. The higher risk for upper cervical injuries is probably due to a proportionately larger head and underdeveloped neck musculature in infants and younger children.

The utility of the International Standards for Neurological Classification of Spinal Cord Injury (ISNCSCI) in young children is significantly limited, and thus, interpretation of examination results and designation of neurological level, motor level, and injury severity (complete/incomplete) must be made with prudence, particularly in children under 5 years of age (22–26). While some studies have shown acceptable levels of interrater agreement between experienced examiners (27), others have documented less than adequate interrater agreement (25,28). Studies in pediatric populations have found the reliability of the ISNCSCI motor and sensory examinations when applied to children and youths 5 years of age and older to be good overall (24). Reliability of the anorectal examination is not as strong with questionable utility in young children and children injured at a young age because they may not have been toilet trained prior to their injury (24).

Motor vehicle crashes are the most common cause of SCI in children and adolescents, with violence and sports being the next most common etiologies (21,22). Violence causes SCI in children of all ages, but is a particularly important cause in adolescents, especially among African-Americans and Hispanics (21,22). Unique etiologies of SCI in children and adolescents include lap-belt injuries, birth injuries, child abuse (29,30), C1-2 subluxation due to tonsillopharyngitis (31), and transverse myelitis (32). Another cause of spinal cord dysfunction that may be mistakenly diagnosed as transverse myelitis is ischemic infarction of the spinal cord as a result of a nucleus pulposus embolism (33). Additionally, children with skeletal dysplasias, juvenile rheumatoid arthritis, and Down syndrome are susceptible to cervical SCI.

Lap-belt injuries most commonly occur in children weighing between 40 and 60 lb (34–36) because the lap-belt rises above the pelvic brim and acts as a fixed anterior fulcrum resulting in flexion/distraction forces in the mid-lumbar spine. The three components of lap-belt injuries are abdominal wall bruising, intra-abdominal injuries, and spinal cord damage. The abdominal wall bruising is caused by trauma from the lap belt and ranges from abrasions and contusions to full-thickness skin loss (Fig. 29.1). The most common intra-abdominal injuries include tears or perforations of the small or large intestines, with injuries less frequently occurring to the kidneys, liver, spleen, pancreas, bladder, or uterus. Although the injury forces are localized to the mid-lumbar spine, the neurological level varies from conus or cauda equina lesions to mid-thoracic levels. The most common location for vertebral damage is between L2 and L4, with distraction-type injuries (Fig. 29.2). Computerized tomography (CT) scans for trauma routinely miss the fracture, especially if it goes through the ligaments and

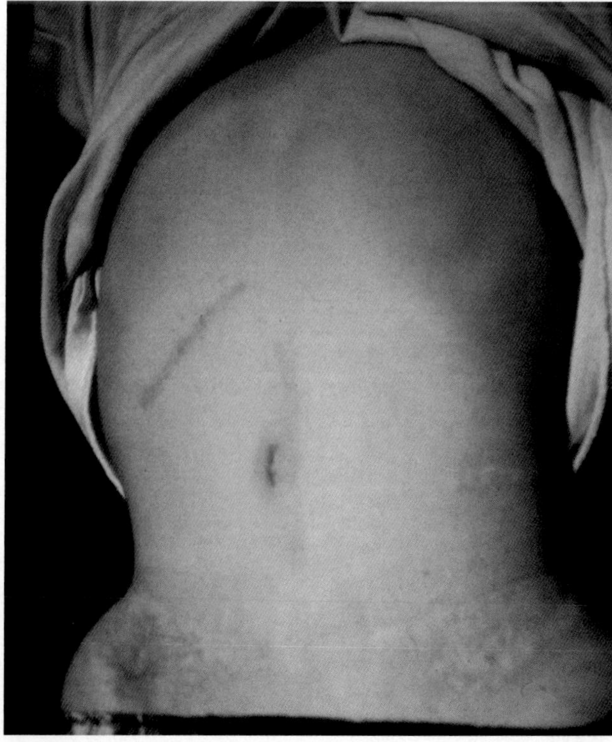

FIGURE 29.1 Scars on lower abdomen related to full thickness skin loss from a lap-belt injury in a 15-year-old male with T6 complete paraplegia.

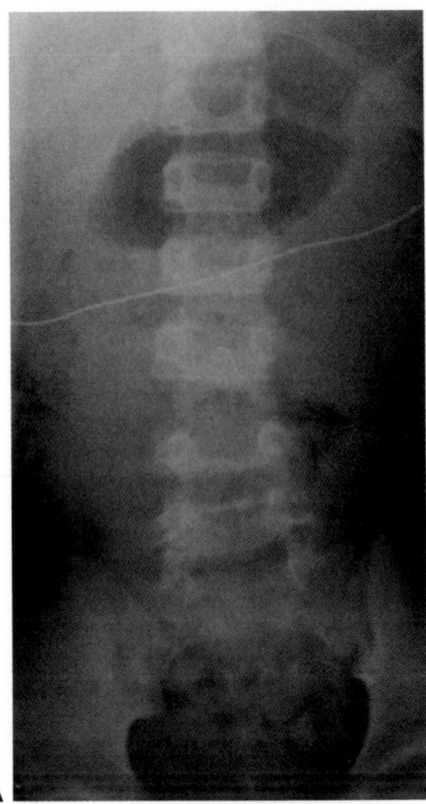
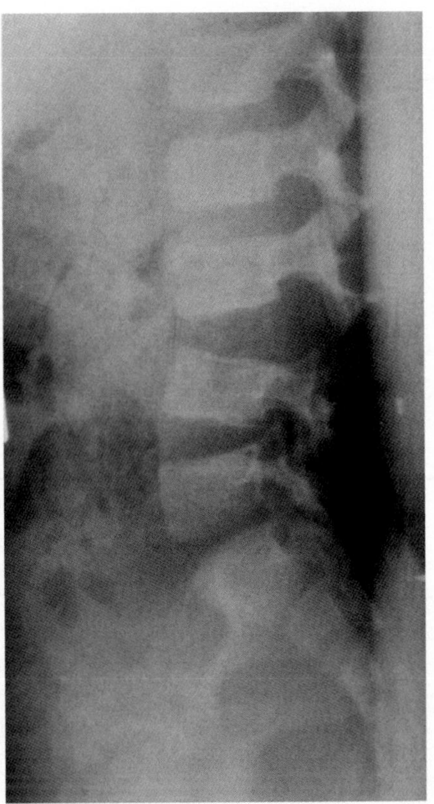

FIGURE 29.2 A,B: Spine radiographs of a 7-year-old male who sustained a complete L2/3 SCI as a result of a lap-belt injury. The radiographs demonstrate a flexion-distraction injury at L3-4.

spontaneously reduces. However, 23% to 30% of patients with SCI related to lap-belt injuries have SCIWORA (Fig. 29.3).

In order to reduce the incidence of lap-belt injuries, children who weigh more than 40 lb and who are 8 years of age and younger (and less than 4 ft 9 inches tall) should ride in booster seats, in the back seat, until the vehicle seat belts fit properly. Seat belts fit properly when the lap belt lays across the upper thighs and the shoulder belt fits across the chest (38).

Neonatal SCI are relatively uncommon with an incidence of approximately one per 60,000 births (39–45). Upper cervical lesions are most common and are related to torsional forces during delivery. In contrast, SCI related to breech deliveries most commonly result in lower cervical or upper thoracic injuries, and they are related to traction forces that occur during delivery. Thoracic or lumbar lesions are uncommon and may result from vascular occlusion associated with umbilical artery catheters or paradoxical air embolism through transitional cardiovascular shunts. Brachial plexus or phrenic nerve injuries and hypoxic encephalopathy may be associated with neonatal SCI. Since affected neonates present initially with a flaccid type of paralysis, the differential diagnosis includes spinal muscular atrophy, amyotonia congenita, congenital myotonic dystrophy, and neural-tube defects.

In children and adolescents with Down syndrome, atlanto-axial instability is related to ligamentous laxity (46,47). An atlanto-dens interval (ADI) greater than 4.5 mm is considered abnormal and occurs in approximately 15% to 20% of individuals with Down syndrome with the majority being asymptomatic. Only those with neurological symptoms require a C1-2 fusion. Restriction of asymptomatic patients with an increased ADI from high-risk activities remains controversial. Additionally, occipital-atlanto instability occurs commonly in children with Down syndrome and must be carefully looked for (46).

Children and adolescents with juvenile rheumatoid arthritis (JRA) may develop C1-2 instability as a result of synovitis of the facet and synovial joints surrounding the odontoid process as well as from destruction of the odontoid process as a result of the inflammatory process (Fig. 29.4) (48). In addition, individuals with polyarticular JRA may experience fusion of the cervical vertebra, particularly C2-3. This may progress to eventual fusion of a significant portion of the cervical spine, placing the patient at risk of a cervical fracture and possible tetraplegic SCI from relatively minor trauma (Fig. 29.5) (49).

Cervical myelopathy may be associated with Larson syndrome and skeletal dysplasias such as achondroplasia and Morquio syndrome (50). Infants with achondroplasia may experience compression of the upper cervical cord and the caudal medulla as a result of a small foramen magnum (51). In addition, individuals with achondroplasia, primarily males, are at risk of developing spastic paraplegia related to spinal stenosis (50). Children with dwarfing syndromes with odontoid dysplasia, such as Morquio mucopolysaccharidosis IV, may develop atlanto-axial instability, and of those with instability over 50% will develop a myelopathy (50).

Pathophysiology

Anatomic and physiologic characteristics of younger children are responsible for SCIWORA and delayed onset of neurological findings. Among children 5 years of age or younger at the time of sustaining an SCI, approximately 64% will have SCIWORA (52). In contrast, SCIWORA is found in

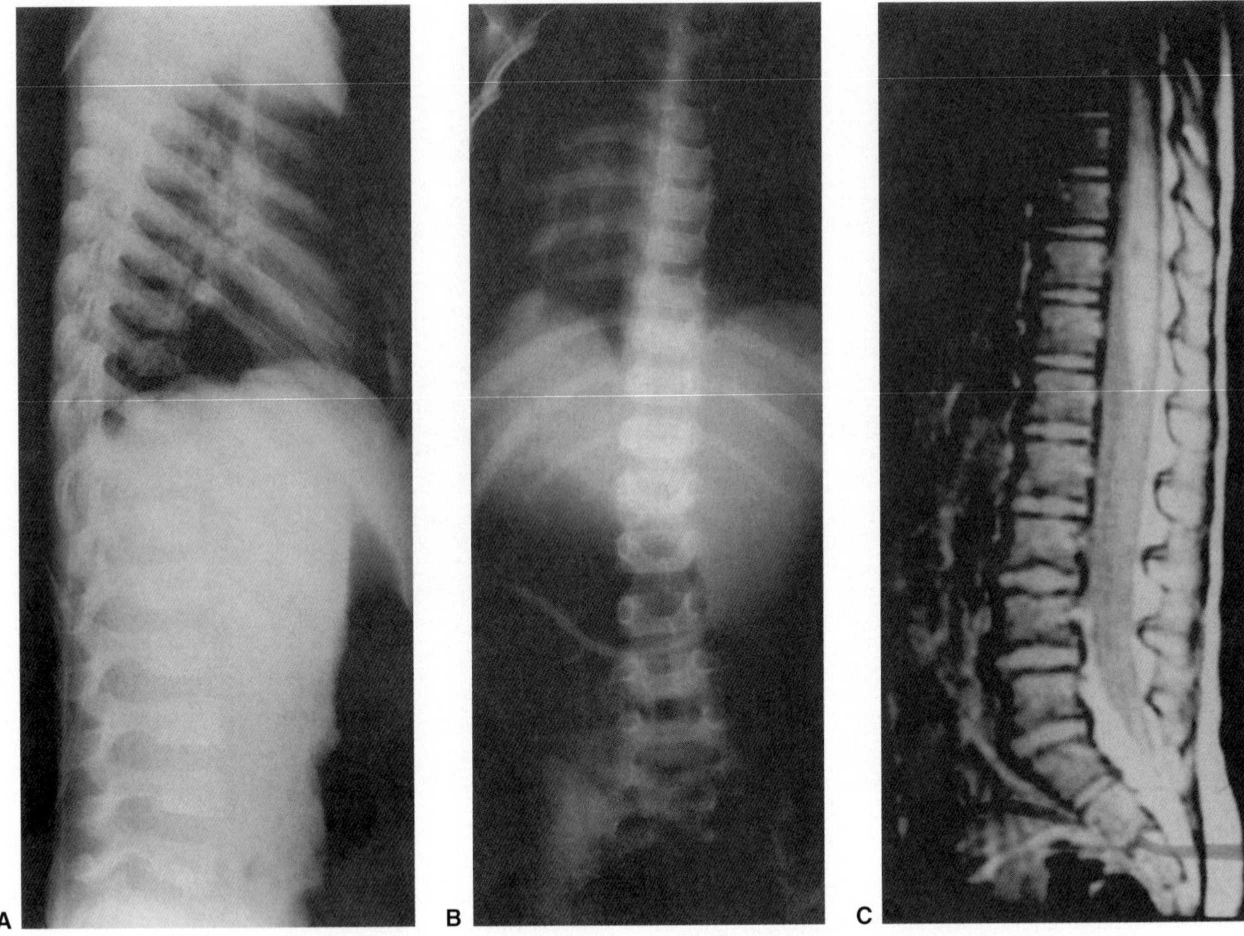

FIGURE 29.3 A–C: Spine radiographs and magnetic resonance imaging (MRI) study of a 2½-year-old male who sustained a complete L2 SCI as a result of a lap-belt injury. There are no abnormalities on the plain radiographs, so the patient has an SCI without radiologic abnormalities (SCIWORA). However, the MRI demonstrates a lucent area in the lumbar spinal cord (C).

approximately 35% of those injured between 6 and 12 years of age and 20% of children injured after 12 years of age. The high incidence of SCIWORA in younger children with SCI is a result of unique anatomic and biomechanical characteristics of the spine (53). This includes increased elasticity of the spine in relation to a less flexible spinal cord, shallow and horizontally oriented facet joints, anterior wedging of the vertebral bodies, vulnerability of the growth zone of vertebral end plates, and poorly developed uncinate processes.

Despite the benign radiologic picture of SCIWORA, affected individuals are more likely to have complete lesions (52,54). Although plain radiographs, tomography, CT, myelography, and dynamic flexion/extension studies are normal, MRI abnormalities are frequently seen in patients with SCIWORA (Fig. 29.3) (55,56). Both extraneural and neural abnormalities may be identified. The primary extraneural MRI findings include rupture of either the anterior or posterior longitudinal ligaments, intradiskal abnormalities, and end-plate fractures. Neural abnormalities include cord disruption, hemorrhage, and edema. The MRI abnormalities correlate with the severity of the neurological deficit and the prognosis for recovery (56). Complete neurological deficits are generally associated with cord disruption and extensive cord hemorrhage, minor cord hemorrhage or edema is more likely associated with incomplete lesions, and no cord abnormalities on MRI correlate with mild partial cord syndromes.

In approximately 25% to 50% of children who sustain an SCI, there is a delay in onset of neurological abnormalities that ranges from 30 minutes to 4 days (19,52,53,57). Many of these children with delayed onset of neurological findings experience transient and subtle neurological symptoms, such as paraesthesias or subjective weakness. The mechanisms that may be responsible for this phenomenon include natural expansion of the cord injury by inflammation, posttraumatic occlusion of radicular arteries, and repeated trauma to the spinal cord as a result of occult spinal instability.

Medical Issues

Urology

Clean intermittent catheterization (IC) is the standard bladder management for children and adolescents with SCI (9,58–62). IC is initiated when the child is approximately 3 years old or earlier if the child is experiencing recurrent UTIs or exhibits renal impairment. Children with adequate hand function begin self-catheterization when they are developmentally 5 to 7 years old (60).

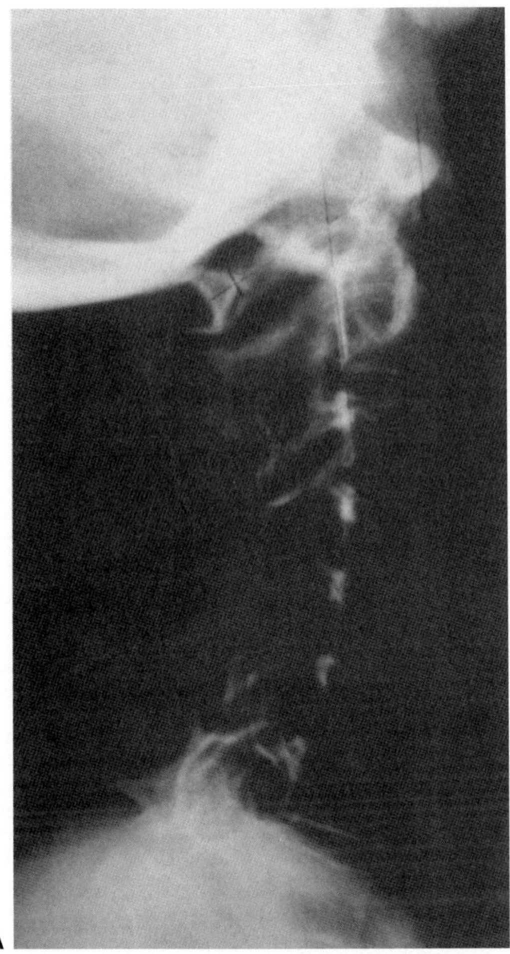

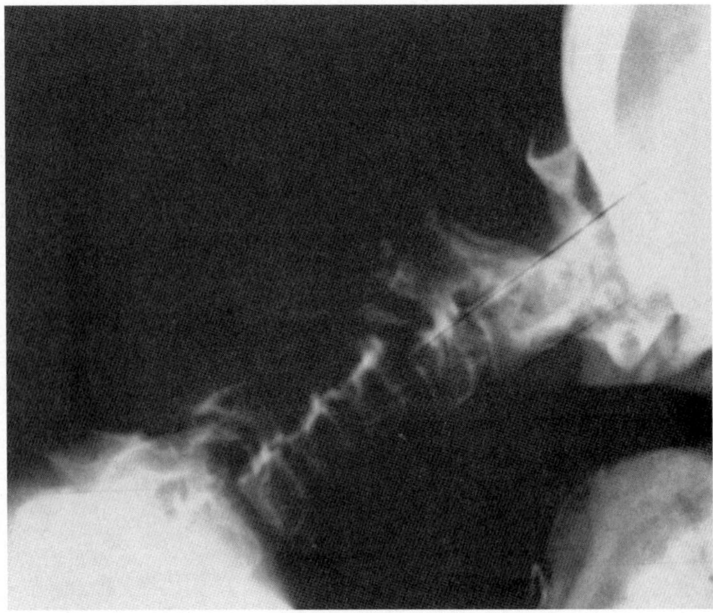

FIGURE 29.4 Flexion and extension cervical spine radiographs of a 14-year-old female with severe polyarticular juvenile rheumatoid arthritis. The radiographs demonstrate erosion of the odontoid process and marked narrowing of the spinal canal on the flexion view (**A**) compared to the extension view (**B**).

The issues of using prophylactic antibiotics to prevent UTIs and the treatment of asymptomatic bacteriuria are no different from adults with SCI (63). Prophylactic antibiotics should be limited to patients who experience recurrent and severe UTIs and in those with obstructive uropathy or compromised renal function, including vesicoureteral reflux and hydronephrosis. Patients with asymptomatic bacteriuria are generally not treated unless they have compromised renal function. Treatment should be limited to those with symptomatic UTIs as reflected by systemic toxicity (fever, chills, dysreflexia, or exacerbation of spasticity), incontinence, or cloudy and foul-smelling urine. The use of fluoroquinolones should be limited in children younger than 18 years of age because of potential adverse effects on articular cartilage and tendons (64).

Similar to adults, continence and independence are important aspects of bladder management for children and adolescents with SCI. Interventions that may be beneficial in managing incontinence include anticholinergics, modification of fluid intake and catheterization schedule, and treatment of urological complications, such as UTIs and urolithiasis. For patients with persistent incontinence, urodynamics should be performed (62). Patients with limited bladder capacity unresponsive to anticholinergics may be candidates for a bladder augmentation (61,66,67).

For individuals who are not independent in performing intermittent catheterization, a continent catheterizable conduit is a potential alternative (61,66,68). A continent catheterizable conduit, the Mitrofanoff procedure, consists of creating a catheterizable conduit using the appendix or a segment of small bowel that connects the bladder to a stoma either in the umbilicus or on the lower abdominal wall (69). This may allow individuals with limited upper extremity function, such as those with C6 or C7 injuries, to catheterize themselves (70,71). In addition, continent catheterizable conduits may facilitate independence in bladder management for individuals who have difficulty accessing their native urethra, such as females who cannot actively abduct their legs, or those who have difficulty transferring to a commode or toilet.

Bowel Management

Similar to the adult SCI population, critical issues for bowel management in pediatric SCI include complete and regular emptying, short duration of the bowel program, continence, aesthetics, and prevention of constipation or diarrhea (62,72–75). The need for regularity in the performance of bowel programs is frequently in conflict with the lack of conformity of children and adolescents. However, anxiety regarding fecal incontinence is a strong incentive for compliance with bowel program regimens. Bowel programs are initiated when children are 2 to 4 years of age, which is a developmentally appropriate age, or earlier if they are experiencing diarrhea or constipation. Children with adequate hand function should be able to perform their own bowel programs when they are developmentally 5 to 7 years old.

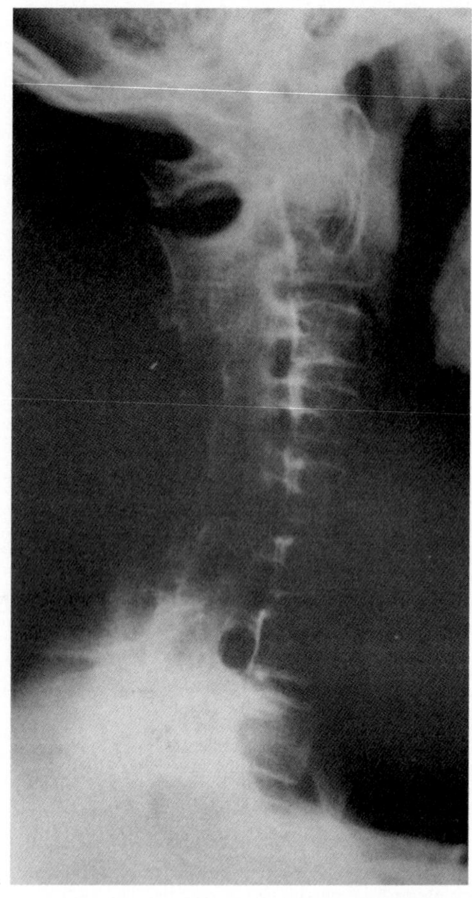

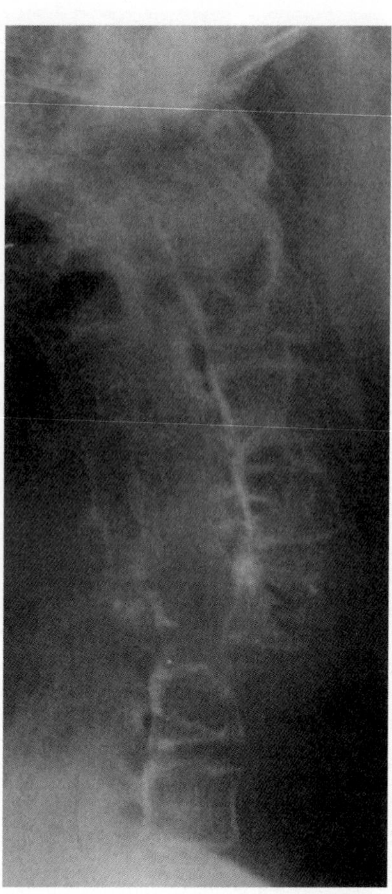

FIGURE 29.5 **A, B:** These are cervical radiographs of a male with polyarticular juvenile rheumatoid arthritis. **A:** Demonstrates spontaneous fusion of his cervical spine from C2 to C7 at 12 years of age (**B**). At 17 years of age he was involved in a motor vehicle crash and sustained a C5-6 fracture-dislocation, resulting in complete C5/6 tetraplegia.

Essential components for a bowel program include privacy, independence, and a regular schedule with respect to frequency and time of the day. The bowel program should take place on a toilet or a commode. A sitting position facilitates defecation, and if neurologically capable the child should be taught and encouraged to increase intra-abdominal pressure. It is important that these basic principles be initiated once a bowel program is initiated, regardless of the age of the child or adolescent. Although there is a lack of published studies, laxatives (such as senna or polyethylene glycol), stool softeners (colace), and laxatives (such as enemeez or magic bullet) are commonly used in infants and children with SCI without incident.

Options for bowel programs include the antegrade continence enema (ACE), enema continence catheters, and pulsed irrigation enemas (76). The ACE procedure allows antegrade evacuation of the bowel by administering an enema directly into the cecum via a surgically created conduit, commonly using the appendix, which is accessible through an abdominal wall stoma (77).

Deep Venous Thrombosis

The literature available about thromboembolic complications in pediatric SCI is limited (78). The incidence of deep venous thrombosis (DVT) in children and adolescents with SCI has been reported to range from 2.5% to 17.5% with a 0% to 2.3% incidence of pulmonary emboli. Data from the Shriners Hospitals for Children SCI and the model system databases reveal that DVTs are extremely rare in children injured between birth and 5 years of age (0%) and in those inured between 6 and 12 years of age (2%). In contrast, DVT were identified in 8% of those injured between 13 and 15 years of age and 9% of those injured between 16 and 21 years of age. Postphlebitic syndrome develops in approximately 25% of children and adolescents with SCI who have developed DVT (79).

Prophylaxis and treatment for DVT in children and adolescents who have sustained an SCI are similar to that for adults (80). Management of DVT includes anticoagulation with low molecular weight heparin (1 mg/kg q12 h subcutaneously) or intravenous heparin (initial bolus of 75 U/kg over 10 minutes followed by continuous infusion of 28 U/kg/h for infants or 20 U/kg/h for children over 1 year). The heparin infusion is adjusted to maintain the activated partial thromboplastin time between 60 and 85 seconds. In individuals under 18 years of age, anticoagulation with low molecular weight heparin should be monitored with antifactor Xa levels (81). Blood should be drawn 4 hours after the subcutaneous administration of the low molecular weight heparin with a target of 0.5 to 1.0 antiXa U/mL for twice daily dosing and 1 to 2 antiXa U/mL for daily dosing. Oral anticoagulation with warfarin sodium, 0.2 mg/kg, is initiated concurrently with heparinization. Dosage adjustments are made to maintain a prothrombin time of 2 to 3 INR (international normalized ratio), and the duration of anticoagulation is generally 12 weeks.

DVT prophylaxis should include graduated elastic stockings and anticoagulation. Because of the low incidence of DVT in children injured prior to adolescence, it may be reasonable to limit the use of anticoagulants to those youth with other factors that may increase the risk of DVT, such as lower extremity or pelvic trauma and fractures. For children who are too small to wear commercially available graduated elastic stockings, use of custom-made lower extremity garments, such as Jobst stockings may be a consideration. Using elastic wraps to wrap the legs is limited because unevenness of wrapping may result in constrictions with venous obstruction, increasing the risk of DVT. Additionally, some elastic wraps contain latex that is contraindicated because of the risk of latex allergy in this patient population. Alternatives for prophylactic anticoagulation are the same as that for adults. Low molecular weight heparin can be administered subcutaneously every 12 hours (0.5 and 0.75 mg/kg for infants younger than 2 months) or daily (1 mg/kg) (82,83). The target for prophylaxis with low molecular weight heparin is 0.2 to 0.4 antiXa U/mL.

Hypercalcemia

Hypercalcemia affects 10% to 23% of individuals with SCI and most commonly involves adolescent and young adult males during the first 3 months after injury (84,85). Hypercalcemia results from increased bone resorption as a result of the immobilization associated with an SCI. The increased bone turnover characteristic of growing children and adolescents and the large and active bone mass particularly in adolescent males is the basis for the increased incidence of hypercalcemia in the pediatric SCI population. The excessive calcium load is not adequately excreted by the kidneys, because hypercalcemia depresses renal function, resulting in decreased calcium excretion and impairment in renal concentrating ability. Parathyroid hormone is usually depressed because of the hypercalcemia.

Patients with hypercalcemia typically present with an insidious onset of abdominal pain, nausea, vomiting, lethargy, malaise, polydipsia, polyuria, and dehydration. Affected patients may exhibit behavioral changes or an acute psychosis. In a series of 87 individuals younger than 16 years old, 18 (24%) experienced hypercalcemia (85). Five of the patients with hypercalcemia had a clinical presentation consistent with an acute abdomen, and two of them underwent exploratory laparotomies. Patients with hypercalcemia can also be asymptomatic.

Serum calcium and ionized calcium are elevated above age-applicable norms. Serum phosphorus is normal, and alkaline phosphatase is either normal or slightly elevated above age-appropriate norms.

The mainstay of managing hypercalcemia is pamidronate and hydration with intravenous normal saline. Pamidronate is very effective in managing hypercalcemia and should be administered intravenously at a dose of 1 mg/kg (maximum dose of 60 mg) administered over 4 hours (86). Usually a single dose of pamidronate is adequate for resolution of the hypercalcemia.

Complications of hypercalcemia include nephrocalcinosis, urolithiasis, and renal failure. Tori and Hill found that 10 of their 18 (55%) pediatric patients with hypercalcemia experienced urinary stones compared to an 18% incidence of stones in patients without hypercalcemia (84). In addition, 2 of their 18 patients developed renal failure and nephrocalcinosis.

Autonomic Dysreflexia

The pathophysiology, clinical presentation, and management of autonomic dysreflexia in children and adolescents with SCI are similar to the adult SCI population (87). Differences between the pediatric and adult SCI population relate to developmental variations of blood pressure in children and adolescents, appropriate blood pressure cuff sizes, their ability to communicate, and varying dependency upon their parents or guardians (88,89).

For children and adolescents, blood pressure is a function of age and body size. Blood pressure increases as children grow older with older adolescents reaching adult norms. Similar to adults with SCI, children and adolescents with cervical and upper thoracic SCI have lower baseline blood pressures compared to the general population. Because of lower blood pressures in children and adolescents with SCI as a consequence of both their age and their neurological level, it is important that baseline blood pressures be determined on a regular basis. Blood pressure elevations of 20 to 40 mm Hg above baseline may be considered a sign of autonomic dysreflexia. Blood pressure measurement in children and adolescents is confounded by the need to use appropriately sized blood pressure cuffs and anxiety that children may experience with health care professionals. Anxiety associated with obtaining blood pressures may make it difficult to obtain accurate measurements both for baseline determinations as well as during an episode of autonomic dysreflexia. A calm and reassuring environment for the child or the adolescent in the presence of their parents may be helpful.

Because of varying cognitive and verbal communication abilities of individuals as they progress through infancy, childhood, and adolescence, symptoms of autonomic dysreflexia may not be expressed or may be communicated less clearly compared to adults (88,89). For example, in preschool-aged children, even though they are verbal, autonomic dysreflexia may present with vague symptoms rather than complaints of a pounding headache. Medical alert identification should be utilized. Despite the life-threatening nature of autonomic dysreflexia, knowledge about it among children with SCI and their parents is lacking (90). Appropriate education should be provided for those adults who have significant interactions and responsibility for children with SCI, such as teachers, school nurses, coaches, and community-based health care providers. Education about autonomic dysreflexia should include diagnosis as well as emergency management.

Children and adolescents should assume increasing responsibility for their care as they grow older, including prevention, diagnosis, and treatment of autonomic dysreflexia. This would include consistent wearing of medical alert identification, maintaining an information sheet or card about autonomic dysreflexia, and responsibility for educating health care providers or other supervising adults about its diagnosis and management.

Management of children and adolescents experiencing autonomic dysreflexia should be conducted efficiently in a calm and reassuring atmosphere. Symptomatic measures are successful in managing the majority of episodes of autonomic dysreflexia. For those not responsive to conservative measures, nitropatse should be applied or nifedipine (0.25 mg/kg) administered by chew and swallow for those who can follow directions or sublingually for younger children and infants. Patients with recurrent autonomic dysreflexia may be managed with prazosin (minipress 25 to 150 mcg/kg/24 hours/every 6 hours) or terazosin (hytrin 1 to 5 mg daily).

Hyperhidrosis

Hyperhidrosis refers to excessive sweating that is primarily seen in individuals with tetraplegia or thoracic paraplegia (91–93). In a series of 154 individuals with SCI, 27%

were affected by hyperhidrosis (91). The exact pathogenesis of hyperhidrosis has not been elucidated. It is probably the result of sympathetic overactivity of the rostral portion of the spinal cord immediately below the zone of injury (91). Similar to autonomic dysreflexia, the increased sympathetic output may be a response to noxious stimuli below the zone of the SCI. Noxious stimuli may include bladder irritation from a UTI or urolithiasis (92), postinjury myelopathic changes including posttraumatic syringomyelia (94), and tethering of the spinal cord at the injury site (95), or it may be unexplained.

Sweat glands are innervated by the sympathetic nervous system. The sympathetics that innervate the sweat glands of the face and neck originate from T1-7, those for the trunk from T4-12, and those for the legs from T9-L2 (93). This pattern of sympathetic innervation of the sweat glands is the basis for excessive sweating in the face and neck, which are above the zone of injury, as a result of noxious stimuli occurring below the zone of injury.

Hyperhidrosis should be treated if it is embarrassing, impairs function, or increases the risk of developing pressure ulcers. The foundation of management is avoidance and alleviation of precipitating factors. If conservative measures are unsuccessful, medications such as propantheline (96) or transdermal scopolamine (93) should be considered.

Temperature Regulation

The severity of temperature regulation defects is dependent upon the level and completeness of the SCI (97). SCIs at T6 or above interfere with the central control of the major splanchnic sympathetics and voluntary muscles of the lower body, producing a poikilothermic state. The patient is unable to increase core temperature by vasoconstriction and shivering below the zone of the SCI. Similarly, the patient is unable to decrease core body temperature by vasodilitation and sweating below the zone of injury. Therefore, this group of patients is at risk of hypothermia or hyperthermia as a result of exogenous stresses, such as environmental temperatures, and endogenous factors, such as exercise (98). Infants and young children with SCI are particularly vulnerable to the extremes of environmental temperatures because of their relatively large surface area and their variable communication, and cognitive and problem-solving abilities. At the other extreme are adolescents with SCI who may be susceptible to hypothermia or hyperthermia because of erratic judgment.

Fever

Fever frequently occurs during the first 3 months after an SCI, and is problematic because of multiple causes and loss of sensation (88,99,100). Although fever in the acute SCI period is not unique to children with SCI, children tend to become febrile more readily and with higher temperature elevations compared to adults. UTIs are responsible for most episodes of fever, with other common causes being pressure ulcers, surgical site infections, DVT, heterotopic ossification (HO), pathological fractures, pulmonary disorders, and epididymitis. Patients with intra-abdominal disorders may present with subtle signs and symptoms, necessitating a high index of suspicion in the presence of fever, anorexia, abdominal distension, nausea, and vomiting (101). Multiple sources of fever are seen in 15% of febrile patients, whereas no etiology is found during 8% to 11% of febrile episodes and may reflect thermoregulatory abnormalities (99,100).

Evaluation of a febrile child with an SCI must encompass a thorough history and physical examination as well as appropriate laboratory and imaging studies guided by the clinical evaluation. The history should include recent blood transfusions and surgical procedures. The physical examination must encompass a general evaluation to identify problems such as otitis media or pneumonia. The evaluation must also be geared to SCI-specific problems, such as identifying a swollen extremity with limited range consistent with a fracture or HO or a swollen scrotum due to epididymitis.

The choice of laboratory and imaging studies must be based on clinical findings, but typically includes a urine analysis and culture, a complete blood count with differential, erythrocyte sedimentation rate, and C-reactive protein. Liver function tests, serum amylase and lipase, plain abdominal radiographs, abdominal and pelvic ultrasound, gallium scan, and computer tomography may be helpful in evaluating the patient for potential intra-abdominal disorders.

Cardiovascular and Fitness

Cardiovascular disorders cause significant morbidity and mortality in adults with SCIs (102). Individuals with SCI are at increased risk of cardiovascular disease because of their sedentary lifestyles and a greater incidence of metabolic syndrome (103,104). Youth with SCI have lower resting metabolic rates and decreased total lean tissue mass predisposing them to obesity (72). The evaluation of fitness is complicated in youth with SCI because the traditional measure of obesity, body mass index, underestimates body fat in children with SCI (104,105). Because of a reasonably long life span, it is important for youth with SCI to reduce their risk of cardiovascular complications by adopting a lifestyle that incorporates fitness and proper nutrition. Nutritional interventions are complicated for youth with SCI because their resting energy expenditure is significantly less compared to the general population (106,107).

Exercise is an integral component in preventing cardiovascular complications, but is challenging in youth with SCI because of physical limitations, superimposed on preferences and compliance. Aside from younger children with paraplegia who may be physically active by crawling and ambulating, older children and adolescents are similar to the adult SCI population with limited exercise options. Youth with cervical and upper thoracic injuries have decreased cardiovascular adaptions to exercise, manifested by decreased cardiac output and aerobic capacity, hyperthermia, and exertional hypotension (98,108–110). Children and adolescents with SCIs need to participate in adapted physical education and recreational activities, with goals of cardiovascular fitness, increased aerobic capacity, muscle strengthening, and endurance (111,112). Programming must take into account the child's preinjury interests and be developmentally based (112). Fitness programs should engender independence, be integrated into the child or adolescent's lifestyle and their family and community activities, and most importantly, be fun. Two innovations that can improve cardiovascular fitness are FES (functional electrical stimulation [FES]) cycles or upper extremity ergometry with video gaming (the Gamecycle).

Children and adolescents with SCI should be assessed for their risk of cardiovascular disorders, which includes factors such as obesity, sedentary lifestyle, smoking, hyperlipidemia, hypertension, and family history. Screening for lipid abnormalities should be pursued in children with a high-risk family history.

Pain

Similar to the adult SCI population, chronic pain is a significant problem among children and adolescents with SCI (113,114–116). Pain can be very disabling and negatively affect school, work, and social interactions. Pain may originate from the area of trauma in a radicular pattern (compression of a nerve root at the level of injury), from mechanical instability of an unhealed fracture, or consist of central pain or dysesthesia (114–116). Evaluation of pain in infants and younger children may be complicated by their variable communication abilities.

Self-abusive behavior, or self-mutilation, is occasionally seen in infants, children, adolescents, and adults with SCI and may be a manifestation of dysesthesia (117). Self-abusive behavior most commonly presents with biting of fingertips, which can result in finger amputations.

Management of dysesthesia, as well as self-mutilation, should incorporate physical modalities, psychological interventions, and medications (118,119). Physical modalities may include physical therapy, hydrotherapy, and transcutaneous electrical neural stimulation (TENS). Children and parents need to be reassured that dysesthesia generally resolves within 3 to 6 months. The medications primarily used in the pediatric SCI population include amitriptyline (0.1 mg/kg/dose at night), carbamazepine (10 to 20 mg/kg/day in two to four divided doses), and gabapentin, which can be used in children older than 12 years of age (900 to 1,800 mg/day in three divided doses)(176,184,185,115,120,121). Other medications that may be beneficial include phenytoin (3 to 5 mg/day in one to two dicvded doses) or clonidine (5 to 7 mcg/kg/day in divided doses every 6 to 12 hours).

Latex Allergy

Children and adolescents with SCI are susceptible to immediate-type, immunoglobulin E-mediated, allergic reactions to latex (122,123). Approximately 6% to 18% of children and adolescents with SCI have evidence for latex allergies (124). Among adults with SCI who had chronic indwelling catheters, 7 of 15 (47%) had evidence of latex allergy (125).

Latex allergy is presumably the result of frequent and extensive contact with latex-containing products, especially medical supplies and equipment. Additional risk factors may include young age of initial exposure and longer duration of exposure to latex-containing products. Reactions can be elicited by direct contact with latex via cutaneous, mucosal, intravenous, or serosal routes or by airborne dissemination of latex antigens that have adhered to glove powder.

Allergic reactions to latex may manifest as localized or generalized urticaria, wheezing, angioedema, or as anaphylaxis. Intraoperative allergic reactions to latex may be life threatening, and they may be difficult to diagnose because of surgical drapes covering the patient's skin, which may exhibit an urticarial rash.

Diagnosis of latex allergy is established by a history consistent with an immediate-type allergic reaction or with in vitro assays or skin tests. Individuals with either a positive history or a positive laboratory or skin test should be considered allergic to latex. Clinical manifestations may be subtle, such as the child who develops a blotchy facial rash when he or she blows up a balloon. Latex allergy should be suspected in individuals who have unexplained intraoperative allergic reactions, or in individuals allergic to kiwi, bananas, avocados, or chestnuts (126). Skin tests are probably the most sensitive method of identifying latex allergy, but are limited by the lack of availability of standardized preparations and the potential for precipitating a severe allergic reaction (122). Laboratory tests exhibit varying sensitivity and specificity depending upon the specific antigens and assay used.

Because of the potential severity of latex allergy, individuals at risk, such as those with SCI or myelomeningocele, should be cared for in a latex-free environment. This approach should minimize the risk of sensitizing patients, in addition to preventing allergic reactions in patients with known as well as those with undiagnosed latex allergies. Patients and their families and caregivers must be educated about the potential for latex allergy and the necessity to avoid all latex-containing products. Individuals allergic to latex should wear a medical alert identification and carry autoinjectable epinephrine.

Pulmonary

Similar to the adult SCI population, pulmonary complications are major problems during both the acute and chronic phase of SCI (12,102,127). Children with high cervical injuries require aggressive and early ventilatory support and will generally require lifelong ventilatory support, phrenic nerve, or diaphragmatic pacing (128–130). Candidates for a phrenic nerve pacemaker are those with an SCI at C3 or higher. In children, bilateral phrenic nerve stimulation must be performed to avoid excessive mediastinal shifts. Tracheostomies are needed because of upper airway obstruction that occurs in young children during phrenic nerve pacing. In addition, some children may fail to thrive when they are entirely dependent upon phrenic nerve pacing; therefore, supplemental nighttime ventilation via the tracheostomy may be required (129). Noninvasive ventilatory support systems such as BiPAP (biphasic positive airway pressure) and airway secretion management may be applicable in the pediatric SCI population (131,132).

Individuals who sustained tetraplegic SCI as newborns or infants may be at particular risk of incipient respiratory failure. This may be manifested as a sleep disordered breathing disorder with sleep apnea, headache, restless sleep, snoring, morning confusion, daytime sleeping, and mental dullness (133,134). A high index of suspicion must be maintained in these young children with tetraplegia, and sleep studies should be considered. Risk factors for sleep-induced respiratory failure include intercostal and diaphragmatic paralysis, use of medications such as baclofen or diazepam, and obesity (134).

Spasticity

Compared to the adult SCI population, a smaller percentage of children with SCI experience spasticity, which may reflect the higher percentage of children with SCI being paraplegic (135). Nonetheless, spasticity remains a major problem for a significant number of children with SCI (136,137). The general principles of managing spasticity in children with SCI are no different than that in the adult SCI population (136). Clinical evaluation must include a thorough history and physical examination with special attention to potential inciting factors. Factors that exacerbate or perpetuate spasticity include noxious stimuli below the zone of injury, and frequently they are not clinically apparent. Therefore, a high index of suspicion and a thorough evaluation are necessary, particularly in view of the age-dependent variability in the ability to communicate. An example of a noxious stimulus that may exacerbate spasticity and that is more common in the pediatric SCI population includes hip subluxation.

The goals of managing spasticity are to improve function, prevent complications, and to alleviate pain, inconvenience, and embarrassment (135). In treating spasticity, both the advantages and disadvantages of spasticity must be accounted for. Components of managing spasticity include prevention, nonpharmacologic interventions, medications, and invasive procedures. Prevention is the foundation of a therapeutic program and encompasses avoidance of precipitating factors and establishment of good bladder, bowel, and skin programs. Nonpharmacologic interventions include relief of inciting factors and a regular program of stretching, range of motion, and positioning.

Because of the unknown effects of anti-spasticity medication on cognitive development in growing children, their use should be limited for spasticity that impacts the child's functioning and that is unresponsive to conservative management. Orally administered baclofen is the initial drug of choice and is initiated at 0.125 mg/kg/dose BID to TID (5 mg BID to TID in children 12 years and older). Doses are increased every 3 to 5 days in increments of 0.125 mg/kg/dose (5 mg/dose in children 12 years and older). The usual maximum daily dose is 1 to 2 mg/kg/d administered TID to QID (80 mg/d in children 12 years and older). Although baclofen remains the drug of choice for managing spasticity in adolescents, the potential for drug experimentation particularly among adolescents must be considered (138).

Other drugs that may be beneficial include diazepam, clonidine, dantrolene, gabapentin, and tizanidine. Dantrolene is generally not used to manage spasticity in children and adolescents with SCI. Although not approved for use for spasticity, gabapentin (900 to 1,800 mg/d ÷ TID for children older than 12 years of age) may help to control spasticity. Although tizanidine is not approved for use in pediatrics, in clinical practice it is used by some clinicians and demonstrates efficacy similar to that in adults with SCI (139). Because of the potential for hepatotoxicity, liver function studies should be performed, particularly during the first 6 months of therapy.

For spasticity unresponsive to standard management, therapeutic options include intrathecal baclofen, selective dorsal root rhizotomies, epidural spinal cord stimulation, and localized injection of botulinum toxin (140–142). Baclofen can be administered intrathecally by a pump that is implanted in a subcutaneous pocket in the anterior abdominal wall. Intrathecal baclofen has been utilized increasingly in children and adolescents with SCI with encouraging results (143). In addition to SCI, experience with intrathecal baclofen in the pediatric population has been expanded to children and adolescents with cerebral palsy (144). Disadvantages of intrathecal baclofen are cost of both the initial implantation and pump refills, and the rare occurrence of serious adverse reactions (145). For spasticity in the lower extremities, 5 to 10 U/kg of botulinum toxin can be administered in each extremity with a maximum of 20 U/kg.

Pressure Ulcers

Similar to the adult SCI population, pressure ulcers are one of the most common complications for children and adolescents with SCI (146). The true incidence of pressure ulcers in either the pediatric or adult SCI populations is not known. In a retrospective study of individuals who sustained their SCI when they were less than 13 years of age, 55% developed at least one pressure ulcer during a mean follow-up period of 10.3 years (146). The peak age for prevalence of pressure ulcers was 8 years of age. Issues that are unique to the pediatric population include variable degrees of compliance in both preventive and therapeutic endeavors associated with different developmental stages of children and adolescents (146,147). Toddlers and younger children may be at risk for skin breakdown as a result of inadvertent trauma from careless activities and play characteristic of these age groups. These younger patients have limited cognitive abilities to follow the usual preventive measures that older individuals follow, such as pressure reliefs. Preventive measures may include wristwatches with automatic resetting timers to remind children to perform pressure reliefs. Additionally, pressure ulcer prevention activities must be developmentally based, and responsibility must be progressively shifted from the parents to the children as they grow up. Because children become physically larger as they grow up, new equipment must be appropriately matched to the child's size. Properly fitting wheelchairs and adequate cushions must be prescribed with pressure mapping to reduce the risk of pressure ulcer development.

Rehabilitation

Rehabilitation must be developmentally based, and as a consequence goals must respond to the dynamic evolutionary forces that accompany growing patients into adulthood (148–153). Goals of rehabilitation should be to maintain health and restore productivity with the ultimate goal that the patient feels that they have a satisfying life. The challenge in caring for children and adolescents with SCI is to address the changing objectives of each developmental stage, with the ultimate goal being that the patient becomes an adult with a high quality of life (154). Pediatric focused care must establish a solid foundation from which satisfactory quality of life flourishes throughout childhood and into adulthood.

Traditional interventions include mobility, activities of daily living, bowel, bladder and skin programs, recreation, psychological and vocational counseling, and social services. Conventional rehabilitation must be expanded to encompass effective mobility and access in the community as well as recreational, educational, and vocational interventions that facilitate a productive and satisfying life. As children and adolescents grow, new equipment is needed because of both increasing size and changing needs. Using mobility as an example, infants and young toddlers may crawl, progress to parapodia, and utilize strollers for wheeled mobility. Preschool and early school–aged children may crawl at home but use a variety of orthotics for ambulation and/or standing in school; they should be independent in appropriate types of wheelchairs. Except for individuals who have less severe neurological impairments allowing community ambulation, older children and adolescents would primarily, if not exclusively, utilize wheelchairs for all their mobility. These older patients may have needs for standing or sports-specific wheelchairs, with older adolescents needing access to motor vehicles for community mobility.

Ambulation

Long-term community ambulation is dependent upon several factors, including neurological level and American Spinal Injury Association (ASIA) Impairment Scale (AIS) score, age, body size, compliance, and preferences. Individuals who are most likely to be community ambulators are those who are young, have L3 or lower lesions, or have AIS scores of D (155,156). Although individuals of all ages with SCI want to walk, children are more likely to be active ambulators compared to adolescents and adults, because of their smaller size, increased energy level, and less concern for cosmetics (156–159).

Parapodia allow children with SCI to stand without the need for upper extremity weight bearing, so that they can perform activities with both hands (156,160). Parapodia may also allow children to ambulate. The requirements for utilizing parapodia include head control and the absence of significant contractures of the lower extremities. Patients who utilize parapodia are either therapeutic or household ambulators; nonetheless, parapodia provide users with some independence in mobility as well as an opportunity to be upright and face their peers at eye level.

Parapodia can be initiated in children as young as 9 to 12 months of age, which is the developmentally appropriate time to initiate standing, and they are useful in providing the young child the opportunity to be upright, prior to the use of other orthotics. Parapodia also have the advantage of not requiring intensive therapy. Although parapodia are accepted by preschoolers and early school–aged children, most children elect to stop using parapodia by 7 to 10 years of age. The most commonly used parapodium is the Rochester parapodium (Fig. 29.6). The child can ambulate by swiveling by twisting their upper trunk and swinging their arms. Alternatively, with walkers or forearm crutches they can perform a swing-to or a swing-through gait.

Reciprocating gait orthoses (RGO) are utilized in individuals with paraplegia with L2 or higher level lesions (Fig. 29.7) (156,158,160). In comparison to other orthotics, such as hip knee ankle foot orthoses (HKAFO) or knee ankle foot orthoses (KAFO), which may be used in this group of patients, RGOs provide a reciprocating gait and are more energy efficient (161). RGOs may be initiated in children as young as 15 to 18 months old. Patients with active hip flexors or who are young and well motivated are most likely to be community ambulators (158–160). However, the vast majority of RGO users will be therapeutic or household ambulators.

Standing, with or without ambulation, may have immense psychological and functional benefits for children and adolescents with SCI (158). In addition to parapodia, there are a variety of static and mobile standing devices that are suitable for children, including standing wheelchairs, standing frames, and mobile standing devices (158). Because of their size, standing wheelchairs would only be appropriate for older children and adolescents. Mobile standing devices would be most acceptable for preschool-aged to preadolescent children. They are primarily utilized for household, school, or vocational activities.

Another option for upright mobility in children with SCI is FES systems, which have been demonstrated to be feasible and practical (162). Utilizing implanted FES systems, adolescents are able to stand at home two to four times a week, allowing them to perform common activities while standing such as reaching high places (163). Compared to KAFOs, implanted FES systems were equal or better in promoting independence and were preferred for the majority of activities (164), although implanted systems are not currently available. Contraindications for lower extremity FES systems include hip dislocation, lower extremity contractures, severe scoliosis, and myocutaneous flaps. Therefore, it is important to prevent these

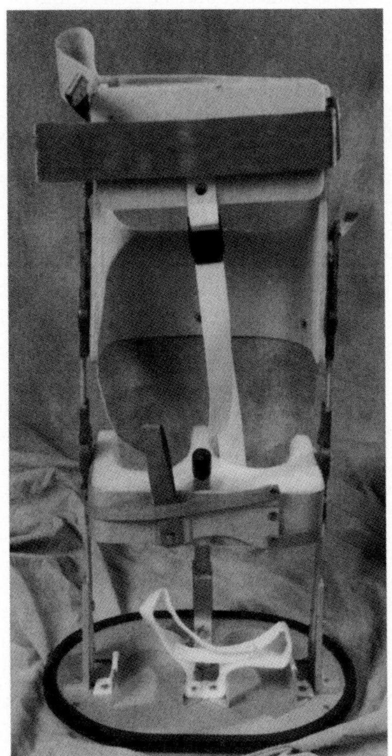
A

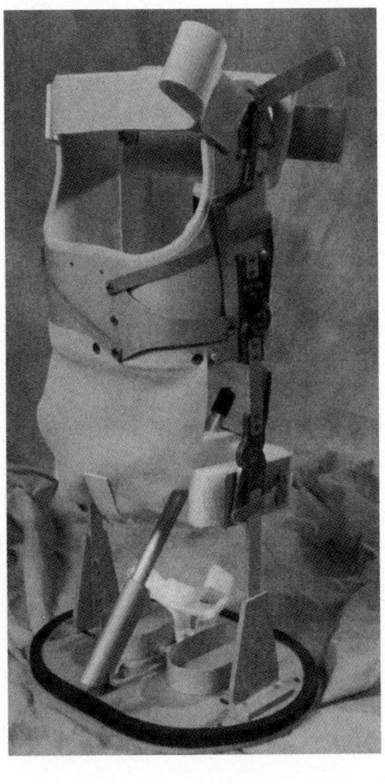
B

FIGURE 29.6 Rochester parapodium; front (A) and back (B) views.

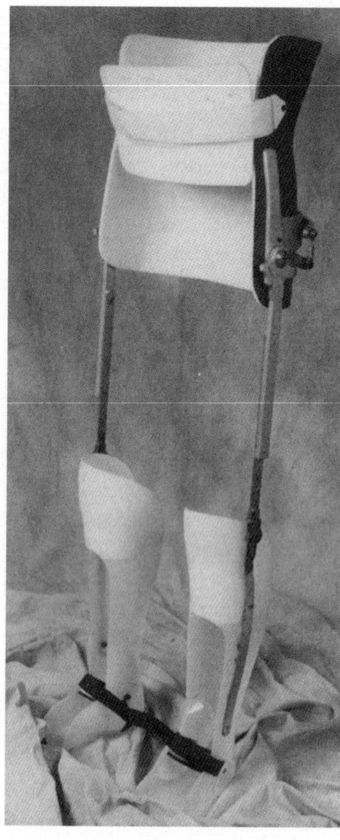

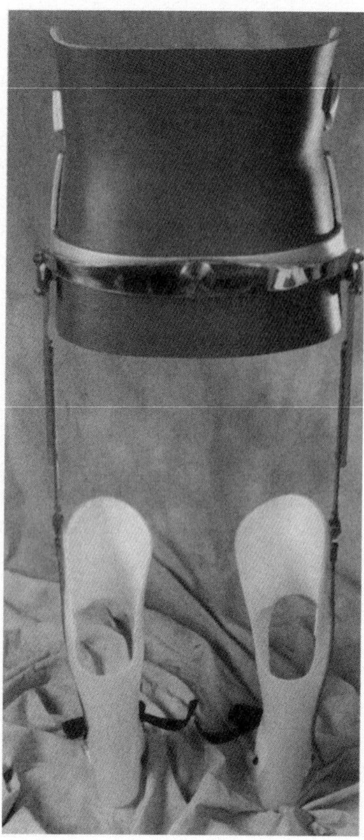

FIGURE 29.7 Reciprocating gait orthosis; front (A) and back (B) views.

complications in children and adolescents with SCIs, who may benefit in the future from innovative treatments such as FES. The Parastep system that is clinically available currently utilizes surface stimulation.

Regardless of the type of upright mobility device used, particular attention to and careful monitoring of the shoulder, elbow, and wrist must occur to prevent overuse syndromes and pain. Children, particularly as they get older, should engage in a routine upper limb exercise program for maintenance of the use of their arm for weight bearing during upright mobility exercises.

Upper Extremity Function

There are a variety of both static and dynamic orthotics, including custom fabrication for toddlers (Fig. 29.8), available to improve hand function of individuals with tetraplegia (165). While low tech, the universal cuff (Fig. 29.8) with or without a dorsal-based support remains the most versatile and beneficial splint. The wrist-driven flexor–hinge splint is also useful for when grasp and release is needed, but children and adolescents typically abandon it due to poor cosmesis and difficulty in donning. Surgical reconstruction, including tendon transfers, of the upper extremities to restore active hand function has been shown to be beneficial in children as young as 4 years of age with SCI (166,167). Surgical reconstruction of the upper extremities has been performed to restore elbow extension, wrist extension, finger flexion, and thumb pinch.

Implantable FES systems have been used to restore grasp and release in youth with C5 or weak C6 lesions who would not be candidates for reconstructive surgeries (168). The use of the Freehand System in adolescents resulted in improved satisfaction and independence, but unfortunately was removed from the market (165). Evidence from animal studies and clinical trials in humans supports the use of this implantable technology in children as young as 6 years of age (169). Currently on the market and available to children and adults is the Bioness System, which provides stimulated pinch and grasp through a surface electrical stimulation system.

ACTIVITY-BASED REHABILITATION

In adults with SCI, cycling has been shown to effectively reduce secondary complications. Cycling with FES results in increases in muscle cross-sectional area, lean body mass, voluntary and electrically induced muscle force, muscle endurance, cardiovascular fitness, and bone mineral density (170–176). Cycling with FES and passive cycling in children have resulted in improved bone mineral density, muscle volume, stimulated quadriceps strength, and lower resting heart rate (177). Therefore, cycling with or without FES can have positive health benefits and is a viable home exercise option for children with SCI.

Psychosocial and Sexuality

Sexuality issues include sexual development, onset or resumption of menses, sexual performance, and fertility. Sexuality should be addressed from a developmental perspective beginning at the time of initial rehabilitation and be reinforced during follow-up visits. The topic should be initiated at the time of injury, irrespective of the child's age, so that parents have

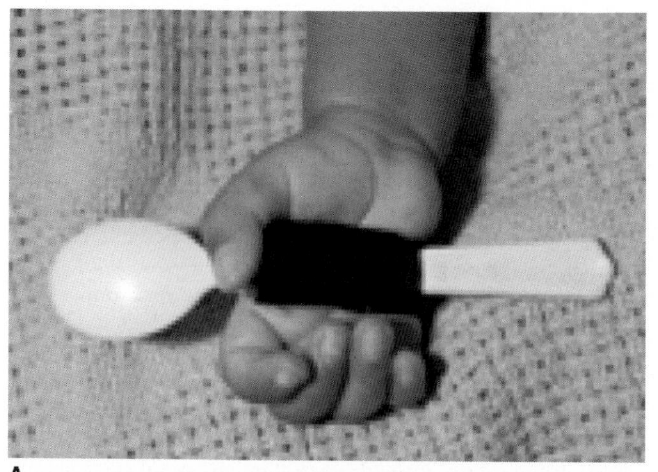

A

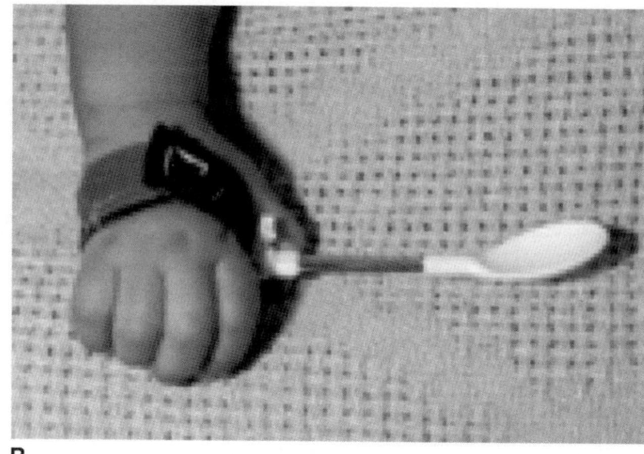

B

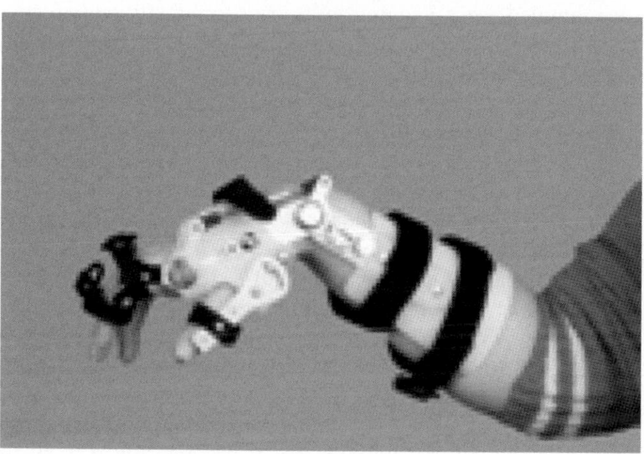

C

FIGURE 29.8 **A,B,C:** Static (A and B) and dynamic (C) orthotics.

accurate expectations of future sexuality and fertility issues. School-aged children and adolescents should be provided developmentally appropriate sexuality information, including pubertal development, fertility, and sexual functioning. When children participate in sexuality educational programs in school, they may have questions about the impact of SCI on their sexual function and menstruation. Adolescents may have specific questions about erection, ejaculation, sexual intercourse, fertility, pregnancy, and birth control. In the absence of a traumatic brain injury, sexual development and puberty should not be affected. Menarche usually occurs within the normal age range (178). Females who had menarche prior to their injury will usually have resumption of menstruation within 6 months of sustaining their SCI.

As for all children with special needs, federal laws protect the educational rights of children and adolescents with SCI. The public laws, the Education for All Handicapped Children Act (EAHCA, 1975) and the Individuals with Disabilities Education Act (IDEA, 1990), require that they be educated in the least restrictive environment. Education plays a critical role in the lives of children and adolescents with SCI in several ways (9,154,179). Along with play, education is the main occupation for children and adolescents. It is very important that they return to school as soon as possible after injury, and ideally they should return to the school that they had attended prior to their injury. Returning to school permits the individual with an SCI to reestablish friendships and peer interactions. In addition, education is a major determinant for adult employment, which in turn is a crucial ingredient of life satisfaction for adults with SCI. Returning to school can be a traumatic event for both the patient as well as the teachers and students. From the patient's perspective, this transition back into school may be greatly facilitated if he or she can visit his or her school and classrooms prior to discharge from SCI rehabilitation. From the students' and teachers' perspective, the previously described visit may be very beneficial. If that is not possible, the teachers and students may benefit from viewing a video of the patient as well as educational materials about SCI. A teaching manual about SCI designed for schoolteachers and nurses may also be useful (179).

Children and adolescents with SCI should receive psychological evaluation and counseling in an ongoing manner, appropriate for their developmental stage. Although the incidence of depression in children and adolescence with SCI is not significantly different compared to norms, depression in the pediatric SCI population is associated with quality of life (180). In adults with pediatric onset SCI, 27% exhibited depressive symptoms with 3% having probable major depressive disorder; these findings are similar to that found in the adult SCI population (181). Because of the significant impact that families have on their children or adolescents with SCI, counseling and support must be provided for parents, siblings, and other significant family members (179). Support and peer groups are also beneficial for patients, parents, and other family members.

Attendant care should be considered for children with tetraplegia even though family members are available for daily care. Availability of attendant care allows the parents to maintain their parental role, including limit setting and provision of support and guidance for their children. It is frequently difficult for parents to fulfill both the roles of parent and caregiver, and parents can easily become burned out if they are required to wear both hats. At a minimum, parents need respite care, particularly if their children have high tetraplegia with complicated and intense needs.

Play and recreation must be an integral component of the rehabilitation program for children and adolescents with SCI (112). Play and recreation-based therapy should be consistent with preinjury interests of the patient. Play is critical for young children in rehabilitation because it is their primary activity of daily living. Play techniques must be incorporated into the rehabilitation program. Recreation and play provides older children and adolescents with time away from rehabilitation staff. They need to be provided appropriate outlets and access to typical childhood and adolescent activities, such as television, movies, music, talk, and sports. They need to be educated about and exposed to community activities and wheelchair sports that are available in their community.

Similar to the adult SCI population, substance abuse and psychological problems are major issues for children and adolescents with SCI (182). Adolescents with SCI may be at greater risk of suicide because of the tremendous impact of an SCI superimposed upon the usual turbulence of adolescence.

Spine and Musculoskeletal

Halo Fixators

Proper halo ring application is important in preventing pin loosening and pin tract infections. Children 12 years of age and younger present unique issues with halo pin fixation. Multiple pins (ten as compared to four in adults) with low torque (2 inch-lb) have been demonstrated to be safe in infants (183). For children between 2 and 12 years of age, torque may range from 4 to 6 inch-lb. For patients older than 12 years of age, pins should be torqued to 8 inch-lb. For children under 6 years of age, CT scanning of the skull is recommended for pin placement because of the variability in skull thickness (184,185). If halo fixation fails because of loosening and/or infection, a Minerva-type cervicothoracolumbosacral orthosis is effective. Because use of Crutchfield tongs in patients younger than 12 years of age may be associated with skull penetration and dural fluid leaks, a halo ring for traction is an effective and the preferred alternative.

Spine Boards

In children younger than 8 to 10 years of age, the head is proportionately larger than their bodies. As a consequence, when children of this age group are immobilized on a standard spine board, their neck will be inadvertently flexed (Fig. 29.9A,B). Therefore, when spinal stabilization is needed in an emergency situation, younger children should be immobilized on child-specific spine boards (Fig. 29.9C) (186). However, if a standard spine board must be used in a younger child, excessive cervical flexion can be avoided by raising the torso 2 to 4 cm, on blankets or foam, leaving the head at the board level (Fig. 29.9D).

Spine Deformities

Spine deformities are very common in pediatric SCI, particularly if the injury is sustained prior to skeletal maturity (187,188) (Fig. 29.10). Among children injured prior to puberty, 98% developed scoliosis with 67% requiring surgical correction (187). In contrast, when the injury occurred after skeletal maturity, the risk of scoliosis was 20% with 5% requiring surgery. The spine deformities may be caused by muscle weakness or imbalance, residual deformity, or it can be iatrogenic, for example, as a result of a laminectomy (189). Problems that can complicate spine deformities include pelvic obliquity, impaired use of the upper extremities secondary to poor sitting balance, pressure ulcers, pain, poor fitting of lower extremity orthotics, and gastrointestinal and cardiopulmonary abnormalities. Because of the high incidence of scoliosis, radiographs of the thoracic–lumbar–sacral spine should be obtained every 3 to 6 months prior to puberty and every 6 to 12 months from puberty to skeletal maturity, and every 2 years thereafter.

Prophylactic bracing with thoracolumbosacral orthoses (TLSO) may be beneficial in delaying the need for spine surgery. In one study of 123 youth with SCI, surgical fusion was reduced to 50% in those who were braced when their curve was 20 degrees or less compared to 86% in those not wearing a brace (190). Additionally, the time to surgical correction was significantly delayed a mean of 4 years in those braced compared to those who were not braced; this delay in surgery is significant in reference to spinal growth before a fusion is performed. In contrast, there was a smaller reduction in those needing surgery from 86% to 60% and only 1 year delay of surgery in those who were braced compared to those who were not braced when the initial curve at presentation was 20 to 40 degrees. Major drawbacks of bracing include interference with mobility and independent functioning, such as self-catheterization (191,192). Irrespective of the degree of scoliosis, bracing with a TLSO may benefit patients with poor trunk support and a flexible curve, facilitating sitting and upper extremity functioning.

Surgical correction for spine deformities should be undertaken when the curve progresses beyond 40 degrees in children older than 10 years (189). For younger children, curves up to 80 degrees are tolerated if they are somewhat flexible and temporarily decrease while in a TLSO; otherwise, a growing spinal system is recommended while waiting for enough spinal growth to perform a fusion.

Hip Deformities

Hip dislocation, subluxation, and contractures are extremely common in pediatric SCI, especially among children injured at younger ages (189,193,194) (Fig. 29.11). In one series, hip instability was observed in 100% of children injured when they were less than 5 years of age and in 83% of those injured when they were younger than 10 years of age. In another series, hip instability was found in 60% of children injured when they were 8 years of age or younger (195). Development of hip instability occurs in patients with tetraplegia or paraplegia, in males and females, and in patients with flaccid as well as spastic SCI (196).

Indications for surgical management of hip instability are not entirely clear. With the development of FES systems for standing and walking and the future possibility for spinal cord regeneration, aggressive prophylactic surgical treatment of hip

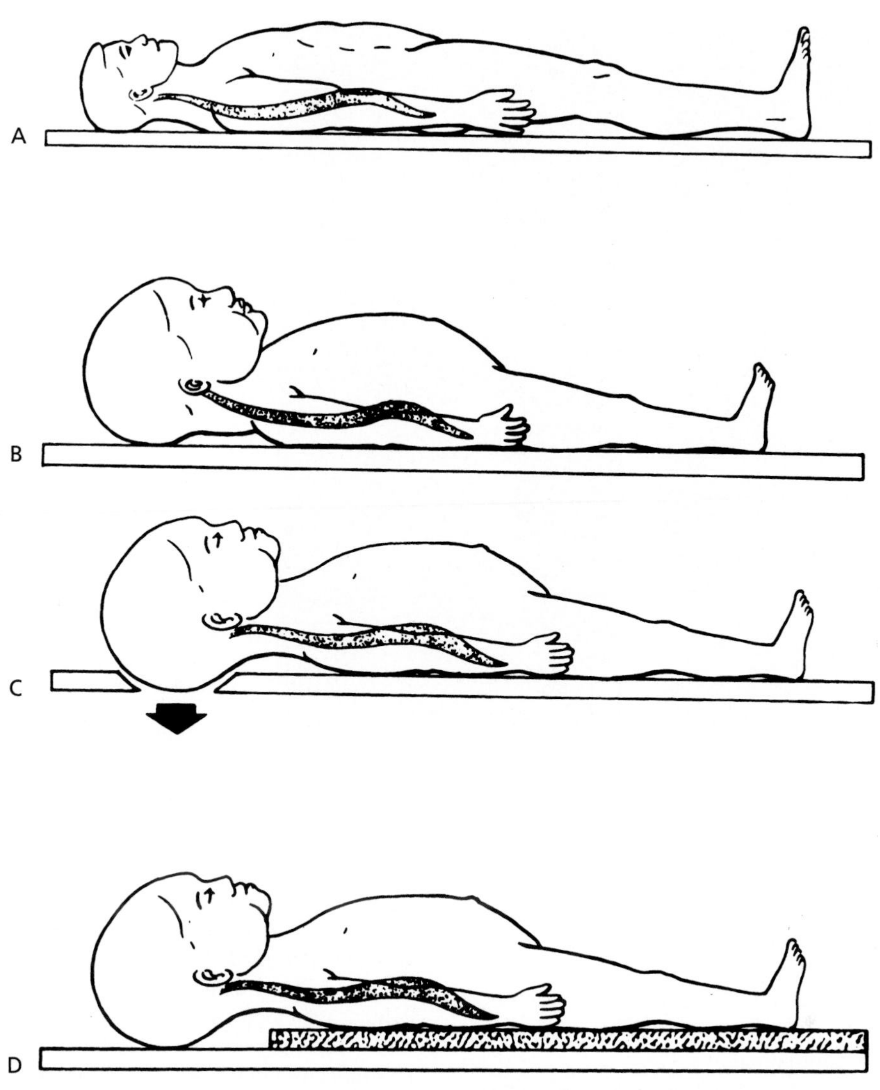

FIGURE 29.9 **A:** shows an adult immobilized on a standard backboard. **B:** Demonstrates a young child on a standard backboard; the relatively large head results in a kyphotic position of the neck. In (**C**), the child is on a modified backboard with a cut-out to recess the occiput, providing safe cervical positioning. In (**D**), the double mattress pad raises the chest, providing for safe cervical positioning. Herzenberg JE, Hensinger RN, Dedrick DK, et al. Emergency transport and positioning of young children who have an injury of the cervical spine. The standard backboard may be hazardous. *J Bone Joint Surg.* 1989;71A:15–22.

instability should be considered (197). If a patient has spasticity and therefore opportunity for future restoration with biologic repairs or FES, then the hips are aggressively prevented from being allowed to dislocate, including adequate control of severe spasticity with medication and/or a baclofen pump. Many times, it is the subluxing hip that is causing the irritation that is exacerbating the spasticity. Surgical management of hip instability may include surgical release of hip contractures, a capsulorrhaphy, varus osteotomies, and acetabular augmentations (anterior or posteriorly) (189,198).

Heterotopic Ossification

The incidence of HO in pediatric SCI is approximately 3% compared to approximately 20% in adults with SCI (189,199). Similar to adults, the hip is most commonly involved in children and adolescents with SCI. The average onset of HO is reported as 14 months for pediatric SCI compared to adults with SCI where the typical onset is 1 to 4 months after injury (200). Prophylaxis for HO utilizing etidronate disodium (didronel) (201) is not routinely used in the pediatric SCI population because of the relatively low risk of HO. In addition, etidronate disodium may be contraindicated in prepubertal children because of the potential development of rachitic-like changes (202). If there is evidence of early HO formation diagnosed by a positive bone scan, ultrasound, MRI or CT, anti-inflammatory drugs such as indomethacin (1 to 3 mg/kg/day in two to three divided doses, maximum dose of 200 mg/day) or tolmetin (20 mg/kg/day in two to three divided doses) for 3 to 6 months may be beneficial.

Indications for surgical interventions include if there are significant functional deficits related to the loss of range. Resection of HO probably should be undertaken approximately 1 to 1.5 years after its onset, in order to avoid progression of femoral neck osteoporosis and intra-articular fibrosis if surgery is postponed until the bone scan and alkaline phosphatase are normal (199,203). Postoperative use of radiation therapy may be contraindicated in younger children because of long-term consequences of radiation. Indomethacin (1 to 3 mg/kg/day in two to three divided doses, maximum dose of 200 mg/day) is used in the postoperative period (204).

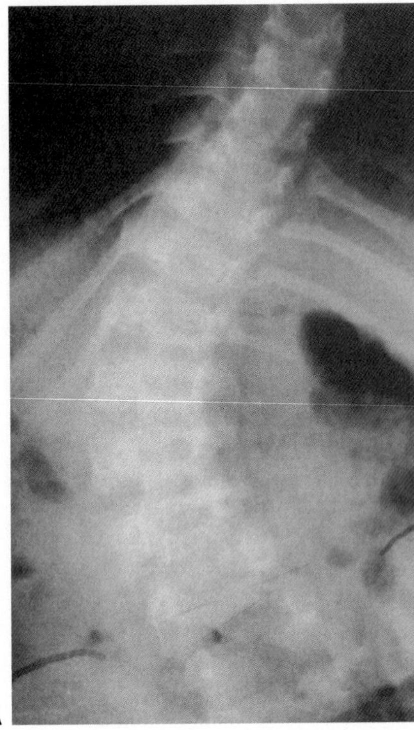

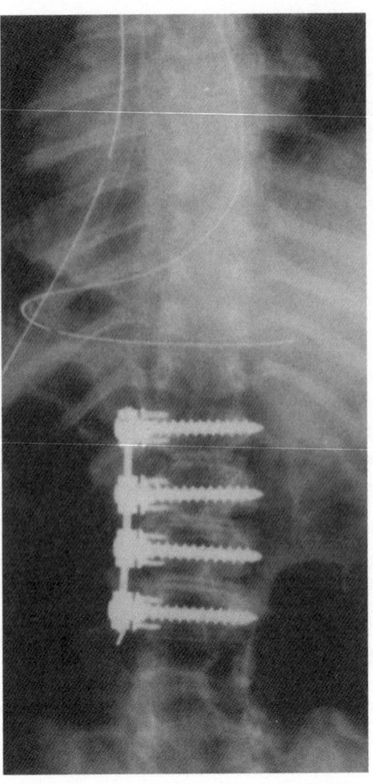

FIGURE 29.10 A,B Spine radiographs of a 8-year-old male who sustained an incomplete T4 SCI (ASIA impairment scale score of D) when he was 2 years old. **A:** Demonstrates a 52 degree thoracolumbar curve. (**B**) is a radiograph obtained after he underwent an anterior spine fusion with instrumentation when he was 8½ years old.

Osteopenia and Pathologic Fractures

Osteopenia begins immediately after sustaining an SCI and plateaus between 6 to 12 months post injury. Children and adolescents with SCI have bone densities of approximately 60% of normal age- and sex-matched controls (205). A combination of standing, stepping, or cycling with FES may increase bone mineral density by approximately 25%.

Pathological long bone fractures occur as a consequence of loss of bone mineral density. Pathological fractures occur in approximately 14% of children and adolescents with SCI (189). The etiology in 40% of the patients included gait training, range of motion, and minor trauma. The etiology of the pathological fractures in the remaining 60% of the patients was not identified. Patients with pathological fractures typically present with fever and a swollen extremity. The most common sites of fracture are the supracondylar region of the femur and the proximal tibia. Initial radiological findings may be subtle, and the diagnosis of a pathological fracture in growing children may require a high index of suspicion (Fig. 29.12) (189). At the other extreme is over diagnosis of a growth plate

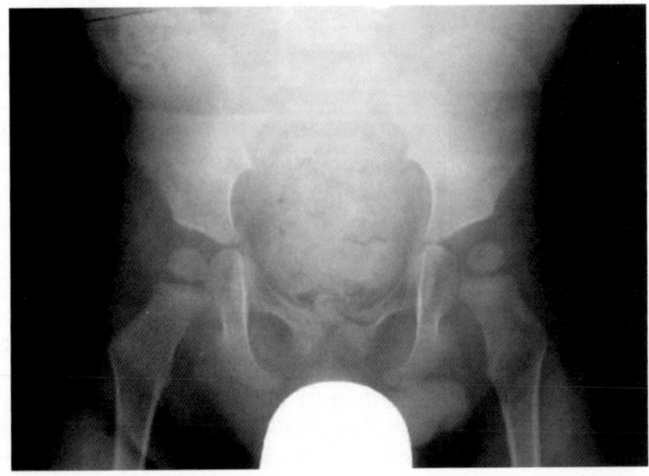

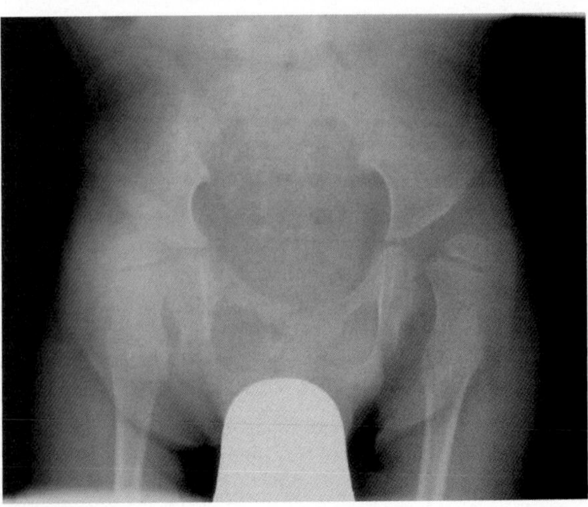

FIGURE 29.11 A,B: Pelvic radiographs of a male who has a complete C5 neonatal SCI. Radiographs obtained at 20 months of age (Fig. 29.11A) demonstrate some uncovering of the left femoral head, which is dislocated on radiographs obtained when he was 5 years of age (Fig. 29.11B).

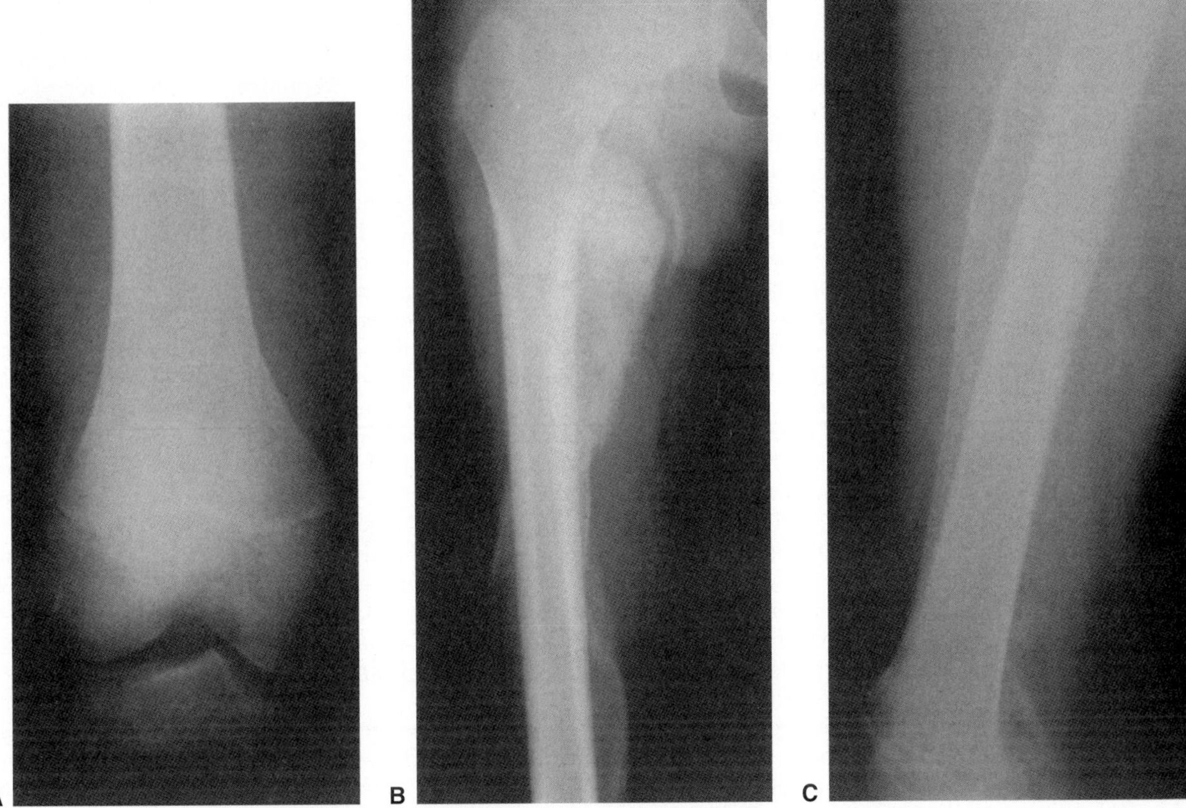

FIGURE 29.12 **A–C:** 15-year-old male with a T10 complete SCI, who sustained a supracondylar femoral fracture 9 months after his injury. There was no apparent cause of the fracture. **A:** demonstrates a slight defect of the medial aspect of the femoral metaphysis. **(B,C)** are radiographs taken 2 months later, and they demonstrate exuberant callus formation of the entire femur.

fracture with radiographic finding consistent with a malignant bone tumor; in which case a pediatric radiologist and orthopedist should be consulted (206,207).

Treatment of pathological fractures should consist of removable splints (189,208). If casts are necessary, they must be well padded over all bony prominences and bivalved to enable inspection to prevent pressure ulcers. Because the bone is osteoporotic, it generally will not hold internal or external fixation very well; however, intramedullary nailing may be very helpful in preventing further deformity or shortening and allows for earlier mobilization. Fortunately, exuberant callous develops within 3 to 4 weeks, at which time the splinting or casting can be minimized with resumption of range of motion (Fig. 29.12). Ambulation with orthotics should be postponed for 6 to 8 weeks after sustaining a fracture.

Prevention is critical, but may be particularly challenging in the pediatric SCI population because of risk taking behavior observed in children and adolescents of different ages. Caretakers must focus on safety in risky activities. Bone mineral loss should be minimized by encouraging weight bearing with orthotics or FES. Good nutrition and adequate sunlight are essential. Appropriate training and adequate equipment for transfers are essential components of pediatric SCI rehabilitation. In the future, medications such as bisphosphonates and other modalities such as vibration may have a role in preventing pathological fractures.

NEURAL-TUBE DEFECTS

Spina bifida and anencephaly are the two most common forms of neural-tube defects, also referred to as spinal dysraphism (209,210). Spina bifida can be classified based on whether neural tissue is exposed (210). Myelomeningoceles are open lesions that either have absent skin covering or are covered only by a thin membrane. Spina bifida lesions with intact skin covering, referred to as occult spinal dysraphism, include lipomeningocele, diastematomyelia, dermal sinus, meningocele, tight filum terminale, and myelocystocele. The diagnosis of spina bifida occulta should be reserved for the common spinal abnormality that is only identified on plain radiographs as a failure of fusion of the spinous processes of the lower lumbar or sacral spine without neurologic abnormalities. Myelomeningoceles are the most common form of nonfatal neural-tube defects, and they are characterized by significant defects of both the brain and the spinal cord.

Epidemiology

The incidence of myelomeningocele has demonstrated trends in respect to time, geography, and race/ethnicity. These trends may be related to the changing nutritional status, periconceptual use of folic acid, availability of prenatal diagnosis, and elective pregnancy termination (211). In the United States, the incidence of myelomeningocele has decreased from 5.9 cases per 10,000 births in 1984 to 3.0 cases per 10,000 in 1999–2000 (212). In the United States from 1983 through 1990, the rates of myelomeningocele varied among racial/ethnic groups with the lowest incidence in Asians/Pacific Islanders (2.3/10,000) and the highest rates for Hispanics (6.0/10,000) (213). However, by 1990, the rates for myelomeningocele were nearly identical for blacks, Hispanics, and whites. There appears to be a higher incidence of neural-tube defects in lower socioeconomic populations (214). Worldwide there has also been significant difference in the incidence of neural-tube defects, with higher rates in certain countries, such as China (215).

Mortality is highest during infancy and is primarily related to problems with hindbrain function, CNS infection, and hydrocephalus (216). Analysis of survival data is complicated by different treatment approaches utilized over the past four decades. Since the introduction of folic acid fortification in the United States in 1998, survival of infants born with spina bifida has improved, suggesting that folic acid may play a role in reducing neurological severity in addition to preventing their occurrence (217). Over the past 50 years, survival has significantly increased as a result of improved treatment approaches. In a recent report, 56% of patients survived to their 20th birthday (218). In another report, 85% of individuals survived to 16 years of age. Of those who survived to 16 years of age, a survival rate past 34 years of age of 75% was found in those with shunted hydrocephalus compared to 94% survival rate for those without hydrocephalus or those with hydrocephalus not requiring a shunt (219).

The etiology of myelomeningocele is unknown, although presumably involves both genetic and environmental factors (220). Maternal diabetes mellitus (221) and maternal use of valproic acid (221) and carbamazepine (223) are associated with an increased risk of neural-tube defects. Other factors that may be associated with the development of neural-tube defects include maternal obesity (224), fever, and hyperthermia (225). The increased incidence of neural-tube defects in lower socioeconomic groups suggests that nutritional deficiencies, including folic acid, may play a role in the etiology of neural-tube defects (214). The risk of neural-tube defects is increased in individuals homozygous for a common mutation in the gene for methylenetetrahydrofolate reductase (226). These observations support the potential role of folic acid deficiency in the etiology of neural-tube defects.

The role of genetic factors in the etiology of neural-tube defects is supported by the observed increased risk for individuals who have previously had an affected baby, first-degree relatives, and individuals who have neural-tube defects themselves. The recurrence risk ranges from 1% to 5% in a family with one affected child and up to 10% in families with two affected children (220,227).

Pathophysiology

Neural-tube defects are caused by failure of the neural tube to close between the third and fourth week of gestation, resulting in abnormalities of the brain and spinal cord (228). The major abnormalities of the brain include hydrocephalus in 80% to 90% of children with myelomeningoceles and the Chiari II malformation in virtually all affected individuals (229). The main characteristics of the Chiari II malformation are a small posterior fossa, caudal displacement of the cerebellar vermis and brain stem into the cervical spinal canal, kinking of the cervicomedullary junction, and beaking of the tectum. The hydrocephalus is caused primarily by obstruction of cerebrospinal fluid (CSF) movement due to the complex deformities of the posterior fossa and brain stem, related to the Chiari II malformation.

The defect of the spine and spinal cord can occur from the thoracic to the sacral levels, with the lumbosacral region involved in approximately 66% to 75% of the cases (230). At the level of the defect, the spinal canal is open dorsally with defects of the posterior elements of several contiguous vertebrae (231). At the level of the myelomeningocele defect, the spinal cord exhibits varying degrees of dysplasia, is present as a flat neural plate, and is covered by a thin membrane. Damage to the spinal cord and resulting neurologic abnormalities are probably a result of several factors. These include spinal cord dysplasia, tethering of the spinal cord at the myelomeningocele defect, toxicity of amniotic fluid, mechanical trauma from the uterine wall during later gestation, labor and delivery, and damage to the neural plate during its surgical repair (232).

Clinical Presentation

An affected neonate should undergo repair of the myelomeningocele shortly after birth in order to reduce the risk of infection and ventriculitis (233). If the myelomeningocele sac is leaking, closure should be undertaken within the first 24 hours of life, otherwise the closure can be performed within the first 2 to 3 days of life (231,233,234). The goals of the initial closure are to cover the defect with skin, untether the spinal cord, and reconstruct the neural tube and dura. After closure of the myelomeningocele defect, the patient needs to be monitored closely for the development of hydrocephalus. This eventually develops in 80% to 90% of cases, necessitating a ventriculoperitoneal shunt (210,235).

The primary manifestations of myelomeningocele are a result of the brain and spinal cord abnormalities. Children with myelomeningocele exhibit a variety of cognitive defects (236). Children who have experienced meningitis or ventriculitis related to an infected shunt or CSF leakage at birth are more likely to have cognitive defects (237). Approximately 30% of individuals with myelomeningocele have below normal intelligence, primarily perceptual motor abnormalities with normal verbal skills. They frequently have disorders of visual spatial organization and may experience learning disabilities, hearing and visual impairments, and seizures (238). Individuals with myelomeningocele may exhibit "cocktail chatter" that is characterized by excessive talking and superficiality of content (239). Children with myelomeningocele frequently demonstrate defects in coordination and dexterity of hand function (240).

Because most individuals with myelomeningocele have hydrocephalus and require ventriculoperitoneal shunts, they are at risk of shunt infections and shunt malfunction. In younger children, shunt malfunction is manifested by symptoms of increased intracranial pressure, including nausea, vomiting, and severe headache. In contrast, the symptoms of shunt malfunction in adolescents and young adults may be subtler. They may present with indolent symptoms of irritability, decreased perceptual motor function, shortened attention span, intermittent headaches, poor school performance, weakness, or worsening scoliosis.

The Chiari II malformation may result in hindbrain dysfunction (229). In infants and younger children, symptoms may include feeding and swallowing abnormalities, stridor, vocal cord paralysis, weak cry, apnea, sleep-disordered breathing (241), nystagmus, opisthotonus, and weakness and spasticity of the upper extremities. Older children and adolescents are more likely to present with progressive scoliosis, decreased upper extremity function, neck pain, and depressed respiratory function. Symptoms of the Chiari II malformation usually resolve with adequate shunting of the hydrocephalus; however, some patients may require a posterior fossa decompression (229,242).

Hydrosyringomyelia in association with the Chiari II malformation is a common finding in individuals with myelomeningocele (229,242). The clinical manifestations are similar to those of development hydrosyringomyelia associated with Chiari I malformations, which is discussed later in this chapter.

The main manifestations of spinal cord dysfunction are motor paralysis, sensory loss, and bladder, bowel, and sexual dysfunction. The extent of the neurological deficit is dependent upon the location of the myelomeningocele. In contrast to SCIs where the degree of motor deficits either approximate or exceed the sensory deficits, individuals with myelomeningocele have sensory deficits that are generally more severe than the motor deficits. The nature of the spinal cord abnormality in myelomeningocele is more severe involvement of the dorsal aspect of the spinal cord including the posterior spinal nerve roots with relative sparing of the anterior spinal nerve roots. In dermatomes with impaired sensation, the function of muscles under voluntary control is limited. Although the vast majority of individuals with myelomeningocele have flaccid paralysis, approximately 10% to 30% exhibit spasticity (243).

There are several classification systems utilized to characterize spinal cord dysfunction in individuals with myelomeningocele (243–245). These classification systems are generally used in order to predict ambulation potential. It is important to accurately and serially document motor and sensory levels and the presence and degree of spasticity. This is particularly important for early identification of complications such as retethering of the spinal cord, hydrosyringomyelia, and hydrocephalus.

A major aspect of the myelomeningocele abnormality at birth is tethering of the spinal cord at the site of the defect. One of the major goals of the initial surgical correction in the neonate is to untether the spinal cord. However, there is a tendency for the spinal cord to become adherent to the myelomeningocele repair site (231). This results in retethering of the spinal cord and a low-lying spinal cord that is found in the majority of individuals with myelomeningocele (246). During growth, the retethered spinal cord cannot migrate cephalad as it normally would. In some patients, the retethered spinal cord may impair remaining spinal cord function, manifested by the onset or worsening of weakness, sensory loss, spasticity, progressive scoliosis, changes in bowel or bladder function, pain, or orthopaedic deformities in the lower extremities. Since the majority of patients with low-lying spinal cords are asymptomatic, the decision to surgically untether the spinal cord must be based on the presence of well-documented clinical changes.

The clinical manifestations and management of the neurogenic bladder and bowel in individuals with myelomeningocele are not significantly different from children and adolescents with SCIs. However, individuals with myelomeningocele may have congenital anomalies of the genitourinary system that require additional monitoring or treatment (247). Males with myelomeningocele are at increased risk of cryptorchidism (248).

Urodynamic testing should be performed during the neonatal period, once the baby has been stabilized after repairing the myelomeningocele defect (249,250). Newborns at risk of developing urinary tract deterioration demonstrate high bladder pressures (leak point pressure of 40 cm H_2O or more) or detrussor–sphincter dyssynergia. These high-risk neonates should be managed with intermittent catheterization and anticholinergics as soon as they are identified by urodynamic testing. Compared to SCI, another major difference in individuals with myelomeningocele is the fact that they have neurogenic bladder dysfunction from conception. This may significantly retard the growth of the bladder, especially in children with high-pressure, low-volume bladders. Bladder augmentation may be required if the bladder capacity is inadequate despite anticholinergic therapy (250).

Intermittent catheterization is standard management of the neurogenic bladder for individuals with myelomeningocele (59,60,249,250,251). However, the ability to perform self-catheterization may be complicated by visual-motor deficits that are commonly found in patients with myelomeningocele and developmental delays that may also be present (60,252).

Bowel incontinence is a major problem for children with myelomeningocele, particularly for those without bulbocavernosus or anocutaneous reflexes (253). Aggressive interventions, including education and regular, consistently timed reflex-triggered bowel evacuations are effective (253). Patients with bowel program complications unresponsive to more conservative measures may be candidates for ACEs (77,254), pulsed irrigation enemas (76), enema continence catheters (255), or biofeedback (256).

Secondary manifestations or complications may be present at birth and be considered congenital defects, or they may be acquired postnatally. Congenital defects, such as clubfeet, dislocated hips, or extension contractures of the knees, are secondary complications of the primary spinal cord defect with resulting in utero paralysis. Postnatally acquired secondary complications result in significant morbidity and occasionally mortality. Prevention and early management of secondary complications are integral in the overall management of youth with myelomeningocele. Meningitis, ventriculitis, tethered cord, and shunt malfunction have already been discussed.

Orthopaedic Issues

Children and adolescents with myelomeningocele experience a variety of orthopaedic complications, particularly disorders of the lower extremities and spine (210,230,257). Orthopaedic deformities are the result of several factors, including paralysis, unopposed muscle function, congenital malformation, and spasticity (257). Orthopaedic deformities may be present at birth and result from paralysis present in utero, effecting the position of the fetus. Examples of this include club feet, dislocated hips, or extension contractures of the knees (230). Other orthopaedic abnormalities such as congenital vertebral and rib anomalies, present in as many as 15% of patients, may be present at birth and are primary defects associated with myelomeningocele. Postnatally acquired orthopaedic complications, such as dislocated hips, hip and knee contractures, and pathological fractures, may develop as a consequence of the neuromuscular defects associated with myelomeningocele. Lastly, scoliosis, kyphosis, and lordosis may be a consequence of both congenital vertebral anomalies and neuromuscular defects (258). The management of these orthopaedic complications is generally complicated and should be directed by clinicians experienced in caring for children and adolescents with myelomeningocele. Depending upon the neurological level, many children and adolescents with myelomeningocele will ambulate to varying degrees, so that management of the lower extremity deformities must take this into account.

Contractures and dislocation of hips are very common in children with myelomeningocele, particularly in those patients with thoracic and upper to mid-lumbar lesions, where up to 90% of patients may be affected (259). In thoracic level lesions, the hip dislocation occurs because all of the hip musculature is denervated (257). In contrast, for lumbar level lesions, hip dysplasia results from muscle imbalance with active hip flexors and adductors but paralyzed extensors and abductors. Management of hip dysplasia in the myelomeningocele population is controversial, particularly because hip dysplasia is usually not painful and may not significantly affect the ability to walk (260). For patients with thoracic and upper to mid-lumbar level lesions, treatment of the hip dysplasia is usually reserved for those with pelvic obliquity, who would be at higher risk of developing pressure ulcers. Children with lower lumbar lesions have good ambulation potential. Their dislocated hips should be surgically corrected by 4 years of age, including both skeletal corrections and muscle transfers, to prevent recurrent dislocation.

Hip contractures are common complications in patients with myelomeningocele and can interfere with ambulation, particularly if they exceed 30 to 40 degrees. Surgical releases are frequently complicated by recurrences. Management of hip contractures must be individualized and based on the neurological level, presence of hip dysplasia, and ambulation status. Hip contractures in patients with thoracic and upper lumbar levels are generally managed by surgical releases and aggressive postoperative bracing and physical therapy. For individuals with mid- to lower lumbar lesions, contractures are managed by a combination of surgical releases and appropriate tendon transfers. However, contracture releases should be limited to those with significant potential for continued ambulation. Hip and knee contractures in older children are most likely a consequence of disinterest in ambulation and increased use of wheeled mobility; therefore, contracture releases in this group of patients may not result in improved ambulation, and recurrence of the contractures is very common.

The major abnormalities of the knees are extension and flexion contractures and a valgus rotation deformity (257). Extension contractures are relatively uncommon and are usually the result of breech deliveries. They may also be seen in patients with mid-lumbar level lesions who have strong quadriceps without strong knee flexors. Most of these cases can be managed with physical therapy and splinting. For extension knee contractures that are resistant to conservative management, a modified V-Y quadricepsplasty should be performed. Knee flexion contractures less than 20 degrees are generally well tolerated, but more severe contractures may limit ambulation potential. Physical therapy and splinting may be effective in children under 2 years of age, otherwise surgical correction is indicated. Valgus rotation deformities of the knee result from iliotibial band tightness and the forces of ambulation. For younger children, treatment includes muscle transfers, distal iliotibial band sectioning, and KAFO. Distal femoral osteotomies may be necessary if the deformity becomes fixed.

Deformities of the ankle and feet are common in children and adolescents with myelomeningocele, and they tend to be resistant to conservative measures and generally require surgical correction (257). Approximately 50% of patients with myelomeningocele have club feet, as a result of muscle paralysis and in utero positioning. These clubfeet tend to be rigid, are resistant to casting, and usually require surgical repair (257). In patients with low lumbar lesions, calcaneovalgus deformities result from unopposed contraction of the anterior tibial muscle, toe extensors, or the peroneal muscles. The deformity is usually progressive, results in a crouch gait, and predisposes to pressure ulcers of the feet from shoe or brace wear. Surgical correction consists of transferring the anterior tibial tendon to the os calcis (257). Cavus deformities of the foot are frequently accompanied by claw toe deformities in individuals with sacral level lesions, predisposing to pressure ulcers under their toes or metatarsal heads.

Pathological fractures are most prevalent in children 3 to 7 years of age, and they are particularly common after cast immobilization or during skeletal traction (261). The fractures are usually in an epiphyseal or metaphyseal location. They can present with exuberant callus formation raising concerns of a tumor to the inexperienced clinician. The fractures typically present with a swollen, warm, and erythematous extremity in a febrile child. They should be managed with splinting and weight bearing should be initiated within 2 to 3 weeks to prevent further osteoporosis and to reduce the risk of further fractures (257).

Scoliosis is a very common complication of myelomeningocele, affecting the majority of patients (258,262). It may be caused by a number of factors, including congenital vertebral anomalies, neuromuscular weakness, pelvic obliquity, and hip contractures (235,258). Almost all patients with thoracic level lesions develop scoliosis with a decreased incidence with lower level lesions (258,263). Progressive scoliosis may be associated with uncompensated hydrocephalus, hydrosyringomyelia, or retethered spinal cord (264). Surgical correction of hydrocephalus, hydrosyringomyelia, or a retethered spinal cord may slow or halt progression of the scoliosis in patients with less severe curvatures (less than 40 degrees), but generally do not have an effect on more severe curves (264,265).

Management of scoliosis should include close monitoring of the motor and sensory exam, degree of spasticity, and deep tendon reflexes of both the upper and lower extremities. Serial radiographs at least annually should be performed. Imaging studies to exclude hydrocephalus, hydrosyringomyelia, and retethered cord should be performed on patients with progressive scoliosis especially if associated with progressive weakness or spasticity. Patients with curves greater than 25 degrees or those with unbalanced curves should wear bivalved molded body jackets when they are awake and up sitting, standing, or walking. Particular care must be taken to avoid development of pressure ulcers under the body jacket. Timing of the surgical repair and the extent and type of spine fusion depends upon

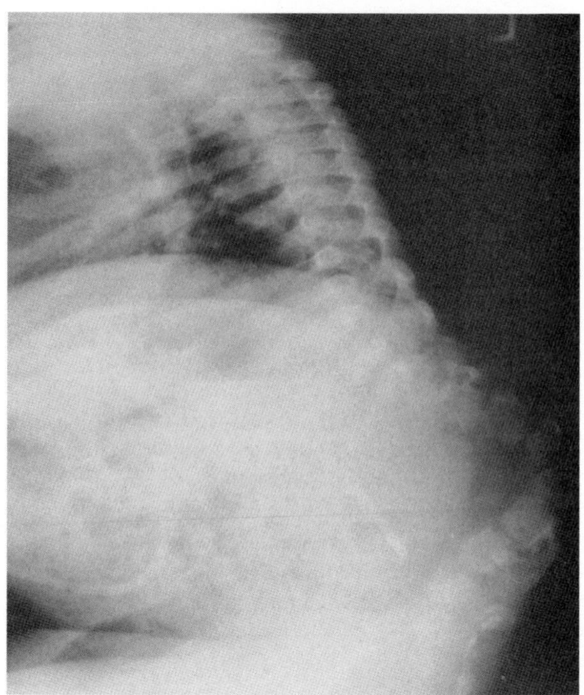

FIGURE 29.13 Severe kyphosis in a child with myelomeningocele.

the child's age (preferably after age 10), location and flexibility of the curve, neurological level, and ambulation status. The lumbosacral joint should generally not be fused in children who are ambulatory. Hip contractures should be corrected prior to spine surgery in order to avoid excessive torque to the spine fusion postoperatively (262).

Kyphosis affects 8% to 15% of patients with myelomeningocele, particularly those with thoracic level lesions, and is commonly severe (less than 90 degrees) (230,231,262) (Fig. 29.13). The kyphosis may interfere with sitting or wearing orthotics, and is a common cause for skin breakdown. Progression of the kyphosis may also compromise ventilation because abdominal contents are pushed up into the thorax. Surgical correction of kyphotic deformities is complex and technically demanding, and is associated with significant morbidity and mortality (231,262). Surgical correction usually requires the resection of a portion of the spine and dural sac. It is critical that adequate functioning of the ventriculoperitoneal shunt be assured in the preoperative evaluation.

Medical Issues

Individuals with myelomeningocele frequently have reduced stature that is caused by a variety of factors (266). These include spine and other orthopaedic deformities, decreased growth in paralyzed extremities, nutritional deficiencies, precocious puberty, and growth hormone deficiency. Approximately 10% to 20% of individuals with myelomeningocele experience precocious puberty (267–269). Precocious puberty is presumably related to brain abnormalities, more commonly affects females and those with hydrocephalus (267).

Children with myelomeningocele frequently become obese, particularly as they become adolescents (268,270) because of their sedentary lifestyle and limited ability and access to fitness activities (270). In addition, this population has a relatively high incidence of metabolic syndrome placing them at great risk of long-term cardiovascular complications (103). With an increasing life expectancy, it is imperative that effective fitness and nutritional programs be initiated during childhood and adolescence with the goal of reducing cardiovascular complications in adulthood.

Individuals with myelomeningocele are at particularly high risk of latex allergy with 18% to 64.5% being affected (271). The high incidence of latex allergy in the myelomeningocele population may be related to the multiple surgeries beginning at a young age that this group of children undergo (272). Sensitization to latex may be reduced in the myelomeningocele population by minimizing exposure to latex (273).

Similar to individuals with SCI, children and adolescents with myelomeningocele are susceptible to developing pressure ulcers (274). Prevention and management of pressure ulcers in patients with myelomeningocele may be complicated by associated cognitive and behavioral disturbances.

Psychosocial and Sexuality

In addition to the psychosocial and sexuality issues that are integral to the development of all children and adolescents, individuals with myelomeningocele face additional burdens because of their chronic physical, psychological, and cognitive deficits (275). This is compounded by the onset of disability at birth and the varying expectations that parents have for their child's future (398). Sexuality and reproductive health issues must be addressed in a developmentally appropriate fashion for children and adolescents as well as for their parents (277). This should include sexual abuse and exploitation, fertility, and sexual functioning.

Although most children with myelomeningocele should be educated in a regular school setting, their psychosocial/sexuality development may be limited by cognitive defects, visuomotor disturbances, learning disabilities, and frequent absences related to health care needs (235). Adult outcomes, including employment and independence, are areas that must be an integral component of the comprehensive care for this population of children (278,279).

Prevention

Folic acid has been demonstrated to be effective in preventing neural-tube defects if taken in the periconceptual period (280–283). It has been estimated that periconceptual use of folic acid can reduce the risk of neural-tube defects by 50% in the general population and 72% in high-risk individuals who have previously had an affected pregnancy (282,283). The United States Public Health Service recommends that all women of childbearing age consume 0.4 mg of folic acid daily, but care should be taken to keep total folate consumption to less than 1 mg/d (282). Women who have had a prior neural-tube defect affected pregnancy should consume 4.0 mg of folic acid daily from at least 1 month before conception through the first 3 months of the pregnancy (282,283).

Prenatal screening for myelomeningocele is accomplished by maternal serum alpha-fetoprotein testing between the 16th and 18th week of gestation (284,285). Confirmation of the diagnosis can be established with high resolution ultrasound or elevated levels of alpha-fetoprotein or acetylcholinesterase in the amniotic fluid (284,286). Prenatal diagnosis provides the parents the opportunity to consider termination of the pregnancy. It alternatively assists parents and health care providers in planning the most appropriate prenatal and postnatal care, such as in utero surgery, elective Cesarean section, and delivery in a medical center that is experienced in caring for newborns with myelomeningoceles (285).

Experimental evidence suggests that some of the neurolgic deficits associated with myelomeningocele may be caused by prolonged exposure of the dysplastic spinal cord to the intrauterine environment, as a result of toxicity of the amniotic fluid or physical trauma (232,287). In utero repair of the myelomeningocele sac has been performed on fetuses at 22 to 28 weeks of gestation and a preliminary report has demonstrated a decreased incidence shunt-dependent hydrocephalus, reversal of the Chiari II malformation, and possibly improved leg function (288,289). However, fetal surgery may result in significant adverse events, including premature labor and birth. In order to compare the safety and efficacy of intrauterine repair with standard postnatal repair, the "Management of Myelomeningocele Study," a National institute of Child Health and Human Development funded study, was initiated in 2003 (288,289).

Elective prelabor Cesarean section has been advocated as a means to prevent further damage to the dysplastic spinal cord as a result of uterine contractions and passage through the birth canal (290,291). The most appropriate circumstances for this approach may be fetuses with lower extremity movement noted on ultrasound, minimal to no hydrocephalus, and neural elements that protrude dorsally (290). However, currently there is insufficient evidence to support prophylactic Cesarean delivery of infants with myelomeningocele (292).

Lipomeningocele

Lipomeningoceles are a form of occult spinal dysraphism with intact skin covering the defect (293). In lipomeningocele, the spinal cord remains within the spinal canal with the junction between the cord and the lipoma also residing within the canal (Fig. 29.14). Individuals with lipomeningoceles are generally normal at birth. Neurologic symptoms first appear during the second year of life, and most patients exhibit some neurologic deficits by early childhood. The typical presenting complaint is that of a cosmetic deformity, a subcutaneous fat collection in the lower back and upper buttocks. Approximately 50% of affected individuals have cutaneous markings, such as a midline dimple, hairy patch, or a hemangiomatous nevus. Surgery is performed with the goal of untethering the spinal cord. Removal of the entire lipoma is generally not performed because the neural tissue extends into the lipoma and aggressive surgical excision of the lipoma may result in a significantly greater neurological deficit.

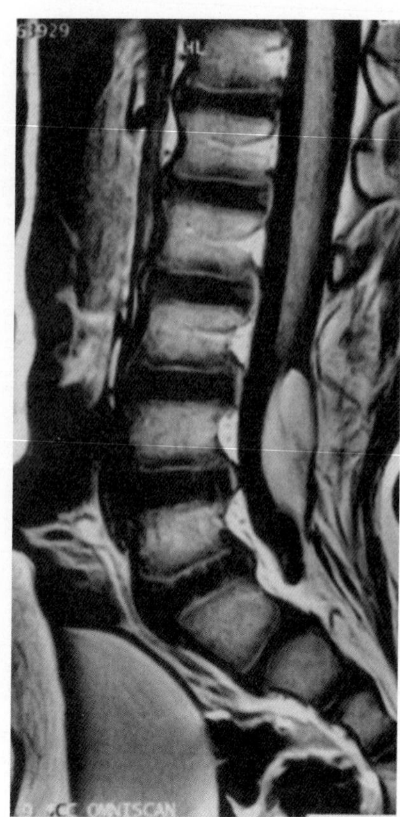

FIGURE 29.14 Magnetic resonance image of a child with a lipomeningocele, demonstrating tethering of the spinal cord and an intraspinal lipoma.

Sacral Agenesis

Sacral agenesis is not a neural-tube defect and is a relatively uncommon congenital anomaly with varying degrees of deficiencies of the sacrum and associated neurological abnormalities (294, 295) (Fig. 29.15). Sacral agenesis is associated with maternal diabetes mellitus, with 1% of infants born to diabetic mothers having sacral agenesis (296). Approximately 12% to 16% of infants with sacral agenesis are born to mothers with diabetes mellitus. Patients generally present either during infancy or between 4 and 5 years of age with persistent urinary incontinence and chronic constipation (295). The majority of affected children also have neurologic deficits of their lower extremities; 40% had weakness and 86% had altered deep tendon reflexes. Interestingly, sensation was usually intact caudally for several segments below the motor level for most individuals with sacral agenesis (294). About two-thirds of affected patients have severe orthopaedic deformities of their lower extremities, including webbed knees requiring amputation with clubfeet being the most common problem (Fig. 29.15).

HYDROSYRINGOMYELIA

Hydrosyringomyelia, or cystic formation in the spinal cord, may also be referred to as syringomyelia, hydromyelia, or syrinx (297). Although hydrosyringomyelia may be associated with spinal cord trauma, tumors, or arachnoiditis, this section will be limited to developmental hydrosyringomyelia. Hydromyelia refers to a dilated central canal communicating with the fourth ventricle and lined by ependyma. In contrast, syringomyelia refers to tubular cavitation within the spinal cord, which is lined by glial cells. From a clinical perspective, there is

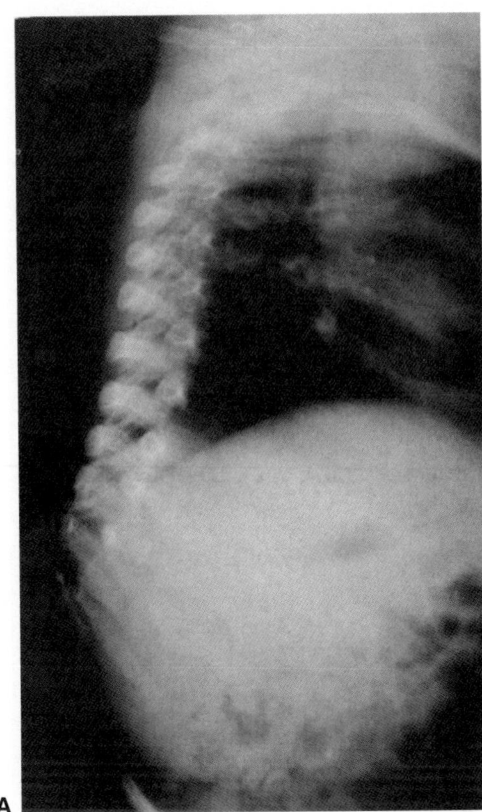

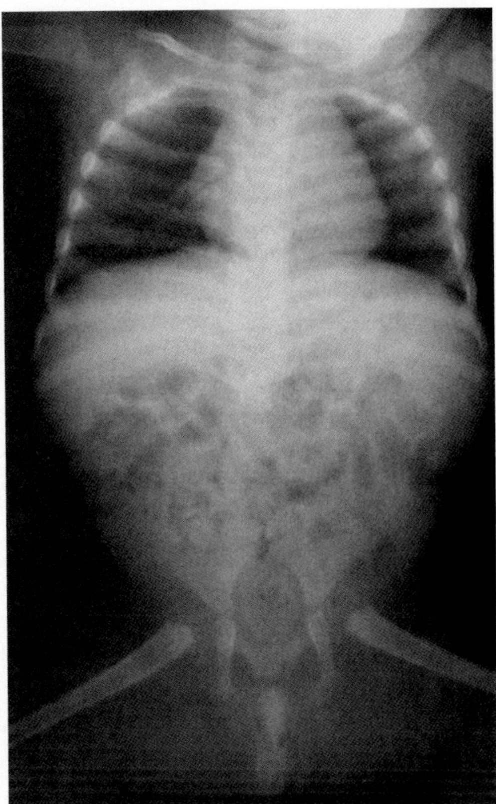

FIGURE 29.15 Radiographs of a child with sacral agenesis demonstrating abrupt loss of the vertebral column at T12-L1

no clear distinction between syringomyelia and hydromyelia, and in this section they will be discussed as one entity, and referred to as hydrosyringomyelia or syrinx.

Developmental hydrosyringomyelia is frequently associated with a Chiari I malformation, in which there is caudal displacement of the cerebellar tonsils below the foramen magnum (Fig. 29.16). It is postulated that the syrinx is caused by altered CSF dynamics at the craniospinal junction as a result of the Chiari I abnormality. The syrinx is most commonly located in the cervical or cervicothoracic spinal cord, but may involve the entire spinal cord. The syrinx may also extend into the brain stem, in which case it is referred to as syringobulbia.

Although hydrosyringomyelia may become symptomatic at any age, typically it does not become clinically apparent until adulthood (298). Nonetheless, many affected patients become symptomatic during childhood or adolescence, and with the ready availability of MRI diagnosis at an earlier age is facilitated (297). The classic presentation of hydrosyringomyelia includes occipital or neck pain, suspended and dissociated sensory loss in a cape distribution, hypotonic weakness of the upper extremities, and spastic weakness in the lower extremities. The occipital and cervical pain may be caused by compression or stretching of upper cervical roots by the Chiari I malformation or distortion of descending fibers of the trigeminal nerves. The usual location of a syrinx in the central part of the spinal cord preferentially affects fibers crossing through the central white matter, compromising temperature and pain sensation with relative sparing of the posterior columns. As the syrinx expands, anterior horn cells, corticospinal tracts, and the posterior columns become affected. The typical location of the syrinx in the cervical or cervicothoracic spinal cord is responsible for the flaccid upper extremity weakness and spastic lower extremity weakness.

Other symptoms of hydrosyringomyelia include dysesthesia in the peripheral dermatomes of the sensory or motor dysfunction. Symptoms related to posterior column dysfunction are relatively common. In one series of 58 patients with hydrosyringomyelia, 76% had abnormalities of proprioception with involvement of the arms alone in 25%, legs alone in 25%, and both the arms and legs in 50% (299). In this same series of 58 patients, 32 (55%) had nystagmus, 50 (86%) had ataxia or limb incoordination primarily due to proprioceptive defects, 5 (9%) had bladder dysfunction, and 2 experienced erectile dysfunction. Eighteen of the fifty-eight patients had symptoms referable to syringobulbia, including swallowing problems, nystagmus, tongue fibrillation, and impaired pharyngeal sensation. Other symptoms referable to brain stem involvement and impingement on the dorsal nuclei of the vagus nerve include either episodic or chronic stridor.

Orthopaedic abnormalities associated with hydrosyringomyelia include scoliosis, pes cavus, and Charcot's joints (297,300,301). In children and adolescents, scoliosis is a relatively common manifestation of hydrosyringomyelia and frequently is progressive, necessitating bracing and surgical intervention (297,300,302). For patients with scoliosis, characteristics that may indicate an underlying hydrosyringomyelia include a left thoracic curve, progressive curves in males, and an abnormal neurological exam such as asymmetric or absent umbilical reflexes.

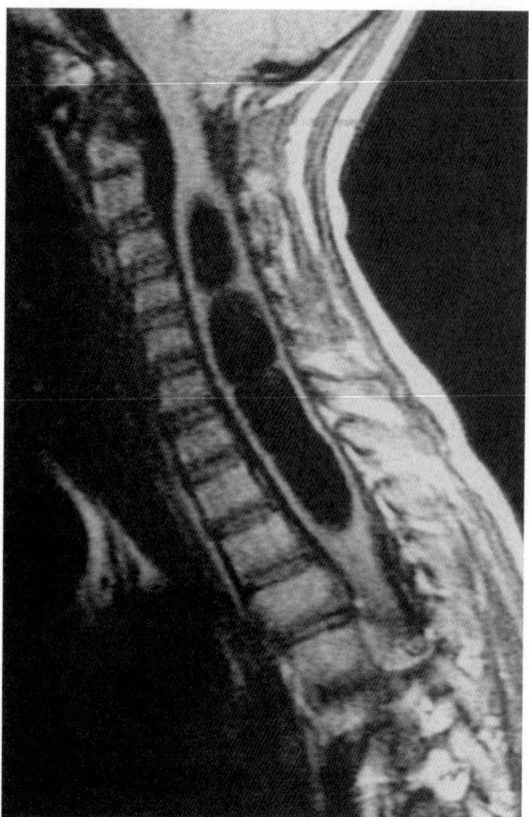

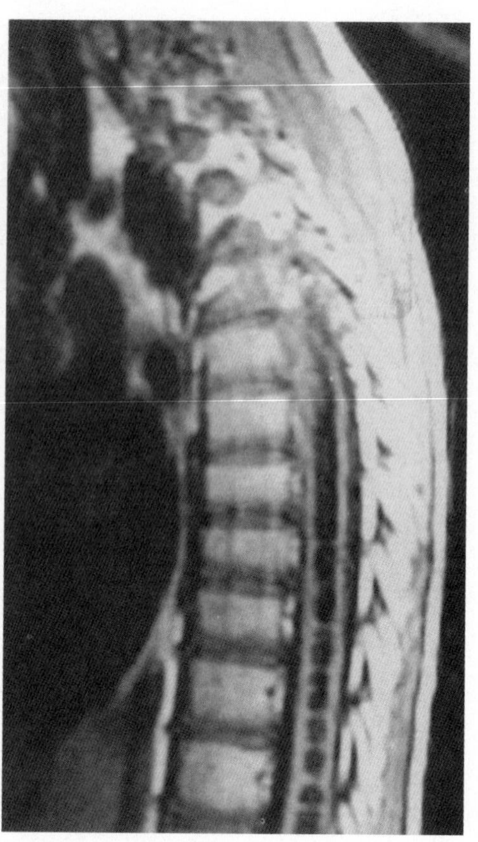

FIGURE 29.16 Magnetic resonance imaging study of a child with hydrosyringomyelia involving the cervical (**A**) and the thoracic (**B**) spinal cord. (**A**) also demonstrates the Chiari I malformation with caudal displacement of the cerebellar tonsils below the foramen magnum.

MRI would be the most appropriate imaging technique to diagnose hydrosyringomyelia and associated neurological abnormalities, such as Chiari I malformation (303). The use of MRI with gadolinium contrast is indicated to exclude intraspinal tumors. Conventional metrizamide myelography with delayed CT imaging can also be utilized to diagnose hydrosyringomyelia, although MRI is the preferred imaging modality. Plain radiographs of the head, neck, and spine should also be obtained in order to identify associated abnormalities, such as scoliosis, a shallow posterior fossa, widening of the spinal canal, basilar invagination, or Klippel-Feil anomaly.

In general, hydrosyringomyelia is a neurodegenerative process with relentless progression, which is usually protracted over time. It is imperative that a patient's clinical course be followed closely in a serial fashion in order to identify progression of neurological findings. Management of hydrosyringomyelia, including indications, timing of interventions and the specific treatment modality, is not entirely clear-cut. For the occasional patient with hydrocephalus, a ventriculoperitoneal shunt should be performed initially. For patients who are asymptomatic, careful clinical observation is essential. However, the decision to observe without surgical interventions must be weighed against the natural history of hydrosyringomyelia, which is one of progressive loss of neurological function and recovery of neurological deficits that is variable after surgical interventions. Currently, the treatment of choice would be posterior fossa decompression with the goal of restoring adequate CSF dynamics at the craniospinal junction (299,303,304). Among patients undergoing posterior fossa decompression, approximately 70% will demonstrate either improvement or stabilization of their neurological status; whereas, complete resolution of neurological deficits is rarely observed. Another treatment option is direct decompression of the syrinx utilizing either a one-time aspiration of the syrinx or a shunt from the syrinx to the subarachnoid space, pleura, or peritoneum (304,305). Close clinical follow-up is essential after surgical interventions have been performed, with MRIs being useful in monitoring the progression of the syrinx.

ACKNOWLEDGEMENTS

The authors would like to acknowledge the assistance of Jim Cockerill.

References

1. Bray GP. Rehabilitation of the spinal cord injured: a family approach. *J Appl Rehabil Counsel* 1978;9:70–78.
2. Anderson CJ, Johnson KA, Klaas SJ, et al. Pediatric spinal cord injury: transition to adulthood. *J Voc Rehabil* 1998;10:103–113.
3. Smith QW, Frieden L, Nelson MR, et al. Transition to adulthood for young people with spinal cord injury. In: Betz RR, Mulcahey MJ, eds. *The child with a spinal cord*

injury. Rosemont, IL: American Academy of Orthopaedic Surgeons, 1996:601–612.

4. Vogel LC, Klaas SJ, Lubicky, JP, et al. Long-term outcomes and life satisfaction of adults with pediatric spinal cord injuries. *Arch Phys Med Rehabil* 1998;79:1496–1503.
5. Anderson CJ, Vogel LC. Employment outcomes of adults who sustained spinal cord injuries as children or adolescents. *Arch Phys Med Rehabil* 2002;83:791–801.
6. Anderson CJ, Krajci KA, Vogel LC. Life satisfaction in adults with pediatric-onset spinal cord injury. *J Spinal Cord Med* 2002;25:184–190
7. Anderson CJ, Vogel LC. Decreased work experience in adolescents with spinal cord injuries compared with peers: implications for adult employment. *Dev Med Child Neurol* 2000;42:515–517.
8. Mulcahey MJ, DiGiovanni N, Calhoun C, et al. Children's and parents' perspectives of activity performance and participation following spinal cord injury. *Am J Occup Ther* 2010;64(4):605–613.
9. Massagli, TL, Dudgeon, BJ, Ross, BW. Educational performance and vocational participation after spinal cord injury in childhood. *Arch Phys Med Rehabil* 1996;77:995–999.
10. Vogel LC. Long-term prophylactic medical care. In: Betz RR, Mulcahey MJ, eds. *The child with a spinal cord injury*. Rosemont, IL: American Academy of Orthopaedic Surgeons, 1996:679–688.
11. Betz RR, Mulcahey MJ, eds. *The child with a spinal cord injury*. Rosemont: American Academy of Orthopaedic Surgeons, 1996.
12. Massagli TL. Medical and rehabilitation issues in the care of children with spinal cord injury. *Phys Med Rehabil Clin N Am* 2000;11:169–182.
13. Vogel LC, Betz RR, Mulcahey MJ. The child with a spinal cord injury. *Dev Med Child Neurol* 1997;39;202–207.
14. Nobunaga AI, Go BK, Karunas RB. Recent demographic and injury trends in people served by the Model Spinal Cord Injury Care Systems. *Arch Phys Med Rehabil* 1999;80:1372–1382.
15. Price C, Makintubee S, Herndon W, et al. Epidemiology of traumatic spinal cord injury and acute hospitalization and rehabilitation charges for spinal cord injuries in Oklahoma, 1988–1990. *Am J Epidemiol* 1994;139:37–47.
16. Bracken MB, Freeman DH, Hellenbrand K. Incidence of acute traumatic hospitalized spinal cord injury in the United States, 1970–1977. *Am J Epidemiol* 1981;113:615–622.
17. Colorado Department of Public Health and Environment. *1995 Annual Report of the Spinal Cord Injury Early Notification System*. Denverco: Colorado Department of Transportation Printing Office; 1996.
18. Hadley MN, Zabramski JM, Browner CM, et al. Pediatric spinal trauma. Review of 122 cases of spinal cord and vertebral column injuries. *J Neurosurg* 1988;68:18–24.
19. Hamilton MG, Myles ST. Pediatric spinal injury: review of 174 hospital admissions. *J Neurosurg* 1992;77:700–704.
20. Kewalramani LS, Kraus JF, Sterling HM. Acute spinal-cord lesions in a pediatric population: epidemiological and clinical features. *Paraplegia* 1980;18:206–219.
21. Vogel LC, DeVivo MJ. Etiology and demographics. In: Betz RR, Mulcahey MJ, eds. *The child with a spinal cord injury*. Rosemont, IL: American Academy of Orthopaedic Surgeons, 1996:3–12.
22. Vogel LC, DeVivo MJ. Pediatric spinal cord injury issues: etiology, demographics, and pathophysiology. *Top Spinal Cord Inj Rehabil* 1997;3:1–8.
23. Shavelle RM, DeVivo MJ, Vogel LC, et al. Long-term survival after childhood spinal cord injury. *J Spinal Cord Med* 2007;30:S48–S54.
24. Mulcahey MJ, Gaughan J, Betz RR, et al. The international standards for neurological classification of spinal cord injury: reliability of data when applied to children and youth. *Spinal Cord* 2007;45:452–459.
25. Mulcahey MJ, Gaughan J, Betz RR, et al. Rater reliability on the ISCSCI motor and sensory scores obtained before and after formal training in testing technique. *J Spinal Cord Med* 2007;30:S146–S149.
26. Vogel L, Samdani A, Chafetz R, et al. Intra-rater reliability of the anorectal examination and classification of injury severity in children with spinal cord injury. *Spinal Cord* 2009;47(9):687–691.
27. Savic G, Bergstrom EM, Frankel HL, et al. Inter-rater reliability of motor and sensory examinations performed according to American Spinal Injury Association standards. *Spinal Cord* 2007;45:444–451.
28. Jonsson M, Tollback A, Gonzales H, et al. Inter-rater reliability of the 1992 international standards for neurological and functional classification of incomplete spinal cord injury. *Spinal Cord* 2000;38:675–679.
29. Gabos PG. Tuten HR, Leet A, et al. Fracture-dislocation of the lumbar spine in an abused child. *Pediatrics* 1998;101:473–477.
30. Piatt JH, Steinberg M. Isolated spinal cord injury as a presentation of child abuse. *Pediatrics* 1995;96:780–782.
31. Wilberger JE Jr. Clinical aspects of specific spinal injuries. In: Wilberger JE Jr, ed. *Spinal cord injuries in children*. Mount Kisco, NY: Futura Publishers, 1986:69–95.
32. Knebusch M, Strassburg HM, Reiners K. Acute transverse myelitis in childhood: nine cases and review of the literature. *Dev Med Child Neurol* 1998:40;631–639.
33. Toro G, Roman GC, Navarro-Roman L, et al. Natural history of spinal cord infarction caused by nucleus pulposus embolism. *Spine* 1994;19:360–366.
34. Apple DF, Murray HH. Lap belt injuries in children. In: Betz RR, Mulcahey MJ, eds. *The child with a spinal cord injury*. Rosemont, IL: American Academy of Orthopaedic Surgeons, 1996:169–177.
35. Garrett JW, Braunstein PW. The seat belt syndrome. *J Trauma* 1962;2:220–238.
36. Johnson DL, Falci S. The diagnosis and treatment of pediatric lumbar spine injuries caused by rear seat lap belts. *Neurosurgery* 1990;26:434–441.
37. Centers for Disease Control. Motor-vehicle occupant fatalities and restraint use among children aged 4–8 Years—United States, 1994–1998. *MMWR Morb Mortal Wkly Rep* 2000;49:135–137.
38. http://www.nhtsa.dot.gov/portal/site/nhtsa/menuitem.9f8c7d6359e0e9bbbf30811060008a0c/.
39. Bresnan MJ, Abroms IF. Neonatal spinal cord transection secondary to intrauterine hyperextension of the neck in breech presentation. *J Pediatrics* 1974;84:734–737.
40. Hankins GDV. Lower thoracic spinal cord injury—a severe complication of shoulder dystocia. *Am J Perinatol* 1998;15:443–444.

41. MacKinnon JA, Perlman M, Kirpalani, et al. Spinal cord injury at birth: diagnostic and prognostic data in twenty-two patients. *J Pediatrics* 1993;122:431–437.
42. Medlock MD, Hanigan WC. Neurologic birth trauma. Intracranial, spinal cord, and brachial plexus injury. *Clin Perinatol* 1997;24:845–857.
43. Menticoglou SM, Perlman M, Manning FA. High cervical spinal cord injury in neonates delivered with forceps: report of 15 cases. *Obstet Gynecol* 1995;86:589–594.
44. Rossitch E, Oakes WJ. Perinatal spinal cord injury: clinical, radiographic and pathologic features. *Pediatr Neurosurg* 1992;18:149–152.
45. Ruggieri M, Smarason AK, Pike M. Spinal cord insults in the prenatal, perinatal, and neonatal periods. *Dev Med Child Neurol* 1999;41:311–317.
46. Tredwell SJ, Newman DE, Lockith G. Instability of the upper cervical spine in Down syndrome. *J Pediatr Orthop* 1990;10:602–606.
47. Ward WT. Atlanto-axial instability in children with Down syndrome. In: Betz RR, Mulcahey MJ, eds. *The child with a spinal cord injury*. Rosemont, IL: American Academy of Orthopaedic Surgeons, 1996:89–96.
48. Nathan FF, Bickel WH. Spontaneous axial subluxation in a child as the first sign of juvenile rheumatoid arthritis. *J Bone Joint Surg* 1968;50A:1675–1678.
49. Vogel LC, Lubicky JP. Cervical spine fusion not protective of cervical spine injury and tetraplegia. *Am J Orthopaedics* 1997;26:636–640.
50. Goldberg MJ. Orthopedic aspects of bone dysplasias. *Orthop Clin N Am* 1976;7:445–455.
51. Yang SS, Corbett DP, Brough AJ, et al. Upper cervical myelopathy in achondroplasia. *Am J Clin Path* 1977;68:68–72.
52. Pang D, Wilberger JE. Spinal cord injury without radiographic abnormalities in children. *J Neurosurg* 1982;57:114–129.
53. Osenbach RK, Menezes AH. Spinal cord injury without radiographic abnormality in children. *Pediatr Neurosci* 1989;15:168–175.
54. Dickman CA, Zambramski JM, Hadley MN, et al. Pediatric spinal cord injury without radiographic abnormalities: report of 26 cases and review of the literature. *J Spinal Disord* 1991;4:296–305.
55. Felsberg GJ, Tien RD, Osumi AK, et al. Utility of MR imaging in pediatric spinal cord injury. *Pediatr Radiol* 1995;25:131–135.
56. Grabb PA, Pang D. Magnetic resonance imaging in the evaluation of spinal cord injury without radiographic abnormality in children. *Neurosurgery* 1994;35:406–413.
57. Choi JU, Hoffman HJ, Hendrick EB, et al. Traumatic infarction of the spinal cord in children. *J Neurosurg* 1986;65:608–610.
58. Fernandes ET, Reinberg Y, Vernier R, et al. Neurogenic bladder dysfunction in children: review of pathophysiology and current management. *J Pediatr* 1994;124:1–7.
59. Lapides J, Diokno AC, Silber SJ, et al. Clean intermittent self-catheterization in the treatment of urinary tract disease. *J Urol* 1972;107:458–461.
60. McLaughlin JF, Murray M, Van Zandt K, et al. Clean intermittent catheterization. *Dev Med Child Neurol* 1996;38:446–454.
61. Pontari MA, Bauer SB. Urologic issues in spinal cord injury: assessment, management, outcome, and research needs. In: Betz RR, Mulcahey MJ, eds. *The child with a spinal cord injury*. Rosemont, IL: American Academy of Orthopaedic Surgeons, 1996:213–231.
62. Vogel LC, Pontari M. Pediatric spinal cord injury issues: medical issues. *Top Spinal Cord Inj Rehabil* 1997;3:20–30.
63. National Institute on Disability and Rehabilitation Research Consensus Statement. The prevention and management of urinary tract infections among people with spinal cord injuries. *J Am Paraplegia Soc* 1992;15: 194–204.
64. Schaad UB. Pediatric use of quinolones. *Pediatr Infect Dis J* 1999;18:469–470.
65. Pannek J, Diederichs W, Botel U. Urodynamically controlled management of spinal cord injury in children. *Neurourol Urodyn* 1997;16:285–292.
66. Gray GJ, Yang C. Surgical procedures of the bladder after spinal cord injury. *Phys Med Rehabil Clin N Am* 2000;11:57–72.
67. Kass EJ, Koff SA. Bladder augmentation in the pediatric neuropathic bladder. *J Urol* 1983;129:552–555.
68. Vogel LC. Unique management needs of pediatric spinal cord injury patients. *J Spinal Cord Med* 1997;20:17–20.
69. Mitrofanoff P. Trans-appendicular continent cystotomy in the management of the neurogenic bladder. *Chir Pediatr* 1980;21:297–305.
70. Chaviano AH, Matkov TG, Anderson CJ, et al. Mitrofanoff continent catheterizable stoma for pediatric patients with spinal cord injuries. *Top Spinal Cord Inj Rehabil* 2000;6(suppl):30–35.
71. Pontari MA, Weibel B, Morales V, et al. Improved quality of life after continent urinary diversion in pediatric patients with quadriplegia after spinal cord injury. *Top Spinal Cord Inj Rehabil* 2000;6(suppl):25–29.
72. Consortium for Spinal Cord Medicine. *Neurogenic bowel management in adults with spinal cord injury*. Washington, DC: Paralyzed Veterans of America, 1998.
73. Goetz LL, Hurvitz EA, Nelson VS, et al. Bowel management in children and adolescents with spinal cord injury. *J Spinal Cord Med* 1998;21:335–341.
74. Kirshblum SC, Gulati M, O'Connor KC, et al. Bowel care practices in chronic spinal cord injury patients. *Arch Phys Med Rehabil* 1998;79:20–23.
75. Stiens SA, Bergman SB, Goetz LL. Neurogenic bowel dysfunction after spinal cord injury: clinical evaluation and rehabilitative management. *Arch Phys Med Rehabil* 1997;78:S86–S102.
76. Puet TA, Jackson H, Amy S. Use of pulsed irrigation evacuation in the management of the neuropathic bowel. *Spinal Cord* 1997;35:694–699.
77. Ellsworth PI, Webb HW, Crump JM, et al. The Malone antegrade colonic enema enhances the quality of life in children undergoing urological incontinence procedures. *J Urol* 1996;155:1416–1418.
78. Radecki RT, Gaebler-Spira D. Deep vein thrombosis in the disabled pediatric population. *Arch Phys Med Rehabil* 1994;75:248–250.
79. David M, Andrew M. Venous thromboembolic complications in children. *J Pediatr* 1993;123:337–346.
80. Consortium for Spinal Cord Medicine. Prevention of thromboembolism in spinal cord injury. *J Spinal Cord Med* 1997;20:259–283.

81. Monagle P, Chalmers E, Chan A, et al; American College of Chest Physicians. Antithrombotic therapy in neonates and children: American College of Chest Physicians Evidence-Based Clinical Practice Guidelines (8th Edition). *Chest* 2008;133:887S–968S
82. Dix D, Andrew M, Marzinotti V, et al. The use of low molecular weight heparin in pediatric patients: a prospective cohort study. *J Pediatr* 2000;136:439–445.
83. Massicotte P, Adams M, Marzinotto V, et al. Low-molecular-weight heparin in pediatric patients with thrombotic disease: a dose finding study. *J Pediatr* 1996;128:313–318.
84. Maynard FM. Immobilization hypercalcemia following spinal cord injury. *Arch Phys Med Rehabil* 1986;67:41–44.
85. Tori JA, Hill LL. Hypercalcemia in children with spinal cord injury. *Arch Phys Med Rehabil* 1978;59:443–447.
86. Kedlaya D, Branstater ME, Lee JK. Immobilization hypercalcemia in incomplete paraplegia: successful treatment with pamidronate. *Arch Phys Med Rehabil* 1998;79:222–225.
87. Consortium for Spinal Cord Medicine. Acute management of autonomic dysreflexia: adults with spinal cord injury presenting to health-care facilities. *J Spinal Cord Med* 1997;20:284–309.
88. Hickey KJ, Vogel LC, Willis KM, et al. Prevalence and etiology of autonomic dysreflexia in children with spinal cord injuries. *J Spinal Cord Med* 2004;27:S54–S60.
89. McGinnis KB, Vogel LC, McDonald CM, et al. Recognition and management of autonomic dysreflexia in pediatric spinal cord injury. *J Spinal Cord Med* 2004;27:S61–S74.
90. Schottler J, Vogel L, Chafetz R, et al. Patient and caregiver knowledge of autonomic dysreflexia among youth with spinal cord injury. *Spinal Cord* 2009;47: 681–686.
91. Anderson LS, Biering-Sorensen F, Muller PG, et al. The prevalence of hyperhidrosis in patients with spinal cord injuries and an evaluation of the effect of dextropropoxyphene hydrochloride in therapy. *Paraplegia* 1992;30:184–191.
92. Fast A. Reflex sweating in patients with spinal cord injury: a review. *Arch Phys Med Rehabil* 1977;58:435–437.
93. Staas WE, Nemunaitis G. Management of reflex sweating in spinal cord injured patients. *Arch Phys Med Rehabil* 1989;70:544–546.
94. Glasauer FE, Czyrny JJ. Hyperhidrosis as the presenting symptom in post-traumatic syringomyelia. *Paraplegia* 1994;32:423–429.
95. Falci SP, Lammertse DP, Best L, et al. Surgical treatment of posttraumatic cystic and tethered spinal cords. *J Spinal Cord Med* 1999;22:173–181.
96. Canaday BR, Stanford RH. Propantheline bromide in the management of hyperhidrosis association with spinal cord injury. *Ann Pharmcother* 1995;29:489–492.
97. Formal C. Metabolic and neurologic changes after spinal cord injury. *Phys Med Rehabil Clin N Am* 1992;3:783–796.
98. Petrofsky JS. Thermoregulatory stress during rest and exercise in heat in patients with a spinal cord injury. *Eur J Appl Physiol* 1992;64:503–507.
99. Beraldo PSS, Neves EGC, Alves CMF, et al. Pyrexia in hospitalized spinal cord injury patients. *Paraplegia* 1993;31:186–191.
100. Sugarman B, Brown D, Musher D. Fever and infection in spinal cord injury patients. *JAMA* 1982;248: 66–70.
101. Sheridan R. Diagnosis of the acute abdomen in the neurologically stable spinal cord-injured patient: a case study. *J Clin Gastroenterol* 1992;15:325–328.
102. DeVivo MJ, Krause JS. Lammertse DP. Recent trends in mortality and causes of death among persons with spinal cord injury. *Arch Phys Med Rehabil* 1999;80:1411–1419.
103. Nelson MD, Widman LM, Abresch RT, et al. Metabolic syndrome in adolescents with spinal cord dysfunction. *J Spinal Cord Med* 2007;30:S127–S139.
104. Liusuwan A, Wiman L, Abresch RT, et al. Altered body composition affects resting energy expenditure and interpretation of body mass index in children with spinal cord injury. *J Spinal Cord Med* 2004;27:S24–S28.
105. McDonald CM, Abresch-Meyer AL, Nelson MD, et al. Body mass index and body composition measures by dual X-ray absorptiometry in patients aged 10 to 21 years with spinal cord injury. *J Spinal Cord Med* 2007;30: S97–S104.
106. Patt PL, Agena SM, Vogel LC, et al. Estimation of resting energy expenditure in children with spinal cord injuries. *J Spinal Cord Med* 2007;30:S83–S87.
107. Liusuwan RA, Widman LM, Abresch RT, et al. Body composition and resting energy expenditure in patients aged 11 to 21 years with spinal dysfunction compared to controls: comparisons and relationships among the groups. *J Spinal Cord Med* 2007;30:S105–S111.
108. Widman LM, Abresch RT, Styne DM, et al. Aerobic fitness and upper extremity strength in patients aged 11 to 21 years with spinal cord dysfunction as compared to ideal weight and overweight controls. *J Spinal Cord Med* 2007;30:S88–S96.
109. King ML, Freeman DM, Pellicone JT, et al. Exertional hypotension in thoracic spinal cord injury: case report. *Paraplegia* 1992;30:261–266.
110. Hopman MT, Oeseburg B, Binkhorst RA. Cardiovascular responses in persons with paraplegia to prolonged arm exercise and thermal stress. *Med Sci Sports Exerc* 1993;25:577–583.
111. Liusuwan RA, Widman LM, Abresch RT, et al. Behavioral intervention, exercise, and nutrition education to improve health and fitness (BENEfit) in adolescents with mobility impairment due to spinal dysfunction. *J Spinal Cord Med* 2007;30:S119–S126.
112. Johnson KA, Klaas SJ. Recreation involvement and play in pediatric spinal cord injury. *Top Spinal Cord Inj Rehabil* 2000;6(suppl):105–109.
113. Anderson JM, Schutt AH. Spinal cord injury in children: a review of 156 cases seen from 1950 through 1978. *Mayo Clin Proc* 1980;55:499–504.
114. Lau C, McCormack G. Chronic pain management in pediatric spinal cord injury. In: Betz RR, Mulcahey MJ, eds. *The child with a spinal cord injury*. Rosemont, IL: American Academy of Orthopaedic Surgeons, 1996;653–670.
115. Bryce TN, Ragnarsson KT. Pain after spinal cord injury. *Phys Med Rehabil Clin N Am* 2000;11:157–168.
116. Siddall PJ, Taylor DA, Cousins MJ. Classification of pain following spinal cord injury. *Spinal Cord* 1997;35:69–75.

117. Vogel LC, Anderson CJ. Self-injurious behavior in children and adolescents with spinal cord injuries. *Spinal Cord* 2002;40:666–668.
118. Balazy TE. Clinical management of chronic pain in spinal cord injury. *Clin J Pain* 1992;8:102–110.
119. Umlauf RL. Psychological interventions for chronic pain following spinal cord injury. *Clin J Pain* 1992;8:111–118.
120. Bowsher D. Central pain following spinal and supraspinal lesions. *Spinal Cord* 1999;37:235–238.
121. Sandford PR, Lindblom LB, Haddox JD. Amitriptyline and carbamazepine in the treatment of dysesthetic pain in spinal cord injury. *Arch Phys Med Rehabil* 1992;73:300–301.
122. Landwehr LP, Boguniewicz M. Current perspectives on latex allergy. *J Pediatr* 1996;128:305–312.
123. Slater JE. Latex allergy. *J Allergy Clin Immunol* 1994;94:139–149.
124. Vogel LC, Schrader T, Lubicky JP. Latex allergy in children and adolescents with spinal cord injuries. *J Pediatr Orthop* 1995;15:517–520.
125. Monasterio EA, Barber DB, Rogers SJ, et al. Latex allergy in adults with spinal cord injury: a pilot investigation. *J Spinal Cord Med*, 2000;23:6–9.
126. Fisher AA. Association of latex and food allergy. *Cutis* 1993;52:70–71.
127. McKinley WO, Jackson AB, Cardena D, et al. Long-term medical complications after traumatic spinal cord injury: a regional model systems analysis. *Arch Phys Med Rehabil* 1999;80:1402–1410.
128. Editorial. Phrenic nerve pacing in quadriplegia. *Lancet* 1990;336:88–90.
129. Weese-Mayer DE, Hunt CE, Brouillette RT, et al. Diaphragm pacing in infants and children. *J Pediatr* 1992;120:1–8.
130. Onders RP, Elmo MJ, Ignagni AR. Diaphragm pacing stimulation system for tetraplegia in individuals injured during childhood or adolescence. *J Spinal Cord Med* 2007;30:S25–S29.
131. Nelson VS. Noninvasive mechanical ventilation for children and adolescents with spinal cord injuries. *Top Spinal Cord Inj Rehabil* 2000;6(suppl):12–15.
132. Tromans AM, Mecci M, Barrett FH, et al. The use of the BiPAP biphasic positive airway pressure system in acute spinal cord injury. *Spinal Cord* 1998;36:481–484.
133. Bach JR. Inappropriate weaning and late onset ventilatory failure of individuals with traumatic spinal cord injury. *Paraplegia* 1993;31:430–438.
134. Flavell H, Marshall R, Thornton AT, et al. Hypoxia episodes during sleep in high tetraplegia. *Arch Phys Med Rehabil* 1992;73:623–627.
135. Vogel LC. Spasticity: diagnostic workup and medical management. In: Betz RR, Mulcahey MJ, eds. *The child with a spinal cord injury*. Rosemont, IL: American Academy of Orthopaedic Surgeons, 1996:261–268.
136. Alpiner NM. Spasticity: pathophysiology and objective assessments. In: Betz RR, Mulcahey MJ, eds. *The child with a spinal cord injury*. Rosemont, IL: American Academy of Orthopaedic Surgeons, 1996:233–253.
137. Hurvitz EA. Nelson VS. Functional evaluation of spasticity and its effect on rehabilitation. In: Betz RR, Mulcahey MJ, eds. *The child with a spinal cord injury*. Rosemont, IL: American Academy of Orthopaedic Surgeons, 1996:255–260.
138. Perry HE, Wright RO, Shannon MW, et al. Baclofen overdose: drug experimentation in a group of adolescents. *Pediatrics* 1998;101:1045–1048.
139. Mathias CJ, Luckitt J, Desai P, et al. Pharmacodynamics and pharmacokinetics of the oral antispastic agent tizanidine in patients with spinal cord injury. *J Rehabil Res Dev* 1989;26:9–16.
140. Apple DF, Murray HH. Spasticity: surgical management. In: Betz RR, Mulcahey MJ, eds. *The child with a spinal cord injury*. Rosemont, IL: American Academy of Orthopaedic Surgeons, 1996:269–283.
141. Jankovic J, Brin MF. Therapeutic uses of botulinum toxin. *N Engl J Med* 1991;324:1186–1194.
142. Penn RD, Savoy SM, Corcos D, et al. Intrathecal baclofen for severe spinal spasticity. *N Engl J Med* 1989;320:1517–1521.
143. Armstrong RW, Steinbok P, Farrell K, et al. Continuous intrathecal baclofen treatment of severe spasms in two children with spinal cord injury. *Dev Med Child Neurol* 1992;34:731–738.
144. Albright AL, Barron WB, Fasick MP, et al. Continuous intrathecal baclofen infusion for spasticity of cerebral origin. *JAMA* 1993;270:2475–2477.
145. Teddy P, Jamous A, Gardner B, et al. Complications of intrathecal baclofen delivery. *Br J Neurosurg* 1992;6: 115–118.
146. Hickey KJ, Anderson CJ, Vogel LC. Pressure ulcers in pediatric spinal cord injury. *Top Spinal Cord Inj Rehabil* 2000;6(suppl):85–90.
147. Bonner L. Pressure ulcer prevention. In: Betz RR, Mulcahey MJ, eds. *The child with a spinal cord injury*. Rosemont, IL: American Academy of Orthopaedic Surgeons, 1996:285–292.
148. Banta JV. Rehabilitation of pediatric spinal cord injury: the Newington Children's Hospital experience. *Conn Med* 1984;48:14–18.
149. Flett PJ. The rehabilitation of children with spinal cord injury. *J Paediatr Child Health* 1992;28:141–146.
150. Mulcahey MJ. Unique management needs of pediatric spinal cord injury patients: rehabilitation. *J Spinal Cord Med* 1997;20:25–30.
151. Mulcahey MJ, Betz RR. Considerations in the rehabilitation of children with spinal cord injuries. *Top Spinal Cord Inj Rehabil* 1997;3:31–36.
152. Nelson MR, Tilbor, AG, Frieden L, et al. Introduction to pediatric rehabilitation. In: Betz RR, Mulcahey MJ, eds. *The child with a spinal cord injury*. Rosemont, IL: American Academy of Orthopaedic Surgeons, 1996:461–470.
153. Zager RP, Marquette CH. Developmental considerations in children and early adolescents with spinal cord injury. *Arch Phys Med Rehabil* 1981;62:427–431.
154. Jaffe KM, McDonald CM. Rehabilitation following childhood injury. *Pediatr Ann* 1992;21:438–447.
155. Hussey RW, Stauffer ES. Spinal cord injury: requirements for ambulation. *Arch Phys Med Rehabil* 1973;54:544–547.
156. Vogel, LC, Lubicky JP. Ambulation in children and adolescents with spinal cord injuries. *J Pediatr Orthop* 1995;15:510–516.
157. Creitz L, Nelson VS, Haubenstricker L, et al. Orthotic prescriptions. In: Betz RR, Mulcahey MJ, eds. *The child with a spinal cord injury*. Rosemont, IL: American Academy of Orthopaedic Surgeons, 1996:537–553.

158. Vogel LC, Lubicky JP. Pediatric spinal cord injury issues: ambulation. *Top Spinal Cord Inj Rehabil* 1997;3:37–47.
159. Vogel LC, Mendoza MM, Schottler JC, et al. Ambulation in children and youth with spinal cord injuries. *J Spinal Cord Med* 2007;30:S158–S164.
160. Vogel LC, Lubicky JP. Ambulation with parapodia and reciprocating gait orthoses in pediatric spinal cord injury. *Dev Med Child Neurol* 1995;37:957–964.
161. Katz DE, Haideri N, Song K, et al. Comparative study of conventional hip-knee-ankle-foot orthoses versus reciprocating-gait orthoses for children with high-level paraparesis. *J Pediatr Orthop* 1997;17:377–386.
162. Johnston TE, Betz RR, Smith BT, et al. Implanted functional electrical stimulation: an alternative for standing and walking in pediatric spinal cord injury. *Spinal Cord* 2003;41:144–152.
163. Moynahan MA, Mullin C, Cohn J, et al. Home uses of a FES system for standing and mobility in adolescents with spinal cord injury. *Arch Phys Med Rehabil* 1996;77:1005–1013.
164. Bonaroti D, Akers J, Smith BT, et al. Comparison of functional electrical stimulation to long leg braces for upright mobility in children with complete thoracic level spinal injuries. *Arch Phys Med Rehabil* 1999;80:1047–1053.
165. Mulcahey MJ. Upper extremity orthoses and splints. In: Betz RR, Mulcahey MJ, eds. *The child with a spinal cord injury*. Rosemont, IL: American Academy of Orthopaedic Surgeons, 1996:375–392.
166. Mulcahey MJ. Rehabilitation and outcomes of upper extremity tendon transfer surgery. In: Betz RR, Mulcahey MJ, eds. *The child with a spinal cord injury*. Rosemont, IL: American Academy of Orthopaedic Surgeons, 1996:419–448.
167. Mulcahey MJ, Betz RR, Smith BT, et al. A prospective evaluation of upper extremity tendon transfers in children with cervical spinal cord injury. *J Pediatr Orthop* 1999;19:319–328.
168. Mulcahey MJ, Betz RR, Smith BT, et al. Implanted FES hand system in adolescents with SCI: an evaluation. *Arch Phys Med Rehabil* 1997;78:597–607.
169. Akers JM, Smith BT, Betz RR. Implantable electrode lead in a growing limb. *IEEE Trans Rehabil Eng* 1999;7:35–45.
170. Scremin AM, Kurta L, Gentili A, et al. Increasing muscle mass in spinal cord injured persons with a functional electrical stimulation exercise program. *Arch Phys Med Rehabil* 1999;80:1531–1536.
171. Hjeltnes N, Aksnes AK, Birkeland KI, et al. Improved body composition after 8 wk of electrically stimulated leg cycling in tetraplegic patients. *Am J Physiol* 1997;273:R1072–R1079.
172. Chilibeck PD, Jeon J, Weiss C, et al. Histochemical changes in muscle of individuals with spinal cord injury following functional electrical stimulated exercise training. *Spinal Cord* 1999;37:264–268.
173. Mohr T, Andersen JL, Biering-Sorensen F, et al. Long-term adaptation to electrically induced cycle training in severe spinal cord injured individuals. *Spinal Cord* 1997;35:1–16.
174. Belanger M, Stein RB, Wheeler GD, et al. Electrical stimulation: can it increase muscle strength and reverse osteopenia in spinal cord injured individuals? *Arch Phys Med Rehabil* 2000;81:1090–1098.
175. Chen SC, Lai CH, Chan WP, et al. Increases in bone mineral density after functional electrical stimulation cycling exercises in spinal cord injured patients. *Disabil Rehabil* 2005;27:1337–1341.
176. McDonald JW, Becker D, Sadowsky CL, et al. Late recovery following spinal cord injury. Case report and review of the literature. *J Neurosurg* 2002;97:252–265.
177. Johnston TE, Smith BT, Oladeji O, et al. Outcomes of a home cycling program using functional electrical stimulation or passive motion for children with spinal cord injury: a case series. *J Spinal Cord Med* 2008;31: 215–221.
178. Anderson CJ, Mulcahey MJ, Vogel LC. Menstruation and pediatric spinal cord injury. *J Spinal Cord Med* 1997;20:56–59.
179. Anderson CJ. Psychosocial and sexuality issues in pediatric spinal cord injury. *Top Spinal Cord Inj Rehabil* 1997;3:70–78.
180. Anderson CJ, Kelly E, Klaas SJ, et al. Anxiety and depression in children and adolescents with spinal cord injuries. *Dev Med Child Neurol* 2009;51:826–832.
181. Anderson CJ, Vogel LC, Chlan KM, et al. Depression in adults who sustained spinal cord injuries as children or adolescents. *J Spinal Cord Med* 2007;30:S76–S82.
182. Callen L. Substance use and abuse. In: Betz RR, Mulcahey MJ, eds. *The child with a spinal cord injury*. Rosemont, IL: American Academy of Orthopaedic Surgeons, 1996:671–677.
183. Mubarak SJ, Camp JF, Vuletich W, et al. Halo application in the infant. *J Pediatr Orthop* 1989;9:612–614.
184. Garfin SR, Roux R, Botte MJ, et al. Skull osteology as it affects halo pin placement in children. *J Pediatr Orthop* 1986;6:434–436.
185. Letts M, Kaylor D, Gouw G. A biomechanical analysis of halo fixation in children. *J Bone Joint Surg* 1988;70B:277–279.
186. Herzenberg JK, Hensinger RN, Dedrick DK, et al. Emergency transport and positioning of young children who have an injury of the cervical spine. The standard backboard may be hazardous. *J Bone Joint Surg* 1989;71A:15–22.
187. Dearolf WW III, Betz RR, Vogel LC, et al. Scoliosis in pediatric spinal cord-injured patients. *J Pediatr Orthop* 1990;10:214–218.
188. Lancourt JE, Dickson JH, Carter RE. Paralytic spinal deformity following traumatic spinal-cord injury in children and adolescents. *J Bone Joint Surg* 1981;63A:47–53.
189. Betz RR, Orthopaedic problems in the child with spinal cord injury. *Top Spinal Cord Inj Rehabil* 1997;3:9–19.
190. Mehta S, Betz RR, Mulcahey MJ, et al. Effect of bracing on paralytic scoliosis secondary to spinal cord injury. *J Spinal Cord Med* 2004;27:S88–S92.
191. Sison-Williamson MM, Bagley A, Hongo A, et al. Effect of thoracolumbosacral orthoses on reachable workspace volumes in children with spinal cord injury. *J Spinal Cord Med* 2007;30:S184–S191.
192. Chavetz RS, Mulcahey MJ, Betz RR, et al. Impact of prophylactic thoracolumbosacral orthosis bracing on functional activities and activities of daily living in the pediatric spinal cord injury population. *J Spinal Cord Med* 2007;30:S178–S183.

193. Miller F, Betz RR. Hip joint instability. In: Betz RR, Mulcahey MJ, eds. *The child with a spinal cord injury*. Rosemont, IL: American Academy of Orthopaedic Surgeons, 1996:353–361.
194. Rink P, Miller F. Hip instability in spinal cord injury patients. *J Pediatr Orthop* 1990;10:583–587.
195. Vogel LC, Gogia RS, Lubicky JP. Hip abnormalities in children with spinal cord injuries. *J Spinal Cord Med* 1995;18:172.
196. Betz RR, Beck T, Huss GK, et al. Hip instability in children with spinal cord injury. *J Am Paraplegia Soc* 1999;17:119.
197. Betz RR, Mulcahey MJ, Smith BT, et al. Implications of hip subluxation for FES-assisted mobility in patients with spinal cord injury. *Orthopedics* 2001;24:181–184.
198. McCarthy JJ, Weibel B, Betz RR. Results of pelvic osteotomies for hip subluxation or dislocation in children with spinal cord injury. *Top Spinal Cord Inj Rehabil* 2000;6(suppl):48–53.
199. Garland DE. A clinical perspective on common forms of acquired heterotopic ossification. *Clin Orthop* 1991;263:13–29.
200. Garland DE, Shimoya ST, Lugo C, et al. Spinal cord insults and heterotopic ossification in the pediatric population. *Clin Orthop* 1989;245:303–310.
201. Banovac K, Gonzalez F, Renfree KJ. Treatment of heterotopic ossification after spinal cord injury. *J Spinal Cord Med* 1997;20:60–65.
202. Silverman SL, Hurvitz EA, Nelson VS, et al. Rachitic syndrome after disodium etidronate therapy in an adolescent. *Arch Phys Med Rehabil* 1994;75:118–120.
203. Freebourn TM, Barber DB, Able AC. The treatment of immature heterotopic ossification in spinal cord injuries with combination surgery, radiation therapy and NSAID. *Spinal Cord* 1999;37:50–53.
204. Wick M, Muller EJ, Hahn MP, et al. Surgical excision of heterotopic bone after hip surgery followed by oral indomethacin application: is there a clinical benefit for the patient? *Arch Orthop Trauma Surg* 1999;119:151–155.
205. Betz RR, Triolo RJ, Hermida VM, et al. The effects of functional neuromuscular stimulation on the bone mineral content in the lower limbs of spinal cord injured children. *J Am Paraplegia Soc* 1991;14:65–66.
206. McCarthy JJ, Betz RR. Hip disorders in children who have spinal cord injury. *Orthop Clin North Am* 2006;37:197–202.
207. Lauer R, Johnston TE, Smith BT, et al. Bone mineral density of the hip and knee in children with spinal cord injury. *J Spinal Cord Med* 2007;30:S10–S14.
208. Miller F. Pathologic long-bone fractures: diagnosis, etiology, management, and prevention. In: Betz RR, Mulcahey MJ, eds. *The child with a spinal cord injury*. Rosemont, IL: American Academy of Orthopaedic Surgeons, 1996:331–338.
209. Botto LD, Moore CA, Khoury MJ, et al. Neural-tube defects *N Engl J Med* 1999;341:1509–1519.
210. Sarwark JF, Lubicky JP, eds. *Caring for the child with spina bifida*, Rosemont, IL: American Academy of Orthopaedic Surgeons, 2002.
211. Yen IH, Khoury MJ, Erickson JD, et al. The changing epidemiology of neural tube defects, United States 1968–1989. *Am J Dis Child* 1992;146:857–861.
212. CDC. Spina bifida and anencephaly before and after folic acid mandate—United States, 1995–1996 and 1999–2000. *MMWR Morb Mortal Wkly Rep* 2004;53:362–365.
213. Centers for Disease Control (CDC). Spina bifida incidence at birth—United States, 1983–1990. *MMWR Morb Mortal Wkly Rep* 1992;41:497–500.
214. Wasserman CR, Shaw GM, Selvin S, et al. Socioeconomic status, neighborhood social conditions, and neural tube defects. *Am J Public Health* 1998;88:1674–1680.
215. Lian ZH, Yang HY, Li Z. Neural tube defects in Beijing-Tianjin area of China. Urban-rural distribution and some other epidemiologic characteristics. *J Epidemiol Community Health* 1987;41:259–262.
216. McLone DG. Continuing concepts in the management of spina bifida. *Pediatr Neurosurg* 1992;18:254–256.
217. Hunt GM. A study of deaths and handicap in a consecutive series of spina bifida treated unselectively from birth. *Z Kinderchir* 1983;(suppl II)38:100–102.
218. Bol KA, Collins JS, Kirby RS. Survival of infants with neural tube defects in the presence of folic acid fortification. *Pediatrics* 2006;117:803–813.
219. Davis BE, Daley CM, Shurtleff DB, et al. Long-term survival of individuals with myelomeningocele. *Pediatr Neurosurg* 2005;41:186–191.
220. Mitchell LE. Epidemiology of neural tube defects. *Am J Med Genetics Part C (Semin Med Genet)* 2005;135C:88–94.
221. Becerra JE, Khoury MJ, Cordero JF, et al. Diabetes mellitus during pregnancy and the risks for specific birth defects: a population based case-control study. *Pediatrics* 1990;85:1–9.
222. Lammer EJ, Sever LE, Oakley GP. Teratogen update: valproic acid. *Teratology* 1987;35:465–473.
223. Rosa FW. Spina bifida in infants of women treated with carbamazepine during pregnancy. *N Engl J Med* 1991;324:674–677.
224. Shaw GM, Velie EM, Schaffer D. Risk of neural tube defect—affected pregnancies among obese women. *JAMA* 1996;275:1093–1096.
225. Graham JM, Edwards MJ, Edwards MJ. Teratogen update: gestational effects of maternal hyperthermia due to febrile illnesses and resultant patterns of defects in humans. *Teratology* 1998;58:209–221.
226. Christensen B, Arbour L, Tran P, et al. Genetic polymorphisms in methylenetetrahydrofolate reductase and methionine synthase, folate levels in red blood cells, and risk of neural tube defects. *Am J Med Genet* 1999;84:151–157.
227. Toriello HV, Higgins JV. Occurrence of neural tube defects among first-, second-, and third-degree relatives of probands: results of a United States study. *Am J Med Genet* 1983;15:601–606.
228. Urui S, Oi S. Experimental study of the embryogenesis of open spinal dysraphism. *Neurosurg Clin N Am* 1995;6:195–202.
229. Rauzzino M, Oakes WJ. Chiari II malformation and syringomyelia. *Neurosurg Clin N Am* 1995;6:293–309.
230. Swank M, Dias L. Myelomeningocele: a review of the orthopaedic aspects of 206 patients treated from birth with no selection criteria. *Dev Med Child Neurol* 1992;34:1047–1052.
231. Pang, D. Surgical complications of open dysraphism. *Neurosurg Clin N Am* 1995;6:243–257.

232. Drewek MJ, Bruner JP, Whetsell WO, et al. Quantitative analysis of the toxicity of human amniotic fluid to cultured rat spinal cord. *Pediatr Neurosurg* 1997;27:190–193.
233. Hahn YS. Open myelomeningocele. *Neurosurg Clin N Am* 1995;6:231–241.
234. Charney EB, Weller SC, Sutton LN, et al. Management of the newborn with myelomeningocele: time for a decision-making process. *Pediatrics*. 1985;75:58–64.
235. Steinbok P, Irvine B, Cochrane DD, et al. Long-term outcome and complications of children born with meningomyelocele. *Childs Nerv Syst* 1992;8:92–96.
236. Hunt GM, Poulton A. Open spina bifida: a complete cohort reviewed 25 years after closure. *Dev Med Child Neurol* 1995;37:19–29.
237. McLone DG, Czyzewski D, Raimondi AJ, et al. Central nervous system infections as a limiting factor in the intelligence of children with myelomeningocele. *Pediatrics* 1982;70:338–342.
238. Cull C, Wyke MA. Memory functions of children with spina bifida and shunted hydrocephalus. *Dev Med Child Neurol* 1984;26:177–183.
239. Swisher LP, Pinsker EJ. The language characteristics of hyperverbal, hydrocephalic children. *Dev Med Child Neurol* 1971;13:746–755.
240. Jansen J, Taudorf K, Pedersen H, et al. Upper extremity function in spina bifida. *Childs Nerv Syst* 1991;7:67–71.
241. Kirk VG, Morielli A, Brouillette RT. Sleep-disordered breathing in patients with myelomeningocele: the missed diagnosis. *Dev Med Child Neurol* 1999;41:40–43.
242. Park TS, Cail WS, Maggio WM, et al. Progressive spasticity and scoliosis in children with myelomeningocele. *J Neurosurg* 1985;62:367–374.
243. Bartonek A, Saraste H, Knutson LM. Comparison of different systems to classify the neurological level of lesion in patients with myelomeningocele. *Dev Med Child Neurol* 1999;41:796–805.
244. McDonald CM, Jaffe KM, Shurtleff DB, et al. Modifications to the traditional description of neurosegmental innervation in myelomeningocele. *Dev Med Child Neurol* 1991;33:473–481.
245. McDonald CM. Rehabilitatioin of children with spinal dysraphism. *Neurosurg Clin N Am* 1995;6:393–412.
246. Shurtleff DB, Duguay S, Duguay G, et al. Epidemiology of tethered cord with meningomyelocele. *Eur J Pediatr Surg* 1997;7(suppl I):7–11.
247. Shurtleff DB, Selection process for the care of congenitally malformed infants. In: Shurtleff DB, ed. *Myelodysplasias and exstrophies: significance, prevention and treatment.* Orlando, FL: Grune and Stratton, 1986:89–115.
248. Jutson JM, Beasley SW, Bryan AD. Cryptorchidism in spina bifida and spinal cord transection: a clue to the mechanism of transinguinal descent of the testis. *J Pediatr Surg* 1988;23:275–277.
249. Joseph DB, Bauer SB, Colodny AH, et al. Clean, intermittent catheterization of infants with neurogenic bladder. *Pediatrics* 1989;84:78–82.
250. Stone AR. Neurologic evaluation and urologic management of spinal dysraphism. *Neurosurg Clin N Am* 1995;6:269–277.
251. Uehling DT, Smith J, Meyer J, et al. Impact of an intermittent catheterization program on children with myelomeningocele. *Pediatrics* 1985;76:892–895.
252. Hannigan KF. Teaching intermittent self-catheterization to young children with myelodysplasia. *Dev Med Child Neurol* 1979;21:365–368.
253. King JC, Currie DM, Wright E. Bowel training in spina bifida: importance of education, patient compliance, age, and anal reflexes. *Arch Phys Med Rehabil* 1994;75:243–247.
254. Herndon CDA, Rink RC, Cain MP, et al. In situ Malone antegrade continence enema in 127 patients: a 6-year experience. *J Urol* 2004;172:1689–1691
255. Shandling B, Gilmour RF. The enema continence catheter in spina bifida: successful bowel management. *J Pediatr Surg* 1987;22:271–273.
256. Loening-Baucke V, Desch L, Wolraich M. Biofeedback training for patients with myelomeningocele and fecal incontinence. *Dev Med Child Neurol* 1988;30:781–790.
257. Karol LA. Orthopedic management in myelomeningocele. *Neurosurg Clin N Am* 1995;6:259–268.
258. Piggott H. The natural history of scoliosis in myelodysplasia. *J Bone Joint Surg* 1980;62B:54–58.
259. Shurtleff DB. Mobility. In Shurtleff DB, ed. *Myelodysplasias and exstrophies: significance, prevention and treatment*. Orlando, FL: Grune and Stratton, 1986:313–356.
260. Feiwell E, Downey DS, Blatt T. The effect of hip reduction on function in patients with myelomeningocele, *J Bone Joint Surg* 1978;60A:169–173.
261. Northrup H, Volcik KA. Spina bifida and other neural tube defects. *Curr Probl Pediatr* 2000;30:317–332.
262. Lubicky JP. Spinal deformity in myelomeningocele. In: Bridwell KH, DeWald RL, eds. *The textbook of spinal surgery*. 2nd ed. Philadelphia, PA: Lippincott-Raven Publishers, 1997:903–931.
263. Mackel JL, Lindseth RE. Scoliosis in myelodysplasia. *J Bone Joint Surg* 1975;57A:1031.
264. Tomlinson RJ, Wolfe MW, Nadall JM, et al. Syringomyelia and developmental scoliosis. *J Pediatr Orthop* 1994;14:580–585.
265. Hall P, Lindseth R, Campbell R, et al. Scoliosis and hydrocephalus in myelocele patients. *J Neurosurg* 1979;50:174–178.
266. Rotenstein D, Reigel DH. Growth hormone treatment of children with neural tube defects: results from 6 months to 6 years. *J Pediatr* 1996;128:184–189.
267. Elias ER, Sadeghi-Nead A. Precocious puberty in girl with myelodysplasia. *Pediatrics* 1994;93:521–522.
268. Hunt GM. Open spina bifida: outcome for a complete cohort treated unselectively and followed into adulthood. *Dev Med Child Neurol* 1990;32:108–118.
269. Trollman R, Strehl E, Dorr HG. Precocious puberty in children with myelomeningocele: treatment with gonadotropin-releasing hormone analogues. *Dev Med Child Neurol* 1998;40:38–43.
270. Roberts D, Shepherd RW, Shepherd K. Anthropometry and obesity in myelomeningocele. *J Paediatr Child Health* 1991;27:83–90.
271. Kelly KJ, Pearson ML, Kurup VP, et al. A cluster of anaphylactic reactions in children with spina bifida during general anesthesia: epidemiologic features, risk factors, and latex hypersensitivity. *J Allergy Clin Immunol* 1994;53–61.
272. Niggemann B, Kulig M, Bergmann R, et al. Development of latex allergy in children up to 5 years of age—a

retrospective analysis of risk factors. *Pediatr Allergy Immunol* 1998;9:36–39.
273. Szepfatusi Z, Seidl R, Bernert G, et al. Latex sensitization in spina bifida appears disease-associated. *J Pediatr* 1999;134:344–348.
274. Harris MB, Banta JV. Cost of skin care in the myelomeningocele population. *J Pediatr Ortho* 1990;10:355–361.
275. Hayden PW, Davenport SLH, Campbell MM. Adolescents with myelodysplasia: impact of physical disability on emotional maturation. *Pediatrics* 1979;64:53–59.
276. Loomis JW, Javornisky JG, Monahan JJ, et al. Relations between family environment and adjustment outcomes in young adults with spina bifida. *Dev Med Child Neurol* 1997;39:620–627.
277. Sawyer SM, Roberts KV. Sexual and reproductive health in young people with spina bifida. *Dev Med Child Neurol* 1999;41:671–675.
278. Bodzioch J, Roach JW, Schkade J. Promoting independence in adolescent paraplegics: a 2-week "camping" experience. *J Pediatr Orthop* 1986;6:198–201.
279. Tew B, Laurence KM, Jenkins V. Factors affecting employability among young adults with spina bifida and hydrocephalus. *Z Kinderchir* 1990;45:34–36.
280. American Academy of Pediatrics. Committee on Genetics. Folic acid for the prevention of neural tube defects. *Pediatrics* 1999;104:325–327.
281. De Wals P, Tairou F, Van Allen MI, et al. Reduction in neural-tube defects after folic acid fortification in Canada. *N Engl J Med* 2007;357:135–142.
282. Centers for Disease Control. Recommendations for the use of folic acid to reduce the number of cases of spina bifida and other neural tube defects. *MMWR Morb Mortal Wkly Rep* 1992;41(RR-14):1–7.
283. MRC Vitamin Study Research Group. Prevention of neural tube defects: results of the Medical Research Council Vitamin Study. *Lancet* 1991;338:131–137.
284. Burton BK. α-Fetoprotein screening. *Adv Pediatr* 1986;33:181–196.
285. Hobbins JC. Diagnosis and management of neural-tube defects. *N Eng J Med* 1991;324:690–691.
286. Babcook CJ. Ultrasound evaluation of prenatal and neonatal spina bifida. *Neurosurg Clin N Am* 1995;6: 203–218.
287. Meuli M, Meuli-Simmen C, Hutchins GM, et al. The spinal cord lesion in human fetuses with myelomeningocele: implications for fetal surgery. *J Pediatr Surg* 1997;32:448–452.
288. Bruner JP. Intrauterine surgery in myelomeningocele. *Semin Fetal Neonatal Med* 2007;12:471–476.
289. Sutton LN. Fetal surgery for neural tube defects. *Best Pract Res Clin Obstet Gynaecol* 2008;22:175–188.
290. Shurtleff DB, Lemire RJ. Epidemiology, etiologic factors, and prenatal diagnosis of open spinal dysraphism. *Neurosurg Clin N Am* 1995;6:183–193.
291. Luthy DA, Wardinsky T, Shurtleff DB, et al. Cesarean section before the onset of labor and subsequent motor function in infants with meningomyelocele diagnosed antenatally. *N Eng J Med* 1991;324:662–666.
292. Merrill DC, Goodwin P, Burson J, et al. The optimal route of delivery for fetal meningomyelocele. *Am J Obstet Gynecol* 1998;179:235–240.
293. Sutton LN. Lipomyelomeningocele. *Neurosurg Clin N Am* 1995;6:325–338.
294. Renshaw TS. Sacral agenesis. *J Bone Joint Surg* 1978;60-A:373–383.
295. Wilmshurst JM, Kelly R, Borzyskowski M. Presentation and outcome of sacral agenesis: 20 years' experience. *Dev Med Child Neurol* 1999;41:806–812.
296. Guzman L, Bauer SB, Hallett M, et al. Evaluation and management of children with sacral agenesis. *Urology* 1983;22:506–510.
297. Isu T, Iwasaki Y, Akino M, et al. Hydrosyringomyelia associated with a Chiari I malformation in children and adolescents. *Neurosurgery* 1990;26:591–597.
298. Cahan LD, Bentson JR. Considerations in the diagnosis and treatment of syringomyelia and the Chiari malformation. *J Neurosurg* 1982;57:24–31.
299. Logue V, Edwards MR. Syringomyelia and its surgical treatment—an analysis of 75 patients. *J Neurol Neurosurg Psychiatry* 1981;44:273–284.
300. Isu T, Chono Y, Iwasaki Y, et al. Scoliosis associated with syringomyelia presenting in children. *Childs Nerv Syst* 1992;8:97–100.
301. Williams B. Orthopaedic features in the presentation of syringomyelia. *J Bone Joint Surg* 1979;61B:314–323.
302. Farley FA, Song KM, Birch JG, et al. Syringomyelia and scoliosis in children. *J Pediatr Orthop* 1995;15:187–192.
303. Batzdorf U. Syringomyelia related to abnormalities at the level of the craniovertebral junction. In: Batzdorf U, ed. *Syringomyelia: current concepts in diagnosis and treatment*. Baltimore, MD: Williams and Wilkins, 1991: 163–182.
304. Williams B, Page N. Surgical treatment of syringomyelia with syringopleural shunting. *Br J Neurosurg* 1987;1:63–80.
305. Barbaro NM, Wilson CB, Gutin PH, et al. Surgical treatment of syringomyelia. *J Neurosurg* 1984;61:531–538.

CHAPTER 30 ■ CERVICAL AND THORACIC SPONDYLOTIC MYELOPATHY

ZOHER GHOGAWALA, NDUKA AMANKULOR, AND ROBERT F. HEARY

INTRODUCTION

Cervical spondylotic myelopathy (CSM) results from degenerative cervical spondylosis, which is one of the most common indications for cervical spine surgery in the United States. Over 112,400 cervical spine operations for degenerative spondylosis are performed annually in the United States. This represents a 100% increase in utilization over the past decade with hospital charges now exceeding 2 billion dollars per year (1). Nearly 1/5 cervical spine operations in the United States are performed to treat CSM (2). Surgical decompression of the spinal cord and fusion of the spinal column can permit recovery of spinal cord function and limit further dysfunction in many cases. Many patients with mild CSM symptoms are not treated surgically. Recent reports suggest that CSM surgery has a high complication rate (13.4% to 17%) (3,4). Moreover, there may be significant differences in the morbidity between ventral and dorsal surgery for CSM. For example, some specific complications (e.g., swallowing difficulty) have a greater incidence in ventral (anterior) procedures over dorsal (posterior) procedures (3). For these and other historical reasons, there is significant uncertainty as to the optimal surgical approach (ventral versus dorsal) for treating CSM especially in older patients. Both operations are in widespread use in contemporary US surgical practice.

CERVICAL SPONDYLOTIC MYELOPATHY—DEFINITION AND PATHOPHYSIOLOGY

CSM is the most common cause of spinal cord dysfunction in the United States and in the world (5) and the most common cause of gait dysfunction in persons over the age of 55 years. The condition presents insidiously and is defined in terms of its clinical signs and symptoms. The most common symptoms include subtle changes in gait and/or balance, neck stiffness, pain radiating to arms, and loss of manual dexterity (i.e., diminished handwriting, "numb, clumsy hands"). Symptoms are commonly asymmetric in the legs. Loss of sphincter control and urinary incontinence is rare early in the course, although some patients complain of urinary urgency, frequency, and hesitancy. The most common signs of CSM include hyperreflexia, lower extremity spasticity, extensor Babinski responses, Hoffmans sign in the fingers, ankle clonus, weakness (of arms greater than legs), and alteration of joint position sense. Wasting of the intrinsic hand muscles is a classical finding in CSM (8). The classical definition of myelopathy is the presence of long tract signs. Patients with CSM may also present acutely with a central cord syndrome, typically following an acute hyperextension injury.

CSM is caused by dynamic repeated compression of the spinal cord from degenerative arthritis of the cervical spine (6). Axonal stretch-associated injury appears to be the leading factor in explaining myelopathy in animal models (6). Spinal cord ischemia from compression of larger vessels and impaired microcirculation is another proposed mechanism (7,8). The natural history of CSM is variable. There is most commonly an initial phase of deterioration followed by a static period lasting a number of years during which the degree of disability may not change significantly. A small percent of patients have rapid onset of symptoms with a long quiet period, with most having a stepwise deterioration of clinical function with intervening periods of quiescence. Older patients are noted to deteriorate more frequently.

Many patients with mild CSM symptoms can be carefully followed in the clinic without surgery. Surgery to decompress and fuse the spine is often advocated for severe or progressive symptoms with mixed results. About two-thirds of patients improve with surgery, while surgery is not successful in 15% to 30% of cases (9). Some series report that 10% to 20% of cases worsen clinically after surgery (9).

CERVICAL STENOSIS WITHOUT PROGRESSIVE MYELOPATHY

The average normal cervical spinal canal diameter is reported to be 17 to 18 mm (10). Not all patients with significant cervical spinal canal narrowing and compression of the spinal cord (diameter of the cervical spinal cord is normally 10 mm) develop myelopathy. In fact, many patients are asymptomatic and can be followed in the clinic without intervention (11). For those that develop symptoms, many of these patients generally benefit from conservative treatment (12). Some patients present with neck pain or intermittent episodes of cervical radiculopathy, resulting in arm or shoulder pain on the basis of neural foraminal narrowing from cervical spondylosis (13). Conservative treatments for neck pain often include non-steroidal antiinflammatory drugs, muscle relaxants, and physical therapy (14). Traction should be avoided. Conservative interventions have not been studied in enough detail to assess efficacy or effectiveness adequately (15). Cervical spine epidural steroid injections are sometimes advocated for the management of cervical spondylotic radiculopathy. Cervical epidural injections are generally considered safe, although a recent review found that serious complications have been reported in many series (16). No randomized clinical trial (RCT) has been performed to determine their long-term efficacy.

MILD CERVICAL SPONDYLOTIC MYELOPATHY

There have been no large RCTs demonstrating that surgery is superior to nonsurgical care for treating CSM. There are small studies that have reported conflicting information. A small RCT consisting of 48 patients with mild to moderate CSM (mJOA score greater than 12) did not demonstrate improvement from surgery after 2 years of follow-up (17). In contrast, another nonrandomized trial (43 patients) did demonstrate better overall functional outcomes improvement in CSM patients following surgery (18). It is generally agreed that patients with mild, stable symptoms may be managed without surgery, although the majority of patients with progressive myelopathy symptoms demonstrate significant improvement in validated outcome measures following surgery (19). In a recent Cochrane review on the role of surgery for cervical myelopathy, Nikolaidis et al. (20) found no conclusive evidence to support surgical treatment, although limitations included small trials and risks of bias in the studies. In a previous review, Fouyas et al. (21) reported that often the disease may remain static for lengthy periods, and sometimes improve without treatment.

RADIOGRAPHIC STUDIES

Plain cervical spine radiographs are widely available and can demonstrate disc space narrowing, osteophytes, loss of cervical lordosis, etc. Saggital films can also assess alignment, which may influence potential surgical procedures. Flexion-extension views may help to diagnose instability and can be safely performed providing there is no evidence of radiographic gross instability (8). However, given the nearly universal presence of spondylotic changes seen on radiographs in the elderly and the difficulty differentiating symptomatic from asymptomatic patients, their usefulness is limited.

Magnetic resonance imaging (MRI) has been the imaging study of choice as the initial screening process in patients in whom CSM is suspected (8). MRI, however, may detect pathology unrelated to the patient's symptoms or detect pathology in asymptomatic patients. Correlating symptoms with MRI findings are therefore important. CT scanning is an additional imaging modality and is superior to MRI in defining the boney anatomy and foraminal stenosis. Therefore, computed tomography (CT) scanning is often used to complement MRI to provide additional boney detail to characterize the lesion responsible for neural encroachment. Myelography and/or CT/myelography are now primarily used only for patients who cannot undergo MRI (i.e., cardiac pacemakers) or in whom MRI is inconclusive.

DIFFERENTIAL DIAGNOSES

Several conditions may present with similar signs and symptoms of CSM and should be sought prior to surgical interventions. The most common conditions to consider include motor neuron disorders (amyotrophic lateral sclerosis), multiple sclerosis (MS), peripheral neuropathies, radiculopathy, normal pressure hydrocephalus, subacute combined degeneration (vitamin B_{12} deficiency), tumors, rheumatoid arthritis, syriongomyelia, and hereditary spastic paplegia. Electrodiagnostic and laboratory studies should be performed to help differentiate these disorders from CSM. Aside from nerve conduction studies and electromyography, somatosensory-evoked potentials can help exclude central disorders including MS.

Laboratory studies should include a CBC to rule out infectious etiology, chemistry panel, vitamin B_{12}, methalmalonic acid and homocysteine levels, and HIV testing in appropriate candidates.

HISTORY—SURGICAL APPROACHES

Surgical treatment for CSM (Fig. 30.1) was developed before studies on the pathophysiology of spinal cord dysfunction were published. Historically, CSM was treated by removing bone from the back of the cervical spine with a dorsal approach known as laminectomy (without fusion). The first cervical laminectomy for spinal cord injury was performed in 1828 (22,23).

While laminectomy without fusion is still performed today, several factors have limited its widespread usage. First, the development of instability or kyphosis in some cases has led many spine surgeons to add fusion to the procedure (laminectomy with fusion) or to perform a laminoplasty (which enlarges the spinal canal without fusing or removing the laminae possibly reducing late failures). Second, the inability to remove ventral osteophytes using the dorsal laminectomy has led to the development of ventral approaches. Fessler et al. (24) suggested, in 1985, that ventral corpectomy surgery (removal of a vertebral body from the front of the spine) might be superior to dorsal decompression. This study compared contemporary ventral surgery patient outcomes to historical results obtained in dorsal surgery patients treated many years earlier. Subsequent studies, however, including a very recent prospective nonrandomized study of 316 patients, have failed to demonstrate differences in disease-specific outcomes between ventral and dorsal surgery (4).

Despite the mixed results from both retrospective and prospective studies examining ventral and dorsal surgery, ventral decompression might be more effective in relieving the symptoms of myelopathy in two specific clinical circumstances. Patients with preoperative kyphosis (greater than 13 degrees) have poorer modified Japanese Orthopedic Association (mJOA) (a validated disease-specific outcome measurement) scores after dorsal surgery (laminoplasty) according to one prospective study (25). Another recent study concluded that for patients with preoperative intramedullary signal changes on MRI, ventral decompression was associated with a significantly greater improvement in motor function compared with dorsal approaches (26).

Enthusiasm for ventral surgery, however, has been tempered by the high early postoperative complication rates. In fact, the complication rate from ventral corpectomy (29.3%) appears to be significantly higher than for dorsal surgical approaches (7.1%) (27,28). Early experience with multilevel corpectomy was associated with high rates of graft dislodgement and fusion failures (29,30). This led to the development of multilevel discectomies, with fusion, using plating, which has reduced the

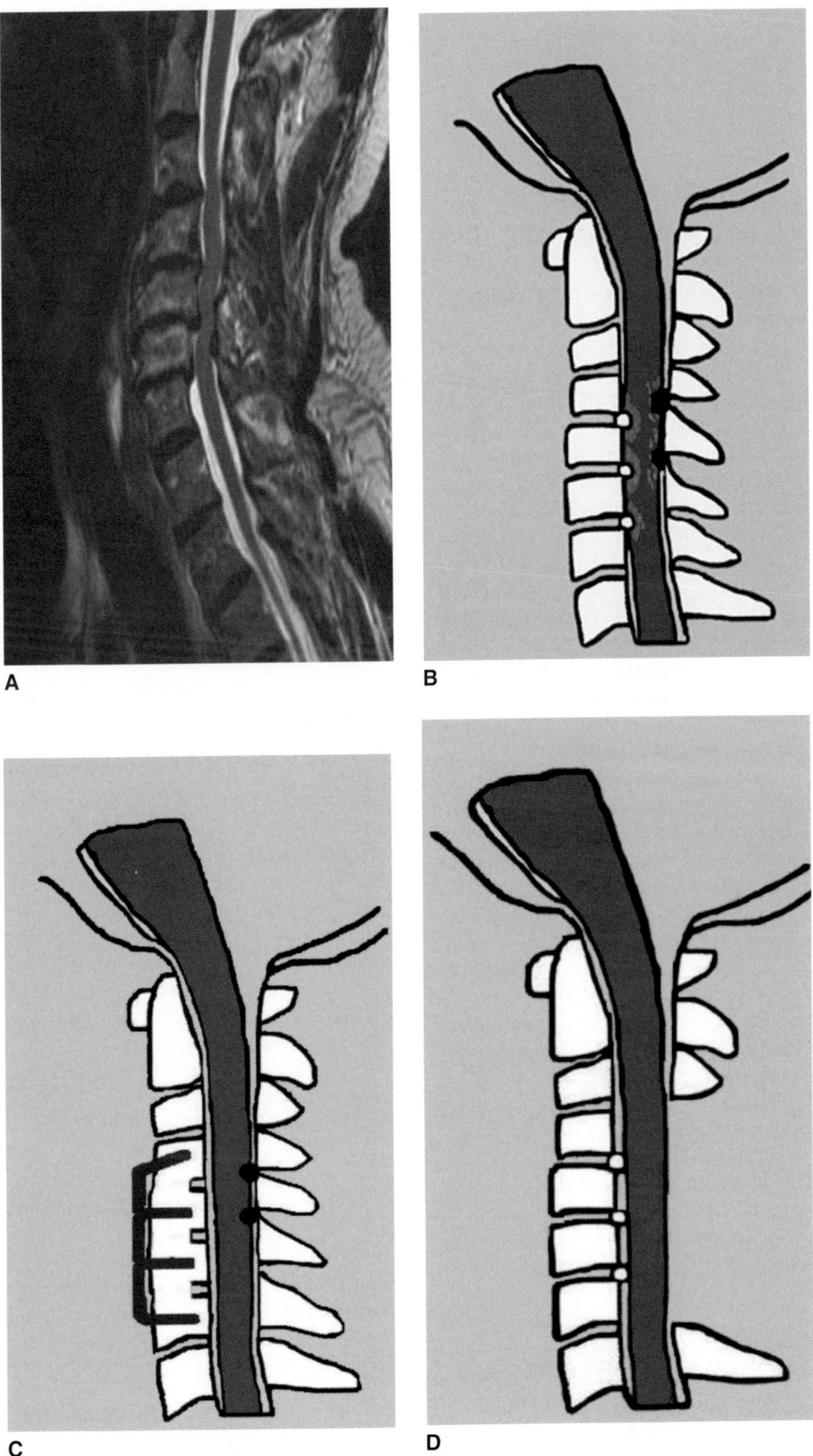

FIGURE 30.1 MRI and schematic images depicting cervical spinal compression and its surgical treatment. (A) Sagittal cervical spine MRI depicting spinal cord compression and distortion in a real patient with cervical spondylotic myelopathy. (B) Schematic representation of ventral osteophytes (*white*) and dorsal ligamentum (*black*) compression of spinal cord with sites of injury (*red*). (C) Schematic ventral surgery—multilevel discectomy, fusion, and plating (*blue*) with removal of ventral osteophytes (*white*). (D) Schematic dorsal surgery—laminectomy with removal of dorsal ligamentum (*black*).

complication rate (31). The multilevel discectomy and fusion procedure have the added advantage of improving cervical lordosis as well as reducing the risk of graft migration. However, pseudoarthrosis and subsidence of grafted bone remain challenges in treating patients with multilevel ventral surgery (32).

CLINICAL GUIDELINES FOR SURGICAL MANAGEMENT

Professional physician organizations such as the American Association of Neurological Surgeons-Congress of Neurological Surgeons Joint Section of Disorders of the Spine and Peripheral Nerves have systematically reviewed the literature and have published clinical guidelines for the surgical management of CSM (33). These guidelines were created to assist surgeons in formulating an appropriate treatment plan, but they also identify major deficiencies in the current literature. In most situations, these clinical guidelines have been unable to issue definitive guidance because high-quality clinical research comparing treatment approaches is lacking largely due to the inherent difficulties in performing clinical trials involving surgical procedures and disorders characterized by significant heterogeneity.

Patients with mild myelopathy symptoms may be managed without surgery. Surgical decompression (ventral or dorsal) is performed in more severe cases of myelopathy. Published series contain heterogeneous patient populations and varying approaches, and the reported outcomes measures differ, making comparisons difficult (9). Several studies have attempted to identify patient characteristics that predict improvement after surgery (34–44). The significance of many of these variables as outcome predictors remains controversial, and their impact on the choice of surgical approach is unclear.

The higher complication rate associated with 3 or more levels of ventral surgery (especially corpectomy) has led some surgeons to perform ventral surgery only in those patients with 2 or fewer levels of disease. Cervical spondylotic disease at 3 or more levels is usually treated with a dorsal approach (36). In current US practice, older patients (75 years or older) are more likely to be treated using dorsal surgery according to the nationwide inpatient sample (2). This is of particular relevance because both older age (more than 74 years) and dorsal surgical approach have been identified as risk factors for developing complications after cervical spine surgery (2). Determining if choice of approach (ventral versus dorsal) might limit complications, especially in older patients, would be especially important.

CURRENT SURGICAL TREATMENT OF CERVICAL SPONDYLOTIC MYELOPATHY

Decompression of the spinal canal to a diameter of at least 13 mm with restoration of cerebrospinal fluid pulsation around the spinal cord is the goal regardless of the approach. It is generally advisable to avoid excessive tension when taping of the shoulders for positioning patients to avoid brachial plexus stretch injury. The use of the operative microscope is generally advocated for ventral approaches. Spinal monitoring (Somatosensory-evoked potentials SSEP and/or Electromyography EMG) is suggested by many surgeons, although no rigorous studies have been done to determine the efficacy of routine spinal monitoring to prevent neurological complications.

Ventral Approaches

Presence of cervical kyphosis or kyphotic deformity has been identified as one of the major reasons to choose a ventral surgical approach when treating CSM. There are two major approaches.

Mutli-level Discectomy and Fusion

Ventral decompression and fusion (2,45) can be performed using a multilevel discectomy with fusion and plating as described recently (31,46). Surgeons use allograft or autograft bone spacers at each disc space and remove all compressive osteophytes using the operating microscope. Fixation is typically performed with either semiconstrained or dynamic titanium plates both of which have been shown to optimize fusion and minimize complications (47,48). In many cases, restoration of cervical lordosis is possible using this technique (Fig. 30.2). In some cases with marked kyphosis, an improvement in sagittal plane alignment is possible; however, the final imaging may still reveal a straightened or kyphotic alignment in the cervical spine.

Cervical Corpectomy and Fusion

The degree of cervical deformity, anatomy of compression by disc/osteophyte, or presence of focal ossification of posterior longitudinal ligament (OPLL) might lead many surgeons to choose to remove a portion or the entire vertebral body in order to achieve the surgical goals. The technique for cervical corpectomy and fusion has been described by Cooper and others (49,50). Complications from multilevel corpectomy and fusion are common and therefore supplementation with dorsal fusion is advocated by some surgeons (see combined ventral and dorsal approaches below) (50). An additional concern with corpectomy procedures is that the correction of sagittal plane malalignment is less feasible than that with the multilevel discectomy and fusion approach.

Dorsal Approaches

Multilevel disease (3 or more levels), developmental narrow spinal canal (12 mm anterior–posterior canal diameter at the base of C2), OPLL, and advanced age (age more than 74 years) are among the many reasons to choose a dorsal approach when treating CSM.

Laminectomy

Cervical laminectomy is effective in relieving the symptoms of CSM in selected patients with preserved cervical lordosis, but is associated with a progressive kyphotic deformity in 21% to 42% of patients (51,52). Cervical foraminotomies are often also performed for treating radiculopathy in addition to myelopathy. In order to attempt to limit the development of postoperative kyphosis, laminectomies without fusion are usually limited to patients with preserved preoperative lordosis. Cases of congenital stenosis are the most ideal for this approach.

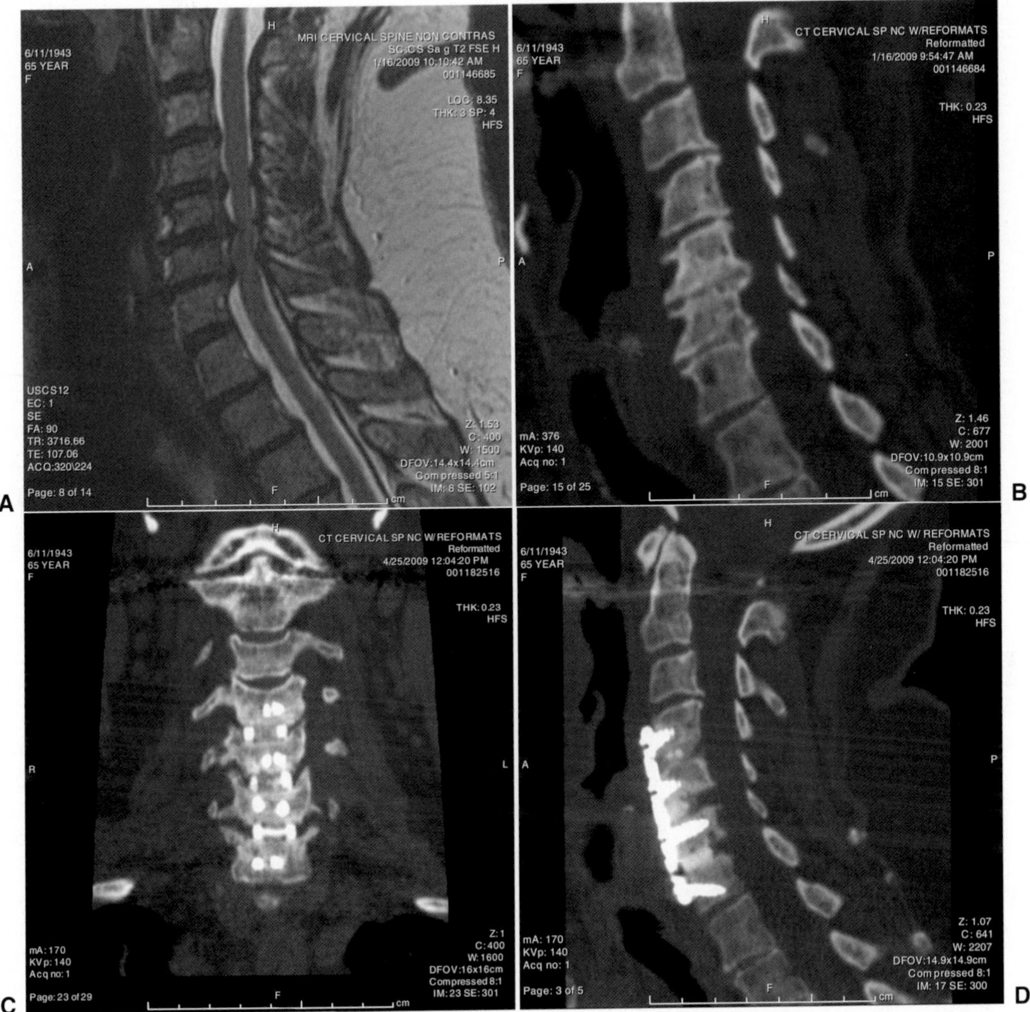

FIGURE 30.2 Multi-level discectomy and fusion for treating CSM. (**A**) Sagittal cervical spine MRI depicting spinal cord compression. (**B**) Sagittal cervical spine CT depicting loss of cervical lordosis and compressive osteophytes at two spinal levels: C5-6 and C6-7. (**C**) Postoperative coronal cervical spine CT image demonstrating allografts at three levels: C4-5, C5-6, and C6-7. (**D**) Postoperative sagittal CT image demonstrating satisfactory removal of compressive osteophytes and restoration of cervical lordosis.

Laminectomy and Fusion

Dorsal decompression and fusion is performed using midline cervical laminectomy with the application of lateral mass screws and rods for rigid fixation as described recently (53). Local autograft bone and/or allograft are used as needed to perform a lateral mass fusion. To improve sagittal alignment, we routinely decompress the spinal cord first and then extend and dorsally translate the spine, using a Mayfield 3-pin head fixation device, to correct alignment. This maneuver can only be safely performed while observing the fully decompressed spinal cord during the maneuver to assure that no further neural compression will occur. This technique requires confirmation, at the conclusion of the reduction, that the spinal cord has remained adequately decompressed.

Laminoplasty

Laminoplasty has been well described in the Japanese literature and has been studied carefully by Heller and colleagues (54). The open-door technique is most widely used in the United States. This procedure involves cutting through the lamina of the cervical spine on one side (the "open" side) at multiple levels, and then cutting a groove on the opposite side of the lamina to create a "hinge" to allow the cross-sectional diameter of the cervical spine to be expanded. The "open" side is then secured using titanium plates to maintain the expanded cervical cross-sectional area. There is a wide choice of titanium plates available that are anatomically contoured for cervical laminar fixation. The surgeon can choose between ceramic or allograft laminar spacers, if it is believed that they add value to the procedure. Some systems also contain "hinge plates" to salvage displaced hinges in the event of excessive bone removal. Typically, 4- or 5-mm self-tapping bone screws are used to fix the plate to the lamina and to the lateral mass at each operated level (Fig. 30.3).

Combined Ventral and Dorsal Approaches

Patients with significant cervical kyphotic deformity and/or patients in whom three or more corpectomies are being contemplated are often treated with a combined ventral and dorsal approach in order to achieve decompression of the spinal cord, correction of the spinal deformity, and maximize

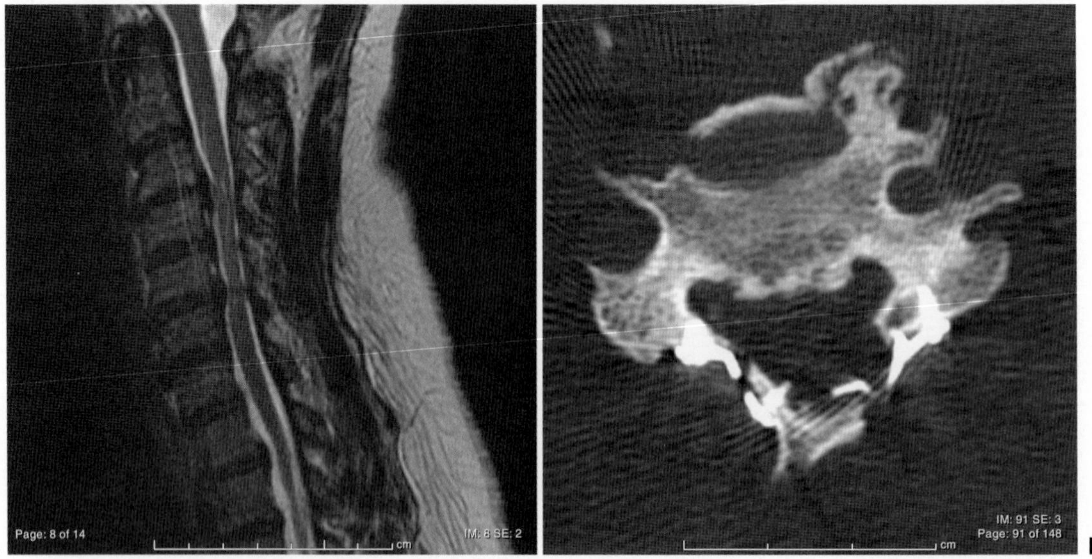

FIGURE 30.3 Open-door laminoplasty for treating CSM. (**A**) Sagittal cervical spine MRI depicting congenital canal narrowing and OPLL. (**B**) Postoperative cervical spine CT axial image demonstrating expansion of spinal canal using open-door laminoplasty with titanium hinge plates and screws.

the likelihood of a successful arthrodesis (55). These operations can be performed in a single day or staged depending on various patient factors as well as surgeon preference. Many surgeons use rigid or semirigid cervical collars for at least 12 weeks postoperatively in these patients.

OUTCOMES OF SURGERY FOR CERVICAL SPONDYLOTIC MYELOPATHY

Most surgical case series have shown improvement following surgery for CSM in approximately 70% of patients (19). Although large RCTs have not been performed comparing surgical to nonsurgical management for treating CSM, one prospective, nonrandomized trial demonstrated better overall functional outcomes in patients treated with surgery (18). Surgical management has become the accepted standard of care for progressive CSM making any future RCTs comparing surgery to non-surgical treatment unlikely to be feasible and potentially unethical.

Several disease-specific outcomes measures have been used to assess the efficacy of surgery for CSM. The modified JOA scale (17 point maximum score) has been frequently used in many studies and has been shown, in most studies, to improve by 2.5 to 4 points after CSM surgery (25,35,38). This disease-specific outcomes measure has been used previously to identify risk factors for poor outcome after surgery for CSM. For example, Suda et al. (25) identified local cervical kyphosis greater than 13 degrees as a significant predictor of poor outcome in patients treated with one type of dorsal surgery (open-door laminoplasty) in a study using the mJOA scale.

CSM has a substantial negative effect on health-related quality of life. A recent VA study found a mean physical component summary score of 27.8 ± 8.3 (over 2 standard deviations below the age-adjusted mean for normal healthy individuals) using the generic SF-36 HR-QOL instrument (56). Surgery for CSM appears to improve quality of life, measured with the SF-36, suggesting that the tool might be valuable to study the differential effects (if they exist) of surgical approach on quality of life in CSM patients (19). Since CSM does not have a known effect on survival, any study attempting to compare two surgical strategies for CSM should consider the effect of surgical intervention on quality of life.

A recent, prospective, non-randomized study of 316 patients with CSM found that surgery resulted in significant improvement using established disease-specific (mJOA) and HR-QOL (SF-36) outcomes instruments (4). The high complication rate observed in this large study (17%) underscores the need to define which procedures (ventral versus dorsal) result in what types of complications and in which patients (4). In addition, this study demonstrates the well-known scenario that prospective studies will invariably report higher complication rates than retrospective reviews of surgical outcomes.

RISK OF COMPLICATIONS FROM SURGERY

In a large, retrospective, cohort review of US hospital discharges associated with cervical spine surgery using the Nationwide Inpatient Sample from 1992 to 2001, Wang et al. (2) found that cervical spondylosis with myelopathy (19% of 932,009 admissions) was associated with higher complication rates compared with other types of cervical spine surgery. Dorsal surgery was utilized more frequently in older patients and was independently associated with higher complication rates. Age greater than 74 years was also an independent predictor for developing complications. Similarly, another recent study found the complication rate in patients older than 75 years was 38% compared with 6% in younger patients (57). This particular analysis, however, did not directly compare ventral and dorsal surgery complication rates and was not limited to CSM patients. Boayke et al., on the other hand, used the Nationwide Inpatient Sample from 1993 to 2002 (58,115 admissions) to compare complication rates between ventral and dorsal fusion procedures for CSM. Their retrospective analysis identified a complication rate of 11.9% for ventral surgery versus 16.4% for dorsal fusion surgery (3).

In a retrospective review of 83 patients treated for CSM using either corpectomy and strut grafting (ventral surgery) or laminoplasty (dorsal surgery), Yonenobu et al. (27) found no significant difference in patient outcome as measured by the Japanese Orthopaedic Association scale. However, patients treated with a laminoplasty (dorsal) experienced fewer complications (7.1%) than patients in the corpectomy (ventral) group (29.3%). Similarly, Edwards found no differences in outcome between patients treated with corpectomy versus laminoplasty, although the laminoplasty (dorsal) group had fewer complications (28).

There are two types of surgical complications that are commonly observed after operations for treating CSM: *dysphagia* (more commonly after ventral surgery) and *C5 nerve root paresis* (temporary but sometimes permanent weakness of the shoulder, seen after both ventral and dorsal surgery but more commonly after dorsal surgery). Edwards reported a 31% rate of persistent dysphagia or dysphonia (hoarseness) after ventral surgery and noted that this complication is often underreported (58). Published rates of C5 paresis range from 12% (ventral procedures) to 30% (dorsal procedures) (59). This complication is often disabling for several months and might be related to traction on the C5 root caused by spinal cord shift after decompression (60). No study to date has prospectively compared C5 paresis rates after ventral and dorsal surgery. Administrative hospital discharge databases are not likely to capture these complication rates accurately nor can they estimate their severity or impact on a patient's quality of life (2). Prospective studies using quality of life instruments are more likely to provide useful information for clinicians and patients on the complication rates after ventral and dorsal surgery and on the overall impact of these complications on patients' lives. Furthermore, since most cases of dysphagia and C5 paresis gradually resolve, the varying definitions for these conditions have led to the marked discrepancies seen in reporting each of these disabling postoperative situations.

Deformity and Late Failures

The development of progressive kyphotic deformity after cervical laminectomy has been reported by several groups (51,52). In some cases, the deformity results in clinical deterioration and poor outcomes (61). Re-operation to correct deformity is sometimes required. The re-operation rate after initial cervical laminectomy is not known, although studies using administrative state inpatient databases should provide useful information in the near future to gain an understanding of the clinical magnitude of the problem.

A NEED FOR RANDOMIZED CONTROLLED TRIALS

While an RCT comparing these two approaches has been advocated by many, the heterogeneity of the patient population along with individual surgeon bias favoring either ventral (anterior) or dorsal (posterior) surgery has discouraged the performance of an RCT to date. Our previous work suggests that most American cervical spine experts (both orthopedic and neurological) believe that there is sufficient clinical equipoise to justify a comparative trial if the study population is carefully defined (62). Several other important reasons justify a trial at this time. First, the complication rate for CSM surgery is very high (17% in one recent prospective study) (4) and particularly so in patients greater than 74 years of age (2), a growing segment of the US population (63). Second, the outcomes in 30% of cases are unsatisfactory (9). Third, the costs of dorsal decompression and fusion appear to be significantly higher than those for ventral surgery, suggesting that even if the approaches had similar outcomes, understanding the differential in hospital costs would be relevant (64).

THORACIC SPINAL STENOSIS

Thoracic spinal stenosis (TSS) causing myelopathy is rare, due mainly to the limited range of motion of the thoracic spine provided by the ribs, sternum, and apophyseal joints (65). The pathogenesis of TSS is similar to that found in other parts of the spine: degenerative changes of the disc with frequent bulging of the disc, hypertrophy of the posterior elements, thickening, and possible calcification of the ligamentum flavum and development of ventral epidural osteophytes (66). Primary TSS with myelopathy should be considered in patients who present with isolated lower extremity weakness and/or incoordination or isolated problems with bowel and bladder dysfunction, particularly when no findings are seen in the cervical or lumbosacral regions on advanced neuroimaging studies.

The clinical evaluation of thoracic myelopathy requires a high index of suspicion and a thorough physical examination. Contrasting with cervical myelopathy, no upper extremity involvement is seen. However, lower extremity weakness, numbness, loss of propioception, and only occasionally bowel and bladder dysfunction and clonus with a positive Babinski sign may be seen with thoracic myelopathy. The differential diagnosis includes MS (affecting the spine), diffuse idiopathic skeletal hyperostosis (DISH), spinal vascular malformations, tumors, infections, hemangiomas, and spinal arachnoid cysts. Thoracic spine x-rays are generally non-diagnostic. MRI is an excellent screening tool for TSS, as well as to rule out other causes; however, if it is not diagnostic, a CT scan, potentially with an accompanying myelogram, may be required to identify the specific areas of stenosis.

In patients presenting with evidence of a progressive myelopathy and neuroimaging confirmation, surgery is recommended. In the great majority of situations, a laminectomy may be performed for patients who have a concentric narrowing of the canal or a predominantly posterior component to their stenosis. On rare occasions, if significant compression from a ventral orientation is present, an anterior or a transpedicular posterior approach may be necessary.

A report of seven patients (four men, three women; mean age 49 years), with TSS and corresponding myelopathy, was published by Dimar et al. (67) This case series reports the surgical treatment consisting of posterior decompression and instrumented fusion (five cases), anterior vertebrectomy and fusion (one), and anterior vertebrectomy with autograft strut followed by wide posterior decompression and instrumented fusion (two). Five patients had significant improvement in their myelopathy and were ambulating normally, one had a modest improvement in ambulation, and one remained wheelchair bound. All patients achieved acceptable radiographic fusions. The concern in all these cases is the development of late spinal instability and recurrent spinal stenosis if solid fusion is not achieved with the initial procedure. Other case series have been reported (68,69). Many neurosurgeons will perform a decompressive laminectomy alone, without fusion, when there is dorsal compression and no evidence of spinal instability.

SUMMARY

CSM is the most common cause of spinal cord dysfunction in the United States. Decompressive surgery for CSM can stabilize or sometimes improve its disabling symptoms; however, there is controversy surrounding the choice of approach: ventral (anterior) versus dorsal (posterior). These two main surgical approaches have been utilized in the United States for nearly 50 years. To date, no RCT has been performed to compare the effectiveness of these competing approaches. In addition, comparative effectiveness studies evaluating the addition of arthrodesis when performing dorsal surgery have not been done. Recent published data demonstrate that complications from CSM surgery (and re-operations for late failures) are prevalent and differ between ventral and dorsal approaches. Definitive studies that can help to establish scientifically based guidelines are likely to improve the results of CSM treatment. In contrast to CSM, TSS causing myelopathy is rare, requires a high index of suspicion for diagnosis, and is typically approached with decompressive laminectomy.

References

1. Patil PG, Turner DA, Pietrobon R. National trends in surgical procedures for degenerative cervical spine disease: 1990–2000. *Neurosurgery* 2005;57(4):753–758.
2. Wang MC, Chan L, Maiman DJ, et al. Complications and mortality associated with cervical spine surgery for degenerative disease in the United States. *Spine* 2007;32(3):342–347.
3. Boakye M, Patil CG, Santarelli J, et al. Cervical spondylotic myelopathy: complications and outcomes after spinal fusion. *Neurosurgery* 2008;62(2):455–461; discussion 61–62.
4. Fehlings MG, Sasso RC, Kopjar B, et al. Anterior vs. posterior surgery of cervical spondylotic myelopathy: a large prospective multi-center clinical trial. In: 24th Annual Meeting of the AANS/CNS Section on Disorders of the Spine and Peripheral Nerves, Orlando, FL, 2008.
5. Young WF. Cervical spondylotic myelopathy: a common cause of spinal cord dysfunction in older persons. *Am Fam Physician* 2000;62(5):1064–1070, 1073.
6. Henderson FC, Geddes JF, Vaccaro AR, et al. Stretch-associated injury in cervical spondylotic myelopathy: new concept and review. *Neurosurgery* 2005;56(5):1101–1113; discussion 1113.
7. al-Mefty O, Harkey HL, Marawi I, et al. Experimental chronic compressive cervical myelopathy. *J Neurosurg* 1993;79(4):550–561.
8. Baron EM, Young WF. Cervical spondylotic myelopathy: a brief review of its pathophysiology, clinical course, and diagnosis. *Neurosurgery* 2007;60(1 Suppl 1):S35–S41.
9. Rowland LP. Surgical treatment of cervical spondylotic myelopathy: time for a controlled trial. *Neurology* 1992;42(1):5–13.
10. Bohlman HH, Emery SE. The pathophysiology of cervical spondylosis and myelopathy. *Spine* 1988;13(7):843–846.
11. Bednarik J, Kadanka Z, Dusek L, et al. Presymptomatic spondylotic cervical cord compression. *Spine* 2004;29(20):2260–2269.
12. Lees F, Turner JW. Natural history and prognosis of cervical spondylosis. *Br Med J* 1963;2(5373):1607–1610.
13. Rao R. Neck pain, cervical radiculopathy, and cervical myelopathy: pathophysiology, natural history, and clinical evaluation. *J Bone Joint Surg* 2002;84-A(10):1872–1881.
14. Mazanec D, Reddy A. Medical management of cervical spondylosis. *Neurosurgery* 2007;60(1 Supp1 1):S43–S50.
15. Aker PD, Gross AR, Goldsmith CH, et al. Conservative management of mechanical neck pain: systematic overview and meta-analysis. *BMJ* 1996;313:1291–1296.
16. Abbasi A, Malhotra G, Malanga G, et al. Complications of interlaminar cervical epidural steroid injections: a review of the literature. *Spine* 2007;32(19):2144–2151.
17. Kadanka Z, Bednarik J, Vohanka S, et al. Conservative treatment versus surgery in spondylotic cervical myelopathy: a prospective randomised study. *Eur Spine J* 2000;9(6):538–544.
18. Sampath P, Bendebba M, Davis JD, et al. Outcome of patients treated for cervical myelopathy. A prospective, multicenter study with independent clinical review. *Spine* 2000;25(6):670–676.
19. Latimer M, Haden N, Seeley HM, et al. Measurement of outcome in patients with cervical spondylotic myelopathy treated surgically. *Br J Neurosurg* 2002;16(6):545–549.
20. Nikolaidis I, Fouyas IP, Sandercock PA, et al. Surgery for cervical radiculopathy or myelopathy. *Cochrane Database Syst Rev* 2010;(1):CD001466.
21. Fouyas IP, Statham PF, Sandercock PA. Cochrane review on the role of surgery in cervical spondylotic radiculomyelopathy. *Spine (Phila Pa 1976)* 2002;27(7):736–747.
22. Wiggins GC, Shaffrey CI. Dorsal surgery for myelopathy and myeloradiculopathy. *Neurosurgery* 2007;60(1 Supp1 1):S71–S81.
23. Smith AG. Account of a case in which portions of three dorsal vertebrae were removed for the relief of paralysis from fracture, with partial success. *N Am Med Surg* 1829;8:94–97.
24. Fessler RG, Steck JC, Giovanini MA. Anterior cervical corpectomy for cervical spondylotic myelopathy. *Neurosurgery* 1998;43(2):257–265; discussion 65–67.
25. Suda K, Abumi K, Ito M, et al. Local kyphosis reduces surgical outcomes of expansive open-door laminoplasty for cervical spondylotic myelopathy. *Spine* 2003;28(12):1258–1262.
26. Suri A, Chabbra RP, Mehta VS, et al. Effect of intramedullary signal changes on the surgical outcome of patients with cervical spondylotic myelopathy. *Spine J* 2003;3(1):33–45.
27. Yonenobu K, Hosono N, Iwasaki M, et al. Laminoplasty versus subtotal corpectomy. A comparative study of results in multisegmental cervical spondylotic myelopathy. *Spine* 1992;17(11):1281–1284.

28. Edwards CC 2nd, Heller JG, Murakami H. Corpectomy versus laminoplasty for multilevel cervical myelopathy: an independent matched-cohort analysis. *Spine* 2002;27(11):1168–1175.
29. Sasso RC, Ruggiero RA Jr, Reilly TM, et al. Early reconstruction failures after multilevel cervical corpectomy. *Spine* 2003;28(2):140–142.
30. Wang JC, Hart RA, Emery SE, et al. Graft migration or displacement after multilevel cervical corpectomy and strut grafting. *Spine* 2003;28(10):1016–1012.
31. Stewart TJ, Schlenk RP, Benzel EC. Multiple level discectomy and fusion. *Neurosurgery* 2007;60(1 Suppl 1):S143–S148.
32. Zdeblick TA, Hughes SS, Riew KD, et al. Failed anterior cervical discectomy and arthrodesis. Analysis and treatment of thirty-five patients. *J Bone Joint Surg* 1997;79(4):523–532.
33. Mummaneni PV, Kaiser MG, Matz PG, et al. Cervical surgical techniques for the treatment of cervical spondylotic myelopathy. *J Neurosurg Spine* 2009;11(2):130–141.
34. Bucciero A, Vizioli L, Carangelo B, et al. MR signal enhancement in cervical spondylotic myelopathy. Correlation with surgical results in 35 cases. *J Neurosurg Sci* 1993;37(4):217–222.
35. Chiles BW 3rd, Leonard MA, Choudhri HF, et al. Cervical spondylotic myelopathy: patterns of neurological deficit and recovery after anterior cervical decompression. *Neurosurgery* 1999;44(4):762–769.
36. Ebersold MJ, Pare MC, Quast LM. Surgical treatment for cervical spondylitic myelopathy. *J Neurosurg* 1995;82(5):745–751.
37. Fukushima T, Ikata T, Taoka Y, et al. Magnetic resonance imaging study on spinal cord plasticity in patients with cervical compression myelopathy. *Spine* 1991;16 (10 Suppl):S534–S538.
38. Kohno K, Kumon Y, Oka Y, et al. Evaluation of prognostic factors following expansive laminoplasty for cervical spinal stenotic myelopathy. *Surg Neurol* 1997;48(3):237–245.
39. Mehalic TF, Pezzuti RT, Applebaum BI. Magnetic resonance imaging and cervical spondylotic myelopathy. *Neurosurgery* 1990;26(2):217–226
40. Morio Y, Yamamoto K, Kuranobu K, et al. Does increased signal intensity of the spinal cord on MR images due to cervical myelopathy predict prognosis? *Arch Orthop Trauma Surg* 1994;113(5):254–259.
41. Okada Y, Ikata T, Yamada H, et al. Magnetic resonance imaging study on the results of surgery for cervical compression myelopathy. *Spine* 1993;18(14):2024–2029.
42. Wada E, Ohmura M, Yonenobu K. Intramedullary changes of the spinal cord in cervical spondylotic myelopathy. *Spine* 1995;20(20):2226–2232.
43. Watabe N, Tominaga T, Shimizu H, et al. Quantitative analysis of cerebrospinal fluid flow in patients with cervical spondylosis using cine phase-contrast magnetic resonance imaging. *Neurosurgery* 1999;44(4):779–784.
44. Yone K, Sakou T, Yanase M, et al. Preoperative and postoperative magnetic resonance image evaluations of the spinal cord in cervical myelopathy. *Spine* 1992;17(10 Suppl):S388–S392.
45. Smith GW, Robinson RA. The treatment of certain cervical-spine disorders by anterior removal of the intervertebral disc and interbody fusion. *J Bone Joint Surg* 1958;40-A(3):607–624.
46. Hillard VH, Apfelbaum RI. Surgical management of cervical myelopathy: indications and techniques for multilevel cervical discectomy. *Spine J* 2006;6(6 Suppl):242S–251S.
47. Brodke DS, Zdeblick TA. Modified Smith-Robinson procedure for anterior cervical discectomy and fusion. *Spine* 1992;17(10 Suppl):S427–S430.
48. Kwon BK, Vaccaro AR, Grauer JN, et al. The use of rigid internal fixation in the surgical management of cervical spondylosis. *Neurosurgery* 2007;60(1 Suppl 1):S118–S129.
49. Cooper PR. Anterior cervical vertebrectomy: tips and traps. *Neurosurgery* 2001;49(5):1129–1132.
50. Douglas AF, Cooper PR. Cervical corpectomy and strut grafting. *Neurosurgery* 2007;60(1 Suppl 1):S137–S142.
51. Lu JJ. Cervical laminectomy: technique. *Neurosurgery* 2007;60(1 Suppl 1):S149–S153.
52. Mikawa Y, Shikata J, Yamamuro T. Spinal deformity and instability after multilevel cervical laminectomy. *Spine* 1987;12(1):6–11.
53. Huang RC, Girardi FP, Poynton AR, et al. Treatment of multilevel cervical spondylotic myeloradiculopathy with posterior decompression and fusion with lateral mass plate fixation and local bone graft. *J Spinal Disord Tech* 2003;16(2):123–129.
54. Heller JG, Edwards CC 2nd, Murakami H, et al. Laminoplasty versus laminectomy and fusion for multilevel cervical myelopathy: an independent matched cohort analysis. *Spine* 2001;26(12):1330–1336.
55. Mummaneni PV, Haid RW, Rodts GE Jr. Combined ventral and dorsal surgery for myelopathy and myeloradiculopathy. *Neurosurgery* 2007;60(1 Suppl 1):S82–S89.
56. King JT Jr, McGinnis KA, Roberts MS. Quality of life assessment with the medical outcomes study short form-36 among patients with cervical spondylotic myelopathy. *Neurosurgery* 2003;52(1):113–120; discussion 21.
57. Holly LT, Moftakhar P, Khoo LT, et al. Surgical outcomes of elderly patients with cervical spondylotic myelopathy. *Surg Neurol* 2008;69(3):233–240.
58. Edwards CC 2nd, Karpitskaya Y, Cha C, et al. Accurate identification of adverse outcomes after cervical spine surgery. *J Bone Joint Surg* 2004;86-A(2):251–256.
59. Bose B, Sestokas AK, Schwartz DM. Neurophysiological detection of iatrogenic C-5 nerve deficit during anterior cervical spinal surgery. *J Neurosurg Spine* 2007;6(5):381–385.
60. Saunders RL. On the pathogenesis of the radiculopathy complicating multilevel corpectomy. *Neurosurgery* 1995;37(3):408–412; discussion 12–13.
61. Yonenobu K, Okada K, Fuji T, et al. Causes of neurologic deterioration following surgical treatment of cervical myelopathy. *Spine* 1986;11(8):818–823.
62. Ghogawala Z, Coumans JV, Benzel EC, et al. Ventral versus dorsal decompression for cervical spondylotic myelopathy: surgeons' assessment of eligibility for randomization in a proposed randomized controlled trial: results of a survey of the Cervical Spine Research Society. *Spine* 2007;32(4):429–436.
63. Riggs BL, Melton LJ 3rd. The worldwide problem of osteoporosis: insights afforded by epidemiology. *Bone* 1995;17(5 Suppl):505S–511S.

64. Ghogawala Z, Wasserberger E, Potter R, et al. Ventral surgery versus dorsal decompression with fusion for cervical spondylotic myelopathy: A cost analysis. 76th Annual Meeting of the American Association of Neurological Surgeons, Chicago, IL, 2008 (abstr).
65. Wood KB, Garvey TA, Gundry C, et al. Magnetic resonance imaging of the thoracic spine. Evaluation of asymptomatic individuals. *J Bone Joint Surg* 1995;77(11): 1631–1638.
66. Kalfas IH. Laminectomy for thoracic spinal canal stenosis. *Neurosurg Focus* 2000;9(4):1–4.
67. Dimar JR, Bratcher KR, Glassman SD, et al. Identification and Surgical Treatment of Primary Thoracic Spinal Stenosis. *Am J Orthop* 2008; 37(11):564–568.
68. Jaspan T, Holland IM, Punt JA. Thoracic spinal canal stenosis. *Neuroradiology* 1987;29(2):217.
69. Barnett GH, Hardy RW, Little JR, et al. Thoracic spinal canal stenosis. *J Neurosurg* 1987;66(3):338–344.

CHAPTER 31 ■ PRIMARY AND METASTATIC TUMORS OF THE SPINAL CORD AND SPINAL CANAL

STEPHEN M. SELKIRK AND ROBERT LOUIS RUFF

INTRODUCTION

This chapter describes the variety of primary spinal cord tumors and spinal column metastases. We have chosen to first provide a broad oversight of tumors and end with a discussion of the benefits of rehabilitation for people with the most common type of tumor involving the spinal cord, namely epidural metastatic cancer. The most common tumors that arise within the spinal cord are primary tumors. However, the common tumors to involve the spinal canal and secondarily compromise the spinal cord are metastatic cancers or secondary tumors. Secondary tumors are about 25 times more common than primary spinal cord tumors (1).

This chapter is further organized based upon tumor location. Fig. 31.1 shows that tumors can be classified based upon the region of the spinal canal that they initially involve, as one of the following: intradural intramedullary tumors that arise within the spinal cord parenchyma (B in figure), intradural extramedullary tumors that grow within the spinal canal but outside the cord parenchyma (C in figure), and extradural spinal cord tumors arising outside the spinal canal that are primarily metastatic (A and D in figure). Intradural and extradural tumors are about equal in prevalence. Intradural tumors are represented by a great number of distinct tumor types, whereas metastatic disease to the spinal cord represents the vast majority of extradural tumors (Table 31.1).

In general, the initial manifestations of intramedullary tumors that arise in the spinal cord are signs of myelopathy with motor and sensory loss. The spinal cord, as is true of other parts of the central nervous system (CNS), does not possess pain sensation. Pain develops later as the tumors expand and irritate the coverings of the spinal cord (pia mater and primarily the dura mater). In contrast, the initial manifestation of tumors that arise outside of the spinal cord is usually back pain. The back pain may radiate in a radicular fashion if there is nerve root traction or can be perceived as pain traveling up and down the spine (Lhermitte phenomenon). The back pain associated with extramedullary tumors often has an electric-like or tingling character and can be worsened or elicited by maneuvers that raise spinal canal pressure such as the Valsalva maneuver (1,2).

INTRADURAL TUMORS

Intradural tumors are an uncommon but important subset of tumors affecting the CNS. For every one intradural tumor, four intracranial tumors will be diagnosed. Given that most intradural tumors are benign or slow growing, however, an accurate diagnosis is essential to minimizing disability over time. Further complicating this issue is that biopsy is generally not a routine component of diagnostic algorithms; apparent tumors must be distinguished from vascular, inflammatory, or infectious lesions based on more indirect testing and clinical history. Frequently, these lesions result in clinicians considering multiple diagnoses concurrently and most often it necessitates the collective input of the neurologist or spinal cord physician, neuroradiologist, and neurosurgeon to establish the correct course of action.

Intradural tumors arise beneath the dura mater and can be divided into extramedullary and intramedullary lesions based on anatomical location outside of or within the spinal cord parenchyma, respectively. Intradural tumors represent only approximately 10% to 15% of CNS neoplasms. Extramedullary tumors comprise nearly two thirds of these and intramedullary tumors encompass the remaining third.

In contrast to extramedullary tumors, the management of intradural tumors almost always includes a surgical procedure, as a definitive diagnosis requires tissue analysis. Surgical resection should include intraoperative monitoring with somatosensory evoked potentials and motor evoked potentials. The extent of resection is based on multiple factors including the diagnosis made from surgically obtained frozen section. This factor will also guide postoperative adjuvant treatment.

Intradural Intramedullary Spinal Cord Tumors

The majority of intradural intramedullary spinal cord (IISC) tumors arise from ependymal cells (56%) or astrocytes (29%), while the remainder includes much less common tumor types such as hemangioblastomas, lipomas, epidermoids, teratomas, meningioblastomas, and oligodendrogliomas. Perhaps the most important factor suggesting an intradural intramedullary process rather than an epidural metastatic lesion is the time course of symptom development. While the most common presenting symptom remains back pain, particularly when supine, an insidious process developing over months rather than weeks suggests an intradural intramedullary process. As described for extramedullary lesions, magnetic resonance imaging (MRI) remains the *sine qua non* for the identification of IISC lesions and should include a survey of the entire neuraxis to identify multifocal disease. Tumors of the spinal cord, as a general rule, are hypointense to isointense on T1-weighted images and hyperintense on T2-weighted images. T2-weighted images can also identify associated

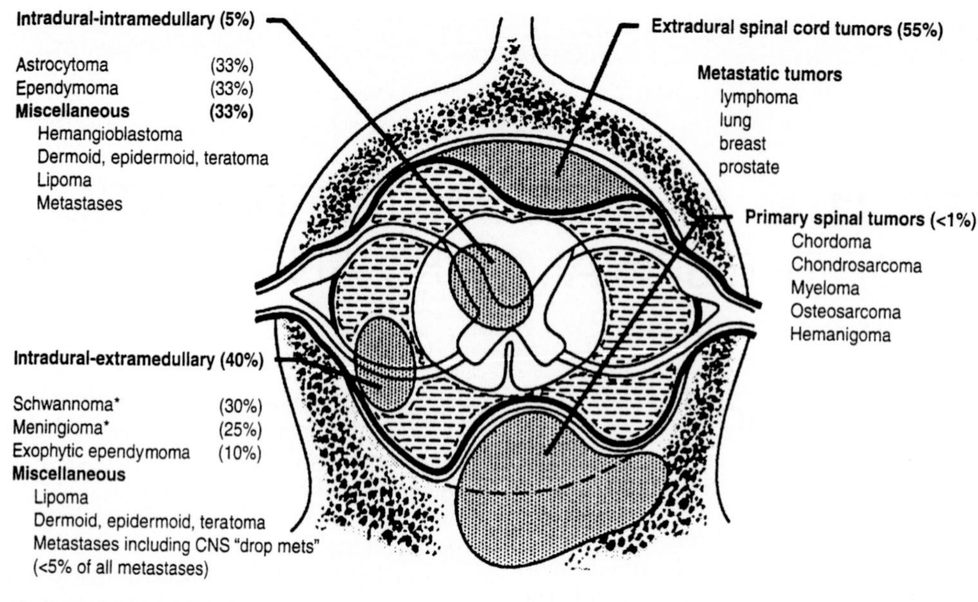

FIGURE 31.1 Intraspinal location and relative incidence of spinal tumors. Primary and metastatic tumors of the spine and spinal cord. Adapted from Tumors of the central nervous system. In: *American cancer society of clinical oncology*. 2nd ed. Atlanta, GA: ACS, 1995:400–410.

syrinx and surrounding edema. At times, the subtype of the IISC tumor can be indentified if it conforms to classical MRI findings. Other modalities such as cerebrospinal fluid (CSF) evaluation are generally useful only to rule out other causes of spinal cord lesions, rather than confirming the diagnosis of an IISC tumor. Modern surgical techniques have resulted in impressive gains in outcome over the last 25 years for patients with IISC tumors (3). In most cases, early and aggressive tumor resection has the greatest likelihood of preserving neurological function (4).

Ependymomas

Ependymomas are a common IISC tumor in adults, peaking in frequency between the second and fourth decade, affecting males and females equally. Ependymomas arise from ependymal cells lining the central canal and exist primarily as two

TABLE 31.1

CLASSIFICATION OF THE TUMORS AFFECTING THE SPINAL CORD AND COLUMN

Intradural intramedullary	Intradural extramedullary	Extradural
Ependymoma	Schwannoma	Metastatic tumors Lymphoma Lung Breast Prostate
Astrocytoma	Meningioma	Primary bony spinal lesions Plasmacytoma Hemangioma Osteoblastoma Osteochondroma Giant cell tumor Osteosarcoma Ewing sarcoma
Hemangioblastoma Metastases Others (rare): Ganglioma Subependymoma Intramedullary schwannoma Germinoma Lymphoma Primitive neuroectodermal	Filum ependymoma Drop metastases	

distinct histological subtypes, which localize to divergent anatomical locations. The myxopapillary subtypes arise in the cauda equina and can extend to the conus medullaris, but for surgical reasons these tumors are considered extramedullary. The classic or cellular subtypes arise primarily in the cervical region (68%) or less commonly the upper thoracic spine. Reactive tumor cells commonly result in disturbances of CSF formation producing cysts, necrosis, hemorrhage, or syrinx formation within the expanding mass (Fig. 31.2). Associated syrinx has been reported in as many as 65% of patients with ependymoma (5). The histological differentiation from astrocytoma usually occurs at surgical resection and is based on the presence of perivascular pseudorosettes or true rosettes under microscopic examination. Nearly all ependymomas are benign, compressing the spinal cord rather than infiltrating adjacent tissue. They are generally well circumscribed, slow growing, and only rarely result in CNS seeding or recurrence (6). These characteristics result in extended survival and minimal recurrence rates in patients. The 15-year survival has been reported to be as high as 60% to 75%, while progression-free survival at 15 years ranges from 35% to 45% (7,8). Favorable factors include smaller tumor size, myxopapillary subtype, and younger age at diagnosis (8,9).

The nature of ependymomas allows for a well-defined surgical plane between tumor and surrounding parenchyma usually permitting partial resection in 83% and complete resection in 65% (3). Immediately after surgery neurological status can worsen but 1-year postresection data suggest that the majority of patients are better or stable from a neurological standpoint (3). Low grade, completely resected tumors only require MRI monitoring (10,11). An inability to fully resect the tumor or evidence of dissemination requires local radiation in the 4,500 to 5,500 centiGray (cGy) range, with additional lower doses to the remainder of the neuraxis. The primary management of ependymomas does not include adjuvant chemotherapy; however, etoposide has demonstrated efficacy in patients with recurrent disease (12,13).

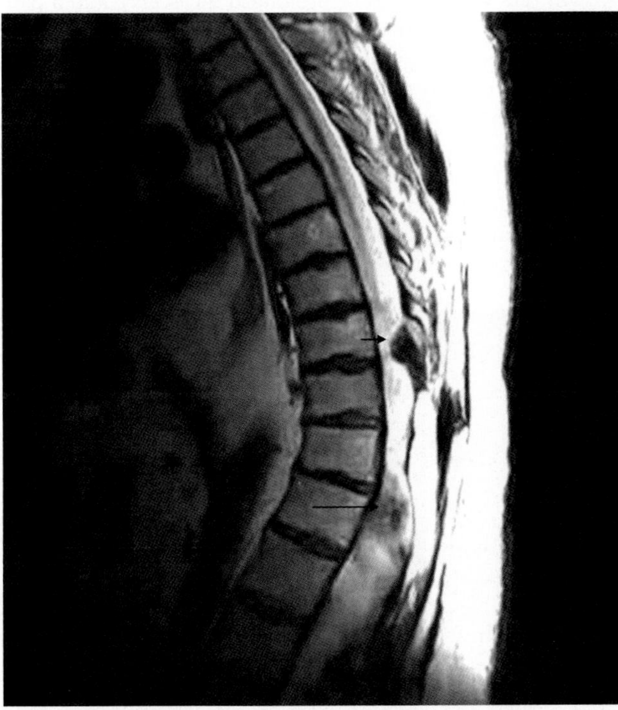

FIGURE 31.2 This patient presented for annual follow-up after surgical resection of an ependymoma. He complained of worsening back pain. T2-weighted images demonstrate an irregular lesion at the previous surgical site (T11-12) consistent with tumor recurrence (*long arrow*). There is a small postsurgical epidural cyst seen at T9 (*short arrow*). Surgery resulting in complete resection is curative, but subtotal resection can result in recurrence.

Astrocytomas

Only 3% of CNS astrocytomas arise in the spinal cord. The prevalence of astrocytomas in the spinal cord is about 1 to 2.5 per 100,000 per year peaking in the first three decades of life (14). In the pediatric population, astrocytomas comprise 90% of IISC tumors in patients less than 10 years of age and 60% in patients between 11 and 18 years of age (15). Astrocytomas, like ependymomas, predominately occur in the cervical or high thoracic region. The histological features of spinal cord astrocytomas do not differ from those arising intracranially. They represent a heterogeneous group ranging from low-grade tumors to high-grade glioblastomas. In the pediatric population, nearly all are benign, with only 10% being glioblastomas or malignant astrocytomas. This is mirrored in the adult, as spinal astrocytomas are usually low grade, that is, World Health Organization grades I and II (16,17). High-grade tumors aggressively disseminate throughout the CSF, rapidly progress clinically, and are associated with dismal survival rates (18,19). Up to 40% of patients will have associated tumoral cysts or syrinx (20,21).

The preponderance of benign subtypes results in patients presenting with slowly progressive symptoms over the course of months to years. As expected, the less common, high-grade tumors present with more rapidly developing signs and symptoms. The most common presentation is pain, typically paravertebral pain but not uncommonly radicular pain (22). Weakness and sensory disturbances also occur frequently, but bowel and bladder symptoms usually only occur in more advanced invasive disease unless the tumor is localized to the conus medullaris. In addition, centrally located invasive cervical astrocytomas can present as classic central cord syndrome, with upper extremity weakness greater than or preceding lower extremity weakness. As with other tumors of the spinal cord, MRI is the diagnostic modality of choice because of its superior sensitivity and its ability to clarify surrounding anatomy, cystic structures, and edema. Astrocytomas are often difficult to differentiate from ependymomas based on MRI alone as both tumor types are isointense or hypointense on T1-weighted images and readily enhance after gadolinium administration regardless of the tumor grade. Differentiating features include the degree of invasiveness, which is greater for astrocytomas, as well as the lack of well-defined tumor margins. Finally, astrocytomas usually appear eccentric within the cord, whereas ependymomas take on a more central location (Fig. 31.3).

As it is for ependymomas, the initial management of spinal astrocytomas is surgical, the goal of which is significant debulking and tissue procurement for confirmation of diagnosis. Unfortunately, the infiltrative nature of this tumor often times results in subtotal resection and a high risk for recurrence. For low- and medium-grade tumors, adjuvant postoperative radiation improves survival and recurrence rate (23,24). High-grade tumors of the spinal cord and intracranial tumors are treated in a similar manner. Patients are administered 5,000 cGy local radiation in 30 fractions over 6 weeks followed by chemotherapy. These regimens have been poorly studied in patients with spinal cord astrocytomas and evidence for this intensity

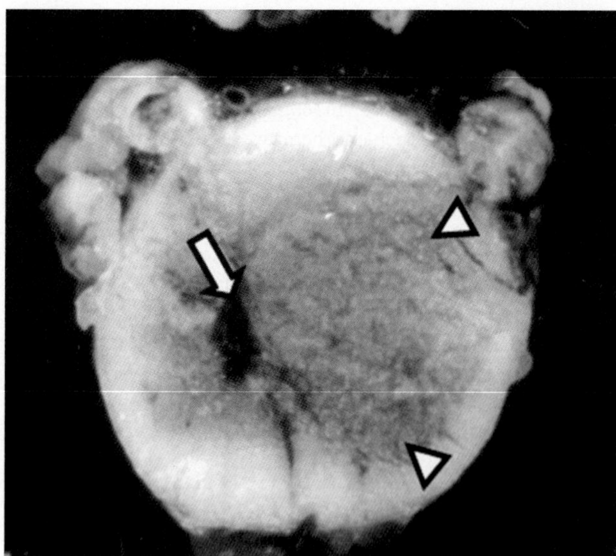

FIGURE 31.3 Pathological transverse section of the lower cervical spinal cord of a patient who succumbed to a spinal cord astrocytoma. Note that the tumor was extending into the ventral and dorsal roots (*arrowheads*). A small cyst or syrinx developed at the medial margin of the tumor (indicated by *arrow*). The tumor was diagnosed 7 years prior to death. The slow expansion permitted the spinal cord tracts to accommodate to the initial expansion of the tumor. The patient became tetraparetic 3 years prior to death. Death was due to systemic sepsis evolving secondary to pneumonia.

of treatment is derived from studies in patients with intracranial tumors. Chemotherapy regimens consist of temozolomide or procarbazine/CCNU/vincristine (25–27).

Hemangioblastomas

Hemangioblastomas are benign tumors derived from hemangioblasts (multipotent cells common to hematopoietic and endothelial cells) representing about 3% of IISC tumors. Approximately 75% of these arise spontaneously with peak incidence between the ages of 30 and 35 and a male predilection (2:1). Spontaneously occurring tumors occur evenly distributed throughout the cord. They are nonencapsulated but well circumscribed and nearly all have a pial attachment and are located dorsally or dorsolaterlly. These tumors are highly vascular and grossly bright red appearing. Histologically, they are benign appearing, cystic, and capillary rich with few actively dividing cells (28).

The presentation of patients is in keeping with the benign nature of the tumor and its anatomical predominance in the dorsal root entry zone. Many times patients present with poorly defined, prolonged symptoms, which in some cases have been present for several years (29,30). Sensory changes represent the most common presenting signs, followed by weakness and pain (31), and 95% of patients will have associated syrinxes (29). MRI accurately defines this tumor type (Fig. 31.4) and the relation to the cord as they vibrantly enhance postcontrast administration (32). T2-weighted studies can define any associated syrinx with a high degree of sensitivity. Although arteriography can define the extensive vasculature of the tumor, in general the additional information is not useful in terms of clinical prognosis or treatment plan.

Although the majority of hemangioblastomas are sporadic, up to 25% arise in patients with von Hippel-Lindau disease (VHL) and therefore, all patients diagnosed with this tumor type should be screened for this disease. Patients with VHL have an autosomally inherited mutation in the tumor suppressor VHL gene predisposing them to a variety of tumors. These patients tend to present at earlier ages and have multiple tumors along the neuraxis. Unlike sporadic hemangioblastomas, this tumor type in patients with VHL tends to arise in the cervical spine more frequently than other locations. Often times, imaging will incidentally identify asymptomatic hemangioblastomas in patients with VHL. Studies on the natural history of this tumor subtype demonstrate a highly variable growth rate with periods of prolonged quiescence and a paucity of good predictors of progression. Therefore, making treatment decisions about asymptomatic hemagioblastomas represents a serious dilemma. Some have suggested reserving surgical resection until symptom onset (28).

Treatment of hemangioblastomas consists of microsurgical resection. Long-term outcomes after resection are generally very good as 90% of patients remain either clinically stable or show neurological improvement (32). Complete resection usually prevents recurrence and provides resolution of edema

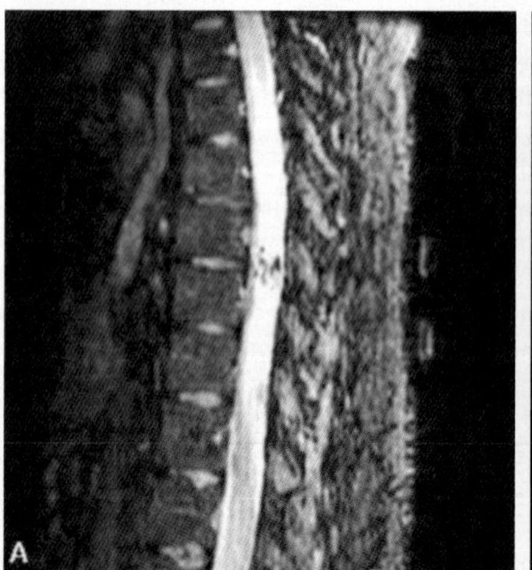

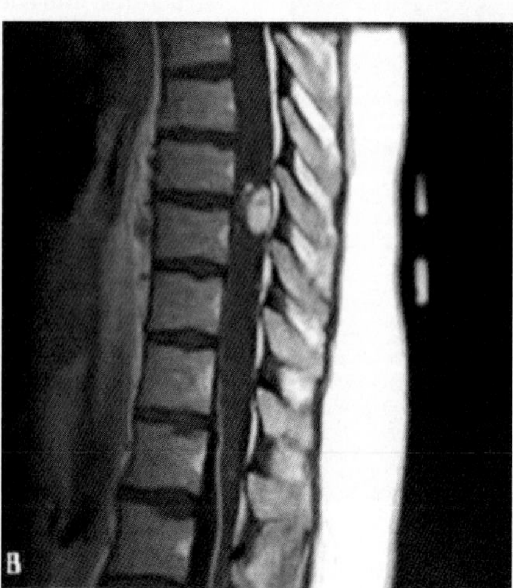

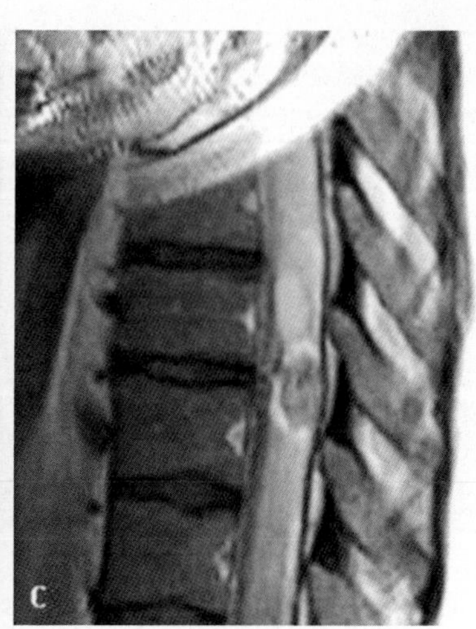

FIGURE 31.4 Spinal cord hemangioblastomas occur sporadically or in association with VHL disease. This patient presented with abdominal pain and after tumor identification was diagnosed with VHL disease. T2-weighted MR images (**A**) and fluid-attenuated inversion recovery images (**B**) are useful in defining peritumoral edema, cystic areas, and associated syringomyelia. These tumors enhance on T1-weighted postcontrast images (**C**).

and associated syrinx. Poor outcomes are associated with the degree of preoperative neurological disability, tumors greater than 500 mm^3, and an anterior location. Postoperative follow-up should include a 3-month MRI with contrast to confirm total tumor resection, as residual tumor will result in recurrence and may require additional surgery (33). Patients with sporadic tumor can have a final MRI 12 months after surgical resection and be considered cured while patients with VHL should have serial annual or biannual screening MRI as recurrence at different regions along the neuraxis is common (34). Radiation therapy is reserved for tumors that are surgically inaccessible (29) due to a relative lack of responsiveness. Chemotherapy plays no role in treatment at this time.

Intramedullary Spinal Cord Metastasis

Metastatic disease to the spinal column, as mentioned previously, is present in the majority of cancer patients who come to autopsy. However, invasion into the spinal cord parenchyma is an uncommon phenomenon, noted in only 0.1% to 2% of cases and representing only 1% of all intramedullary spinal cord tumors (35). The most common source of intramedullary spinal cord metastasis (ISCM) is by far small cell lung cancer, comprising 54% to 85% of cases. Although theoretically any primary source can metastasize to the spinal cord, breast cancer (11% to 13%), melanoma (9%), lymphoma (4%), renal cell carcinoma (9%), and colorectal cancer represent the remainder of cases (36).

ISCM are distributed evenly throughout the cord with 15% of patients presenting with multifocal cord involvement and 57% with concomitant brain metastasis. The diagnosis of metastatic cancer is almost always well established in patients at the time of presentation making the diagnosis less complicated. Typical clinical presentation is a rapidly progressive myelopathy picture, which, in contrast to extradural metastasis, most commonly presents with the patient complaining of sensory deficits (42.5%). Pain, which is the most common symptom with extradural metastasis, is less common, although it is the presenting symptom in a significant number of patients (37). Signs of ISCM include weakness (93%), sensory changes (78% to 87%), and bowel/bladder dysfunction (62%). Notably signs can be asymmetric in almost half of patients (35). The average age of presentation is 58 years with a slight male predominance (64%). The diagnosis of ISCM is based on MRI, which can accurately distinguish an intramedullary lesion from an extramedullary lesion but not from other intramedullary processes. CSF studies are not useful and nuclear radioisotope scans do not usually provide information that alters the treatment course.

Interestingly, ISCM has a predilection to the spinal gray matter of the posterior horns. This anatomical location represents a highly vascularized region relative to adjacent white matter supporting the hypothesis that the hematogenous route is the primary mechanism of cellular dissemination. The localization to the posterior horns also accounts for the fact that the majority of patients present with sensory disturbance, in contrast to patients with extradural metastasis who most often present with pain.

Patients who are diagnosed with ISCM usually have disseminated disease with a preexisting poor prognosis limiting treatments to palliative modalities. This consists of external radiation and dexamethasone administration and results in diminished pain and improvement in neurological dysfunction in 85% of patients (35). The high rate of successful palliation is likely secondary to the radiosensitive nature of the majority of the primary sources (small cell lung, lymphoma, and breast). Currently, surgical procedures and adjuvant chemotherapy as applied to ICSM lack efficacy data to support using them. The average time from diagnosis to death is 3 months.

Uncommon Intramedullary Tumors

Intramedullary gangliogliomas occur predominately in children and young adults and represent less than 1% of all spinal cord tumors (38,39). These tumors usually spread over more vertebral segments than astrocytomas or ependymomas and are universally eccentrically located. They have a mixed pattern of hypo- and hyperintense signal on T1-weighted MRI without peritumoral edema and patchy enhancement postcontrast administration, thereby allowing for radiographic differentiation. Spinal cord subependymomas are rare tumors as less than 50 have been reported. These tumors lack differentiating clinical or image-based characteristics; consequently, diagnosis is made after tissue is examined histologically. Even less common are reports of spinal intramedullary schwannoma, primary intramedullary germinoma, lymphoma, and primitive neuroectodermal tumors (40,41).

Intradural Extramedullary Spinal Cord Tumors

Intradural extramedullary spinal cord (IESC) tumors represent about two thirds of intradural spinal tumors. The vast majority of these tumors are benign and amenable to full surgical resection. Nerve sheath tumors, meningiomas, and myxopapillary ependymomas of the filum terminale account for nearly 95% of cases.

Nerve Sheath Tumors

Neurofibromas and schwannomas account for 40% of extramedullary tumors and are generally considered together. They affect men and women equally with peak incidence in the fifth decade (42). Schwannomas are nerve sheath tumors derived from the myelin-producing Schwann cells of the peripheral nervous system (PNS). They are almost always benign, confined to the outside of the nerve, and exert mass effect leading to symptoms. Less than 1% transition to a malignant schwannoma or neurofibrosarcoma. Grossly they do not enlarge the nerve itself; rather they are usually perched eccentrically with a discreet attachment to the nerve. The majority of schwannomas arise from the dorsal nerve root in contrast to neurofibromas, which are derived from ventral nerve roots. The representative literature suggests a predilection to the cervical spine but a significant percentage arise in the thoracic and lumbar spine as well (43,44).

Neurofibromas are associated with neurofibromatosis 1 (NF1) and result from the bi-allelic inactivation of the associated NF1 gene encoding the neurofibromin protein. Multiple neurofibromas establish the diagnosis of NF1, but even solitary lesions should raise suspicion. Neurofibromas arise from non-myelinating Schwann cells of the PNS that have failed to form Remak bundles (45). They are histologically characterized by the presences of copious fibrous tissue and prominent nerve fibers within the tumor mass. Grossly, they result in a fusiform enlargement of the nerve. These tumors are also usually benign but tend to become intimately connected to nerve fibers so that surgical resection is difficult. A small percentage of these are malignant, and half of malignant neurofibromas occur in patients with a diagnosis of NF1.

The most common presentations of nerve sheath tumors are pain (36%) and paresthesias (36%) followed by motor weakness (24%). Further symptom breakdown demonstrates that tumors confined within the dura most commonly present with pain while those with a combination of intra and extradural components more commonly present with complaints of paresthesias (46). Pain is frequently radicular in distribution secondary to the dorsal or dorsal-lateral localization of the mass.

Treatment of nerve sheath tumors is surgical. Complete surgical resection of neurofibromas and schwannomas not associated with NFI is curative and adjuvant therapy is not indicated. However, complete separation from the nerve itself is difficult often times resulting in sacrifice of all or part of the nerve root involved. Approximately 80% of patients show neurological improvement after surgery (46). In contrast, all malignant nerve sheath tumors should be irradiated after resection and treated with chemotherapy based on established protocols for soft tissue sarcomas (47). Benign nerve sheath tumors that are not amenable to surgery or are only partially removed should likely be irradiated as well. However, there is also evidence that frequent MRI monitoring, particularly in older, asymptomatic patients, should be considered as generally these tumors are slow growing. This is especially true for patients with NF1 who are at high risk for malignant conversion of existing tumor or secondary malignancy from radiation given a genetic predisposition to cellular transformation (47). Recurrence rates vary greatly in case series from 19% at 5 years and 43% at 10 years to 1.5% in other studies (42,44).

Meningiomas

Meningiomas are derived from the arachnoid cap cells of the arachnoid villi located on the meninges and are the most common primary CNS tumor. Spinal meningiomas are derived from the cap cells in dura juxtaposed to nerve root sleeves resulting in their lateral or ventrolateral anatomical position. The majority of meningiomas are intradural but about 10% are intra- and extradural or entirely extradural (48). Purely extradural tumors have a male predominance (49). Spinal meningiomas occur predominately in females (75% to 85%) with bimodal peak incidence in the fifth and seventh decades (50–52). Eighty percent of these tumors are located in the thoracic spine and the majority (99%) are solitary. Multiple meningiomas of the spine are most common in patients with neurofibromatosis (53).

The primary treatment of spinal meningiomas is surgical resection. Large case series have determined that recurrence after total resection is nearly nonexistent and outcomes are excellent (54,55). As with nerve sheath tumors, only partially resected or surgically inaccessible symptomatic meningiomas should be irradiated. Chemotherapy is usually not employed.

Filum Ependymoma

Spinal ependymomas have been described previously with the section on intramedually tumors. Fifty percent of spinal ependymomas, however, arise from the intradural portion of the filum terminale. From a histology standpoint, these tumors arise from neuroectoderm and are classified as intramedullary, but from a surgical and clinical perspective, it is more commonsensical to classify them with extramedullary masses. These tumors can arise at any age but peak incidence is in the third to fifth decade (56). Similar to spinal ependymomas at other locations, filum ependymomas are encapsulated but well circumscribed usually arising from the proximal segment of the filum with possible extension into the conus. The majority of these tumors are of the myxopapillary histological subtype, which establishes the outer core surrounding a hyalinized, relatively acellular center (57). Early studies had suggested that these tumors were benign and the most amenable to complete resection; however, the intimate relationship to the cauda equina and adjacent CSF results in increased rates of subtotal surgical removal and recurrence relative to ependymomas located elsewhere in the cord.

Differentiating disk pathology from filum tumor based on clinical data is difficult. Patients with filum ependymomas tend to present with protracted histories of subtle symptoms progressing over years. Back pain radiating asymmetrically into the legs is the most common complaint at presentation. Worsening pain with valsalva is a distinguishing characteristic of filum tumor. As for other tumors described herein, MRI is the diagnostic tool of choice and surgical removal the most appropriate treatment modality. Overall surgical outcomes are good. Postoperative neurological worsening is usually accompanied by subsequent improvement over a 6-month period (52). Subtotal resection of filum ependymomas results in a 20% risk of tumor reemergence (58), which is treated with repeat surgery or radiation.

Drop Metastasis

Drop metastases are an uncommon complication of intracranial tumors. These lesions are located intradurally and extramedullary and seed the spine via the CSF after transformed cells from the primary mass exfoliate into the subarachnoid space. It is hypothesized that disruption of the primary tumor and surrounding blood-brain barrier via surgical manipulation may increase the risk for subsequent drop metastases. Reports of intramedullary drop metastasis are extremely limited (59). As a whole, the number of patients with symptomatic seeding of the spinal cord from intracranial tumors is low. For patients with intracranial glioblastoma multiforme, several large series of patients have reported that 1% to 2% will develop drop metastases (59,60). This is far less than the percentage of patients at autopsy with seeding of the CSF. This is likely due to the fact that drop metastases occur late in the disease course in patients with aggressive primary tumors resulting in death prior to symptom onset from the metastases (61). In contrast, patients with medulloblastoma develop drop metastases more frequently. Eleven percent of patients have MRI detectable disease spread to the spinal cord at the time of initial diagnosis and 22% have MRI detectable spread at follow-up (62). Drop metastases localize to the lumbar or lower thoracic spine in the majority of cases (63). Patients presenting with pain and a history of intracranial tumor diagnosis should undergo MRI to detect spread to the spine. These patients can be treated with radiation or surgery depending on the status of their primary tumor, its responsiveness to various interventions, and the extent of spinal cord involvement. Having said this, the diagnosis carries a poor prognosis, as death occurs 2 to 3 months after identification (64).

Extradural Spinal Cord Tumors

Extradural spinal cord tumors include primary boney tumors and secondary metastatic lesions to the spine. The most common sources of these metastatic lesions are lymphoma, lung breast, and prostate, with obvious gender predilections. Overall, lung is the most common primary source when the genders are combined. In the pediatric population, multiple myeloma is the most common malignant tumor and vertebral hemangiomas are the most common benign lesions. The management of these tumors has evolved swiftly. MRI has allowed for early diagnosis with detailed information regarding the surrounding anatomy, while advances in surgical technology, focal radiation techniques, and chemotherapeutics have evolved to significantly improve survival rates. Most often, patients with vertebral tumors present with insidious and progressive pain. The extent of neurological disability is directly related to the time between pain onset and diagnosis, underscoring the need for early and accurate diagnosis followed by swift intervention (65).

Primary Bony Spinal Lesions

Plasma Cell Neoplasms

Multiple myelomas or plasmacytomas are the most common primary malignant lesions of the adult spinal column. Plasma cell neoplasms are more common in the African American population, affecting males more than females. Patients with solitary plasmacytomas present with pain. Nearly half of solitary plasmacytomas progress to multiple myeloma within 5 years warranting close monitoring to detect disease progression at the earliest time point. Vertebroplasty with adjuvant radiotherapy is the treatment of solitary lesions. Chemotherapy, although not curative, can significantly prolong life (66).

Hemangiomas

Hemangiomas are vascular lesions arising from newly formed blood vessels. Case series have demonstrated that most spinal hemangiomas are identified incidentally, while 20% present with pain and 8% present with neurological deficits (67). These tumors are more common in women, localized more often to the thoracic or upper lumbar spine, and are solitary the majority of the time. Most tumors are confined to the vertebral body and are clinically insignificant. Extension of tumor into the epidural space results in direct compression of the spinal cord and usually pain. Retrospective studies defined pain as the imperative symptom indicating a need for intervention and follow-up surveillance. Treatment is surgical with preoperative angiography and embolization. Patients who undergo complete surgical resection secondary to pain and/or neurological disability universally recover and remain free from recurrence. Retrospective studies demonstrate that in patients with incomplete resection, recurrence is highly dependent upon the dose of adjuvant radiation administered (68).

Osteoblastic Lesions

Osteoblastic lesions are benign tumors of unknown origin. Osteoblastomas are by definition larger than 1.5 cm in diameter, whereas smaller tumors are termed osteoid osteomas. These tumors usually occur in individuals less than 40 years of age, and present with back pain. This pain classically worsens at night but is relieved with small doses of aspirin. They can induce scoliosis resulting in structural changes directly, the severity of which is related to the patient age at onset and duration of symptoms. Histologically, these tumors are comprised of osteoid and interconnected bone trabeculae intermixed with highly vascular connective tissue. Computed tomography (CT) scan is the diagnostic tool of choice as it allows for precise localization. Complete surgical excision is necessary if pain or scoliosis is present.

Osteochondromas

Osteochondromas are the most common benign bone tumor. They consist of cartilage and bone and develop as an outgrowth connected to the vertebrae by a stalk. These tumors occur most often in the cervical spine, are more common in men, and peak in the third decade of life. Plain films or CT can easily identify the lesion. Treatment consists of surgical excision and only rarely do they undergo malignant transformation.

Giant Cell Tumors

Giant cell tumors of the spine are uncommon. These tumors are characterized by the presence of multinucleated giant cells that are derived from, or related to osteoclasts. When they do occur in the spine, they usually localize to the sacrum and present with pain. They are usually benign but locally highly aggressive and invasive. Ten percent are reportedly malignant. Diagnosis can be made with plain film evaluation as lesions have a characteristic soap bubble appearance. Upon breaching a threshold size, these tumors are difficult to completely resect without sacrificing bowel and bladder innervation. Sacrectomy with wide excision can be curative if the loss of bowel and bladder function is acceptable to the patient. Usually, subtotal resection dictates the need for adjuvant radiation (69).

Osteosarcomas

Osteosarcomas account for 35% of primary bone tumors, are derived from osteoblasts, and result in the formation of tumoral bone. They rarely involve the spine but when present, occur in young patients who initially complain of pain. The development of osteosarcomas is related to previous radiotherapy, but in a large series of patients with spinal osteosarcoma, less than 3% of patients had a history of previous radiation exposure (70). The prognosis is poor for patients with this tumor type and therefore treatment is usually aggressive. Surgical total spondylectomy with adjuvant radiation and chemotherapy is recommended but only a small percentage of patients survive long-term (71).

Ewing Sarcomas

Ewing sarcomas comprise about 6% of all primary malignant bone tumors, but only 3.5% of these tumors involve the spine. They have a male predilection and occur usually in children before the age of 20. Spinal Ewing sarcoma localize to the sacrum and lumbar spine almost exclusively. Plain films of the spine reveal lytic destructive lesions. Optimal treatment includes presurgical embolization with an attempt at maximum resection during decompression of the cord (72). Adjuvant chemotherapy and radiotherapy are advocated as well. Localized disease treated with chemotherapy is associated with 70% long-term survival while metastatic disease results in only 10% long-term survival.

Spinal Cord Compression in Metastatic Cancer

Of the estimated 500,000 patients dying of cancer annually, likely 1 in 20 of these patients will be diagnosed with spinal cord compression (73). The risk for spinal cord involvement is dependent upon the primary source and is highest for breast, prostate, and lung cancer. Together these three sources account for 50% to 60% of all cases involving spinal cord compression with renal cell carcinoma, myeloma, non-Hodgkin lymphoma, and colon cancer accounting for most of the remaining cases (74). However, nearly all forms of systemic cancer have been reported to seed the epidural space and a measureable percentage of cases are of unknown primary origin. Spinal cord compression usually manifests in patients with a preexisting diagnosis; nonetheless, in 20% of patients, it is the presenting symptom of cancer. Thirty percent of these patients will eventually be diagnosed with lung cancer, 34% will have a hematologic malignancy (multiple myeloma or non-Hodgkin lymphoma), 10% with prostate cancer, 6% with renal cell carcinoma, and 13% will not have a diagnosed primary source (75). The majority of metastatic lesions occur in the thoracic spine. Metastasis from lung has more frequent involvement of the lower cervical and upper thoracic canal due to cancer in lung apex (pancoast tumors), whereas in contrast prostate cancer involves the epidural space of the lumbar and thoracic spinal column.

Pathophysiology

Spinal cord dysfunction occurs when malignant cells seed and then multiply within the spinal epidural space resulting in epidural spinal cord compression (ESCC). Malignant cells can enter the epidural space via expansion of a paravertebral tumor through an intravertebral foramen and into the spinal canal compressing the cord (76). More commonly, cells reach the vertebral bodies via hematogenous spread, followed by proliferation in the bone and spread into the epidural space. Myelopathy presumably results with epidural expansion of the cancer or when boney destruction is sufficient to cause collapse and displacement into the epidural space. Direct compression of the cord by either mechanism results in acute oligodendrocyte and myelin loss followed by secondary axonal transection and glial scar formation. Anterior invasion compresses and eventually occludes venous drainage resulting in loss of the blood–spinal cord barrier and edema. As compression continues, arterial supply is eventually compromised and infarction ensues (77). Thus ischemia secondary to compression rather than compression itself can lead to spinal cord dysfunction and irreversible neurological damage. Treatment of ESCC must begin emergently in order to prevent irreversible damage to the spinal cord (65). Consequently, the likelihood of an individual with ESCC responding to treatment with a good outcome is increased if treatment starts before myelopathy has developed. In addition, the likelihood of a good outcome is greater if treatment starts within hours of the recognition of ESCC (65).

Hematogenous dissemination of malignant cells to the vertebral column was thought to occur via Batson vertebral venous plexus since Batson proposed the theory in 1940. More recent theories center on arterial dissemination and rely primarily on experimental animal data (78).

Clinical Presentation

Pain is a nearly ubiquitous symptom in patients with ESCC with some studies demonstrating up to 95% of patients noting back pain prior to diagnosis (74). The median time from pain onset to diagnosis is as long as 8 weeks in some series (76). Pain can be caused by damage to bony vertebral structures causing localized pain or by nerve compression causing radicular pain. In addition, irritation of the dura can produce Lhermitte phenomena. Pain that radiates in a radicular distribution, Lhermitte phenomena, and pain that is elicited by valsalva in a person with known metastatic cancer to the spinal column or perisurgical region can indicate ESCC before myelopathy or radiculopathy develop (2). Often pain may be referred and present as hip pain (girdle discomfort) or scapular pain with thoracic level or cervical level involvement, respectively (79). Localized pain develops as cells extend into the soft tissue structures or stretch the periosteum. It usually develops first and is concomitant with the level of spinal cord involvement, which is directly related to the volume of bone and the extent of blood flow to various segments of the cord. The majority of ESCC occur in the thoracic cord (60%), followed by lumbosacral (30%) and cervical (10%). As the mass expands, nerve roots are compressed, resulting in a radicular pain quality with increasing intensity. Radicular pain is usually unilateral in the cervical and lumbar regions but bilateral with thoracic invasion (74). Radicular pain is characteristically worsened by movement and valsalva and usually worse at night as the recumbent position lengthens the spine and distends the epidural venous plexus. Finally, mechanical pain, characterized by worsening with movement and improvement with lying still, is caused by vertebral body collapse and in general is a foreboding symptom associated with extensive bony invasion by cancer cells.

Weakness is the second most common presenting sign in patients diagnosed with ESCC and is present in up to 75% of patients at diagnosis (2,80). Remarkably in one series, 68% of patients were nonambulatory at the time of diagnosis (76). Weakness from ESCC is more often asymmetrical when presenting in an upper motor neuron pattern and symmetrical with a lower motor neuron pattern. Other symptoms of spinal cord compression are highly variable and more dependent upon location and extent of involvement at the time of presentation. Sensory symptoms are present in at least one half of patients at the time of diagnosis, but rarely precede motor dysfunction (76,81). A pattern of distal sensory loss progressing proximally is common. Isolated ataxia has been reported with early involvement of the spinocerebellar tract but this is rare (76). Equally uncommon is isolated autonomic dysfunction; bowel and bladder dysfunction, however, is reported as being present in about 50% of patients at diagnosis (80).

Diagnosis

Although a thorough history and complete neurological evaluation are important, any patient presenting with new onset back pain and a preexisting diagnosis of cancer should have diagnostics studies to exclude ESCC. Studies in the Netherlands, where access to MRI is limited secondary to economic constraints, have demonstrated that no sign or symptom in a patient with cancer presenting with back pain can preclude the need for the definitive radiological study, that is, MRI (82). The sensitivity and specificity of MRI for the diagnosis of ESCC is 93% and 97%, respectively (83). It is superior to CT in terms of defining surrounding anatomy and its routine use adds information beyond what a CT scan can provide, thereby leading to changes in the parameters used in radiation therapies in 40% to 53% of cases (84). MRI also allows for evaluation of the entire spine in a short time window, which is important as one third of patients will have compression at multiple sites along the cord. These findings always affect surgical decision making and therefore imaging of the entire spine should be routine (2,85).

Other imaging techniques are limited in diagnostic potential. Plain film studies have a 15% false-negative rate and require extensive bony erosion before a compressive lesion can be identified (80). Classical findings include pedicle thinning, increased size of the neural foramina, altered osseous density, compression fractures, and paraverterbral masses (85). However, these are late findings. Radionuclide bone scans offer increased sensitivity compared to plain films but are unable to identify whether epidural tumor if present (86). Positron emission tomography (PET) using fluorodeoxyglucose is superior to radionuclide bone scans as it is reliant upon metabolic activity rather than indirectly identifying metastasis through increased bone turnover. However, PET scans lack the appropriate resolution for diagnosis. Finally, CT scan with myelography, which was the radiologic study of choice prior to MRI for the diagnosis of ECSS, is now reserved for patients who cannot undergo MRI because of implanted devices, but is preferred for the guidance of percutaneous needle biopsies.

Treatment

Given the poor median survival of patients diagnosed with ESCC, the definitive treatment is defined in terms of ameliorating symptoms rather than complete eradication of tumor cells in the spine. Early studies demonstrating the efficacy of corticosteroids in reducing neurological deficits in patients with CNS lesions were performed in the early 1960s (87). For patients with ESCC, steroids are the first-line treatment and result in a rapid reduction in edema and inflammation resulting in an equally expeditious improvement of neurological deficits. The only randomized study demonstrating the efficacy of corticosteroid administration was reported in 1994 and tested steroid plus radiotherapy versus radiation therapy alone. Results showed a significant increase in the ability to ambulate at 3 (81% versus 63%) and 6 months (59% and 33%) post treatment in the steroid plus radiotherapy group (88). This study solidified the use of steroids as first-line treatment. Controversy persists, however, regarding the precise steroid regimen to use in order to optimize symptom relief and minimize side effects. Complicating the issue are animal studies, which demonstrate a dose-dependent effect (89), while human studies failed to recapitulate an association between dose and relief of pain, maintenance of ambulation, or improvement of bladder function (90). Spinal cord damage becomes irreversible soon after clinical onset, producing a justified sense of urgency by practitioners and resulting in a tendency to use steroids at the high end of the dosing spectrum (65). This is particularly justified in patients who are not ambulatory at presentation or have rapidly progressive neurological deterioration. In these patients, a loading dose of 96 mg of dexamethasone intravenously followed by 96 mg/d for 3 days and then a 10-day taper is justified. For patients ambulating and with less progressive signs or symptoms, a 10-mg loading dose followed by a 16-mg oral dose and then a taper may be acceptable.

Radiation therapy directed against the compressive lesion has been the standard treatment for ESCC for over 60 years, but efficacy has never been tested in a randomized controlled study. All evidence of efficacy versus supportive care is derived from retrospective analysis, which has demonstrated a clear benefit to patient from radiotherapy (91). Similar to the use of corticosteroids, the most efficacious dose and treatment course has not been established, but the use of the modality itself is widely agreed upon. Clinical trials have been performed comparing different dosing and radiation schedules; however, interpretation of these studies is complicated by the variation in radiosensitivity of different primary tumors and comparison to nonstandard treatments. In general patients with a poor prognosis for survival due to extensive systemic tumor, burden should be treated with a short course of high-dose radiotherapy ranging from 8 Gy in one fraction to 20 Gy in five fractions. Patients with controlled systemic disease and minimal to moderate neurological dysfunction should receive a more protracted course of 40 Gy in 20 fractions as this regimen results in less local recurrence of symptoms. In order to reduce the recurrence of ESCC at the border of the radiation treatment port, it is essential that the radiation ports extend at least two vertebral bodies beyond the ESCC margins recognized on imaging studies (92).

Prior to the widespread use of radiation therapy, laminectomy was the only available treatment. Later retrospective trials and one randomized prospective trial failed to demonstrate the efficacious of laminectomy either alone or in conjunction with radiotherapy and therefore it is no longer part of a treatment strategy for patients with ECSS. More recently, direct decompressive surgery, utilizing an anterior approach, immediate circumferential decompression, and spinal cord stabilization, has been shown to benefit patients beyond radiation therapy alone. In fact, the initial randomized trial comparing direct decompressive surgery and postoperative radiotherapy with only radiotherapy was halted prematurely after demonstrating statistical significance at only 50% of its target recruitment goal (93). The combination therapy resulted in more patients able to walk after treatment, decreased need for pain medication and steroids, and more patients maintaining ambulation for longer times. In addition, more patients unable to walk at study start were able to walk after treatment. One caveat to this study was that the recruitment of patients was limited to those with less radiosensitive tumor types. Current indications for surgery include relapse after radiotherapy or progression during radiotherapy, unknown primary tumor, and evidence of instability of the spine or fractures. Particularly salient here, the complication rates from surgical management of ESCC was nearly double (94) for patients 65 years of age and older (71% versus 43%).

Finally, the use of chemotherapy is limited to patients with recurrence who cannot undergo surgery or radiotherapy. In general, tumor responsiveness and the prolonged time to obtain decompression of the spinal cord make this modality less useful. However, for cancers that are exquisitely sensitive to chemotherapy, this treatment modality can be of benefit (95).

Natural Progression

Untreated ESCC results in progressive incapacitating pain, weakness leading to paraplegia, and bowel/bladder dysfunction. Median survival of patients with ESCC is dependent upon the primary tumor type as well as the extent of metastatic disease and ambulatory ability at presentation. As stated previously, the goal of treatment is to alleviate symptoms and prevent further neurological decline. The median survival for patients even with radiosensitive tumors is as at best 5 to 7 months while patients with lung cancer have a median survival of only 1.5 months (73). In a study of veterans with ESCC, the median survival of patients with ESCC was 104 weeks for patients who could walk after completion of ESCC treatment and only 6 weeks for nonambulatory patients (65). In that study, 14 of the 30 nonambulatory patients (47%) died of myelopathic complications, such as pneumonia, infected pressure sores, and urosepsis, which are also the leading causes of death in the first year after traumatic SCI. In another study, patients ambulating after therapy had a median survival of 9 months while those nonambulatory survived only 1 to 2 months (96). More relevant to the proceeding section, patients with ESCC spend two times as many days hospitalized in the last year of life compared to cancer patients without ESCC (73) underlying the complexity of this diagnosis in terms of ongoing medical management and the need for an early and comprehensive rehabilitation program. In contrast, patients who were able to walk after the completion of ESCC treatment remained ambulatory up to 5 weeks before they died (65).

Patients who survive for relatively extended periods are at high risk for recurrent ESCC. In fact, patients surviving 3 years posttreatment of ESCC universally redeveloped compression from metastatic cells (76). Taken together, somewhere between 8% and 20% of patients with a diagnosis of ESCC will develop recurrent compression with one half developing compression at the identical spinal cord level and half at a different level (97). For patients treated with radiation therapy, having radiation therapy ports that extended two vertebral segments beyond the caudal and cephalad margins of the ESCC can reduce the likelihood of ESCC recurrence at the initial site (92). Although there is some controversy regarding how to best treat recurrent disease, current treatment paradigms recommend a second dose of radiotherapy for initial recurrence and then chemotherapy and surgery for future recurrences with the goal of maintaining ambulation as long as possible.

SPINAL CORD COMPRESSION AS AN ONCOLOGIC EMERGENCY

Spinal cord compression is life threatening only when innervation of the diaphragm is affected by lesions at C3 or above. However, as previously described, it can lead to considerable and irreversible morbidity that negatively impacts upon a patient's quality of life. Progression of neurological disability can be swift, and therefore emergent intervention is compulsory. Steroids are the first-line treatment and result in a rapid reduction in edema and inflammation resulting in an equally expeditious improvement of neurological deficits. This intervention should be followed by emergent consultation with a radiation oncologist. Surgical consultation is limited to those patients requiring tissue biopsy or stabilization of the spinal column, while chemotherapy is only useful if the primary source represents a known chemosensitive cell type.

REHABILIATION OF PATIENTS WITH CANCERS OF THE SPINAL CORD

Overall, there should be some degree of urgency in recognizing and treating patients with primary and secondary cancers of the spinal cord as inaction can lead to significant and severe, irreversible neurological disability. Given the short median survival of patients with ESCC and the degree of neurological disability that can accompany primary spinal cord tumors, an early referral to a multidisciplinary rehabilitation center is vital. For cancer patients, the appropriate rehabilitation program should be short in duration and focus on improvements in mobility, transfer techniques, and self-care. The efficacy of rehabilitation in patients with a poor prognosis and ESCC has been documented repeatedly. McKinley et al. (98) reported on 32 patients with a median expected survival of 3 months who underwent rehabilitation and achieved functional improvements in mobility and self-care and maintained these improvements for at least 3 months after being discharged. Furthermore, 84% of these patients achieved discharge to home rather than a nursing facility. Two other reports demonstrated the benefits of a 2-week directed rehabilitation program focusing on transfers, skin care, and bladder/bowel management in nonambulatory patients with ECSS (99,100). Fig. 31.5 shows that among patients who were not able to walk after completion of ECSS treatment that providing

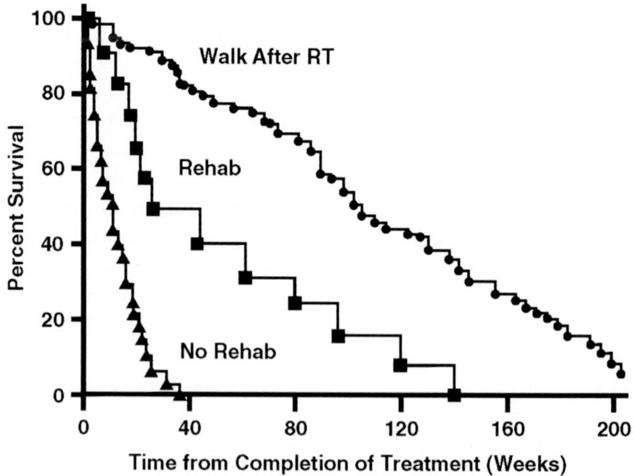

FIGURE 31.5 Rehabilitation prolongs survival of patients with ESCC who are not able to walk after completing radiation therapy for ESCC (From Zaidat OO, Ruff RL. Treatment of spinal epidural metastasis improves patient survival and functional state. *Neurology* 2002;58:1360–66; and Ruff RL, Adamson VW, Ruff SS, et al. Directed rehabilitation reduces pain and depression while increasing independence and satisfaction with life for patients with paraplegia due to epidural metastatic spinal cord compression. *J Rehabil Res Dev* 2007a;44:1–10). The three curves include the following: (a) subjects who could not walk after completion of ESCC treatment and who did not receive rehabilitation (No Rehab) median survival of 6 weeks, (b) patients who could not walk after completion of ESCC treatment who received a 2-week course of rehabilitation (Rehab) median survival of 26 weeks, and (c) patients who could walk after completion of spinal epidural metastasis treatment (Walk after RT) median survival of 104 weeks (Zaidat OO, Ruff RL. Treatment of spinal epidural metastasis improves patient survival and functional state. *Neurology* 2002;58:1360–66).

a 2-week course of directed rehabilitation improved survival. Median survival was 26 weeks in patients undergoing rehabilitation versus 6 weeks in the control group (99,100). Lower pain levels, less depression, and improved quality of life were also associated with the rehabilitation program. These gains were durable and maintained until time of death (100).

FUTURE DIRECTIONS

As alluded to throughout this text, the field of cancer research and its translation to clinical medicine is moving forward at a rapid pace. Emerging forms of highly directed radiotherapy hold promise for the treatment of many different forms of spinal cord tumors. These spinal stereotactic radiosurgery (SRS) systems allow for accurate delivery of higher dose radiation to tumor cells while minimizing exposure of normal, uninvolved tissues. SRS systems are considered experimental as large randomized trials have yet to demonstrate efficacy versus standard radiotherapy regimens. Published reports using CyberKnife (Accuray Incorporated, Sunnyvale, CA), however, have shown a decrease in pain in treated patients, improvement in neurological deficits, or lack of progression in nearly 80% of patients treated with minimal adverse effects (101). The ability to understand the genetics of primary tumors such as astrocytomas holds great promise in directing and personalizing therapeutics as does the field of cancer vaccines and similar molecular-based techniques. By and large, these advances have great potential to diminish suffering, improve quality of life, and prolong lifespan in patients with spinal cord tumors.

References

1. Lada R, Kaminski HJ, Ruff RL. Metastatic spinal cord compression. Chapter 11. In: Vinken PJ, Bruyn GW, Vecht C, eds. *Handbook of clinical neurology. Vol. 69 (Revised Series Volume 25) Neuro-oncology part III. Neurological disorders in systemic cancer*. Amsterdam, The Netherlands: Elsevier Biomedical Publishers, 1997:167–189.
2. Ruff RL, Lanska D. Epidural metastases in prospectively evaluated veterans with cancer and back pain. *Cancer* 1989;63:2234–2241.
3. Yukihiro M, Yoshihito S, Yoshito K, et al. Surgical results of intramedullary spinal cord tumor with spinal cord monitoring to guide extent of resection. *J Neurosurg Spine* 2009;10:404–413.
4. Shrivastava RK, Epstein FJ, Perin NI, et al. Intramedullary spinal cord tumors in patients older than 50 years of age: management and outcome analysis. *J Neurosurg Spine* 2005;2:249–255.
5. Chang UK, Choe WJ, Chung SK, et al. Surgical outcome and prognostic factors of spinal intramedullary ependymomas in adults. *J Neurooncol* 2002;57:133–139.
6. Akyurek S, Chang EL, Yu TK, et al. Spinal myxopapillary ependymoma outcomes in patients treated with surgery and radiotherapy at MD Anderson Cancer Center. *J Neurooncol* 2007;82:323–325.
7. Gomez Dr, Missett BT, Wara WM, et al. High failure rate in spinal ependymomas with long-term follow-up. *Neuro Oncol* 2005;7:254–259.
8. Abdel-Wahab M, Etuk B, Palermo J. Spinal cord gliomas: a multi-institutional retrospective analysis. *Int J Radiat Oncol Biol Phys* 2006;64:1060–1071.
9. Marks JE, Adler SJ. A comparative study of ependymomas by site of origin. *Int J Radiat Oncol Biol Phys* 1982;8:37–43.
10. Wen BC, Hussey DH, Hitchon PW, et al. The role of radiation therapy in the management of ependymomas of the spinal cord. *Int J Radiat Oncol Biol Phys* 1991;20: 781–786.
11. Shaw EG, Evans RG, Scheithauer BW, et al. Radiotherapuetic management of adult intraspinal ependymomas. *Int J Radiat Oncol Biol Phys* 1986;12: 323–327.
12. Chamberlain MC. Salvage chemotherapy for recurrent spinal cord ependymoma. *Cancer* 2002;95:997–1002.
13. Chamberlain MC. Etoposide for recurrent spinal cord ependymoma. *Neurology* 2002;58:1310–1311.
14. McCormick PC, Stein BM. Intramedullary tumors in adult. *Neurosurg Clin N Am* 1990;1:609–630.
15. Innocenzi G, Raco A, Cantore G, et al. Intramedullary astrocytomas and ependymomas in the pediatric age group: a retrospective study. *Childs Nerv Syst* 1996;12:776–780.
16. Epstein FJ, Farmer JP, Freed D. Adult intramedullary astrocytomas of the spinal cord. *J Neurosurg* 1992; 77:355–359.
17. Cooper PR. Outcome after operative treatment of intramedullary spinal cord tumors in adults: intermediate and long-term results in 51 patients. *Neurosurgery* 1989;25:855–859.
18. Sarabia M Millan JM, Escudero L, et al. Intracranial seeding from an intramedullary malignant astrocytoma. *Surg Neurol* 1986;26:573–576.
19. Ciappetta P, Salvati M, Capoccia G, et al. Spinal glioblastomas: report of seven cases and review of the literature. *Neurosurgery* 1991;28:302–306.
20. Reimer R and Onofrio BM. Astrocytomas of the spinal cord in children and adolescents. *J Neurosurg* 1985;63:669–675.
21. Epstein F, Epstein N. Surgical management of holocord intramedullary spinal cord astrocytomas in children. *J Neurosurg* 1981;54:829–832.
22. Fischer G, Brotchi J, Chignier G, et al. Clinical material. In: Fischer G, Brotchi J, eds. *Intramedullary spinal cord tumors*. Stuttgart (Germany): Thieme, 1996:10–20.
23. Minehan KJ, Shaw EG, Scheithauer BW, et al. Spinal cord astrocytomas: a pathological and treatment considerations. *J Neurosurg* 1995;83:590–595.
24. O'Sullivan C, Jenkin RD, Doherty MA, et al. Spinal cord tumors in children: long-term results of combined surgical and radiation treatment. *J Neurosurg* 1994;81:507–512.
25. Isaacson R. Radiation therapy and the management of intramedullary spinal cord tumors. *J Neurooncol* 2000;47:231–238.
26. Shirato H, Kamada T, Hida K, et al. The role of radiotherapy in the management of spinal cord glioma. *Int J Radiat Oncol Biol Phys* 1995;33:323–328.
27. Balmaceda C. Chemotherapy for intramedullary spinal cord tumors. *J Neurooncol* 2000;47:293–307.
28. Lonser RR, Oldfield EH. Spinal cord hemangioblastomas. *Neurosurg Clin N Am* 2006;17:37–44.

29. Wanebo JE, Lonser RR, Glenn GM, et al. The natural history of hemangioblastomas of the central nervous system in patients with von Hippel-Lindau disease. *J Neurosurg* 2003;98:82–94.
30. Lonser RR, Vortmeyer AO, Butman JA, et al. Edema is a precursor to central nervous system peritumoral cyst formation. *Ann Neurol* 2005;58:392–399.
31. Roonprapunt C, Silvera VM, Setton A, et al. Surgical management of isolated hemangioblastomas of the spinal cord. *Neurosurgery* 2001;49:321–328.
32. Lonser RR, Weil RJ, Wanebo JE, et al. Surgical management of spinal cord hemangioblastomas in patients with von Hippel-Lindau disease. *J Neurosurg* 2003;98:106–116.
33. Conway JE, Chou D, Clatterbuck RE, et al. Hemangioblastomas of the central nervous system in von Hippel-Lindau syndrome and sporadic disease. *Neurosurgery* 2001;48:55–63.
34. Lonser RR, Glenn GM, Walther M, et al. von Hippel-Lindau disease. *Lancet* 2003b;361:2059–2067.
35. Chi JH, Parsa AT. Intramedullary spinal cord metastasis: clinical management and surgical considerations. *Neurosurg Clin N Am* 2006;17:45–50.
36. Mut M, Schiff D, Shaffrey ME. Metastasis to nervous system: spinal epidural and intramedullary metastases. *J Neurooncol* 2005;75:43–56.
37. Aryan HE, Farin A, Nakaji P, et al. Intramedullary spinal cord metastasis of lung adenocarcinoma presenting as Brown-Sequard syndrome. *Surg Neurol* 2004;61:72–76.
38. Hamburger C, Buttner A, Weis S. Ganglioglioma of the spinal cord: report of two rare cases and review of the literature. *Neurosurgery* 1997;41:1410–1415.
39. Kalyan-Raman UP, Olivero WC. Ganglioglioma: a correlative clinicopathological and radiological study of ten surgically treated cases with follow-up. *Neurosurgery* 1987;20:428–433.
40. Gorman PH, Rigamonti D, Joslyn JN. Intramedullary and extramedullary schwannoma of the cervical spinal cord—case report. *Surg Neurol* 1989;32:459–462.
41. Miller DJ, McCutcheon IE. Hemangioblastomas and other uncommon intramedullary tumors. *J Neurooncol* 2000;47:253–270.
42. Levy WJ, Latchaw J, Hahn JF, et al. Spinal neurofibromas: a report of 66 cases and a comparison with meningiomas. *Neurosurgery* 1986;18:331–334.
43. Celli P. Treatment of relevant nerve roots involved in nerve sheath tumors: removal or preservation? *Neurosurgery* 2002;51:684–692.
44. Klekamp J, Samii M. Surgery of spinal nerve sheath tumors with special reference to neurofibromatosis. *Neurosurgery* 1998;42:279–289.
45. Zheng H, Chang L, Patel N, et al. Induction of abnormal proliferation by nonmyelinating Schwann cells triggers neurofibroma formation. *Cancer Cell* 2008;13:117–28.
46. Jinnai T, Koyama T. Clinical characteristics of spinal nerve sheath tumors: analysis of 149 cases. *Neurosurgery* 2005;56:510–515.
47. Merimsky O, Lepechoux C, Terrier P, et al. Primary sarcomas of the central nervous system. *Oncology* 2000;58:210–214.
48. Solero CL, Fornari M, Giombini S, et al. Spinal meningiomas: review of 174 operated cases. *Neurosurgery* 1989;25:153–160.
49. Calogero JA, Moossy J. Extradural spinal meningiomas. Report of four cases. *J Neurosurg* 1972;37:442–447.
50. Klekamp J, Samii M. Surgical results of spinal meningiomas. *Acta Neurochir Suppl* 1996;65:77–81.
51. Gezen F, Kahraman S, Canakci Z, et al. Review of 36 cases of spinal cord meningioma. *Spine* 2000;25:727–731.
52. McCormick PC, Post KD, Stein BM. Intradural extramedullary tumors in adults. *Neurosurg Clin N Am* 1990b;1:591–608.
53. Chaparro MJ, Young RF, Smith M, et al. Multiple spinal meningiomas: a case of 47 distinct lesions in the absence of neurofibromatosis or identified chromosomal abnormality. *Neurosurgery* 1993;32:298–301.
54. Cohen-Gadol AA, Zikel OM, Koch CA. Spinal meningiomas in patients younger than 50 years of age: a 21-year experience. *J Neurosurg* 2003;98:258–263.
55. Roux FX, Nataf F, Pinaudeau M, et al. Intraspinal meningiomas: review of 54 cases with discussion of poor prognosis factors and modern therapeutic management. *Surg Neurol* 1996;46:463–464.
56. Fearnside MR, Adams CB. Tumours of the cauda equine. *J Neurol Neurosurg Psychiatry* 1978;41:24–31.
57. Tarlov IM. Perineural cysts of the spinal nerve roots. *Arch Neurol Psychiatry* 1938;40:1067–1074.
58. Sonneland PR, Scheithauer BW, Onofrio BM. Myxopapillary ependymoma. A clinicopathologic and immunocytochemical study of 77 cases. *Cancer* 1985;56:883–893.
59. Stanley P, Senac MO Jr, Segall HD. Intraspinal seeding from intracranial tumors in children. *Am J Roentgenol* 1985;144:157–61.
60. Stark AM, Nabavi A, Mehdorn HM, et al. Glioblastoma multiforme—report of 267 cases treated at a single institution. *Surg Neurol* 2005;63:162–169.
61. Cairns H, Russell DS. Intracranial and spinal metastases in gliomas of the brain. *Brain* 1931;54:377–420.
62. Meyers SP, Wildenhain SL, Chang JK, et al. Postoperative evaluation for disseminated medulloblastoma involving the spine: contrast-enhanced MR findings, CSF cytologic analysis, timing of disease occurrence, and patient outcomes. *Am J Neuroradiol* 2000;2:1757–1765.
63. Lam CH, Cosgrove GR, Drislane FW, et al. Spinal leptomeningeal metastasis from cerebral glioblastoma. Appearance on magnetic resonance imaging. *Surg Neurol* 1991;35:377–380.
64. Grabb PA, Albright AL, Pang D. Dissemination of supratentorial malignant gliomas via the cerebrospinal fluid in children. *Neurosurgery* 1992;30:64–71.
65. Zaidat OO, Ruff RL. Treatment of spinal epidural metastasis improves patient survival and functional state. *Neurology* 2002;58:1360–66.
66. Tuscano JM. Multiple myeloma: epidemiology and therapeutic options. *Manag Care* 2008;17:9–15.
67. Pastushyn A, Slin'ko EL, Mirzoyeva GM. Vertebral hemangiomas: Diagnosis, management, natural history and clinicopathological correlates in 86 patients. *Surg Neurol* 1998;50:535–547.
68. Fox MW, Onofrio BM. The natural history and management of symptomatic and asymptomatic vertebral hemangiomas. *J Neurosurg* 1993;78:36–45.
69. Camins MB, Rosenblum BR. Osseous lesions of the cervical spine. *Clin Neurosurg* 1991;37:722–739.

70. Dahlin DC, Coventry MB. Osteogenic sarcoma. A study of six hundred cases. *J Bone Joint Surg* 1967;49: 101–110.
71. Sundaresan N, Rosen G, Huvos AG, et al. Combined treatment of osteosarcoma of the spine. *Neurosurgery* 1988;23:714–719.
72. Sharafuddin MJ, Haddad FS, Hitchon PW, et al. Treatment options in primary Ewing's sarcoma of the spine: report of seven cases and review of the literature. *Neurosurgery* 1992;30:610–618
73. Loblaw DA, Laperriere NJ, Mackillop WJ. A population based study of malignant spinal cord compression in Ontario. *Clin Oncol* 2003;15:211–217.
74. Schiff D. Spinal cord compression. *Neurol Clin* 2003;21:1–14.
75. Schiff D, O'Neill B, Suman V. Spinal epidural metastasis as the initial manifestation of malignancy: clinical features and diagnostic approach. *Neurology* 1997;49:452–456.
76. Gilbert R, Posner J. Epidural spinal cord compression from metastatic tumor: diagnosis and treatment. *Ann Neurol* 1978;3:40–51.
77. Kato A, Ushio Y, Hayakawa T, et al. Circulatory disturbance of the spinal cord with epidural neoplasm in rats. *J Neurosurg* 1985;63:260–265.
78. Arguello F, Baggs RB, Duerst RE, et al. Pathogenesis of vertebral metastasis and epidural spinal cord compression. *Cancer* 1990;65:98–106.
79. Levack P, Graham J, Collie D, et al. Don't wait for a sensory level—listen to the symptoms: a prospective audit of the delays in diagnosis of malignant cord compression. *Clin Oncol* 2002;14:472–480.
80. Bach F, Larsen B, Rhode K, et al. Metastatic spinal cord compression: occurrence, symptoms, clinical presentations and prognosis in 398 patients with spinal cord compression. *Acta Neurochir (Wien)* 1990;107:37–43.
81. Helweg-Larsen S, Sorensen P. Symptoms and signs in metastatic spinal cord compression: a study from first symptom until diagnosis in 153 patients. *Eur J Cancer* 1994;30A:396–398.
82. Kienstra GEM, Terwee CB, Dekker FW, et al. Prediction of spinal epidural metastases. *Arch Neurol* 2000;57:690–695.
83. Li KC, Poon PY. Sensitivity and specificity of MRI in detecting malignant spinal cord compression and in distinguishing malignant from benign compression fractures of vertebrae. *Magn Reson Imaging* 1988;6:547–556.
84. Colletti PM, Siegal HJ, Woo MY, et al. The impact on treatment planning of MRI of the spine in patients suspected of vertebral metastasis: an efficacy study. *Comput Med Imaging Graph* 1996;20:159–162.
85. Portenoy R, Lipton R, Foley K. Back pain in the cancer patient: an algorithm for evaluation and management. *Neurology* 1987;37:134–138.
86. Gosfield E, Alavi A, Kneeland B. Comparison of radionuclide bone scans and magnetic resonance imaging in detecting spinal metastases. *J Nucl Med* 1993;34:2191–2200.
87. Cantu RC. Corticosteroids for spinal metastases. *Lancet* 1968;2:912.
88. Sorenson PS, Helweg-Larsen S, Mouridsen H, et al. Effect of high-dose dexamethasone in carcinomatous metastatic spinal cord compression treated with radiotherapy: a randomized trial. *Eur J Cancer* 1994;30A:22–27.
89. Delattre J, Arbit E, Thaler H, et al. A dose-response study of dexamethasone in a model of spinal cord compression caused by epidural tumor. *J Neurosurg* 1989;70:920–925.
90. Vecht C, Haaxma-Reiche H, van Putten W, et al. Initial bolus of conventional versus high dose dexamethasone in metastatic spinal cord compression. *Neurology* 1989;39:1255–1257.
91. Barron K, Hirano A, Sraski S, et al. Experiences with metastatic neoplasm involving the spinal cord. *Neurology* 1959;9:91–106.
92. Kaminski HJ, Diwan VG, Ruff RL. Second occurrence of spinal epidural metastases. *Neurology* 1991;41:744–746.
93. Patchell RA, Tibbs PA, Regine WF, et al. Direct decompressive surgical resection in the treatment of spinal cord compression caused by metastatic cancer: a randomized trial. *Lancet* 2005;366:643–648.
94. Chen YJ, Chang G, Chen H, et al. Surgical results of metastatic spinal cord compression secondary to non-small cell lung cancer. *Spine* 2007;32:E413–E418.
95. Posner JB, Howieson J, Cvitkovic E. "Disappearing" spinal cord compression: oncolytic effect of glucocorticoids and other chemotherapeutic agents on epidural metastases. *Ann Neurol* 1977;2:409–413.
96. Maranzano E, Bellavita R, Rossi R, et al. Short-course versus split-course radiotherapy in metastatic spinal cord compression: results of a phase III randomized, multicenter trial. *J Clin Oncol* 2005;23:3358–3365.
97. van der Sande J, Kroger R, Boogerd W. Multiple spinal epidural metastases: an unexpectedly frequent finding. *J Neurol Neurosurg Psychiatry* 1990;53:1001–1003.
98. McKinley WO, Conti-Wyneken AR, et al. Rehabilitative functional outcome of patients with neoplastic spinal cord compression. *Arch Phys Med Rehabil* 1996;77: 892–895.
99. Ruff RL, Adamson VW, Ruff SS, et al. Directed rehabilitation reduces pain and depression while increasing independence and satisfaction with life for patients with paraplegia due to epidural metastatic spinal cord compression. *J Rehabil Res Dev* 2007;44:1–10.
100. Ruff RL, Ruff SS, Wang X. Persistent benefits of rehabilitation on pain and life quality for non-ambulatory patients with spinal epidural metastasis. *J Rehabil Res Dev* 2007;44:271–278.
101. Degen JW, Gagnon GJ, Voyadzis J, et al. Cyberknife stereotactic radiosurgical treatment of spinal tumors for pain control and quality of life. *J Neurosurg Spine* 2005;2:540–549.

CHAPTER 32 ■ SPINAL AND SPINAL CORD INFECTIONS

ILYA KUPERSHTEIN AND MICHAEL VIVES

INTRODUCTION

Spinal infections involve a wide spectrum of disease processes. They can carry with them significant morbidity and even mortality. Spinal infections were first described centuries ago. "Pott Paraplegia" was introduced by Percival Potts in 1779 when he described lower extremity paralysis and abnormal spinal curvature (1). With newer diagnostic and therapeutic technologies, spinal infections can be diagnosed at an earlier stage, and with strong antibiotic regimens, the prognosis has improved over the past few decades. Despite these developments, the treatment of spinal infections remains challenging (2). The presentation of the spinal infection can range from an indolent, chronic course, to dramatic and progressive loss of neurologic function. This chapter discusses the risk factors that predispose patients to developing spinal infections, their presentation, workup, and treatment recommendations. The chapter is organized anatomically, with spinal column infections discussed first, followed by infections affecting epidural structures, and finally intramedullary spinal infectious processes.

SPINAL COLUMN INFECTIONS

Pyogenic Vertebral Osteomyelitis and Discitis

Evidence of vertebral osteomyelitis has been discovered as far back as Egyptian mummies. Pyogenic infections are caused by bacteria, which elicit purulence. Different terms have been used interchangeably: adult discitis, septic discitis, spondylitis, and spondylodiscitis. Pyogenic vertebral osteomyelitis in adults usually involves the disc and endplate initially, followed by progressive involvement of the adjacent vertebral bodies. The term "spondylodiscitis" is therefore commonly used since it describes the pathology more accurately. Vertebral osteomyelitis accounts for about 2% to 4% of all pyogenic osteomyelitis (3).

Etiology

Different risk factors can contribute to the development of pyogenic osteomyelitis. Immunocompromised patients, advanced age, poor nutritional status, and intravenous (IV) drug abuse are risk factors for developing spondylodiscitis. The mode of inoculation may include hematogenous spread, contiguous involvement, or direct inoculation following trauma or therapeutic interventions. Most pyogenic infections occur in the lumbar spine. Hematogenous spread is most common and *Staphylococcus aureus* is the most likely agent, accounting for more than 50% in pyogenic infections. Contiguous spread is much less likely; however, it has been reported in retropharyngeal and retroperitoneal abscesses. Posttraumatic etiology is rare and it usually involves open spine fractures or gunshot wounds.

Pathogenesis

Bacterial or pyogenic infections are the most common spinal infections encountered in the United States. Common inciting organisms include *S. aureus* and *Staphylococcus epidermidis.* Patients who have sickle cell are predisposed to infections with Salmonella. Patients who are immunocompromised can develop gram-negative infections with *Escherichia coli*, *Proteus mirabilis*, and Enterococcus, while IV drug abusers have a higher incidence of *Pseudomonas aeruginosa* infections (4). Brucellosis, a gram-negative coccobacilli, can also cause vertebral osteomyelitis, especially at the L4 level, and is associated with bony sclerosis that causes a "Parrots beak" osteophyte.

There has been some controversy in the past as to the mode of inoculation in hematogenous spread of infection. Recent literature suggests that the area of initial insult occurs in the vertebral endplates, which are supplied by low flow end arterioles (5). These bacteria release proteolytic enzymes that cause destruction of the disc space and could lead to contiguous spread of infection to the adjacent vertebral bodies. With bacterial vertebral osteomyelitis, there should be a high index of suspicion for an associated epidural abscess, especially in the setting of progressive neurologic deficit (6).

Clinical Presentation

The most common presenting symptom is lower back pain (2). The time course for the development of pain, its location, and whether improvement or progression has occurred should be established. Depending on the virulence of the organism, the symptoms could range from acute onset to an insidious chronic course. In fact, delay in diagnosis of greater than 3 months has been reported (7). It is imperative to obtain a full history to be able to formulate a diagnosis and to better tailor a treatment plan based on the patient's other factors. Constitutional symptoms such as fevers, chills, or night sweats are suggestive of an infectious etiology. Persistence of pain even with rest and anti-inflammatory medications differentiate spinal infections and tumors from mechanical back pain. During the history, the presence of radiculopathic or myelopathic symptoms should be noted.

Elements of the past medical history that may be significant include diabetes, HIV, previous history of abscesses, tuberculosis (TB), IV drug use, and cancer (with chemotherapy or radiation). Other medical problems that require long-term IV access (via central or Peripherally inserted Central Catheter [PICC] lines) or indwelling Foley catheters can predispose to seeding of the spine. A history of previous spine surgeries or recent invasive spinal procedures such as discography, epidural injections, and facet injections should also be elicited.

Physical exam begins with the vital signs to determine if a patient has an elevated temperature. However, fever is only seen in 50% of patients (7). Blood pressure and heart rate are obtained to evaluate for signs of septic shock. A thorough neurological exam is performed to recognize any motor or sensory deficit. Pathologic reflexes raise suspicion of an upper motor neuron lesion.

Laboratory Findings

A complete blood count with differential is usually ordered to evaluate the leukocyte count and the presence of a left shift and bandemia, which are signs of systemic infection. However, the white blood cell (WBC) count is only increased in 40% of patients on presentation and could be normal in a chronic setting of infection (6). Erythrocyte sedimentation rate (ESR) is a much more sensitive test for infection and is usually elevated in more than 90% of cases (6). The specificity of the test is much lower, however, and patients can have increased sedimentation rate with other inflammatory conditions such as rheumatoid arthritis, malignancies, and pressure ulcers. C-reactive protein (CRP) is an acute phase protein produced by the liver and adipocytes. It is also not a specific test for spinal infections, but can be used in conjunction with ESR as a screening tool. ESR and CRP are also good indicators of treatment response. Routine monitoring of these indices with progressive decrease from initial values suggests treatment success (7,8). Serum nutrition markers can help to establish the current state of the host and their ability to fight infections. Malnutrition is defined as albumin level less than 3.5 g/dL, a total lymphocyte count less than 1,500 cells/mm^3, and a serum transferrin level of less than 150 mcg/dL (9).

Imaging

Plain radiographs are the most basic of the imaging modalities and are readily obtainable. The downside of plain radiographs is poor visualization of certain areas of the spine. Moreover, radiographic changes due to spondylodiscitis tend to lag 2 to 4 weeks behind the clinical presentation, and occasionally even longer (10). The initial findings on x-ray are decreased disc space height, rarefaction of the endplates, and blurring of paravertebral soft tissue contours (see Fig. 32.1) Deformity and malalignment are not seen until late in the disease process.

Computed tomography (CT) scans provide better visualization of the bony vertebral elements. Endplate destruction and other changes are seen sooner with CT scans then with plain radiographs. Coronal and sagittal reconstructions can give better appreciation of structural deformity and overall bony involvement that developed secondary to the disease process. Although not ideal, soft tissue collections and paravertebral soft tissue changes can be evaluated better on the CT scan than on the plain x-ray.

Radionuclide studies are another imaging modality that may be helpful and have their own advantages. Bone scan with Technetium-99 will have positive results prior to radiographs showing the disease process. Also, bone scan allows the discovery of other involved sites since it images the whole skeleton. An increased uptake on bone scan is not specific to

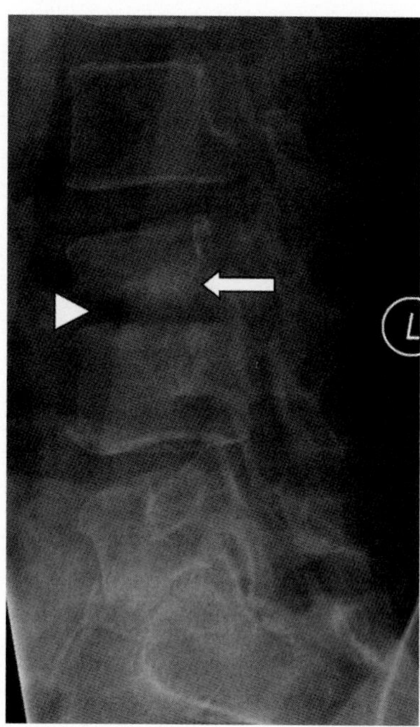

FIGURE 32.1 Lateral plain radiograph demonstrating spondylodiscitis of L3-4 (*arrowhead*). Note the destruction of the inferior endplate of L3 (*white arrow*).

a spinal infection, however, since any bone turnover process can produce a positive result. WBC labeled scan is used extensively and with excellent specificity in the appendicular skeleton; however, its specificity drops dramatically in the axial skeleton. Gallium scans have reported 90% sensitivity and 85% specificity for detecting spinal infections. In the setting of normal Technetium-99 and Gallium scans, the chance of having spinal infection is extremely low (11).

Magnetic resonance imaging (MRI) with gadolinium is the modality of choice in vertebral osteomyelitis and discitis. This imaging modality allows for very early detection of vertebral body and disc space changes. T1-weighted images will show a decreased signal in involved vertebrae secondary to the marrow being replaced. T2-weighted images will show an increase in the vertebral signal intensity due to bony edema. As a result of the previously described pathogenesis, the hallmark MRI findings in pyogenic infections include destruction of the endplates, involvement of the disc, and subchondral bone straddling the disc space (see Fig. 32.2). MRI with contrast also allows for better evaluation of soft tissues and for concomitant paraspinal or epidural abscess collection. Positive MRI findings should be differentiated from other entities including malignancies, which often do not involve the disc space (12).

Treatment

The first step in treatment is an accurate diagnosis. Identifying the insulting organism is imperative prior to formulating the treatment plan and the antibiotic regimen. Therefore, antibiotics should be held if at all possible prior to a biopsy. Biopsy can be performed either by CT-guided percutaneous method or by an open approach in the operating room. Either way, administration of antibiotics prior to a biopsy decreases the chances of isolating the organism in the culture medium (13).

The treatment spectrum can vary from medical management with antibiotics and bracing, all the way to complex surgical debridement and reconstruction with fusion. The precise

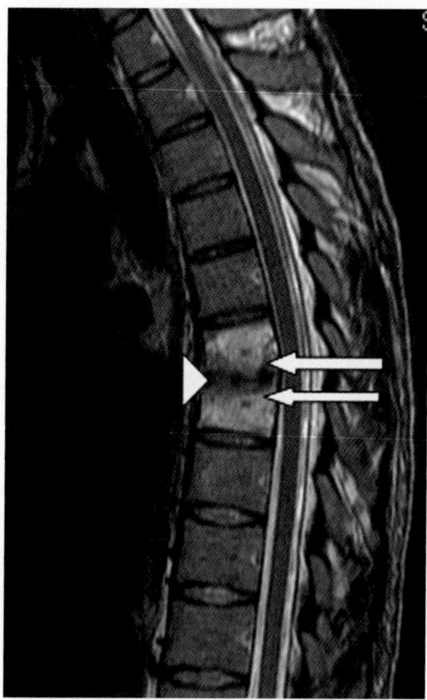

FIGURE 32.2 Sagittal T2-weighted MRI of the thoracic spine demonstrating spondylodiscitis. Note the disc involvement (*arrowhead*), endplate destruction (*long white arrows*), and high signal in the adjacent vertebral bodies (*short arrow*).

treatment algorithm is based on the patient's medical state, level of progression of the disease, and any associated neurological deficits (3).

After identifying the organism, at least 4 to 6 weeks of IV antibiotics are usually recommended. Some advocate following this with a course of oral antibiotics. Surveillance of the ESR and CRP can help guide the exact duration of antibiotic administration. Treatment of spinal infections also requires a multidisciplinary approach. Nutritional support may be necessary, since many of these patients are substantially malnourished. Physical therapy may assist in mobilizing the patient and prevent other complications that can develop if a patient remains immobile, which include deep vein thrombosis, pneumonia, pulmonary embolism, and decubitus ulcers (14).

Surgical indications include intractable pain, spinal instability, deformity that has the potential to impair function, neurologic deficits at presentation or progressive neurologic deficits, overwhelming sepsis, and failure of medical management. The goals of surgical intervention are identifying the underlying organism, pain relief, debridement of necrotic tissue, decompression of neural elements, and stabilization of the vertebral column. Since the focus of infection is typically in the anterior spinal column, an anterior approach provides the best access for achieving surgical goals. There has been debate in the literature about using instrumentation to stabilize the spine in the presence of infection due to concerns that the implants could become seeded and harbor glycocalyx-producing organisms. Some have argued in favor of a two-stage reconstruction with initial anterior debridement followed by a second posterior stabilization through a clean wound (13). However, more recent clinical series have supported the use of instrumentation at the initial setting, with no significant increase in the rate of recurrence of infection (15,16). Therefore, the current trend involves the use of instrumentation during the anterior approach to provide better stability for the spine and increase fusion rates, but only after aggressive debridement of grossly infected bone and tissues (17). Even in the setting of anterior instrumentation, additional posterior stabilization is occasionally required to provide adequate stability of the spine.

Different markers can be followed to evaluate the success of treatment. Pain usually subsides and fevers and leukocyte counts return to normal. However, as discussed previously, these markers are not specific to this disease process and are often normal even at presentation prior to treatment. ESR and CRP are more sensitive markers and can be routinely monitored. CRP has been shown to be a more reliable and predictive marker with values declining faster as the treatment progresses (7,8). Antibiotic therapy is typically continued a minimum of 6 weeks postoperatively, with the exact duration adjusted according to the laboratory values listed above.

Outcome

Patients who undergo surgical intervention tend to have improved pain when examined after a period of recovery. In one study, 64% of the patients who were treated nonoperatively reported residual back pain while only 26% of patients who underwent surgical intervention had the same complaint (6). Certain risk factors predispose to poor recovery, such as rheumatoid arthritis, age, systemic steroid use, and diabetes. Outcome also is affected by the extent of the disease at the time of diagnosis and treatment (18).

Nonpyogenic Osteomyelitis (Tuberculosis)

TB infection of the spine is referred to as Pott disease. Even though the disease was first described in the 18th century, most of the developments in treatment of the disease occurred during the second half of the 20th century. Patient groups that are at a higher risk of developing TB are immigrants, immunocompromised individuals, homeless people, and substance abusers (19). Since the 1980s, there has been an increased prevalence of TB in the United States. Some possible explanations include increased prevalence of HIV, longer survival rates of patients with chronic diseases, and increased homelessness. Current estimates show that up to 1.7 billion people or almost a third of the world population is, or has been, infected with TB (14). The skeletal system is affected in 3% to 5% of patients with TB. Out of those cases, up to 50% will have involvement of the spine. The thoracic spine is the most common anatomic location (20). Up to 25% of patients will have a multifocal disease process, however (21).

Etiology and Pathogenesis

Mycobacterium tuberculosis is the organism responsible for TB infection. Most originate from a pulmonary source and spread via hematogenous or lymphatic routes. TB infections are often a result of reactivation of a quiescent pulmonary lesion. Subsequently, the organisms seed the spine and are predisposed to take root in the vertebral bodies. TB mycobacterium lacks proteolytic enzymes and therefore tends to spare the disc space (13). Mycobacteria can be associated with an abscess and form caseation necrosis.

Clinical Presentation

TB can present as a chronic process with a long subclinical course. Patients can have symptoms of pain, chills, night sweats, fatigue, and weight loss. The most common structural deformity with the more chronic disease process is kyphosis of the thoracic spine. Neurological involvement may lead to radiculopathy, sensory loss, motor weakness, pathologic reflexes, and bowel and bladder problems (22).

TB infections of the spine are subclassified into three types: peridiscal, anterior, and central. The most common type is called peridiscal where adjacent vertebral bodies are affected but the intervertebral discs and adjacent endplates are spared until late in the disease. Anterior lesions are primarily located under the anterior longitudinal ligament and can spread to multiple adjacent levels along this potential space, without frank involvement of the intervening discs. On the other hand, central lesions remain in the vertebral body and can mimic malignancy (14).

Laboratory Findings

When suspecting Pott disease, the blood workup obtained should be similar to that drawn when dealing with pyogenic infections. The WBC count may be normal. As is the case with pyogenic infections, ESR and CRP are more sensitive markers; however, they are nonspecific and may be only mildly elevated. Skin testing for tuberculin purified protein derivative offers additional information in some cases. Patients can have a positive test with previous exposure to TB, but with no active infection or with an atypical mycobacterial infection. Conversely, the skin test can be falsely negative in immunocompromised, elderly, or malnourished patients (13).

Imaging

X-rays are the initial imaging modality of choice; however, early bony changes are not easily visualized on plain radiographs. Chest x-ray should be obtained to evaluate for pulmonary lesions, which are usually the primary source of infection. Occasionally, soft tissue masses can be appreciated on x-rays and calcification of an abscess is associated with TB (22). The contiguous spread of the TB infection beneath the parietal pleura can cause large paravertebral abscesses in thoracic disease, and those occurring in the lumbar area can cause psoas abscesses (23). CT scan helps to evaluate the bony pathology more accurately than plain radiographs. However, MRI with contrast is the modality of choice and can visualize the combined bony and soft tissue pathology. In recent literature, MRI has been shown to help differentiate TB infections from pyogenic etiology (24). Demonstration of the marked involvement of the endplate and disc in pyogenic infections and the relative sparing of these structures in TB (especially in the setting of multiple contiguous levels of bony involvement or a large anterior soft tissue collection) are the MRI parameters typically used to differentiate the two conditions (see Fig. 32.3A).

Treatment

The initial management involves similar principles as previously described. First, it is imperative to obtain an organism on biopsy and antibiotics should be held prior to the procedure. Mycobacteria grow more slowly in a culture medium, sometimes taking up to 6 weeks. Newer laboratory techniques utilizing the polymerase chain reaction (PCR) can more rapidly identify TB (25). Once identified, multidrug chemotherapy is frequently successful but can require 6 to 12 months of treatment. Isoniazid, rifampin, pyrazinamide, and either streptomycin or ethambutol make up the standard drug regimen. Bracing of the spine is generally recommended, especially in thoracic lesions. Indications for surgical treatment include unstable pathologic fracture, progressive neurological symptoms due to compression of the neurologic elements, intractable pain, or failure of medical management. As previously discussed, the pathology is typically anterior, so surgery usually involves debridement and reconstruction through an anterior approach. Supplemental posterior fixation is often advocated to increase the rigidity of the construct and promote solid fusion. There is general agreement that persistent colonization

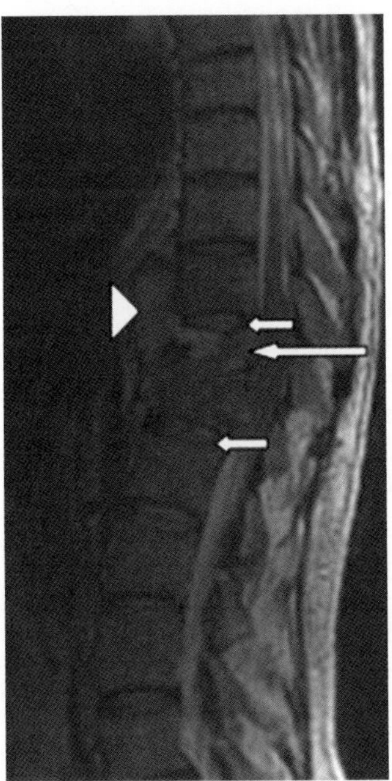

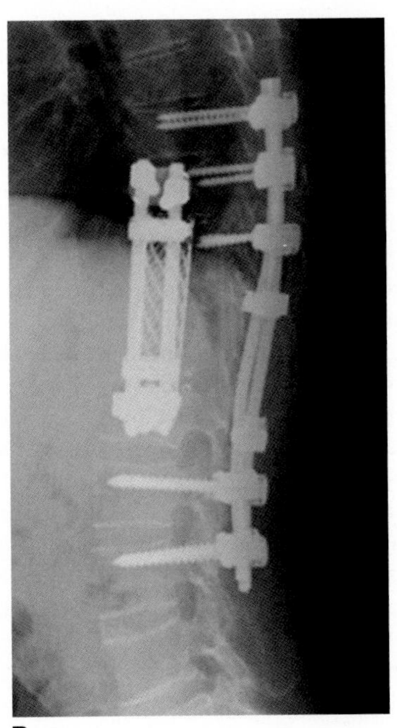

FIGURE 32.3 (**A**) Sagittal T2-weighted MRI demonstrating Pott disease (TB) of the thoracolumbar junction. Note the large anterior collection (*arrowhead*), vertebral collapse (*long arrows*), and relative preservation of the intervertebral disc (*short arrow*). (**B**) Same patient as in (**A**) after undergoing anterior debridement, spinal cord decompression, and anterior-posterior reconstruction with a titanium cage filled with autograft and allograft plus anterior and posterior instrumentation.

of metallic implants by mycobacterium is uncommon when the grossly infected tissue is debrided (26), so instrumented fusion is generally performed (see Fig. 32.3B). Bracing after surgery is usually recommended for a period of up to 3 months.

Outcome

The outcome of Pott disease is dependent on multiple considerations. The host factors will determine how the patient is able to respond to medical and surgical treatments. Most patients recover with appropriate treatment. Elderly patients and patients with paraplegia tend to have a poor prognosis (22). Recovery from neurological deficit is affected by multiple factors including age, medical comorbidities, duration and severity of neurological involvement, time to initiation of treatment, and extent of damage to the spinal cord (20).

Spinal Fungal Infections

Fungal infections of the spine are rare and can present as chronic conditions secondary to a long indolent course. The most common species are aspergillosis, cryptococcosis, blastomycosis, coccidiomycosis, and candidiasis. Some species are found in certain geographical areas, while others are present in normal human flora (27). Patients with fungal infections are usually immunosuppressed, and optimization of host factors plays a role in healing and the ability to recover from infection. Delay in diagnosis may result from failure to evaluate tissue specimens for fungal organisms. Although the treatment involves antifungal medications, such as amphotericin B or ketoconazole, surgical intervention is often necessary (27). Aggressive debridement and reconstruction through combined anterior and posterior approaches may be required in cases with extensive involvement of the anterior column.

EXTRAMEDULLARY INFECTIOUS PROCESSES

Epidural Abscess

Epidural abscess is a collection of purulent material in the epidural space. The most common etiology is bacterial. Pyogenic bacteria from the Staphylococcus or Streptococcus family are the most common. Gram-negative rods, however, may be the causative organism in up to 20% of cases. About 7% of spine infections are associated with epidural abscess. Inciting organisms can spread by hematogenous route, contiguous spread from spondylodiscitis, or bydirect inoculation, from either open fractures or iatrogenic contamination (13). The initial location of insult is usually the metaphyseal area of the vertebral body next to the endplates. Most epidural abscesses occur in the thoracic (51%) and lumbar (35%) spine and tend to be in the posterior epidural space where adipose tissue is present. Cervical epidural abscesses are less common and may be located in the anterior epidural space contiguous with discitis/osteomyelitis. There are different theories on the actual cause of neurological deficits. Some theories that have been discussed in the literature include direct compression from purulent material, instability, vascular insult involving septic emboli, or reactive inflammatory edema (28).

Clinical Presentation

Patients typically present with a constellation of symptoms. The classic clinical triad includes back pain, fevers, and neurological deficits (29). The complete triad, however, is present in only a minority of patients (30). Patients can present with acute onset of symptoms or a chronic history with a new acute exacerbation. Neurological deficits may be present in the setting of an abscess compressing the spinal cord (28). Risk factors for neurologic compromise include diabetes, rheumatoid arthritis, increased age, systemic steroid use, and IV drug abuse (31).

A detailed neurological exam is essential to identify the deficits and help anatomically localize the lesion. Neurological deficits can include decrease in sensation, motor strength, and gait difficulty. If the abscess is compressing the cauda equina, it can cause symptoms of saddle paresthesia and bowel or bladder incontinence. It is important to note that bladder retention could develop prior to bladder incontinence and therefore is the earlier sign of cauda equina syndrome.

Laboratory Findings

Routine laboratory work should be obtained. There can be an increase in WBC count with a left shift and bandemia. ESR and CRP will usually be elevated and these markers can be used to help assess the response to treatment. Blood cultures can help isolate the organism in some cases.

Imaging

Plain x-rays should be obtained to evaluate the overall bony alignment and for any bone changes. Vertebral body destruction and disc space narrowing will not be seen in the acute setting of the disease. CT can further help to evaluate bony architecture of the involved segments, and soft tissue windows can be scrutinized for evidence of mass effect on the thecal sac. MRI with gadolinium is the gold standard in diagnosing an abscess in the epidural space. MRI will provide information on the extent of the abscess and the segments that are involved. The T1 postgadolinium images can be particularly helpful for defining the extent of the abscess. Compressive effects on neurological elements including the spinal cord and nerve roots are also best seen with MRI.

Treatment

The primary goals of treatment are preservation or improvement of neurologic function, eradication of the infection, restoration or maintenance of stability, and relief of pain. Surgical intervention is the mainstay of treatment. Some have suggested that antibiotics alone may be effective in patients who are neurologically intact, particularly if the abscess is located in the lumbar area, where the cauda equina is more tolerant of compressive insults (32). Progressive neurological deficits or failure to respond to medical treatment warrant prompt decompression of the involved segments followed by antibiotic therapy (28). If the abscess is anatomically located anterior to the spinal cord in the cervical or thoracic spine, then an anterior approach may be necessary. Posteriorly located abscesses can be removed by laminectomy. If there is structural compromise from spondylodiscitis anteriorly, however, then laminectomy alone may predispose to progressive deformity. Instrumented fusion may be necessary under these conditions, following similar principles as previously described (15,16).

Outcome

The outcome in cases of epidural abscess is largely dependent on the duration of symptoms and the extent of neurological deficit prior to surgical intervention. Host factors play an important role in helping the patient to recover from the infection. Immunocompromised and malnourished patients can have problems with wound healing and recurrence of the infection.

Postoperative Infections

The incidence of surgical site infection varies with the magnitude of the procedure and has been traditionally quoted to be as low as 1% to 2% after laminectomy or discectomy, but increases to as high as 12% with the use of instrumentation (33). There has been literature published supporting the idea of increased risk of spinal infections in postoperative patients with metastatic disease of the spine (4). Most postoperative infections result from inoculation of the surgical site from skin flora at the time of the surgical procedure, although hematogenous seeding from another source can also occur. Specific surgical factors that increase the risk of infection include long implant constructs, use of an operating microscope, longer duration of surgery, and increased blood loss. Patient-related factors include immune status, malnutrition, obesity, advanced age, smoking, diabetes, and spinal cord injury.

Clinical Presentation

The most common clinical symptoms of postoperative spinal wound infections include increasing pain and tenderness around the surgical site. Fever and chills may be present, but may not develop until late in the course of an infection. The postsurgical incision should be carefully evaluated for erythema, drainage, fluctuence, and wound dehiscence. Postsurgical spinal infections can be subclassified into deep and superficial infections. Superficial infections are above the fascia. A deep infection below a tight fascial closure can progress despite a benign appearing wound.

Diagnostic Studies

Blood work may be helpful in establishing the diagnosis of a postoperative spinal infection. Leukocytosis is suggestive of a postoperative spinal infection; however, the WBC is often within normal limits. During the course of normal healing, the ESR usually peaks about 5 days after surgery, but may remain elevated for more than a month postoperatively even in the absence of an infection (34). The CRP normally peaks about 2 days postoperatively and trends toward normal 2 weeks after surgery (35). In cases of suspected infection, these tests should be obtained. In situations where an infection is not readily apparent, repeat testing should be performed with the expectation of a return to the normal range in a noninfected wound.

Imaging studies have variable utility in early postoperative spinal infections. Plain radiographs can detect mechanical failure of implants or their fixation, which might explain the patients worsening pain. The findings on advanced imaging studies such as CT or MRI may be difficult to distinguish from normal postoperative changes. While superficial wound cultures are not universally recommended, some have advocated swabbing the wound after sterile skin preparation (36).

Treatment

A suspected superficial wound infection may be successfully treated with antibiotics, although extreme vigilance should be maintained for signs of progression. For more established infections, surgical irrigation and debridement are the mainstays of treatment (37). Both superficial and deep wound cultures should be obtained at the time of surgery. The treatment is similar as with other infections. IV antibiotic therapy is started after surgery and is continued for 6 to 8 weeks, using the ESR and CRP laboratory parameters for guidance as already discussed. Management of the previously placed instrumentation and bone graft in the presence of a postoperative infection has been debated, since these entities may act as sources of persistent infection. Conversely, the stability afforded by the implants and the eventual fusion that they ultimately create presumably helps eradicate the infection. The current trend involves retaining well-fixed instrumentation and organized bone graft with no increased risk of recurrence of the infection (15–17).

After irrigation and debridement, several options for wound management exist. If the infection does not appear substantial and has been addressed early, primary closure over drains can be performed. Grossly infected wounds can be packed and brought for serial irrigation and debridement until the wound bed appears healthy, followed by delayed closure. Recently, vacuum-assisted closure devices have been used to manage such problematic wounds with good success (38).

Arachnoiditis

Irritation or inflammation of the subarachnoid space can lead to reactive proliferation of connective tissue and scarring leading to arachnoid thickening, opacification, and adhesion formation. These changes can obliterate the subarachnoid space, and in severe cases the nerve rootlets of the cauda equina or the spinal cord itself can be compressed by bands of connective tissue or loculated pockets of cerebrospinal fluid (CSF). Infectious agents were formerly believed to be the primary cause of this phenomenon, but it is now recognized that a variety of mechanisms can trigger these changes. Intrathecal administration of oil-based contrast agents during myelography has been implicated as a cause of adhesive arachnoiditis (39). Intrathecal or epidural anesthetic agents can also induce the later development of arachnoiditis in rare cases (40). Irritation of the subarachnoid space during spinal surgery or from subarachnoid hemorrhage can also trigger these changes.

Arachnoiditis has a nonspecific clinical picture. The lumbar spine is the area most commonly affected and such patients typically complain of back and lower extremity pain, sensory loss, or weakness. Findings on MRI that are consistent with arachnoiditis include abnormal morphology and position of the nerve roots such as central clumping or adherence to the periphery. In severe situations, the thecal sac may be markedly distorted (41). The mainstay of treatment is control of chronic symptoms. Surgical exploration with resection of the adhesions has not proven to be generally beneficial (42).

SPINAL CORD INFECTIONS

In comparison with the infections of the spinal column reviewed above, infections involving the spinal cord itself are quite rare. This section will cover abscess formation of the spinal cord and acute transverse myelitis (ATM), an intrinsic inflammatory condition of the spinal cord of elusive etiology. Finally, involvement of the spinal cord in HIV, and other rare viral and fungal afflictions of the spinal cord (many of which are seen in the HIV population) will be reviewed.

Intramedullary Abscesses

Etiology

Spinal cord infections are rare with only about 100 case reports in the literature (43). The first case of spinal cord abscess was described by Hart in 1830. There appears to be a bimodal distribution in patient population affected by this uncommon condition with peaks in the pediatric and elderly age groups. In the pediatric population, spinal cord infections have been associated with congenital abnormalities such as a dermal sinus (44). The adult and elderly population usually develops an intramedullary abscess via hematogenous spread. The most common sources are pulmonary, cardiac from endocarditis, and genitourinary tract. The source is not always determined, however. In the study by Candon et al. (15), a primary source of infection was only found in 45% of the patients.

Pathogenesis/Clinical Presentation

An intramedullary abscess is usually caused by *Staphylococcus* or *Streptococcus* species, but up to 25% of patients will have negative intraoperative cultures. Patients are usually classified into three groups based on the duration of symptoms: acute, subacute, and chronic (45). Patients in the acute stage have symptoms lasting less than 1 week. Subacute presentation is between 1 and 6 weeks of symptoms, and chronic cases have symptoms lasting longer than 6 weeks. Signs and symptoms are dependent on the location of the lesion. The most common anatomic location that has been reported is the thoracic spine, but other locations throughout the spinal cord have been reported as well (15). Patients with acute abscesses present with spinal cord dysfunction including weakness, sensory changes, bowel, and bladder impairment. Fever and regional spinal pain may also be present (46).

Imaging/Treatment

MRI with contrast is the imaging modality of choice (10). After the location of the lesion has been visualized and evaluated, surgical intervention is usually necessary. Evacuation of the abscess is usually accomplished by a laminectomy and midline myelotomy (46,47). Intraoperative ultrasound can be used to help localize the site of the planned myelotomy. Parenteral antibiotics are usually given for 6 to 8 weeks. However, even with meticulous yet aggressive treatment of this disease, up to 70% of patients are left with neurological sequelae (45,48).

Neurosyphilis

Syphilis has been known to be a great imitator. The word comes from the Greek language "syphlos" meaning crippled. Neurosyphilis occurs when the syphilitic infection affects the central nervous system (CNS). It is often incorrectly referred to as a "tertiary syphilis." In fact, neurosyphilis can occur in any stage of the disease process including the primary stage (49).

Etiology

Syphilis is a sexually transmitted disease caused by *Treponema pallidum*. It is a systemic disease and can have active manifestations that affect multiple parts of the body. On the other hand, it can be asymptomatic and exist in a latency stage for many years. Neurosyphilis is more common in males and HIV positive patients (50). Syphilis infection is classified into primary, secondary, tertiary, or quaternary stage. Early forms of neurosyphilis primarily affect the meninges, CSF, and cerebral or spinal cord vasculature. Late forms of neurosyphilis primarily affect the brain and spinal cord parenchyma (49).

Clinical Presentation

Patients can present with various symptoms, which can also vary in magnitude. Some of the more common symptoms include personality changes, ataxia, stroke, ophthalmic symptoms, urinary symptoms, "lightning pain," headaches, dizziness, hearing loss, and seizures. These symptoms can be vague and nonspecific to neurosyphilis; therefore, a thorough history and physical exam can assist a clinician with developing the differential diagnosis. On physical examination, a physician can find signs of hyporeflexia, sensory impairment, papillary changes, dementia, Romberg sign, Charcot joints, and hypotonia (51).

Laboratory Findings

Confirmatory laboratory studies include positive rapid plasma reagin and venereal disease research laboratory (VDRL) tests. These tests are inexpensive and easily obtainable; however, they are not entirely specific to syphilis. Microscopy of fluid from the primary lesion using darkfield illumination can diagnose treponemal disease. Since there are other treponemal species that are not a cause of syphilis, correlation between clinical symptoms and microscopy is essential when formulating the diagnosis. There are more specific antibodies and immunofluorescence tests, which include *Treponema pallidum* hemagglutination assay and fluorescent treponemal antibody absorption (52). Neurosyphilis is diagnosed with high leukocyte count in the CSF (greater than 20 WBCs per μL) in the setting of a syphilis infection or a reactive CSF VDRL test result (53).

Imaging

Plain x-rays might not show any pathology especially in early stages of the disease. CT is helpful in providing better information about the bony elements, and since neurosyphilis primarily involves the meninges and the spinal cord parenchyma, CT is not the optimal test to evaluate those changes. However, neurosyphilis can produce a Charcot spine with reactive bony changes, which will be visible on plain radiographs and CT scans.

MRI can show inflammatory changes in the meninges and diffuse swelling in the spinal cord itself. Syphilis causes gummatous and ischemic lesions and most of the changes occur in the posterior column of the spinal cord or the brain (54).

Treatment

Since the beginning of the antibiotic era, little has changed in the treatment of syphilis. Penicillin administered intravenously is still the main treatment (55). In situations where a patient is allergic to penicillin, successful desensitization treatments have been performed followed by a course of penicillin therapy (56). Bony lesions that develop usually are a result of defective protective sensation. External immobilization utilizing bracing is used to limit excessive motion.

Outcome

Although syphilis can be cured, the neurological effects of neurosyphilis might not resolve. Therefore, it is imperative to diagnose and treat the disease process as early as possible, prior to the irreversible changes that can occur in the CNS.

Tabes Dorsalis

Tabes Dorsalis is a manifestation of untreated syphilis. It is caused by demyelination of the posterior columns of the spinal cord. Clinical findings can include weakness, hyporeflexia, paresthesias, sharp shooting pain, ataxia, Charcot joints, and visual impairment. If left untreated, it can progress to paralysis, dementia, and blindness. Once permanent damage to the CNS occurs, it cannot be reversed. IV penicillin is the treatment of choice along with pain medications as needed. Physical therapy is often used to address muscle weakness and improve function (57).

Transverse Myelitis

ATM is an uncommon syndrome characterized by intrinsic inflammation of both sides of a spinal cord segment, resulting in a horizontal level. Involvement may be at any region, from the cervical to the lumbosacral spine, but the thoracic cord is the most commonly affected (58). In one study conducted in New Mexico over a 30-year period, the incidence was determined to be 4.6 per million per year (59). The etiology can be infectious, autoimmune, postvaccinal, and often the specific cause cannot be isolated. The infectious causes can be numerous including multiple viral and bacterial species. Up to 40% of the cases are attributed to viral etiology (60). Some will report a flu-like condition with low-grade fevers leading up to the onset of neurological symptoms. The presenting patients can be classified into two groups: acute presentation with severe neurological symptoms and a subacute progressive onset over days and weeks. The group with acute catastrophic presentation tends to have poor prognosis, while subacute courses have a more favorable outcome (61). In some cases, loss of vision from optic nerve inflammation may accompany the spinal cord involvement. This combination of acute optic neuritis and transverse myelitis (TM) is a unique disease called neuromyelitis optica or Devic syndrome. See Chapter 34 for a more detailed discussion (62,63).

Multiple Sclerosis (thoroughly covered in Chapter 34) may initially present as a TM. This presentation of MS must be differentiated from the topic discussed here, ATM, and the nosology is reviewed by Scott (64). TM as an initial clinical presentation of MS is infrequent, occurring in only 1.5% of all MS cases (65). There have been many studies investigating the long-term risk of developing MS in patients presenting with TM (61,64,66–68), and it is very much dependent on whether the TM presentation is complete or partial (64). Patients who present with acute complete TM, defined as symmetrical and moderate or severe loss of function relative to a distinct spinal cord level, truly have MS less than 2% of the time at 5 years.

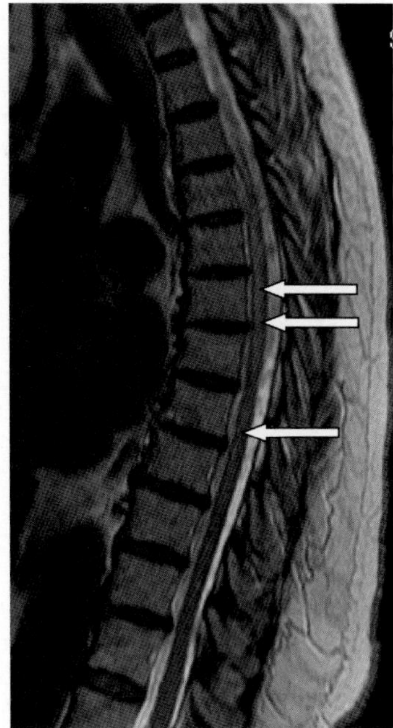

FIGURE 32.4 Thoracic MRI of a patient who presented with rapid onset of back pain and paraplegia 3 weeks after a viral illness. This T2-weighted sagittal cut shows diffuse increased signal intensity in the cord, consistent with edema (*white arrows*). MRI of the brain did not reveal any lesions consistent with multiple sclerosis.

Conversely, those with acute partial TM go on to be confirmed to have clinically definite MS 20% to 30% of the time at 5 years (64). MRI of the brain is the differentiating test, and if it is highly suggestive of MS (see Chapter 34) at the time of the presentation of myelitis, that the risk of actually having clinically definite MS has been estimated 50% at 2 years (69,70).

Prior to considering the diagnosis of ATM, MRI should be evaluated for extrinsic pathologies causing cord compression or intramedullary tumor. Lesions ascribed to ATM typically show cord swelling with or without diffuse increased signal centrally within the cord on T2-weighted images (Fig. 32.4). While not diagnostic, CSF examination typically reveals a mononuclear pleocytosis, often with up to 100 to 200 cells, and an increased protein level. Intrathecal IgG synthesis, defined as an IgG index greater than 0.8 and/or the presence of oligoclonal bands in the CSF was present in 61% of patients with acute TM in one study (71). In cases of necrotizing myelopathy, the spinal cord may swell sufficiently to result in a spinal block with an extremely elevated CSF protein level (Froin's reaction). Treatment is largely supportive, with controversy regarding the benefit of corticosteroid therapy (61,72,73). Subsets of patients have benefited from plasma exchange, IV immunoglobulin, or cyclophosphamide being included in their treatment regimen (74).

Involvement of the Spinal Cord in HIV

Spinal cord afflictions in patients with HIV may occur as a direct manifestation of the HIV infection, or due to opportunistic infections by other organisms during late stages of the disease. The brain is the most common part of the CNS involved, but involvement of the spinal cord often follows (75). Spinal cord dysfunction may go undetected in the presence of a confusing picture including brain involvement and peripheral neuropathy. During autopsies, up to 10% of patients with acquired immunodeficiency syndrome (AIDS) will have opportunistic infections involving the spine. The most prevalent spinal cord disease in AIDS, however, is a direct result of the HIV-1 infection and has been termed vacuolar myelopathy (VM) (75,76).

Vacuolar Myelopathy

VM is the most common myelopathy associated with AIDS and is found in up to 50% of autopsies in this patient group (75). VM occurs in the late stages of the HIV disease process when the CD4+ count is less than 200. It affects the dorsal and lateral columns of the spinal cord. The disease is often asymptomatic until it becomes severe (77). There are different theories on pathogenesis of this disease, but none are proven and more studies are needed to isolate the cause. Imaging in this condition is fairly nonspecific. MRI can show mild atrophy of the spinal cord or nonspecific areas of high signal on T2-weighted images. Analysis of CSF may show nonspecific increased protein and mild pleocytosis or it may be normal (76).

Pathologic examination of these lesions at autopsy demonstrates multiple segmental vacuolar myelin swellings with macrophage infiltration (75). The pathologic features resemble those seen in subacute combined degeneration, and a link to low serum vitamin B_{12} has been explored, but not yet definitively established (78). The current treatment is supportive and prognosis is often poor. Antiretroviral agents, B_{12}/folate supplements, corticosteroids, and IV gamma globulins have all been utilized as preventative measures but without significant late effect.

Herpes Viruses

Viral infections of the spine are rare. Different subgroups of the herpes virus can, however, affect the spinal cord in immunocompromised patients. These include Cytomegalovirus (CMV), Varicella Zoster virus, and Herpes Simplex virus (HSV). The general treatment approach for these infections is administration of antiviral medication and supportive care.

Cytomegalovirus

One of the more common viral pathogens is CMV, which is usually associated with advanced AIDS. CMV can cause a rapidly ascending polyradiculoneuropathy or a necrotizing radiculomyelitis, classically of the cauda equina (75). The clinical presentation can include pain, urinary retention, flaccid paralysis and areflexia. The treatment is with antiviral medications, such as gancyclovir or cidofavir. The prognosis of these infections in severely immunocompromised individuals remains poor with a high mortality rate (75,79).

Varicella Zoster Virus

Varicella zoster virus (VZV) causes chickenpox, often in childhood, after which the virus can remain in spinal cord or cranial nerve cell bodies in a latent phase. The virus can then reactivate in the elderly or in an immunocompromised host. CNS manifestations can occur from a primary infection or reactivation. In reactivations, VZV myelitis usually involves the posterior horn cells first due to spread of the infection from spinal ganglia via the posterior roots (80). CSF can be analyzed by PCR for viral DNA and VZV-specific antibodies. Treatment is initiated as early as possible with antiviral medication; steroids can be used in attempt to decrease inflammation (81).

Herpes Simplex Virus 1 and 2

HSV infections of the spinal cord are rare. In the immunocompromised patient population, however, there have been case reports of HSV causing necrotizing TM. This usually occurs in advanced stages of AIDS with CD4+ counts of less than 50 (82). Prompt initiation of therapy with antiviral medications is essential.

HTLV-1

The human T-cell lymphotropic virus type I (HTLV-I) is a retrovirus that was identified as the cause for tropical spastic paraparesis (TSP)-associated myelopathy in the Caribbean and HTLV-1–associated myelopathy (HAM) in Japan. The abbreviation TSP/HAM is thus now generally used to describe this neurologic syndrome associated with HTLV-1. It typically manifests as a chronic, progressive myelopathic syndrome. The pathogenesis remains unclear with some patients developing severe symptoms, while most remaining healthy despite becoming lifelong carriers of the virus (83). The average latency period is 11 years and the most common symptoms and signs at presentation are chronic progressive spastic paraparesis with hyperreflexia, ankle clonus, and bilateral Babinski signs (84). The most common findings on spinal cord MRI are thoracic spinal cord atrophy. Laboratory tests that are helpful in making the diagnosis include serum antibodies and CSF fluid can show mild pleocytosis, mild to moderate increase in protein, and HTLV-1 antibodies (83). There is no established treatment for this disorder but corticosteroids may transiently relieve some symptoms (83–85). Medications focused on modulating myelopathic symptoms, such as neuropathic pain and spasticity, should be prescribed.

Polio and Postpolio Syndrome

Poliovirus, an enterovirus that can affect the spinal cord, is currently rare in the Western world due to effective vaccination programs. Most infections result in inapparent infection or mild systemic symptoms. Paralytic poliomyelitis is a rare complication due to the virus' predilection to affect the anterior horn cells of the spinal cord. Flaccid weakness with wasting, fasciculations, and areflexia are present with sparing of sensory and sphincter functions (86). Postpolio syndrome describes the development of new muscle weakness and fatigue in skeletal or bulbar muscles beginning 25 to 30 years after an acute attack of paralytic poliomyelitis (87). Current evidence suggests that this syndrome is due to evolution of a subclinical ongoing motor neuron dysfunction with attrition of the oversprouting motor neurons and failure of reinnervation (88). These conditions are extensively covered in Chapter 35.

Fungal and Parasitic Infections of the Spinal Cord

Patients with HIV can develop fungal infections of the spinal cord, including cryptococcosis, aspergillosis, mucormycosis, and candidiasis (75). Parasitic infections are a rare subset of the spinal cord infections. Toxoplasmosis is the most common and usually effects patients with established AIDS. Although toxoplasmosis usually involves the brain and basal ganglia, it can involve the spinal cord and cause spinal cord edema at the level of the lesion (89). Schistosomes have also been known to affect the CNS. The presentation is usually rapidly progressive symptoms with neurologic deficits. Some cases demonstrate eosinophilia in CSF fluid, which can help diagnose a parasitic infection (90). MRI is the imaging study of choice, which can help identify the pathology and the extent of spinal cord edema. Diagnosis is based on biopsy and the clinical presentation. Treatment typically involves antiparasitic drugs, corticosteroids, and surgery (91).

SUMMARY

Spinal infections have predated modern medicine, yet continue to cause morbidity and mortality today. Infections of the spinal column, including pyogenic spondylodiscitis, Pott disease, and epidural abscess can occur via hematogenous spread or direct inoculation. Correlation of the clinical presentation, laboratory studies, and imaging findings help support the diagnosis. Identification of the causative organism and targeted antibiotic therapy are the mainstays of treatment. Surgical intervention may be necessary to decompress the neurologic elements, restore stability, or debride grossly infected tissue that has been refractory to medical management. Infections of the spinal cord itself are less common. Many of these cases involve immunocompromised patients, typically with advanced cases of HIV/AIDS. While these infections can range from bacterial infections to rare parasites, common viral pathogens are the predominant agents in this patient population. Treatment in these cases is more commonly centered on antiviral therapeutics and symptomatic/supportive care.

References

1. Garceau GJ, Brady TA. Pott's paraplegia. *J Bone Joint Surg Am* 1950;32:87–102.
2. Al-Nammari SS, Lucas JD, Lam KS. Hematogenous methicillin-resistant Staphylococcus aureus spondylodiscitis. *Spine* 2007;32:2480–2486.
3. Khan IA, Vaccaro AR, Zlotolow DA. Management of vertebral diskitis and osteomyelitis. *Orthopedics* 1999;22:758–765.
4. Weinstein MA, McCabe JP, Cammisa FP Jr. Postoperative spinal wound infection: a review of 2,391 consecutive index procedures. *J Spinal Disord* 2000;13:422–426.
5. Wood II GW. Anatomic, biologic, and pathophysiologic aspects of spinal infections. *Spine* 1989;3:385–396.
6. Hadjipavlou AG, Mader JT, Necessary JT, et al. Hematogenous pyogenic spinal infections and their surgical management. *Spine* 2000;25:1668–1679.
7. Sapico FL, Montgomerie JZ. Pyogenic vertebral osteomyelitis: report of nine cases and review of the literature. *Rev Infect Dis* 1979;1:754–776.
8. Mok JM, Pekmezci M, Piper SL, et al. Use of C-reactive protein after spinal surgery: comparison with erythrocyte sedimentation rate as predictor of early postoperative infectious complications. *Spine* 2008;33:415–421.
9. Francis O. T. Akenami. Severe malnutrition is associated with decreased levels of plasma transferrin receptor. *Br J Nutr* 1997;77:391–397.
10. Rothman SL. The diagnosis of infections of the spine by modern imaging techniques. *Orthop Clin North Am* 1996;27:15–31.
11. Adatepe MH, Powell OM, Isaacs GH, et al. Hematogenous pyogenic vertebral osteomyelitis: diagnostic value of radionuclide bone imaging. *J Nucl Med* 1986;27:1680–1685.
12. Vaccaro AR, Shah SH, Schweitzer ME, et al. MRI description of vertebral osteomyelitis, neoplasm, and compression fracture. *Orthopedics* 1999;22:67–73.
13. Hilibrand AS, Quartararo LG, Moulton MJR. Spinal infections, chapter 55. In: Koval K, ed. *Orthopaedic knowledge update* 7. American Academy of Orthopaedic Surgeons (Rosemont, Illinois), 2002:661–672.
14. Jacofsky D, Currier B. Infections of the spine chapter 43. In: Fardon D, Garfin S, eds. *Orthopaedic knowledge update: spine 2*. American Academy of Orthopaedic Surgeons, 2002:431–442.
15. Candon E, Frerebeau P. Bacterial abscesses of the spinal cord. Review of the literature (73 cases). *Rev Neurol (Paris)* 1994;150:370–376.
16. Robinson Y, Tschoeke SK, Finke T, et al. Successful treatment of spondylodiscitis using titanium cages: a 3-year follow-up of 22 consecutive patients. *Acta Orthop* 2008;79:660–664.
17. Carragee E, Iezza A. Does acute placement of instrumentation in the treatment of vertebral osteomyelitis predispose to recurrent infection: long-term follow-up in immune-suppressed patients. *Spine* 2008;33:2089–2093.
18. Eismont FJ, Bohlman HH, Soni PL, et al. Pyogenic and fungal vertebral osteomyelitis with paralysis. *J Bone Joint Surg Am* 1983;65:19–29.
19. Buskin SE, Gale JL, Weiss NS, et al. Tuberculosis risk factors in adults in King County, Washington, 1988 through 1990. *Am J Public Health* 1994;84:1750–1756.
20. Moon MS. Tuberculosis of the spine. Controversies and a new challenge. *Spine* 1997;22:1791–1797.
21. Moon MS, Moon JL, Kim SS, et al. Treatment of tuberculosis of the cervical spine: operative versus nonoperative. *Clin Orthop Relat Res* 2007;460:67–77.
22. Pertuiset E, Beaudreuil J, Lioté F, et al. Spinal tuberculosis in adults. A study of 103 cases in a developed country, 1980–1994. *Medicine (Baltimore)*. 1999;78:309–320.
23. Mückley T, Schütz T, Kirschner M, et al. Psoas abscess: the spine as a primary source of infection. *Spine* 2003;28:E106–E113.
24. Harada Y, Tokuda O, Matsunaga N. Magnetic resonance imaging characteristics of tuberculous spondylitis vs. pyogenic spondylitis. *Clin Imaging* 2008;32:303–309.
25. Wang D. Diagnosis of tuberculous vertebral osteomyelitis (TVO) in a developed country and literature review. *Spinal Cord* 2005;43:531–542.

26. Ozdemir HM, Us AK, Ogun T. The role of anterior spinal instrumentation and allograft fibula for the treatment of pott disease. *Spine* 2003;28:474–479.
27. Kim CW, Perry A, Currier B, et al. Fungal infections of the spine. *Clin Orthop Relat Res* 2006;444:92–99.
28. Bluman EM, Palumbo MA, Lucas PR. Spinal epidural abscess in adults. *J Am Acad Orthop Surg* 2004;12:155–163.
29. Rigamonti D, Liem L, Sampath P, et al. Spinal epidural abscess: contemporary trends in etiology, evaluation, and management. *Surg Neurol* 1999;52:189–197.
30. Davis DP, Wold RM, Patel RJ, et al. The clinical presentation and impact of diagnostic delays on emergency department patients with spinal epidural abscess. *J Emerg Med* 2004;26:285–291.
31. Darouiche RO. Spinal epidural abscess. *N Engl J Med* 2006;355:2012–2020.
32. Savage K, Holton PD, Zalavras CG. Spinal epidural abscess: early outcome in patients treated medically. *Clin Orthop Relat Res* 2005;439:56–60.
33. Bassewitz HL, Fishgrund JS, Herkowitz HN. Postoperative spine infections. *Semin Spine Surg* 2000;12:203–211.
34. Jonsson B, Soderholm R, Stromqvist B. Erythrocyte sedimentation rate after lumbar spine surgery. *Spine* 1991;16:1049–1050.
35. Meyer B, Schaller K, Rohde V, et al. The C-reactive protein for detection of early infections after lumbar microdiscectomy. *Acta Neurochir (Wein)* 1995;136:145–150.
36. Hong HS, Chang MC, Liu CL, et al. Is aggressive surgery necessary for acute postoperative deep spinal wound infection? *Spine* 2008;33:2473–2478.
37. Glassman SD, Dimar JR, Puno RM, et al. Salvage of instrumental lumbar fusions complicated by surgical wound infection. *Spine* 1996;21:2163–2169.
38. Mehbod AA, Ogilvie JW, Pinto MR, et al. Postoperative deep wound infections in adults after spinal fusion: management with vacuum-assisted wound closure. *J Spinal Disord Tech* 2005;18:14–17.
39. Brodsky AE. Post laminectomy and post fusion stenosis of the lumbar spine. *Clin Orthop* 1976;115:130.
40. Sklar EM, Quencer RM, Green BA, et al. Complications of epidural anesthesia: MR appearance of abnormalities. *Radiology* 1991;181:549–554.
41. Ross JS, Masaryk TJ, Modic MT, et al. MR imaging of lumbar arachnoiditis. *Am J Roentgenol* 1987;149:1025–1032.
42. Wiesel SW. The multiply operated lumbar spine. *Instr Course Lect* 1985;34:68–77.
43. Benzil DL, Epstein MH, Knuckey NW. Intramedullary epidermoid associated with an intramedullary spinal abscess secondary to a dermal sinus. *Neurosurgery* 1992;30:118–121.
44. Gerlach R, Zimmermann M, Hermann E, et al. Large intramedullary abscess of the spinal cord associated with an epidermoid cyst without dermal sinus. Case report. *J Neurosurg Spine* 2007;7:357–361.
45. Menezes AH, Graf CJ, Perret GE. Spinal cord abscess: a review. *Surg Neurol* 1977;8:461–467.
46. Martin RJ, Yuan HA. Neurosurgical care of spinal epidural, subdural, and intramedullary abscesses and arachnoiditis. *Orthop Clin North Am* 1996;27:125–136.
47. Akalan N, Ozgen T. Infection as a cause of spinal cord compression: a review of 36 spinal epidural abscess cases. *Acta Neurochir (Wien)* 2000;142:17–23.
48. Chan CT, Gold WL. Intramedullary abscess of the spinal cord in the antibiotic era: clinical features, microbial etiologies, trends in pathogenesis, and outcomes. *Clin Infect Dis* 1998;27:619–626.
49. Marra CM. Update on Neurosyphilis. *Curr Infect Dis Rep*. 2009;11:127–134.
50. Ghanem KG, Moore RD, Rompalo AM, et al. Neurosyphilis in a clinical cohort of HIV-1-infected patients. *AIDS* 2008;22:1145–1151.
51. Yasaki S, Ohshima J, Yonekura J, et al. A case of early syphilis presenting general paresis-like symptoms and bilateral tonic pupils. *Rinsho Shinkeigaku* 1992;32: 994–999.
52. Marra CM, Tantalo LC, Maxwell CL, et al. Alternative cerebrospinal fluid tests to diagnose neurosyphilis in HIV-infected individuals. *Neurology* 2004;63:85–88.
53. Marra CM, Maxwell CL, Smith SL, et al. Cerebrospinal fluid abnormalities in patients with syphilis: association with clinical and laboratory features. *J Infect Dis* 2004;189:369–376.
54. Peng F, Hu X, Zhong X, et al. CT and MR findings in HIV-negative neurosyphilis. *Eur J Radiol* 2008;66:1–6.
55. Stoner BP. Current controversies in the management of adult syphilis. *Clin Infect Dis* 2007;44(Suppl 3):S130–S146.
56. Soriano V, Niveiro E, Fernández J, et al. Successful desensitization to penicillin after diagnostic reassessment. *Allergol Immunopathol (Madr)* 2003;31:94–96.
57. Jay CA. Treatment of neurosyphilis. *Curr Treat Options Neurol* 2006;8:185–92.
58. Dawson DM, Potts F. Acute nontraumatic myelopathies. *Neurol Clin* 1991;9:585–603.
59. Jeffery DR, Mandler RN, Davis LE. Transverse myelitis. Retrospective analysis of 33 cases with differentiation of cases associated with multiple sclerosis and parainfectious events. *Arch Neurol* 1993;50:532–535.
60. Tyler KL, Gross RA, Cascino GD. Unusual viral causes of transverse myelitis: hepatitis A virus and cytomegalovirus. *Neurology*. 1986;36:855–858.
61. Ropper AH, Poskanzer DC. The prognosis of acute and subacute transverse myelopathy based on early signs and symptoms. *Ann Neurol* 1978;4:51–59.
62. Sebastian del la Cruz F, Lopez-Dolado F. Devic's optic neuromyelitis: analysis of 7 cases. *Rev Neurol* 1999;28: 476–482.
63. Wingerchuk DM, Hogancamp WF, O'Brian PC, et al. The clinical course of neuromyelitis optica (Devic's syndrome). *Neurology* 1999;53:1107–1114.
64. Scott TF. Nosology of idiopathic transverse myelitis syndromes. *Acta Neurol Scand* 2007;115:371–376.
65. Fischer C, Mauguiere F, Ibanez V, et al. Visual, early auditory and somatosensory evoked potentials in multiple sclerosis (917 cases). *Rev Neurol* 1986;142:517–523.
66. Berman M, Feldman S, Alter M, et al. Acute transverse myelitis: Incidence and etiologic considerations. *Neurology* 1982;31:966.
67. Lipton HL, Teasdall RD. Acute transverse myelopathy in adults: a follow-up study. *Arch Neurol* 1973;28: 252–257.
68. Miller DH, et al. The early risk of multiple sclerosis following isolated acute syndromes of the brainstem and spinal cord. *Ann Neurol* 1989;26:635–639.

69. Lee KH, et al. Magnetic resonance imaging of the head in the diagnosis of multiple sclerosis: a prospective 2 year follow-up with comparison of clinical evaluation, evoked potentials, oligoclonal banding, and CT. *Neurology* 1991;41:657–660.
70. Perumal J, Zabad R, Caon C, et al. Acute transverse myelitis with normal brain MRI: long term risk of MS. *J Neurol* 2008;255:89–93.
71. Harzheim M, Schlegel U, Urbacj H, et al. Discriminatory features of acute transverse myelitis: a retrospective analysis of 45 patients. *J Neurol Sci* 2004;217:217–233.
72. Sebire G, Hollenberg H, Meyer L, et al. High dose methylprednisolone in severe acute transverse myelopathy. *Arch Dis Child* 1997;76:167–168.
73. Lahat E, Pillar G, Ravid S, et al. Rapid recovery from transverse myelopathy in children treated with methylprednisolone. *Pediatr Neurol* 1998;199:279–282.
74. Greenberg BM, Thomas KP, Krishnan C, et al. Idiopathic transverse myelitis: corticosteroids, plasma exchange, or cyclophosphamide. *Neurology* 2007;68:1614–1617.
75. Budka H. Neuropathology of myelitis, myelopathy, and spinal infections in AIDS. *Neuroimaging Clin N Am* 1997;7:639–650.
76. Di Rocco A. Diseases of the spinal cord in human immunodeficiency virus infection. *Semin Neurol* 1999;19:151–155.
77. Gonzales MF, Davis RL. Neuropathology of acquired immunodeficiency syndrome. *Neuropathol Appl Neurobiol.* 1988;14:345.
78. Kieburtz KD, Giang DW, Schiffer RB. Abnormal vitamin B_{12} metabolism in human immunodeficiency virus infection: association with neurological dysfunction. *Arch Neurol* 1991;48:312–314.
79. Guiot HM, Pita-García IL, Bertrán-Pasarell J, Alfonso G. Cytomegalovirus polyradiculomyelopathy in AIDS: a case report and review of the literature. *P R Health Sci J* 2006;25:359–362.
80. Quencer RM, Poswt MJ. Spinal cord lesions in patients with AIDS. *Neuroimag Clin N Am* 1997;7:359–373.
81. Gilden D Varicella zoster virus and central nervous system syndromes. *Herpes* 2004;11(Suppl 2):89A–94A.
82. Corti M, Soto I, Villafañe MF, et al. Acute necrotizing myelitis in an AIDS patient. *Medicina (B Aires)* 2003;63:143–146.
83. Bangham CR. HTLV-1 infections. *J Clin Pathol* 2000;53:581–586.
84. Carod-Artal FJ, Mesquita HM, Ribeiro Lda S. Neurological symptoms and disability in HTLV-1 associated myelopathy. *Neurologia* 2008;23:78–84.
85. Kincaid O, Lipton HL. Viral myelitis: an update. *Curr Neurol Neurosci Rep* 2006;6:469–474.
86. Berger JR, Ryan SJ. Medical myelopathies. In: Herkowitz HN, Garfin SR, Balderston RA, et al., eds. *The spine*. 4th ed. Phildelphia, PA: W.B. Saunders, 1999: 1413–1430.
87. Dalakas MC. The post-polio syndrome as an evolved clinical entity. *Ann N Y Acad Sci* 1995;753:68–80.
88. Dalakas MC. Pathogenetic mechanisms of post-polio syndrome. *Ann N Y Acad Sci* 1995;753:167–185.
89. Porter SB, Sand MA. Toxoplasmosis of the central nervous system in the acquired immunodeficiency syndrome. *N Engl J Med* 1993;327:1643–1648.
90. Osoegawa M. Diagnosis and treatment of CNS parasite infection with special reference to parasitic myelitis. *Rinsho Shinkeigaku* 2004;44:961–964.
91. Ferrari TC. Involvement of central nervous system in the schistosomiasis. *Mem Inst Oswaldo Cruz.* 2004;99(5 Suppl 1):59–62.

CHAPTER 33 ■ VASCULAR, NUTRITIONAL, AND OTHER NONTRAUMATIC CONDITIONS OF THE SPINAL CORD

STEPHEN S. KAMIN

INTRODUCTION

The spinal cord can be affected by ischemic, nutritional, and other nontraumatic insults of many types. This chapter addresses many of these diverse causes of spinal cord dysfunction. Although much less prone to vascular disease than the brain, the spinal cord may also be the site of ischemia. This may occur by classical mechanisms of thrombosis or embolism, as well as on a hemodynamic basis or in association with dural arteriovenous malformations (AVMs). Nutritional causes of myelopathy, both deficiency states such as subacute combined degeneration and exposure to toxins in foodstuffs, as in lathyrism, are reviewed. Systemic diseases such as lupus erythematosus and Sjögren syndrome (SS) may lead to myelopathy and will be examined. A large number of inherited diseases involve the spinal cord. Only hereditary spastic paraparesis (HSP) presents exclusively or predominantly as a typical myelopathy and therefore is the only such disease discussed here. Iatrogenic injury to the cord as a result of radiation therapy will be reviewed. Finally, myelopathy due to decompression sickness (DCS) will also be presented in this chapter.

SPINAL CORD STROKE

The rapid development of paraplegia with complete sensory loss and bowel and bladder dysfunction is a devastating occurrence, which may result from ischemia of the spinal cord. Given the frequency of brain infarction, spinal cord stroke is a surprisingly rare phenomenon. The precise mechanism of spinal cord stroke often cannot be determined, but such strokes are frequently seen in the setting of aortic disease or manipulation of the aorta or in the aftermath of profound systemic hypotension. To understand the clinical picture and likely mechanisms of spinal stroke, some knowledge of the vascular anatomy of the spinal cord is necessary.

Blood Supply of the Spinal Cord

The blood supply of the spinal cord was first described by Adamkiewicz in 1882 (1). The cord is supplied by a single, midline anterior spinal artery and two posterior spinal arteries (2). All arise from the vertebral arteries in the neck and run the length of the spinal cord. At the level of the conus medullaris, they form an anastomotic network that encircles the cord. Small branches of the radicular arteries contribute at each segmental level. Only a few such arteries contribute to the blood supply to a significant extent, generally 6 to 10 anteriorly and 10 to 23 posteriorly. In the lower thoracic and lumbar area, the blood supply is via a single large radicular artery known as the artery of Adamkiewicz. This usually arises between T9 and L2, most frequently at T11 on the left. It can be distinguished on angiography by the distinctive hairpin turn that it makes before entering the thecal sac.

The anterior spinal artery supplies approximately the anterior two thirds of the cord. This includes most of the gray matter of the cord and the anterior and lateral white matter columns. The posterior spinal arteries supply the remainder, including the tips of the posterior horns and the posterior columns. Paramedian vessels arise from the anterior spinal artery and penetrate the deeper portions of the cord, especially the gray matter. Anastomotic vessels between the anterior and the posterior spinal arteries give off many small penetrating vessels, which circumferentially supply the white matter. This pattern parallels that seen in the brainstem.

This pattern of blood supply, with primary inflow to the spinal arteries from the vertebral arteries rostrally and the artery of Adamkiewicz caudally, with minor contributions from radicular arteries along the rest of the length of the cord, leads to a watershed or borderzone area in the upper to midthoracic level, which is often reflected in the clinical syndromes of spinal cord ischemia. The concept, however, has recently been brought into question by Weidauer et al. (3), who found no radiographic evidence of such a borderzone effect. There is also a borderzone region within the gray matter of the cord, as the penetrating arteries are end arteries with little anastomosis between them. This contributes to the pathophysiology behind traumatic central syndrome as discussed in Chapter 6.

Spinal Stroke Syndromes

Various patterns of neurological deficit can be seen in spinal cord ischemia, depending on the specific arteries involved. The most dramatic and devastating picture is that of total transection of the cord. This presents with flaccid paraplegia or tetraplegia, loss of all sensation below the level of the lesion, and bowel and bladder dysfunction. The onset is usually abrupt and progression is rapid. There is often radicular pain at the onset, which may last for hours or rarely days. If the infarct is in the cervical area, there is tetraplegia. Pain is generally interscapular and may radiate to the shoulder. In lower lesions, paraplegia results. Pain may radiate to the abdomen or the anterior thighs. In lesions of the conus medullaris, the pain is referred to the buttocks. The tendon stretch reflexes and abdominal reflexes are abolished initially, but hyperreflexia may develop in days or weeks, along with Babinski signs. Sensory loss involves all modalities, and the intensity and level of the sensory loss may change during the course of the stroke. Sphincter dysfunction is generally complete, with initially a flaccid anal sphincter followed by the development of excessive tone if the stroke syndrome involves the upper motor neurons exclusively. This will lead to the clinical symptoms of urinary retention and constipation. Other autonomic disturbances may also occur, including vasodilatation with hypotension, bowel pseudo-obstruction, loss of thermoregulatory reflexes, and pulmonary edema. The prognosis for functional improvement in this syndrome is poor, and medical complications are frequent.

The "classic" spinal stroke syndrome is the syndrome of the anterior spinal artery (4). This presents with flaccid paraplegia or tetraplegia and dissociated sensory loss below the level of the lesion. Pain and temperature sensations are affected but vibration and joint position sense are relatively preserved. This reflects the pattern of blood supply to the cord, with the anterior spinal artery supplying only the anterior two thirds. Sphincter disturbance is usually present.

A partial Brown-Sequard syndrome occasionally occurs early in the course of anterior spinal artery infarction (5). This may reflect occlusion of a paramedian penetrating vessel. Other partial syndromes also frequently occur. The anterior horn may be preferentially affected due to the greater susceptibility of gray matter to ischemia as compared to white matter due to the greater metabolic demands of cell bodies (6). This produces flaccid weakness without sensory or sphincter disturbance, often described as "pseudopoliomyelitic." If it occurs in the cervical region, there is isolated arm weakness.

The posterior spinal artery syndrome is rare and difficult to recognize (7). It usually begins with spinal pain and paresthesias in the legs. Examination reveals loss of vibration and joint position sense in the legs and areflexia. There is often variable weakness and sphincter dysfunction due to more anterior extension of the infarction, but the degree of involvement is never as profound as in the anterior spinal artery syndrome.

Central cord infarctions may result from borderzone ischemia in the central gray matter of the cord. They do not differ clinically from other spinal cord strokes and can only be diagnosed radiographically or pathologically. They often are merely longitudinal extensions of complete transverse infarcts.

Mechanisms of Spinal Cord Infarction

In many cases, the precise mechanism of spinal cord infarction cannot be determined. For instance, Masson's review of 28 cases revealed aortic disease in 8, diverse causes in 3, and no identified cause in 17 (8). Similarly, Salvador de al Barrera et al. (9) found no definite etiology in 36.1% of 36 cases. There are, however, a number of situations that predispose to such infarcts and a specific mechanism may be inferred.

Hypotensive Infarction

Borderzone or "watershed" infarction of the cord may occur as a result of profound hypotension. As discussed above, the vascular supply of the cord makes certain segments, particularly in the mid-thoracic region, more prone to ischemia when the perfusion pressure is reduced. Consequently, in the setting of a marked fall in blood pressure due to cardiac arrest or massive hemorrhage, infarction may ensue. The usual presentation is acute flaccid paraplegia with sensory loss and areflexia corresponding to the transverse infarction picture discussed earlier. This may in fact be the most common cause of cord infarction. In a review of 11 cases of spinal stroke at the Stokes Mandeville Spinal Injuries Center in Britain, 10 of the cases were due to hypotension and only one due to aortic occlusion (10). An additional four patients who suffered hypotension during surgery were described later (11). Similar events have also been reported in children (6). The degree and duration of hypotension necessary to produce infarction in humans is unknown. In this series, one patient was in cardiac arrest for 5 minutes and another had a minimum pressure recorded of 47/25, which persisted for 2.5 hours. On the other hand, one patient had a lowest recorded pressure of 90/60, but the intraoperative records were incomplete. Kobrine et al. (12) found in experimental monkeys that both spinal cord and cerebral blood flow began to decrease when the mean arterial pressure was 50 torr and was unmeasurable at a pressure of 25 torr. They felt that autoregulation was more robust in the brain than the cord, making the cord more sensitive to hypotension. How this information relates to humans with atherosclerosis is uncertain, but it is likely that superimposed arterial narrowing may further compromise the circulation of the cord and increase the risk of ischemia even at higher levels of blood pressure.

Stroke in Association with Aortic Surgery

It has been known for many years that operation on the aorta presents a significant risk of postoperative paraplegia (13). In experimental dogs, paraplegia can be induced in 50% of animals whose aorta is occluded distal to the left subclavian artery (14). DeBakey et al. (15) reported a 5.5% incidence of paraplegia after resection of aneurysms of the descending aorta. Crawford et al. (16) reported an incidence of 6.8% even with the use of extracorporeal bypass. In correction of coarctation of the aorta, Brewer et al. (17) reported an incidence of paraplegia of 0.41% of 12,532 cases. There was no clear correlation between the risk of paraplegia and the number of intercostal arteries sacrificed or the duration of aortic occlusion. Investigators have generally felt that if the aorta was occluded below the level of the renal arteries, cord infarction would not occur (18). However, even in this situation, paraplegia can on occasion occur (19). Endovascular procedures pose a lower risk than open surgical procedures (20).

It is difficult to determine the precise mechanism of infarction in these cases. Systemic hypotension occurred in some cases. In others, occlusion of radicular arteries by the aortic lesion may lead to infarction, especially in the setting of relative hypotension. Aortic dissection may result in paraplegia by such a mechanism in the absence of surgical intervention. Although aortic surgery is now the most common cause of cord infarction, intraoperative hypotension, either systemic or local due to cross-clamping of the aorta may well play a significant role. Likewise, hypotension during other surgical procedures has also been reported to cause spinal cord infarction (21). Coarctation of the aorta may also lead to spontaneous paraplegia. In some cases, the mechanism appeared to be ischemic, while in others it was compressive due to epidural or subarachnoid hemorrhage (22). Only in the endovascular cases is the mechanism fairly certain to be embolization of atherosclerotic debris dislodged by the catheter. However, the mechanism of the delayed cases continues to be uncertain.

Embolism

Fibrocartilaginous material from intervertebral discs is probably the most common source of emboli to the spinal cord. Such emboli are hypothesized to originate from Schmorl nodules and to reach the cord via the basicentral vein of the vertebral body. These emboli most often affect the cervical region. They may be associated with trauma, often of a minor nature, or with pregnancy and the puerperium (23–27). Meyer et al. (28) report a pathologically confirmed case of fibrocartilaginous embolization 2.5 hours after epidural injection of steroids at C6-7. Presumably, disc material was inadvertently aspirated into the needle used for the injection and then directly introduced into the anterior spinal artery. Atheromatous emboli are very rare (22). Cholesterol embolism has also been reported (28).

Venous Infarction

Occlusion of the venous drainage of the cord may also lead to infarction, although reports of such cases are rare. Hughes reported a pathologically proven case that demonstrated hemorrhagic infarction of the central cord from T3 to T6 (29). Clarke and Cumming reported a classic anterior spinal artery syndrome in association with thrombosis of the left common femoral and internal iliac veins. An arteriogram was negative, so infarction was felt to be secondary to the venous lesion (30). Rao et al. (31) reviewed 15 cases from the literature in 1982. Pain in the back, abdomen, or neck was common at the onset, occurring in 10 patients. The infarctions were generally extensive, six involving the whole cord. Two of these also involved the medulla. The underlying conditions predisposing to venous infarction included chronic infections, polycythemia vera, ulcerative colitis, and pancreatic cancer. In some cases, there was in situ venous thrombosis and in others emboli occurred.

Other Causes

Spinal cord infarction has been reported as a consequence of vertebral artery dissection. Crum et al. (32) reported one case and reviewed seven others from the literature. Minor cervical trauma or chiropractic manipulation was the cause in some cases. The anterior spinal artery syndrome occurred in two cases and the posterior spinal artery syndrome in three. A combination of spinal cord and medullary infarction was seen in two patients. Unilateral dissection could cause either unilateral or bilateral infarctions, but unilateral infarction always resulted from unilateral dissection.

Vasculitis has rarely been reported to cause spinal cord infarction. In the preantibiotic era, meningovascular syphilis was often presumed to be the cause of spinal stroke, but there are few proven cases (33,34). Other chronic meningitides such as tuberculosis and cryptococcosis can also lead to spinal stroke (35). Two cases of spinal cord infarction due to polyarteritis nodosa were reported by Corbin (36). Other rare causes include cervical spondylosis (37), epidural injections (38), and hypercoagulable states (39).

Spinal Arteriovenous Malformations (Foix-Alajouanine Syndrome)

In 1926, Foix and Alajouanine described two patients who developed subacute myelopathy leading to death. At autopsy, they discovered necrosis of the spinal cord and numerous thick-walled tortuous vessels lying on the surface of the cord (40). Lhermitte identified these vessels as being associated with an AVM, which usually resides on the dura (41). It was generally believed that the rapidly progressing myelopathy resulted from thrombosis of these abnormal vessels within the spinal cord (42,43). Consequently, this process, which came to be known as the Foix-Alajouanine syndrome, was felt to be irreversible and to carry a very poor prognosis. For instance, Aminoff and Logue at Queen Square and Maida Vale analyzed 60 cases (44,45). Within 6 months of onset, 19% of patients required bilateral support to walk or required a wheelchair for mobility. Within 3 years, 50% were at that stage of disability. Only 30% were walking independently at 3 years.

Spinal AVMs are classified into four types (46). Type I AVMs, also called dural AV fistulas, are the most common. They generally lie on the dorsal aspect of the lower thoracic cord and conus medullaris. There is usually a single feeding vessel. Type II lesions are intramedullary lesions with a true AVM nidus within the spinal cord. Type III lesions are so-called juvenile malformations and are rare. Type IV AVMs are intradural, extramedullary lesions and are also relatively uncommon. The remainder of this section will focus on type I and, to a lesser extent, type II lesions.

The clinical course of spinal AVMs is most often gradual, especially in type I lesions. This was the case in 23 of 27 patients in the series of Rosenblum et al. (47) and 40 of 71 of Tobin and Layton's patients (48). Although a stepwise course of deterioration is often considered classic, this occurs in only a minority of patients (48,49). Acute onset of symptoms is more common in the intramedullary type II lesions (50% as per Rosenblum et al. [47]), probably due to hemorrhage. It may be many years from onset of symptoms before the correct diagnosis is made. A third of the patients in the series of Symon et al. (50) had symptoms for 3 years or more before diagnosis.

The most common initial symptoms are sensory disturbance, pain, and leg weakness (see Table 33.1), although experts disagree on the relative frequency of the initial symptoms identified. The Mayo Clinic group in 1976 found that sensory complaints were the most common initial symptom, followed by leg weakness and pain. The Dutch researchers reported gait disturbance most frequently, followed by sensory disturbances. Pain was distinctly less common, occurring in only 13% of patients at onset (49). It is not clear why these differences are reported. As these are initial, prediagnosis symptoms, it is unlikely that this results from improvements in diagnostic ability. Sphincter disturbance is much less common at onset. It is important to realize that the location of pain is not a reliable guide to the site of the vascular malformation (51). By the time of diagnosis, leg weakness, sensory disturbance, and sphincter dysfunction are almost universal. The major physical signs (see Table 33.2) include leg weakness, usually of an upper motor neuron type (48), although Aminoff and Logue found muscle atrophy in two thirds of patients and increased reflexes in only 45% (51). Similarly, Jellema et al. found upper motor neuron signs in 33 of 80 patients, with coexistent or preceding lower motor neuron signs in 11 of these (49). A pure lower motor neuron syndrome occurred

TABLE 33.1

FOIX-ALAJOUANINE SYNDROME INITIAL SYMPTOMS

Symptom	%
Sensory	97
Radicular	21
Spinal level	37
Leg weakness	56
Pain	49
Radicular	17
Nonradicular	10
Back pain	23
Sphincter disturbance	35
Bladder	25
Bowel	10
Ataxic gait	20

Adapted from Mercier E, Quere I, Campello C, et al. The 20210A allele of the prothrombin gene is frequent in young women with unexplained spinal cord infarction. *Blood* 1998;92:1840–1841.

in 29 patients, reflecting the frequent involvement of the conus medullaris. A sensory level is often found, although the frequency varies in different series, ranging from 18% (49) to 55% (51). Radicular sensory loss or the Brown-Sequard syndrome occurs occasionally. Note that none of these signs or symptoms is at all specific for the diagnosis of a spinal AVM. The only pathognomonic finding is a bruit over the spine, and this is not common. It was found in two of eight cases in the Mayo series in which it was listened for (48,52). A cutaneous angioma may overlie the AVM, and this may be more common than a spinal bruit (53).

Definitive diagnosis of spinal AVMs requires radiographic demonstration of the vascular anomaly. Angiography provides the most detailed information on the vascular anatomy but

TABLE 33.2

FOIX-ALAJOUANINE SYNDROME NEUROLOGICAL SIGNS

Sign	%
Abnormal gait	76
Weakness	75
Reflex abnormality	
Hyperreflexia	56
Hyporeflexia	14
Both	10
Sensory	
Radicular	13
Nonradicular	54
Spinal level	55
Sphincter	
Bladder	52
Bowel	24
Babinski sign	31

Adapted from Mercier E, Quere I, Campello C, et al. The 20210A allele of the prothrombin gene is frequent in young women with unexplained spinal cord infarction. *Blood* 1998;92:1840–1841.

is technically challenging. Myelography usually demonstrates serpiginous filling defects dorsal to the cord, but small lesions can be missed. It is often necessary to turn the patient onto his back in order to demonstrate the abnormality. Magnetic resonance imaging (MRI) has now nearly replaced myelography in the initial diagnosis of spinal AVMs (54), but there are no good studies on the sensitivity of this technique. Gilbertson et al. (55) published the most thorough comparison of the radiographic techniques for spinal AVF diagnosis in 1995, but even this paper comes from the relatively early period of spinal MR imaging.

The pathophysiology of the Foix-Alajouanine syndrome is now felt to be related to increased venous pressure from the AVM, rather than to a primary thrombotic process. (56,57). Even intracranial fistulas may occasionally produce the syndrome by such a mechanism (58). Consequently, the neurological deficits are potentially reversible with elimination of the fistula. As early as 1979, Logue (45) reported motor improvement from surgical extirpation of dural AVMs in 15 of 24 patients whom he treated at Queen Square. Five of seven patients who required a wheelchair for mobility regained some ability to walk. Surgery was relatively ineffective in reversing sphincter disturbance. Only 5 of 23 patients with abnormal bladder function improved and only two regained normal bladder function. Eleven of twenty-two patients had modest improvement in sensation. Eight of twelve patients with pain were pain free postoperatively. Sexual function was unaffected by surgery. Similar or better results were reported by Symon et al. (50). Interestingly, all three patients with intracranial fistulas reported by Wrobel et al. (58) had some improvement with surgery. Longer-term results are not as impressive, as late deterioration often occurs (59). In addition to surgical obliteration of the fistula, endovascular embolization with polyvinyl alcohol beads or with cyanoacrylate ("super glue") is also effective (60–62), although recanalization may occur (63,64). In balancing efficacy and risk, Anson and Spetzler (46) believed that surgery was the preferred treatment in most cases. However, with improvements in technique, endovascular procedures have become the initial treatment of choice, although some patients will later require surgery (65). On the other hand, patients initially treated with surgery rarely need later intervention. Treatment was most successful in relieving motor deficits and gait disturbance. Bowel and bladder dysfunction was equally likely to improve or to worsen after treatment. Leg pain and muscle spasms became worse in a majority of patients. Unfortunately, many studies do not stratify the outcomes by treatment modality or have only short follow-up times (66,67). Thus, despite the growing popularity of the less invasive endovascular treatments, it is unclear that this is the optimal approach to the treatment of these lesions.

NUTRITIONAL MYELOPATHIES

Subacute Combined Degeneration

The association between progressive myelopathy and pernicious anemia has been recognized since the latter part of the 19th century (68). This condition was named "subacute combined degeneration" by Russell et al. (69) because of the consistent involvement of both posterior columns and corticospinal tracts (CSTs). The condition was identified quite early as resulting from a nutritional deficiency, although the missing factor, vitamin B_{12}, was not isolated until 1948 (70). In 1926, Minot and Murphy devised a treatment based on a diet including at least half a pound of liver per day, for which they won the Nobel Prize (71). One can imagine the unpalatable nature of this treatment.

The selective deficiency of vitamin B_{12} in pernicious anemia is caused not by a dietary deficiency of B_{12}, but by the absence of intrinsic factor, which is necessary for the absorption of minute amounts of the vitamin in the terminal ileum. Castle called this situation "starvation in the midst of plenty" (72). Subacute combined degeneration (SCD) also occurs in other settings leading to defects of B_{12} absorption, such as extensive gastric resection, ileal resection, tapeworm infestation, and other causes of intestinal malabsorption. Dietary deficiency of B_{12} may also lead to subacute combined degeneration. The condition takes a long time to develop, as normal body stores of B_{12} are approximately 5 mg, and daily loss of the vitamin is only 1 to 2.6 mcg a day. Thus, total depletion may take several years to occur (73,74).

The clinical presentation of SCD is quite stereotyped and consistent (73,75). Sensory symptoms, usually numbness or tingling in the legs, are almost always the first complaint. Weakness and unsteadiness of gait occur later. The arms are rarely affected. Sphincter disturbance is uncommon. The earliest neurological sign is loss of vibration and joint position sense in the legs. Alterations of other sensory modalities occur only in more severe and long-standing cases. Reflex changes are variable early on, but reflexes are invariably diminished in more severe cases. Extensor plantar responses are generally seen in severe cases (9/14 in Ref. (73)). Lhermitte sign was seen in 25% of cases seen at the Queen Square Hospital in London (76). Overall, neurological signs and symptoms are more common in patients with dietary vitamin B_{12} deficiency and pernicious anemia than in those with other causes of B_{12} deficiency (75).

Vitamin B_{12} deficiency has other physiological effects in addition to SCD. Megaloblastic anemia is common, but it is important to recognize that neurological involvement may precede the anemia. In the large pathological series from the Massachusetts General Hospital (73), all 41 cases had anemia. However, SCD without anemia has been well described (77,78). Dementia and affective disorders are also common in B_{12} deficiency. They occurred in 46% of cases in the series of Shorvon et al. (75). Optic neuritis can also be present (79).

The diagnosis of SCD rests on the determination of vitamin B_{12} levels in a patient with a consistent history and neurological examination. Borderline low levels may cause some confusion, and demonstration of elevated homocysteine and methylmalonic acid levels is very useful. These are the main substrates of the enzymes for which B_{12} serves as a cofactor and are therefore typically elevated in B_{12} deficiency. A rather complex algorithm for laboratory evaluation is outlined by Green and Kinsella (80). Electrophysiological testing may reveal abnormalities. Sensory nerve conduction velocities may be slowed and somatosensory evoked potentials are almost always abnormal. Tibial P37 responses are delayed (81) and median nerve P14 latencies and P9-P14 and N13-P14 interpeak latencies are prolonged (82). This is consistent with slowed central conduction at the cervical cord level. Central motor conduction times (CMCT) are usually normal. Evoked responses may improve or normalize with treatment in a minority of patients (81).

MRI findings have now been reported in a number of cases of SCD and correlate very well with the clinical picture. Hyperintense lesions on T2-weighted scans are typical and are often confined to the posterior columns (81,83–85). Contrast enhancement has been reported (86). High signal has also been seen in the brain stem (83).

The pathological findings in SCD are very consistent (73). The earliest change is swelling of the myelin sheaths leading to a vacuolated appearance of the white matter tracts of the cord. Each vacuole represents a single axon. Later, macrophages infiltrate and many lipid-laden macrophages are present. In chronic lesions, there is also a dense fibrillary gliosis. The posterior columns are always affected and may be the only site of degeneration. Lateral and anterior funiculi may also be involved. These findings correlate very well with the clinical presentation of a primarily posterior column type of sensory loss with sensory ataxia. The lower cervical segments are the most severely affected levels in about half of the cases and thoracic segments are comparably affected in most of the rest. Abnormalities of the dorsal root ganglia and peripheral nerves are not prominent. The pathological changes in experimental animals subjected to a B_{12} deficient diet are identical (74). It took 3 to 4 years to produce the syndrome in monkeys, quite similar to the situation in human cases.

It is generally felt that the biochemical basis of SCD is a defect in the synthesis of methionine from homocysteine. However, the enzyme methionine synthase also requires folate as a cofactor, and folate much less often produces neurological impairment. Shorvon et al. (75) identified neurological and psychological abnormalities in 65% of their patients with isolated folate deficiency (compared to 68% of those with B_{12} deficiency), but these were almost exclusively affective disorders and dementia. They identified no cases of SCD due to folate deficiency. However, a number of case reports of SCD induced by folate deficiency have appeared in the literature (87–90). Folate supplementation may reverse the neurological abnormalities, although it is generally not considered advisable to supplement folate without also supplementing B_{12} in this clinical situation (90).

An interesting iatrogenic cause of SCD is nitrous oxide anesthesia. The first cases actually resulted from nitrous oxide abuse by health care workers, particularly dentists (91–93). Schilling himself (of Schilling test fame) reported the first case of SCD induced by nitrous oxide anesthesia in a patient with unrecognized B_{12} deficiency (94). Other cases have followed (84,95–98).

Treatment of SCD rests on the repletion of the body stores of vitamin B_{12} (80). This is most rapidly accomplished with intramuscular injection of 100 to 1,000 μg of B_{12} a day for 5 days, followed by 100 to 1,000 μg injected intramuscularly monthly thereafter. Oral therapy is also effective, even for patients with pernicious anemia, as approximately 1% of dietary B_{12} is absorbed by passive diffusion independent of intrinsic factor. Therefore, an oral dose of 1,000 μg of B_{12} a day will provide 10 μg of absorbed B_{12}, an amount greater than daily requirements.

Vitamin E Deficiency

Spinocerebellar degeneration due to vitamin E deficiency is often initially mistaken for subacute combined degeneration. Vitamin E is a fat-soluble vitamin that may be deficient in patients with chronic malabsorption syndromes or liver disease with cholestasis. Its absorption depends on the presence of bile salts, which are reabsorbed in the terminal ileum. Harding et al. (99) published the classic description of patients with spinocerebellar degeneration due to malabsorption. Additional cases have since been reported (100–104). Patients generally present with sensory ataxia due to loss of joint position sense from posterior column involvement. They also typically have absent tendon stretch reflexes and leg weakness. True cerebellar ataxia is present, presumably due to involvement of the spinocerebellar tracts. Dysarthria has also been reported, and one patient had ophthalmoplegia, implicating brain stem structures as well. Supplementation with vitamin E may lead to substantial improvement in symptoms.

Although pathological studies are not available in humans, monkeys with experimental vitamin E deficiency show loss of axons and myelin in the dorsal columns (105). There is also marked loss of large myelinated fibers in the sural nerve. This correlates well with the main clinical feature of sensory ataxia in humans. MRI of a human case (104) showed T2-hyperintense lesions in the posterior columns, again correlating well with the clinical picture.

A similar condition has been reported in children with chronic liver failure (106) or cystic fibrosis (107) and in experimental animals (105,108,109). The inherited condition abetalipoproteinemia or Bassen-Kornzweig disease is characterized by vitamin E deficiency with acanthocytosis and spinocerebellar ataxia (110). Cases of neuroacanthocytosis without beta-lipoprotein deficiency typically present with chorea and self-mutilation rather than spinocerebellar ataxia (111,112).

Copper Deficiency

A clinical entity that has been recently identified is myeloneuropathy resembling SCD due to copper deficiency. It has been long known that copper deficiency in domestic farm animals produces a myelopathic neurological syndrome known a swayback, but until 2001 analogous cases had never been seen in humans. In that year, Schleper and Stuerenburg (113) reported a case of subacute myelopathy in a woman with a history of gastric resection. She had an 18-month history of progressive paresthesias, spastic paresis, and sensory ataxia. There was also a microcytic anemia. MRI showed T2-hyperintense lesions in the posterior columns of the cervical spinal cord. The serum copper level was 4.9 μg/L (normal 6 to 35). Treatment with parenteral copper relieved her paresthesias but did not improve her neurological function.

Since then, numerous cases of myelopathy due to copper deficiency have been reported. Kumar published the largest series of cases in 2006 (114). In 25 patients seen at the Mayo Clinic, the clinical presentation was of gait difficulty and paresthesias of the legs. All patients had severe sensory ataxia and some also had mild spasticity, brisk reflexes, and Babinski signs. Nine had spastic bladder. Symptoms and signs were present in the arms in all but two patients. Copper levels ranged from undetectable to 4.5 μg/L. Anemia or leucopenia (a known consequence of copper deficiency) was seen in all but five patients. MRI showed T2-hyperintense lesions in the cervical or thoracic cord or both in 11 patients. The posterior columns were almost always involved. None of the lesions enhanced with gadolinium. Fifteen patients also had lesions in the brain, the significance of which was unclear. Axonal neuropathy (generally of mixed sensorimotor type) was seen in 21 of the 24 patients who had electrophysiological testing. The most common cause of copper deficiency was gastric resection or bypass surgery. Malabsorption, zinc ingestion, and iron ingestion were implicated in some patients. In eight cases, the cause was not determined.

Treatment by parenteral or oral copper replacement promptly restored normal copper levels in 18 of 20 patients for whom there was adequate follow-up. Hematological abnormalities resolved in all patients. Symptomatic improvement often occurred, but residual neurological deficits persisted in all patients. All but one patient had no further deterioration, however. Copper deficiency myeloneuropathy is probably an underdiagnosed condition and should always be considered in patients with subacute gait disturbances and myelopathic signs.

Toxic Myelopathy

In addition to the myelopathies caused by nutritional deficiency states discussed above, myelopathies can also be produced by the ingestion of toxins in food. These are not accidental contaminations but rather naturally occurring toxins in staple foods. Toxic myelopathies are not often seen in the United States but are not rare in tropical areas where the diet depends nearly exclusively on certain crops. Interested readers are referred to a thorough review of the topic by Spencer (115).

The most well known of these nutritional toxicities is lathyrism (116,117). This term refers to several different syndromes produced by the ingestion of chickling peas of the genus Lathyrus. Effects on bones and blood vessels (osteolathyrism and angiolathyrism) are seen only in experimental animals. The human disease, neurolathyrism, is characterized by the subacute onset of weakness in the legs. Pain and paresthesias may also occur. The affected person develops a spastic gait and often needs canes to walk. Sphincter disturbance and erectile dysfunction are common in some series. Sensory loss is less common. In a review of 35 cases from the Uttar Pradesh state of northern India in 1975 (118), 71% of patients presented with motor symptoms. Thirty-four percent had paresthesias and only 6% had bladder disturbance at onset. The disease developed over less than a week in three cases, 1 to 2 weeks in 13, and 1 to 6 months in 19. The condition is generally permanent. Pathological studies reveal degeneration of the white matter of the spinal cord, predominantly the CSTs.

Use of these peas as one third to one half of the diet for 2 months or more is sufficient to produce the syndrome. This generally occurs in conditions of severe disruption of the food supply, as in times of war, flood or famine. As recently as the 1980s, it was still endemic in parts of India, Bangladesh, and Ethiopia. This condition was recognized by Hippocrates in 46 BC, who wrote "At Ainos, all men and women who ate peas continuously became impotent in the legs and that state persisted."

Several different compounds present in various Lathyrus species have been proposed as causes of lathyrism. These include beta-cyano-L-alanine (119), beta-diaminobutyric acid (120), and *N*-oxalylamino-L-alanine (BOAA) (121). This last is generally postulated as the actual compound at fault. Feeding BOAA to macaque monkeys does produce a clinically similar upper motor neuron disease, but no pathological studies have been reported (122). It may exert its effect by neuroexcitatory mechanisms.

A similar condition known as "konzo" occurs in Africa in populations where the staple food is manioc or cassava root. This is a plant that contains a number of cyanogens, compounds that release cyanide under acidic conditions. It has been known for centuries by those who use this crop that the roots must be soaked and prepared carefully to extract these compounds before eating. However, during droughts or civil unrest, the people often resort to varieties with higher concentrations of cyanogens and may not prepare the roots as carefully. This has led to outbreaks of konzo in Tanzania (123), Congo (124), and elsewhere in Africa. Victims have elevated levels of thiocyanate, the main metabolite of cyanide, in blood and urine. In one district of Zaire in 1991, Tylleskar et al. (125) found 110 cases in a population of 6,764. In 90% of cases, the disease was full blown in less than 1 day and never progressed over more than 3 days. The gait was always affected, with 25% needing canes and 11% unable to walk. Ninety-seven percent had hyperreflexia, 85% clonus, and 17% Babinski signs. Visual disturbance was also reported by 12% at the onset of the disease. A follow-up of a cohort of patients after 14 years showed no change in their neurological condition (126). All patients in whom testing had been done had negative titers of HTLV-I antibodies (127).

Interestingly, cassava eaters in West African countries such as Nigeria develop a quite different neurological syndrome termed "tropical ataxic neuropathy" (128). This is characterized by sensory ataxia often associated with visual loss and sensorineural deafness. The most common symptoms are numbness and paresthesias (81%), visual loss (71%), ataxic gait (56%), weakness (35%), and hearing disturbance (34%). Neurological signs include posterior column sensory loss (81%), leg and gait ataxia (67%), a positive Romberg test (60%), optic atrophy (55%), and deafness (32%). Upper motor neuron signs are much less common (13%). It is not known why the ingestion of the same food causes two such different syndromes in different parts of Africa.

A very similar condition of ataxia and deafness was also reported by Montgomery et al. in Jamaica (129). Spinal fluid was normal in all 25 cases and poor nutrition was reported in 19 of 21 cases in which this information was available. In contrast, a spastic paraparesis was seen in 181 patients. These latter patients rarely had deafness. Spinal fluid was often abnormal, with up to 49 white cells, and protein was elevated in 35%. There was no apparent association with nutritional status. Autopsies were available only on spastic cases and showed demyelination and perivascular lymphocytic infiltrates. It is my opinion that most of these latter were cases of tropical spastic paraparesis/HTLV-I associated myelopathy (TSP/HAM), a condition that was not recognized in 1964.

MYELOPATHY IN COLLAGEN VASCULAR DISEASE

Systemic Lupus Erythematosus

Neurological abnormalities are common in systemic lupus erythematosus (SLE). The very first description of the disease by Kaposi in 1872 included two patients with delirium (130). The classic review of the subject by Johnson and Richardson (131) reported 24 autopsied cases from the Massachusetts General Hospital. Thirteen patients had seizures, ten cranial nerve disorders, three hemiparesis, two peripheral neuropathy, and eight mental disorders. One patient had paraparesis from spinal cord involvement. They also reviewed 14 other cases of spinal cord disease from the literature.

A more recent review (132) identified 34 cases of myelopathy in the literature and described two more. Patients generally presented with paraparesis (67%) and numbness of the legs (53%). Bladder dysfunction was present in 31% and back pain in 31%. The ultimate degree of deficit was generally severe. Fifty-eight percent became paraplegic, and sphincter function was lost in 91%. Loss of reflexes was as common as hyperreflexia. The sensory level was most often thoracic (69%). Outcome was poor overall. On follow-up, 37% of patients had died and 40% had little or no improvement. Only 20% returned to normal.

Although myelopathy is one of the less common neurological manifestations of SLE, it is not truly rare. In one study from a single center (133), 3% of their patients had spinal cord disease. In 5 of 10, it was the first manifestation of lupus. Other authors have also reported acute myelopathy as the presenting manifestation of lupus (134,135). A prospective study of 500 patients with SLE produced four who already had myelopathy and 12 more who developed it during the follow-up period (136). Interestingly, 15 of these 16 had anticardiolipin antibodies. The remaining patient had a false-positive VDRL and an elevated activated partial thromboplastin time (aPTT). This obviously suggests a possible mechanism for this rather mysterious condition. In Al-Husaini and Jamal's review, 11 of 17 patients for whom information was available had a false-positive serological test for syphilis (132). On the other hand, Mok et al. (133) and Sanna et al. (137) found no association with antiphospholipid antibodies.

Cerebrospinal fluid (CSF) is usually abnormal in lupus-associated myelopathy (138). In 20 patients who had lumbar punctures, 16 had elevated protein, generally greater than 100 mg/dL. Glucose was reduced in four cases. In contrast, of 21 lupus patients with neurological disease other than myelopathy, only one had a low glucose. A leukocytic pleocytosis was seen in 15 of 20 patients, ranging from 7 to 16,100 cells. A significant number of red cells was seen in five. Even higher proportions of CSF abnormalities were reported in Al-Husaini and Jamal's review, primarily in cases reported after 1973 (132).

Pathological studies are rare and show a variety of changes. Vascular changes were reported in 11 of 12 cases and eight of these had myelomalacia, necrosis, or infarction, suggesting a vascular etiology of the myelopathy. In contrast, Johnson and Richardson (131) in their case reported a vacuolar degeneration of all the white matter tracts with lipid-laden macrophages. Provenzale and Bouldin (139) reported similar findings, which they dubbed "subpial leukomyelopathy," in seven cases. Only three cases had cord infarcts.

The most appropriate treatment of lupus-associated myelopathy is unknown. Corticosteroids have been used most often and may be beneficial. Propper and Bucknall (140) reported that of 26 cases, seven patients had a partial or full recovery. This included five of eight patients on "high-dose steroids" and two of eighteen on "low-dose" treatment. Berlanga et al. (141) treated one patient with monthly intravenous cyclophosphamide (CPP) with recovery, after a relapse occurred on tapering the patient's steroids. Slovick (142) employed plasma exchange and reported improvement beginning within 1 day of instituting treatment. Mok et al. treated three patients with mycophenolate mofetil. One had a complete response sustained for a year. The other two had partial response but both relapsed after 5 to 8 months (143).

Sjögren Syndrome

The other collagen vascular disease, which has been most frequently associated with myelopathy is SS. Central nervous system (CNS) disease occurs in up to 20% of all patients with SS (144,145). Disease is usually multifocal and the spinal cord is often involved. The course of this disease is usually relapsing and remittent. Alexander et al. reported 20 patients with CNS manifestations of SS (146), of whom 17 had myelopathy. Thirteen had paraparesis, most often acute or subacute in onset. Ten patients had neurogenic bladder, two of whom had no other evidence of spinal cord disease. Two had the Brown-Sequard syndrome. All the patients had evidence of brain disease. Pathology in one case revealed an angiitis of arterioles and venules and necrosis of the cord (147).

The multifocal, relapsing-remitting nature of the manifestations in SS raises the diagnostic possibility of multiple sclerosis in patients not already diagnosed with SS. MRI has been reported in one case of myelopathy, showing increased signal on T2-weighted images and enhancement with gadolinium (148). Spinal fluid analysis also resembles the picture of multiple sclerosis. Oligoclonal bands were seen in 89% of patients with SS (146) and an increased IgG index is also common. There is often a mild lymphocytic pleocytosis. Alpha-fodrin antibodies are more common in SS than in MS, although false positives and false negatives both occur (149). Of course, the presence of the sicca complex (dry eyes and dry mouth) can generally distinguish SS from MS, and two thirds of SS patients have serological evidence of the disease.

Steroids have generally been employed in the treatment of CNS SS. This appears to be beneficial, but the occurrence of spontaneous remissions makes this conclusion uncertain. Plasma exchange (150), chlorambucil (151), and cyclophosphamide (149) have also been used.

A further complicating issue in the diagnosis of Sjögren's associated myelopathy is that many patients with HTLV-I infection also have the sicca syndrome. In two Japanese studies (HTLV-I is endemic in certain parts of Japan), 12 of 31 (152) and 6 of 10 patients (153) with HAM had SS by standard criteria. One such patient was treated with a combination of steroids, lamivudine and tenofovir, followed by mycophenolate mofetil, with excellent results (154).

Sarcoidosis

Spinal sarcoidosis is a rare manifestation of a rare form of sarcoidosis. Neurological involvement in sarcoidosis occurs in about 5% of cases (155). Spinal involvement is present less than 1% of cases, and only a few dozen examples have been reported in the literature (156). The presentation is not distinctive, consisting of progressive paraparesis or quadriparesis. Most lesions occur in the cervical region. The vast majority of cases have MR imaging results indicating an intramedullary mass lesion, which is often mistaken for a tumor. Intradural, extramedullary lesions are exceedingly rare (157). Diagnosis is often through biopsy of the lesion. Frozen sections are often misleading and the diagnosis may not be made until review of the permanent specimens. Although recovery after surgical removal of extramedullary granulomas can occur, deterioration accompanies extensive resection of intramedullary lesions in half of all cases. Steroid treatment leads to improvement in about 75% of patients (158).

HEPATIC MYELOPATHY

Liver failure is a well-recognized cause of CNS dysfunction. In the presence of spontaneous or surgically produced portosystemic shunts, a reversible syndrome of cognitive dysfunction known as hepatic encephalopathy is common. This syndrome is weakly correlated with hyperammonemia, although it is likely that ammonia is not the actual toxic substance. Protein restriction and treatment with lactulose and nonabsorbable antibiotics such as neomycin generally improve or reverse the encephalopathy. There is also an irreversible hepatocerebral degeneration manifesting as an extrapyramidal syndrome similar to Wilson disease.

Much less well recognized is a generally irreversible myelopathy, which has been named "hepatic myelopathy" or "portal-systemic myelopathy." This syndrome, first described by Zieve et al. in 1960 (159,160), is characterized by progressive spastic weakness of the legs. Sensory loss and sphincter disturbance are rare. As of 1999, 50 cases have been reported in the English language literature (161). The great majority of patients had undergone surgical portosystemic shunting, although a few cases have also occurred in patients with spontaneous shunts (162,163). The author has seen one case in a patient with no evidence of portosystemic shunting. The mean interval from shunting to onset of paraparesis is 28.7 months with a range of 4 of 120 months (161). The great majority (80%) has also had episodes of hepatic encephalopathy, often recurrently. The degree of neurological impairment and its rate of development are variable. Many patients are fairly severely affected and most require assistance are ambulation.

The diagnosis of hepatic myelopathy is clinical, based on the recognition of myelopathy in the appropriate setting. Other identifiable causes of myelopathy must be excluded. Likely causes in this patient population include vitamin B_{12} or folate deficiency, neurosyphilis, HIV and HTLV-I infection, and compressive lesions of the spinal cord. Only a few reports of MRI have been published (161,163–165). None showed any abnormality. Nardone et al. recently reported abnormal CMCT by transcranial magnetic stimulation in 6 patients. In two, CNCTs improved after liver transplantation (166).

Pathological information is available in only 15 cases of hepatic myelopathy (see references in (161)). This uniformly showed demyelination of the lateral CSTs and occasionally the ventral CSTs and posterior columns. There was variable axonal loss. The lesions are found throughout the length of the spinal cord, becoming more prominent at lower levels.

The pathogenesis of hepatic myelopathy is not well understood. There appear to be no experimental models of the condition. Since portosystemic shunting is almost always present, it is likely to be crucial in the development of myelopathy. It is generally assumed that some toxic substance plays a role (160,164,165,167–170), although the exact nature of this substance is unclear. Hemodynamic factors (171,172) or nutritional deficiencies are also possibilities.

Treatment of hepatic myelopathy has generally been unrewarding. The usual interventions for hepatic encephalopathy, including protein restriction, lactulose, and neomycin, usually have no effect on the neurological deficit. A small number of cases have improved (173–176). Five cases of liver transplantation in patients with hepatic myelopathy have been reported. In four cases, the myelopathy improved over a period of several months (177,178) and in the other there was no change (179).

PARANEOPLASTIC NECROTIZING MYELOPATHY

When myelopathy occurs in the setting of a systemic malignancy, the cause is almost always extrinsic compression of the spinal cord by metastases to the spine. Rarely, neurological syndromes may occur in the absence of direct metastatic involvement of the nervous system and without metabolic derangements. These are known as paraneoplastic syndromes, or in the older literature "remote effects of cancer" (180). The mechanism of these syndromes is generally immunological, with antibodies to tumor cell surface proteins that cross-react with components of normal neural elements. The most common of these are paraneoplastic cerebellar degeneration due to anti-Purkinje cell antibodies or antineuronal nuclear antibodies, and paraneoplastic limbic encephalitis or encephalomyelitis, also due to antineuronal nuclear antibodies. These occur most often in cases of small cell cancer of the lung, ovarian cancer, and lymphomas, but have been reported in numerous other malignancies.

A much rarer paraneoplastic syndrome is necrotizing myelopathy. A review by Ojeda in 1984 identified 22 cases in the literature and reported two additional cases (181). Since then, a handful of further cases have been reported (182–190). This is a fulminant condition characterized by rapidly progressive flaccid paralysis. The patients may be paraplegic or tetraplegic, depending on the site of cord involvement. Reflexes are lost and sensation is diminished to all modalities. Eventually, respiratory function may be compromised and the patient dies either of respiratory failure or of medical complications. The longest reported survival from onset of paralysis is 150 days, but the median is 30 days, with a range of 5 to 150 days. The syndrome has been associated with a variety of tumors, the most common being lymphoma (nine cases), lung cancer (six cases), and breast cancer (four cases). CSF studies have shown increases in protein, which can be dramatic (up to 2.7 g/dL), generally normal glucose, and small numbers of lymphocytes (2 to 27) or neutrophils (2 to 48) and erythrocytes (0 to 800). One case had an increase in CSF IgG and T-helper cells (186). One case of recurrent myelitis at the time of recurrence of breast cancer was associated with the aquaporin-4 antibody seen in neuromyelitis optica (187). Treatment has generally been of no benefit, but one case improved with steroids (183). MRI has been reported in only a few cases and shows T2 hyperintensity with swelling of the cord (188).

Pathological examination reveals massive hemorrhagic necrosis of the gray and white matter of the spinal cord. There is no predilection for particular tracts or structures. Spinal blood vessels are generally normal, although fibrin thrombi have been reported in venules and arterioles. The longitudinal extent of involvement is variable, ranging from a few segments to the whole cord. Most often, cervical and thoracic levels are involved.

HEREDITARY SPASTIC PARAPARESIS

HSP is a diverse group of inherited disorders characterized by progressive spastic paresis of the legs. The condition was reviewed by McDermott et al. (191) in 2000. It was first described by Strümpell in 1880 and has acquired the eponym Strümpell-Lorrain syndrome (192). Over the next 100 years, various authors have reported a number of cases that formed a rather heterogeneous group, with variable age of onset, rapidity of progression, and involvement of other neural systems. Harding (193) was the first investigator to impose some order on this rather messy condition in 1981.

Harding divided HSP into "pure" cases with no other significant neurological findings and "complicated" ones, which had a variety of other neurological deficits such as amyotrophy, seizures, sensory neuropathy, and dementia. Within the pure group, there also appeared to be a natural division between those with onset before the age of 35 years and slow progression (type I) and those with later onset and more rapid worsening (type II). However, there was still significant overlap between groups and the borders are rather fuzzy. As with the spinocerebellar ataxias, recent information on the genetics of these conditions has shown that there is a good deal of clinical heterogeneity within genetically district groups, as is discussed below (192).

HSP is quite rare, with estimates of 2.0 to 9.6 per 100,000 in various European countries. Patients usually present with difficulty walking. There is often delay in walking in cases with childhood onset. Spasticity and bladder dysfunction are also common. Patients may be asymptomatic and abnormalities are only revealed on examination. The main physical findings are spasticity and hyperreflexia of the legs and less frequently the arms. Weakness is generally much less prominent. Less frequently there may be sensory abnormalities, usually of vibration sense. Of note, cranial nerve involvement does not occur in pure cases, although complicated cases may have retinal degeneration, optic atrophy, sensorineural hearing loss, or dysarthria.

A review by Durr et al. (194) of 23 index cases of pure autosomal dominant HSP and 119 other family members revealed 70 cases. Of these, 12 were unaware of their deficits. Insidious onset of stiffness of the legs was the most frequent initial symptom (52/70). Hyperreflexia was present in the legs in all patients and in the arms in 32%. Spasticity in the legs was mild in 14, moderate in 24, and severe in 16. There was proximal muscle weakness in the legs in 66%. Vibration sense was decreased in 65%. Sphincter dysfunction was present in 49%. The mean age at onset was 29 years and the distribution was unimodal. There was a good deal of variation within families.

Results of diagnostic testing are not specific but can be used to exclude alternative diagnosis such as cervical spondylosis or primary progressive multiple sclerosis. There may be cervical cord atrophy on MRI, as seen in 5/12 of Durr's cases. Mild brain atrophy occurs occasionally as well (194).

CSF is generally normal (191). Electrophysiological testing has revealed involvement of systems other than motor pathways, even in "pure" cases. Durr found evidence of axonal neuropathy in three members of one family. Visual evoked potentials were abnormal in 2/14, brainstem potentials in 4/14, and somatosensory responses in 9/14.

There are very few pathological reports of HSP. Most were published by Schwarz and Liu (195,196). In pure cases, the primary feature is axonal degeneration in CST and dorsal columns. The changes are most prominent in the thoracolumbar CST and cervical dorsal columns, particularly in the fasciculus gracilis. Spinocerebellar pathways are affected in about 50% of cases.

The genetics of HSP is very diverse. Cases can be autosomal dominant, autosomal recessive, or X-linked. As of 2004, 22 distinct chromosomal loci had been identified for HSP. Many are heterogeneous both clinically and in terms of the specific mutations involved. Eight of the genes have been cloned. Spastin (SPG4), the most common of the mutated genes, is a housekeeping ATPase involved in many cellular functions (197). Two X-linked forms have well-characterized mutations. One form affects proteolipid protein and is thus allelic to Pelizaeus-Merzbacher disease (198,199). It causes a complicated form of HSP with cerebellar ataxia and mental retardation. The other X-linked form affects L1CAM, a cell adhesion molecule (200). Other mutations in this gene produce X-linked hydrocephalus, X-linked agenesis of the corpus callosum and MASA syndrome (mental retardation, aphasia, shuffling gait, and adducted thumbs). Clearly, much more remains to be learned about these conditions. Further work on HSP will no doubt help shed light on the genetic and cellular basis of various neurodegenerative syndromes. Currently, there is no treatment of the disease process, although specific treatments to diminish spasticity and improve function (rehabilitation) can be prescribed.

RADIATION MYELOPATHY

Therapeutic radiation of the CNS is a common treatment modality in oncology. The brain or spinal cord may be irradiated as a treatment of primary or metastatic tumor. The nervous system, especially the spinal cord, may also be an innocent bystander exposed during radiation of nearby malignancies. Although the CNS is generally felt to be relatively resistant to the deleterious effects of radiation because of the low rate of turnover of cells, it is of course not completely immune to injury. Particularly at higher doses, damage to the spinal cord may result from therapeutic radiation.

Two major clinical syndromes occur as a result of irradiation of the spinal cord. Early radiation myelopathy occurs 6 weeks to 6 months after radiation, with a mean of 10 to 16 weeks. The symptoms include numbness and paresthesias of the limbs and the electric shock-like symptom known as Lhermitte sign. The symptoms may be intermittent. They typically resolved within a few months. The pathology is generally felt to be demyelination of the white matter tracts, particularly the posterior columns. An analogous phenomenon occurs after brain irradiation. Somatosensory evoked potentials showed prolongation of the N20 latency 3 months after irradiation of the neck for nasopharyngeal carcinoma. Latencies returned to normal at 9 months (201). In experimental animals, a delayed loss of oligodendrocytes can be observed as a result of radiation (202). There is no clear dose-response effect in this syndrome. As this is a benign, spontaneously reversible condition, treatment is not indicated.

The more serious, and fortunately much rarer, condition is delayed radiation myelopathy. This generally presents as the gradual development of weakness and sensory loss below the level of irradiation. Sphincter disturbance may also occur. Hyperreflexia and extensor plantar responses are generally present. The condition may progress to a picture of complete cord transection. The onset of the delayed syndrome ranges from 6 months to 4 years from the time of radiation, with an average of 12 to 23 months, depending on the population reported on (203). Rarely, there may be acute onset of symptoms. Survival from onset of symptoms has varied widely in different studies, ranging from an average of 6.4 months to a minimum of 24 months (204).

Schultheiss et al. (204) have proposed three clinical criteria for the diagnosis of radiation myelopathy. First, no other etiology, such as direct involvement by tumor, must be present. Second, the signs and symptoms should be consistent with the picture outlined above. Finally, the dose and latency should be consistent with a radiation effect. Onset before 6 months is rare and should raise the question of other etiologies. The dosage effects on spinal cord are not fully determined, but the condition is rare with total radiation doses of less than 5,000 cGy. Conventional fractionation with fractions of about 200 cGy yields an estimated incidence of about 0.2% at a total dose of 4,500 cGy. The level at which 5% of patients would develop myelopathy may be between 5,700 and 6,100 cGy. The 50% incidence level is probably between 6,800 and 7,300 cGy. Hyperfractionation, with multiple daily fractions of 40 to 50 cGy, appears to be more dangerous, as cellular repair mechanisms may not be effective with such short intertreatment intervals. Recently, a case of radiation myelopathy due to radioactive ^{131}I treatment for thyroid carcinoma metastatic to the spine was reported (205).

Given these dosage constraints, clinicians are understandably reluctant to reirradiate the spinal cord. This is not of purely theoretical importance, as cord compression due to epidural metastases is frequently a recurrent problem. A review from the Mayo Clinic reports on 54 such patients who were reirradiated (206). Total dosages received over both courses of radiation ranged from 3,650 to 8,089 cGy with a median of 5,425 cGy. Forty patients were ambulatory at the start of reirradiation and 42 were walking at the end. There was later deterioration in five patients after 6.5 to 22.5 months. Only one of these patients underwent diagnostic imagining at that time, and he had new epidural metastasis. It is not known if the other four patients had recurrent metastatic disease or radiation myelopathy. However, these results certainly suggest that reirradiation can generally be done safely if the clinical situation so warrants. More recent reports are in accord with these findings (207–209).

Pathological studies have demonstrated two main classes of lesions in radiation myelopathy. The most extensive review was presented by Schultheiss et al. (210). In 50 cases, they identified 19 with purely white matter lesions, 9 with purely vascular lesions, and 22 with a mixture of both. The white matter lesions were characterized by demyelination, with fat-laden macrophages and sometimes with focal necrosis or axon loss. Vascular lesions included hemorrhage, thrombosis, fibrinoid necrosis, and infarction. A mononuclear cell inflammatory response occurred in approximately half the cases and was seen equally in white matter and vascular cases. Cases with white matter lesions had a shorter latency to onset than the vascular cases: 13.6 months in pure white matter cases, 10.7 months in mixed, and 29.2 months in pure vascular lesions. These data indicate dual mechanisms in the pathogenesis of radiation myelopathy, with both direct injury to oligodendroglia and damage to blood vessels.

The treatment of radiation myelopathy is unsatisfactory. Steroids may offer some transient benefit by decreasing cord edema (211). Prolonged improvement is rare (212,213). Based on the presumed vascular nature of the process, a few investigators have tried anticoagulation, with a few case reports of benefit (214,215). Interestingly, this approach has also shown some promise in treating radiation necrosis of the brain (214). A French group reported stabilization or improvement of six of nine patients treated with hyperbaric oxygen (216).

DECOMPRESSION MYELOPATHY

With increasing numbers of people participating in sport scuba diving, DCS is a condition that more physicians are likely to see. It has been known for nearly 150 years that rapid return to the surface after underwater activity can lead to serious health effects, often referred to as "the bends." At depth, nitrogen dissolves in the bloodstream and bubbles out of solution as the ambient pressure decreases on surfacing. This condition was first described in 1854 in workers excavating the piers of bridges (217–219). Indeed, Washington Roebling, engineer and builder of the Brooklyn Bridge, was himself disabled and ultimately died of what was then called "caisson disease," after the pressurized underwater chambers, or caissons, in which the workers did their jobs.

Neurological decompression injury is classified as type II DCS. The most common manifestation is myelopathy. A review of 117 cases of neurologic injury reported to the National Diving Accident Network in 1981 and 1982 revealed 70 cases of type II DCS (220). The most common presenting symptoms were progressive paresthesias (24 cases) and numbness of the limbs (39), followed by weakness (16), nausea (12), dizziness and vertigo (9), headache (6), and ataxia (4). Both arms and legs can be affected. Symptoms generally began more than half an hour after surfacing, and in 28% at least 6 hours after the dive.

The mechanism of decompression myelopathy has not been fully elucidated. The most widely accepted mechanism is venous congestion (221). Arterial occlusion by air embolus does not seem to be present. Pathological studies on experimental animals have revealed white matter hemorrhages (222) and bubbles in the parenchyma of the cord (223). A case-control study by Wilmshurst and Bryson (224) found that right-to-left shunts were significantly more common in cases of decompression myelopathy that in control divers without injury (52% versus 12%), lending some credence to the role of paradoxical gas embolism. One human case of recovered DCS that came to autopsy showed degeneration of the fasciculus gracilis from C1 to T4 and of the lateral CSTs from C1 to L4 (223). MR imaging in 10 cases showed white matter lesions consistent with the clinical picture (225).

The primary treatment of DCS is recompression therapy, and it is generally successful in mild to moderate cases. The US Navy has developed standard protocols for treatment. Hyperbaric oxygen or a 50/50 mixture of helium and oxygen is also effective (226). In the study by Dick and Massey (220), patients with mild symptoms recovered whether they were treated or not. Treatment of cases of intermediate severity was effective, but 4 of 16 such patients had neurological residua for up to 1 month. Severe cases rarely respond to therapy. Although symptoms may slowly improve, they generally persist for at least 6 months. Residual symptoms included weakness, sensory loss, irritability, and emotional lability (220). In an Israeli review of 68 cases, 78% of patients recovered fully. However, 22% had persistent neurological signs and symptoms (226). Even strict adherence to the standard decompression schedules devised by the US Navy does not preclude the development of DCS. In the Israeli study, 41% of the dives were well within the dive table standards.

This chapter has highlighted the multifarious mechanisms of nontraumatic spinal cord injury. Many of these conditions are quite rare. However, in the appropriate clinical context, or in cases where an obvious cause of spinal cord injury is not evident, investigation for rarer causes of myelopathy may be revealing and can lead to effective treatment.

References

1. Adamkiewicz A. Die blutgefasse des menschlichen ruckenmarkes. II. Die gefasse der ruckenmarksoberflache. *SitzungsberichtederMathematisch-Naturwissenschaftlichen Classe der Kaiserlichen Akademie der Wissenschaften Wien* 1882;85:101–130.
2. Turnbull IA. Blood supply of the spinal cord. In: Vinken PJ, Bruyn GW. *Handbook of clinical neurology*. Vol. 12 ed. Amsterdam, The Netherlands: North Holland, 1972:478–491.
3. Weidauer S, Nichtweiss M, Lanfermann H, et al. Spinal cord infarction: MR imaging and clinical features in 16 cases. *Neuroradiology* 2002;44:851–857.
4. Garcin R, Godlewski S, Rondot P. Etude clinique des medullopathies d'origine vasculaire. *Revue Neurologique* 1962;106:558–591.
5. Lapresle J, Decroit JP. Pathologie vasculaire de la moelle (a' l'exception de la pathologie malformative). *Encycl Med Chir Neurologie* 1984;17067, A10, 4.
6. Gilles FH, Nag D. Vulnerability of human spinal cord in transient cardiac arrest. *Neurology* 1971;21:833–839.
7. Gutowski NJ, Murphy RP, Beale DJ. Unilateral upper cervical posterior spinal artery syndrome following sneezing. *J Neurol Neurosurg Psychiatry* 1992;55:841–843.
8. Masson C, Pruvo JP, Meder JF, et al. Spinal cord infarction: clinical and magnetic resonance imaging findings and short term outcome. *J Neurol Neurosurg Psychiatry* 2004;75:1431–1435.
9. Salvador de al Barrera S, Barca-Buyo A, Montoto-Marqués A, et al. Spinal cord infarction: prognosis and recovery in a series of 36 patients. *Spinal Cord* 2001;39:520–525
10. Silver JR, Buxton PH. Spinal stroke. *Brain* 1974;97: 539–550.
11. Singh U, Silver JR, Welply NC. Hypotensive infarction of the spinal cord. *Paraplegia* 1994;32:314–322.
12. Kobrine AI, Evans DE, Rizzole HV. Relative vulnerability of the brain and spinal cord to ischemia. *J Neurol Sci* 1980;45:65–72.

13. Ross RT. Spinal cord infarction in disease and surgery of the aorta. *Can J Neurol Sci* 1985;12:289–295.
14. Blalock A, Park EA. Surgical treatment of experimental coarctation (atresia) of aorta. *Ann Surg* 1944;119:445.
15. Debakey ME, Cooley DA, Crawford ES, et al: Aneurysms of the thoracic aorta: analysis of 179 patients treated by resection. *J Thorac Cardiovasc Surg* 1959;36:393.
16. Crawford ES, Fenstermacher JM, Richardson W, et al. Reappraisal of adjuncts to avoid ischemia in the treatment of thoracic aortic aneurysms. *Surgery* 1970;67:182.
17. Brewer LA III, Fosburg RG, Mulder GA, et al. Spinal cord complications following surgery for coarctation of the aorta. A study of 66 cases. *J Thorac Cardiovasc Surg* 1972;64:368–381.
18. Adams HD, Van Geertruyden HH. Neurologic complications of aortic surgery. *Ann Surg* 1956;144:574.
19. Askew AR, Wilmshurst CC. Abdominal aortic aneurysm presenting with splenic rupture and subsequent paraplegia. *Vasc Surg* 1973;7:253.
20. Makaroun MS, Dilavou ED, Kee ST, et al. Endovascular treatment of thoracic aortic aneurysms: results of the phase II multicenter trial of the GORE TAG thoracic endoprosthesis. *J Vasc Surg* 2005;41:1–9.
21. Weinberg L, Harvey WR, Marshall RJ. Post-operative paraplegia following spinal cord infarction. *Acta Anesthesiol Scand* 2002;46:469–472.
22. Fosburg RG, Brewer LA III. Arterial vascular injury to the spinal cord. In: Vinken PJ, Bruyn GW, eds. *Handbook of clinical neurology*. Vol 26. Amsterdam, The Netherlands: North-Holland Publishing Co., 1976:63–79.
23. Strigley JR, Lambert CD, Bilbao JM, et al. Spinal cord infraction secondary to intervertebral disc embolism. *Ann Neurol* 1981;9:296–301.
24. Fergin I, Pyoff N, Adahi M. Fibrocartilaginous venus emboli to the spinal cord with necrotic myelopathy. *J Neuropathol Exp Neurol* 1965;24:63–74.
25. Naina JL, Donohue WL, Pricharch JS. Fatal nucleus pulposus embolism of spinal cord after trauma. *Neurology* 1961;11:83.
26. Jurkovic I, Eiben E. Fatal myelomalacia caused by massive fibrocartilaginous venous emboli from nucleus pulposus. *Acta Neuropatho* 1970;15:284–247.
27. Han JJ, Massagli TL, Jaffe KM. Fibrocartilaginous embolism—an uncommon cause of spinal cord infarction: a case report and review of the literature. *Arch Phys Med Rehabil* 2004;85:153–157.
28. Meyer HJ, Monticelli F, Kiesslich J. Fatal embolism of the anterior spinal artery after local cervical analgesic infiltration. *Forensic Sci Int* 2005;149:115–119.
28. Laguna J, Cravioto H. Spinal cord infarction secondary to occlusion of the anterior spinal artery. *Arch Neurol* 1973;28:134–136.
29. Hughes JT. Venous infarction of the spinal cord. *Neurology* 1971;21:794–800.
30. Clarke CE, Cumming WJ. Subacute myelopathy caused by spinal venous infarction. *Postgrad Med J* 1987;63: 669–671.
31. Rao KR, Donnenfeld M, Chusid JD, et al. Acute myelopathy secondary to spinal venous thrombosis. *J Neurolo Sci* 1982;56:107–113.
32. Crum B, Mokri B, Fulgham, J. Spinal manifestations of vertebral artery dissection. *Neurology* 2000;55:304–306.
33. Williamson RI. Spinal thrombosis and hemorrhage due to syphilitic disease of the vessels. *Lancet* 1894;2:14.
34. Spiller WG. Thrombosis of the cervical anterior median spinal artery: syphilitic acute anterior poliomyelitis. *J Nerv Ment Dis* 1909;36:601.
35. Caplan LR. Case records of the Massachusetts General Hospital: case 5-1991. *N Engl J Med* 1991;324:322–332.
36. Corbin, JL. Anatomie et Pathologie Arterielle de la Moelle. Paris: Masson, 1961.
37. Okuno S, Touho H, Ohnishi H, et al. Cervical infarction associated with vertebral artery occlusion due to spondylotic degeneration: case report. *Acta Neurochir (Wien)* 1998;140:981–985.
38. Ludwig MA, Burns SP. Spinal cord infarction following cervical transforaminal epidural injection: a case report. *Spine* 2005;30:E266–E268
39. Mercier E, Quere I, Campello C, et al. The 20210A allele of the prothrombin gene is frequent in young women with unexplained spinal cord infarction. *Blood* 1998;92: 1840–1841.
40. Foix C, Alajouanine T. La myelite necrotique subaigue. *Rev Neurol* 1926;2:1–42.
41. Lhermitte J, Fribourg-Blanc A, Kyriaco N. La gliose angeiohypertrophique de la moelle epiniere (myelitie necrotique de Foix-Alajouanine). *Rev Neurol* 1931;2:37–53.
42. Pia HW, Vogelsang H. Diagnose und therapie spinaler angiome. *Dtsch Z Nervenheilk* 1965;187:74–96.
43. Wirth FP Jr, Post KD, Di Chiro G, et al. Foix-Alajouanine disease. Spontaneous thrombosis of a spinal cord arteriovenous malformation: a case report. *Neurology* 1970;20:1114–1118.
44. Aminoff MJ, Logue V. The prognosis of patients with spinal vascular malformations. *Brain* 1974;97:211–218.
45. Logue V. Angiomas of the spinal cord: review of the pathogenesis, clinical features, and results of surgery. *J Neurol Neurosurg Psychiatry* 1979;42:1–11.
46. Anson JA, Spetzler RF. Classification of spinal arteriovenous malformations and implications for treatment. *BNI Q* 1992;8:2–8.
47. Rosenblum B, Oldfield EH, Doppman JL, et al. Spinal arteriovenous malformations: a comparison of dural arteriovenous fistulas and intradural AVM's in 81 patients. *J Neurosurg* 1987;67:795–802.
48. Tobin WD, Layton DD Jr. The diagnosis and natural history of spinal cord arteriovenous malformations. *Mayo Clinic Proc* 1976;51:637–646.
49. Jellema K, Canta LR, Tijssen CC, et al. Spinal dural arteriovenous fistulas: clinical features in 80 patients. *J Neurol Neurosurg Psychiatry* 2003;74:1438–1440.
50. Symon L, Kuyama H, Kendall B. Dural arteriovenous malformations of the spine. Clinical features and surgical results in 55 cases. *J Neurosurg* 1984;60:238–247.
51. Aminoff MJ, Logue V. Clinical features of spinal vascular malformations. *Brain* 1974;97:197–210.
52. Matthews WB. The spinal bruit. *Lancet* 1959;2: 1117–1118.
53. Doppman JL, Wirth FP Jr, Di Chiro G, et al. Value of cutaneous angiomas in the arteriographic localization of spinal cord arteriovenous malformations. *N Engl J Med* 1969;281:1440–1444.
54. Minami S, Sagoh T, Nishimura K, et al. Spinal arteriovenous malformation: MR imaging. *Radiology* 1988;169:109–115.

55. Gilbertson JR, Miller GM, Goldman MS, et al. Spinal dural arteriovenous fistulas: MR and myelographic findings. *Am J Neuroradiol* 1995;16:2049–2057.
56. Aminoff MJ, Barnard RO, Logue V. The pathophysiology of spinal vascular malformations. *J Neurological Sci* 1974;23:255–263.
57. McCutcheon IE, Doppman JL, Oldfield EH. Microvascular anatomy of dural arteriovenous abnormalities of the spine: a microangiographic study. *J Neurosurg*1996;84:215–220.
58. Wrobel CJ, Oldfield EH, Di Chiro G, et al. Myelopathy due to intracranial dural arteriovenous fistulas draining intrathecally into spinal medullary veins. Report of three cases. *J Neurosurg* 1988;69:934–939.
59. Tacconi L, Lopez Izquierdo BC, Symon L. Outcome and prognostic factors in the surgical treatment of spinal dural arteriovenous fistulas. A long-term study. *Br J Neurosurg* 1997;11:298–305.
60. Merland JJ, Reizine D. Treatment of arteriovenous spinal cord malformations. *Semin Intervent Radiol* 1987;4: 281–290.
61. Merland JJ, Reizine D. Embolization techniques in the spinal cord. In: Dondelinger RF, Rossi P, Kurdziel JC, et al., eds. *Interventional radiology*. New York, NY: Thieme Medical, 1990:433–442.
62. Mourier KL, Gelbert F, Rey A, et al. Spinal dural arteriovenous malformations with perimedullary drainage, indications and results of surgery in 30 cases. *Acta Neurochir (Wien)* 1989;100:136–141.
63. Morgan MK, Marsh WR. Management of spinal dural arteriovenous malformations. *J Neurosurg* 1989;70:832–836.
64. Hall WA, Oldfield EH, Doppman JL. Recanalization of spinal arteriovenous malformations following embolization. *J Neurosurg* 1989;70:714–720.
65. Jellema K, Tijssen CC, van Rooij WJJ, et al. Spinal dural arteriovenous fistulas. Long-term follow-up of 44 treated patients. *Neurology*. 2004;62:1839–1841.
66. van Dijk JMC, TerBrugge KG, Willinsky RA, et al. Multidisciplinary management of spinal dural arteriovenous fistulas. Clinical presentation and long-term follow-up in 49 patients. *Stroke* 2002;33:1578–1583.
67. Song JK, Gobin P, Duckwiler GR, et al. N-butyl 2-cyanoacrylate embolization of spinal dural arteriovenous fistulae. *Am J Neuroradiol* 2001;22:40–47.
68. Lichtheim. Zur Kenntniss der perniciösen Anämie, Verhandl Deutsch Kong innere Med. Cong. F. *Innere Med*, 1887;6:84–99.
69. Russell JSR. The relationship of some forms of combined degenerations of the spinal cord to one another and to anaemia. *Lancet* 1898;2:5–14.
70. Smith EL. Purification of anti-pernicious anaemia factors from liver. *Nature* 1948;161:638–639.
71. Minot GR, Murphy WP. Treatment of pernicious anemia by special diet. *JAMA* 1926;87:470–476.
72. Adams RD, Victor M. *Principles of neurology*. 4th ed. New York, NY: McGraw Hill, 1989:833.
73. Pant SS, Asbury AK, Richardon EP Jr. The myelopathy of pernicious anemia: a neuropathological reappraisal. *Acta Neurol Scand* 1968;44(Suppl 35):5–36.
74. Agamanolis DP, Victor M, Harris JW, et al. An ultrastructural study of subacute combined degeneration of the spinal cord in vitamin B_{12}-deficient rhesus monkeys. *J Neuropath Exp Neurol* 1978;37:273–299.
75. Shorvon SD, Carney MWP, Chanarin I, et al. The neuropsychiatry of megaloblastic anaemia. *Br Med J* 1980;281:1036–1038.
76. Gautier-Smith PC. Lhermitte's sign in subacute combined degeneration of the cord. *J Neurol Neurosurg Psychiatry* 1973;36:861–863.
77. Perold JG. Vitamin B_{12} neuropathy in the absence of anaemia. A case report. *South Afr Med J* 1981;59:570.
78. Hensing JA. Subacute combined degeneration, neutrophilic hypersegmentation, and the absence of anemia. A case report. *Ariz Med*.1981;38:768.
79. Wilhelm H, Grodd W, Schiefer U, et al. Uncommon chiasmal lesions: demyelinating disease, vasculitis, and cobalamin deficiency. *Ger J Ophthalmol* 1993; 2(4–5):234–240.
80. Green R, Kinsella LJ. Current concepts in the diagnosis of cobalamin deficiency. *Neurology* 1995;45:1435–1440.
81. Hemmer B, Glocker FX, Schumacher M, et al. Subacute combined degeneration: clinical, electrophysiological, and magnetic resonance imaging findings. *J Neurol Neursurg Psych* 1998;65:822–827.
82. Di Lazzaro V, Restuccia D, Fogli D, et al. Central sensory and motor conduction in vitamin B12 deficiency. *Electroencephalogr Clin Neurophysiol* 1992;84: 433–439.
83. Katsaros VK, Glocker FX, Hemmer B, et al. MRI of spinal cord and brain lesions in subacute combined degeneration. *Neuroradiology* 1998;40:716–719.
84. Beltramello A, Puppini G. Cerini R, et al. Subacute combined degeneration of the spinal cord after nitrous oxide anaesthesia: role of magnetic resonance imaging [letter]. *J Neurol Neurosurg Psychiatry* 1998;64:563–564.
85. Larner AJ, Zeman AZ, Allen CM, et al. MRI appearances in subacute combined degeneration of the spinal cord due to vitamin B_{12} deficiency [letter]. *J Neurol Neurosurg Psychiatry* 1997;62:99–100.
86. Kuker W, Thron A. Subacute combined degeneration of the spinal cord: demonstration of contrast enhancement [letter]. *Neuroradiology* 1999;41:387.
87. Ravakhah K, West BC. Case report: subacute combined degeneration of the spinal cord from folate deficiency. *Am J Med Sci* 1995;310:214–216.
88. Pincus JH. Folic acid deficiency, a cause of spinal cord system degeneration. In: Botz MI, Reynolds EH, eds. *Folic acid in neurology, psychiatry and internal medicine*. New York, NY: Raven, 1979:427–433.
89. Donnelly S, Callaghan N. Subacute combined degeneration of the spinal cord due to folate deficiency in association with a psychotic illness. *Ir Med J* 1990;83:73–74.
90. Lever EG, Elwes RD, Williams A, et al. Subacute combined degeneration of the cord due to folate deficiency: response to methyl folate treatment. *J Neurol Neurosurg Psychiatry* 1986;49:1203–1207.
91. Layzer RB, Fishman RA, Schafer JA. Neuropathy following abuse of nitrous oxide. *Neurology* 1978;28:504–506.
92. Layzer RB, Myeloneuropathy after prolonged exposure to nitrous oxide. *Lancet* 1978;2:1227–1230.
93. Sahenk Z, Mendel JR, Couri D, et al. Polyneuropathy from inhalation of N_2O cartridges through a whipped cream dispenser. *Neurology* 1978;28:485–487.
94. Schilling RF. Is nitrous oxide a dangerous anesthetic for vitamin B_{12}-deficient subjects? *JAMA* 1986, 255:1605–6.

95. Stacy CB, Di Rocco A, Gould RJ. Methionine in the treatment of nitrous-oxide-induced neuropathy and myeloneuropathy. *J Neurol* 1992;239:401–403.
96. Flippo TS, Holder WD Jr. Neurologic degeneration associated with nitrous oxide anesthesia in patients with vitamin B_{12} deficiency. *Arch Surg* 1993;128:1391–1395.
97. Sesso RM, Iunes Y, Melo AC. Myeloneuropathy following nitrous oxide anesthaesia in a patient with macrocytic anaemia. *Neuroradiology* 1999;41:588–590.
98. Marie, RM; Le Biez E, Busson P, et al. Nitrous Oxide Anesthesia-Associated Myelopathy. *Arch Neurol* 2000;57:380–382.
99. Harding AE, Muller DP, Thomas PK, et al. Spinocerebellar degeneration secondary to chronic intestinal malabsorption: a vitamin E deficiency syndrome. *Ann Neurol* 1982;12:419–424.
100. Bertoni JM, Abraham FA, Falls HF, et al. Small bowel resection with vitamin E deficiency and progressive spinocerebellar syndrome. *Neurology* 1984;34:1046–1052.
101. Brin MR, Fetell MR, Green PH, et al. Blind loop syndrome, vitamin E malabsorption, and spinocerebellar degeneration. *Neurology* 1985;35:338–342.
102. Harding AE, Matthews S, Jones S, et al. Spinocerebellar degeneration associated with a selective defect of vitamin E. absorption. *N Engl J Med* 1985;313:32–35.
103. Gutmann L, Schockcor W, Gutmann L, et al. Vitamin E-deficient spinocerebellar syndrome due to intestinal lymphangiectasia. *Neurology* 1986;36:554–556.
104. Vorgerd M, Tegenthoff M, Kuhne D, et al. Spinal MRI in progressive myeloneuropathy associated with vitamin E deficiency. *Neuroradiology* 1996;38(Suppl 1):S111–S113.
105. Nelson JS, Fitch CD, Fischer VW, et al. Progressive neuropathologic lesions in vitamin E-deficient rhesus monkeys. *J Neuropathol Exp Neurol* 1981;40:166–186.
106. Sencer W. Neurological manifestations in malabsorption syndrome. *J Mt Sinai Hosp* 1957;24:331–345.
107. Geller A, Gilles F, Schwachman H. Degeneration of fasiculus gracilis in cystic fibrosis. *Neurology* 1977;27:185–187.
108. Pentschew A, Schwarz K. Systemic axonal dystrophy in vitamin E deficient adult rats: with implication in human neuropathology. *Acta Neuropathol (Berl)* 1962;1:313–334.
109. Towfighi J. Effects of chronic vitamin E deficiency on the nervous system of the rat. *Acta Neuropathol (Berl)*. 1981;54:261–268.
110. Adam RD, Victor M. *Principles of neurology*. 4th ed. New York, NY: McGraw-Hill, 1989:1059.
111. Herbert PN, Assmann G, Gotto AM, et al. Familial lipoprotein deficiency. In: Stanbury JH, Wyngaarden DS, Fredrickson DS, eds. *The metabolic basis of inherited disease*. 5th ed. New York, NY: McGraw Hill, 1983:589–621.
112. Miller RJ, Davis CJF, Illingworth DR, et al. The neuropathy of abetalipoproteinemia. *Neurology* 1980;30:1286–1291.
113. Schleper B, Stuerenburg HJ. Copper deficiency-associated myelopathy in a 46-year-old woman. *J Neurol* 2001;248:705–706.
114 Kumar N. Copper deficiency myelopathy (human swayback). *Mayo Clin Proc* 2006;81:1371–1384.
115. Spencer PS. Food toxins, AMPA receptors, and motor neuron diseases. *Drug Metab Rev* 1999;31:561–587.
116. Barrow MV, Simpson CF, Miller EJ. Lathyrism: a review. *Q Rev Biol* 1974;49:101–128.
117. Roman GC, Spencer PS, Schoenberg BS. Tropical myeloneuropathies: the hidden endemias. *Neurology* 1985;35:1158–1170.
118. Ludolph AC, et al. Studies on the etiology and pathogenesis of motor neuron disease. I. Lathyaism: clinical findings—established cases. *Brain* 1987;110:149–165.
119. Ressler C. Isolation and identification from the common vetch of the neurotoxin beta-cyano-L-alamine, a possible factor in neurolathyrism. *J Biol Chem* 1962;237:733–735.
120. Ressler C, Redstone PA, Erenburg RH. Isolation and identification of a neuroactive factor from Lathyrus latifolius. *Science* 1961;134:188–190.
121. Rao, SLN, Adiga PR, Sama PS. The isolation and characterization of beta-N-oxalytalpha, beta-diaminopropionicacid, a neurotoxin from the seeds of Lathyrus sativus. *Biochemistry* 1964;3:432–436.
122. Spencer PS, Roy DN, Ludolph A, et al. Lathyrism: evidence for role of the neuroexcitatory aminoacid BOAA. *Lancet* 1986;2:1066–1067.
123. Howlett WP, Brubaker GR, Mlingi N, et al. Konzo, an epidemic upper motor neuron disease studied in Tanzania. *Brain* 1990;113:223–235.
124. Tylleskar T, Banea M, Bikangi N, et al. Dietary determinants of a non-progressive spastic paraparesis (Konzo): a case-referent study in a high incidence area of Zaire. *J Epidemiol* 1995;24:949–956.
125. Tylleskar T, Banea M, Bikangi N, et al. Epidemiological evidence from Zaire for a dietary etiology of konzo, an upper motor neuron disease. *Bull World Health Organ.* 1991;69:581–589.
126. Cliff J, Nicala D. Long-term follow-up of konzo patients. *Trans R Soc Trop Med Hyg* 1997;91:447–449.
127. Tylleskar T, Legue FD, Peterson S, et al. Konzo in the Central African Republic. *Neurology* 1994;44: 959–961.
128. Osuntokun BO. An ataxic neuropathy in Nigeria, a clinical, biochemical and electrophysiological study. *Brain* 1968;215–248.
129. Montgomery RD, et al. Clinical and pathological observations in Jamaica neuropathy. *Brain* 1964;87:425–462.
130. Kaposi M. Neue Beitrage zur Kenntnis des Lupus erythematosus. *Arch Dermatol U Syph* 1872;4:36.
131. Johnson RT, Richardson EP. The neurological manifestions of systemic lupus erythematosus. A clinical-pathological study of 24 cases and review of the literature. *Medicine* 1968;47:337–369.
132. Al-Husaini A, Jamal GA. Myelopathy as the main presenting feature of systemic lupus erythematosus. *Eur Neurol* 1985;24:94–106.
133. Mok CC, Lau CS, Chan EY, et al. Acute transverse myelopathy in systemic lupus erythematosus: clinical presentation, treatment, and outcome. *J Rheumatol* 1998;25:467–73.
134. Lopez-Dupla M, Khamashta MA, Sanchez AD, et al. Transverse myelitis as a first manifestation of systemic lupus erythematosus: a case report. *Lupus* 1995;4: 239–242.
135. Zenone T, Steineur MP, Sibille M, et al. Myélopathie révélatrice d'un lupus. Deux observations et revue de la literature. *Rev Méd Interne* 2000;21:1114–1120.

136. Lavalle C, Pizarro S, Drenkard C, et al. Transverse myelitis. A manifestation of systemic lupus erythematosus strongly associated with antiphospholipid antibodies. *J Rheumatol* 1993;17:34–51.
137. Sanna G, Bertolaccini ML, Cuadrado MJ, et al. Neuropsychiatric manifestations in systemic lupus erythematosus: prevalence and association with antiphospholipid antibodies. *J Rheumatol* 2003;30: 985–992.
138. Andrianakos AA, Duffy J, Suzuki M, et al. Transverse myelopathy in systemic lupus erythematosus. Report of three cases and review of the literature. *Ann Intern Med* 1975;83:616–624.
139. Provenzale J, Bouldin TW. Lupus-related myelopathy: report of three cases and review of the literature. *J Neurol Neurosurg Psychiatry* 1992;55:830–835.
140. Propper DJ, Bucknall RC. Acute transverse myelopathy complicating systemic lupus erythematosus. *Ann Rheum Dis* 1989;48:5125.
141. Berlanga B, Rubio FR, Moga I, et al. Response to intravenous cyclophosphamide treatment in lupus myelopathy. *J Rheumatol* 1992;19:829–830.
142. Slovick DI. Treatment of acute myelopathy in systemic lupus erythematosus with plasma exchange and immunosuppression [letter]. *J Neurol Neurosurg Psychiatry* 1986;49:103–105.
143. Mok CC, Mak A, To CH. Mycophenolate mofetil for lupus related myelopathy *Ann Rheum Dis* 2006;65: 971–973
144. Molina R, Provost TT, Arnett FC, et al. Primary Sjogren's syndrome in men-clinical, serologic, and immunogenetic features. *Am J Med* 1986;80:23–31.
145. Alexander EL, Arnett FC, Provost TT, et al. Sjogren's syndrome: association of anti-Ro (SS-A) antibodies with vasculitis, hematologic abnormalities, and serologic hyperreactivity. *Ann Intern Med* 1983;98:155–159.
146. Alexander EL, Malinow K, Lejewski JE, et al. Primary Sjogren's syndrome with central nervous system disease mimicking multiple sclerosis. *Ann Intern Med* 1986;104:323–330.
147. Rutan G, Martinez AJ, Fieshko JT, et al. Primary biliary cirrhosis, Sjogren's syndrome, and transverse myelitis. *Gastroenterology* 1986;90:206–210.
148. Urban E, Jabbari B, Robles H. Concurrent cerebral venous sinus thrombosis and myeloradiculopathy in Sjogren's syndrome. *Neurology* 1994;44:554–556.
149. de Seze J, Delalande S, Fauchais AL, et al. Myelopathies secondary to Sjogren's syndrome: treatment with monthly intravenous cyclophosphamide associated with corticosteroids. *J Rheumatol* 2006;33:709–11.
150. Konttinen YT, Kinnunen E, Von Bonsdorff, et al. Acute transverse myelopathy successfully treated with plasmapheresis and prednisone in a patient with primary Sjogren's syndrome. *Arthr Rheum* 1987;30:339–344.
151. Wright RA, O'Duffy JD, Rodriguez M. Improvement of myelopathy in Sjogren's syndrome with chlorambucil and prednisone therapy. *Neurology* 1999;52:386–388.
152. Izumi M, Nakamura H, Nakamura T, et al. Sjogren's syndrome (SS) in patients with human T cell leukemia virus I associated myelopathy: paradoxical features of the major salivary glands compared to classical SS. *J Rheum* 1999;26:2609–2614.
153. Nakamura H, Eguchi K, Nakamura T, et. al. High prevalence of Sjogren's syndrome in patients with HTLV-I associated myelopathy. *Rheum Dis* 1997;56:167–172.
154. Pot C, Chizzolini C, Vokatch N, et al. Combined antiviral-immunosuppressive treatment in human T-lymphotrophic virus 1–Sjögren-associated myelopathy. *Arch Neurol* 2006;63:1318–1320.
155. Delaney P. Neurologic manifestations in sarcoidosis. Review of the literature, with a report of 23 cases. *Ann Intern Med* 1977;87:336–345.
156. Kanzaki M, Mochizuki H, Kobayashi H, et al. Intraspinal sarcoidosis: clinical features, MR imaging and electrophysiological study. *Neurol Sci* 2004;25:91–94.
157. Schaller B, Kruschat T, Schmidt H, et al. Intradural, extramedullary spinal sarcoidosis: report of a rare case and review of the literature. *Spine J*.2006;6:204–210.
158. Mathieson CS, Mowle D, Ironside JW, et al. Isolated cervical intramedullary sarcoidosis-a histological surprise. *Br J Neurosurg*.2004;18:632–635.
159. Zieve L, Mendelson DF. Goepfert M. Shunt encephalomyelopathy. I. Recurrent protein encephalopathy with response to arginine. *Ann Int Med* 1960;53:33–52.
160. Zieve L, Mendelson DF, Goepfert M. Shunt encephalomyelopathy. II. Occurrence of permanent myelopathy. *Ann Int Med* 1960;53:63.
161. Mendoza G, Marti-Fabregas, Kulisevsky J, et al. Hepatic myelopathy: a rare complication of portacaval shunt. *Eur Neurol* 1994;34:209–212.
162. Baltzan MA, Olszewski J, Zervas N. Chronic Portohepatic encephalopathy. *J Neuropathol Exp Neurol* 1957;16:410–421.
163. Campellone JV, Lacomis D, Giuliani MJ, et al. Hepatic myelopathy. Case report with review of the literature. *Clin Neurol Neurosurg* 1996;98:242–246.
164. Lebovics E, Dematteo RE, Schaffner F, et al. Portal systemic myelopathy after portacaval shunt surgery. *Arch Intern Med* 1985;145:1921–1922.
165. Bain VG, Bailey RJ, Jhamandas JH. Postshunt myelopathy. *J Clin Gastroenterol* 1991;13:562–564.
166. Nardone R, Buratti T, Oliviero A, et al. Corticospinal involvement in patients with a portosystemic shunt due to liver cirrhosis: a MEP study. *J Neurol* 2006;253:81–85.
167. Scobie BA, Summerskill WHJ. Permanent paraplegia with cirrhosis. *Arch Intern Med* 1964;113:805–810.
168. Pant SS, Rebeiz JJ, Richardson EP. Spastic paraparesis following portocavalshunts. *Neurology* 1968;18: 134–141.
169. Mousseau R, Reynolds T. Hepatic paraplegia. *Am J Gastroenterol* 1976;66:343–348.
170. Sherlock S, Summerskill WHJ, White LP, et al. Portal-systemic encephalopathy: neurological complications of liver disease. *Lancet* 1954;453–457.
171. Budillon G, Scala G, Mansi D, et al. Hepatic paraplegia: an uncommon complication of portosystemic shunt. *Acta Neurol (Napoli)* 1979;34:93–100.
172. Giangaspero F, Dondi C, Scarani P, et al. Degeneration of the corticospinal tract following portosystemic shunt associated with spinal cord infarction. *Virchows Arch [A]* 1985;406:475–481.
173. Kissel P, Arnoud G, Tridon P, et al. Sur un cas de myelopathie par shunt portocave. *Rev Neurol (Paris)* 1962;106:782–786.

174. Krake A, Patterson M. Chronic permanent encephalomyelopathy following hepatic shunts. *South Med J* 1964;57:617–621.
175. Liversedge LA, Rawson MD. Myelopathy in hepatic disease and portosystemic venous anastomosis. *Lancet* 1966;1:277–279.
176. Krinashwami V, Radhakrishna T, John BM. Myelopathy in cirrhosis. *J Indian Med Assoc* 1969;53:195–197.
177. Troisi R. Debruyne J, de Hemptinne B. Improvement of hepatic myelopathy after liver transplantation [letter]. *N EnglJ Med* 1999;340:151.
178. Weissenborn K, Bokemeyer M, Krause J, et al. Neurological and neuropsychiatric syndromes associated with liver disease. *AIDS* 2005;19(Suppl 3):S93–S98
179. Counsell C, Warlow C. Failure of presumed hepatic myelopathy to improve after liver transplantation [letter]. *J Neurol Neurosurg Psychiatry* 1996;60:590.
180. Posner JB, Paraneoplastic syndromes. In: Posner JB, ed. *Neurologic complications of cancer*. Philadelphia, PA: Davis FA, 1995;353–385.
181. Ojeda VT. Necrotizing myelopathy associated with malignancy. A clinicopathologic study of two cases and literature review. *Cancer* 1984;53:1115–1123.
182. Gieron MA, Margraf LR, Korthals JK, et al. Progressive necrotizing myelopathy associated with leukemia: clinical, pathologic, and MRI correlation. *Child Neurol* 1987;2:44–49.
183. Dansey RD, Hammond-Tooke GD, Lai K, et al. Subacute myelopathy: an unusual paraneoplastic complication of Hodgkin's disease. *Med Pediatr Oncol* 1988;16:284–286.
184. Storey E, McKelvie PA. Necrotizing myelopathy associated with multiple myeloma. *Acta Neurol Scand* 1991;84:98–101.
185. Hughes M, Ahern V, Kefford R, et al. Paraneoplastic myelopathy at diagnosis in a patient with pathologic stage 1A Hodgkin disease. *Cancer* 1992;70:1598–1600.
186. Kuroda Y, Miyahara M, Sakemi T, et al. Autopsy report of acute necrotizing opticomyelopathy associated with thyroid cancer. *J Neurol Sci* 1993;120:29–32.
187. Mueller S, Dubal DB, Josephson SA. A case of paraneoplastic myelopathy associated with the neuromyelitis optica antibody. *Nat Clin Pract Neurol* 2008;4:284–288.
188. Drach LM, Enzensberger W, Fabian T, et al. Paraneoplastic necrotizing myelopathy in a case of AIDS with lymphoma [letter]. *J Neurol Neurosurg Psychiatry* 1996;60:237.
189. Wilson JWL, Morales A, Sharp D. Necrotizing myelopathy associated with renal cell carcinoma. *Urology* 1983;21:390–392.
190. Anderson DW, Borsaru A. Case report: lymphoma-related resolving paraneoplastic myelopathy with MRI correlation. *Br J Radiol* 2008;81:e103–e105
191. McDermott CJ, White K, Bushby K, et al. Hereditary spastic paraparesis: a review of new developments. *J Neurol Neurosurg Psychiatry* 2000;69:150–160.
192. Strumpell A, Beitrage zur pathologie des ruckenmarks. *Archiv fur Psychiatrie und Nervenkrankheiten* 1880;10:676–717.
193. Harding AE, Hereditary pure spastic paraplegia: a clinical and genetic study of 22 families. *J Neurol Neurosurg Psychiatry* 1981;44:871–883.
194. Durr A, Brice A, Serdaru M, et al. The phenotype of "pure" autosomal dominant spastic paraplegia. *Neurology* 1994;44:1274–1277.
195. Schwarz GA, Hereditary (familial) spastic paraplegia. *Arch Neurol Psychiatry* 1952;68:655–682.
196. Schwarz GA, Liu CN. Hereditary (familial) spastic paraplegia. *Arch Neurol Psychiatry* 1956;75:144–162.
197. Hazan J, Fonknechten N, Mavel D, et al. Spastin, a novel AAA protein, is altered in the most frequent form of autosomal dominant spastic paraplegia. *Nat Genet* 1999;23:296–303.
198. Bonneau D, Rozet J-M, Bulteau C, et al. X-linked spastic paraplegia (SPG2): clinical heterogeneity at a single locus. *J Med Genet* 1993;30:381–384.
199. Johnson AW, McKusick VA. A sex-linked recessive from of spastic paraplegia. *Am J Hum Genet* 1962;14:83–94.
200. Jouet M, Rosenthal A, Armstrong G, et al. X-linked spastic paraplegia (SPG1), MASA syndrome and X-linked hydrocephalus result from mutations in the L1 gene. *Nat Genet* 1994;7:402–407.
201. Tang LM, Chen ST, Hsu WC, et al. A longitudinal study of multimodal evoked potentials in patients following radiotherapy for nasopharyngeal carcinoma. *Neurology* 1996;47:521–525.
202. Li Y-Q, Jay V, Wong C. Oligodendrocytes in the adult rat spinal cord undergo radiation induced apoptosis. *Cancer Res* 1996;56:5417–5422.
203. Palmer JJ. Radiation myelopathy. In: Vinken PJ, Bruyn GW, ed. *Handbook of clinical neurology*. Vol. 26. Amsterdam, The Netherlands: North-Holland Publishing Co., 1976:81–95.
204. Schultheiss TE, Kun LE, Ang KK, et al. Radiation response of the central nervous system. *J Rad Oncol Biol Phys* 1995;31:1093–112.
205. Murakami H, Kawahara N, Yahata T, et al. Radiation myelopathy after radioactive iodine therapy for spine metastasis. *Br J Radiol* 2006;79:e45–e49
206. Schiff D, Shaw EG, Cascino TL. Outcome after spinal reirradiation for malignant epidural spinal cord compression. *Ann Neurol* 1995;37:583–589.
207. Nieder C, Grosu AL, Andratschke NH, et al. Update of human spinal cord reirradiation tolerance based on additional data from 38 patients. *Int J Radiat Oncol Biol Phys* 2006;66:1446–1449
208. Rades D, Stalpers LJA, Veninga T, et al. Spinal reirradiation after short-course RT for metastatic spinal cord compression. *Int J Radiat Oncol Biol Phys* 2005;63: 872–875.
209. Okamoto Y, Murakami M, Yoden E, et al. Reirradiation for locally recurrent lung cancer previously treated with radiation therapy. *Int J Radiat Oncol Biol Phys* 2002;52:390–396
210. Schultheiss TE, Stephens LC, Maor MH. Analysis of the histopathology of radiation myelopathy. *Int J Radiat Oncol Biol Phys* 1988;14:27–32.
211. Schultheiss TE, Stevens LC. Radiation myelopathy. *AJNR* 1992;13:1056–1058.
212. Udaka F, Tsuji T, Shigematsu K, et al. A case of chronic progressive radiation myelopathy successfully treated with corticosteroids. Rinsho Shinkeigaku. *Clin Neurol* 1990;30:439–443.

213. Hirota S, Soejima T, Higashino T, et al. A case of chronic progressive chronic radiation myelopathy treated with long-time corticosteroids administration. *J Clin Radiol* 1998;43:649–652.
214. Glantz MJ, Burger PC, Friedman AH, et al. Treatment of radiation induced nervous system injury with heparin and warfarin. *Neurology* 1994;44:2020–2027.
215. Koehler PJ, Verbiest H, Jager J, et al. Delayed radiation myelopathy; serial MR-imaging and pathology. *Clin Neurol Neurosurg* 1996;98:197–201.
216. Angibaud G, Ducasse JL, Baille G, et al. Potential value of hyperbaric oxygen in the treatment of post radiation myelopathies. *Rev Neurol* 1995;151:661–666.
217. Pol B, Watelle TSJ. Memoire sur les effets de la compression de l' air. *Ann Hyg Publ (Paris) 2 ser 1*. 1854;2:241–279.
218. Bert P. *La Pression barometrique*. Paris: Masson, 1878.
219. Hill L, Caisson sickness and compressed air. *J R Soc Arts* 1911;59,400–412.
220. Dick APK, Massey EW. Neurologic presentation of decompression sickness and air embolism in sport divers. *Neurology* 1985;35:667–671.
221. Hallenbeck JM, Bore AA Elliott DH. Mechanisms underlying spinal cord damage in decompression sickness. *Neurology* 1975;25:308–316.
222. Francis TJ, Griffin JL, Homer LD. et al. Bubble-induced dysfunction in acute spinal cord decompression sickness. *J Appl Physiol* 1990;68:1368–1375.
223. Palmer AC, Calder IM, McCallum RI, et al. Spinal cord degeneration in a case of "recovered" spinal decompression sickness. *Br Med J Clin Ed* 1981;283:888.
224. Wilmshurst P, Bryson P. Relationship between the clinical features of neurological decompression illness and its causes. *Clin Sci*.2000;99:65–75
225. Sparacia G, Banco A, Sparacia B, et al. Magnetic resonance findings in scuba diving-related spinal cord decompression sickness. *Magma* 1997;5:111–115.
226. Aharon-Peretz J, Adir Y, Gordon CR, et al. Spinal cord decompression sickness in sport diving. *Arch Neurol* 1993;50:753–756.

CHAPTER 34 ■ MULTIPLE SCLEROSIS

DENISE I. CAMPAGNOLO AND TIMOTHY L. VOLLMER

INTRODUCTION

Multiple sclerosis (MS) is a chronic inflammatory disorder of the central nervous system (CNS) affecting 2.5 million people worldwide, approximately 400,000 in the United States (1). The main pathologic features of this disease are focal areas of demyelination along with axonal injury. The clinical course is unpredictable, but in most patients neurological disability incrementally increases over time. Although its etiology is unknown, MS is generally considered to result from a cascade of immune attack on CNS structures (optic nerves, brain, spinal cord), occurring preferentially in genetically susceptible individuals. There are likely precipitating environmental factors, probably infectious in nature. MS is the leading cause of neurologic disability in young people and there is no cure. Currently, there are seven approved immunotherapies for MS that can modify the clinical and magnetic resonance imaging (MRI) disease activity.

HISTORICAL PERSPECTIVE

Although the first well-documented case occurred in 1822 (1,2), MS probably existed even earlier but was not recognized as a specific disease entity because of the difficulty in differentiating it from other neurologic disorders of the time. In the 1860s, the French neurologist, Jean-Martin Charcot provided the first detailed descriptions of the clinical features of MS, established diagnostic criteria, and correlated clinical manifestations with autopsy findings (3,4). By the late 19th century, the clinical and pathological features of MS were well recognized, leading Guillain to state that "disseminated sclerosis is, after syphilis, the most frequent disease of the nervous system" (5,6). In the early 20th century, abnormalities of cerebrospinal fluid (CSF) were recognized as significant and the microscope allowed for recognition of inflammation around blood vessels in the CNS. In 1982, MRI became available with the first visualization of T2-weighted white matter lesions (2).

EPIDEMIOLOGY

MS commonly starts in late adolescence or early adult life, with peak onset occurring at a mean age of about 30 years. Like many other putative autoimmune diseases, MS is more common in women (with a ratio of 2:1) than men. However, unlike most other autoimmune disorders, MS has two unique epidemiologic features, an unusual and as yet unexplained worldwide pattern and an effect of migration in altering risk for developing the disease. In terms of the former, MS is more likely to occur in white people with Northern European ancestry than in Native Americans, African Americans, Asians, and members of certain ethnic groups (7–10). Incidence of MS is highest at the extremes of latitude in the Northern and Southern hemispheres. Prevalence studies indicate a crude North-South gradient in North America with prevalence rates of 150 to 200 per 100,000 population described in Canada and the northern United States as compared to less than 50 per 100,000 in the American south (7,8,10), where there are larger populations of African Americans. In Europe, prevalence rates less predictably relate to latitude, although MS is more common in Scandinavia and Great Britain than in Mediterranean countries (11). In the Southern hemisphere, the North-South gradient is reversed with MS being higher in Southern than Northern Australia. A relatively low rate of MS has been reported in Asia. Many exceptions to the rate of MS by latitude have been described and remarkable differences in MS prevalence have been documented in populations in close geographic proximity such as Australia and New Zealand (10–14). Risk of infections and low vitamin D levels due to low sunlight exposure have been implicated as explanations for this global pattern of MS, but to date neither has been proven. With respect to the former, interest remains in several human (Epstein-Barr virus, human herpesvirus 6, retroviruses, *Chlamydia pneumoniae*) and animal (canine distemper) viruses as possible candidate agents (15–17). Unfortunately, reports of isolation or identification of infectious agents in MS tissue have generally proven to be nonreproducible or nonspecific.

MS is a partially genetic disease. Susceptibility to MS has been associated with human leukocyte antigen DR2 allele, with candidate genes DRB1*1501 and DRB5*0101, and genes for IL-2Ra and IL-7Ra in increasing risk of developing MS (18). The relationship between DR2 and MS risk, the higher rate of MS in families where one member already has the disease than in the general population, and the increased risk for MS the closer the relationship to an affected blood relative all indicate that genes probably play an important role as to who gets the disease. However, as yet no specific gene has been shown to have a powerful effect in this regard, and it seems likely that multiple, perhaps interacting, genes confer MS susceptibility.

The most powerful evidence for environmental triggers comes from migration studies. Persons who move from a high- to low-risk geographic area *retain* their high risk if they are 15 years of age or older when they move. Interestingly, if they move from a low- to high-risk area, their risk increases if the move took place within a wider span of ages (11 to 45 years) (19). This indicates that MS risk for individuals or their offspring often changes upward or downward depending on age of migration and whether migration occurs to or from low or high prevalence areas (7,8,10,19). The nature of these potential causative environmental factors is not known at present. It is clear, however, that MS is a complex disorder the development of which requires some combination of hereditary and environmental factors.

MECHANISM OF TISSUE INJURY

The genetic and environmental issues discussed above speak to a triggering event in the acquisition of MS. Regardless of the trigger, it is clear that the immune response plays a critical role in causing CNS demyelination. The most impressive evidence for the immunologic basis of MS comes from the effectiveness, at least transiently, of a number of immunomodulating or immunosuppressive agents, which have markedly different mechanisms of action. Nonetheless, the final common denominator is their impact on immune function. Although all of the details surrounding exactly how the immune response causes tissue injury is unknown, it seems clear that macrophages, T and B cells (which lead to antibody production), are directly involved (20). What remains a question is whether the presence of an infectious agent is required. Cells of the innate immune response, including natural killer (NK) cells or NK T cells, are increasingly being studied as both potential mediators and, on the other hand, regulators of the autoaggressive immune response characteristic of this disorder. A number of alterations in brain, blood, CSF, T-cell subtypes, cytokines, chemokines, immunoglobulins, and adhesion molecules have been implicated as effectors of immunologic tissue damage (20). An animal model of autoimmune CNS demyelination, experimental allergic encephalomyelitis (EAE), has many clinical and pathologic features in common with MS, and much has been learned via study of this murine disease (21). The EAE model, however, also has limitations that prohibit direct extrapolation to human MS (21).

NEUROPATHOLOGIC CHARACTERISTICS OF MS

MS should not be considered a disorder solely of white matter. MS is a disorder of neurons and oligodendrocytes globally throughout the CNS. From the earliest stages of the disease, there are abnormalities in grey matter, axonal transection, as well as demyelination (22). There appears to be at least four distinct neuropathologic patterns of MS lesions as reported by Lucchinetti et al. (23). Pattern I is predominantly T lymphocyte infiltration and macrophage-mediated demyelination, pattern II is like pattern I but with a humoral (IgG) component, pattern III has predominant loss of oligodendrocytes, and pattern IV is characterized by death of oligodendroglia (22). These biopsy and autopsy data, in combination with imaging studies showing both acute and chronic lesions in the same patient, speak to the dynamic nature of this disease. MS plaques or lesions on MRI represent dynamic areas of inflammation; injury to myelin, axons, and glia; attempts at functional and anatomical repair; and unfortunately varying degrees of gliotic scarring and neuronal degeneration for which there are limited therapeutic options.

CLINICAL FEATURES

The diagnosis of MS is based on a thorough history, neurological examination, and laboratory testing. The key to proper diagnosis is demonstrating multiple lesions in the CNS (dissemination in space), occurring at different times (dissemination in time) and the exclusion of other disorders with similar features. Early in the course, when patients have had only one neurological event (termed clinically isolated syndrome or CIS), the diagnosis may not be certain, but with the passage of time this becomes less problematic. MS deficits can occur in an acute episodic pattern (called relapses, attacks, or exacerbations) over days to weeks, or MS deficits can evolve in a more chronic progressive fashion. When attacks occur, symptoms last on average 6 to 12 weeks. Symptoms or signs highly suggestive of MS include optic neuritis, diplopia or partial/complete internuclear ophthalmoplegia (representing a lesion of the medial longitudinal fasciculus in the midbrain), Lhermitte sign (an electrical sensation down the spine and/or limbs with neck flexion), and Uhthoff's phenomenon (heat sensitivity) (24,25). Table 34.1 provides the most common presenting symptoms of MS. These symptoms stem from the predilection for MS lesions to involve motor, sensory, autonomic, and integrative pathways in the brain and spinal cord. Symptoms that stand out as potential "red flags" about the accuracy of the MS diagnosis include generalized areflexia, aphasia, homonymous hemianopsia, diffuse muscle atrophy, multiorgan involvement, or progressive disease explainable by one lesion in the neuraxis or involving only one neurological subsystem.

The differential diagnosis can be quite extensive and takes into consideration the temporal presentation, the presence or absence of dissemination of lesions, system involvement, family history, and age at onset (26,27). Table 34.2 lists the diagnoses that can mimic MS on initial acute presentation. If only one system is involved, there is a family history, or onset begins in childhood one should consider hereditary disorders as those listed in Table 34.2.

Laboratory tests can be of great value to the clinician in supporting the diagnosis of MS and excluding other diseases. Routine blood tests in most patients include a complete blood count, complete metabolic panel, sedimentation rate, ANA, VDRL, B-12 level, thyroid function tests, anticardiolipin

TABLE 34.1

MOST FREQUENT SYMPTOMS SEEN AT ONSET OF MS

Sensory symptoms that begin distally and expand proximally (32%–52%)
Unilateral visual loss (6%–23%)
Motor (6%–14%; after age 50 increases to 47%)
Incoordination (11%–15%)
Diplopia/Vertigo (due to internuclear ophthalmoplegia) (11%–18%)

From Weinshenker BG, Bass B, Rice GP, et al. The natural history of multiple sclerosis: a geographically based study. I. Clinical course and disability. *Brain* 1989;112(Pt 1):133–146.

TABLE 34.2

DIFFERENTIAL DIAGNOSIS OR ENTITIES THAT CAN MIMIC MS

Infectious disorders	Lyme disease Acute disseminated encephalomyelitis (ADEM) Transverse myelitis Viral Infections (i.e., HTLV-1) Epidural abscess Neurosyphyllis
Vascular disease	Vasculitides and primary CNS vasculitis Arteriovenous malformations Vasculopathy
Structural	Neoplasms (brain or spinal cord) Syrinx Spondylosis
Hereditary/degenerative	Spinocerebellar degenerations Leukodystrophies Mitochon drial disorders Cerebral autosomal dominant arteriopathy with subcortical infarcts and leukoencephalopathy
Nutritional Lymphoproliferative and others	B_{12} deficiency Sjogren's syndrome Sarcoidosis Anticardiolipin/antiphospholipid antibody syndrome Primary CNS lymphoma Neuromyelitis optica

antibody titers, and Lyme serology. Neuroimaging studies (MRI of brain and spinal cord if signs and symptoms point there) are generally performed in every patient for diagnostic purposes and to show the extent and degree of lesion activity. MRI is also used in assessing prognosis and appropriateness of therapeutic intervention (28). If a patient has been on an immunomodulating therapy and continues to have frequent relapses or repeat MRI showing increased number of lesions or gadolinium (Gd) enhancement, this would aid in the decision to consider a change in treatments.

The hallmark of MS on MRI scanning is multiple periventricular white matter lesions appearing as areas of increased signal intensity on T2-weighted images. This is a sensitive test for MS, with T2-weighted scans being abnormal in 70% to 95% of patients having clinically definite MS (CDMS) and in approximately 50% of patients with an initial presentation of optic neuritis (28). Lesions often are rounded or ovoid, and usually appear homogenous but may possess a rim of altered signal intensity. Similar lesions occur in the white matter of the brain stem and spinal cord. T2 lesions seen on MRI scans reflect increased water content resulting from edema and inflammation or demyelination. These lesions are not specific for MS. Similar lesions can be seen in patients over 50 with small vessel ischemic disease, as well as patients with systemic lupus erythematosis, sarcoid, Lyme disease, and other inflammatory disorders. Enhancing lesions on T1-weighted MRI studies after Gd administration reflect ongoing or recently active disease, as the Gd tends collect in areas of blood-brain barrier (BBB) breakdown.

The detection of new lesions on MRI scanning is a much more sensitive way of assessing disease activity than the patient's history or the physician's neurological exam (28). MS traditionally has been characterized based on its clinical features, mainly dissemination in space and time. Disability progression often occurs over years. However, MRI shows that pathologic changes in MS are more frequent and dynamic than is appreciated by clinical means. At the time of first presentation (CIS) with neurologic symptoms referable to MS, MRI will often show evidence of earlier lesions during times when patients have been clinically asymptomatic (29).

MRI also has prognostic value in predicting the risk of developing MS in certain patients. The optic neuritis study group follow-up showed that with a normal MRI at presentation, the risk of developing MS after 5 years was 22%, whereas patients with even one lesion on brain MRI (besides the optic nerve involvement), the risk of developing MS more than doubled to 56% (30,31). Intravenous methylprednisolone (MP) treatment was effective at hastening speed of visual recovery, but it remains controversial whether it reduces risk of developing CDMS (30,31).

MRI findings may also correlate with disability. "Black holes" on T1-weighted imaging (suggesting brain or spinal cord atrophy), high lesion load on T2-weighted imaging controlled for disease duration, and the repeated documentation of large numbers of enhancing lesions have been associated with greater disability (28,32–34).

Evoked potentials (EPs) record speed and amplitude of electrical signals obtained from the brain or spinal cord in response to a provided stimulus. For visual evoked potentials (VEPs), the stimulus is visual in the form of a black and white checkerboard pattern that reverses every few seconds. Brainstem auditory evoked potentials are recorded after auditory stimuli (clicks) are delivered through a headset. Lastly, somatosensory evoked potentials (SSEPs) are obtained in response to an electrical stimulus delivered to the distal upper or lower extremities. Collectively, these multimodal EPS can be of use for demonstrating a clinically silent lesion, thus confirming a pattern of CNS involvement consistent with demyelination (i.e., prolonged latency). These would aid in documentation of dissemination in space. In the case of VEPs, they provide objective evidence of a subjective complaint such as visual loss, although the correlation between symptoms of visual impairment and VEPs is poor (35). A latency of greater than 10 milliseconds between the eyes is abnormal even when the absolute values are within normal range. However, if patients are drowsy, inattentive, or have ocular pathology, these will affect the results. For SSEPs, typically lower extremity studies provide information about the entire spinal cord. These tests can be helpful but certainly not necessary to make the diagnosis of MS and are not used with the same frequency as MRI (36).

CSF analysis is not done as routinely as in the past with the general availability and sensitivity of MRI testing but does play an important role in problematic or atypical cases. Determination of CSF cells, protein, and glucose and testing for oligoclonal bands (OCBs) and increased IgG (IgG index or synthesis rate) are routinely carried out when a spinal tap is performed. Typically, oligoclonal bands or an increase in CSF IgG is found in the presence of a normal or slightly elevated protein in about 90% of MS patients. Oligoclonal bands unique to the CSF and not seen in the serum confirm increased immunoglobulin production in the CNS (37). The finding of OCBs or elevated IgG synthesis or index in the CSF of CIS patients has a high predictive value for conversion to CDMS (38).

DIAGNOSTIC CRITERIA FOR MULTIPLE SCLEROSIS

Several diagnostic criteria for MS have been developed over the years; all have drawn upon various configurations of symptoms and test results to make the diagnosis. The first of these were the "Schumaker criteria," which relied primarily on the results of the neurological examination, as that is all that were available at that time (39). Thus dissemination in time was determined by the patient's history, specifically by the recurrence of exacerbations and/or progressively worsening symptoms. Dissemination in space relied on the examination findings and at least two different parts of the CNS responsible for them. The last component was exclusion of other diseases that mimic MS. In this period, prior to the advent of MRI, patients were sometimes followed for years in order to fulfill the above Schumaker criteria before making a diagnosis of MS.

By the early 1980s, MRI was available for clinical use and the introduction of the MRI has had direct impact on diagnosis of MS. In 1983, Poser et al. proposed a new set of criteria for diagnosing MS that combined findings from the clinical examination and patient history with the results of MRI, CSF testing, and VEPs. In the Poser criteria, clinical symptoms alone were enough to diagnose MS (40). There had to be two exacerbations, and clinical evidence requires documented abnormalities on examination. Thus the examination confirmed dissemination in the CNS; these clinical criteria therefore established the accepted dissemination in space and time. In the absence of clinical findings, the Poser criteria used paraclinical evidence supporting the presence of "lesions" demonstrated by neuroimaging, EP studies, urologic testing, or other modalities. Laboratory supported diagnosis requires one of two possible immune disturbances in CSF: IgG oligoclonal bands or intrathecal IgG production. Poser criteria included the diagnosis of "definite MS" and "probable MS," which are clinically or laboratory supported. The Poser criteria broadened the definition of relapse to include brief symptoms such as Lhermitte sign, provided they recurred multiple times over a period of days to weeks. In general, a definite diagnosis required two separate disease attacks to document dissemination in time consistent with multiphasic disease process and proven dissemination in space as outlined above (40).

The McDonald Criteria

In 2001, the International Panel on the Diagnosis of Multiple Sclerosis, headed by Dr. W. Ian McDonald, published a new set of criteria, which became known as the McDonald criteria (41). These criteria still accepted a diagnosis of MS on the basis of clinical findings and the patient's history alone. For the first time, however, the criteria listed combinations of imaging and test results that could be used to establish the MS diagnosis when the clinical findings were not clear, such as in the setting of one bout of optic neuritis (one example of CIS). The McDonald criteria introduced the use of the MRI to establish the nature, number, and location of the demyelinating lesions that would be specific for a patient with MS. The McDonald criteria provide guidelines that allow lesion patterns to assess the likelihood of MS.

The McDonald criteria (41) underscore the presence of lesions in these white matter areas as critical imaging data that allow for the diagnosis of MS. These criteria were widely adopted for clinical trials. Generally, however, clinicians use the McDonald criteria only as guidelines, even after they were revised in 2005, because some patients who would not meet the criteria would nonetheless benefit from treatment at the time of discovery of the first demyelinating lesion.

In 2006, Swanton et al. (42) suggested simplifying the McDonald 2005 criteria to require at least one positive T2-weighted lesion in at least two of the four key CNS regions: brain (periventricular, juxtacortical, posterior fossa) and spinal cord, as proof of dissemination in space, and the presence of a new T2-positive lesion any time after a baseline image had been taken as proof of dissemination in time. These new guidelines only changed the MRI components of the criteria and did not suggest any changes for PPMS.

In 2007, the same group published a study in which they compared the ability of their simplified MRI criteria to predict whether CIS patients would develop CDMS (43). The importance of this study was most apparent in the light of published clinical trials that showed that disease modifying agents (see therapy section) can benefit select patients at the time of their first demyelinating event, before they would have fulfilled the McDonald 2005 criteria. The new criteria had a specificity of 87% and an improved sensitivity of 72% for predicting CDMS after CIS as compared to the 88% specificity and 60% sensitivity for the McDonald 2005 criteria (43). None of these criteria, however, are perfect, as approximately 6% of patients who would meet all MRI criteria for CDMS will never have a second neurological event, and therefore never attain the CDMS diagnosis, they remain probable MS (44). The diagnosis and decision to begin therapies remains in the hands of skilled and knowledgeable physician with expertise in MS. Brain and spine MRI have become the most important diagnostic tests to help confirm lesions separated in space and time.

In 2010, the International Panel reconvened to review the effectiveness of the McDonald criteria (45) (see Table 34.3). They considered the information from a number of studies that had been performed during the previous few years, and used the data to make revisions. The MRI criteria for dissemination in space allowed for consideration of spinal cord lesions, because these can be helpful in distinguishing MS in difficult cases. The changes in 2010 criteria as compared to the previous criteria allowed for a much quicker time to diagnosis. Finally, the Panel found that for the diagnosis of primary progressive MS (MS that progresses from the time of onset, with or without superimposed relapses), there had to be at least one year of progression retrospectively or prospectively determined) plus two out of three other criteria as described in Table 34.3.

Classification of MS

MS has been classified into four categories based on the temporal profile of clinical disease activity as depicted in Fig. 34.1 (46). Relapsing-remitting MS (RRMS) patients have

TABLE 34.3

DIAGNOSTIC CRITERIA FOR MS

	McDonald 2010 (42)	**2006 criteria** by Swanton et al. (43)
Dissemination in space (DIS)		
No. of criteria to be met	1	1
No. of T2 lesions *or* Gd-enhancing lesions	≥ 1 T2 lesion in at least 2 of the 4 MS typical regions (listed below)	1 or more per region in at least 2 regions (listed below)
CNS regions for lesion localization typical for MS		
Brain, periventricular	≥1	≥1
Brain, juxtacortical	≥1	≥1
Brain, posterior fossa	≥1[a]	≥1[a]
Spinal cord	≥1[a]	≥1[a]
Dissemination in time		
Gd-enhancing lesion	Detection of asymptomatic Gd+ enhancing AND nonenhancing lesions at any time	N/A
Or, T2-weighted lesions	Detection of a new T2 lesion and/or Gd+ lesion(s) on follow up MRI, irrespective of its timing with reference to baseline scan	New T2 on follow-up MRI, compared with baseline scan taken at any point after symptom onset.
Or, second clinical attack at least 1 mo after first attack	Yes	NA
Or, progression	1 y of disease progression plus 2 of the 3 following criteria: a. Evidence of DIS in the brain based on >1 T2 lesions in at least 1 area characteristic for MS b. evidence for DIS in spinal cord based on T2 lesions in cord c. positive CSF (oligoclonal bands and/or elevated IgG index)	NA

[a]If patient's symptoms could be brain stem or spinal cord syndrome, lesions in CNS regions corresponding to symptoms are not counted

acute attacks (also called relapses or exacerbations) followed by periods of stability but not slow deterioration between attacks. RRMS is seen in 85% of patients early in the course of their disease. Secondary progressive MS (SPMS) is seen later in the evolution of the disease in many patients (50%), often after an initially relapsing-remitting phase. Patients in this category show deterioration between attacks. Unfortunately, it is often difficult to assess whether deterioration between attacks represents disease progression or a transient change due to diurnal variation, fatigue, depression, fever, or medications. PPMS is seen in about 10% of patients who have no obvious relapse or remission but a progressive course from disease onset. Progressive relapsing MS (PRMS) is even less common being seen in about 5% of patients and characterized by progression of disease from onset with occasional relapses superimposed on the progressive course.

Another way to classify MS is based on age at onset of symptoms. Most cases of MS are diagnosed before 40 years of age. Late-onset MS (LOMS) has been defined as MS with onset after age 50. One of the notable differences between typical MS and LOMS is that many more LOMS patients have the PP form of the disease (greater than 30%) (47).

In the past, this classification scheme was used for inclusion in therapeutic trials with the idea of enrolling patients with a similar type of clinical disease course. As a result, Food and Drug Administration (FDA) approval of new drugs for MS is based on this classification. Unfortunately, this classification is not as useful in a practice setting since the distinction between types is not always so clear cut, particularly between RRMS and SPMS. Further, disease type does not necessarily correlate with degree of disability. Theoretically, patients may have RRMS and be more severely disabled than patients with SPMS with disease of the same duration. Mounting evidence suggests that rather than being different entities, these different types of MS have the same underlying pathogenic mechanisms, but that the phenotype is only reflective of the number, location, and severity of CNS active inflammatory lesions (thus still relapsing with corresponding MRI gad enhancements) versus those with little in the way of active inflammation any longer, but with now only evidence of the neuronal and axonal damage that is common to all types of MS. These concepts would allow for classification of persons with MS into essentially two broad clinically useful categories, those who are still relapsing and those who are not, knowing that clinical manifestations are much less sensitive than MRI data as to true disease activity (29).

Disability caused by MS is measured using scales such as the Kurtzke expanded disability status scale (EDSS) and the MS functional composite (MSFC). The EDSS remains the most commonly used rating scale for disability in clinical trials. The EDSS measures disability on an ordinal 0 (normal) to 10 (death) scale, with 0.5 step increments. This measures a wide disability range; 1 to 3.5 (minimal deficits), 4 to 6.5

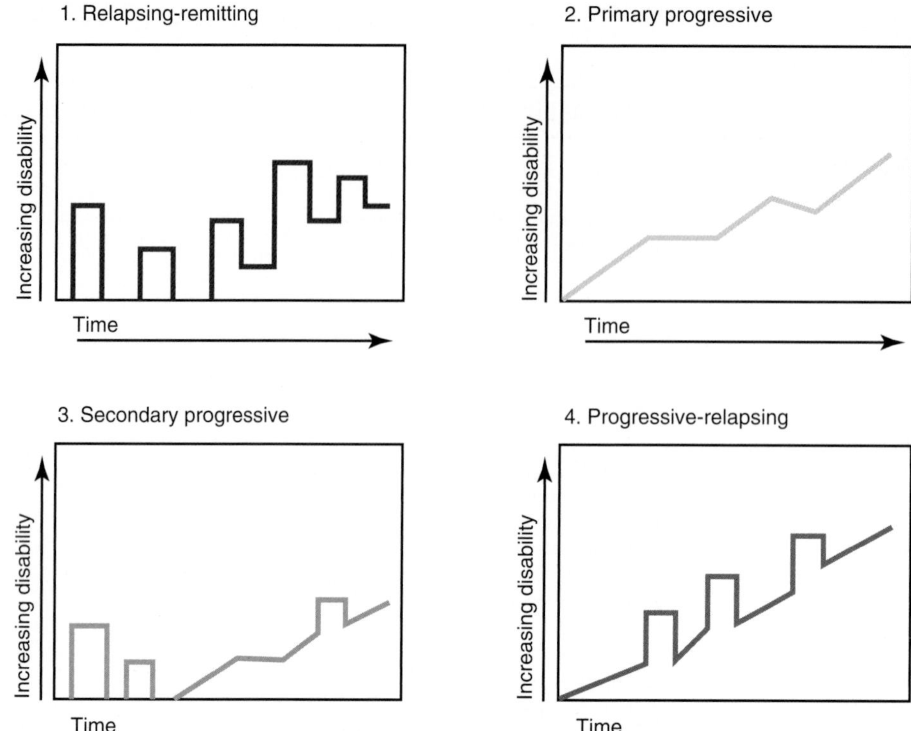

FIGURE 34.1 Types and courses of MS. 1. RRMS is characterized by clearly acute attacks with full recovery or with sequelae and residual deficit upon recovery. Periods between disease relapses are characterized by lack of disease progression. 2. Primary PPMS is characterized by disease showing progression of disability from onset, without plateaus or remissions or with occasional plateaus and temporary minor improvements. 3. SPMS begins with an initial RR course, followed by progression of variable rate, which may also include occasional relapses and minor remissions. 4. PRMS shows progression from onset but with clear acute relapses with or without recovery. (From Lublin FD, Reingold FC. Defining the clinical course of multiple sclerosis: Results of an international survey. *Neurology* 1996;46(64):907–911. Used from Lippincott Williams & Wilkins, with permission.)

(moderate), 7 to 9.5 (severe), and 10 (death) (48) (see Table 34.4). The MSFC measures cognition, ambulation, and hand/arm function and gives a single composite score derived from these three measures (49).

PROGNOSIS

Natural history studies (25) are quite informative about prognosis in patients with MS although these studies need to be reevaluated now that effective therapies are available for modifying disease course. In these studies, approximately 50% of MS patients required a cane or other assistive device for ambulation 15 years after disease onset. It is now possible to decrease MS exacerbations, slow the rate of deterioration, and diminish MRI lesion formation with appropriate therapy and it is conceivable that this will translate into a better prognosis, particularly if treatment is begun early after the diagnosis is made (Figs. 34.2–34.6).

Natural history studies also indicate that MRI findings are a much better barometer of disease activity than clinical evaluations, and suggest that MS is neither as intermittent nor as benign as was previously thought. In some studies, frequency type and severity of exacerbations, degree of persistent neurological deficit, age, sex, symptom profile, and MRI findings may have prognostic value as to future course as outlined in Table 34.5 (33,34,50). During pregnancy, especially the third trimester, relapse rate reduces by as much as 70% as compared to before pregnancy (51). This relapse rate reduction is greater that that seen with even the most effective immunotherapies. In the first 3 months postpartum, however, exacerbations are commonly seen, returning to prepregnancy rates, likely related to the loss of the hormones of pregnancy. Exacerbations are also common following viral and possibly bacterial infections. On the other hand, surgery, anesthesia, trauma, and stress have not been clearly shown to aggravate MS, and the pregnancy itself is a time of reduced disease activity. Although life expectancy is generally not greatly impacted, one study from the Danish MS Registry estimated that MS reduced life span by approximately 10 years (52).

TABLE 34.4

KURTZKE EXPANDED DISABILITY STATUS SCALE

Score	Explanation
0	Normal neurologic exam
1–1.5	No disability, minimal signs
2–2.5	Impairment, minimal disability
3–3.5	Mild disability
4–5.5	Ambulatory from >500 to >100 m
6.0	Unilateral assistance for 100 m
6.5	Bilateral assistance for 20 m
7–7.5	Wheelchair bound; <20 m steps
8–8.5	Bedbound; communicates and eats
9.5	Bedbound; cannot communicate or eat
10	Death

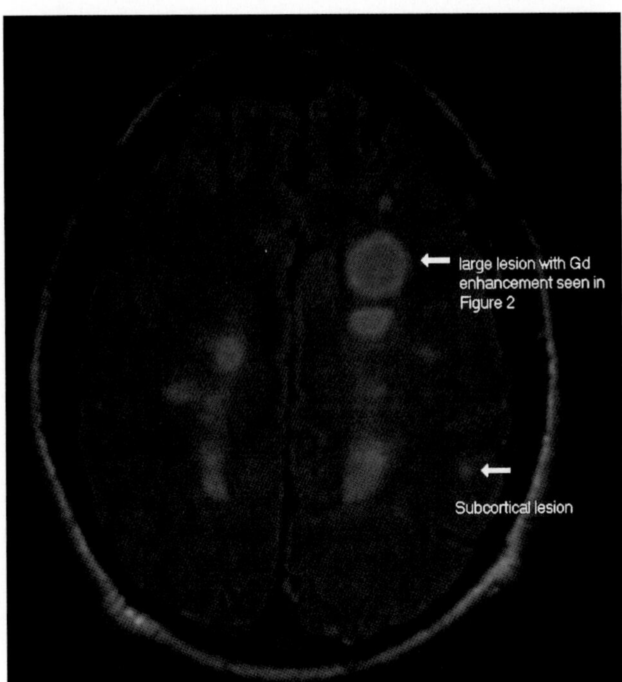

FIGURE 34.2 Fluid attenuated inversion recovery (FLAIR) axial image demonstrating multiple periventricular lesions typical of MS, the largest (*upper arrow*) in the left centrum semiovale. A subcortical lesion is also demonstrated (*lower arrow*). FLAIR sequences generate heavy T2-weighted images where water appears dark instead of bright as in regular T2 images. Thus, FLAIR images make MS lesions more conspicuous than on T2 images.

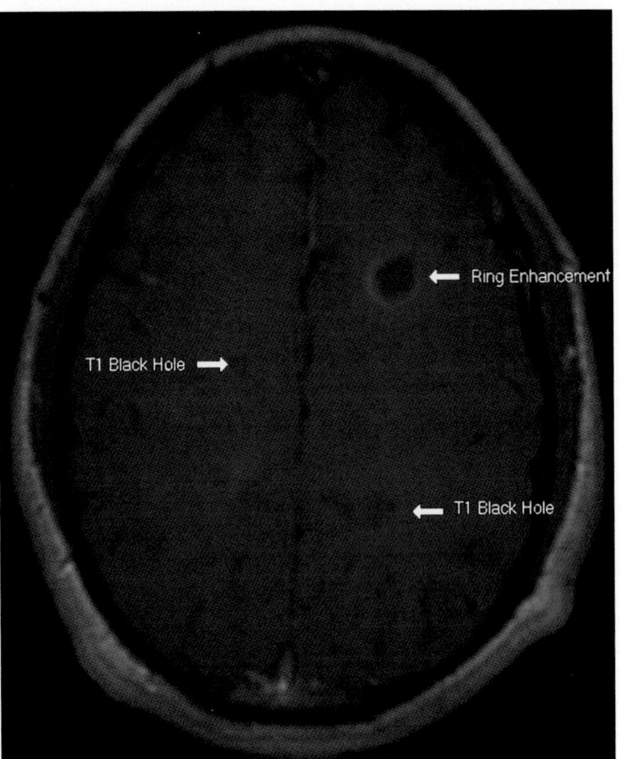

FIGURE 34.3 After Gd administration, T1-weighted image demonstrating ring enhancement (*upper most arrow*) in the dominant left-sided lesion seen in Fig. 34.2. This represents active demyelination and permeability of the BBB. In addition, two T1 hypointense lesions are noted; these are commonly referred to as "T1 black holes" and can be acute (edematous) or chronic (reflecting severe demyelination, axonal loss, and matrix destruction).

MS MIMICS AND VARIANTS

Neuromyelitis optica (NMO or Devic Disease) is a rare CNS inflammatory disorder that involves a necrotizing inflammatory process directed at the spinal cord and optic nerves. An emerging consensus is that NMO is a distinct neuropathological disease from MS (53). The patients present with acute myelitis and/or optic neuritis, and these conditions produce distinctive MRI findings. Spinal cord lesions typically traverse more then three vertebral spinal segments (not typical in MS). Brain MRIs can show lesions in the hypothalamus and periventricular areas, and orbital MRIs confirm optic nerve demyelination. The pathology involves humoral attack against the BBB antigen aquaporin 4 (the principal water channel in the CNS). Anti-aquaporin 4 IgG is detectable on serum laboratory testing with a sensitivity of 76% and a specificity of 94%. Clinical outcome is poor if the condition is left untreated, with blindness and tetraplegia expected. Respiratory failure and ventilator dependency is often seen. Aggressive immunosuppression has been the mainstay of treatment until recently when the monoclonal antibody rituximab (a B-cell depleting agent) has shown good efficacy in a small study (54,55).

Two variants are Balo's concentric sclerosis and Marburg variant. Balo's involves a specific MRI appearance of alternating hypointense and isointense concentric rings on T1 sequences. Marburg variant is a fulminant single phase presentation with an often fatal course due to brainstem involvement.

Transverse myelitis (TM) is an inflammatory condition of the spinal cord that at times can be the initial presentation of MS. The condition is discussed in more detail in

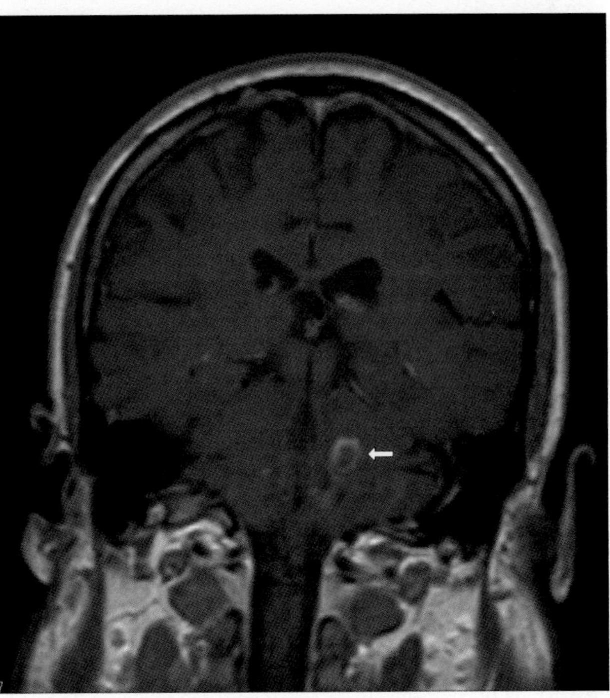

FIGURE 34.4 After Gd administration, coronal T1-weighted image demonstrating ring enhancement of a left cerebellar lesion, representing active demyelination and permeability of the BBB.

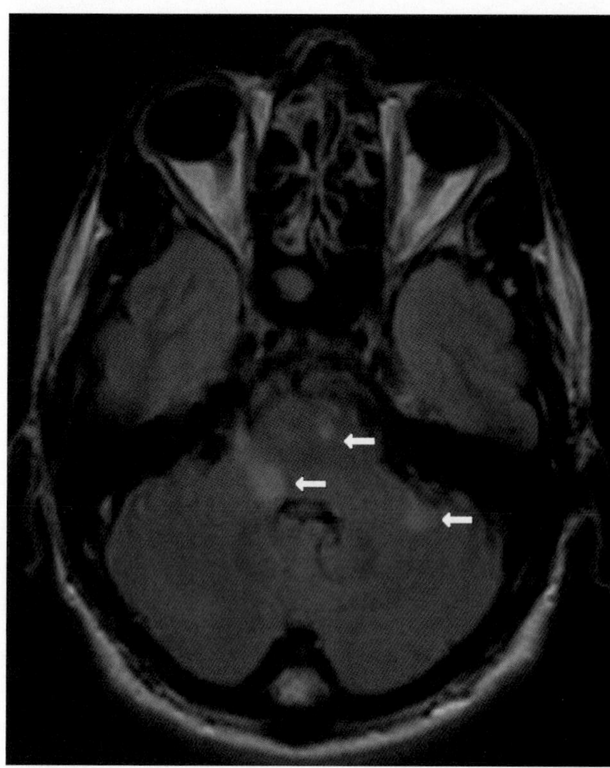

FIGURE 34.5 Axial FLAIR demonstrating MS lesions in the ventral pons, right middle cerebellar peduncle, and left cerebellum. These are three typical areas of posterior fossa involvement in MS.

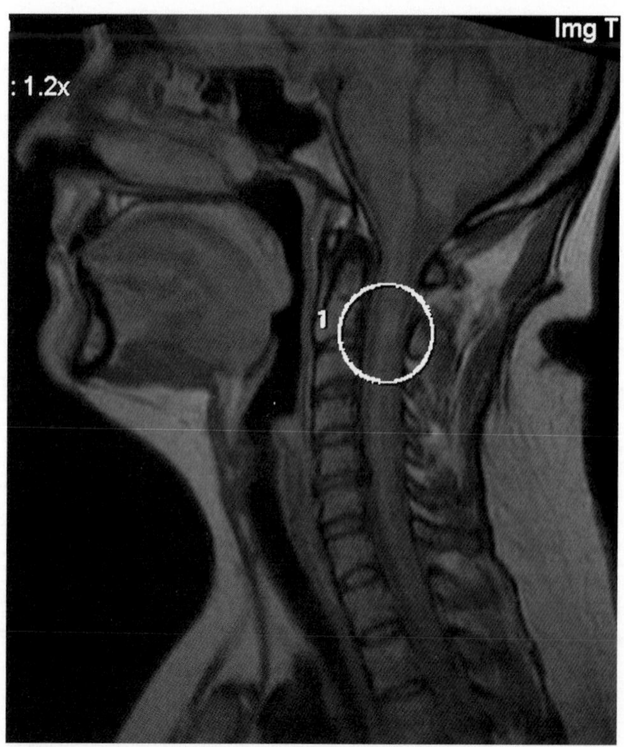

FIGURE 34.6 Hyperintense T2 spinal cord MS lesion (*1 circled*) in the high cervical cord. MS lesions typically traverse 1 or 2 contiguous spinal levels and less than 50 of the cord cross-sectional area.

TABLE 34.5

CLINICAL FACTORS WITH PROGNOSTIC VALUE IN MS

Favorable	Unfavorable
Younger age at onset	Older age at onset
Female	Male
Normal MRI at presentation	High lesion load on MRI at presentation
Complete recovery from first relapse	Lack of recovery from first relapse
Low relapse rate	High relapse rate
	Early cerebellar involvement
Long interval to second relapse	Short interval to second relapse
Low disability at 2 and 4 y	Early development of mild disability
	Insidious motor onset

the chapter on Infectious Diseases of the Spinal Cord (see Chapter 32) because isolated TM is usually a post infectious sequela. It is useful to review the terminology that is currently used to describe the two distinct presentations of TM. Patients presenting with incomplete patchy involvement of at least one spinal segment, with mild to moderate weakness, patchy sensory loss, occasional bladder involvement are at highest risk (80% to 90% within 3 years) for developing MS. Brain MRI is needed to determine if lesions are present. These cases are termed acute partial TM. In contrast, those patients who present with acute complete TM have moderate to severe weakness, typical bladder involvement, and significant disability, but low risk of conversion to CDMS (less than 2% at 5 years) (56). These patients typically have an antecedent infection and they are discussed further in Chapter 32.

TREATMENT

The treatment of MS can be divided into three broad categories: (a) treatment of acute relapses, (b) immunotherapies for relapse prevention/disease modification, and (c) symptomatic management. Use of specific medications under each of these categories is usually not mutually exclusive with relation the timing their implementation.

A MS relapse as defined by the McDonald criteria is an episode of neurological disturbance lasting at least 24 hours, corresponding to a new focal area of inflammation/demyelination within the CNS, and reliably distinguished from pseudorelapse or symptom fluctuations brought on by body temperature elevations (40). Fleeting or paroxysmal symptoms (such as trigeminal neuralgia or tonic spasms) that last more then 24 hours can also be diagnosed as a relapse. Treatment for acute relapses aims to hasten remission of symptoms from that exacerbation. The gold standard for treatment of acute relapses is corticosteroids, which speed recovery but do not affect long-term progression of disease activity. A typical steroid treatment for an acute relapse is 1 g methyprednisolone (MP) IV daily for 3 days as recommended by the 2002 North American guidelines (57) and the 2004 European Consensus Group on therapy. An oral equivalent dose can be utilized but gastrointestinal and psychiatric side effects (insomnia; psychosis) were shown to be higher. Intravenous MP is preferred over ACTH, which had been used more frequently in the past (57). Although MP is most commonly used, there is insufficient evidence to determine a clear "best" choice of steroid, nor is there sufficient evidence to determine if a steroid taper is necessary after the high-dose bolus. It is generally recommended to have patients on oral calcium and vitamin D supplementation, as well as H2 blockade therapy while on steroids. Also anxiolytic medication and/or sleep aids are needed for some patients while on steroids.

Other therapeutic options for treatment of acute relapse are (a) plasmaphoresis, which involves removal, filtering, and return of blood plasma from the patient's bloodstream and (b) the use of intravenous immunoglobulin (IVIg), which remains controversial (58). In one controlled study, the concurrent use of a planned comprehensive rehabilitation team intervention during IV steroid treatment has been shown to be more effective than IV steroid therapy alone during relapses (59).

Disease Modifying Therapies

This class of medication aims to prevent relapse and disease progression and therefore disability. To date, there is no cure for MS, and up until 1993, no drugs were proven to be effective in modifying disease progression in MS. Since that time, seven immunomodulating disease modifying therapies (DMTs) have been FDA approved and proven to be useful, albeit palliative, in decreasing clinical and MRI exacerbations, or slowing the rate of clinical and MRI deterioration. These include the (a) human proteins or human protein derivatives interferon β1a (Avonex; Rebif) and β1b (Betaseron; Extavia), glatiramer acetate (Copaxone), (b) an immunosuppressive drug mitoxantrone (Novantrone), and (c) a monoclonal antibody natalizumab (Tysabri), and (d) a sphingosine 1-phosphate (S1P) receptor modulator. In general, the human proteins are preferable as first-line drugs because of their excellent risk-benefit profile. One of them should generally be administered as soon as the diagnosis of MS is made. There is now evidence that suggests that the interferons and glatiramer delay conversion to CDMS in those high-risk CIS patients over a period of 2 to 5 years as compared to placebo. Both interferon β1b and 1a and glatiramer acetate (which is not an interferon and whose mode of action is different from interferon β) are approved by the FDA for this indication (60,61) (see Table 6).

In 2006, the National Multiple Sclerosis Society published treatment guidelines that underscore the importance of the early and accurate diagnosis of early MS symptoms, initiation of a DMT as soon as the diagnosis of MS is made, and the continued treatment with a DMT with reevaluation in the setting of intolerance or treatment failure (60,61). Each DMT has proven efficacy. Making exact comparisons among pivotal trials for each agent is difficult because each of the pivotal trials was carried out using dissimilar protocols. The choice of which product to prescribe should be made in conjunction with the patient, considering lifestyle issues, efficacy, and side effect profile. Both interferon treatments (interferon β1a [Avonex, Rebif] and interferon β1b [Betaseron; Extavia]) and glatiramer acetate (GA; Copaxone) can be used for patients upon diagnosis of MS as results from three head-to-head trials to date suggest comparable effectiveness between these four compounds. Two studies have demonstrated differences in efficacy (62,63). Side effects with GA include mild injection site reaction and rare immediate postinjection reactions, which are systemic reactions with chest pain, dyspnea, and anxiety. There is no direct cardiac effect. With the interferons, the main side effects include flu-like symptoms, fatigue, increased spasticity, and headaches. Management of patients with interferons includes monitoring for antidrug neutralizing antibodies (NABs). Multiple independent studies have demonstrated decreased efficacy in patients developing NABS. Indeed, neurologists have adapted a consensus statement supporting regular monitoring for NABs in all patients on interferon therapy (64).

Immunosuppressant drugs have been used for more than 20 years with limited benefit in the treatment of progressive MS. Mitoxantrone (Novantrone) is the only agent approved for the treatment of SPMS. It is an anthracenedione antineoplastic agent that intercalates with DNA and exerts a potent immunomodulating effect that suppresses humoral immunity, reduces T cell numbers, decreases T helper cell activity, and enhances T suppressor cell function. It has been shown to slow worsening of disability. The main limiting factor regarding this drug is a dose-related idiopathic cardiotoxicity and life time dose limiting the length of time that it can be used in MS.

Natalizumab (Tysabri), a monoclonal antibody against VLA4, a leukocyte adhesion molecule, demonstrated the largest effect on relapse reduction, MRI changes and delaying the accumulation of physical disability in the pivotal trials that lead to its FDA approval in fall of 2004. Three months later, it was voluntarily withdrawn from the market by the manufacturer after the first reported cases of progressive multifocal leukoencephalopathy (PML), a typically fatal brain disease. These initial cases only occurred in patients receiving combined therapy with a second immunomodulating agent. Reintroduction of the drug in 2006 and its current availability is through a risk minimization program. Since the rerelease of natalizumab as a monotherapy, there have conitinue to be cases of PML occurring and the incidence of PML is stated in the label (65).

In September 2010 the FDA approved fingolimod (Gilenya) as a first in class, oral immunomodulating therapy for relapsing forms of MS. Efficacy appears to be interferon-like, the side effects relate to the presence of S1P receptors on sites other than the central nervous system. Thus monitoring is recommended for bradycardia, macular edema, infections, decreased pulmonary function, hepatic effects (66).

Treatment of MS-Related Symptoms

Symptomatic therapy for weakness, spasticity, tremors, diplopia, paroxysmal attacks (including trigeminal neuralgia), impotence, pain, bladder and bowel dysfunction, depression, fatigue, and pseudobulbar emotional incontinence are available and should be deployed to maximize patient function and comfort. Treatment of spasticity related to MS is no different from treatment of spasticity in other spinal cord–related diseases. The only caution is that MS-related fatigue can make tolerance of sedating antispasticity medication more difficult. Medications such as baclofen (both oral and intrathecal), tizanidine, and diazepam are most commonly used. Spasticity treatments are discussed further in Chapter 15.

TABLE 34.6

DISEASE MODIFYING THERAPIES

Drug (brand name) and its FDA-approved indication(s)	Dose and route of administration	Known or presumed mode of action	Side effects/reported serious adverse events
Interferon β 1a (Avonex), RRMS; CIS 1a (Rebif), RRMS 1b (Betaseron), RRMS; CIS	30 μg once weekly by IM injection 44 μg three times weekly by SQ injection 250 μg every other day by SQ injection	As a group the interferons inhibit T-cell migration across BBB by 1. reducing matrix metalloproteinase production 2. reducing efficiency of antigen presentation 3. reducing inflammatory cytokine production	As a group the interferons cause flu-like symptoms; potential liver function impairment; lymphopenia; potential depression; site reactions; Nabs
Glatiramer acetate (Copaxone), RRMS; CIS	20 mg daily by SQ injection	Increase regulatory T and B cells and reduce inflammatory cytokine production	Site reactions; immediate postinjection reactions
Mitoxantrone (Novantrone) worsening RRMS; SPMS; PRMS	12 mg/m² every 3 mo lifetime dose 140 mg/m² by IV infusion	Known immunosuppressive: Inhibits DNA synthesis thus depletes white blood cells as a group including T cells; reduces inflammatory cytokines	Leukemias; idiopathic cardiotoxicity; infections; low WBCs; infections; hair thinning; blue-green urine 24 h postinfusion
Natalizumab (Tysabri) RRMS Monotherapy only through prescribing program	300 mg each month IV infusion	Binds and blocks adhesion molecule on activated lymphocytes, thus preventing transmigration across BBB	Rare: possibly fatal PML; infusion allergic reactions; headache; arthralgias; Nabs; anti-JCV antibody testing will stratify risk of PML
Fingolimod (Gilenya) Relapsing forms of MS	0.5 mg hard capsule; one PO daily	Sequesters lymphocytes and neutrophils (not monocytes) in lymph nodes	Bradyarrhythmias and atrioventricular blocks, infections, macular edema, respiratory effects, hepatic effects

RRMS, relapsing remitting multiple sclerosis; SPMS, secondary progressive multiple sclerosis; PRMS, progressive relapsing multiple sclerosis; CIS, clinically isolated syndrome; Mg, milligrams; BBB, blood brain barrier; WBCs, white blood cells; Nabs, need to check for neutralizing antibodies that reduce efficacy of the medication; IV, intravenous; PO, orally; PML, progressive multifocal leukoencephalopathy; JCV, John Cunningham Virus, the causative virus for PML.

Fatigue is seen in up to 80% of patients and can often interfere with daily activities. Treatment options include medications such as amantadine (Symmetrel) (100 to 300 mg daily), methylphenidate (Ritalin) (10 to 30 mg daily), modafinil (Provigil) (100 to 400 mg daily), armodafinil (Nuvigil) (150 to 300 mg), and selective serotonin reuptake inhibitors. All of these medications are used "off label" for fatigue and often require preauthorization through third-party payors. In evaluating patients with fatigue, the possibility of a sleep disorder such as sleep apnea or drug abuse should be ruled out. Appropriate use of assistive devices (scooters, walkers, wheelchairs) that help to conserve energy expenditure should also be discussed with patients (67).

Bladder, bowel, and sexual dysfunction associated with MS are treated similarly to other spinal cord diseases and will be addressed in Chapters 13 and 23, respectively. Urodynamic studies may be extremely helpful in guiding treatment and can sometimes be a diagnostic test related to initial diagnosis when urgency or incontinence are initial MS symptoms. See Chapter 13 for more information on urodynamics.

Tremors and incoordination in MS may be helped with medications such as clonazepam, isoniazid, propranolol, and ondansetron or with the use of weighted bracelets and arm rests. Unfortunately, tremors are difficult to treat and medication can cause sedation or side effects. There is conflicting evidence as to the possible usefulness of deep brain stimulation, as used in Parkinson disease, for the worst cases of tremor.

Paroxysmal motor and sensory attacks frequently occur during the course of MS. If associated with an acute attack of MS, corticosteroids may accelerate their resolution. Symptomatic relief is usually readily achievable using carbamazepine, gabapentin, or baclofen. Brief courses of these medications may suffice but often long-term therapy is required (67).

Pain can be treated by first identifying its cause. Musculoskeletal pains are common in MS patients, often due to mechanical imbalances and associated degenerative changes. CNS pain can be treated with analgesics, amitriptyline or other tricyclic antidepressants, carbamazepine, and gabapentin. Muscle spasms can be treated as for spasticity.

Diplopia often resolves spontaneously or with the use of corticosteroids for an acute attack of MS. Persistent diplopia can be treated with eye patching, and severe nystagmus causing oscillopsia may improve with gabapentin or eye prisms.

Depression can be treated with antidepressant drugs, psychotherapy, and avoidance of drugs associated with causing depression whenever possible. Amitriptyline is particularly useful for pseudobulbar emotional incontinence, and benzodiazepines are of value in treating panic attacks (43).

Cognitive Impairment

It has only been over the past several years that it has been recognized that MS can cause problems with cognition, planning, and judgment. Approximately one third of patients with MS will have some problems in these areas, particularly in areas of executive functioning (68). In the vast majority of patients, these deficits are mild to moderate, with some noticeable impact on everyday activities but not severe enough to prevent functioning at work. However, in about 5% to 10% of patients, cognitive dysfunction may be so severe that the person cannot function without supervision. This can be the case even with mild physical disability. Abstract reasoning and problem solving, verbal fluency, visuospatial skills, speed of information processing, attention, and concentration, especially sustained attention and memory are the cognitive functions thought to be affected in MS. These changes occur as a result of the cerebral demyelination and axonal damage that occurs in MS, resulting in brain atrophy (68). Secondary effects of MS can contribute to cognitive dysfunction; for example, a urinary tract infection may lead to increased spasticity and worse cognitive processing. Depression, fatigue, and anxiety can affect a patient's attention and ability to concentrate and focus (68).

To accurately assess cognitive dysfunction, a full neuropsychological battery is often necessary. Pharmacologic management of cognitive dysfunction has focused on disease modifying agents that alter the course of the disease so as to slow the neuropathologic changes underlying cognitive deficits. Symptomatic treatments for improving cognition have met with limited success. Donepezil (Aricept) has been used to treat Alzheimer dementia, and has been used to help cognitive problems in MS with mixed results (69,70). Cognitive rehabilitation has been promising both to help patients with compensatory strategies such as lists, computers, and with cognitive exercises and drills.

Emotional changes have also been observed in MS. These include depression, suicidal ideation, grieving, emotional lability (pseudobulbar affect), euphoria, antisocial behavior, sexual inappropriateness, and psychotic states. Medications used to treat MS such as steroids can produce both depression and hypomanic states. Interferon therapy can also contribute to depression. Patients can be depressed as a reaction to altered life circumstances and increased disease activity. Women often will notice worsening of depression during menstruation, suggesting a hormonal effect. Assessment of emotional changes in MS is a complex undertaking. Standard treatments such as psychotherapy and pharmacologic management of symptoms such as depression are often helpful (68). A combination of detromethorphan and quinidine (Nuedexta) has been FDA approved for loss of emotional control (71).

Dysphagia and Dysarthria

Speech impairment has long been recognized as a feature in MS. Scanning speech and dysarthria are often noted. Areas of demyelination that occur in the periventricular white matter of the brain, brainstem, cerebellum, and spinal cord can interrupt the transmission of the message between the brain and the muscles in the lips, tongue, soft palate, vocal cords, and diaphragm. Since these muscles control the quality of speech and voice, dysarthria and dysphonia may result. These problems can temporarily worsen with exacerbations and fatigue. Other problems that patients notice are impairments of loudness, pitch control, decreased vital capacity, and hypernasality. Spastic dysarthria is due to bilateral lesions of the corticobulbar tracts. Patients with a harsh, strained voice quality often exhibit hypertonicity in facial muscles and palatal muscles. Ataxic dysarthria results from bilateral or generalized lesions of the cerebellum. When vocal tremor is noted, patients also exhibit intention tremor of the head, trunk, arms, and hands. Patients with rapid alternating movements of the tongue and lips often exhibit nystagmus or jerky eye movements. Mixed dysarthria can be due to a combination of generalized lesions of demyelination in the cerebral white matter and the cerebellum or spinal cord. Patients can then exhibit impaired loudness control, vocal tremor, and impaired articulation and pitch control (67).

To treat dysarthria, medications to help with spasticity, ataxia, tremor and fatigue in conjunction with therapy by a speech language pathologist are recommended. Medications such as baclofen, tizanidine, and diazepam are helpful for spasticity. Spasticity can affect speech and voice in many ways during respiration, phonation, articulation, and resonance. Too much muscle tone can restrict range of motion of the diaphragm reducing breath support. Excess tone in the vocal cords can result in a harsh, strained voice quality. Choosing the appropriate treatment strategies and objectively monitoring the effect of specific medications on speech and voice are ideally accomplished by a team approach by the physician and speech-language pathologist (67).

Symptomatic Therapy to Improve Walking

In January 2010 the FDA approved a potassium channel blocker, dalfampridine (Ampyra), to improve walking in adult patients with MS. Improvement was demonstrated by increased walking speed in two placebo-controlled clinical trials, as measured by a timed 25 foot walk (72,73). The maximum recommended dose is 10 mg twice daily, 12 hours apart with or without food (74). Not all patients respond to dalfampridine, in the first controlled study 34.8% of participants were considered responders, and in the second study 42.9%. The magnitude of improvement in speed also was variable with most responders improving their walking speed by 25% to 30% of their baseline walking speed. Dalfampridine (Ampyra) is contraindicated in patients with a history of seizures, or who have moderate to severe renal impairment (74).

REHABILITATION IN MS

When dealing with an unpredictable, often disabling disease like MS, it is important to create an environment in which patients can function as optimally as possible. Occupational therapy can be of great value in enhancing the patient's quality of life through adaptive equipment, home modifications, hand control vehicles, and maximizing the use of available motor skills for ADL. It is important for the occupational therapist to work on energy conservation strategies and routines to make the best use of limited energy reserves. Further cognitive changes with MS make mental exercises and compensatory strategies to maintain cognitive function vital. Since ataxia (incoordination) is common, OTs teach patients how to avoid rapid multi-joint movements that would promote imbalance and falls. Equipment evaluations including those to accommodate for visual changes are critical (75). Physical therapy can help enhance quality of life and ADL performance with muscle stretching, strengthening programs, balance exercises, gait training, bracing, ambulation and transfer training, deployment of safety measures, and use of assistive devices. The physical therapist works with the patient to develop a customized exercise routine. It is generally accepted that for people with MS, moderate exertion focused on maintaining consistent quality of movement is recommended. This is in contrast to people without MS where the focus is on maximal exertion to point of muscle fatigue to build strength (76). The rating of perceived exertion scale is used to help people with MS understand proper intensity of their exercise program (77). Options for exercise for MS patients should include water- or land-based activities, group or individual exercise, written instructions are always recommended, with incorporation of local classes or activities (such as Yoga, Tai Chi, or Pilates) with appropriate modifications to patients' level of functioning. Due to the effects of temperature on conduction block, some MS patients will be sensitive to elevations in their core body temperature related to strenuous exercise, or exercise in hot weather. This becomes particularly important with respect to pool-based exercise programs that are typically conducted in pools that are specifically kept warm for arthritis patients. It has traditionally been recommended that the temperature of the water for MS patients be less than 85°F; however more recently, it has been shown that individual patients may do well with temperature of the water as high as 94°F (78). The use of walking aides, braces, robotically assisted devices (79), and functional electrical stimulations are addressed in other chapters. Speech therapy is necessary for MS-related hypophonation, dysphagia, communication devices, and cognitive assessment and cognitive retaining strategies.

Inpatient Rehabilitation for Persons with MS

The indication for admission to an inpatient rehabilitation service does not differ in MS patients as compared to persons with other neurological diseases. The primary goal of an admission is to reduce levels of disability (80,81). The efficacy of such an admission for patients with PPMS has been systematically studied and those who participated in a short inpatient rehabilitation significantly improved their level of disability and handicap as compared to a wait-listed control group (80). We already mentioned benefits of a coordinated rehabilitation program after steroid treated relapse (59). Not all studies are positive, however, so there is still uncertainty about the benefits (82). As with other persons with severe disability, it is important to prevent serious complications such as pressure ulcers, urosepsis, aspiration, and severe depression in MS patients by identifying those patients at risk and deploying appropriate preventive measures. There are no published reports of the incidence of deep venous thromboses (DVTs) in MS patients. The authors feel this is an under-recognized complication especially in those with moderate to severe disability. In young patients holding the diagnosis of MS, who also have a history of multiple thrombotic events (miscarriages, DVTs, strokes, etc.), the antiphospholipid syndrome (APS or Hughes syndrome) should be considered as an alternate or concomitant diagnosis. APS has been associated with autoimmunity and has clinical features that mimic MS (83).

FUTURE DIRECTIONS

It can be anticipated that as the genetic susceptibility for MS is clarified, genomic research will result in refinement of treatment options and clarify which patients are genetically appropriate for such treatments. Another area of research is biomarker identification with the goals of being able to better diagnose and monitor disease activity and disease response to treatment. Also promising is the development of multiple other oral agents to treat MS. At the time of this writing, there are four oral immunotherapies in phase III clinical trials (laquinimod, cladribine, fumarate, and teriflunomide). Fingolimod is already approved. It has yet to be seen if oral therapies improve adherence. Similarly, the impending emergence of therapies based on use of monoclonal antibodies, such as FDA approved natalizumab and those in clinical trial (rituximab, ocrelizumab, and alemtuzumab), also may enhance adherence due to infrequent infusion schedule. However, safety issues still need to be clarified with these medications.

The first oral agent to improve walking, dalfampridine (Ampyra) has been approved by the FDA (discussed above) (72–74). Nerisperidine (Sanofi-Aventis) is similar compound in phase II clinical trial, with both sodium and potassium-channel blocking ability. This combination channel blocking prevents neuronal hyperexcitability, thereby potentially lessening seizure risk as compared to potassium channel blockade alone (84). In addition to pharmacologic intervention to improve walking, robot-assisted gait training has begun to be examined for MS patients with walking impairment (79).

The field of MS research may be challenged by the long held but possibly erroneous concepts about MS. Emerging MRI data indicate that MS is as much a disease of gray matter as it is one of white matter (85,86). Similarly, the concept that immune attack in MS is directed toward myelin is being challenged by MRI and immunological studies demonstrating autoimmune attack directed at neurons and axons. This supports the idea that MS is an autoimmune disease of the CNS, not just of myelin. Finally, the very nomenclature we use to subtype MS may have little or no relevance to underlying biology or outcomes. Whether patients respond to immunological therapies seems to relate more to markers of inflammatory disease such as relapses, Gd enhancements on MRI, or rapid disease progression, than if they are classified as RRMS, SPMS, or PPMS. Certainly, the biologically irrelevant category of PRMS has already entered the dust bin of history. In summary, progress in our understanding of MS may depend more on our ability to discard outmoded concepts of MS as it does on new scientific discovery.

References

1. Grima DT, Torrance GW, Francis G, et al. Cost and health related quality of life consequences of multiple sclerosis. *Mult Scler* 2000;6(2):91–98.
2. Firth D. The case of Auygustus d'Este (1794–1848): the first account of disseminated sclerosis. *Proc R Soc Med* 1941;34:381–384.
3. Murray TJ. Multiple sclerosis. In: *The history of a disease*. New York, NY: Demos Medical Publishing, 2005.
4. Fredrikson S, Slavenka K-H. The 150-year anniversary of multiple sclerosis: does its early history give an etiological clue? *Perspect Biol Med* 1989;32:237–243.
5. Charcot J-M. Séance du 14 mars. *C R Seances Soc Biol Fil* 1868;20:13–14.
6. Brain WR. Critical review: disseminating sclerosis. *QJM* 1930;23:343–391.
7. Kurtzke JF. MS epidemiology worldwide. One view of current status. *Acta Neurol Scand Suppl* 1995;161:23–33.
8. Kurtzke JF, Beebe GW, Norman JE. Epidemiology of multiple sclerosis in U.S. veterans: III. Migration and the risk of MS. *Neurology* 1985;35:672–678.
9. Sadovnick AD, Ebers GC. Epidemiology of multiple sclerosis: a critical overview. *Can J Neurol Sci* 1993;20:17–29.
10. Cook SD. The epidemiology of multiple sclerosis: clues to the etiology of a mysterious disease. *Neuroscientist* 1996;2:172–180.
11. Lauer K. Multiple sclerosis in the old world: the new old map (editorial). In: Firnhaber W, Laure L, eds. *Multiple sclerosis in Europe. An epidemiological update*. Darmstadt, Germany: LTV Press, 1994:14–27.
12. McLeod JG, Hammond SR, Hallpike JF. Epidemiology of multiple sclerosis in Australia with NSW and SA survey results. *Med J Aust* 1994;160:117–122.
13. Lauer K. Environmental associations with the risk of multiple sclerosis: the contribution of ecological studies. *Acta Neurol Scand Suppl* 1995;161:77–88.
14. Hillert J. Human leukocyte antigen studies in multiple sclerosis. *Ann Neurol* 1994;36:S15–S17.
15. Cook SD, Rohowsky-Kochan C, Bansil S, et al. Evidence for multiple sclerosis as an infectious disease. *Acta Neurol Scand Suppl* 1995;161:34–42.
16. Ascherio A, Munger KL. Environmental risk factors for multiple sclerosis. Part I: the role of infection. *Ann Neurol* 2007;61(4):288–299.
17. Ascherio A, Munger KL. Environmental risk factors for multiple sclerosis. Part II: noninfectious factors. *Ann Neurol* 2007;61(6):504–513.
18. Hafler DA, Compston A, Sawcer S, et al. Risk alleles for multiple sclerosis identified by a genome wide study. *N Engl J Med* 1997;357(9):851–862.
19. Kurtzke JF. Multiple sclerosis in time and space—geographic clues to cause. *J Neurovirol* 2000;6(Suppl 2): S134–S140.
20. Rose JW, Carlson NG. Pathogenesis of multiple sclerosis. Continuum lifelong learning. *Neurology* 2007;13(5):35–62.
21. Bettelli E. Building different mouse models for human MS. *Ann N Y Acad Sci.* 2007;1103:11-8.
22. Dutta R, Trapp BD. Pathogenesis of axonal and neuronal damage in multiple sclerosis. *Neurology* 2007;68 (22 Suppl 3):S22–S31.
23. Lucchinetti C, Bruck W, Parisi J, et al. A quantitative analysis of oligodendrocytes in multiple sclerosis lesions. A study of 113 cases. *Brain* 1999;122 (Pt 12): 2279–2295.
24. Weinshenker BG, Bass B, Rice GP, et al. The natural history of multiple sclerosis: a geographically based study. I. Clinical course and disability. *Brain* 1989;112(Pt 1):133–146.
25. Weinshenker BG. The natural history of multiple sclerosis. *Neurol Clin* 1995;13:119–146.
26. Burks, J, Johnson, K. *Multiple sclerosis diagnosis, medical management, and rehabilitation*. New York, NY: Demos Medical Publishing, 2000:83–93, 385–391, 405–417.
27. Kesselring J. Differential diagnosis. In: Kesselring J, ed. *Multiple sclerosis*. Chapter 11. Cambridge, UK: Cambridge University Press, 1997.
28. Frohman EM, Goodin DS, Calabresi PA, et al. The utility of MRI in suspected MS: report of the Therapeutics and Technology Assessment Subcommittee of the American Academy of Neurology. *Neurology* 2003;61(5):602–611
29. O'Riordan JI, Thomson AJ, Kingsley DP, et al. The prognostic value of brain MRI in clinically isolated syndromes of the CNS: a 10 year follow up. *Brain* 1998;121:495–503.
30. Kaufman DI, Trobe JD, Eggenberger ER, et al. Practice parameter: the role of corticosteroids in management of acute monosymptomatic optic neuritis. Report of Quality Standards Subcommittee of the American Academy of Neurology. *Neurology* 2000;54(11):2039–2044.
31. Beck RW. The optic neuritis treatment trial: three year follow-up results. *Arch Ophthalmol* 1995;113:136–137.
32. Simon J, Jacobs LD, Campion MK, et al. A longitudinal study of brain atrophy in relapsing multiple sclerosis. *Neurology* 1999;53:139–148.
33. Filippi M, Horsfield MA, Morrissey SP, et al. Quantitative brain MRI lesion load predicts the course of clinically isolated syndromes suggestive of multiple sclerosis. *Neurology* 1994; 44:635–641.
34. Khoury SJ, Guttman CRG, Orav EJ, et al. Longitudinal MRI in multiple sclerosis: correlation between disability and lesion burden. *Neurology* 1994;44:2120–2124.
35. Jones SJ. Clinical assessment of central nervous system axons: evoked potentials. In: Waxman SG, Kocsis JD, Stys PK, eds. *The axon—structure, function and pathophysiology*. New York, NY: Oxford Press, 1995:629–643.
36. Fraser C, Klistorner A, Graham S, et al. Multifocal visual evoked potential latency analysis: predicting progression to multiple sclerosis. *Ach Neurol* 2006;63(6):847–850.
37. Cohen JA, Ruddick RA, eds. *Multiple sclerosis therapeutics*. 2nd ed. London, UK: Martin Dunitz Ltd., 2003.
38. Jacobs LD, Kaba SE, Miller CM, et al. Correlation of clinical. Magnetic resonance imaging, and cerebrospinal fluid findings in optic neuritis. *Ann Neurol* 1997;41: 392–398.
39. Schumacher GA, Beebe GW, Kibler RF, et al. Problems of experimental trials of therapy in multiple sclerosis: report by the panel on the evaluation of experimental trials of therapy in multiple sclerosis. *Ann N Y Acad Sci* 1965;122:552–568.
40. Poser CM, Paty DW, Scheinberg L, et al. New diagnostic criteria for multiple sclerosis: guidelines for research protocols. *Ann Neurol* 1983;13(3):227–231.
41. McDonald WI, Compston A, Edan G, et al. Recommended diagnostic criteria for multiple sclerosis: guidelines from

the International Panel on the diagnosis of multiple sclerosis. *Ann Neurol* 2001;50(1):121–127.
42. Swanton JK, Fernando K, Dalton, CM, et al. Modification of MRI criteria for multiple sclerosis in patients with clinically isolated syndromes. *J Neurol Neurosurg Psychiatr* 2006;77(7):830–833.
43. Swanton JK, Rovira A, Tintore M, et al. MRI criteria for multiple sclerosis in patients presenting with clinically isolated syndromes: a multicentre retrospective study. *Lancet Neurol* 2007;6:677–686.
44. Brex PA, Ciccarelli O, O'Riordan JI, et al. A longitudinal study of abnormalities on MRI and disability from multiple sclerosis. *N Engl J Med* 2002;346:158–164.
45. Polman CH, Reingold SC, Banwell B, et al. Diagnostic criteria for multiple sclerosis: 2010 Revisions to the McDonald criteria. *Ann Neurol* 2011;69(2):292–302.
46. Lublin FD, Reingold SC. Defining the clinical course of multiple sclerosis: results of an international survey. *Neurology* 1996;46:907–911.
47. Martinelli V, Rodegher M, Moiola L, et al. Late onset multiple sclerosis: clinical characteristics, prognostic factors, and differential diagnosis. *Neurol Sci* 2004;25:S350–S355.
48. Kurtzke JF. Rating neurologic impairment in multiple sclerosis: an expanded disability status scale (EDSS). *Neurology* 1983;33:1444–1452.
49. Rudick R, Cutter G, Baier M, et al. Use of the multiple sclerosis functional composite to predict disability in relapsing MS. *Neurology* 2001;56:1324–1330.
50. Richards RG, Sampson FC, Beard SM, et al. A review of the natural history and epidemiology of multiple sclerosis: implications for resource allocation and health economic models. *Health Technol Asses* 2002;6(10):1–73.
51. Confavreux C, Hutchinson M, Hours MM, et al. Pregnancy in multiple sclerosis group. Rate of pregnancy-related relapse in multiple sclerosis. *N Engl J Med* 1998;339:285–291.
52. Brønnum-Hansen H, Stenager E, Hansen T, et al. Survival and mortality rates among Danes with MS. *Int MS J* 2006;13:67–71.
53. Wingerchuk DM, Lennon VA, Pittock SJ, et al. Revised diagnostic criteria for neuromyelitis optica. *Neurology* 2006;66(10):1485–1489.
54. Cree BAC, Lamb S, Morgan K, et al. An open label study of the effects of rituximab in neuromyelitis optica. *Neurology* 2005;64:1270–1272
55. Jacob A, Weinshenker BG, Violich I, et al. Treatment of neuromyelitis optica with rituximab: retrospective analysis of 25 patients. *Arch Neurol* 2008;65(11):1443–1448.
56. Scott TF. Nosology of idiopathic transverse myelitis syndromes. ACTA *Neurol Scand* 2007;115:371–376.
57. Sellebjerg F, Barnes D, Filippini G, et al. EFNS guideline on treatment of multiple sclerosis relapses: report of an EFNS task force on treatment of multiple sclerosis relapses. *Eur J Neurol* 2005;12(12):939–946.
58. Fazekas F, Lublin FD, Li D, et al. Intravenous immunoglobulin in relapsing-remitting multiple sclerosis. A dose finding trial. *Neurology* 2008;71:265–271.
59. Craig J, Young CA, Ennis M, et al. A randomized controlled trial comparing rehabilitation against standard therapy in multiple sclerosis patients receiving intravenous steroid treatment. *J Neurol Neurosurg Psychiatry* 2003;74(9):1225–1230.
60. National MS Society. Treatment recommendations for physicians:www.nationalmssociety.org/docs/HOM/ExpOp_Rehab.pdf; January 29, 2008.
61. Thrower BW. Clinically isolated syndrome: predicting and delaying multiple sclerosis. *Neurology* 2007;68(24 Suppl 4):S12–S15.
62. Durelli L, Verdun E, Barbero P, et al. Every other day interferon beta 1b versus once weekly interferon beta 1a for multiple sclerosis: results of a 2-year prospective randomized multicenter study (INCOMIN) *Lancet* 2002;359:1453–1460.
63. Schwid SR, Thorpe J, SHarief M, et al. Enhanced benefit of increasing interferon beta 1a dose and frequency in relapsing remitting multiple sclerosis: The Evidence Study. *Arch Neurol* 2005;62:785–792.
64. Polman CH, Deisenhammer F, Giovannoni G, et al. Neutralizing antibodies to interferon beta: Assessment of their clinical and radiographic impact: an evidence report: report of the Therapeutics and Technology Assessment Subcommittee of the American Academy of Neurology. *Neurology* 2007;69(15):1553–1555.
65. http://www.tysabri.com/tysbProject/tysb.portal/_baseurl/threeColLayout/SCSRepository/en_US/tysb/home/index.xml
66. http://www.pharma.us.novartis.com/product/pi/pdf/gilenya.pdf
67. Schapiro RT. *Managing the symptoms of multiple sclerosis*. 5th ed. New York, NY: Demos Medical Publishing LLC, 2007.
68. Prakash RS, Snook EM, Lewis JM, et al. Cognitive impairments in relapsing-remitting multiple sclerosis: a meta-analysis. *Mult Scler* 2008;14:1250–1261.
69. Krupp LB, Christodoulou C, Melville P, et al. Donepezil improved memory in multiple sclerosis in a randomized clinical trial. *Neurology* 2004;63:1579–1585.
70. Krupp LB, Christodoulou C, Melville P, et al. A multicenter randomized clinical trial of donepezil to treat memory impairment in multiple sclerosis. Proceedings from the 62nd annual American Academy of Neurology meeting, Toronto Canada; S21.004.
71. http://www.nuedexta.com/pdf/Prescribing%20Information.pdf
72. Goodman AD, Brown TR, Krupp LB, et al. on behalf of the Fampridine MS-F203 investigators. Sustained-release oral fampridine in multiple sclerosis: a randomized, double-blind, controlled trial. *Lancet* 2009;373:732–738.
73. Goodman AD, Brown TR, Cohen JA, et al.; Fampridine MS-F202 Study Group. Dose comparison trial of sustained-release fampridine in multiple sclerosis. *Neurology* 2008:71:1134–1141.
74. http://ampyra.com/local/files/PI.pdf
75. Forwell SJ, Zackowski KM. Occupational therapist. *Int J MS Care* 2008;10(3):94–98.
76. Sutliff MH. Physical therapist. *Int J MS Care* 2008;10(4): 127–131.
77. Morrison EH, Cooper DM, White IJ, et al. Ratings of perceived exertion during aerobic exercise in multiple sclerosis. *Arch Phys Med Rehabil* 2008;89(8):1570–1574.
78. Peterson C. Exercise in 94°F water for a patient with multiple sclerosis. *Phys Ther* 2001;81(4):1049–1058.
79. Beer S, Aschbacher B, Manoglou D, Gamper E, Kool J, Kesselring J. Robot-assisted gait training in

multiple sclerosis: a pilot randomized trial. *Mult Scler* 2008;14(2):231–236.
80. Freeman JA, Langdon DW, Hobart JC, Thompson AJ. The impact of inpatient rehabilitation on progressive multiple sclerosis. *Ann Neurol* 2005;42(2):236–244.
81. Khan F, Turner-Stokes L, Ng L, Kilpatrick T. Multidisciplinary rehabilitation for adults with multiple sclerosis. *Cochrane Database Syst Rev* 2007;(2):CD006036
82. Storr LK, Sørensen PS, Ravnborg M. The efficacy of multidisciplinary rehabilitation in stable multiple sclerosis patients. *Mult Scler* 2006;12(2):235–242.
83. Asherson RA, Cervera R, Merrill JT, et al. Antiphospholipid antibodies and the antiphospholipid syndrome: clinical significance and treatment. Semin Thromb Hemost 2008;34(3):256–266.
84. http://clinicaltrial.gov/ct2/show/NCT00811902
85. Pirko I, Lucchinetti CF, Sriram R, Bakshi R. Gray matter involvement in multiple sclerosis. *Neurology* 2007;68(9):634–642.
86. Zivadinov R, Reder AT, Filippi M, et al. Mechanisms of action of disease-modifying agents and brain volume changes in multiple sclerosis. *Neurology* 2008;71(2): 136–144.

CHAPTER 35 ■ ADULT MOTOR NEURON DISEASE

NANETTE C. JOYCE, GREGORY T. CARTER, AND LISA S. KRIVICKAS

Adult motor neuron disease (MND) is often considered synonymous with amyotrophic lateral sclerosis (ALS); however, it is a heterogenous group of disorders holding in common the nearly selective destruction of motor neurons within the neuraxis (1). MND can be acquired through familial inheritance, immune-mediated, infectious, toxic, malignant, or sporadic causes. Included are diseases that exclusively affect lower motor neurons (LMNs) or upper motor neurons (UMNs), in addition to ALS with its relentless destruction of both.

There is no universally accepted classification system for MND. These diseases are often stratified based on whether the dysfunction is localized to the LMN, UMN, or both. However, this strategy is complicated by progressive muscular atrophy (PMA), primary lateral sclerosis (PLS), and progressive bulbar palsy (PBP). These MNDs blur the boundaries, as their course often progresses from a pure UMN or LMN syndrome to frank ALS. Whether these conditions exist as distinct diseases or represent part of the spectrum of ALS is still debated. At least one form of PLS, with a benign course, restricted to UMN involvement, has been reported (2,3). Others classify MNDs under the umbrella terms *typical* and *atypical* MND. Typical MND includes sporadic and hereditary juvenile or adult ALS with both UMN and LMN involvement. Other MNDs such as PMA, PLS, and PBP, whose phenotypes deviate from this pattern, are classified as atypical MNDs.

In the United States, ALS is also referred to as Lou Gehrig disease after the beloved Yankees baseball star whose fans watched as the ravaging effects of ALS ran its course. Arguably, he remains the most famous celebrity diagnosed with ALS. His story is sadly poignant as a nearly classic case of ALS. On July 4th, 1939 he announced his retirement from baseball in front of a packed Yankees Stadium. In 1941, at the age of 36 and only 2 years after his diagnosis, Lou Gehrig "the iron horse" succumbed to the disease. While it is beyond the scope of this chapter to provide a detailed review of all motor neuron disorders, a select group of diseases is introduced as illustrative of the larger group as a whole to provide the reader with a framework for the evaluation, diagnosis, management, and rehabilitation of adults with MND. The primary focus is, however, a discussion regarding ALS—the most common adult MND—as the diagnostic and therapeutic strategies used to treat patients living with ALS can often be applied broadly across all adult MNDs.

OVERVIEW OF THE MAJOR ADULT MOTOR NEURON DISEASES

Typical Motor Neuron Disease

Amyotrophic Lateral Sclerosis

ALS is a rapidly progressive neurodegenerative disease caused by the loss of both UMNs and LMNs in the motor cortex, brain stem, and spinal cord, resulting in spasticity, diffuse muscular atrophy, and weakness. Most cases of ALS are presumably acquired and occur sporadically. However, approximately 10% of all ALS cases are familial ALS (FALS) and usually inherited as an autosomal dominant trait, although, recessive, X-linked and mitochondrial cases have been reported. In 1993, the first disease-causing gene was identified in a family with FALS and was localized to chromosome 21q22.1, encoding for the antioxidant enzyme Cu/Zn superoxide dismutase (SOD1) (4,5). More than 135 disease-causing SOD1 mutations have since been identified, representing approximately 20% of all FALS cases (4–6). A single-base substitution is the most common SOD1 mutation, and in the United States, the most common nucleotide substitution is alanine to valine at position four (A4V) (7). Evidence suggests that these mutations result in a toxic gain of function due to the abnormal tertiary structure, misfolding, of the SOD1 protein rather than direct impairment in the antioxidant function of the enzyme, leading to cell apoptosis (5,6,8).

Multiple disease-causing genes have now been identified, including fused in sarcoma (FUS), vesicle-associated membrane protein-associated protein B/C, angiogenin, TAR DNA-binding protein (TARDBP), and CHMP2B in addition to others (9–11). Phenotype association studies are beginning to suggest correlations between genotype, age of onset, rate of disease progression, and location of disease onset (9).

The etiology of sporadic ALS (SALS) is as yet unknown. Data have implicated a multifactorial process with a complex array of pathogenic cellular mechanisms that end in a final common pathway of motor neuron apoptosis. At least nine cellular mechanisms have been implicated including excitotoxicity from excessive glutamate activity, oxidative stress with accumulation of reactive oxygen species, mitochondrial and astroglial dysfunction, impaired axonal transport, neurofilament aggregation, protein misfolding with endoplasmic reticulum stress and buildup of cytoplasmic inclusions, inflammatory dysfunction with abnormal microglial and dendritic cell activation, and deficits of neurotrophic factors leading to dysfunction of signaling pathways resulting in early cell apoptosis (12). Both abnormal FUS and TDP-43 proteins have been identified not only in FALS patients but also in those with sporadic disease (13). This commonality offers hope for new insight into the underlying pathogenesis of sporadic disease and suggests the possibility of a single upstream inciting event.

Epidemiology of Amyotrophic Lateral Sclerosis. ALS most commonly strikes people between 50 and 74 years of age with a reported mean age of onset between 58 and 63 years (14–16). The incidence of ALS is reported to be approximately 1 to 3 per 100,000. In a recent population study done in the Netherlands, the incident cases peaked between the ages of 70 and 74 and then rapidly decreased suggesting that ALS may not be strictly a disease of aging (17). The overall prevalence rate is between 5 and 10 per 100,000, making it one of the most common neuromuscular diseases worldwide (17,18). Although many population-based studies have attempted to identify causal associations, most positive findings have been only weakly associated and repeat studies have revealed conflicting findings. Perhaps the most consistent association is seen with tobacco use. A recently published study by Wang et al., published in 2011, used pooled data from five large prospectively followed cohorts, including over 1 million subjects (19). They identified 832 ALS diagnoses and from this cohort compared smoking-related exposure. They found that smoking increased the risk of ALS when compared to those who had never smoked with relative risks of 1.44 with $p < 0.001$ for current smokers and 1.42 with $p < 0.02$ for previous smokers. In addition, they found that the earlier the exposure, the higher the risk of ALS ($p = 0.03$).

Further, population studies suggest that the incidence of ALS is increasing, although this is probably due in large part to people living longer and better recognition of the diagnosis (20,21). Studies searching for an environmental trigger have been spurred by disease clustering, most profoundly demonstrated in the Western Pacific Region of the world where the prevalence in some regions is currently three times higher than elsewhere but has been reported as 50 times higher during the 1950s to 1960s (22). Other sporadic cluster cases have been reported, but without obvious environmental or causative factors (18). Consistently men appear to be more commonly affected than women, with a male to female ratio of about 1.5:1.0 (14,17).

Poor prognostic factors include older age at the time of onset, female sex, bulbar or pulmonary dysfunction early in the clinical course of the disease, and short time from symptom onset to diagnosis (14–18). More women than men present with bulbar symptoms, and the progression of bulbar palsy appears to be more rapid in women (23,24). Young men with ALS may have a longer life expectancy, but the overall median 50% survival rate is approximately 2 years postdiagnosis, except in patients with primary bulbar symptoms, in whom the 50% survival rate is only 1 year. Survival rates vary to a degree depending on the patient's decision to use or not use noninvasive or invasive mechanical ventilation and a feeding tube. Nonetheless, by 5 years postdiagnosis, the overall survival rate is only 28% (14,16,18). Atypical, "ALS-like," MNDs have been reported infrequently as a remote complication of several malignancies, including lymphoma and small cell carcinoma of the lung (25,26). These likely represent paraneoplastic syndromes and not a true manifestation of ALS (27). Irrespective, patients with atypical MND should be screened for malignancy.

Atypical Motor Neuron Diseases

Primary Lateral Sclerosis (UMN: Sporadic)

PLS is a rare sporadic disorder characterized by progressive spasticity. Symptoms most commonly begin in the lower limb and may progress to involve the upper limbs and occasionally the bulbar region (28). Disease onset is most common in the fifth decade. Etiology of the disease is unknown. PLS can be clinically difficult to distinguish from hereditary spastic paraplegia (HSP) and is most reliably identified by the lack of familial inheritance (29). Asymmetric limb onset and spasticity involving the upper limbs or bulbar region may be diagnostically helpful in distinguishing PLS from the symmetric lower limb involvement typically observed in HSP (30). Limb wasting is rare in PLS and occurs in only 2% of patients (31). Debate remains that PLS is an ALS spectrum disorder and not its own disease entity. However, purely UMN cases have been reported to persist. The likelihood of progression to frank ALS is reduced if a patient remains free of muscle wasting or other LMN symptoms for 4 years after diagnosis, and in these cases, life expectancy is greatly increased (28,31).

Hereditary Spastic Paraplegia (UMN: Hereditary)

HSP is a disorder of UMNs and presents most commonly with progressive spasticity, weakness of the lower limbs, hypertonic urinary bladder, and impaired vibration sense. It is a genetically heterogenous group with inheritance patterns including autosomal dominant, recessive, and X-linked forms (32,33). To date, 32 HSP loci and 11 HSP-related genes have been identified (34). Symptoms are characteristically symmetric and progress with a caudal to rostral pattern due to progressive degeneration of the corticospinal tract. Mild involvement of the dorsal columns occurs with progression of the disease (32). Age of onset varies and population-based studies in Ireland showed a prevalence of 1.27 per 100,000 (34).

Diagnosis is based on the clinical characteristics of the disease, neurologic examination demonstrating involvement of the corticospinal tract in both lower extremities, family history, and identification of a pathogenic mutation in a disease-causing gene (29).

HSP is also classified by clinical characteristics and can be divided into "pure" or "complex" presentations. "Pure" HSP is considered the more classic pattern with spasticity, urinary disturbance, and vibration sense impairment (32,33).

"Complex" HSP is characterized by a combination of the above symptoms with concomitant neurologic disorders such as seizures, impaired cognition, dementia, extrapyramidal disturbance, or peripheral neuropathy in the absence of other coexisting disorders such as diabetes mellitus, etc. (32,33).

Progressive Muscular Atrophy (LMN: Sporadic)

PMA is a rare sporadic neurodegenerative disease selectively affecting the anterior horn cells of the spinal cord without UMN involvement. The etiology has yet to be discovered. Significant similarities between the natural history of PMA and ALS have been observed and debate continues as to whether PMA should be considered its own clinical entity or a variant in the ALS disease spectrum (35–38). Kim et al. followed 91 patients diagnosed with PMA within a cohort of 962 patients; all others were diagnosed with ALS. Those with PMA were more likely men, were older, and lived longer than those diagnosed with ALS. Twenty-two percent of the ninety-one patients developed UMN signs within a sixty-one–month period progressing to an ALS phenotype.

Another prospective study followed 37 patients diagnosed with PMA (38). The median age of onset was 57 and distal limb weakness with muscle atrophy was the most common presenting symptom. The upper limbs were affected slightly more often than the lower limbs with either asymmetric or symmetric presentation. Bulbar symptoms were not typically evident at diagnosis but developed over the course of the disease in 43% of the patients. The onset of bulbar symptoms was a poor prognostic indictor. Other poor prognostic indicators included an FVC less than 90% predicted at the time of diagnosis and decline in the FVC within the first 6 months after diagnosis. Over the 18 months of the study, 35% of patients developed UMN signs. The 5-year survival rate was 45% with median survival of 56 months.

In addition, postmortem studies have identified degeneration of the corticospinal tract and ubiquitinated inclusions characteristic of ALS in 50% of the PMA patients studied (35).

Spinal and Spinobulbar Muscular Atrophy (LMN: Hereditary)

There are many forms of SMA, all of which involve selective destruction of anterior horn cells (39). The various forms of SMA are clinically dissimilar, with some rare forms affecting distal or bulbar muscles only. The most common forms are often referred to as types I, II, and III (39). These are mostly disorders of childhood and are usually inherited as autosomal recessive traits. SMA-I, also known as Werdnig-Hoffman disease (WHD) or acute, infantile-onset SMA, is a severe disorder most often resulting in death before the age of two. SMA-II, also referred to as early-onset, intermediate SMA or chronic WHD, is less severe, with signs and symptoms becoming apparent in the first 6 to 18 months of life. SMA-III, also known as Kugelberg-Welander disease, is a chronic, late-onset disorder, associated with significantly less morbidity. Signs and symptoms of SMA-III usually become apparent between the ages of 5 and 15. In prior studies looking at SMA-II and SMA-III over a 10-year period, subjects with SMA-II showed marked weakness and progressive decline of strength (39). Subjects with SMA-III had a relatively static or very slowly progressive course and were far stronger (39). In both SMA-II and SMA-III, proximal weakness was greater than distal weakness. Joint contractures, progressive scoliosis, and restrictive lung disease (RLD) were present in most of the individuals with SMA-II, but these complications were rare in those with SMA-III (39).

There are two forms of SMA that have onset in the adult age group. One is an adult-onset form of SMA, which may be referred to as SMA-IV, with age of onset of 17 to 55 years with either recessive or dominant forms of inheritance (40,41). The disease clinically appears much like SMA-III, although it may be more progressive. The other form is SBMA or Kennedy disease. This disorder, which was first described as recently as 1968, is a sex-linked, recessive MND characterized by progressive spinal and bulbar muscular atrophy, gynecomastia, and reduced fertility (42,43). In relation to PMA, adult-onset SMA progresses more slowly. In addition, the bulbar and respiratory muscles are not usually involved in adult SMA but may be involved in PMA.

Patients with adult-onset SMA, SBMA, and SMA-III can have normal life spans, and many of the rehabilitative modalities discussed in this chapter are applicable to this population. Further, with the rapid advancement of rehabilitation technology, many patients with SMA-II are now living well into adulthood and successful pregnancies have been reported in this disease (44).

SMA is caused by a mutation in the survival motor neuron 1 gene (SMN1), which has been mapped to chromosome 5q13.2. Mutations in exons 7 and 8 of the SMN1 are present in more than 98% of patients with autosomal recessive childhood-onset SMA (40,41,45). Phenotypic severity appears to be influenced by the copy number of the nearly identical survival motor neuron 2 gene (SMN2) (46,47). Although, the most abundant protein generated by SMN2 is truncated and rapidly degraded due to splicing of exon 7 from the transcribed ribonucleic acid (RNA), a small percent of normal survival motor neuron protein is produced. In support of this theory, patients with SMA-III were found to have three to four copies of the SMN2 gene compared to one copy of the gene in SMA-I (47). Researchers are currently pursuing strategies to manipulate the SMN2 gene into producing increased levels of normal protein (48).

In addition, mutations in the neuronal apoptosis inhibitory protein (NAIP) gene also appear to affect disease severity. Deletions of NAIP have been found in approximately 67% of patients with SMA-I, 42% of those with SMA-II, and few were found in patients with adult-onset SMA, although the percentage is not known (40,41,46).

SBMA has been mapped to the androgen receptor gene on the long arm of the X chromosome (40,42). The mutation, which consists of an expansion of CAG trinucleotide repeats, occurs in the first exon of the gene, producing decreased sensitivity of androgen receptors on motor neurons. The disease has some clinical variability, although phenotypic expression does not correlate with the length of CAG trinucleotide repeats. This is in contrast to myotonic muscular dystrophy and fragile X syndrome, in which an increased number of tandem triplet repeats correlates directly with disease severity (42). Commercially available blood tests (DNA analysis) are available for SMA and SBMA. SBMA can occur without any family history or gynecomastia, and all men with atypical ALS should be tested for SBMA (42,49,50).

Prevalence rates for SMA types II and III are estimated to range from as high as 40 per million among children to around 12 per million in the general population, with adult-onset SMA and SBMA being far less common (39).

Poliomyelitis and Postpolio Syndrome (LMN: Infectious)

Prior to the development of the polio vaccine, poliomyelitis was the most common cause of acute flaccid paralysis and disability in the United States. Acute poliomyelitis is an infectious disease that targets the anterior horn cells of the spinal cord and brain stem. The responsible pathogen is the poliovirus, a small RNA virus belonging to the enterovirus group of the picornavirus family. Transmission occurs via fecal-oral route and there are three antigenically distinct strains, each with the potential to cause disease. Type I accounts for approximately 85% of cases progressing to paralytic illness. Approximately 1% of patients who contract the virus develop acute flaccid paralysis (51).

In the northern hemisphere, epidemics were most common during the summer months. Peak incidence in the United States occurred during epidemics in the first half of the 20th century culminating in 1952 with approximately 58,000 reported cases (51,52). Children under age 15 were most commonly affected.

In patients with acute infection, symptoms consist of fever, malaise, myalgia, sore throat, and gastrointestinal upset. Aseptic meningitis with headache, back pain, and stiff neck develops with increasing severity of the disease. In those who progress to paralytic disease, localized fasciculations with intensely painful myalgias occur after 2 to 5 days of illness (51). Asymmetric weakness and atrophy affecting the legs more often than either the arms or bulbar muscles progress to flaccid paralysis. Dysautonomia including labile blood pressure, cardiac arrhythmia, and gastrointestinal and urinary dysfunction can require emergent medical intervention and is associated with higher rates of mortality (51). Respiratory failure often develops rapidly if infection involves the medullary respiratory center and/or weakness of respiratory muscles. Paralysis remains static for several days to weeks, followed by slow recovery over months to years. Improvement of strength after acute paralytic polio occurs both by recovery of some neurons and by sprouting from remaining axons innervating locally denervated muscle fibers (53). The enlarged motor units can be up to eight times the normal size. Recovery is often incomplete with residual weakness and disability (53).

Late effects of poliomyelitis occur commonly in patients with history of paralytic polio. In a prospective study of 85 patients with signs of late effects of polio, the most common complaints were pain, muscular weakness, and fatigue (54). Loss of function, due to degenerative joint disease with and without nerve entrapment, was diagnosed in 53% of patients. The increased incidence of symptomatic osteoarthritis was attributed to compensatory mobility patterns secondary to limb weakness, side-to-side growth disparity, and overuse of unaffected limbs.

Of the 85 patients, only 26% met criteria for the diagnosis of postpolio syndrome. Gradual or sudden onset of new progressive weakness and decreased muscular endurance after a period of at least 15 years of functional stability is suggestive of PPS. The etiology of PPS is unknown. Proposed mechanisms for the development of PPS include distal degeneration of surviving enlarged neurons due to increased metabolic demand, degeneration of terminal axonal sprouts resulting in muscle fiber denervation, neuromuscular junction dysfunction as demonstrated by increased jitter on single-fiber e1ectromyographic (EMG), and loss of neurons through the normal aging process (51,53,54). Careful medical evaluation should be undertaken to exclude other possible and potentially treatable causes of the patient's complaints.

In the 1930s, the March of Dimes was established due to public outcry (175). Their aggressive campaign raised public funds to support research and development of a vaccine. Two decades later, on April 12, 1955, Dr. Jonas Salk announced the results from the largest field trial in medical history (51,52). After injecting nearly 700,000 secondgraders with either a trivalent inactivated polio vaccine or a placebo, he observed that the vaccine had nearly eliminated subsequent infection in the treated cohort. Since 1979, there have been no cases of wild-type poliovirus infection reported within the United States.

The World Health Organization, UNICEF, Rotary International, and the U.S. Centers for Disease Control launched the Global Polio Eradication Effort in the late 1980s. Though the incidence has steadily declined, there remain a couple of countries where wild poliovirus is still endemic. However, in the first 6 months of 2010, only 452 new cases of poliomyelitis were reported worldwide, located primarily in West Africa and the Indian subcontinent (52).

DIAGNOSTIC EVALUATION OF MOTOR NEURON DISEASE

The diagnosis of ALS and other forms of adult MND is primarily a process of exclusion. Based on a history and physical examination, that identifies signs and symptoms of MND, a differential diagnosis is developed directing a workup designed to exclude processes mimicking ALS. Only in FALS with known mutations, Kennedy disease, and the few adult-onset SMA cases in which SMN mutations are detected is a definitive diagnostic test available. For most patients with signs and symptoms of MND, electrodiagnostic testing (EDX), laboratory testing, neuroimaging studies, and occasionally a muscle biopsy are used to exclude other diagnoses. The Awaji-updated El Escorial criteria (EEC), as described later in this chapter, are used to assess the certainty of a diagnosis of ALS as other disease processes are excluded.

Clinical Presentation

Patients with ALS most often seek evaluation complaining of focal weakness (60%), rarely of generalized weakness or cramps and very rarely of generalized fasciculations or respiratory failure (55). Although fasciculations are a prominent feature in most patients with ALS, patients who only complain of fasciculations and have an otherwise normal neurologic examination usually have benign fasciculation syndrome and are unlikely to develop ALS.

Symptom onset may be anywhere within the motor system. A study of 613 patients by Norris et al. (56) identified the following locations of initial symptoms: legs, 41%; arms, 34%; bulbar muscles, 24%; generalized weakness, 1%; and respiratory muscles, 1 of 613 patients. In an effort to address growing concerns within the ALS community regarding clinical trial success and design, the heterogeneity of ALS patients, and how this heterogeneity may influence outcomes in research, phenotype studies have been undertaken and eight common patterns of presentation and disease progression have been defined. Chio et al. (57) prospectively studied 1,332 patients classified by phenotype. They found distinctive and distinguishable clinical and prognostic characteristics within each group. The classic phenotype presented with upper or lower limb onset and mild pyramidal signs. This was the most common phenotype in men and second in women. Four percent of patients had concomitant frontotemporal dementia (FTD) and median survival was 2.6 years. Bulbar ALS showed equal incidence across sex. Nine percent of bulbar patients had FTD, the highest figure among phenotypes. Median survival was 2.0 years. Flail arm, with proximal limb atrophy, was relatively rare and more common in men. FTD in this group was rare and median survival was 4.0 years. Flail leg presents with progressive distal lower limb weakness and has a similar incidence between men and women. Four percent of these patients had FTD, and median survival was 3.0 years. Pyramidal ALS with spastic para/tetraparesis, one or more abnormal reflexes, and/or pseudobulbar affect, in tandem with LMN signs had the earliest onset and was equally common among men and women. Median survival was 6.3 years. The rarest phenotype was respiratory ALS with the worst median survival of 1.4 years. Pure lower motor neuron was twice as common in men. They were the youngest cohort at diagnosis (56.2 years). No patient suffered FTD and median survival was 7.3 years. Pure upper motor neuron had the slowest disease course, with a 10-year survival of 71.1%.

Evaluation

The evaluation of a patient suspected of having MND begins with a detailed history, general physical examination, and neurologic examination. On neurologic examination, one is looking for evidence of UMN and LMN dysfunction. The mental status, nonmotor cranial nerve function, sensory examination, and cerebellar examination results should be normal.

Patients with UMN pathology often complain of loss of dexterity or a feeling of stiffness in the limbs. They may note weakness, caused by spasticity, resulting from disinhibition of brain stem control of the vestibulospinal and reticulospinal tracts. Findings on examination include spasticity and hyperreflexia with abnormal spread of reflexes, clonus, or the presence of brisk reflexes despite muscle atrophy in the presence of LMN loss. The gold standard used to diagnose UMN pathology is the presence of pathologic reflexes, such as the Babinski sign, the Hoffman sign, a brisk jaw jerk, and a palmomental reflex. If the toe extensors are paralyzed, visualization of contraction of the tensor fascia lata when an attempt is made to elicit a Babinski response has the same significance as great toe extension. The corneomandibular reflex, where stimulation of the cornea provokes contralateral jaw displacement in people with corticobulbar disease, may be a more sensitive and specific indicator than the jaw jerk of UMN pathology in ALS (58).

Patients with LMN pathology usually present complaining of muscle weakness. They may also note muscle atrophy, fasciculations, and muscle cramping. Cramping may occur anywhere in the body, including the thighs, arms, and abdomen. Cramping of abdominal or other trunk muscles should raise a red flag, urging the clinician to consider a diagnosis of ALS.

Findings on examination include weakness, atrophy, hypotonia, hyporeflexia, and fasciculations. Head drop is a manifestation of neck extensor muscle weakness and has a limited differential diagnosis. ALS and myasthenia gravis are the two most common causes of head drop. Atrophy often appears first in the hand intrinsic muscles (Fig. 35.1). Although fasciculations are not a necessary criterion for the diagnosis of ALS, one should question the diagnosis when none are observed.

Signs and symptoms suggesting bulbar muscle weakness include dysarthria, dysphagia, drooling, and aspiration. These signs and symptoms may be caused by UMN or LMN dysfunction involving the bulbar muscles. Signs of spastic dysarthria, indicating UMN pathology, include a strained and strangled quality of speech, reduced rate, low pitch, imprecise consonant pronunciation, vowel distortion, and breaks in pitch. LMN dysfunction creates flaccid dysarthria in which speech has a nasal or wet quality, pitch and intensity are monotone, phrases are abnormally short, and inspiration is audible. Complaints of difficulty chewing and swallowing, nasal regurgitation, or coughing when drinking liquids are common symptoms of dysphagia in ALS.

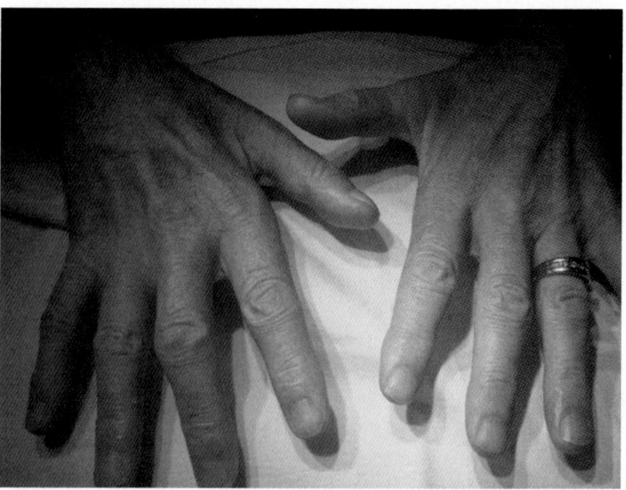

FIGURE 35.1. Hand atrophy with mild side-to-side asymmetry in a patient with amyotrophic lateral sclerosis.

On physical examination, the following tests may be used to assess facial and bulbar muscle function: ability to bury the eyelashes, pocket air in the cheeks, whistle, jaw opening and lip closure strength, and phonation of a variety of syllables such as puh, kuh, tuh, and ah. The tongue should be examined for fasciculations, atrophy, and range of motion in both protrusion and side-to-side wag (Fig. 35.2). Palate elevation should also be assessed, as it can cause early obstructive sleep apnea in patients in addition to impairing swallow. The gag reflex and jaw jerk should be assessed to look for UMN dysfunction. Pseudobulbar affect is a UMN syndrome caused by motor neuron loss in the corticobulbar tracts with disinhibition of limbic motor control, sometimes called emotional incontinence. Patients with pseudobulbar affect experience inappropriate laughter or crying that is not concordant with their mood and can be embarrassing.

In patients who present with respiratory failure, the earliest signs are often nocturnal and include poor sleep with frequent awakening, an increase in nightmares, early morning headaches, excessive daytime fatigue or sleepiness, and orthopnea. Frequent sighing, a weak cough, and difficulty clearing bronchial or pulmonary secretions are other signs of respiratory muscle weakness. Later signs of respiratory dysfunction are dyspnea with exertion, truncated speech, respiratory paradox, dyspnea when eating, rapid shallow breathing, visible accessory muscle contraction, and flaring of the nasal alae. With advanced, untreated RLD, patients may have an elevated hematocrit level, low serum chloride concentration, respiratory acidosis with a compensatory metabolic alkalosis, hypertension, and cor pulmonale.

Some patients seek initial medical attention because of fractures or sprains that do not heal. In reality, these patients probably sustained their initial injury because of a fall or other injury (e.g., sprained ankle) that occurred because of underlying muscle weakness; they were then unable to recover to their premorbid level of function because of that weakness. Other common musculoskeletal complaints include neck and back pain, shoulder pain due to a frozen shoulder, elbow flexion and ankle plantar-flexion contractures, and claw hand. Patients may experience osteoporotic fractures or stress fractures because of immobilization-induced bone density loss.

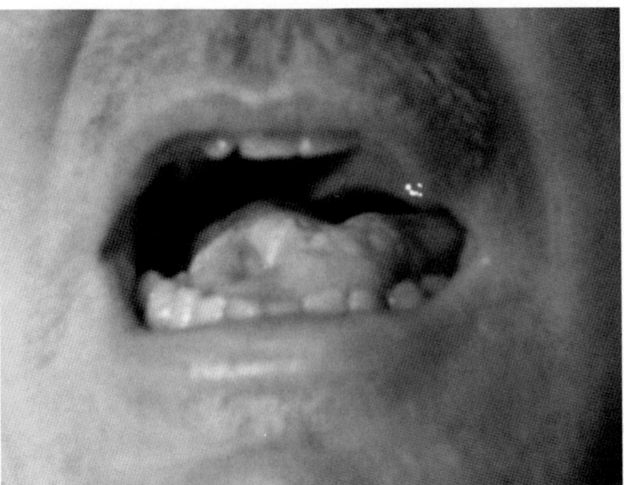

FIGURE 35.2. Tongue atrophy in amyotrophic lateral sclerosis. The patient was unable to protrude the tongue beyond the teeth and had lost the ability to elevate the palate.

Differential Diagnosis

After obtaining a history and examining the patient, the clinician is able to generate a differential diagnosis, which guides further diagnostic testing. The differential diagnosis differs depending on whether the presentation is primarily LMN, UMN, bulbar, or mixed LMN and UMN (See Table 35.1).

El Escorial-Awaji Criteria

The EEC for diagnosing ALS were developed by a task force of the World Federation of Neurology in 1990 to ensure inclusion of more homogeneous patient populations in ALS clinical trials (59). These criteria have been used to enroll patients in most of the recent clinical trials. The criteria were revised in 1998 to improve the speed and certainty of diagnosis (60) and again in December of 2006, during an international consensus conference in Awaji-shima, Japan (61). The goal of the Awaji revisions were to allow even earlier diagnosis. This change was made as a response to studies that found that 22% of ALS patients may die without reaching a diagnosis more certain than "possible" ALS.

The EEC with the Awaji-shima consensus recommendations classify the certainty level of the diagnosis of ALS as falling into one of three categories: definite, probable, and possible. The Awaji recommendations included a reaffirmation of the general principles of the EEC (61). Diagnosis in ALS is clinically based and neurophysiological examination is used only when the diagnosis is suspected clinically. Needle EMG, considered an extension of the clinical examination in detecting features of denervation and reinnervation, should have the same significance as clinical findings and, therefore, renders the category of "probable with laboratory support" obsolete (61). In addition, they recommended that fasciculation potentials be considered evidence of ongoing denervation in the absence of fibrillation potentials and positive sharp waves (PSWs). Although fasciculation potentials are seen in benign conditions, abnormal fasciculations can be identified based on a complex morphology and instability when studied with high bandpass filter and a trigger delay line (61). The use of the Awaji criteria is still being debated; however, in response to critics, prospective investigations to validate these criteria continue to be completed (62,63). One such study, by Noto et al. (63), found that the Awaji criteria increased sensitivity in the diagnosis of bulbar onset patients when compared to EEC.

TABLE 35.1

DIFFERENTIAL DIAGNOSIS OF SUSPECTED MND

UMN and LMN findings
ALS
Cervical myelopathy
Syringomyelia
Spinal cord tumor and AVM
Lyme disease
MND associated with electrical injury
Bulbar findings
Progressive bulbar palsy
Myasthenia gravis
Multiple sclerosis
Brain stem glioma
Stroke
Syringobulbia
Spinobulbar muscular atrophy
UMN findings
Primary lateral sclerosis
Multiple sclerosis
Adrenoleukodystrophy
Hereditary spastic paraplegia
Human T-lymphocyte virus–associated myelopathy
LMN findings
Progressive muscular atrophy
Spinal muscular atrophy
Spinobulbar muscular atrophy
Acute inflammatory demyelinating polyradiculoneuropathy
Chronic inflammatory demyelinating polyradiculoneuropathy
Multifocal motor neuropathy with conduction block
Poliomyelitis
Postpolio syndrome
West Nile virus
Hexosaminidase A deficiency
Monomelic amyotrophy
Brachial amyotrophic diplegia
Lambert-Eaton myasthenic syndrome
Plexopathy
Lead intoxication
Benign fasciculations

The EEC and AC divide the motor system into four regions: bulbar, cervical, thoracic, and lumbosacral. Each requires evidence of UMN and LMN pathology and progressive spread of symptoms or signs within a region or to other regions. There should be a lack of both electrophysiologic and neuroimaging evidence of other disease processes that may explain the clinical signs. The diagnostic certainty depends on how many regions reveal UMN and LMN pathology. Figure 35.3 summarizes the schema for placing patients in the three diagnostic categories. Clinical weakness, atrophy, and fasciculations are considered evidence of LMN pathology. Pathologic spread of reflexes, clonus, spasticity, and pseudobulbar features are considered evidence of UMN pathology.

Electrodiagnostic Testing

The various forms of MND, including SMA, Kennedy disease, PMA, SALS, and FALS, share several electrodiagnostic features but differ in some aspects due to varying rates of disease

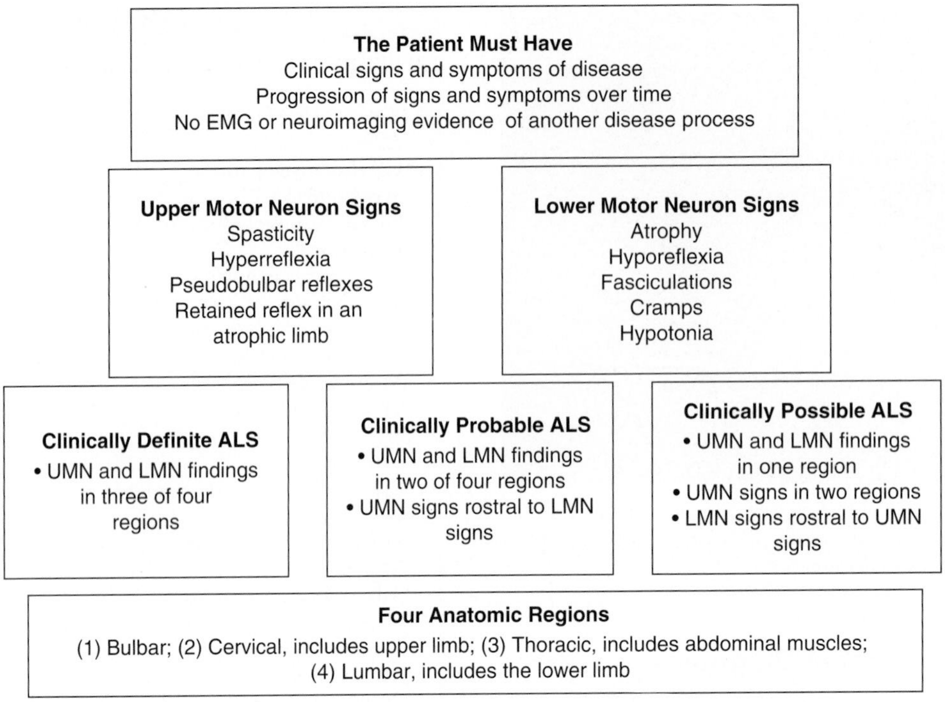

The Patient Must Have
Clinical signs and symptoms of disease
Progression of signs and symptoms over time
No EMG or neuroimaging evidence of another disease process

Upper Motor Neuron Signs
Spasticity
Hyperreflexia
Pseudobulbar reflexes
Retained reflex in an atrophic limb

Lower Motor Neuron Signs
Atrophy
Hyporeflexia
Fasciculations
Cramps
Hypotonia

Clinically Definite ALS
- UMN and LMN findings in three of four regions

Clinically Probable ALS
- UMN and LMN findings in two of four regions
- UMN signs rostral to LMN signs

Clinically Possible ALS
- UMN and LMN findings in one region
- UMN signs in two regions
- LMN signs rostral to UMN signs

Four Anatomic Regions
(1) Bulbar; (2) Cervical, includes upper limb; (3) Thoracic, includes abdominal muscles; (4) Lumbar, includes the lower limb

FIGURE 35.3. Modified El Escorial criteria from the Awaji-Shima International Conference. ALS, amyotrophic lateral sclerosis; UMN, upper motor neuron; LMN, lower motor neuron.

progression. General EDX characteristics of MND include normal sensory nerve conduction study (NCS) results, normal or low motor amplitudes depending on disease stage, and normal distal motor latencies and conduction velocities. However, with profound loss of motor amplitude, conduction velocities may drop as low as 25% lower than the lower limit of normal because of loss of the fastest conducting fibers (64). The needle electrode examination (NEE) reveals a decreased recruitment pattern, either small or large motor unit action potentials (MUAPs) with or without evidence of remodeling depending on the specific disease process, and spontaneous activity including PSWs, fibrillation potentials, fasciculations, and complex repetitive discharges (CRDs). The prominence of the various forms of spontaneous activity varies with the different forms of MND.

Electrodiagnosis in Spinal Muscular Atrophies

The EDX features of the autosomal recessive SMA types I through IV are determined by the rate of anterior horn cell degeneration and the stage in the course of the disease. Sensory NCS results are normal in all forms of SMA. Compound muscle action potentials (CMAPs) are decreased in proportion to the degree of muscle atrophy. Motor velocities are most likely to be abnormally slow in SMA-I because of the extensive loss of motor axons.

The most profound loss of MUAPs is seen in SMA-I. With maximal effort, only a few MUAPs may fire at a rapid rate. Small MUAPs are common because reinnervation cannot compensate for the rapid loss of anterior horn cells. Myopathic-appearing low-amplitude, polyphasic, short-duration units may also be seen because of muscle fiber degeneration. In the other types of SMA, one sees large-amplitude MUAPs (up to 10 or 15 mV), because the number of fibers per motor unit increases as motor unit remodeling occurs. These large units tend to be polyphasic with increased duration. Satellite potentials appear as remodeling occurs. Myopathic-appearing MUAPs are also seen in some older patients with SMA-III, and their etiology is not well understood.

On NEE in SMA-I, fibrillation potentials and PSWs are diffuse and seen in many muscles, including the paraspinals. Fasciculation potentials are relatively uncommon, but spontaneously firing MUAPs at 5 to 15 Hz, even during sleep, are a unique EDX feature of both SMA-I and SMA-II (65). In the more chronic forms of SMA, fibrillation potentials and PSWs are even more common and increase in frequency as age increases. CRDs are often seen in SMA-II and SMA-III, and fasciculations are more common than in type I (66,67).

Electrodiagnosis in Kennedy Disease

Motor NCS abnormalities are similar to those seen in other forms of MND. Although patients generally do not have sensory complaints, absence or reduction of sensory nerve action potentials (SNAPs) is a common finding (68,69). NEE shows large-amplitude and long duration MUAPs consistent with the rather indolent disease course. Fibrillation potentials and PSWs may be very prominent and present in all muscles examined. Fasciculation potentials are abundant in limb, facial, and tongue muscles.

Electrodiagnosis in Adult Nonhereditary Motor Neuron Disease

For many years, Lambert's criteria have been the standard for the EMG diagnosis of ALS (70,71). The following four criteria must be met to make a definite diagnosis of ALS: (a) PSWs or fibrillation potentials in three of five limbs, counting the head as a limb. For a limb to be considered affected, at least two muscles innervated by different peripheral nerves and roots should show active denervation; (b) normal sensory NCS results; (c) normal motor conduction studies; however, if the CMAP amplitude is very low, conduction velocity may drop as low as 70% of the lower limit of normal; and (d) reduced recruitment of MUAPs on needle examination. More recently, Cornblath et al. (72) studied 61 patients with ALS and found that even with low CMAPs, motor distal latencies and F-wave latencies did not exceed 125% of the upper limit of normal and motor conduction velocities did not fall below 80% of the lower limit of normal.

The EDX findings in PMA are identical to those in ALS; the distinction between the two diagnoses is made by the presence or absence of UMN signs on physical examination. By definition, the EDX examination is normal in PLS, and if sensory abnormalities are identified during nerve conduction studies in the setting of a purely UMN syndrome, an evaluation for HSP should be considered. In PBP, active denervation is found only in muscles of the head and neck.

NCS in ALS are characterized primarily by asymmetric decreases in CMAP amplitudes. The mild slowing of motor conduction velocity and the prolongation of F-wave latencies are attributed to loss of the fastest conducting axons and disease-specific changes in ion channels of the distal nerve. An interesting phenomenon observed in many patients is that of the split hand; CMAP amplitudes are decreased to a greater extent on the radial side of the hand than on the ulnar side. CMAPs obtained from the abductor pollicis brevis and first dorsal interosseous are much lower than those obtained from the abductor digiti minimi. When evaluating a motor nerve, more than two stimulation sites should be assessed to exclude the presence of conduction block. Multifocal motor neuropathy with conduction block, a treatable polyneuropathy, is occasionally misdiagnosed as ALS. The ulnar nerve easily can be stimulated at the wrist, below the elbow, above the elbow, in the axilla, and in the supraclavicular fossa. In limbs with UMN signs, H reflexes may be elicited from muscles in which they cannot normally be obtained. While normal sensory findings should be expected in patients with ALS, 17% of patients evaluated in a prospective multicenter study had SNAP abnormalities, and if found should not exclude a diagnosis of ALS (73). The sympathetic skin response is absent in 40%, suggesting subclinical autonomic nervous system involvement (74). Repetitive stimulation studies may show a decrement in CMAP with stimulation at 3 Hz, which is similar to that seen in myasthenia gravis. A decrement is particularly likely to be detected in patients with rapidly progressing disease and in muscles with an abundance of fasciculations (64).

The NEE is the most important part of the EDX examination in cases of suspected ALS. In patients with advanced ALS, fibrillation potentials and PSWs are prominent in most muscles, but they may be sparse early in the course of the disease. Occasionally, CRDs and doublets or triplets are seen in patients with ALS, but these are not typical findings in ALS. The thoracic paraspinals should be examined around the T8 root level during NEE, as they are not involved in tandem cervical and lumbar stenosis and can help exclude this as a diagnostic possibility. In addition, when the EEC are employed, the finding of denervation in the thoracic and either the cervical or the lumbar region is sufficient for a definite diagnosis, making examination of the tongue or facial muscles (which many patients find unpleasant) unnecessary. Although fasciculations and denervation of the tongue are considered almost pathognomonic for ALS, they are seldom found in patients who do not have clinical evidence of bulbar muscle involvement.

The recruitment pattern is decreased in involved muscles with rapid firing of MUAPs. If the disease is progressing relatively slowly, MUAP amplitudes and durations become increased, but if the course is very rapid, denervation outpaces reinnervation, and enlarged MUAPs do not have time to develop. The density and distribution of fasciculations and fibrillations do not correlate with disease course or prognosis, and therefore, serial EDX examinations, once a definite diagnosis has been made, are not useful for monitoring disease progression.

Neurophysiologists have begun to explore the use of transcranial magnetic stimulation as a method of identifying subclinical UMN dysfunction. Results are contradictory with respect to the sensitivity and specificity of various findings as evidence of UMN dysfunction, and these techniques must be considered experimental at present. Abnormalities suggesting UMN pathology include a motor evoked potential (MEP) much lower in amplitude than the CMAP recorded from the same muscle, prolonged central motor conduction time, decreased MEP thresholds, and prolongation of the contralateral silent periods and transcallosal inhibition when compared to healthy controls (75–78).

Neuroimaging

Imaging studies are used to exclude possibilities other than MND from the differential diagnosis. Magnetic resonance imaging (MRI) is the primary imaging modality used in the evaluation of patients with suspected ALS. Almost all patients should have an MRI of the cervical spine to rule out cord compression, a syrinx, or other spinal cord pathology. The location of symptoms will dictate whether other regions of the spinal cord should be imaged. In patients presenting with the PMA phenotype, an MRI of the involved region of the spinal cord with gadolinium should be considered to look for a metastatic polyradiculopathy. In those presenting with bulbar symptoms, a brain MRI should be performed to rule out stroke, tumor, and syringobulbia.

Although MRI is generally not performed to confirm a diagnosis of ALS, a few associated abnormalities have been reported. Rarely, spinal cord and motor cortex atrophy is apparent. Corticospinal tract hyperintensity with T2 imaging has been observed in a few younger patients with a predominance of UMN signs (55).

Laboratory Evaluation and Other Diagnostic Tests

In most neuromuscular clinics, a routine panel of laboratory tests is performed for all patients suspected of having ALS. A suggested set of such tests is provided in Table 35.2. The rationale behind performing this extensive battery of tests is to assess the general health of the patient and to exclude treatable conditions. The differential diagnosis, developed after the history and physical examination, may suggest that more specialized testing be performed. Table 35.3 suggests additional tests that may be warranted when the presentation is with the PMA, the PLS, or the PBP phenotype. When there is a family history of MND, testing for the most common gene abnormalities, SOD1, FUS, and TARDBP should be considered.

TABLE 35.2

SUGGESTED LABORATORY STUDIES

Hematology
- Complete blood count
- Sedimentation rate

Chemistry
- Electrolytes, BUN, creatinine
- Glucose
- Hemoglobin A_{1C}
- Calcium
- Phosphorous
- Magnesium
- Creatine kinase
- Liver function tests
- Serum head level
- Urine heavy metal screen
- Vitamin B_{12}
- Folate

Endocrine
- T4, thyroid-stimulating hormone

Immunology
- Serum immunoelectrophoresis
- Urine assay for Bence Jones proteins
- Antinuclear antibody
- Rheumatoid factor
- GM1 antibody panel

Microbiology
- Lyme titre
- Venereal Disease Research Laboratories test

Optional
- Human immunodeficiency virus test—if risk factors present
- Anti-Hu antibody—if suspicion of malignancy

TABLE 35.3

SPECIALIZED LABORATORY EVALUATION BASED ON PATIENT PRESENTATION

Phenotype	Test	Diagnosis to be excluded
PMA	DNA:CAG repeat on X chromosome	SBMA
	DNA:SMN gene	SMA
	Hexosaminidase A	Hexosaminidase A Deficiency
PLS	Voltage-gated Ca^{2++} channel Ab	Lambert-Eaton Myasthenic Syndrome
	CSF examination	Polyradiculopathy-infectious or neoplastic
	Very-long-chain fatty acids	Adrenoleukodystrophy
	HTLV-1 Ab	HTLV myelopathy
PBP	Parathyroid hormone	Hyperparathyroidism
	CSF examination	Multiple sclerosis
	Acetylcholine receptor Ab	Myasthenia gravis
	DNA:CAG repeat on X chromosome	SBMA

Ab, antibody; CSF, cerebrospinal fluid; PBP, primary bulbar palsy; PLS, primary lateral sclerosis; PMA, progressive muscular atrophy; SBMA, spinobulbar muscular atrophy; SMA, spinal muscular atrophy; SMN, survival motor neuron gene; HTLV1, human T-cell lymphotropic viruses.

PHARMACOLOGIC MANAGEMENT OF MOTOR NEURON DISEASE

Although there is not yet a cure for ALS, significant research advances are being made in an attempt to identify drugs and compounds that will slow disease progression. Although the findings thus far are not overly impressive, offering patients pharmacologic treatment of their disease has psychological benefits that may outweigh the actual slowing of disease progression that currently can be achieved. Offering the patient the opportunity to participate in clinical trials provides hope in the face of a seemingly desperate situation. Riluzole (Rilutek) is the only drug approved by the Food and Drug Administration (FDA) specifically for treatment of ALS.

Riluzole inhibits the presynaptic release of glutamate and reduces neuronal damage in experimental models of ALS. It was approved by the FDA for treatment of ALS in 1995 after the completion of two clinical trials that showed that it slowed disease progression (79,80). Both of these studies demonstrated prolonged tracheostomy-free survival for patients taking riluzole as opposed to placebo, although the benefit was modest. In the larger of the two studies, the relative increased probability of survival at 1 year for patients taking riluzole was 18%, and this benefit diminished after 15 months (80). Median survival benefit was 60 days. Unfortunately, no functional benefit was derived; strength declined at a similar rate in those taking riluzole and placebo.

The recommended dose of riluzole is 50 mg twice daily. It is generally well tolerated with the most common side effects being asthenia, nausea, diarrhea, and gastrointestinal upset. Elevation of hepatic enzymes is a more serious side effect. The alanine aminotransferase (ALT) level should be monitored monthly for the first 3 months and every 3 months thereafter. The drug should be discontinued if the ALT level reaches five times the upper limit of normal. Other serious, but rare, complications are renal tubular impairment and pancreatitis (81,82).

The retail cost of riluzole is approximately $1,000 per month. Because of the marginal survival benefit provided by the drug, if either side effects or the cost has an adverse effect on the patient's quality of life, the drug should be discontinued. A practice advisory published by the American Academy of Neurology recommends that riluzole be prescribed for patients with ALS who are not ventilator dependent (83). There is no evidence of benefit in patients who are ventilator dependent or in patients with more slowly progressing forms of MND such as SMA or postpolio syndrome.

Because oxidative stress is one of the proposed pathogenic factors in ALS, many physicians recommend a variety of antioxidants. Vitamin E, vitamin C, and coenzyme Q are the most frequently used. Double-blind placebo controlled studies of vitamin E as an add-on to riluzole have not shown any additional disease-modifying benefit in patients with ALS, although, large population-based studies continue to identify a reduction in the risk of developing ALS in those who take vitamin E (84–86). A phase II trial of coenzyme Q10 did not reveal sufficient evidence of efficacy to proceed to a phase III trial (87). No placebo controlled trials have been completed to assess the effects of vitamin C on disease progression in ALS;

however, one small study evaluating a cocktail of antioxidant compounds failed to demonstrate either efficacy or harm (88). If patients are taking these supplements, safe recommended daily dose ranges are 1,000 to 3,000 mg of vitamin C, 400 to 800 IU of vitamin E, 60 to 240 mg of coenzyme Q.

Another over-the-counter compound taken by many patients with ALS and often recommended by their physicians is creatine. Creatine is an amino acid compound naturally found in skeletal muscle and other tissues. For years, it has been used as an ergogenic aid by athletes. It is part of the cellular energy buffering and transport system supplying adenosine triphosphate to muscle. Two recent studies have generated interest in using creatine to improve strength in patients with neuromuscular diseases. Creatine given to transgenic ALS mice improved motor performance, prolonged survival, and slowed loss of motor neurons (89). A small study by Groeneveld et al. (90) found no benefit from oral creatine in patients with ALS; however, the study was insufficiently powered and dosing may have been too low to achieve a therapeutic effect. A phase I dose escalation study was recently completed defining the pharmacokinetics and determining adequate dosing (91). A clinical trial is currently ongoing.

AMYOTROPHIC LATERAL SCLEROSIS CLINICAL TRIALS

The number of clinical drug trials for ALS has increased dramatically in recent years and multiple national and international research collaboratives have been formed to rapidly screen therapeutic candidates. However, the lack of successful drug translation for ALS has continued to be a frustration for scientists, physicians, and patients hoping for more effective treatment strategies. Recent trials have tested a number of growth factors, glutamate antagonists, calcium channel blockers, and amino acids. At present, more than 50 trials are currently listed as recruiting ALS patients on the Clinicaltrials.Gov, National Institutes of Health Web site.

At present, there are ongoing phase III clinical trials assessing the efficacy of dexpramipexole and ceftriaxone. Dexpramipexole is an enantiomer of pramipexole, a drug commonly used in the treatment of Parkinson disease and restless leg syndrome. Pramipexole has been proposed to exert a broad spectrum of neuroprotective properties, primarily through antioxidant effects, inhibiting apoptotic enzymes and preserving mitochondrial structure and activity. More recent work has suggested that pramipexole possesses antiexcitotoxic properties. Pramipexole has high intrinsic dopaminergic receptor activity and, consequently, dose-limiting side effects, including orthostatic hypotension and hallucination. Dexpramipexole has lower affinity for dopaminergic receptors and therefore fewer side effects (92). Initial phase I studies demonstrated safety and a nonsignificant reduction of 17% in the slope of decline of the ALSFRS-R. Promising results on the phase II study, which included 102 patients and produced dose-dependent slowing of decline over three months and a trend toward improved survival at 6 months, spurred on the phase III study (93).

Ceftriaxone was identified to increase both brain expression of astroglial glutamate transporter GLT1 and its biochemical and functional activity delaying loss of neurons and muscle strength. Its central nervous system penetration and long half-life are well known, obviating the need for extensive safety trials.

Based on evidence from studies in both the SOD1 animal model and human FALS and SALS postmortem-derived tissue showing that diseased astrocytes are toxic to neurons, stem cell therapies are being developed to replace astrocytes by direct transplantation or by transplantation of neural stem cells possessing the potential to differentiate *in vivo* into astrocytes (94). Another stem cell therapy in early phase development uses adult stem cells to produce neurotrophins in an attempt to influence the microenvironment of motor neurons and interrupt cellular signals for apoptosis (95).

Other emerging therapies include antisense oligonucleotides that in preclinical studies have increased survival in G93A rats, small interfering RNA, and zinc finger proteins (96). Sangamo's (CA, USA) zinc finger technology targets VEGF and promotes neuron survival in ALS animal models. A phase I trial in 40 ALS patients has been completed (96).

In the future, a cocktail approach to slowing disease progression may be the ideal treatment strategy. Such a multidrug regimen might include one or more glutamate antagonist, antioxidants, neurotrophic factors, and gene modulating and stem cell therapies. However, clinical trials evaluating drug synergies have only recently been initiated.

The Muscular Dystrophy Association (*www.mdausa.org*), the Amyotrophic Lateral Sclerosis Association (www.alsa.org), and the National Institutes of Health (www.clinicaltrials.gov) maintain updated Web sites providing information on drug development and clinical trials. These sites are excellent resources for patients interested in enrolling in a clinical trial.

REHABILITATION AND PALLIATIVE CARE

At present, *incurable*, adult MNDs are not completely *untreatable*. The goals of rehabilitation and palliative care for these patients are to maximize functional capacities, prolong or maintain independent function and locomotion, inhibit or prevent physical deformity, and provide access to full community integration for good quality of life. In ALS, this also includes addressing end-of life-issues and ensuring that the patient has a comfortable death.

The comprehensive management of all of the varied clinical problems associated with adult MNDs is an arduous task. For this reason, the multidisciplinary approach is much more effective and takes advantage of the expertise of many clinicians, rather than placing the burden on one. Management is best carried out by a team consisting of physicians; physical, occupational, and speech therapists; social workers; vocational counselors; and psychologists, among others. Ideally, due to the significant mobility problems associated with these diseases, the physician and all the key clinic personnel should be available at each visit. Tertiary care medical centers in larger urban areas can usually provide this type of service. This may be an independent clinic or sponsored by one or more of the consumer-driven organizations sponsoring research and clinical care for people with MNDs, including the Muscular Dystrophy Association or the Amyotrophic Lateral Sclerosis Association.

The rehabilitative and palliative care strategies discussed in this section may be applied to any form of adult MND; however, the focus of this discussion is primarily on ALS.

Initial Rehabilitation Clinical Evaluation

Initial confirmation of the diagnosis is critical and is a primary responsibility of the consulting neuromuscular disease specialist. Due to the ominous prognosis of ALS, a confirmatory second opinion should always be sought. A physiatrist is well suited to direct the rehabilitation team and oversee a comprehensive, goal-oriented treatment plan (97,98). Irrespective, a single primary physician who coordinates all rehabilitative care should be identified early in the process, either a specialist or the family physician if he or she is willing and knowledgeable of the disease.

At initial evaluation, the patient should be thoroughly educated about the expected outcome and the problems that may be encountered. Enrollment in an experimental drug trial, as discussed previously in this chapter, should be encouraged and facilitated. It not only furthers science but also provides some hope for the patient and ensures frequent follow-up. The physician should then assess the patient's goals and orchestrate a rehabilitative and ultimately a palliative program that matches those goals. In ALS, palliative care should be aimed at maximizing a patient's comfort and quality of life, not necessarily extending his or her life.

Spectrum of Clinical Problems and Treatment Paradigms

Weakness and Fatigue. Skeletal muscle weakness is the *sine qua non* of all adult MND, including ALS, and is the ultimate cause of most clinical problems associated with these diseases. There have been few well-controlled studies looking at exercise-induced strength gains in this population. However, in slowly progressive neuromuscular diseases, a 12-week moderate-resistance (30% of maximum isometric force) exercise program resulted in strength gains ranging from 4% to 20% without any notable deleterious effects (99). Nonetheless, in the same population, a 12-week high-resistance (training at the maximum weight a subject could lift 12 times) exercise program showed no further added beneficial effect compared with the moderate-resistance program and there was evidence of overwork weakness in some of the subjects (100). Bello-Haas et al. studied the effects of resistance training on quality of life and function in 27 ALS patients. Although the sample size was small, no negative effects were observed due to the intervention, and patients in the treatment arm had significantly higher ASLFRS scores at 6 months (101).

Due to the active ongoing muscle degeneration in most cases of ALS, and to a lesser extent in SMA and SBMA, the risk for overwork weakness is great and exercise should be prescribed cautiously and with a common sense approach. Patients should be advised not to exercise to exhaustion, which can produce more muscle damage and dysfunction (102). Patients participating in an exercise program should be cautioned of the warning signs of overwork weakness, which includes feeling weaker rather than stronger within 30 minutes after exercising or excessive muscle soreness 24 to 48 hours after exercising. Other warning signs include severe muscle cramping, heaviness in the extremities, and prolonged shortness of breath (102).

Early intervention with gentle, low-impact aerobic exercise such as walking, swimming/pool exercise, and stationary bicycling will improve cardiovascular performance, increase muscle efficiency, and thus help fight fatigue (103,104). Fatigue in ALS is multifactorial and is due in part to impaired muscular activation (105,106). Other contributing factors include generalized deconditioning from immobility and clinical depression (104). Aerobic exercise not only improves physical functioning but is beneficial in fighting depression and improving pain tolerance.

Restrictive Lung Disease. The terminal event in ALS is usually directly related to respiratory failure. RLD usually develops in ALS but may also be present in SMA and SBMA. Although the term RLD is frequently used, this is not *lung disease* per se but is due to weakness of the diaphragm, chest wall, and abdominal musculature (107). Weakness in the bulbar musculature, which can lead to aspiration, confounds the problem in ALS and SBMA. Patients should be educated early in the disease process so they can make informed decisions down the line (107,108). Routine pulmonary function tests, including maximal sniff inspiratory pressure (SNIP), forced vital capacity (FVC), and maximal inspiratory and expiratory pressures, should be monitored closely (109,110). Dysphagia symptoms closely parallel vital capacity and significantly complicate the clinical course (111,112).

Ultimately, most patients develop hypoventilation, which leads to elevated CO_2 levels (107). Measuring only O_2 saturation levels with pulse oximetry may be inadequate. End-tidal CO_2 levels should be measured periodically, depending on the clinical condition of the patient. Arterial blood gas evaluations are usually not necessary and will not add any needed information. A thorough review of systems will help define any problems. Patients who are hypoventilating will often become hypercapnic and hypoxic at night and complain of a morning headache, restlessness, nightmares, and poor-quality sleep. This may cause daytime somnolence. Insufficient respiration with hypoxia may occur later, particularly if the lungs are damaged by chronic aspiration.

Noninvasive ventilation should be considered when the SNIP value is 40 cm H_2O or less, the FVC is equal to or less than 50% predicted, or the maximal inspiratory pressure is measured at −60 cm H_2O or lower (110). Bach (111) showed significant success with the use of 24-hour noninvasive positive pressure ventilation (PPV) by mouth, and early intervention with noninvasive ventilation has been shown to improve survival by 11 months compared to controls (113). Noninvasive PPV can be done easily in the home and should be considered the preferred modality of assisted ventilation in ALS. Bimodal positive airway pressure is the preferred form of noninvasive PPV in ALS. It can be used via a mouthpiece with or without a lip seal, a nasal mask, or a full face mask. Patients may benefit initially from using noninvasive PPV mainly at night.

There are various methods of improving respiratory hygiene that may also help the patient with ALS, including devices that produce an artificial cough via a face mask by rapidly going from a positive to a negative airway pressure to help bring up secretions (108). This technique has been around since the polio epidemics more than 40 years ago and is now available through several commercial names, including the Cofflator (Respironics, Pittsburgh, PA) or the In-Exsufflator (JH Emerson Co, Cambridge, MA).

If better airway access becomes absolutely necessary and the informed patient wishes more aggressive care, a tracheostomy is then considered. In most centers, only very few patients elect to have a tracheostomy. End-of-life discussions, defining circumstances for discontinuation of ventilator support, should occur before invasive mechanical ventilation is initiated.

Dysphagia/Dysarthria. Clinical signs and symptoms of dysphagia and dysarthria may closely parallel one another (114). Early signs include changes in voice patterns (voice becoming hoarse) and persistent coughing after swallowing liquids, which can indicate microaspiration. Early findings of dysphagia, identified by videofluoroscopic studies, include abnormalities in the oral swallowing phase with decreased function of bolus transport by both the anterior and the posterior part of the tongue (115). A speech therapist should be consulted early for clinical swallowing evaluations and recommendations on dietary modification such as thickening liquids and preparing food that forms into a bolus easily. A modified barium swallow or fiberoptic endoscopic examination of swallowing safety is helpful for accurately determining the presence of aspiration and defining which food textures the patient can safely swallow (116).

Malnutrition is very common in ALS, occurring in 16% to 55% of ALS patients (117). Dysphagia and an underlying hypermetabolic state, the cause of which is not fully understood, are blamed for the nutritional disorder (117). Rapid weight loss corresponds with a more rapid disease course. BMI has been identified as an independent predictor of survival; those patients whose BMI is between 30 and 35 have the longest survival (118). Endoscopic gastrostomy (PEG) tube circumvents the problems of dysphagia and has inconsistently been shown to prolong survival (119). PEG or radiographically inserted gastrostomy tube should be strongly considered when the patient loses more than 10% of his or her baseline body weight or is taking longer than 1 hour to eat a meal (110). It is best to have the gastrostomy tube placed before the patient becomes malnourished or his or her FVC drops to less than 50% of the predicted value, because it will be considerably easier for the surgeon or interventional radiologist to perform the procedure. Patients should be reassured that they will still be able to eat food orally for enjoyment, provided that their caregivers have had some training to manage episodes of choking. Nonetheless, using the gastrostomy tube as the primary route of nutritional intake will ensure adequate fluids and nourishment.

Some patients may decline a PEG tube. This choice is left up to the patients, but they must be fully informed that at some point, they may be unable to swallow. At that time, PEG placement may be impossible or at the very least technically difficult and involve intubating the patients to facilitate ventilation during the procedure. If intubation is required for the procedure, the patients must understand prior to the procedure that they may not be able to be weaned from the ventilator. Thus, it is not really an option to wait until they cannot swallow and then change their mind. Because the gastrointestinal tract generally maintains adequate function in ALS, parenteral hydration and feeding is not necessary and is associated with high nursing needs, cost, and some degree of medical comorbidity. It should not be discussed as a viable option. The patient who can no longer swallow and does not have a feeding tube will eventually die from dehydration and malnutrition. Some patients do elect this route and they can be made comfortable.

Dysarthria in ALS does not respond well to conventional articulation training. However, some adaptive strategies such as maintaining a slow speaking rate with an emphasis on increasing the precision of speech production may be helpful and can be taught by a speech-language pathologist (104,120). As the disease progresses, dysarthria should be approached by prescribing communicative aids, rather than traditional ongoing speech therapy. An alphabet supplementation or word board works well early when patients still have reasonable arm function. After that, developing yes and no or other binary commands with eye-gaze systems may be useful, particularly if the patient is using mechanical ventilation. There have been major recent advancements made in devices such as speech synthesizers or multipurpose, multiaccess, computer-based augmentative communication systems. Although expensive, these devices greatly enhance patients' ability to communicate when they can no longer phonate. These types of devices may often be borrowed or rented from Assistive Technology Centers, which are often found at tertiary care medical centers.

Patients with ALS and bulbar symptoms usually have difficulty controlling and swallowing the amounts of saliva that are normally present in the oral cavity. Drugs with strong anticholinergic effect, such as benztropine (Cogentin), glycopyrrolate (Robinul), or some of the tricyclic antidepressants (amitriptyline), are very effective at drying up secretions. In refractory cases, injection of botulinum toxin A or B into the salivary glands can effectively control secretions (121). Radiation to the salivary glands may also be helpful, although problematic complications are common (104).

Spasticity. Spasticity in ALS is probably induced both at the motor cortex and at the spinal cord level. The γ-aminobutyric acid analogue baclofen acts to facilitate motor neuron inhibition at spinal levels and is the agent of choice. Initial doses are 5 to 10 mg twice to three times a day, titrating up to doses of 20 mg four times a day. Occasionally, higher doses (up to 160 mg/day) are more effective but caution is advised. Side effects include weakness, fatigue, and sedation. An intrathecal baclofen pump may be beneficial to some patients with PLS. A new agent tizanidine, α2-agonist similar to clonidine, inhibits excitatory interneurons and may also be helpful. Dosing range is 4 to 8 mg three to four times a day, with a similar side effect profile to that of baclofen. Benzodiazepines may also be helpful but can cause respiratory depression and somnolence. Dantrolene, by blocking Ca^{2+} release in the sarcoplasmic reticulum, is effective at reducing muscle tone but will also cause generalized muscle weakness and is not recommended. Slow (30-second sustained), static muscle stretching may be helpful, particularly in the more symptomatic muscle groups such as the gastrocnemius, and may be done in bed. Positional splinting is also a helpful adjunctive modality, but skin must be monitored frequently for pressure areas.

Depression. Reactive clinical depression is expected in patients diagnosed with MND, and although depression occurs among ALS patients, it is not inevitable (122). Once the diagnosis is confirmed, the patient should be counseled with respect to the prognosis to allow time for grieving, anger, and ultimately "acceptance" of their disease, which is important for the mental well-being of the patients and their family (123,124).

The practitioner should keep in mind that the time around diagnosis is often associated with high levels of anxiety that can undermine quality of life (124). Antidepressant medicine should be offered to patients when needed, since it can provide assistance with mood elevation, appetite stimulation, and sleep (125).

Good family, social, and religious support systems are all helpful and should be encouraged. The patient should be referred to a support group. The most prominent consumer-driven organizations facilitating support groups for people with ALS are the MDA and the ALS Association. In addition, referral to a psychiatrist or clinical psychologist with experience in treating depression associated with terminal and/or chronic disease might be necessary (125). Depression in the spouse, significant other, family, or friends should not be overlooked. Partners and caregivers often rate the patients' quality of life significantly lower than the patients themselves (126). This misperception may be a reflection of their own mood. Caregiver burden, related to loss of function in the patient, increases throughout the course of ALS and is positively related to increases in caregiver depression and anxiety (126).

Pain and Immobility. Although not frequently characterized as a major component of ALS, most of these patients do experience significant pain. The pain is due largely to immobility, which can cause adhesive capsulitis, mechanical back pain, pressure areas on the skin, and more rarely neuropathic pain (104). Frequently, severe weakness in the neck flexors and extensors will cause a "floppy head" associated with severe neck pain and tightness. This may be helped by cervical orthosis such as the Headmaster-type collar, which is a light weight wire-frame collar with padding over the pressure points.

Wheelchairs should have adequate lumbar support and good cushioning (gel foam). The chair should be properly fitted to avoid pressure ulcers and provide adequate support for the spine. Simply giving the patient a prescription for a wheelchair often ends up with the patient getting a standard manual chair that does not fit properly. A power wheelchair, although expensive, can be justified because it will help prolong independent mobility and thus markedly improve quality of life (127).

A good pressure-relieving mattress (air or dense foam) should be used on the bed at home, along with foam wedges to facilitate proper positioning. This will help prevent pressure ulcers and contractures. Daily passive- and active-assisted range of motion is critical. Maintaining mobility and functional independence as long as possible will have positive physical and psychological benefits. Ankle-foot orthoses molded in the neutral position may prolong ambulation and avoid injury if there is unilateral or bilateral footdrop. Lightweight, low-profile, leaf spring or prefabricated carbon fiber AFOs can offer dorsiflexion assist without adding significant additional weight on a weakened limb. Wheeled walkers (Gran Tour in particular) or quad (four-point) canes may also help, depending on the pattern of weakness. Other useful equipment includes handheld shower nozzles, bathtub benches, grab bars, raised toilet seats, hospital beds, commode chairs, aids in activities of daily living (e.g., sock aid and grabbers), and wheelchair ramps. An occupational therapist will help define which, if any, of these devices will be useful to the patient. Other simple suggestions such as moving the patient's bedroom to the first floor, removing any loose rugs, or covering slippery floors are helpful and can be done during an in-home evaluation by the therapist. The ALS patient's function will change rapidly. It should be the goal of the rehabilitation team to anticipate those changes and initiate equipment acquisition to meet the patient's needs seamlessly as they develop.

Pharmacologic management of pain in ALS includes the use of nonsteroidal anti-inflammatory drugs (NSAIDs), particularly if there is evidence of an active inflammatory process such as tenosynovitis or arthritis. Regular dosing of acetaminophen (1,000 mg every 6 hours) may be used along with an NSAID or alone if NSAIDs are not tolerated. Tricyclic antidepressants and antiepileptic drugs such as gabapentin (Neurontin) can sometimes be helpful for pain, particularly if there is a neuropathic component. Gabapentin also has the added benefit of some antispasticity properties. Narcotic medicine should be reserved for refractory pain. Concern for narcotic addiction is pointless in patients with a terminal disease and the medications should be given on a regular dosing schedule and titrated to the point of comfort (128). Concomitant use of the antiemetic, antihistamine hydroxyzine (Vistaril), given along with the narcotic, will enhance the effectiveness (i.e., 30-mg codeine plus 50-mg hydroxyzine every 6 waking hours). Unlike narcotic medications, hydroxyzine is not a cortical depressant but has direct skeletal muscle relaxant and analgesic properties known to potentiate the analgesic effect of narcotic medication. The exact mechanism of this potentiation is unknown (128). Combination elixirs can be prepared by the pharmacy for ease of administration. Oral or sublingual morphine (Roxanol) (l0 to 30 mg every 4 hours) is also effective for comfort care and may also help relieve "air hunger" in the terminal stages of the disease. Another option is taking the total dose of immediate-release morphine required to alleviate pain and giving half of that every 12 hours in a controlled-release preparation such as MS Contin. Intramuscular delivery route should be avoided due to muscle wasting.

Fentanyl or morphine patches may deliver inconsistent dosing, particularly if there is excessive perspiration. A patient-controlled analgesic pump mechanism may not work in advanced stages of ALS due to the inability of the patient to control the delivery. The main problems with narcotic medication in ALS are respiratory depression and constipation. These side effects may be quite acceptable in the final phases of life when respiratory insufficiency or severe pain requires increased doses of morphine and lorazepam. Patients and caregivers should be made aware of these issues.

Autonomic Dysfunction. Although dysautonomia is not generally a predominant feature of ALS, it can cause some unique clinical problems. Patients may complain of feeling quite hot, along with problems of esophageal and gastric dysmotility and cardiac arrhythmias (129). This can cause problems when patients are exercising, particularly if they become overheated and dehydrated. Recommendations include dressing in fabric that wicks away perspiration, such as polypropylene; eating several small meals a day, or if a PEG is being used, switching from bolus feeds to a continuous drip, along with plenty of fluid; and taking care not to exercise to exhaustion.

Incontinence. Urinary disorders have not typically been considered a significant problem in ALS. However, in a prospective study of 54 subjects, 41% were identified as having urinary disorders and 35% had a postvoid residual of greater than 50 mL (130). The likelihood of urinary disorders increased with severity of disease and the presence of spasticity (130). Urologic evaluation should be considered in the patient with prominent spasticity. Incontinence can also become a problem with immobility and difficulty getting to the toilet. Patients should avoid drinking large amounts of fluids after dinner to avoid nighttime incontinence. Men may wear a condom catheter at night. Absorbent undergarments may also be used, but skin should be monitored closely for maceration and protected with topically applied moisture-repelling agents. Sympathomimetic agents such as pseudoephedrine (30 to 60 mg up to four times a day) may help increase urinary outlet sphincter tone. However, this may also increase blood pressure and could induce urinary retention, particularly if used in conjunction with anticholinergic agents in men with prostatic enlargement. An indwelling Foley or suprapubic catheter is a reasonable choice later in the course of the disease when mobility problems become significant. Bowels are best regulated by a routine protocol on a time-based regimen (e.g., every morning). Fiber/bulk agents should be given routinely, along with fluids. Suppositories and mini enemas may be used as needed.

Dementia. The current emerging consensus among researchers and physicians is that the prevalence of cognitive impairment in ALS is higher than previously believed. Cognitive impairment in ALS may appear along a clinical continuum, ranging from mild impairment to frontotemporal lobar dementia (FTLD) (131). Cognitive impairment occurs in sporadic and familial forms of ALS. Patients may present with cognitive deficits before, after, or at the onset of MND (131). In ALS patients with cognitive impairment, imaging studies show frontal atrophy and hypometabolism in the frontotemporal regions and the anterior cingulate gyrus (132). The prevalence of cognitive dysfunction severe enough to fulfill the Neary criteria for FTLD has been reported to occur in 10% to 14% of patients evaluated in two large population-based studies (133,134). Symptoms of FTD include disinhibition, impulsivity, changes in sleep and eating patterns, decreased attention, decreased executive functioning and planning, apathy, and poverty of speech progressing to mutism. Memory is relatively preserved in these patients. Half of the ALS patients followed in the above studies had normal cognitive function. The remaining 30% to 40% had evidence of cognitive impairment without fulfilling the Neary criteria for FTLD. Those patients without frank dementia had a higher frequency of impairment in language and memory domains when compared to normal controls (133,134).

There have been few studies evaluating treatments addressing the symptoms of cognitive impairment in ALS. SSRIs and tricyclic antidepressant may help control associated behavioral symptoms (131). Diminishing the effects of hypoxia on cognition by the use of noninvasive ventilation should be considered, and evaluation assessing the presence of nocturnal hypoxemia should be initiated early in the disease process. Finally, one must consider the effects of cognitive impairment on the patient's capacity to participate in end-of-life decisions. The presence of cognitive impairment may be problematic for the validity of living wills and other legal documents pertaining to patient's wishes for medical care (131).

End-of-Life Issues. ALS is a disease that poses some unusual ethical and humanitarian considerations. Although it is considered a fatal condition, unlike most cancers or other grave, incurable illnesses, it may take years to die, even though the disease continues to debilitate the person in the process.

Despite the most aggressive treatment available, ALS will progress. Early in the disease, a social worker should be consulted to help arrange durable power of attorney to a responsible family member, usually the spouse. In most states, this can be done by a paralegal for a nominal fee. A living will should then be drafted, which clearly outlines the patient's wishes regarding extent of medical intervention desired (135). This is particularly important with respect to entering hospice level care. Presumably by the time hospice level care is being considered, patients have had ample time for grieving, anger, and ultimately acceptance of their fate. However, in our experience, many patients with ALS still are hesitant about going into hospice because it implies that the disease has reached *end stage* (136).

The patient should also be referred to a support group. Support groups are often a great resource, not only for psychological support but also for problem solving and equipment recycling of items such as hospital beds.

Most of this section of this chapter has centered around *comprehensive clinical care* of the patient with adult-onset MND, emphasizing "everything that modern medicine has to offer." The physician must consider that the patient with advanced ALS may not want all of this, which is not necessarily a wrong decision. Life-*sustaining therapy*, defined as any artificial device or intervention that compensates for the failure of an organ system that would normally result in death, is the patient's choice, not the physician's (136–139). The most obvious example of this would be mechanical ventilation, but this also includes artificial hydration and nutrition. Legally and ethically speaking, a mentally competent patient can refuse any prescribed treatment. It is the physician's responsibility to ensure that the patient understands the consequences of this. The physician should always respect and foster the patient's autonomy and self-direction with respect to these types of interventions. This does not extend to the point of physician-assisted suicide, in which the physician takes active steps to end the patient's life. This is an illegal act that carries grievous ethical concerns that are beyond the scope of this chapter. Despite this, a recent study documented that approximately 56% of patients with ALS surveyed in Washington and Oregon states would consider assisted suicide (137). As of October 1997, the Oregon Death with Dignity Act legalizes physician-assisted suicide in that state, although the actual impact of that bill on the care of patients with ALS has not yet been reported. Nonetheless, this stunningly high percentage of patients with ALS who would consider this strongly implies that the quality of care in advanced ALS is inadequate. If the patient is requesting this, then the physician should reassess the situation, making sure that everything has been done to maximize patient comfort and quality of life.

Further, quality of life studies have identified a lack of adequate communication between the physician and the patient and a poor perception (both positive and negative) on the part of the physician of the level of quality of life in these patients (127). It takes a great deal of time to explain all of the end-of-life issues, including the available treatment options and choices. Without this investment of time on the clinician's part, the patient is unaware of the services that may be available to ease his or her suffering.

The most appropriate level of care for patients with ALS may change frequently and these patients should be followed closely. Unfortunately, patients with advanced ALS are often told "there is nothing that can be done," when in fact optimizing in-home care with hospice can maximize quality of life for these patients and provide for a comfortable, painless passing. Krivickas et al. (140) documented that most patients with ALS probably do not receive enough in-home care. Of 98 patients with advanced ALS studied, only 9 received hospice home care, 24 received nonhospice home care, and 7 received both hospice and nonhospice home care. The remaining 58 patients received no in-home care at all. Even among those having home care assistance, primary nonmedical ALS primary caregivers spent an average of 11 hours/day caring for patients. Among ALS primary caregivers studied, 42% and 48% felt physically and psychologically unwell, respectively. The authors concluded that home and hospice care received by patients with ALS is inadequate because it starts too late to relieve the burden placed on family caregivers. Because the focus of care in hospice is the family, however defined by the patient, this problem could be easily resolved. Hospice provides an interdisciplinary team of professionals whose mission is to support the patient and the family through his or her remaining days together. Support is given for physical, psychological, emotional, and spiritual needs of the family unit in the home setting, bypassing the need for laborious trips to clinics.

The National Hospice Organization does have some guidelines for entry of patients with ALS into hospice (Table 35.4), which are somewhat arduous but allow for early entry into hospice of most patients with ALS in the advanced stages of the disease (141). These guidelines require physicians to make some estimate of life expectancy, which is very difficult to do in ALS and is something for which most physicians are probably ill prepared. Compared with patients with terminal cancer, patients with ALS have a relatively slow progression in respect to the actual dying process, which decreases the clinician's awareness that hospice care may be appropriate. Most clinicians likely perceive that hospice is for "near terminal" patients, which is correct, except that patients with ALS may be in that state for a prolonged period. During this time, hospice care could ease suffering considerably. Lack of physician knowledge of the services provided by hospice is widespread (142). Physicians not familiar with the care of terminal patients may not be comfortable with the aggressive use of opiates and benzodiazepines advocated by hospice clinicians for the control of symptoms in ALS. The physician may find it difficult to give carte blanche orders for effective titration of these types of medications, which will ease air hunger and anxiety in the patient with end-stage ALS.

Irrespective, in the final stages of the disease, it is medically appropriate to involve a home hospice team. Regular home visits by hospice nurses will ensure proper medication delivery, pain control, and skin and bowel care, as well as provide the physician with a progress report without having to bring the patient to the clinic. They can also provide counseling to avoid panic calls to 911 by family members and unnecessary nighttime visits to the emergency department. Most patients wish to die at home, and in most cases, with a supportive family and the help of hospice, this is a feasible and worthwhile goal.

An informed patient and family will welcome the comprehensive level of terminal care that hospice offers, consoled with the knowledge that dying with dignity in the serenity and security of one's own home is, in some modest but meaningful way, a measure of victory over this otherwise insufferable illness. Finally, we urge clinicians to attend memorial services because it is a healing and rewarding experience.

TABLE 35.4

CRITERIA FOR HOSPICE ADMISSION IN AMYOTROPHIC LATERAL SCLEROSIS

Hospice is appropriate when there has been an overall rapid progression of amyotrophic lateral sclerosis (a critical factor), e.g., disability has progressed significantly in the past 12 mo. The patient or family desires no further aggressive treatment or cardiopulmonary resuscitation.

In addition, at least one of the following must also apply:

1. Increased respiratory distress
    a. vital capacity of less than 30% predicted
    b. significant dyspnea at rest
    c. supplemental oxygen required at rest
    d. patient has refused intubation, tracheostomy, and mechanical ventilation
2. Severely impaired nutrition
    a. tube feeding not elected or discontinued
    b. oral intake insufficient/dysphagia
    c. continued weight loss in spite of tube feedings
    d. dehydration or hypovolemia
3. Life threatening complications
    a. recurrent aspiration pneumonia
    b. decubitus ulcers, multiple, stage 3 to 4, particularly if infected
    c. upper urinary tract infection, e.g., pyelonephritis
    d. sepsis
    e. fever recurrent after antibiotics

ACKNOWLEDGMENT

Supported by Research and Training Center grant no. HB133B980008 from the National Institute on Disability and Rehabilitation Research, Washington, DC, USA.

References

1. Rowland LP. How amyotrophic lateral sclerosis got its name: the clinical-pathologic genius of Jean-Martin Charcot. *Arch Neurol* 2001;58(3):512–515.
2. Mulder DW. The clinical syndrome of amyotrophic lateral sclerosis. *Proc Staff Meet Mayo Clin* 1957;32:427.
3. Stark FM, Moershc FP. Primary lateral sclerosis: a distinct clinical entity. *J Nerv Ment Dis* 1945;102:332.
4. Siddique T, Deng H. Genetics of amyotrophic lateral sclerosis. *Hum Mol Genet* 1996;5(Spec No):1465–1470.
5. Lyons TJ, Lill H, Goto JJ, et al. Mutations in copper-zinc superoxide dismutase that cause amyotrophic lateral sclerosis alter the zinc binding site and the redux behavior of the protein. *Proc Natl Acad Sci* 1996;93(22):12240–12244.

6. Hosler BA, Brown RH. Copper/zinc superoxide dis mutase mutations and free radical damage in amyotrophic lateral sclerosis. *Adv Neurol* 1995;680:41–46.
7. Cudkowicz ME, McKenna-Yasek D, Sapp PE, et al. Epidemiology of mutations in superoxide dismutase in amyotrophic lateral sclerosis. *Ann Neurol* 1997;41(2):210–221.
8. Auclair JR, Boggio KJ, Petsko GA, et al. Strategies for stabilizing superoxide dismutase (SOD1), the protein destabilized in the most common form of familial amyotrophic lateral sclerosis. *Proc Natl Acad Sci USA* 2010;107(50):21394–21399.
9. Millecamps S, Salachas F, Cazeneuve C, et al. SOD1, ANG, VAPB, TARDBP, and FUS mutations in familial amyotrophic lateral sclerosis: genotype-phenotype correlations. *J Med Genet* 2010;47(8):554–560.
10. Tsai CP, Soong BW, Lin KP, et al. FUS, TARDBP, and SOD1 mutations in a Taiwanese cohort with familial ALS. *Neurobiol Aging* 2011;32(3):553.e13–553.e21.
11. Ticozzi N, Tiloca C, Morelli C, et al. Genetics of familial Amyotrophic lateral sclerosis. *Arch Ital Biol* 2011;149(1):65–82.
12. Wijesekera LC, Leigh PN. Amyotrophic lateral sclerosis. *Orphanet J Rare Dis* 2009;4:3.
13. Kabashi E, Bercier V, Lissouba A, et al. FUS and TARDBP but Not SOD1 Interact in Genetic Models of Amyotrophic Lateral Sclerosis. *PLoS Genet* 2011;7(8):e1002214.
14. Norris F, Sheperd R, Denys E, et al. Onset, natural history and outcome in idiopathic adult motor neuron disease. *J Neurol Sci* 1993;118(1):48–55.
15. Pradas J, Finison L, Andres PL, et al. The natural history of amyotrophic lateral sclerosis and the use of natural history controls in therapeutic trials. *Neurology* 1993;43(4):751–755.
16. Ringel SP, Murphy JR, Alderson MK, et al. The natural history of amyotrophic lateral sclerosis. *Neurology* 1993;43(7):1316–1322.
17. Huisman MH, de Jong SW, van Doormaal PT, et al. Population based epidemiology of amyotrophic lateral sclerosis using capture-recapture methodology. *J Neurol Neurosurg Psychiatry* doi:10.1136/jnnp.2011.244939.
18. Chancellor AM, Warlow CP. Adult onset motor neuron disease: worldwide mortality, incidence, and distribution since 1950. *J Neurol Neurosurg Psychiatry* 1992;55(12):1106–1115.
19. Wang H, O'Reilly ÉJ, Weisskopf MG, et al. Smoking and risk of amyotrophic lateral sclerosis: a pooled analysis of 5 prospective cohorts. *Arch Neurol* 2011;68(2):207–213.
20. Neilson S, Robinson I, Alperovitch A. Rising amyotrophic lateral sclerosis mortality in France 1968–1990: increased life expectancy and inter-disease competition as an explanation. *J Neurol* 1994;241(7):448–455.
21. Neilson S, Robinson I, Nymoen EH. Longitudinal analysis of amyotrophic lateral sclerosis mortality in Norway, 1966–1989: evidence for a susceptible subpopulation. *J Neurol Sci* 1994;122(2):148–154.
22. Okumura H. Epidemiological and clinical patterns of western pacific amyotrophic lateral sclerosis (ALS) in Guam and sporadic ALS in Rochester, Minnesota, USA and Hokkaido, Japan: a comparative study. *Hokkaido Igaku Zasshi* 2003;78(3):187–195.
23. Nelson LM, McGuire Y, Longstreth WT Jr, et al. Population-based case-control study of amyotrophic lateral sclerosis in western Washington State. I. Cigarette smoking and alcohol consumption. *Am J Epidemiol* 2000;151(2):156–163.
24. Nelson LM, Matkin C, Longstreth WT Jr, et al. Population-based case-control study of amyotrophic lateral sclerosis in western Washington State. II. Diet. *Am J Epidemiol* 2000;151(2):164–173.
25. Stubgen JP. Neuromuscular disorders in systemic malignancy and its treatment. *Muscle Nerve* 1995;18:636–648.
26. Carter GT, Fritz RC. Pancreatic adenocarcinoma presenting as a monomelic motor neuronopathy. *Muscle Nerve* 1997;20:103–105.
27. Rosenfeld MR, Posner JB. Paraneoplastic motor neuron disease. *Adv Neurol* 1991;56:445–459.
28. Gordon PH, Chang B, Katz IB, et al. The natural history of primary lateral sclerosis. *Neurology* 2006;66(5):647–653.
29. Brugman F, Veldink JH, Franssen H, et al. Differentiation of hereditary spastic paraparesis from primary lateral sclerosis in sporadic adult-onset upper motor neuron syndromes. *Arch Neurol* 2009;66(4):509–514.
30. Singer MA, Statland JM, Wolfe GI, et al. Primary lateral sclerosis. *Muscle Nerve* 2007;35(3):291–302.
31. Tartaglia MC, Rowe A, Findlater K, et al. Differentiation between primary lateral sclerosis and amyotrophic lateral sclerosis: examination of symptoms and signs at disease onset and during follow-up. *Neurology* 2007;64(2):232–236.
32. Salinas S, Proukakis C, Crosby A, et al. Hereditary spastic paraplegia: clinical features and pathogenetic mechanisms. *Lancet Neurol* 2008;7(12):1127–1138.
33. Fink JK. *Hereditary spastic paraplegia overview*. http://www.ncbi.nlm.nih.gov/books/NBK1509/. Accessed August 27, 2011.
34. McMonagle P, Webb S, Hutchinson M. The prevalence of "pure" autosomal dominant hereditary spastic paraparesis in the island of Ireland. *J Neurol Neurosurg Psychiatry* 2002;72:43–46.
35. Ince PG, Evans J, Knopp M, et al. Corticospinal tract degeneration in the progressive muscular atrophy variant of ALS. *Neurology* 2003;60(8):1252–1258.
36. Meyer T, Munch C, van Landeghem FK, et al. Progressive muscle atrophy. A rarely diagnosed variant of ALS. *Nervenartzt* 2007;78(12):1383–1388.
37. Kim WK, Liu X, Sandner J, et al. Study of 962 patients indicates progressive muscular atrophy is a form of ALS. *Neurology* 2009;73(20):1686–1692.
38. Visser J, van den Berg-Vos R, Franssen H, et al. Disease course and prognostic factors of progressive muscular atrophy. *Arch Neurol* 2007;64:522–528.
39. Carter GT, Abresch RT, Fowler WM, et al. Profiles of neuromuscular disease: spinal muscular atrophy. *Am J Phys Med Rehabil* 1995;74(5):S150–S159.
40. Fishbeck KH, Ionasecu V, Ritter AW. Localization of the gene for X-linked spinal muscular atrophy. *Neurology* 1986;36:1595.
41. MacKenzie AE, Jacob P, Surh L, et al. Genetic heterogeneity in spinal muscular atrophy: a linkage analysis-based assessment. *Neurology* 1994;919–924.

42. Amato AA, Prior TW, Barohn RJ, et al. Kennedy's disease: a clinicopathologic correlation with mutations in the androgen receptor gene. *Neurology* 1993;43(4): 791–794.
43. Kennedy WR, Alter M, Sung JH. Progressive proximal spinal and bulbar muscular atrophy of late onset: a sex-linked recessive trait. *Neurology* 1968;18:671.
44. Caner CT, Bonekat HW, Milio L. Successful pregnancies in the presence of spinal muscular atrophy: two case reports. *Arch Phys Med Rehabil* 1994;75(2):229–231.
45. Moulard B, Salachas F, Chassande B, et al. Association between centromeric deletions of the SMN gene and sporadic adult-onset lower motor neuron disease. *Ann Neurol* 1998;43:640–644.
46. Watihayati MS, Fatemeh H, Marini M, et al. Combination of SMN2 copy number and NAIP deletion predicts disease severity in spinal muscular atrophy. *Brain Dev* 2009;31(1):42–45.
47. Zheleznyakova GY, Kiselev AV, Vakharlovsky VG, et al. Genetic and expression studies of SMN2 gene in Russian patients with spinal muscular atrophy type II and III. *BMC Med Genet* 2011;12:96.
48. Humphrey E, Fuller HR, Morris GE. Current research on SMN protein and treatment strategies for spinal muscular atrophy. *Neuromuscul Disord* 2011.
49. Parboosingh JS, Meininger V, McKenna-Yasek D, et al. Deletions causing spinal muscular atrophy do not predispose to amyotrophic lateral sclerosis. *Ann Neurol* 1999;56:710–712.
50. Parboosingh JS, Figlewicz DA, Krizus A, et al. Spinobulbar muscular atrophy can mimic ALS: the importance of genetic testing in male patients with atypical ALS. *Neurology* 1997;49:568–572.
51. Kidd D, Williams AJ, Howard RS. Poliomyelitis. *Postgrad Med J* 1996;72:641–647.
52. Halstead LS. A brief history of postpolio syndrome in the United States. *Arch Phys Med Rehabil* 2011;92: 1344–1349.
53. March of Dimes International Conference on Post-polio syndrome: identifying best practices in diagnosis and care. http//www.marchofdimes.com/files/PPSreport.pdf. Accessed June 9, 2009.
54. Farbu E, Rekand T, Gilhus NE. Post-polio syndrome and total health status in a prospective hospital study. *Eur J Neurol* 2003;10(4):407–413.
55. Mitsumoto H, Chad OA, Pioro EP. *Amyotrophic lateral sclerosis*. Philadelphia, PA: FA Davis Co, 1998.
56. Norris F, Shepherd R, Denys E, et al. Onset, natural history, and outcome in idiopathic adult motor neuron disease. *J Neurol Sci* 1993;118:48–55.
57. Chiò A, Calvo A, Moglia C, et al. Phenotypic heterogeneity of amyotrophic lateral sclerosis: a population based study. *J Neurol Neurosurg Psychiatry* 2011;82(7):740–746.
58. Okuda B, Kodama N, Kowabata K, et al. Corneomandibular reflex in ALS. *Neurology* 1999;52:1699–1701.
59. Brooks B. El Escorial World Federation of Neurology criteria for the diagnosis of amyotrophic lateral sclerosis. Subcommittee on Motor Neuron Diseases/Amyotrophic Lateral Sclerosis of the World Federation of Neurology Research Group on Neuromuscular Diseases and the El Escorial Clinical Limit of Amyotrophic Lateral Sclerosis Workshop Contributors. *J Neuro Sci* 1994;124:96–107.
60. World Federation of Neurology Research Group on Motor Neuron Diseases. *El Escorial revisited: revised criteria for the diagnosis of amyotrophic lateral sclerosis*. World Federation of Neurology Research Group on Motor Neuron Diseases, 1998.
61. de Carvalho M, Dengler R, Eisen A, et al. Electrodiagnostic criteria for diagnosis of ALS. *Clin Neurophysiol* 2008;119(3):497–503.
62. Dengler R. El Escorial or Awaji Criteria in ALS diagnosis, what should we take? *Clin Neurophysiol* 2011.
63. Noto YI, Misawa S, Kanai K, et al. Awaji ALS criteria increase the diagnostic sensitivity in patients with bulbar onset. *Clin Neurophysiol* 2011.
64. Dumitru D. Central nervous system disorders. In: Dumitru D, ed. *Electrodiagnostic medicine*. Philadelphia, PA: Hanley & Belfus, 1995:453–462.
65. Hausmanowa-Petrusewicz I, Friedman A, Kowalski J, et al. Spontaneous motor unit firing in spinal muscular atrophy of childhood. *Electromyo Clin Neurophysiol* 1987;27:259–264.
66. Hausmanowa-Petrusewicz I, Karwanska A. Electromyographic findings in different forms of infantile and juvenile proximal spinal muscular atrophy. *Muscle Nerve* 1986;9:37–46.
67. Swift T. Commentary: electrophysiology of progressive spinal muscular atrophy. In: Gamstorp I, Samat H, eds. *Progressive spinal muscular atrophies*. New York, NY: Raven Press, 1984:135–139.
68. Ferrante MA, Wilbourn AJ. The characteristic electrodiagnostic features of Kennedy's disease. *Muscle Nerve* 1997;20:323–329.
69. Meriggioli MN, Rowin J, Sanders DB, et al. Distinguishing clinical and electrodiagnostic features of x-linked bulbospinal neuronopathy. *Muscle Nerve* 1999;22:1693–1697.
70. Lambert E. Electromyography in amyotrophic lateral sclerosis. In: Norris F, Kurland L, eds. *Motor neuron disease*. New York, NY: Grune & Stratton, 1969:135–153.
71. Lambert E, Mulder D. Electromyographic studies in amyotrophic lateral sclerosis. *Mayo Clin Proc* 1957;332:441–446.
72. Cornblath DR, Kuncl RW, Mellits ED, et al. Nerve conduction studies in amyotrophic lateral sclerosis. *Muscle Nerve* 1992;15(10):1111–1115.
73. Pugdahl K, Fuglsang-Frederiksen A, Johnsen B, et al. A prospective multicentre study on sural nerve action potentials in ALS. *Clin Neurophysiol* 2008;119(5):1106–1110.
74. Dettmers C, Fatepour D. Faust H, et al. Sympathetic skin response abnormalities in amyotrophic lateral sclerosis. *Muscle Nerve* 1993;16:930–934.
75. Ziemann V, Winter M, Reimers CD, et al. Impaired motor cortex amyotrophic lateral sclerosis. Evidence from paired transcranial magnetic stimulation. *Neurology* 1998;49(5):1292–1298.
76. de Carvalho MD, Miranda PC, Luis ML, et al. Conical muscle representation in amyotrophic lateral sclerosis patients: changes with disease evolution. *Muscle Nerve* 1999;22:1684–1692.
77. Schulte-Matter WJ, Muller T, Ziez S, et al. Transcranial magnetic stimulation compared with upper motor neuron signs in patients with amyotrophic lateral sclerosis. *J Neurol Sci* 1999;170:51–56.

78. Desiato MT, Palmicri MG, Giacomini P, et al. The effect of riluzole in amyotrophic lateral sclerosis: a study with cortical stimulation. *J Neurol Sci* 1999;169:98–107.
79. Bensimon G, Lacomblez L, Meininger V, et al. A controlled trial of riluzole in amyotrophic lateral sclerosis. *N Engl Med* 1994;330:585–591.
80. Lacomblez L, Bensimon G, Leigh PN, et al. Dose-ranging study of riluzole in amyotrophic lateral sclerosis. *Lancet* 1996;347:1425–1431.
81. Poloni TE, Alimonti D, Montagna G, et al. Renal tubular impairment during riluzole therapy. *Neurology* 1999;52:670.
82. Drory VE, Sidi I, Korczyn AD, et al. Riluzole-induced pancreatitis. *Neurology* 1999;52:892–893.
83. Practice advisory on the treatment of amyotrophic lateral sclerosis with riluzole. *Neurology* 1997;49:657–659.
84. Graf M, Ecker D, Horowski R, et al. High dose vitamin E therapy in amyotrophic lateral sclerosis as add-on therapy to riluzole: results of a placebo-controlled double-blind study. *J Neural Transm* 2005;112(5):649–660.
85. Desnuelle C, Dib M, Garrel C, Favier A. A double-blind, placebo-controlled randomized clinical trial of alpha-tocopherol (vitamin E) in the treatment of amyotrophic lateral sclerosis. ALS riluzole-tocopherol Study Group. *Amyotroph Lateral Scler Other Motor Neuron Disord* 2001;2(1):9–18.
86. Wang H, O'Reilly ÉJ, Weisskopf MG, et al. Vitamin E intake and risk of amyotrophic lateral sclerosis: a pooled analysis of data from 5 prospective cohort studies. *Am J Epidemiol* 2011;173(6):595–602.
87. Kaufmann P, Thompson JL, Levy G, et al. Phase II trial of CoQ10 for ALS finds insufficient evidence to justify phase III. *Ann Neurol* 2009;66(2):235–244.
88. Vyth A, Timmer JG, Bossuyt PM, et al. Survival in patients with amyotrophic lateral sclerosis treated with an array of antioxidants. *J Neurol Sci* 1996;139(Suppl1):99–103.
89. Klivenyi P, Ferrante RJ, Matthews RT, et al. Neuroprotective effects of creatine in a transgenic animal model of amyotrophic lateral sclerosis. *Nat Med* 1999;5(3):347–350.
90. Groeneveld GJ, Veldink JH, van der Tweel I, et al. A randomized sequential trial of creatine in amyotrophic lateral sclerosis. *Ann Neurol* 2003;53(4):437–445.
91. Atassi N, Ratai EM, Greenblatt DJ, et al. A phase I, pharmacokinetic, dosage escalation study of creatine monohydrate in subjects with amyotrophic lateral sclerosis. *Amyotroph Lateral Scler* 2010;11(6):508–513.
92. Cheah BC, Kiernan MC. Dexpramipexole, the R(+) enantiomer of pramipexole, for the potential treatment of amyotrophic lateral sclerosis. *IDrugs* 2010;13(12):911–920.
93. Robinson R. New Als drug shows dose-dependent efficacy in phase 2 trial. *Neurol Today* 2010;10:1.
94. Haidet-Phillips AM, Hester ME, Miranda CJ, et al. Astrocytes from familial and sporadic ALS patients are toxic to motor neurons. *Nat Biotechnol* 2011.
95. Joyce N, Annett G, Olson S, et al. Mesenchymal Stem Cells for the Treatment of Neurodegenerative Diseases. *Regen Med* 2010;5(6):933–946.
96. Sea K, Gowing G, Joyce N, et al. ALS in California: a report from The First Annual California ALS Research Summit. *Neurodegen Dis Manage* 2011;1(4):281–284.
97. Fowler WM, Carter GT, Kraft GH. Role of physiatry in the management of neuromuscular disease. In: *Physical medicine and rehabilitation clinics of North America.* Philadelphia, PA: WB Saunders, 1998:1–8.
98. Francis K, Bach JR, Delisa JA. Evaluation and rehabilitation of patients with adult motor neuron disease. *Arch Phys Med Rehabil* 1999;80:951–963.
99. Aitkens SG, McCrory MA, Kilmer DO, et al. Moderate resistance exercise program: its effects in slowly progressive neuromuscular disease. *Arch Phys Med Rehabil* 1993;74(7):711–715.
100. Kilmer DD, McCrory MA, Wright NC, et al. The effect of a high resistance exercise program in slowly progressive neuromuscular disease. *Arch Phys Med Rehabil* 1994;75(5):560–563.
101. Bello-Haas VD, Florence JM, Kloos AD, et al. A randomized controlled trial of resistance exercise in individuals with ALS. *Neurology* 2007;68(23):2003–2007.
102. Kilmer DD. The role of exercise in neuromuscular disease. *Phys Med Rehabil North Am* 1998;9(1):115–125.
103. Caner GT. Rehabilitation management of neuromuscular disease. *J Neural Rehabil* 1997;11(2):1–12.
104. Caner CT, Miller RG. Comprehensive management of amyotrophic lateral sclerosis. *Phys Med Rehabil North Am* 1998;9(1):271–284.
105. Sharma KR, Miller RG. Electrical and mechanical properties of skeletal muscle underlying increased fatigue in patients with amyotrophic lateral sclerosis. *Muscle Nerve* 1996;19:1391–1400.
106. Sharma KR, Kelll-Braun JA, Majumdar S, et al. Physiology of fatigue in amyotrophic lateral sclerosis. *Neurology* 1995;45(4):733–740.
107. Krivickas LS. Pulmonary function and respiratory failure. In: Mitsumoto H, Chad DA, Pioro EP, eds. *Amyotrophic lateral sclerosis.* Philadelphia, PA: FA Davis Co, 1998:382–404.
108. Bendiu JO. Management of pulmonary complications in neuromuscular disease. In: *Physical medicine and rehabilitation clinics of North America.* Philadelphia, PA: WB Saunders, 1998:167–185.
109. Carrat P, Cassano A, Gadaleta F, et al. Association between low sniff nasal-inspiratory pressure (SNIP) and sleep disordered breathing in amyotrophic lateral sclerosis: preliminary results. *Amyotroph Lateral Scler* 2011.
110. Miller RG, Jackson CE, Kasarskis EJ, et al. Practice parameter update: the care of the patient with amyotrophic lateral sclerosis: drug, nutritional, and respiratory therapies (an evidence-based review): report of the Quality Standards Subcommittee of the American Academy of Neurology. *Neurology* 2009;73(15):1218–1226.
111. Bach JR. Amyotrophic lateral sclerosis: predictors for prolongation of life by noninvasive respiratory aids. *Arch Phys Med Rehabil* 1995;76(9):828–832.
112. Bach JR. Amyotrophic lateral sclerosis: communication status and survival with ventilatory support. *Arch Phys Med Rehabil* 1993;72(6):343–349.
113. Bourke SC, Tomlinson M, Williams TL, et al. Effects of non-invasive ventilation on survival and quality of life in patients with amyotrophic lateral sclerosis: a randomised controlled trial. *Lancet Neurol* 2006;5(2):140–147.

114. Carter CT, Johnson ER, Bonekat HW, et al. Laryngeal diversion in the treatment of intractable aspiration in motor neuron disease. *Arch Phys Med Rehabil* 1992;73(7):680–682.
115. Kawai S, Tsukuda M, Mochimatsu I, et al. A study of the early stage of dysphagia in amyotrophic lateral sclerosis. *Dysphagia* 2003;18(1):1–8.
116. Langmore SE, Schatz MA, Olsen N. Fiberoptic endoscopic examination of swallowing safety: a new procedure. *Dysphagia* 1988;2:216–219.
117. Genton L, Viatte V, Janssens JP, et al. Nutritional state, energy intakes and energy expenditure of amyotrophic lateral sclerosis (ALS) patients. *Clin Nutr* 2011.
118. Paganoni S, Deng J, Jaffa M, et al. Body mass index, not dyslipidemia, is an independent predictor of survival in amyotrophic lateral sclerosis. *Muscle Nerve* 2011;44(1):20–24.
119. Spataro R, Ficano L, Piccoli F, et al. Percutaneous endoscopic gastrostomy in amyotrophic lateral sclerosis: effect on survival. *J Neurol Sci* 2011;304(1–2):44–48.
120. Miller RG, Rosenberg JA, Gelinas DF, et al. Practice parameter: the care of patients with amyotrophic lateral sclerosis (an evidence-base review). *Muscle Nerve* 1999;22:1104–1118.
121. Guidubaldi A, Fasano A, Ialongo T, et al. Botulinum toxin A versus B in sialorrhea: a prospective, randomized, double-blind, crossover pilot study in patients with amyotrophic lateral sclerosis or Parkinson's disease. *Mov Disord* 2011;26(2):313–319.
122. Kübler A, Winter S, Ludolph AC, et al. Severity of depressive symptoms and quality of life in patients with amyotrophic lateral sclerosis. *Neurorehabil Neural Repair* 2005;19(3):182–193.
123. Meininger V. Breaking bad news in amyotrophic lateral sclerosis. *Palliat Med* 1993;7(Suppl 4):37–40.
124. Nygren I, Askmark H. Self-reported quality of life in amyotrophin lateral sclerosis. *J Palliat Med* 2006;9(2):304–308.
125. Kurt A, Nijboer F, Matuz, et al. Depression and anxiety in individuals with amyotrophic lateral sclerosis: epidemiology and management. *CNS Drugs* 2007;21(4): 279–291.
126. Pagnini F, Rossi G, Lunetta C, et al. Burden, depression, and anxiety in caregivers of people with amyotrophic lateral sclerosis. *Psychol Health Med* 2010;15(6): 685–693.
127. Abresch RT, Seyden NK, Wineinger MA. Quality of life: issues for persons with neuromuscular diseases. In: *Physical medicine and rehabilitation clinics of North America*. Philadelphia, PA: WB Saunders, 1998: 233–248.
128. Fields HL. Relief of unnecessary suffering. In: Fields HL, Liebeskind JC, eds. *Pharmalogic approaches to the treatment of chronic pain: new concepts and critical issues*, vol 1. Seattle: International Association for the Study of Pain Press. 1994:1–11.
129. Pisano F, Miscio G, Mazzuero G, et al. Decreased heart rate variability in amyotrophic lateral sclerosis. *Muscle Nerve* 1995;18:1225–1231.
130. de Carvalho ML, Motta R, Battaglia MA, et al. Urinary disorders in amyotrophic lateral sclerosis subjects. *Amyotroph Lateral Scler* 2011.
131. Irwin D, Lippa CF, Swearer JM. Cognition and amyotrophic lateral sclerosis (ALS). *Am J Alzheimers Dis Other Demen* 2007;22(4):300–312.
132. Phukan J, Elamin M, Bede P, et al. The syndrome of cognitive impairment in amyotrophic lateral sclerosis: a population-based study. *J Neurol Neurosurg Psychiatry* 2011.
133. Gordon PH, Delgadillo D, Piquard A, et al. The range and clinical impact of cognitive impairment in French patients with ALS: a cross-sectional study of neuropsychological test performance. *Amyotroph Lateral Scler* 2011.
134. Rippon GA, Scarmeas N, Gordon PH, et al. An observational study of cognitive impairment in amyotrophic lateral sclerosis. *Arch Neurol* 2006;63(3):345–352.
135. Bernat JL. Ethical and legal issues in the management of amyotrophic lateral sclerosis. In: Belsh JM, Schiffman PL, eds. *Amyotrophic lateral sclerosis: diagnosis and management for the clinician*. Armonk, NY: Futura Publishing, 1996:357–372.
136. Caner GT, Butler LM, Abresch RT, et al. Expanding the role of hospice in the care of amyotrophic lateral sclerosis. *Am J Hosp Palliat Care* 1999;16(6):707–710.
137. Ganzini L, Johnston WS, McFarland BH, et al. Attitudes of patients with amyotrophic lateral sclerosis and their caregivers toward assisted suicide. *N Engl Med* 1998;339(14):967–973.
138. Moore MK. Dying at home: a way of maintaining control for the person with ALS/MND. *Palliat Med* 1993;7(Suppl 4):65–68.
139. Oppenheimer EA. Decision-making in the respiratory care of amyotrophic lateral sclerosis: should home mechanical ventilation be used? *Palliat Med* 1993;7(Suppl 4):49–64.
140. Krivickas LS, Shockley L, Mitsumoto H. Home care of patients with amyotrophic lateral sclerosis (ALS). *J Neurol Sci* 1997;152(Suppl 1):S82–S89.
141. Standards and Accreditation Committee Medical Guidelines Task Force. *Medical guidelines for determining prognosis in selected non-cancer diseases*. The National Hospice Organization. Arlington, VA, 1996:24–26.
142. Enck RE. Hospice: the next step. *Am J Hosp Palliat Care* 1999;16(2):436–437.

CHAPTER 36 ■ ACUTE AND CHRONIC INFLAMMATORY DEMYELINATING POLYNEUROPATHIES

JAY M. MEYTHALER AND NIKKI FOX, D.O.

INTRODUCTION

This chapter provides a review of the major inflammatory demyelinating peripheral nerve conditions, with emphasis on the most common entities, namely acute and chronic inflammatory demyelinating polyneuropathy. These diseases are common causes of nontraumatic paresis in the world. Hence, these patients, along with their functional deficits, are frequently seen in the spinal cord rehabilitation setting.

INCIDENCE AND IMPORTANCE

Guillain-Barré Syndrome

Guillain-Barré syndrome (GBS) is an immunopathy associated with an acute, often fulminate, evolution of a demyelinating inflammatory polyradiculoneuropathy (1–5). GBS, also known as acute inflammatory demyelinating polyneuropathy (AIDP), is the most common cause of acute nontraumatic neuromuscular paralysis in developed countries, afflicting approximately 0.4 to 1.7 per 100,000 people annually (1–3,6,7). In addition, with the reduction of worldwide polio cases, it is estimated to be the most common cause of acute neuromuscular paralysis in the world. There are approximately 3,500 to 5,000 new cases per year in the United States (8–10). This acute disease causes ventilatory-dependent respiratory failure in 25%, mortality in 4% to 15%, chronic fatigue in approximately 68%, and permanent disability in 20% (7,8). GBS is also a significant cause of long-term disability for at least 1,000 persons per year in the United States and many more elsewhere (9). Furthermore, given the young age at which GBS can occur, it is likely that at least 25,000 and perhaps as many as 50,000 Americans live with residual functional deficits from GBS (9).

The economic cost of GBS within the United States in 2004 was estimated to be $1.7 billion, including $0.2 billion (14%) in direct medical costs and $1.5 billion (86%) in indirect costs (11). Most calculations were for community hospital admissions. The majority of indirect costs were secondary to premature deaths, with the mean cost per patient at $318,966 (11,12). The average inpatient per patient costs have been over $31 thousand (11,13).

While the disease is primarily demyelinating in nature, primary axonal varieties of GBS have been described (14,15). There is now evidence supporting axonal subtypes of GBS: acute motor axonal neuropathy (AMAN) and acute motor and sensory axonal neuropathy (AMSAN) are caused by antibodies to gangliosides residing on the axolemma, followed by target macrophages that invade the axon at the node of Ranvier (10). *Campylobacter jejuni* infection appears to be related to axonal forms of this disease, and approximately 25% of patients with GBS have incurred a recent infection with *C. jenuni* (16). Lipo-oligosaccharides from the *C jejuni* bacterial wall contain ganglioside-like structures; injection of these into rabbits has shown to induce neuropathy resembling AMAN (17). Comparing the demyelinating and axonal forms of the diseases, the latter may account for up to two thirds of cases in less developed countries (17).

Other Inflammatory Neuropathies

Chronic demyelinating polyneuropathies have an incidence of at least 1,000 new cases per year within the United States (14). These other inflammatory polyneuropathy syndromes present with many of the same clinical and diagnostic findings of GBS including chronic inflammatory demyelinating polyneuropathy (CIDP), autoimmune neuropathies due to connective tissue diseases, cancer, toxic neuropathies, and hormonal and metabolic neuropathies (15,17–19). CIDP and AIDP are temporally continuous and the difference is that CIDP is an ongoing demyelinating neuropathy lasting at least 8 weeks if not longer. The greatest diagnostic controversy surrounds CIDP and relapsing inflammatory polyneuropathy, which are considered by some to be separate from GBS (14,15,21,22). What is important from a rehabilitation point of view is that the clinical course may vary considerably in these other presentations from those of classically described GBS, so an accurate diagnosis and prognosis is important. Clinically, the major differences between the two entities are the time course, some of the clinical signs, and their response to various treatments (22,23).

Although the incidence of CIDP is lower than GBS secondary to its protracted development, its prevalence is greater (10). CIDP is usually differentiated from the other two most common chronic demyelinating polyneuropathies, multifocal motor neuropathy (MMN) and paraproteinemic neuropathy (23). The paraproteinemic neuropathies, which include the monoclonal gammopathies, account for approximately 10% of neuropathies of unknown etiology (24).

When all inflammatory polyneuropathies are combined, they have an incidence rate, mortality, and direct economic cost similar to that attributed to spinal cord injury (SCI) (9). Yet the amount of attention paid to the disease process of inflammatory polyneuropathies does not even begin to approximate that focused on SCI. While this chapter focuses predominately on GBS, there will be some mention of other inflammatory polyneuropathies, particularly CIDP, MMN, and paraproteinemic neuropathy, as they all cause similar deficits.

CLINICAL PRESENTATION

Guillain-Barré Syndrome

GBS presents as a rapid evolution of areflexia and ascending motor paralysis with or without sensory loss (10). Osler offered the first reasonable clinical description (25), but years later Guillain, Barré, and Strohl published a report in which the syndrome of a radiculoneuritis associated with elevated protein in the cerebrospinal fluid (CSF) without a cellular reaction (26). Still the definition of GBS was based on clinical presentation.

Briefly, GBS is an immunopathy with an acute, often fulminate evolution of a demyelinating inflammatory polyradiculoneuropathy (8). There are three general phases to the disease: a progressive or acute phase, a plateau phase, and a recovery phase. The acute onset is frequently followed by a devastating course that may take a person from being absolutely normal to a bedridden state and on a respirator within 2 or 3 days. The progression usually occurs over 10 to 12 days before a plateau is reached, which is followed by gradual recovery. Some patients may have a stuttering onset while others may present with a rather slow progression that can take place over a few weeks (27). The duration of the illness is usually less than 12 weeks in the majority of patients, with most expected to have a favorable outcome usually defined as ambulation without assistive devices (1). There is almost a 2:1 preponderance toward males (1), although this has been questioned (13). The diagnosis is made on clinical grounds, although CSF evaluation can be suggestive of diagnosis (see Table 36.1).

About 40% to 60% of the patients have some antecedent infectious process (9,15). Most commonly, patients describe a nonspecific or "flu-like" upper respiratory infection (1). Symptoms usually occur approximately 2 to 4 weeks before the onset of weakness. Gastrointestinal illnesses, often relatively mild, are reported as the second most common type of illness (1). Culture and serological techniques have shown that 20% to 30% of cases in North America, Australia, and Europe are preceded by primary infection or reinfection by *C. jejuni* (10). *Campylobacter jejuni* enteritis has been linked to the more severe axonal variety (16,28). Viruses that have been most often implicated are cytomegalovirus and Epstein-Barr virus (1,10,29). *Mycoplasma pneumoniae* has also been recognized as a bacterial cause of the disease (10,28). Surgical procedures and trauma are predisposing events in a small percentage of patients, less than 2% to 3% (27). Flu vaccines

TABLE 36.1

FEATURES REQUIRED FOR THE DIAGNOSIS OF GBS (18)

Features required for diagnosis	Features strongly supportive of the diagnosis
A. Progressive motor weakness of more than one limb of a varying degree. The degree ranges from minimal weakness of the legs, with or without mild ataxia, to total paralysis of the muscles of all four extremities and the trunk, bulbar and facial paralysis, and external ophthalmoplegia. B. Areflexia (loss of tendon jerks). Universal areflexia is the rule, though distal areflexia with definite hyporeflexia of the biceps and knee jerks will suffice if other features are consistent.	A. Clinical features (ranked in order of importance) 1. Progression, symptoms and signs of motor weakness develop rapidly but cease to progress by 4 wk into the illness. Approximately 50% will reach the nadir by 2 wk, 80% by 3 wk, and more than 90% by 4 wk. 2. Relative symmetry. Symmetry is seldom absolute, but usually, if one limb is affected, the opposite is as well. 3. Mild sensory symptoms or signs 4. Cranial nerve involvement. Facial weakness occurs in ~50% and is frequently bilateral. Other cranial nerves may be involved, particularly, those innervating the tongue and muscles of deglutition and sometimes the extraocular motor nerves. On occasion (<5%), the neuropathy may begin in the nerves to the extraocular muscles or other cranial nerves. 5. Recovery. It usually begins 2–4 wk after progression stops. Recovery may be delayed for months. Most patients recover functionally. 6. Autonomic dysfunction. Tachycardia and other arrhythmias, postural hypotension, hypertension, and vasomotor symptoms, when present, support the diagnosis. These findings may fluctuate. Care must be exercised to exclude other bases for these symptoms, such as pulmonary embolism. 7. Absence of fever at the onset of neuritic symptoms. B. CSF features strongly supportive of the diagnosis 1. CSF protein. After the first week of symptoms, CSF protein is elevated (>40 mg/dL) or has been shown to rise on serial lumbar punctures. 2. CSF cells. Counts of 10 or fewer mononuclear leukocytes/mm^3 in CSF.

have been implicated in some cases (18,27), and more recently human immunodeficiency virus (HIV) has been implicated in the development of GBS (10,29). Epidural anesthesia, as well as drugs including thrombolytic agents and heroin, has also been associated with its development (15). Underlying systemic diseases, such as lupus erythematosis, sarcoidosis, Hodgkin disease, and other neoplasms, have been recognized to cause a small number of "symptomatic" cases of GBS (15,19).

Acute GBS typically begins with fine paresthesias in the toes or fingertips and extends proximally over hours to a few days. This is normally followed within days by the major clinical manifestation of ascending symmetrical weakness. The acute phase of GBS begins with a rapid progression of the disease and concludes when no further symptoms or signs of deterioration occur. This phase can last up to 4 weeks (30). Stage two is the plateau phase when symptoms remain the same as the acute phase but do not worsen. This may last from a few days to a few weeks (30). The third or recovery phase may last from a few weeks up to 2 years. It begins as the patient's condition starts to improve and ends when he or she reaches maximum recovery. Residual deficits such as weakness and fatigue may last for months to years (9,30). It is estimated that 20% of patients will have permanent functional deficits, and 10% of AIDP patients convert to CIDP (9,30).

With acute onset of GBS, pain is common (30–34). This presents as either bilateral sciatica or aching in large muscles of the upper legs, flanks, or back (36). Leg weakness may make walking and climbing stairs difficult (19,33). In about one third of all cases, facial and oropharyngeal weakness may develop (15,19,33). In severe cases, the disease progresses to affect respiration and may result in cranial nerve palsies with associated functional losses in eye movements and swallowing (15). Disturbances of clinical autonomic function develop and can vary from sinus tachycardia, bradycardia, facial flushing, fluctuating hypertension and/or hypotension, loss of sweating, or episodic profuse diaphoresis. Cardiac arrhythmias may be a leading cause of death in GBS (15). These disturbances have been demonstrated to occur within several weeks from the initial onset and they often do not manifest until the patient begins to be physiologically stressed in rehabilitative therapies. If a patient is placed in an intensive care unit, pneumonia, sepsis, and acute respiratory distress syndrome have been reported as the most common causes of mortality (9,31,35).

The many clinical variants of GBS, which may cause diagnostic difficulty, include Fisher syndrome (FS) that involves ophthalmoplegia, ataxia, and areflexia with little weakness and accounts for approximately 5% of the cases (19,36). AIDP occurs primarily in adults with most cases existing in the Western world. Other variants of inflammatory demyelinating polyneuropathy that may present initially as AIDP include AMAN, occurring in children and young adults, and AMSAN occurring in both adults and children. AMSAN often presents with FS (10). Some variants present as weakness without paresthesias or sensory loss (3%); isolated weakness of the arm and oropharynx or the leg (3%); bilateral weakness of facial muscles with distal paresthesias (1%); severe ataxia and sensory loss (1%); acute dysautonomia, an autonomic polyneuropathy often combined with sensory features (less than 1%); and "axonal" GBS with rapid, almost complete paralysis and electrically nonexcitable motor nerves, which amounts to 20% of reported cases in the developed world (14,15,19,30–40). The effect of these many "subtypes" on the ultimate functional outcome or disability of these afflicted patients is not sufficiently described in the literature. Approximately 10% of patients will have minor relapses, but these relapses do not appear to affect the prognosis (13,15).

Other Inflammatory Neuropathies

In CIDP, cranial nerve involvement, autonomic dysfunction, and antecedent infections are rare (23,38,41). CIDP and GBS do share features such as elevated CSF protein levels and electrodiagnostic evidence of demyelination, as compared to MMN where the CSF protein is normal and the conduction block is predominately along the distribution of the motor nerves, with little involvement of the sensory nerves (1,10,22).

In paraproteinemic neuropathies, a cause of CIDP, there is an immunoglobulin-mediated demyelinating polyneuropathy associated with anti–myelin-associated glycoprotein (MAG) antibodies. Most of the patients present with a prominent sensory ataxia that has a very slow onset and progression, usually over years rather than months (23,42). Specific types are heavy chain disease, so named for excessive production of immunoglobulin heavy chains, and cryoglobulinemias. There are three types of cryoglobulinemias. Type I is most commonly found in patients with a plasma cell dyscrasia, such as multiple myeloma (MM) or Waldenström macroglobulinemia. Types II and III are closely affiliated with infection of the hepatitis C virus (43,44).

EMG AND LABORATORY FINDINGS

Guillain-Barré Syndrome

Abnormalities of nerve conduction studies (NCS) reflecting demyelination, as well as the delay or absence of late responses, are the most sensitive and specific electrodiagnostic findings in the inflammatory polyneuropathies (40). Demyelination is demonstrated by the presence of slowed conduction velocities, prolonged distal motor latencies, and partial conduction block. Late responses, such as the H reflex and F wave, are often delayed or absent (40,41). However, since a slowing or absence of responses is not specific, the late responses should be used in conjunction with other diagnostic criteria to make the diagnosis (18,40,45,46). Proposed electrodiagnostic criteria for GBS are given in Table 36.2 (18,40). Electrodiagnostic and physiological parameters in GBS associated with a poor outcome are found in Table 36.3. In addition to a summed motor velocity less than 80% of normal, it has been suggested that a summed proximal motor amplitude less than 20% of normal and a low distal compound muscle action potential (CMAP) amplitude less than 20% of the lower limit of normal (LLN) at 3 to 5 weeks may be predictors of a poorer outcome or a more prolonged course of the disease (27,40,46).

A primary axonal variety of GBS has been described, AMAN, which may account for part of the discrepancy between the clinical diagnostic criteria and the electrodiagnostic criteria (10,38). The current proposed electrodiagnostic

TABLE 36.2

PROPOSED ELECTRODIAGNOSTIC CRITERIA FOR GUILLAIN-BARRÉ SYNDROME (GBS OR AIDP)

Proposed electrodiagnostic criteria for GBS

These criteria concern NCS (including proximal nerve segments) in which the predominant process is demyelination.
Must have three of the following four features:

1. Reduction in CV in two or more motor nerves
   a. <80% of LLN if amplitude >80 of LLN.
   b. <70% of LLN if amplitude <80% of LLN.
2. Conduction block or abnormal temporal dispersion in one or more motor nerves either peroneal or distal sites and >20% drop in negative-peak area of peak-to-peak amplitude between proximal and distal sites.
   Criteria for abnormal temporal dispersion and possible conduction block.
   a. >15% change in duration between proximal and distal sites and >20% drop in negative-peak area or peak-to-peak amplitude between proximal and distal sites.
3. Prolonged distal latencies in two or more nerves.
   a. >125% of upper limit or normal (ULN) if amplitude >80% of LLN.
   b. >150% of ULN if amplitude <80% of LLN.
4. Absent F waves or prolonged minimum F-wave latencies (10–15) trials in two or more motor nerves.
   a. >120% of ULN if amplitude >80% of LLN.
   b. >150% of ULN if amplitude <80% of LLN.

TABLE 36.3

NERVE ELECTRODIAGNOSTIC STUDIES (GBS)

Must have three of the following four criteria:

1. Reduction in CV in two or more motor nerves.
   a. <80% of LLN if amplitude is >80% of LLN.
   b. <70% of LLN if amplitude is <80% of LLN.
2. Conduction block or abnormal temporal dispersion in one or more motor nerves: peroneal nerve between ankle and below fibular head, median nerve between wrist and elbow, or ulnar nerve between wrist and below elbow.
   Criteria for partial conduction block:
   a. <15% change in duration between proximal and distal sites and greater than 20% drop in negative-peak (-p) area of peak-to-peak (p-p) amplitude between proximal and distal sites.
   Criteria for abnormal temporal dispersion and possible conduction block:
   a. >15% change in duration between proximal and distal sites and greater than 20% drop in negative-peak (- p) area or peak-to-peak (p-p) amplitude between proximal and distal sites.
3. Prolonged distal latencies in two or more nerves.
   a. >125% of upper limit of normal (ULN) if amplitude is >80% of LLN
   b. >150% of ULN if amplitude is <80% of LLN.
4. Absent F waves or prolonged minimum F-wave latencies (10–15 trials) in two or more motor nerves.
   a. >120% of ULN if amplitude is >80% of LLN.
   b. >150% of ULN if amplitude is <80% of LLN.

criteria for GBS are for the demyelinating versions of the disease and do not include the primary axonal variety (40). This is because 85% of GBS in the Western World is demyelinating (9). Furthermore, approximately 90% of affected individuals will present with abnormal motor nerve conduction studies within the first weeks of affliction, and some patients will present with sensory nerve conduction abnormalities (46).

Regarding protein concentration, a common misconception exists that the CSF protein should initially always be elevated in GBS. On the contrary, in a study by Van Doorn et al., it was shown that within the first week after symptoms presented, the CSF protein level is often normal in inflammatory neuropathies (47). It then increases by greater than 90% toward the end of the second week (47).

Other Inflammatory Neuropathies

In CIDP, electrophysiological studies are similar to those initially described for those in GBS and are found in Table 36.4 (22,39,41).

Patients with MMN may have sensory abnormalities on NCS, but often the sensory studies are within normal limits (40,41,47–49). A subtype of MMN, MMN with Conduction Block, has been described that has elicited demonstrable sensory findings with NCS, such as prolonged latencies, slowed conduction velocities, and prolonged late responses (40,46–48). In this subtype, there is usually a characteristic finding of conduction block, temporal dispersion, or a combination of the two along the distribution of the motor nerves (22,46). These patients are thought to be a variant of CIDP, although the upper extremity prevalence, asymmetry, and lack of response to treatment with prednisone suggest this is possibly a rogue disorder with differing manifestations than that of CIDP (31,46,48).

A confirmatory workup should include an examination of CSF, including CSF pressure and protein content (18,19). These results usually reveal a normal pressure, with few (0 to 100) lymphocytes or no cells at all (9,10,17–19). An important note is that the CSF protein can be elevated in cases of CIDP several times the normal value (10,23,32).

In paraproteinemias, whether IgM, IgA, IgG, Waldenstom, MM; polyneuropathy, organomegaly, endocrinopathy, M protein, and skin changes syndrome (POEMS); or primary light chain amyloidosis (AL), they all share similar CIDP electrophysiological testing results with features of demyelination, axonal degeneration, or both (43,50). POEMS does offer a variation in the electrophysiological studies, namely slowing of conduction velocity (CV) primarily in the intermediate nerve segment, and a greater, more severe decrease in CMAP and sensory nerve action potentials in the legs as compared to the arms. Prolongation of distal latency may be present, but is usually less prominent than that of CIDP. Conduction block is also seen, but less common. EMG shows distal fibrillations and large, polyphasic voluntary motor unit action potentials with decreased recruitment (50).

Electrophysiological studies of primary light chain AL are consistent with axonal polyneuropathy, with severity more so in the sensory nerve distribution than motor. As previously stated, EMG usually reveals fibrillations and neurogenic changes (48,47).

TABLE 36.4

ELECTRODIAGNOSTIC STUDIES (CIDP)

A. Mandatory	B. Supportive
NCS including studies of proximal nerve segments in which the predominant process is demyelination. Must have three of the following four criteria: 1. Reduction in CV in two or more motor nerves. a. <80% of LLN if amplitude >80% of LLN. b. <70% of LLN if amplitude <80% of LLN 2. Partial conduction block or abnormal temporal dispersion in one or more motor nerves: peroneal nerve between ankle and below fibular head, median nerve between wrist and elbow, or ulnar nerve between wrist and below elbow. Criteria suggestive of partial conduction block: <15% change in duration between proximal and distal sites and >20% drop in negative-peak (-p) area or peak-to-peak (p-p) amplitude between proximal and distal sites. Criteria for abnormal temporal dispersion and possible conduction block: >15% change in duration between proximal and distal sites and >20% drop in -p area or p-p amplitude between proximal and distal sites. These criteria are only suggestive of partial conduction block as they are derived from studies or normal individuals Additional studies, such as stimulation across short segments or recording of individual motor unit potentials, are required for confirmation. 3. Prolonged distal latencies in two or more nerves: a. >125% of ULN if amplitude >80% of LLN. b. >150% of ULN if amplitude <80% of LLN. 4. Absent F waves or prolonged minimum F-wave latencies (10–15 trials) in two or more motor nerves: a. >120% of ULN if amplitude >80% of LLN. b. >150% of ULN if amplitude <80% of LLN.	1. Reduction in sensory CV <80% of LLN. 2. Absent H reflexes.

DIFFERENTIAL DIAGNOSIS

The separation of CIDP from GBS is based upon the clinical time course. In CIDP, the duration of progression should be at least 2 months while the disease nadir for GBS should be reached within 4 weeks (21). This leaves a gap of 4 weeks where there has been some clinical confusion (21). Explanations recently published in a retrospective study by Kuitwaard et al. (51) have offered evidence in order to clear up some of this confusion. Some recent publications dissect GBS into recurrent episodes, such as treatment-related fluctuation (GBS-TRF) and FS, non-recurrent episodes, acute-onset CIDP (A-CIDP), subacute IDP, and CIDP as a single entity (51,52). However, this may just add to confusion as it has not been linked to improved treatment.

Recurrent episodes are defined as episodes of GBS separated by at least 2 or 4 months if there had been an incomplete recovery between (51,52). Approximately 10% of patients have had a relapse in the first week or two following treatment (28). These are distinguished from CIDP characterized by extensive asymptomatic periods with return of tendon reflexes, quick onset, facial weakness occurring more often, increase in "antecedent illness," and CSF that returns to baseline within 1-week timeframe. GBS recurrence was found to be more prevalent in patients with FS, those younger than 30 years, and patients with mild disease patterns (51,52). If any of these were present, the risk of recurrence doubled.

GBS treatment-related failure occurs in 65 to 16% of patients with GBS and is thought to be secondary to prolonged autoimmune activation surpassing the effect of intravenous immunoglobulin (IVIg) or plasma exchange (PE) and is characterized by a significant deterioration within 2 months after disease onset (51–53).

CIDP is defined as a condition with a subsequent chronic course. However, most patients thought to have this had exacerbations after a 9-week period, placing it well past the identified 4-week timeframe (52). Subacute immune demyelinating polyneuropathy (IDP), like CIDP, peaks at 4 to 8 weeks and usually responds to treatment with steroids (52). The distinction between the two is not well defined, although CIDP is considered to be possibly monophasic with resolution after one treatment, and subacute IDP is considered "intermediate" with response to steroids (52).

Why are such distinctions important? By further evaluating other possibilities in the discrepancy of time span between GBS and CIDP, it is hoped that these differences will lead to more appropriate treatment methods. Primary clinical use of this "distinction" is to treat GBS in the recurrent form, including GBS-TRF with IVIg alone, and subacute IDP and CIDP with steroids and IVIg or another form of immunosuppression (52–54). CIDP is generally separated from MMN by the fact that the latter is usually characterized by asymmetrical distal upper extremity weakness with motor conduction block and/or temporal dispersion in the afflicted nerves. Another distinct characteristic of CIDP is association with antibodies against GM1 gangliosides (21,23,28,31,48).

CLINICAL AND PATHOPHYSIOLOGIC MODELS

Guillain-Barré Syndrome

The clinical features required for diagnosis of inflammatory polyneuropathies are only a progressive motor weakness of more than one limb and areflexia (15). Hence, the clinical course and the pattern of weakness generally determine the differential diagnosis of these similar syndromes and diseases. The most common diseases/syndromes confused with inflammatory polyneuropathies include spinal cord compression, transverse myelitis, myasthenia gravis, basilar artery occlusion, neoplastic meningitis, vasculitic neuropathy, polymyositis, metabolic myopathies, and paraneoplastic neuropathy (15). Other diagnoses that can be confused with inflammatory neuropathies include hypophosphatemia, heavy-metal intoxication, neurotoxic fish poisoning, botulism, poliomyelitis, and tick paralysis from Lyme disease (15).

Pathologically, GBS and CIDP resemble experimental allergic neuritis (EAN) in animals (8,9,21). Both EAN and GBS share common histopathological features characterized by the presence of perivascular mononuclear cell inflammation, demyelination, and edema. Experiments in various animal models have clearly demonstrated that the sensitization of T lymphocytes of the CD4 subclass to proteins in the myelin sheath is necessary for disease induction (8). It was initially thought that this process was primarily due to this disorder of T-cell sensitization (Fig 36.1). Data currently exist, however, implicating auto antibodies directed against nonprotein determinants (10)

The presence of antiganglioside antibodies, such as antiganglioside GM1, GM1b, GD1a, and G11NAc-GD1 antibodies or antiganglioside GQ1b antibodies, has been associated with axonal damage as well as a poorer outcome (50,56–62). Studies have shown that activation of complement occurs along the site of the damaged nerve. In mouse models, some antiganglioside antibodies appear to be highly toxic to peripheral nerves (58–62). Most antiganglioside antibodies are specific to subgroups of GBS.

The immune target in the patient population with GBS, is by in large, still unknown after decades of research (50). Salvatore et al., along side other studies, have proposed that circulating IgG and IgM antibodies to lipopolysaccharides of *C. jejuni* may in fact cross-react with human gangliosides depicted on nerve fibers (63). This suggests that this molecular resemblance of one organism to another may be responsible for antibody formation in GBS (63).

In the GBS subtype AMAN, IgG antibodies directed against particular ganglioside classes have been correlated with various clinical presentations and disease severity in a certain percent of cases with *C. jejuni* infections (16). Anti-GM1b antibodies are associated with more progressive and debilitating forms, characterized by distal weakness and late recovery (62). Anti–*N*-acetylgalactosaminyl-GD1a (anti–GalNAC-GD1a) is usually detected in pure motor forms without cranial nerve

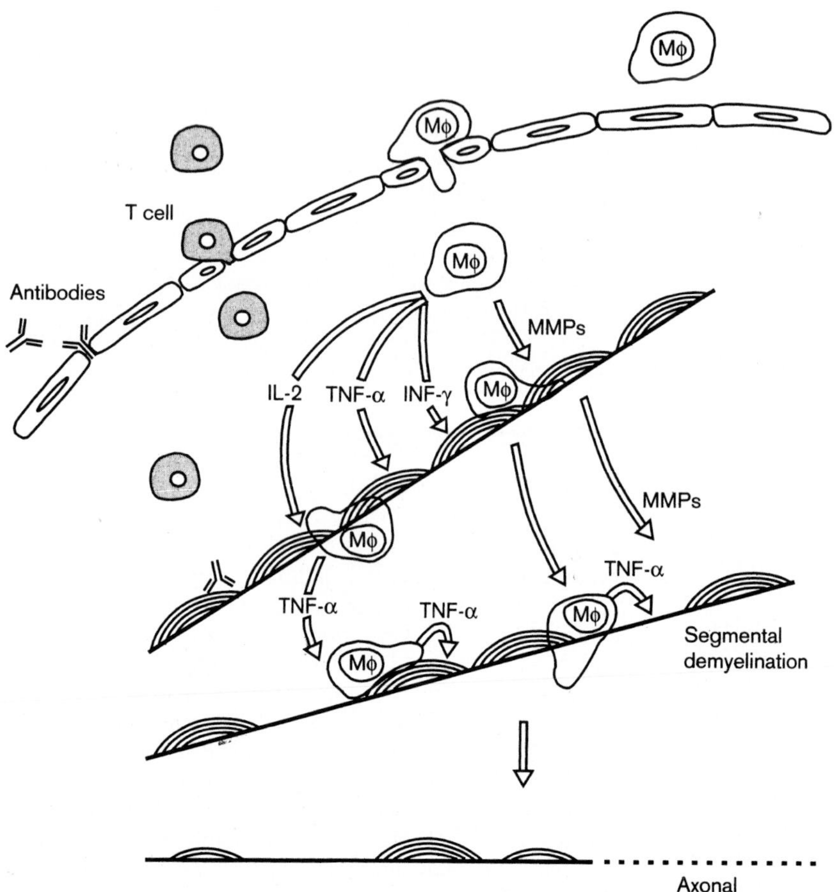

FIGURE 36.1 Diagrammatic scheme of the main cellular elements that seem to play a role in the inflammatory polyneuropathies. (From Dalakas MC. Advances in chronic inflammatory demyelinating polyneuropathy: disease variants and inflammatory response mediators and modifiers. *Curr Opin Neurol* 1999;12:403–409, with permission.)

involvement (62). These gangliosides are well-known components of the axonal membrane, which offers explanation as to why the nodal membrane represents the initial site of damage, following deposition of compliment (63). Last but not least, in a recent study by Wanschitz et al., which investigated the presence of anti–alphaB-crystallin-IgG antibody responses as inflammatory markers at peripheral nerve tissue, it was found that GBS patients had significantly greater values of alpha B-crystallin-IgG indices than others with other neurological diseases (64).

Other Inflammatory Neuropathies

Chronic Inflammatory Demyelinating Polyneuropathy

Cellular and humoral factors have been implicated in CIDP, similar to those involved with GBS, but the precise pathogenic mechanism is still unknown (10,23). Immunological basis was suggested by pathological studies expressing fascicular inflammatory infiltrates, endoneurial edema and increased vascular permeability. Cell-mediated delayed hypersensitivity is supported by the detection of T cells and macrophages (63). However, the role of these antibodies is unclear, but it is theorized that these activated T cells and macrophages release cytokines, upregulate various adhesion molecules on the endothelial walls, and initiate breakdown of the blood-nerve barrier (23,63). Endoneurial edema and increased vascular permeability has also been noted (63). In terms of specific laboratory studies, it has been demonstrated that in CIDP patients often present with high titers of immunoglobulin G or immunoglobulin M antibodies to acidic glycolipids, but not to sulfated glycolipids (10,23).

There have also been antibodies to peripheral myelin protein (Po) noted in CIDP (10,23). The result is theorized to be similar to the models of GBS with a localized increase in putative antibodies, complement, activated T cells, macrophages, and cytokines. Among the cytokines, interferon-gamma, interleukin-2, and tumor necrosis factor-alpha have been implicated in the final common pathway for GBS, CIDP, MMN, and paraproteinemic neuropathies causing demyelination. Approximately 25% of patients with clinical features of CIDP have been shown to also have a monoclonal gammopathy of undetermined significance (MGUS) (10). Cases associated with such monoclonal gammopathy, either IgA or IgG, and cases without have shown similar favorable response to treatment (10).

CIDP usually occurs with certain systemic disorders. Two categories have been described: an idiopathic form and a disorder with concurrent conditions such as diabetes, CIDP-MGUS, rheumatologic disorders, malignancies, endocrine diseases, acute or chronic hepatitis, HIV, and Charcot-Marie-Tooth disease. Classic CIDP displays proximal limb weakness almost as severe as distal limb weakness. This offers one distinction between GBS and CIDP (63).

Multifocal Motor Neuropathy

MMN is a rare peripheral neuropathy (41). It presents as a lower motor neuron syndrome, producing asymmetrical weakness and cramps in single nerve distribution. Primary involvement occurs in the upper limbs. This disease is slowly progressive, without spontaneous remission, and only elicits minor sensory symptoms. It is distinguished from CIDP with regard to its response to IVIg. Autonomic dysfunction is rare. Multifocal acquired demyelinating sensory and motor neuropathy (MADSAM) usually presents as mononeuropathy multiplex of upper limbs. Eventually, distal nerves in lower limbs are also affected, but this occurs later. About 80% have elevated CSF protein (63).

In MMN patients, the response to IVIg is usually better than that of patients with CIDP (41,63). Some may have a recently discovered primary axonal form of MADSAM (63). The majority of patients, regardless of type, present with sensory changes such as numbness and paresthesias (41,63).

Paraproteinemic Neuropathy

Paraproteinemic neuropathy, including monoclonal gammopathy, has been found to be heterogeneous (45). Approximately 10% of patients with peripheral neuropathy have monoclonal paraprotein in the bloodstream (43,50). A monoclonal spike is first detected on serum protein electrophoresis (SPEP). Confirmation of the presence of the M protein is obtained by immunofixation electrophoresis, which determines a heavy chain and light chain type (50). This should be done even if SPEP is within normal limits when monoclonal gammopathy is suspected, as immunofixation is more sensitive.

Approximately two thirds of the population who have a paraproteinemia also have MGUS. Paraproteinemias have typically been associated with IgG M-proteins, IgA M-proteins, IgM M-proteins, Waldenström macroglobulinemia, non-Hodgkin B-cell lymphoma, and chronic B-cell lymphocytic leukemia (24,50).

About 26% of patients with MGUS will eventually develop one of these diseases. The rate of malignant transformation in the general population with paraproteinemic neuropathies is estimated to be 2% per year (19). Even after 25 years postdiagnosis, and being medically stable, a patient can still develop a hematologic malignancy as patients with polyneuropathy and MGUS have a 25% increase in risk of malignant transformation (10,43,50).

Polyneuropathies with IgA and IgG-M paraproteins are considered non-IgM MGUS neuropathies (43,50). IgM is associated more with sensory findings, more severe gait ataxia, and more pathological findings on NCS (50). The pathogenic role of IgA and IgG paraproteins is unknown.

Commonly, paraproteinemic neuropathy is slowly progressive with predominantly IgM-associated paraprotein and sensory involvement. This type reacts against MAG that occurs in about half of the patient population (50). The primary location and concentration of MAG is in the periaxonal Schwann cell membranes and the nodal loops of myelin. The disease leaves patients with minimal disability even after several years, secondary to its slow progression and by its distal clinical characteristics described as distal acquired demyelinating symmetric neuropathy (63). In patients with anti-MAG antibodies, studies of peripheral nerves have revealed primarily a demyelinating process (43). There has not been any identified inflammation, or macrophage recruitment, but M-protein deposition has been identified on myelin sheaths (50,63). In patients with disabling or quickly progressive disease, small clinical trials have demonstrated short-term benefits from IVIg or PE. Recently, fludarabine and rituximab have been reported to be beneficial in some cases by causing immunosuppression (50).

Waldenström Macroglobulinemia

Waldenström macroglobulinemia is uncommon, but characterized by infiltration of lymphocytes and plasma cell dyscrasia of the bone marrow and presents as an IgM monoclonal gammopathy (50). Most patients present with systemic symptoms such as fever, weight loss, and bleeding. It is a slowly progressive distal polyneuropathy with sensorimotor involvement. Electrophysiological studies display findings of an axonal and demyelinating neuropathy. Anti-MAG antibody is present in 50% of cases. If the patient is asymptomatic, they are not usually treated. Once they become symptomatic, alkylating agents or nucleoside analogs are typically initiated (50). Possibly, chlorambucil and PE can be used in conjunction for the treatment of neuropathy. The effectiveness of this combination is uncertain although some benefit has been reported (50).

Multiple Myeloma

MM also is a plasma cell dyscrasia. It is characterized by proliferation of plasma cells and accounts for about 10% of all hematologic malignancies. The annual incidence is about 4/100,000 per year (10,50). Age range is 40 to 80 years regarding onset and usually peaks during the seventh decade. Typical symptoms are bone pain, fatigue, and recurrent infections primarily lung and kidney. The diagnosis is suggested by serum M protein values greater than 3 g/dL, Bence-Jones proteins in the urine, lytic bone lesions, anemia, increased serum calcium, and more than 10% plasma cells in the bone marrow (10,50). Plasmacytosis will usually cause symptoms of nerve root pain due to direct compression from the tumor. Neuropathy associated with MM is heterogeneous if it is without AL. The exact mechanism is controversial at this point. Myeloma neuropathy characteristics are reported to be similar to carcinomatous neuropathy. Presentation is usually as a mild sensorimotor, pure sensory, or a subacute or relapsing-remitting polyneuropathy (50). Nerve biopsies show demyelination and axonal degeneration. Currently, the most accepted models for pathogenesis of the neuropathy are production of humoral substance by the tumor, pathogenic effect of the light chain, or humoral immune-mediated response (10,50,64).

POEMS is a rare cause of demyelinating axonal polyneuropathy (50). Prominent clinical features include sclerotic bone lesions, papilledema, Castleman disease (linked to IL-6 overproduction), polycythemia, and thrombocytosis (50). The major criteria are polyneuropathy, monoclonal plasma cell proliferative disorder, and at least one of the above-mentioned clinical features. POEMS occurs most frequently in the fifth decade of life and presents as a severe symmetric, progressive, sensorimotor polyneuropathy (50). Initial symptoms are paresthesias, tingling, and cold sensation of the feet. Distal motor weakness usually ensues with gradual spread of symptoms proximally. Persons may complain of difficulty rising from a seated position as the proximal leg muscles weaken. Eventually, hand strength is also affected. Clinically, patients may present with amenorrhea if female, gynecomastia in men, hyperprolactinemia, type II diabetes mellitus, hypothyroidism, and adrenal insufficiency. Changes of the skin can occur as hyperpigmentation, skin thickening, and digital clubbing. Other features may be peripheral edema, ascites, or pleural effusions. The pathogenesis is currently unknown, although high levels of cytokines such as IL-6, IL-1, vascular endothelial growth factor, and TNF have been noted (50). Nerve biopsies demonstrate decreased density of myelinated fibers, mild endoneurial and subperineurial edema, and scattered endoneurial mononuclear cells. No standard treatment for POEMS currently exists, although neuropathic symptoms can be treated with irradiation of the plasmacytoma or other lesions with substantial improvement. If systemic, the patient needs to be treated with chemotherapy alkylating agents.

Amyloidosis

Primary light chain AL presents as several protein disorders. It is characterized by extracellular deposition of misfolded proteins (50). These aggregate in soft tissues as insoluble "fibrils." Diagnosis currently requires identification of the misfolded protein via Congo red stain revealing "apple green bifringence."

AL is familial, primary, or secondary. Secondary often occurs after a long history of inflammation. AL is the most common form in the Western hemisphere and can manifest as a multisystem disorder, with idiopathic peripheral neuropathy as one of its initial and most common presentations.

Approximately 17% of patients who have AL experience symptoms of numbness, burning, and lancinating pain in the distal limbs, or legs (50). The spinothalamic tract is affected more so than discriminatory touch. Eventually, weakness sets in and motor deficiencies present distally, with gradual proximal progression into the upper limbs. Carpal tunnel presents in about half of the patient population. Diagnostically, it is determined by detection of amyloid deposition via biopsy of the sural nerve, although absence of amyloid in this area does not exclude the diagnosis. Other areas that also must be histologically sampled are the abdominal fat pad, rectal mucosa, skin, salivary glands, and bone marrow (50).

TREATMENT

Guillain-Barré Syndrome

It is clear that progress is being made in the treatment of GBS and the other inflammatory neuropathies. It has been suggested that improved survival and functional outcome have been related to the use of special care units experienced in handling the complications of the disease and rehabilitation centers skilled with rehabilitating these patients (9,14). Most of these special care units are located in regional medical centers. Many of the GBS patients die of avoidable medical complications such as sepsis, adult respiratory distress syndrome, pulmonary emboli, or cardiac arrest perhaps related to dysautonomia. Intubation is necessary in one third of patients prior to recovery from GBS and has been shown to be required between days 6 and 18 of presentation (7). Even with appropriate medical supportive care, the rate of mortality has stubbornly remained between 5% and 10% for GBS (7,9,15).

Plasmapheresis, also termed PE, and infused immunoglobulins (IVIg) are now the accepted therapies for GBS (10,65–69). North American and European prospective, randomized clinical trials have clearly demonstrated that plasmapheresis shortens the time to achieve independent walking and the time a patient stays on ventilatory support. In addition, plasmapheresis has been reported to improve functional improvement with regard to mobility at 6 months (7,65–69).

General recommendations for GBS patients are that IVIg or PE be administered early in the development of neurological symptoms and preferably before disease nadir (7,69). Typically, PE is administered five to six times and performed every other day over a 1- to 2-week period. This equates to a total exchange of approximately five plasma volumes (7,10). Results from a prospective, randomized Dutch trial of 100 GBS patients treated with IVIg compared to PE suggested that IVIg is at least as good as if not better than PE (69), but timing was critical (7,69). No difference was found between the two treatments regarding improvements in disability after 1 month, duration of mechanical ventilation, death, or remaining disability status after disease resolution. Combining the two treatments demonstrated no significant improvement over administering PE or IVIg alone (7,10,66). Due to the shorter duration of treatment, in general, 5 days for IVIg versus 10 days for plasmapheresis, IVIg has been favored to reduce the length of time in the acute care setting for those who have not developed ventilatory dependence. It is also easier to administer. The usual dosage is 0.4 g/kg daily for 5 consecutive days (53). However, there have been reports of high incidences of relapse following IVIg (55). Although treatment with PE and immunoglobulins has decreased the duration of mechanical ventilation by half, GBS still remains the most common cause of acute neuromuscular ventilatory failure (30).

The use of steroids alone in acute GBS has not been found to be useful (2,7,10,69). In early clinical trials with humans, it was suggested steroids were useful in decreasing the severity of illness (71). However, in a large randomized prospective study of 242 patients treated with 500 mg of methylprednisolone, it was concluded that steroids were ineffective (2,7,69).

Other Inflammatory Neuropathies

IVIg and PE, once thought of as alternative treatments, are now considered mainstream for many other inflammatory neuropathies (7,53,72). Chronic inflammatory polyneuropathies (CIDP), MMN, and some specific types of paraproteinemias have responded to IVIg and PE (21,23,24,72). CIDP has been distinguished by its responsiveness to steroids versus GBS (13,21,31,72). In particular, oral prednisone or prednisolone has been shown to be effective in relapsing or progressive forms (42,63). In one controlled study comparing PE to IVIg in the treatment of CIDP, both were found to be beneficial (14). Recommendations for therapy with IVIg is 0.4 g/kg daily for 5 days (53,54); or alternatively can be administered at this dose on a weekly basis for up to 6 weeks (53,54). Cyclophosphamide can be considered an option in patients who do not respond to IVIg although this regimen should not exceed 12 months or total cumulative dose of 85 g (63). Furthermore, in resistant cases, there has been some success with the use of alpha-interferon, cyclosporine, azothioprine, and cyclophosphamide. In contrast, MMN generally has not been responsive to steroids (23).

Treatment in paraproteinemic neuropathy should be directed at decreasing circulating antibodies. IgM has a half-life of several days; therefore, IVIg and PE are ineffective. These neuropathies have been responsive to prednisone in those patients with nonmalignant IgG or IgA monoclonal demyelinating gammopathies (63). Paraproteinemic neuropathies have also been responsive to anti–B-cell reagents such as fludarabine, chlorambucil, or cytoxan, which reduce the M-protein concentration (24,50). Other current treatment options include alkylating agents, chemotherapeutic agents (dodeoxydoxorubicin), stem cell transplantation, and cardiac transplantation. Randomized studies also showed melphalan and prednisone combinations to be first line regarding prolonging survival, when compared to colchicine (50,73–75).

CLINICAL COURSE

Guillain-Barré Syndrome and CIDP

The course of illness may be more prolonged in adults, particularly older adults, than in children (27). Persons who have suffered GBS may continue to improve for up to 2 years after injury (76,77), although there is little besides general descriptions on the rate or variability of the neurological recovery. Prognostic factors with regard to a poor outcome recently identified in a North American study were older age, requirement for respiratory support, faster rate of progression, abnormal physiological characteristics of peripheral nerve function, or if no PE was performed (27,78). There has been no correlation between recovery from GBS and sex, occupation, the presence of diabetes mellitus, previous steroid usage, or prior immunization (27,79).

The point of maximal neurologic dysfunction is reported as the "disease nadir" (27). The average period from the clinical onset of symptoms to nadir of illness is 8 days (1). The point of time before, or at disease nadir has frequently been considered critical with regard to the success of therapeutic interventions utilizing PE or IVIg (27), but this has never been established and in one study did not correlate with outcome (80). Yet many institutions will not intervene with PE or IVIg if the patient has already begun to obtain neurological recovery or has not deteriorated neurologically for several days. There is still further work needed to delineate whether late intervention after the point of disease nadir is useful in GBS. By definition, GBS should reach its maximal nadir within 4 weeks although most will reach nadir within 2 weeks (10,14,21,22). In contrast, CIDP usually has a duration of progression of greater than 2 months (10,23).

It is our experience, from the rehabilitation perspective, that patients with severe cases of GBS requiring admission to inpatient rehabilitation have an extended period to disease nadir. The development of relapses may be related to a more extended course of the disease in these patients. Frequent neurological evaluations will detect the development of relapses, and intervention with PE and/or IVIg may be of therapeutic benefit (53). The reason why some patients continue to deteriorate is unknown at this point. One suggestion is that such patients may have more prolonged immune attacks, which cause severe axonal degeneration. Unfortunately, current treatment protocols remain insufficient to limit progression of the disease in some patients (47).

SUPPORTIVE CARE ISSUES

There are multiple medical complications that may develop from inflammatory polyneuropathies beyond the obvious motor weakness and sensory loss. Many of these complications may persist for some time, interfering with rehabilitation or lead to permanent functional deficits. These complications require supportive treatment and some will be described below.

Requirement of Ventilatory Support

Significant research exists on the predisposing factors in GBS for the requirement of ventilatory support (23,29). Respiratory failure and pneumonia may be noted in 25% to 30% of patients in the acute phases of illness (first 12 weeks), but many will have adequate recovery of their respiratory function (15,28,30). Up to 30% of these patients will develop pneumonia (15,30). Those who do not have full respiratory recovery may have complications leading to long-term morbidity secondary to antecedent chronic obstructive pulmonary disease, restrictive pulmonary disease from pulmonary scarring secondary to pneumonia, tracheitis from chronic intubation, or respiratory musculature insufficiency (82,83). Although GBS in general is nonfatal, in recent studies it was reported that the approximately 5% to 10% death rate secondary to GBS was due to respiratory or cardiovascular complications (84). In part, this is felt to be due to demyelination of the phrenic nerves (85).

It has been noted that the presence of autonomic dysfunction has a relationship with the requirement of ventilatory support (13,19,32). In epidemiologic studies, it is estimated that 5% to 30% (depending on severity) of patients will require mechanical ventilation, 20% will remain permanently disabled, and half of this number will be severely disabled (84,30).

Intubation should be considered when the vital capacity falls below 15 mL/kg (15,28,30). The requirement of ventilatory support correlates with outcome as evaluated by ambulatory function and motor functional status (13,32). More recently, the requirement of ventilatory support has been associated with the severity of damage to the peripheral nervous system and has been correlated with longer lengths of stay and increased costs for inpatient rehabilitation (26,79). In CIDP, MMN, and paraproteinemic neuropathy, patients rarely become ventilator dependent (23,85).

Dysautonomia

Orthostatic hypotension, unstable blood pressure, or abnormal heart rate indicates dysautonomia in GBS and is felt to seriously affect 20% of GBS patients (30). These indications have been expanded to include bowel and bladder dysfunction (89). Autonomic dysfunction of the cardiovascular system without bladder and bowel dysfunction has a relationship with the requirement of ventilatory support (13,19,32,34,84,90,91). In previous epidemiological studies, dysautonomia has been noted to be present in particularly severe versions of GBS extending the acute care length of stay (13,90,91) and is felt to be clinically related to life-threatening cardiac arrhythmias, cardiovascular collapse, and death in various case reports of GBS in approximately 3% to 10% of studies (31,84,89). In one case series of 100 patients, 11 developed cardiac arrhythmias sufficient to compromise their circulation and 7 of the 11 died (90). Considering the close statistical interaction between dysautonomia that involves the cardiopulmonary system and the requirement for ventilatory support, the use of beta-blockade for prophylaxis in this subgroup should be considered (13). Transcutaneous pacing has been indicated in some cases, as well as use of atropine. Generally, vasoactive medications and respiratory depressants should be used cautiously (47).

Urological and bowel dysfunction may develop early in the disease process but it is felt to resolve in most cases; however, this conclusion appears to be based totally on anecdotal evidence (15,18). Some males will develop residual impotence (15). One report suggests that the incidence of dysautonomia associated with bowel or bladder dysfunction is not statistically related to dysautonomia that involves the cardiovascular system (92). Patients should be evaluated via urodynamic studies (30). Patients should also be monitored for bowel dysfunction, which generally presents as constipation (30).

Regarding other inflammatory polyneuropathies, the incidence of dysautonomia is considered to be much less prevalent, but nevertheless remains a possible complication.

Pain and Sensory Involvement

Most reports of GBS describe pain as a prominent and early clinical feature of the diagnosis and it has been reported to be the sole initial presenting symptom in some cases (93). The types of pain described include paraesthesia, dysaesthesia, axial and radicular pain, meningism, myalgia, joint pain, and visceral discomfort (94). The incidence of pain is felt to be present in 33% to 77% of patients (30,33).

Immobilization

Patients with inflammatory polyneuropathy may be hypotonic or totally immobilized from quadriplegia. The effect of immobilization on the development of functional deficits is not well understood in GBS. Patients have been reported to develop complications of decubitis ulcers, tendon shortening, joint contractures, and malalignment as well as peroneal nerve palsies (15,30). Yet the treatment approach has been similar to many patients who have an upper motor neuron (UMN) lesion such as SCI or traumatic brain injury.

Dysfunction of bone and calcium metabolism can occur in GBS (9,95). Hypercalcemia of immobilization of such a severe nature as to require aggressive medical intervention has been noted in a few case reports (95,96). There have been few reports of heterotopic ossification (HO) occurring in GBS, but if present it may have a significant impact on functional recovery (9,95,97,98,). The pathophysiology of HO to this day is poorly defined in the setting of UMN lesions, and is even more so in lower motor neuron paralytic conditions. However, in a study by Zeilig et al., the development of HO in GBS appears to be related to severe axonal involvement and the subsequent need for mechanical ventilation (76). Patients with HO, even after physical and occupational therapy, retained poor quality of gait with functional deficits in activities of daily living. The most clinically significant finding was loss of range of motion, although this was nonspecific (98). The incidences of hypercalcemia and HO have been minimally studied in GBS and are thought to be the result of prolonged immobilization (95–97).

Anemia

Anemia in persons with GBS with such severe involvement as to require inpatient rehabilitation is more common than that found in the corresponding spinal cord population (99,100).

The anemia was originally believed to be related to immobilization (23). In a retrospective study, 79% of persons admitted to acute inpatient rehabilitation due to GBS had anemia with hematocrit and hemoglobin two standard deviations below the mean (13,99). In two other retrospective studies, GBS patients with a history of receiving plasmapheresis/PE had a higher mean hemoglobin and hematocrit than those that did not (13,99). All these changes reversed with mobilization in one study (13). Plasmapheresis/PE may play a factor by reducing inflammatory immunoglobulins that may interact with bone marrow precursors (13,99). More recent evidence points to the effects of IVIg, which appears to have some bone marrow suppressive effects (92).

It has been suggested that correcting anemia may aid in the treatment of orthostatic hypotension in immobilized patients with GBS (100–103). However, anemia does not appear to be related to rehabilitation outcome or length of stay for those persons with such severe involvement as to require inpatient rehabilitation (99).

Cranial Nerve Involvement

GBS affects not only spinal nerves and peripheral nerves but also cranial nerves in the more severe cases (19,34,104). The most commonly involved cranial nerve is the facial with a resultant Bell palsy, but almost every cranial nerve has been implicated (9). Isolated cranial nerve involvement without distinct signs of GBS is considered a rare variant of this disease (104). Studies have indicated that cranial nerve involvement was associated with an increased total length of hospital stay (acute and rehabilitation combined) for those persons with such severe involvement as to require inpatient rehabilitation (13,79). There has also been an association between cranial nerve involvement and the incidence of dysautonomia that involves the cardiovascular system (105). In previous studies, cranial nerve involvement was associated with a prolonged duration to reach the plateau phase of illness, but they did not independently predict future motor deficit (13,32). Cranial nerve involvement may result in dysphagia, bilateral vocal cord paralysis, optic neuritis, and hearing loss (19,32,106–109).

Cranial nerve involvement may develop in CIDP, but it is rare in both MMN and paraproteinemic neuropathy (23,24).

REHABILITATION

It must be stressed that rehabilitation of the patient should start before admission to the rehabilitation unit. Early attention to cranial nerve involvement including patches or taping of the eyes at night with the use of eye drops or ointment to prevent dryness, bowel care to prevent constipation, oral hygiene, attention to proper nutrition, skin care with the prescription of frequent turning and a proper mattress, DVT prophylaxis, and orthotic management to prevent contractures are some of the issues that should be addressed. In addition, attention to pain and the proper prescription of medications and therapeutics may relieve considerable psychological and emotional distress.

There are no detailed studies in the other inflammatory polyneuropathies that evaluate the usefulness of rehabilitation. Consequently, the rest of the chapter will focus generally on GBS, but it is assumed that many of the same general principles would apply to other inflammatory polyneuropathies.

Approximately 40% of the patients who are hospitalized with GBS will require admission to inpatient rehabilitation (9,76,79,110). With the recent use of increased PE and early transfer to rehabilitation, there are suggestions that the number of patients referred for acute inpatient rehabilitation has increased substantially. Those referred for inpatient rehabilitation are generally considered the more severely involved patients. One study describes an incidence of persistent motor weakness in 54% of these patients ranging from mono- to tetraplegia of 54% (76). Fatigue is described in up to 80% of patients (30). It is clear rehabilitation requires an organized program with defined end points. A common scenario for patients with GBS is 3 to 6 weeks of inpatient rehabilitation, followed by outpatient or a home rehabilitation program for 3 to 4 months (79,110).

At this time, very few studies that encompass long-term rehabilitation outcome have been performed. The majority assess long-term functional status, but not the protocols specifically (9,15). The only studies reported are largely descriptive with no well-defined functional outcomes except for physical findings regarding weakness or alterations in gait (13,76,77,80,98,111). Consequently, most rehabilitation approaches for measuring functional outcome in GBS have been adopted on the basis of experience with other diseases.

Because the course of GBS remains clinically unpredictable at the onset of the disease and patients are being transferred to rehabilitation more quickly, close supervision on an inpatient rehabilitation service is warranted. This evaluation should include detailed, daily physical examinations that document motor and sensory tests to evaluate for relapses and/or complications, as well as measuring vital capacity for patients at risk.

The requirement for ventilatory support has a strong correlation with the functional motor gain and recovery obtained during inpatient rehabilitation as measured by the admit motor and discharge functional independence measure (FIM) Rasch motor converted score on admission to rehabilitation (13,79). Those who had required ventilatory support were generally more functionally limited and recovered less motor function than those who did not require ventilatory support (13,79,110). This agrees with other epidemiologic studies that generally evaluated outcome in GBS by ambulatory function (4,32,111).

Poor proprioceptive function has been associated with a longer length of stay on inpatient rehabilitation (13,79). However, there was no association with proprioceptive changes and functional status as measured by the admit motor and discharge FIM Rasch motor converted score on admission to rehabilitation, so the connection is unclear (79). Also, there appears to be no relationship between the presence of relapses and rehabilitation outcome except for lower FIM Rasch converted motor discharge scores from inpatient rehabilitation (79). This relationship may be related to the more extended course of the disease in these patients, but clearly requires further study.

GBS is a disease that often leads to a functional deficit. About 50% of patients have lingering neurological deficits, 15% to 20% of the patients will have severe persistent residual deficits in function, although about 80% regain ambulatory function within 6 months (110). Up to two thirds may have persistent fatigue and/or reduced endurance (9,47,76,104,110). It is evident that very little is known about the true incidence of disability in these patients. The absence of deep tendon reflexes in upper or lower extremities, along with either severe distal upper extremity weakness or lower extremity weakness, are indicative of an incomplete recovery (80). This may lead to an impairment that is defined as "any loss or abnormality of psychological, physical, or anatomical structure or function" (113). Disability, as defined by the World Health Organization, exists when an impairment prohibits one from accomplishing a task required for personal independence (113). Assessment of disability in GBS has usually been on a crude 6-point ordinal scale or some modification thereof (2,65–69):

- 0: healthy
- 1: minor symptoms or signs
- 2: able to walk 5 m without assistance
- 3: able to walk 5 m with assistance
- 4: chair or bed bound
- 5: requiring assisted ventilation for at least part of the day or night
- 6: dead

One problem with studies utilizing this scale is that the length of time patients have been followed varied between 6 and 12 months, while recovery may continue for up to 18 months. Additionally, the usefulness of this scale in relation to the more traditional scales utilized to measure outcome in rehabilitation has yet to be established. More importantly, this scale may not be sensitive enough to detect subtle changes in function with various treatment options.

In a study by Merkies et al. (114), 20 patients diagnosed with sensory-motor GBS and CIDP were examined through treatment and therapy to investigate responsiveness to selective scales. The rank ordering (from best to worse) was of selected impairment and disability measures using different responsiveness techniques in patients with immune-mediated polyneuropathies. The goals in this study were (a) to emphasize responsiveness as an important feature in the evaluation of outcome measures, (b) to determine whether there are differences in rank ordering using different measures of responsiveness, and (c) to investigate whether responsiveness scores can help physicians to select among valid and reliable impairment and disability measures in immune-mediated polyneuropathies. The results of this study suggested that the overall disability sum score, the Medical Research Counsel sum score, and the Vigorimeter (used to assess hand strength) were the best functional measures (114).

Another important issue that needs to be addressed by rehabilitation research is how patients with an inflammatory polyneuropathy age with a functional deficit (8). It has been shown that the extent of muscle strength recovery following GBS may be a major determinant of the patient's ultimate functional potential (2,15,61).

REHABILITATION THERAPEUTICS

Motor Recovery and Musculoskeletal Complications

There have been few systematic studies on the efficacy of physical therapy in GBS; therefore, the effects of physical training cannot fully be defined (9,15,47,115). Generally, therapy approaches have been adapted from the experiences with other neuromuscular illnesses and diseases. It has been suggested that over exercising the affected motor units in therapy may impede recovery in GBS patients (110,116,117). Clearly, overworking muscle groups in patients with peripheral nerve involvement has been clinically associated with paradoxical weakening (117–120). Fatigue is an important problem and has been reported in 60% to 80% of patients with GBS (30). In one recent study, fatigue was found to be an independent factor from degree of weakness during the initial stages of GBS (115). Garssen et al. analyzed results from a select population of patients who performed 12 weeks of bicycle training, and discovered that fatigue was relieved by the training in 16 neurologically well-recovered patients with GBS, and in four medically stable individuals with CIDP (115). Holistically, changes in fatigue, mobility, and functioning seem not to be influenced by physical fitness alone, but a combination of psychological and physical factors after GBS (47,116).

Motor weakness has been associated with muscle shortening and resultant joint contractures (119). These complications can be prevented with daily range-of-motion exercises (110,120). Depending on the amount of weakness, exercise can be passive, active assistive, or active. Proper positioning in patients is necessary to prevent nerve compressions and skin breakdowns (30). Initial exercise, even in the acute phases, can include a program of gentle strengthening involving isometric, isotonic, isokinetic, manual-resistive, and progressive-resistive exercises carefully tailored to the clinical condition of the patient (120). Repetitive low resistance exercises are also recommended to improve overall endurance (110). Orthotics should be prescribed for proper positioning and optimizing residual motor function (9,110). With regard to medications, amantadine, which has been applied to treatment of fatigue in other populations, has not been shown to decrease fatigue in GBS (47).

Sensory Dysfunction and Pain

There are patients with significant involvement in vibratory sensation and joint position. Proprioceptive losses cause ataxia and incoordination resulting in functional deficits. In one study, proprioceptive losses were not correlated with long-term functional status or the severity of illness (13). This may be due to the small patient numbers in that study (13). Therapy, which utilizes techniques of sensory reintegration and repetitive exercises to redevelop coordination, has been suggested for these patients (9). This will aid in developing motor engrams that are based on the altered sensory perception.

Many patients will relate a history of severe pain in the early stages of recovery from GBS, yet there is a dearth of studies on the nature or duration of this pain. There are no significant studies regarding interventions for deafferent pain syndrome in any of the inflammatory polyneuropathies. Various therapies that utilize desensitization techniques may be clinically useful. Medical intervention usually starts with tricyclic antidepressants, capsaicin, lidocaine patches, and transcutaneous nerve stimulation (9). Second-line agents such as anticonvulsants (carbamazepine, gabapentin) are effective for neuropathic pain (28,121,122). Occasionally, for those who have unremitting pain, the use of narcotics and opiates is indicated for acute management.

Mechanical pain can be treated with paracetamol, NSAIDS, and opiates if necessary. Pain can be particularly cumbersome to control during acute stages of GBS. Often it is located in the back, buttocks, both anterior and posterior compartments of the thighs, and axial skeleton (28). This has been linked in one report to impaired joint mobility in GBS (120). GBS patients with severe pain may have a poor tolerance for activity resulting in a longer hospitalization.

Dysautonomia

Dysautonomia is very prevalent in GBS (30), but is much rarer in the other causes of inflammatory polyneuropathies (13,21,24,31,32,47,81). Recent studies on dysautonomia estimate that up to 20% GBS patients in a hospital setting will have evidence of cardiovascular instability (27,31,89,92). Patients who have excessive sympathetic outflow and hypertension appear to have extreme sensitivity to vasoactive drugs (47,89,123,). These patients are particularly likely to develop episodes of hypotension or hypertension with suctioning (124). This is of concern as some patients are prone to cardiac arrhythmias (13,92,125). Treatment of orthostasis should be directed toward physical modalities such as compression hose, abdominal binders, and proper hydration. There have been suggestions that low-dose beta-blockade should be utilized prophylactically in this patient population (9,47), particularly with those patients referred for rehabilitation soon after disease nadir and before the cardiovascular system is stressed by therapy.

Bowel and bladder dysfunction is generally of the lower motor neuron variety. Recent evidence does not indicate a link of bowel and bladder dysfunction with dysautonomia that involves the cardiovascular system (47,92). Urological dysfunction may develop early in the disease process but is believed to resolve in most cases (15,18). Initial management of the bladder should be directed toward avoiding overdistention with consequent bladder wall disruption (9). Furthermore, up to 30% of patients acquire urinary tract infections (15).

Deep Venous Thrombosis

Deep venous thrombosis (DVT) is believed to be common in GBS (30,82). It has been proposed that approximately 7% of all DVTs that occur are secondary to neurological cases such as GBS (86). However, the incidence of DVT in GBS has never been systematically studied. Predisposing factors such as the severity of disease or the length of immobilization have not been well delineated (87). In one early study, pulmonary embolus (PE) was thought to occur in up to one third of patients who suffered from GBS (87). In a study by Gaber et al. (126), 73 patients with GBS were retrospectively evaluated. Fifty were anticoagulated (warfarin, unfractionated heparin, and low molecular weight heparin were used, doses not specified) (68%) for 5 to 490 days with the mean being 72 days. Anticoagulation was halted in 28 patients when they became ambulatory, and in six who were still wheelchair dependent. Three patients on anticoagulation developed clinical DVT and two who were not anticoagulated for a total DVT incidence of 7% (126). Three patients developed pulmonary emboli, two of which were on prophylactic anticoagulation (126).

The prophylactic treatment for DVT is recommended (15,82) based on judgments that immobilization will lead to an increased incidence of DVT as predicted by Virchow's triad (88). Early mobilization is suggested to be beneficial in similar patient groups. It is currently recommended to utilize either heparin or low molecular weight heparin in immobilized GBS patients (30).

In children with GBS, the risk of DVT is felt to be very low (30). The incidence of DVT in other inflammatory polyneuropathies is unknown but is believed to be increased depending on the severity of the disease and the rapidity of onset of the immobility.

Immobilization

Clearly, prolonged immobilization leads to a reduction of blood volume (101,102,110) and increased episodes of postural hypotension in the rehabilitation setting (79). In other immobilized patients, utilization of a tilt table has been a useful therapeutic tool (9).

These patients tend to lose a significant amount of body mass due to immobilization, particularly muscle mass. When this is combined with a significant sensory loss, patients are susceptible to the development of decubitis ulcers. Proper bed positioning with frequent postural changes is required to prevent the development of decubiti (9,31,110).

The loss of body mass coupled with an already compromised peripheral nervous system makes proper positioning a necessity to protect peripheral nerves, which may be compressed between body prominences and the bed (9,110,119). The nerves that are most frequently involved are the ulnar, peroneal, and the lateral femoral cutaneous sensory nerves (110).

In the patients noted to have immobilization hypercalcemia, early mobilization even in a therapeutic pool was correlated with a therapeutic drop in the serum calcium level (95). The use of aggressive range of motion may also impede the effects heterotopic ossification may have on joint mobility and function (110,111).

Few studies have been performed on the nutritional needs of these patients. In our clinical experience, close nutritional monitoring is warranted, as patients tend to lose weight in the acute stage of illness (9). Patients are hypermetabolic and hypercatabolic due to endocrine, infectious, and inflammatory aspects of Guillain-Barré. High-energy (40 to 45 nonprotein kcal/kg) and high-protein (2.0 to 2.5 g/kg) intake offers a positive effect on protein repletion, nitrogen balance, and aids in fighting off pulmonary infections. High-protein meals may also detour muscle wasting in GBS patients (127). With immobilization and reduced activity, many of those who can eat tend to gain weight after the first few weeks of illness. The consequent weight gain impedes the potential functional gains in transfers and mobility as it may overwhelm any residual motor function.

Psychological-Social Issues

Psychosocial variables have been demonstrated to impact outcome of rehabilitation in many other diagnoses. Symptoms of mild depression are common long after the initial onset and are indicated by persistent mental fatigue, although GBS itself is not believed to result in chronic fatigue syndrome (55,110,115). Clearly, an extended period in the intensive care setting, due to ventilatory support, may result in psychological changes. It is expected that severely involved GBS patients have many of the same psychological and social issues that are suffered by SCI patients (9). This could result in the utilization of already established interventions. It is reasonable to consider that a reactive depression may be the result of deafferent pain syndromes that can result from inflammatory neuropathies (9).

Respiratory

Respiratory failure and pneumonia may be noted in 30% of the acute cases in the first 12 weeks (13,30,80) but are rare in the other causes of inflammatory polyneuropathy (21). Complications from GBS in the rehab setting are incomplete pulmonary recovery including COPD; restrictive lung diseases that include issues secondary to scarring, pneumonia, or atelectasis; and finally tracheitis due to frequent intubation and weakening of respiratory muscles (110). Aggressive respiratory therapy with pulmonary toilet is necessary in the early stages of disease, including acute inpatient rehabilitation, as it would be with any patient with a neuromuscular disease affecting pulmonary function. Other therapy measures include chest percussion, breathing exercises, and resistive inspiratory training (110). Since respiratory failure appears to be the strongest predictor of hospital length of stay, close monitoring is required (13,79,90,91). Patients with cranial nerve involvement are particularly susceptible to pulmonary infections due to aspiration (110). Perhaps this is why cranial nerve involvement and dysautonomia have been so closely linked to ventilatory dependence and severity of GBS (13,79,90,91). The use of cardiac telemetry has been useful in the quick diagnosis of cardiac arrhythmias induced by therapeutic exercise.

Inflammatory polyneuropathy may lead to restrictive pulmonary function, which may persist for some time after ventilatory assistance is discontinued. Restrictive pulmonary conditions in other diseases have been associated with sleep hypercapnea and hypoxia during rapid eye movement sleep, because within the central nervous system, the centrally mediated ventilatory response to hypoxia and hypercapnea is diminished during sleep (110,128–131). Many patients may be assessed on the floor by the use of frequent nighttime observations utilizing a pulse oximeter. In those who develop sleep hypoxia or hypercapnea, treatment with bi-level positive airway pressure may be indicated (9,110). More recently, it has been suggested that theophylline may be of benefit in those patients who present with reduced hypercapnea or hypoxia at night due to central respiratory control mechanisms that accommodate to prolonged blood gas alterations (132), but needs to be balanced against potential cardiac arrhythmia exacerbation.

Clearance of secretions to reduce the work of breathing is necessary (133). Often this will require the use of resistive inspiratory training. Many of these patients will initially have a tracheostomy; therefore, a proper tracheostomy tube capping protocol with frequent rest periods needs to be instituted. It is imperative not to over fatigue the muscles of respiration during the initial period of motor unit recovery, as this can trend the patient toward respiratory failure. Patients are encouraged strongly not to return to smoking if they did so previously (110).

OUTPATIENT AND LONG-TERM FOLLOW-UP

The extent and duration of physically disabling sequelae in the inflammatory polyneuropathies, including the incidence of secondary medical complications, have never been adequately described (9). With regard to motor function, poliomyelitis and GBS have many similar clinical issues. Whether the same long-term problems will develop in this population due to a loss in the number of active motor units is not entirely known. Furthermore, there have been no long-term studies on aging in patients who have suffered GBS (9). It is likely that these patients will suffer a loss of function as they age, similar to those status postpoliomyelitis (134). There are some existing outpatient therapy programs that focus on a patient's endurance, which can aid in the maintenance of functional capacity (110). However, much of the rehabilitation of GBS is based on the experience gleaned from similarly presenting neuromuscular conditions.

The incidence of GBS, which may be two thirds that of SCI, is the most prevalent cause of acute nontraumatic neuromuscular paralysis in the world, now that polio has been contained. When one adds in all the inflammatory polyneuropathies, there is an incidence close to that of SCI. Undoubtedly, a significant portion of the patients discharged directly home can benefit from outpatient rehabilitative services. Furthermore, vocational and psychosocial outcomes have not been addressed appropriately in an adequate number of studies. Counseling and education of both the patients and their families are critical. Upon discharge, most patients continue to have impairments over a 12-month period. Compassion and referral to local support groups such as the GBS Foundation can be helpful for patients and their families (110).

Unfortunately, the services for patients disabled by GBS are as fragmented as those originally described two decades ago for TBI and SCI. This led to the creation of model systems of care, which developed a comprehensive continuum of care, improving the lives of such patients. However, although support systems have been constructed for victims of GBS and other immune-mediated polyneuropathies, there is still a need for the development of model systems of care for patients with these debilitating diseases.

References

1. Alter M. The epidemiology of Guillain-Barre syndrome. *Ann Neurol* 1990;27:S7–S12.
2. Guillain-Barre syndrome steroid group. Double-blind trial of intravenous methyl-prednisolone in Guillain-Barre syndrome. *Lancet* 1993;341:586–590.
3. McLean M, Duclos P, Jacob P, Humphreys P. Incidence of Guillain-Barre syndrome in Ontario and Quebec, 1983–1989, using hospital service databases. *Epidemiology* 1994;5:443–448.
4. Winer JB, Hughes RAC, Osmond C. A prospective study of acute idiopathic neuropathy: Clinical features and their Prognostic value. *J Neurol Neurosurg Psychiatric* 1988;51:605–612.
5. Raphael JC, Masson C, Morice V, et al. Le Syndrome de Guillain-Barre: etude retrospective de 233 observations. *Sem Hop Pares* 1984;60:2543–2546.

6. Prevots D, Sutter R. Assessment of Guillain-Barre syndrome mortality and morbidity in the United States: Implications for acute flaccid paralysis surveillance. *J Infect Dis* 1997;175:S151–55.
7. Hughes RAC, Wijdicks EFM, Barohn R, et al. Practice parameter: immunotherapy for Guillain-Barré syndrome; Report of the Quality Standards Subcommittee of the American Academy of Neurology. *Neurology* 2003;61:736–740.
8. Asbury AK. Guillain-Barre syndrome: historical aspects. *Ann Neurol* 1990;27:S2–S6.
9. Meythaler JM. Rehabilitation of Guillain-Barre syndrome: a review. *Arch Phys Med Rehabil* 1997;78:872–879.
10. Hauser SL, Asbury AK. Guillain Barre' syndrome and other immune-mediated neuropathies. In: *Harrison's principles of internal medicine*. 16th ed. 2005:2514–2516.
11. Frenzen PD. Economic cost of Guillain-Barré syndrome in the United States. *Neurology* 2008;71(1):21–27.
12. Carter GM, Buntin MB, Hayden O, et al. *Analyses for the initial implementation of the inpatient rehabilitation facility prospective payment system*. Santa Monica, CA: RAND, 2002.
13. Meythaler JM, DeVivo MJ, Braswell WC. Rehabilitation outcomes of patients who have developed Guillain-Barre syndrome. *Am J Phys Med Rehabil* 1997;76:411–419.
14. Trojaborg W. Lecture in honor of Professor Emeritus Fritz Buchtal. Acute and chronic demyelinating polyneuropathy: an overview. *Electroencephalogram Clin Neurophysiol Suppl* 1999;50:16S–27S.
15. Ropper AH. The Guillain-Barre syndrome. *N Engl J Med* 1992;326:1130–1136.
16. Rees JH, Soudain SE, Gregson NA, et al. Campylobacter jejuni infection and Guillain-Barre Syndrome. *N Engl J Med* 1995;333:1374–1379.
17. Hughes R, Cornblath D. Guillain-Barré syndrome. *Lancet* 2005;366:1653–1666.
18. Asbury AK, Cornblath DR. Assessment of current diagnostic criteria for Guillain-Barre syndrome. *Ann Neurol* 1990;27:S21–S24.
19. Ropper AH, Wijdicks EFM, Truax BT. *Guillain-Barre syndrome*. Philadelphia, PA: F.A. Davis, 1991.
20. Asbury AK, Arnason BG, Karp HR, et al. Criteria for diagnosis of Guillain-Barre Syndrome. *Ann Neurol* 1978;3:565–566.
21. Van der Meche FG, Van Doorn PA. Chronic inflammatory demyelinating polyneuropathy (CIDP). Electroencephalogram *Clin Neurophysiol Suppl* 1999;50(suppl):493S–498S.
22. Ad Hoc Subcommittee of the American Academy of Neurology AIDS Task Force. Research Criteria for diagnosis of chronic inflammatory demyelinating polyneuropathy (CIDP). *Neurology* 1991;41:617–618.
23. Dalakas MC. Advances in chronic inflammatory demyelinating polyneuropathy: disease variants and inflammatory response mediators and modifiers. *Curr Opin Neurol* 1999;12:403–409.
24. Latov N. Prognosis of neuropathy with monoclonal gammopathy. *Muscle Nerve* 2000;23:150–152.
25. Osler W. *The principles and practice of medicine*. New York: Appleton, 1892:777–778.
26. Guillain G, Barre JA, Strohl A. Sur un syndrome de radiculonevrite avec hyperalbuminose du liquide cephalorachidien sans reaction cellulaire: Remarques sur les caracteres cliniques et graphiques des reflexes tendineurx. *Bull Soc Med Hop Paris* 1916;40:1462–1470.
27. McKhann GM. Guillain-Barre syndrome: clinical and therapeutic observations. *Ann Neurol* 1990;27:S13–S16.
28. Pritchard J. What's new in Guillain-Barre' syndrome? *Postgrad Med J* 2008;84; 532–538. Reprint of paper in Journal: *Pract Neurol* 2006;6:208–217.
29. McFarlin DE. Immunological parameters in Guillain-Barre syndrome. *Ann Neurol* 1990;27:S25–S28.
30. Hughes RAC, Wijdicks EFM, Benson E, et al. Supportive care for patients with Guillain-Barre Syndrome. *Arch Neurol* 2005;62:1194–1198.
31. Atkinson SB, Carr RL, Maybee P, et al. The challenges of managing and treating Guillain-Barré syndrome during the acute phase. *Dimens Crit Care Nurs* 2006;25(6):256–263.
32. Hughes RAC. *Guillain-Barre syndrome*. London, UK: Springer-Verlag, 1990.
33. Ropper AH. Unusual clinical variants and signs of Guillain-Barre syndrome. *Arch Neurol* 1986;43:1150–1152.
34. Ropper AH, Shahani BT. Pain in Guillain Barre syndrome. *Arch Neurol* 1984;41:511–514.
35. Lawn, ND, Wijdicks EF. Fatal Guillain-Barré syndrome. *Neurology* 1999;52:635–638.
36. Fisher M. An unusual variant of acute idiopathic polyneuritis (syndrome of ophthalmoplegia, ataxia, and areflexia). *N Engl J Med* 1956;255:57–65.
37. Young RR, Asbury AK, Corbett JL, et al. Pure pan-dysautonomia with recovery: description and discussion of diagnostic criteria. *Brain* 1975;98:613–636.
38. Feasby TE, Gilbert JJ, Brown WF, et al. An acute axonal form of Guillain-Barre polyneuropathy. *Brain* 1986;109:1115–1126.
39. Melillo EM, Sethi JM, Mohsenin V. Guillain-Barre Syndrome: rehabilitation outcome and recent developments. *Yale J Biol Med* 1998;71:383–389.
40. Cornblath D. Electrophysiology in Guillain-Barre syndrome. *Ann Neurol* 1990;27:S17–S20.
41. Saperstein DS, Amato AA, Wlfe GI, et al. Multifocal acquired demyelinating sensory and motor neuropathy: the Lewis-Sumner syndrome. *Muscle Nerve* 1999;22:560–566.
42. Hughes RAC, Makowska AD, Gregson NA. Pathogenesis of chronic inflammatory demyelinating polyradiculoneuropathy. *J Periph Nerv Syst* 2006;11:30–46.
43. Lunn M. What's new in paraproteinemic demyelinating neuropathy in 2007–2008? *J Peripher Nerv Syst* 2008;13:264–266.
44. Ferri C, Zignego AL, Pileri SA "Cryoglobulins". *J Clin Pathol* 2002;55:4–13.
45. Brosnan CF, Claudio L, Tansey FA, et al. Mechanisms of autoimmune neuropathies. *Ann Neurol* 1990;27:S75–S79.
46. Weiss L, Silver J, Weiss J. *EASY EMG. A guide to performing nerve conduction studies and electromyography*. Chapter 16. 2004:166.
47. Van Dorn PA, Liselotte R, Bart JC. Clinical features, pathogenesis, and treatment of Guillain Barre' syndrome. *Lancet Neurol* 2008;7:939–950.
48. Shapiro, Barbara E, Preston, DC. *Electromyography and neuromuscular disorders. clinical electrophysiologic correlations*. 2nd ed. Chapter: *Polyneuropathy*. 2005:397–399.
49. Said G. Chronic Inflammatory demyelinating polyneuropathy. *J Neurology* 2002;249:245–253.

50. Kwan JY. Paraproteinemic neuropathy. *Neurol Clin* 2007;25:47–69.
51. Kuitwaard K, van Koningsveld R, Ruts L, et al. Recurrent Guillain-Barré syndrome. *J Neurol Neurosurg Psychiatry* 2009;80:56–59.
52. Hadden RDM. Deterioration after Guillain-Barre' syndrome: recurrence, treatment-related fluctuation or CIDP? *J Neurol Neurosurg Psych* 2009;80:3.
53. Hughes RAC, Donfrio P, Dalakas MC, et al., the ICE Study Group. Intravenous immune globulin (10% caprylate-chromatography purified) for the treatment of chronic inflammatory demyelinating polyradiculoneuropathy (ICE study): A randomized placebo-controlled trial. *Lancet Neurol* 2008;7:136–144.
54. Soueidan SA, Dalakas MC. Treatment of autoimmune neuromuscular diseases with high-dose intravenous immune globulin. *Pediatr Res* 1993;33:S95–S100.
55. Hughes RA, Rees JH. Guillain-Barre syndrome. *Curr Opin Neurol* 1994;7:386–392.
56. Baptiste DC, Fehlings MG. Pharmacological approaches to repair the injured spinal cord. *J Neurotrauma* 2006;23:318–334.
57. Samson JC, Fiori MG. Gangliosides and Guillain-Barre syndrome: No casual link. *Br Med J* 1994;308:653.
58. Diez-Tejedor E, Gutierez-Rivas E, Gil-Peralta A. Gangliosides and Guillain-Barre syndrome: the Spanish data. *Neuroepidemiology* 1993;12:251–256.
59. Beghi E. Exposure to exogenous gangliosides and Guillain-Barre syndrome. *Neuroepidemiology* 1995;14:45–48.
60. Grigoletto F. Gangliosides and Guillain-Barre syndrome. Apparent association is a coincidence. *Br Med J* 1994;308:653–654.
61. Yuki N, Yamada M, Sato S, et al. Association of IgG anti-GD1a antibody with severe Guillain-Barre syndrome. *Muscle Nerve* 1993;16:642–647.
62. Kornberg AJ, Pestronik A. The clinical and diagnostic role of anti-GM1 antibody testing. *Muscle Nerve* 1994;17:100–104.
63. Monaco S, Turri E, Zanusso G, et al. Treatment of inflammatory and paraproteinemic neuropathies. *Current Drug Targets-Immune Endocr Metabol Dis* 2004;4:141–148.
64. Julia W, Ehling R, Loscher WN, et al. Intrathecal anti-alphaB-crystallin IgG antibody responses: Potential inflammatory markers in Guillain-Barre' syndrome. *J Neurol* 2008;255:917–924.
65. Guillain-Barre Study Group. Plasmapheresis and acute Guillain-Barre syndrome. *Neurology* 1985;35:1096–1104.
66. Plasma Exchange/Sandoglobulin Guillain-Barre Syndrome Trial Group. Randomized trial of plasma exchange, intravenous immunoglobulin, and combined treatments in Guillain-Barre syndrome. *Lancet* 1997;349:1123–1129.
67. French Cooperative Group on Plasma Exchange in Guillain-Barre syndrome. Efficiency of plasma exchange in Guillain-Barre syndrome: role of replacement fluids. *Ann Neurol* 1987;22:753–761.
68. Vermeulen M, van der Meche FGA, Speelman JD, et al. Plasma and gamma-globulin infusion in chronic inflammatory polyneuropathy. *J Neurol Sci* 1985;70:317–326.
69. van der Meche FGA, Schmitz PIM, the Dutch Guillain-Barre study group. *N Engl J Med* 1992; 326;1123–1129.
70. Watts PM, Taylor WA, Hughes RAC. High-dose methylprednisolone suppresses experimental allergic neuritis in the Lewis rat. *Exp Neurol* 1989;103:101–104.
71. Feasby TE. Inflammatory-demyelinating polyneuropathies. *Neurologic Clin* 1992;10:651–670.
72. Hughes R, Bensa S, Willison H, et al, and the Inflammatory Neuropathy Cause and Tratment (INCAT) Group. Randomized controlled trial of intravenous immunoglobulin versus oral prednisolone in chronic inflammatory demyelinating polyradiculoneuropathy. *Ann Neurol* 2001;50:195–201.
73. Gertz MA, Rajkumar SV. Primary systemic amyloidosis. *Curr Treat Options Oncol* 2002;3:261–271.
74. Kyle RA, Gertz MA, Greipp PR. A trial of three regimens for primary amyloidosis: colchicine alone, melphalan and prednisone, and melphalan, prednisone, and colchicine. *N Engl J Med* 1997;336:1202–1207.
75. Monaco S, Turri E, Zanusso G, et al. Treatment of inflammatory and paraproteinemic neuropathies. *Curr Drug Targets Immune Endocr Metabol Disord* 2004;4:141–8.
76. Zelig G, Ohry A, Shemsesh Y, et al. The rehabilitation of patients with severe Guillain-Barre syndrome. *Paraplegia* 1988;26:250–254.
77. Costa EG. Rehabilitation of patients with Guillain-Barre syndrome. *Revista De Neuro-Psiquiatra* 1970;33:219–232.
78. Mckhann GM, Griffin JW, Cornblath DR, et al. Plasmapheresis and Guillain-Barre syndrome: Analysis of prognostic factors and the effect of plasmapheresis. *Ann Neurol* 1988;23:347–353.
79. Meythaler JM, DeVivo MJ, Clausen GC, et al. Prediction of outcome in Guillain-Barre Syndrome admitted to rehabilitation. *Arch Phys Med Rehabil* 1994;75:1027A.
80. Eberle E, Brink J, Azen S, et al. Early predictors of incomplete recovery in children with Guillain-Barre polyneuritis. *J Pediatrics* 1975;86:356–359.
81. Ponsford S, Willison H, Veitch J, et al. Long-term clinical and neurophysiological follow-up of patients with peripheral neuropathy associated with benign monoclonal gammopathy. *Muscle Nerve* 2000;23:164–174.
82. Garoeth PJ. *Guillain-Barre syndrome*. New York, NY: Thyme Medical Publishers, 1993.
83. Tantalum JS, Boreal CO. Respiratory dysfunction in Guillain-Barre syndrome. *Clin Chest Med* 1994;15:705–714.
84. Alshekhlee A, Hussain Z, Sultan B, et al. Guillain Barre' syndrome: incidence and mortality rates in US hospitals. *Neurology* 2008;70:1608–1613.
85. Beydoun SR, Copeland D. Bilateral phrenic neuropathy as a presenting feature of multifocal motor neuropathy with conduction block. *Muscle Nerve* 2000;23:556–559
86. Gaber TA. Significant reduction of the risk of venous thromboembolism in all long-term immobile patients a few months after the onset of immobility. *Med Hypotheses*. 2005;64:1173–1176.
87. Raman TK, Blake JA, Harris TM. Pulmonary embolism in Landry-Guillain-Strohl syndrome. *Chest* 1971;60:555–557.
88. Shakoor H, Santacruz JF, Dweik RA. Venous thromboembolic disease. *Compr Ther* 2009;35(1):24–36. Review.
89. Zochodne DW. Autonomic involvement in Guillain-Barre syndrome: a review. *Muscle Nerve* 1994;17:1145–1155.
90. Sedano MJ, Calleja J, Canga E, et al. Guillain-Barre syndrome in Cantabria, Spain: an epidemiological and clinical study. *Acta Neurologica Scand* 1994;89:287–292.
91. Taly AB, Gupta SK, Vasanth A, et al. Critically ill Guillain Barre syndrome. *J Assoc Physicians India* 1994;42: 871–874.

92. Meythaler JM, DeVivo M, Johnson A, et al. Incidence of leukopenia and anemia in Guillain Barre syndrome patients admitted to inpatient rehabilitation: effect of IVIG. *Arch Phys Med Rehabil* 1999;80:1188 (Abstract).
93. Ravn H. The Landry-Guillain-Barre syndrome: a survey and a clinical report on 127 cases. *Acta Neurol Scand* 1967;43(S30):8–64.
94. Pentland B, Daonald SM. Pain in the Guillain-Barre syndrome: a clinical review. *Pain* 1994;59:159–164.
95. Meythaler JM, Korkor AB, Nanda T, et al. Immobilization hypercalcemia associated with Landry-Guillain-Barre syndrome: successful therapy with combined Calcitonin and Etidronate Sodium. *Arch Intern Med* 1986;146:1567–1571.
96. Evans RA, Bridgeman M, Hills E, et al. Immobilization hypercalcemia. *Miner Electrolyte Metab* 1984;10:244–248.
97. Gitter AJ, Haselkorn JK. Landry-Guillain-Barre syndrome and heterotopic ossification: Case report. *Arch Phys Med Rehabil* 1990;71:823.
98. Forsberg A, de Pedro-Cuesta J, Widén Holmqvist L. Use of healthcare, patient satisfaction and burden of care in Guillain-Barre syndrome. *J Rehabil Med* 2006;38:230–236.
99. Meythaler JM, DeVivo MJ, Clausen GC, et al. Anemia in Guillain-Barre Syndrome patients admitted to rehabilitation. *Arch Phys Med Rehabil* 1994;75:1051A.
100. Hirsch GH, Menard MR, Anton HA. Anemia after traumatic spinal cord injury. *Arch Phys Med Rehabil* 1991;72:195–201.
101. Johnson PC, Fisher CL, Leach C. Hematological implications of hypodynamic states. In: Murray RH, McCally M, eds. *Hypogravic and hypodynamic environments*. Washington, DC: NASA, 1971:27–34.
102. Lancaster MC. Hematologic aspects of bed rest. In: Murray RH, McCally M, eds. Hypogravic and hypodynamic environments. Washington, DC: NASA, 1971:299–307.
103. Low PA. Autonomic neuropathies. *Curr Opin Neurol* 1994;7:402–406.
104. Dididze M. Clinical variants of Guillain-Barre syndrome: some aspects of differential diagnosis. *Georgian Med News* 2009;166:48–51.
105. Meythaler JM, De Vivo MJ, Johnson A, et al. Incidence of neurogenic bladder in Guillain-Barre Syndrome patients admitted to inpatient rehabilitation. *Arch Phys Med Rehabil* 1998;79:1183–4 (Abstract).
106. Sridharan GV, Tallis RC, Gautman PC. Guillain-Barre syndrome in the elderly. A retrospective comparative study. *Gerontology* 1993;39:170–175.
107. Panosian MS, Quatela VC. Guillain-Barre syndrome presenting as acute bilateral vocal cord paralysis. *Otolaryngol Head Neck Surg* 1993;108:171–173.
108. Nadkarni N, Lisak RP. Guillain-Barre syndrome with bilateral optic neuritis and central white matter disease. *Neurology* 1993;43:842–843.
109. Herinckx C, Deggouj N, Gersdorff M, et al. Guillain-Barré syndrome and hypacusia. Acta Oto-Laryngologica Belgica 1995;49:63–67.
110. Khan F. Rehabilitation in Guillian Barre syndrome. *Aust Fam Physician* 2004;33:1013–1017.
111. Rudolph T, Larsen JP, Farbu E. The long-term functional status in patients with Guillain-Barré syndrome. *Eur J Neurol* 2008;15(12):1332–1337.
112. Dalakas MC. Intravenous immunoglobulin in the treatment of autoimmune neuromuscular diseases: present status and practical therapeutic guidelines. *Muscle Nerve* 1999;22:1479–1497.
113. World Health Organization. International classification of impairments, disabilities, and handicaps: a manual of classification relating to the consequences of disease. Geneva: World Health Organization, 1980.
114. Merkies IS, Schmitz PI, Van Der Meché FG, et al. Comparison between impairment and disability scales in immune-mediated polyneuropathies. *Muscle Nerve* 2003;28:93–100.
115. Garssen MP, Bussman JB, Schmitz PI, et al. Physical training and fatigue, fitness, and quality of life in Guillain Barré syndrome and CIDP. *Neurology* 2004;63: 2393–2395.
116. Bussmann JB, Garssen MP, van Doorn PA, et al. Analysing the favourable effects of physical exercise: relationships between physical fitness, fatigue and functioning in Guillain-Barré syndrome and chronic inflammatory demyelinating polyneuropathy. *J Rehabil Med* 2007;39(2):121–125.
117. Bensman A. Strenuous exercise may impair muscle function in Guillain-Barré patients. *J Am Med Assoc* 1970;214:468–469.
118. Herbison GJ, Jaweed M, Ditunno JF. Exercise therapies in peripheral neuropathies. *Arch Phys Med Rehabil* 1983;64:201–205.
119. Bushbacher L. Rehabilitation of patients with peripheral neuropathies. In: Braddom RL, ed. Physical medicine and rehabilitation. Philadelphia, PA: W.B. Saunders, 1995:972–989.
120. Soryal I, Sinclaire E, Hornby J, et al. Impaired joint mobility in Guillain-Barré syndrome: A primary or a secondary phenomenon? *J Neurol Neurosurg Psychiatric* 1992;55:1014–1017.
121. Calissi PT, Jaber LA. Peripheral diabetic neuropathy: current concepts in treatment. *Ann Pharmacother* 1995;7–8:69–77.
122. Rosner H, Rubin L, Kestenbaum A. Gabapentin adjunctive therapy in neuropathic pain states. *Clin J Pain* 1996;12:56–8.
123. Lichtenfield P. Autonomic dysfunction in the Guillain-Barre syndrome. *Am J Med* 1971;50:772–780.
124. Eiben RM, Gersony WM. Recognition, prognosis and treatment of the Guillain-Barre syndrome (acute idiopathic polyneuritis). *Med Clin N Am* 1963;47:1371–1380.
125. Winer JB, Hughes RAC. Identification of patients at risk of arrhythmia in the Guillain-Barré syndrome. *Q J Med* 1988;68:735–739.
126. Gaber TA, Kirker SG, Jenner JR. Current practice of prophylactic anticoagulation in Guillain-Barré syndrome. *Clin Rehabil* 2002;16:190–193.
127. Roubenoff RA, Borel CO, Hanley DF. Hypermetabolism and hypercatabolism in Guillain-Barré syndrome. *J Parenter Enteral Nutr* 1992;16:464–472.
128. Bach JR. Rehabilitation of the patient with respiratory dysfunction. In: DeLisa JA, ed. Rehabilitation medicine: principles and practice. 2nd ed. Philadelphia, PA: J.B. Lippincott Company, 1993:952–72.

129. Redding GJ, Okamoto GA, Guthrie RD, et al. Sleep patterns in nonambulatory boys with Duchenne Muscular dystrophy. *Arch Phys Med Rehabil* 1985;66:818–821.
130. Shneerson J. Disorders of ventilation. Boston, MA: Blackwell Scientific publications, 1988:43.
131. Smith PEM, Edwards RHT, Calverley PMA. Ventilation and breathing pattern during sleep in Duchenne muscular dystrophy. *Chest* 1989;96:1346–1351.
132. Javaheri S, Parker TJ, Wexler L, et al. Effect of theophylline on sleep-disordered breathing in heart failure. *N Eng J Med* 1996;335:562–567.
133. Alba AS. Concepts in pulmonary rehabilitation. In. Braddom RL, ed. Physical medicine and rehabilitation. Philadelphia, PA: W.B. Saunders, 1995:671–685.
134. Trojan DA, Cashman NR, Shapiro S, et al. Predictive factors for post-poliomyelitis syndrome. *Arch Phys Med Rehabil* 1994;75:770–777.
135. Notermans NC, Franssen H, Eurelings M, et al. Diagnostic criteria for demyelinating polyneuropathy associated with monoclonal gammopathy. *Muscle Nerve* 2000;23:73–79.

INDEX

Page numbers followed by f denote figures; page numbers followed by t denote tables

U